Pediatric and Adolescent Gynecology

Fifth Edition

Pediatric and Adolescent Gynecology

Fifth Edition

S. Jean Herriot Emans, M.D.
Professor of Pediatrics
Harvard Medical School
Chief, Division of Adolescent/Young Adult Medicine
Vice Chair for Clinical Affairs, Department of Medicine
Children's Hospital Boston
Boston, Massachusetts

Marc R. Laufer, M.D.
Associate Professor of
Obstetrics, Gynecology and Reproductive Biology
Harvard Medical School;
Chief of Gynecology
Children's Hospital Boston;
Division of Reproductive Medicine
Department of Obstetrics and Gynecology
Brigham and Women's Hospital;
David B. Perini Quality of Life Clinic
Dana Farber Cancer Instituite;
Boston, Massachusetts

Donald P. Goldstein, M.D.
Clinical Professor of
Obstetrics, Gynecology and Reproductive Biology
Division of Gynecologic Oncology
Department of Obstetrics and Gynecology
Brigham and Women's Hospital
Boston, Massachusetts

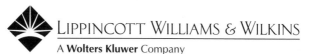

LIPPINCOTT WILLIAMS & WILKINS
A **Wolters Kluwer** Company
Philadelphia · Baltimore · New York · London
Buenos Aires · Hong Kong · Sydney · Tokyo

Acquisitions Editor: Anne M. Sydor
Developmental Editor: Kerry Barrett
Marketing Manager: Kathy Neely
Project Manager: Nicole Walz
Senior Manufacturing Manager: Ben Rivera
Creative Director: Doug Smock
Cover Designer: Larry Didona
Compositor: Maryland Composition, Inc.
Printer: Edwards Brothers

© 2005 by Lippincott Williams & Wilkins
530 Walnut St.
Philadelphia, PA 19106 USA
www.LWW.com

Printed in the United States of America

Fourth edition 1998, Lippincott Raven Publishers
Third edition 1990, Little Brown

9 8 7 6 5 4

Library of Congress Cataloging-in-Publication Data

Pediatric and adolescent gynecology / edited by S. Jean Emans, Marc R. Laufer, Donald
P. Goldstein.—5th ed.
       p. ; cm.
    Includes bibliogrpahical references and index.
    ISBN 10: 0-7817-4493-8   ISBN 13: 978-0-7817-4493-5
  1. Pediatric gynecology. 2. Adolescent gynecology. I. Emans, S. Jean Herriot.
II. Laufer, Marc R. III. Goldstein, Donald Peter.
       [DNLM: 1. Genital Diseases, Female—Adolescent. 2. Genital Diseases, Female—
Child. 3. Genital Diseases, Female—Infant. WS 360 P37076 2005]
RJ478.E46 2005
618.92′098—dc22

                                                                    2004017947

Care has been taken to confirm the accuracy of the information presented and to describe
generally accepted practices. However, the authors, editors, and publisher are not
responsible for errors or omissions or for any consequences from application of the
information in this book and make no warranty, expressed or implied, with respect to the
currency, completeness, or accuracy of the contents of the publication. Application of this
information in a particular situation remains the professional responsibility of the
practitioner.
    The authors, editors, and publisher have exerted every effort to ensure that drug
selection and dosage set forth in this text are in accordance with current
recommendations and practice at the time of publication. However, in view of ongoing
research, changes in government regulations, and the constant flow of information
relating to drug therapy and drug reactions, the reader is urged to check the package
insert for each drug for any change in indications and dosage and for added warnings and
precautions. This is particularly important when the recommended agent is a new or
infrequently employed drug.
    Some drugs and medical devices presented in this publication have Food and Drug
Administration (FDA) clearance or limited use in restricted research settings. It is the
responsibility of the health care provider to ascertain the FDA status of each drug or
device planned for use in their clinical practice.

                                                            10 9 8 7 6 5 4

Dedication

To our spouses (John, Sue, and Connie), families, friends, and colleagues who have encouraged us in our goals of improving health care for girls and young women. This project could not have been completed without their love and support.

Contents

Contributing Authors

Robert L. Barbieri, M.D., *Chair, Department of Obstetrics, Gynecology and Reproductive Biology, Brigham and Women's Hospital; Kate Macy Ladd Professor of Obstetrics, Gynecology and Reproductive Biology, Harvard Medical School, Boston, Massachusetts*

Richard Bourne, J.D., Ph.D., *Associate General Counsel, Office of General Counsel, Children's Hospital Boston, Boston, Massachusetts*

Vicki Burke, R.N., B.S.N., *Staff Nurse, Division of Gynecology, Children's Hospital Boston, Boston, Massachusetts*

S. Jean Emans, M.D., *Chief, Division of Adolescent/Young Adult Medicine, Vice Chair for Clinical Affairs, Department of Medicine; Director, MCHB Leadership Education in Adolescent Health (LEAH) Program; Co-Director, Center for Young Women's Health, Children's Hospital Boston; Professor of Pediatrics, Harvard Medical School, Boston, Massachusetts*

Donald P. Goldstein, M.D., *Emeritus Chief, Division of Gynecology, Department of Surgery, Children's Hospital Boston; Division of Gynecologic Oncology, Department of Obstetrics and Gynecology, Brigham and Women's Hospital; Clinical Professor of Obstetrics, Gynecology and Reproductive Biology, Harvard Medical School, Boston, Massachusetts*

Catherine Gordon, M.D., M.Sc., *Divisions of Adolescent/Young Adult Medicine and Endocrinology, Department of Medicine, Children's Hospital Boston; Assistant Professor of Pediatrics, Harvard Medical School, Boston, Massachusetts*

W. Hardy Hendren, M.D., *Emeritus Chief of Surgery, Children's Hospital Boston, The Distinguished Robert E. Gross Professor of Surgery, Harvard Medical School, Boston, Massachusetts*

Paula Hillard, M.D., *Chief of Gynecology, Division of Adolescent Medicine, Children's Hospital Medical Center of Cincinnati; Professor of Obstetrics and Gynecology and Pediatrics, University of Cincinnati School of Medicine, Cincinnati, Ohio*

Ingrid Holm, M.D., M.P.H., *Divisions of Genetics and Endocrinology, Department of Medicine, Children's Hospital Boston, Assistant Professor of Pediatrics, Harvard Medical School, Boston, Massachusetts*

Jessica A. Kahn, M.D., M.P.H., *Division of Adolescent Medicine, Children's Hospital Medical Center of Cincinnati; Associate Professor of Pediatrics, University of Cincinnati School of Medicine, Cincinnati, Ohio*

Marc R. Laufer, M.D., *Chief of Gynecology, Department of Surgery, Co-Director, Center for Young Women's Health, Children's Hospital Boston; Division of Reproductive Medicine, Department of Obstetrics and Gynecology, Brigham and Women's Hospital; David B. Perini Quality of Life Clinic, Dana Farber Cancer Institute; Associate Professor of Obstetrics, Gynecology and Reproductive Biology, Harvard Medical School, Boston, Massachusetts*

M. Ranee Leder, M.D., *Section on Behavioral-Developmental Pediatrics, Children's Hospital; Assistant Professor of Clinical Pediatrics, The Ohio State University College of Medicine and Public Health, Columbus, Ohio*

Joan Mansfield, M.D., *Divisions of Adolescent/Young Adult Medicine and Endocrinology, Department of Medicine, Children's Hospital Boston; Joslin Diabetes Center; Assistant Professor of Pediatrics, Harvard Medical School, Boston, Massachusetts*

Maurice Melchiono, R.N., M.S., C-FNP, *Adolescent Medicine Nurse Practitioner, Division of Adolescent/Young Adult Medicine, Department of Medicine, Children's Hospital Boston; Co-Director of Nursing Training, MCHB Leadership Education in Adolescent Health (LEAH) Program; Nursing Director, Ambulatory Medicine Programs; Clinical Instructor in Pediatrics, Harvard Medical School, Boston, Massachusetts*

Anne Jenks Micheli, M.S., R.N., *Director, Nursing/Patient Services Perioperative and Allied Areas, Children's Hospital Boston, Boston, Massachusetts*

Amy B. Middleman, M.D., M.P.H, M.S.Ed., *Section on Adolescent Health, Department of Pediatrics, Texas Children's Hospital; Assistant Professor of Pediatrics, Baylor College of Medicine, Houston, Texas*

Angela Maida Nicoletti, M.S, R.N., *Women's Health Nurse Practitioner, Clinical Coordinator of Adolescent Reproductive Health Service, Brigham and Women's Hospital; Clinical Instructor in Obstetrics, Gynecology and Reproductive Biology, Harvard Medical School, Boston, Massachusetts*

Craig A. Peters, M.D., *Department of Urology, Children's Hospital Boston; Associate Professor in Surgery, Harvard Medical School, Boston, Massachusetts*

The Honorable Susan D. Ricci, *Associate Justice, Probate and Family Court, Worcester County, Massachusetts*

Cathryn L. Samples, M.D., M.P.H., *Division of Adolescent/Young Adult Medicine, Department of Medicine, Children's Hospital Boston; Assistant Professor of Pediatrics, Harvard Medical School, Boston, Massachusetts*

Lydia A. Shrier, M.D., M.P.H., *Division of Adolescent/Young Adult Medicine, Department of Medicine, Children's Hospital Boston; Assistant Professor of Pediatrics, Harvard Medical School, Boston, Massachusetts*

Phaedra P. Thomas, R.N., B.S.N., *Nursing Coordinator for Children's Hospital League Resource Center for Young Women's Health, Children's Hospital Boston, Boston, Massachusetts*

Elizabeth R. Woods, M.D., M.P.H., *Associate Chief, Division of Adolescent/Young Adult Medicine, Department of Medicine, Children's Hospital Boston; Associate Professor of Pediatrics, Harvard Medical School, Boston, Massachusetts*

Wendy L. Wornham, M.D., *Department of Medicine, Children's Hospital Boston; Assistant Clinical Professor of Pediatrics, Harvard Medical School; Pediatrician and Medical Director, Lexington Pediatrics, Lexington, Massachusetts*

Foreword

Three decades ago, "pediatric and adolescent gynecology" was not recognized as a major field in medicine. In the 1960s and 1970s, a few pioneering pediatricians were gaining the experience and knowledge needed to diagnose and treat common gynecological problems they encountered in their young patients. In parallel, a small cadre of gynecologists, often working at children's hospitals, were exploring how gynecological disorders presented in children and adolescents. Today, there are thousands of clinicians, many working in interdisciplinary teams composed of pediatricians, gynecologists and nurses, who have broad and deep expertise in both pediatric medicine and gynecology. This vibrant field is served both by an active and growing national society, the North American Society of Pediatric and Adolescent Gynecology, founded in 1986, and a major journal, the *Journal of Pediatric and Adolescent Gynecology*. How did this field grow so quickly?

Often new fields develop at the intersection of two well established areas of medicine when a pressing clinical need becomes apparent. Pediatric and adolescent gynecology was born at the intersection of two existing fields; a medical field, pediatrics, and a surgical field, gynecology. The pressing clinical need was the realization that young patients with pediatric and adolescent gynecology problems are best served by clinicians with expertise in both fields working in interdisciplinary teams. Through close collaboration at Children's Hospital Boston, Drs. Jean Emans and Don Goldstein proved that an interdisciplinary team provides the best care to these patients. In the first edition of *Pediatric and Adolescent Gynecology*, published in 1977, Drs. Emans and Goldstein committed to the written word their insights concerning this new field of medicine. In the 1st Edition, every chapter but one was written by either Drs. Emans or Goldstein. In the 4th Edition, Dr. Marc Laufer, a specialist in pediatric and adolescent gynecology, reproductive endocrinology, and infertility, joined the editorial team, bringing his unique endocrine and surgical perspectives to the book. Due to the explosive growth in medical knowledge and subspecialty expertise, the 4th Edition also heralded the addition of many new contributors with special knowledge in key areas. The 5th Edition represents an extensive revision of this valuable and enduring classic.

Pediatric and Adolescent Gynecology is the classic textbook in its field. It was a catalyst to the growth of the field and it continues to lead the way, helping clinicians be more proficient and knowledgeable in the care of the child and adolescent. It is a joy to read, and can be quickly consulted to answer a specific question about a patient in your office and serve as a thorough review of the field. Simply put, this is the best book about pediatric and adolescent gynecology. If you plan on owning one textbook on pediatric and adolescent gynecology, this is the classic.

Forward by Robert L. Barbieri, M.D.
Kate Macy Ladd Professor of Obstetrics and Gynecology
Chairman, Department of Obstetrics, Gynecology and Reproductive Biology
Brigham and Women's Hospital
Harvard Medical School
Boston, Massachusetts

Preface

It has been more than 25 years since the first edition of this textbook. With the publication of the fifth edition of *Pediatric and Adolescent Gynecology*, we continue to strive to provide pediatricians, obstetrician-gynecologists, family practitioners, internists, nurse practitioners, residents and fellows with a complete text to address the common and rare gynecologic problems of children and adolescents. Drawing from the experience of the three editors and the many contributing authors, we have balanced the medical and surgical approaches to the pediatric and adolescent patient.

Pediatric and adolescent gynecologic problems may present in a varied fashion. Many gynecologic issues can be diagnosed on the basis of the history and physical examination. Step-by-step descriptions of the techniques for examination, ancillary testing, and suggested treatment plans are provided in each chapter of this text. In addition to updating all materials, we have added new chapters on urologic issues for girls and young women, and information regarding complementary and alternative medicine. New additional expert authors have been included in the 5th edition. We are also honored that Catherine Gordon., M.D., M.Sc, has rewritten the puberty chapter; W. Hardy Hendren, M.D. has contributed to the revised chapter on congenital anomalies of the reproductive tract; Craig Peters, M.D. has authored the new urology chapter; Lydia Shrier, M.D., M.P.H. has rewritten the STD chapter; Elizabeth Woods, M.D., M.P.H. the vaginitis chapter; Jessica Kahn, M.D., M.P.H. and Paula Hillard, M.D., have revised the HPV and Pap smear chapter; Angela Nicolletti, MS, RN, NP, the chapter on teen pregnancy; Ranee Leder, M.D. has revised the sexual abuse chapter; and the Honorable Judge Susan Ricci has participated in the legal issues chapter.

As editors and authors, we want to stimulate the physician and nurse practitioner to become knowledgeable and proficient in the gynecologic care of the child and adolescent. The Divisions of Gynecology and Adolescent Medicine at Children's Hospital Boston have worked together for more than 25 years and have been able to complement each other addressing the gynecologic needs of children and adolescents. We are grateful to the pediatricians, family practice physicians, obstetrician gynecologists, nurse practitioners, and others who have referred many patients to our programs. We are also grateful to Dr. Judah Folkman for having the vision to foster the creation of our pediatric and adolescent gynecology program at Children's Hospital Boston. The dialogue between medical and surgical specialties at Children's Hospital Boston, and the Brigham and Women's Hospital fostered by our Chiefs, Drs. Gary Fleisher, Robert Shamberger, Hardy Hendren, and Robert Barbieri, has been an essential factor in providing excellent gynecologic care to children and adolescents.

The field of pediatric and adolescent gynecology has been greatly enhanced by the formation in 1986 of the North American Society of Pediatric and Adolescent Gynecology (NASPAG). The sharing of ideas, research, techniques, and protocols at annual meetings and informally among members as well as the creation and support of the *Journal of Pediatric and Adolescent Gynecology*, has been of significant importance to the future of this field. Advances in other professional organizations including the American Academy of Pediatrics, the American College of Obstetrics and Gynecology, the American Society for Reproductive Medicine, American Professional Society on the Abuse of Children (APSAC), Society for Adolescent Medicine, and others have furthered the mission of provision of excellent care to children and adolescents.

We have also aimed to improve health care educational materials available on the internet. Our Center for Young Women's Health provides educational handouts in English and Spanish at www.youngwomenshealth.org. We encourage you to use this website to provide your clients, friends, and families with age appropriate educational information that can be printed and distributed.

With these efforts we aim to improve the health care and education of girls and young women around the world now and into the future.

S.J.H.E.
M.R.L.
D.P.G.

Acknowledgments

We are indebted to many people who have helped with this and previous editions. We want like to acknowledge and thank: Joyce Adams, M.D., Trina Anglin, M.D., Mary Aruda, R.N., P.N.P., Robert L. Barbieri, M.D., Carol Barnewolt, M.D., Stuart Bauer, M.D., Lauren R. Brown, M.D., Richard Bourne, J.D., Ph.D., Vicki J. Burke, R.N., B.S.N., Arnold Colodny, M.D., Marian Craighill, M.D., M.P.H., John Crigler, M.D., Ann J. Davis, M.D., Janet S. Donovan, R.N., B.S.N, Sara Forman, M.D., Catherine Gordon, M.D., M.Sc., Astrid Heger, M.D., W. Hardy Hendren, III, M.D., Paula A. Hillard, M.D., Ingrid Holm, M.D., Carol Jenny, M.D., Jessica A. Kahn. M.D., M.P.H., Ranee Leder, M.D., Maureen Lynch, M.D., Joan Mansfield, M.D., Maurice Melchiono, R.N., F.N.P., Anne Jenks Micheli, R.N., M.S., Amy Middleman, M.D., M.S.Ed., M.P.H., David Muram, M.D., Samir Najjar, M.D., Angela Nicoletti, R.N., M.S., Sally Perlman, M.D., Craig Peters, M.D., Susan Pokorny, M.D., The Honorable Susan Ricci, Cathryn Samples, M.D., M.P.H., Jane Share, M.D., Lydia Shrier, M.D., M.P.H., Victoria Smith, M.D., Phaedra Thomas, R.N., B.S.N., Jonathan D.K. Trager, M.D., Elizabeth Woods, M.D., M.P.H., and Wendy Wornham, M.D.

Our special thanks to the Children's Hospital Boston's administrative and nursing leadership for the ongoing support of the Adolescent Medicine and Gynecology Programs. We greatly appreciate the dedication and hard work of Alison Clapp, Children's Hospital Boston Librarian, and to Freedom Baird, Michelle Delmonico, Annette Luongo, Avery Putterman, Maria Robinson, Deborah Siegel, and Jessica Tsai for invaluable assistance in preparing the manuscript and artwork. We appreciate the color plate contributed by John C. Browning, M.D., and Clifford O. Mishaw, M.D. (Texas Children's Hospital), and we greatly appreciate the photographic and editorial contributions of Jonathan D.K. Trager, M.D., Assistant Clinical Professor of Dermatology and Pediatrics, The Mount Sinai Medical School, New York, NY.

We are indebted to the Maternal and Child Health Bureau for funding the Interdisciplinary Leadership Education in Adolescent Health Training Program Grant (#5 T71MC 00009-12) (S.J. Emans. PI), to the previous HRSA grant for HIV care and prevention (E. Woods, PI) and the current Research Cooperative Agreement with NICHD (#5 U01 HD040526-04) for the Adolescent Medicine Trials Unit of the Adolescent Medicine Network for HIV/AIDS Interventions (ATN) (C. Samples, PI), and to the Children's Hospital League and many other benefactors for funding www.youngwomenshealth.org. These grants have provided the support for faculty and fellows to disseminate information critical to improving the health of adolescents in the United States and beyond.

We dedicate this book to our families and friends who have lived through the stacks of references and manuscripts.

S.J.H.E.
M.R.L.
D.P.G.

1

Office Evaluation of the Child and Adolescent

S. Jean Emans

OFFICE EVALUATION OF THE CHILD AND ADOLESCENT

Gynecologic assessment and inspection of the external genitalia of the infant and child provide an opportunity to provide preventive health care and to diagnose important clinical conditions. Although gynecologic problems are uncommon in young girls, palpation of the breasts, inspection for hernias, and assessment of the external genitalia should be part of the routine physical examination. When the child presents for an evaluation for a specific problem, there should be a "problem-focused" history and physical exam. The time of a "problem-specific" or a routine exam can be utilized as an opportunity to teach anatomy and to provide recommendations regarding hygiene. The presence of clitoromegaly, a hernia, early signs of puberty, *Candida* vulvitis, vulvar dermatoses, or an abnormality in the configuration of the hymen may be a clue to other problems.

A healthy dialogue between parents and children on issues of sexuality should begin during the prepubertal years. Parents should be encouraged to answer the questions of their young children with simple facts and correct anatomic terminology. Appendix 1 contains a list of resources and Internet sites that may help parents become more comfortable in talking with their children about sexuality.

Obtaining the History

Vaginal discharge or bleeding, pruritus, signs of sexual development, or an allegation of sexual abuse should prompt a more thorough evaluation. The nature of the history depends on the presenting complaint. If the problem is vaginitis, questions should focus on the timing of the onset of symptoms; the type of discharge; perineal hygiene; skin conditions (e.g., eczema, psoriasis); antibiotic therapy;

recent infections in the patient or other members of the family, including strepto-coccal infection and pinworm infestation; masturbation; and the possibility of sexual abuse (see Chapter 24). Behavioral changes and somatic symptoms such as abdominal pain, headaches, and enuresis may suggest the possibility of abuse. Information on the caretakers should always be elicited. If the problem is vaginal bleeding, the history should include information about recent growth and devel-opment, signs of puberty, the use of hormone creams or tablets, trauma, vaginal discharge, and any previous finding of foreign bodies in the vagina or other ori-fices. Although the history is usually obtained chiefly from a parent, the child should first be asked questions about toys or school to put her at ease. Then, ques-tions may be asked about genital complaints, genital contact, and, depending on the complaint, whether she has ever placed something in her vagina. Eye contact with the child should be maintained, and she should be told that she is an impor-tant part of the team. Questions focusing on what has bothered the child, such as itching or discharge, can help her understand why the examination is important. She should be given the opportunity to ask her own questions. A questionnaire can be used to speed the intake process so that the young child does not become fid-gety while the history is being taken. However, the history-taking time can be used advantageously to put the child at ease and to promote the understanding that the clinician is acting in her best interests.

Gynecologic Examination

The gynecologic examination should be carefully explained in advance to the child and parents/guardians. It is extremely important to tell the parent that the size of the vaginal opening is quite variable and that the examination will be painless and in no way alter the hymen. A diagram showing the vulva is often helpful, as many parents still believe that the virginal introitus is totally covered by the hymen (Fig. 1-1). Gynecologic assessment of the child typically involves inspection of the genitalia, not instrumentation of the vagina.

Both parent and child should be told that the instruments to be used are spe-cially designed for little girls and do not enter the vagina. The otoscope or hand lens to be used for external examination should be shown to the child with an assurance that the clinician will use these instruments "to look." The child may wish to look through the lens of the otoscope. If a colposcope will be used for an evaluation of sexual abuse, the child should have a chance to look at the instru-ment, turn the light on and off, and view fingers or jewelry through the binocular eyepieces so that she will feel more comfortable with the examination.

The child can then be offered her choice of gown color and asked whether she wishes to have her parent lift her onto the table or climb "up the big stairs." In our clinic, the parent typically stays in the room to talk with the young child and assist in the examination. Although the father, mother, both parents, or a relative

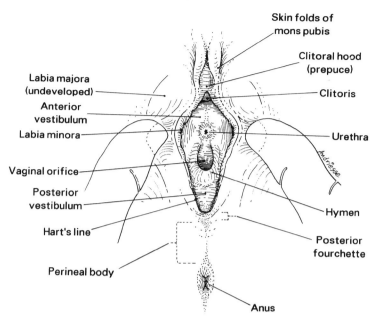

FIG. 1-1. External genitalia of the prepubertal child.

may accompany the child for the assessment, most commonly the mother plays an active role during the examination. The older child should be asked whom she prefers to have in or out of the room during the examination. Most children and many young adolescents prefer their mothers in the room; most middle to late adolescents prefer that their mothers not be present in the examination room.

The majority of children are comfortable on the examining tables with the mother (or father or other caretaker) sitting close by or holding a hand. Some girls are quite fearful, especially if they have previously been sexually abused or had a prior painful genital examination. In this case, the mother or other caretaker can sit on the table with the child or even with her feet in stirrups and have the child's legs straddle her thighs in a (semi) reclined position (Figs. 1-2 to 1-5). A hand mirror can help the child relax and allows her to become an active participant in the examination. The mirror can be used for both education and distraction. If the clinician is confident and relaxed, the patient usually responds with cooperation. An abrupt or hurried approach will precipitate anxiety and resistance in the child. Sometimes it is necessary to leave the room and return when the patient feels ready. Occasionally, a very anxious or fearful child needs to return several days later to have the examination completed. The tempo of the examination depends on the urgency of evaluating a problem and the degree of cooperation that can be elicited. For example, if a child has had a discharge for months, the examination can extend

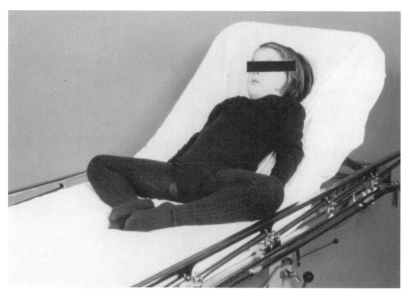

FIG. 1-2. Positioning the prepubertal child in the frog-leg position. She can lie horizontally or with the head of the examining table raised. [Courtesy of Dr. Trina Anglin, Office of Adolescent Health, Health Resources and Services Administration (HRSA), Washington, DC.]

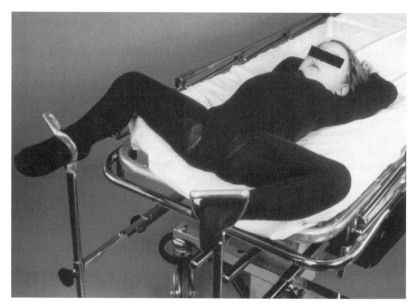

FIG. 1-3. Positioning the child in the lithotomy position with the use of stirrups. (Courtesy of Dr. Trina Anglin, Office of Adolescent Health, Health Resources and Services Administration (HRSA), Washington, DC.)

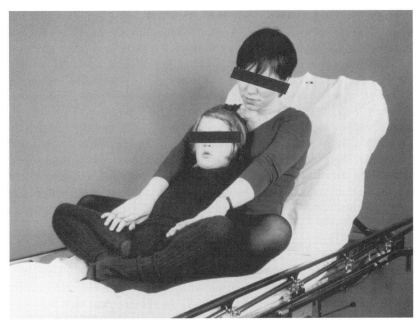

FIG. 1-4. Positioning the child in the frog-leg position with the aid of her mother. (Courtesy of Dr. Trina Anglin, Office of Adolescent Health, Health Resources and Services Administration (HRSA), Washington, DC.)

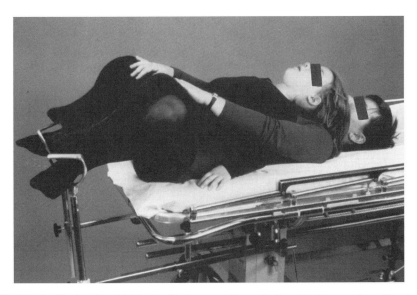

FIG. 1-5. Positioning the child in the lithotomy position with the aid of her mother. (Courtesy of Dr. Trina Anglin, Office of Adolescent Health, Health Resources and Services Administration (HRSA), Washington, DC.)

over several visits, if necessary, so that the clinician can gain the confidence of the child. If a child has significant vaginal bleeding, has experienced trauma, or cooperation cannot be elicited, then an examination with sedation or under anesthesia may be necessary.

The examination of any child with gynecologic complaints should include a general pediatric assessment including the child's weight and height, skin, head and neck, chest wall, heart, lungs, and abdomen. The breasts should be carefully inspected and palpated. The increasing diameter of the areola or a unilateral tender breast bud is often the first sign of puberty. The abdominal examination is often easier if the child places her hands on the examiner's hand; she is then less likely to tense her muscles or complain of being "tickled." The inguinal areas should be carefully palpated for a hernia or gonad; occasionally, an inguinal gonad is the testis of an undiagnosed male pseudohermaphrodite. The skin should be examined for evidence of other skin conditions such as eczema, psoriasis, seborrheic dermatitis, hemangioma, or café au lait spots.

Although the complete gynecologic examination of the child includes inspection of the external genitalia, visualization of the vagina and cervix, and rectoabdominal palpation, the extent of the examination should be tailored to the presenting complaint. Examination of the child is usually possible without sedation or anesthesia if the child has not been traumatized by previous examinations and if the clinician proceeds slowly. The child should be explicitly told that the examination will not hurt. For the initial examination, the young child should be in a supine position with her knees apart and feet touching in the frog-leg position or in the lithotomy position with the use of adjustable stirrups, with or without a caretaker assisting (Figs. 1-2 to 1-5). Asking a child whether she has ever seen a frog and whether she can say "ribbit" will often put her at ease so that she can assume the correct position "like a frog." Other young girls like to refer to this position as "making your legs like a butterfly's wings." A colorful poster on the ceiling or wall is a good distraction. During inspection of the external genitalia, the young girl may be less anxious if she assists the clinician by holding the labia apart. Occasionally, a child does not wish to remove her panties. The examination can still be accomplished in many girls by gently moving the crotch of the underwear to one side to allow inspection. The clinician should note the presence of pubic hair, the size of the clitoris, the configuration of the hymen, signs of estrogenization of the vagina and hymen, and perineal hygiene. The normal clitoral glans in the premenarcheal child is on average 3 mm in length and 3 mm in transverse diameter (1). The normal external genital structures are usually easily visible with gentle lateral traction downward and laterally (Fig. 1-6A). The hymen will often gape open if the child is asked to cough or take a deep breath. If the hymenal orifice and edges of the hymen are not visible, the labia can be gently gripped and pulled forward in a traction maneuver to enable viewing of the anterior vagina (Fig. 1-6B). The vaginal mucosa of the prepubertal girl appears thin and red in contrast with the moist, dull pink, estrogenized mucosa of the pubertal girl. Frequently, the

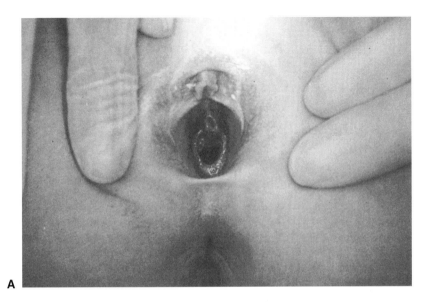

A

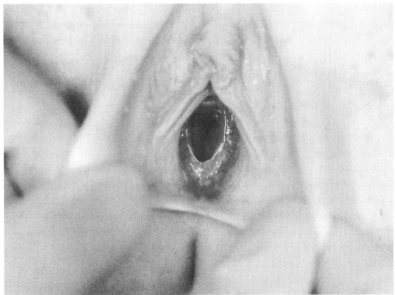

B

FIG. 1-6. Examination of the vulva, hymen, and anterior vagina by gentle lateral retraction **(A)** and gentle gripping of the labia and pulling anteriorly **(B).**

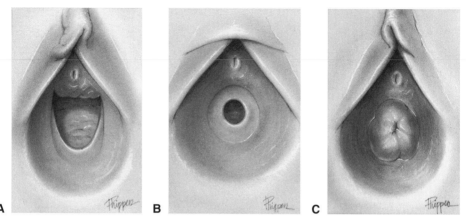

FIG. 1-7. Configurations of hymens in prepubertal girls: **(A)** posterior rim or crescentic hymen, **(B)** circumferential or annular hymen, and **(C)** fimbriated or redundant hymen. (From Pokorny SF. Configuration of the prepubertal hymen. *Am J Obstet Gynecol* 1987;157:950; with permission.)

perihymenal tissue is erythematous. Friability of the posterior fourchette as the labia are separated can occur in children with vulvitis or a history of sexual abuse or if the labia are separated widely and the tissue tears (2).

The configuration of the hymen should be noted and accurately described (Figs. 1-7 and 1-8; see also Color Plate 1). A hand lens or the light and magnification of an otoscope, without a speculum, can be used (Fig. 1-9). Hymens can be classified as posterior rim (or crescent), annular, or redundant (3). In girls with a redundant hymen, the edges of the hymen and the anterior vagina are often difficult to visualize. Congenital abnormalities of the hymen, especially microperforate and septate hymens, are not uncommon (Figs. 1-10 to 1-17; see also Chapter 10 and www.youngwomenshealth.org/hymen.html). It may initially be difficult to establish the presence of an opening in a microperforate hymen. Several techniques are useful: a small amount of warm water or saline can be squirted with a syringe or an Angiocath, or the young girl can be placed in the knee–chest position (Fig. 1-18). Probing can also be done with a small urethral catheter or feeding tube (see Fig. 1-16), or a nasopharyngeal Calgiswab moistened with saline. If there is a small slit-like opening inferior to the urethra, then the small swab needs to be inserted in a fashion parallel to the hymenal tissue. Applying a small amount of lidocaine jelly may reduce discomfort if probing is necessary and if vaginal cultures are not needed as part of the evaluation. Congenital absence of the hymen has not been documented (4,5).

Acquired abnormalities of the hymen usually result from sexual abuse and rarely from accidental trauma (see Chapters 3 and 24; see also Color Plates 9–13, and 15–18). Chapter 24 reviews the most current literature on normal and abnormal

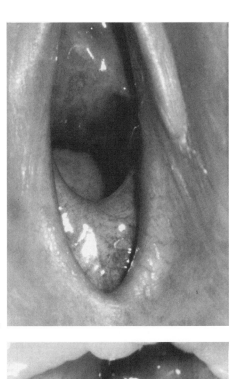

A

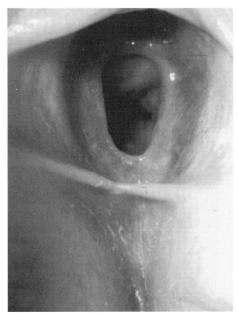

B

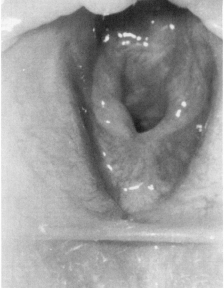

C

FIG. 1-8. Types of hymens (photographed through a colposcope): **(A)** crescentic hymen, **(B)** annular hymen, and **(C)** redundant hymen with crescent appearance after retraction.

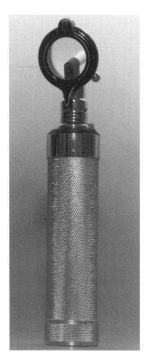

FIG. 1-9. Otoscope (without a speculum) for visualizing hymen and vagina.

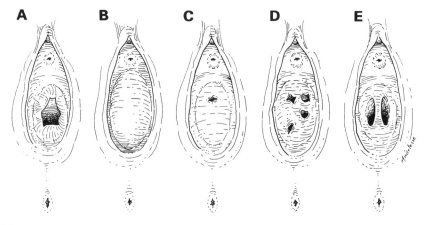

FIG. 1-10. Types of hymens: **(A)** normal, **(B)** imperforate, **(C)** microperforate, **(D)** cribriform, and **(E)** septate.

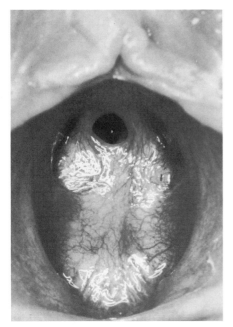

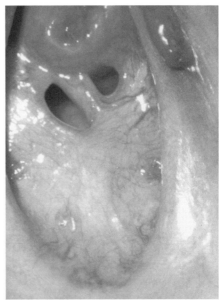

FIG. 1-12. Microperforate septate hymen.

FIG. 1-11. Microperforate hymen.

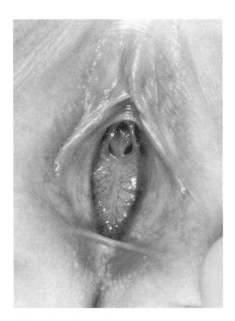

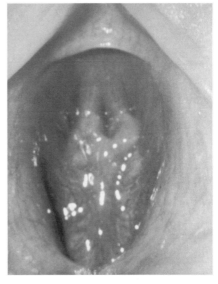

FIG. 1-13. Microperforate septate hymen.

FIG. 1-14. Imperforate hymen.

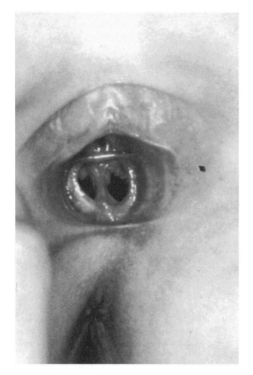

FIG. 1-15. Septate vagina.

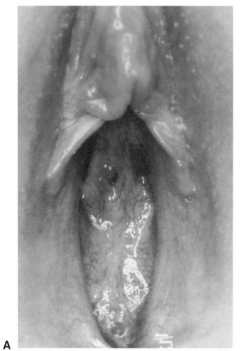

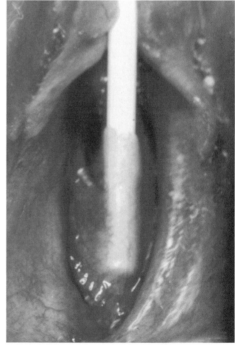

A

B

FIG. 1-16. Microperforate hymen. A: Opening difficult to visualize. B: Opening gently probed.

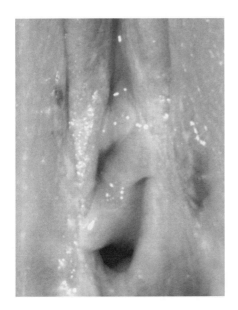

FIG. 1-17. Hymenal tags.

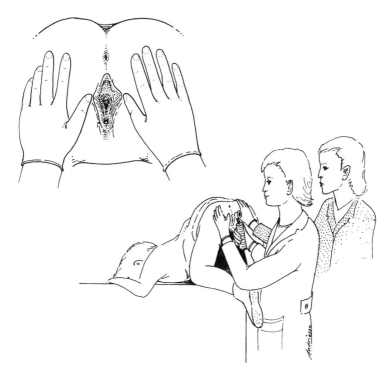

FIG. 1-18. Examination of the prepubertal child in the knee–chest position.

anogenital findings and the signs associated with sexual abuse. Signs of acute trauma from sexual abuse include hematomas, abrasions, lacerations, hymenal transections, and vulvar erythema and irritation. Physical healing from trauma is often complete by 10 to 14 days. Signs of previous sexual abuse may include acute and healed trauma, hymenal remnants, scars, and hymenal transections, which may heal in a V shape or a U shape. It should be remembered that in most girls with a history of substantiated sexual abuse, the findings on genital examination are normal. Clinicians seeing girls for annual physical examinations should be encouraged to inspect the genitalia and the hymen and, if possible, to make drawings in the office notes of the configuration of the hymen. A change from previously noted anatomy could provide an important clue to sexual abuse.

The significance of measuring the diameter of the hymenal orifice is controversial. The transverse and anterior–posterior measurements are influenced by age, relaxation of the child, method of examination and measurement, and type of hymen. The older the child and the more relaxed she is, the larger the opening. The opening is larger with retraction on the labia and when the child is in the knee–chest position than with gentle separation alone when the supine position is used. The orifice of a posterior rim hymen appears larger than the opening of a redundant hymen. Measurements can be obtained with a small clear plastic centimeter ruler or more accurately with a colposcope. Our study of 3- to 6-year-old girls found a mean transverse measurement of 2.9 ± 1.3 mm (range 1 to 6 mm) and mean anterior–posterior measurement of 3.3 ± 1.5 mm (range 1 to 7 mm) (2) (see Chapter 24 for other studies). Although a large hymenal orifice may be consistent with a history of sexual abuse, a more significant finding is the absence of hymenal tissue that has resulted to the enlarged opening.

The anus and labia should always be examined for cleanliness, excoriations, and erythema. Perianal excoriation may be a clue to pinworm infestation. Normal findings, as well as those associated with sexual abuse, are noted in Chapter 24.

For girls with vulvitis or lichen sclerosus (see Color Plates 2, 3, and 4), an external examination may be all that is needed to make a diagnosis and formulate a treatment plan (see Chapter 3). However, if there is discharge, bleeding, or any other complaint that may be of vaginal origin, the clinician should proceed with visualization of the vagina.

In girls over 2 years old, the knee–chest position provides a particularly good view of the vagina and cervix without instrumentation (6). The patient is told that she should lie with her chest on the table and her "bottom in the air." She is reassured that the examiner plans to "take a look at her bottom" but will not put anything inside her. In the knee–chest position, the child rests her head to one side on her folded arms and supports her weight on bent knees (6 to 8 in. apart). With her buttocks held up in the air, she is encouraged to let her spine and stomach "sag downward." Some girls like to hear that they may have slept in this position when they were "little." A pillow can be placed under the girl's abdomen if she desires. A sheet can also be used so that she feels covered. An assistant or the mother helps hold the buttocks apart, pressing laterally and slightly upward. As the child takes deep breaths, the vaginal orifice falls open for examination (see Fig. 1-18). In 80% to 90% of prepubertal girls, an ordinary otoscope head, used without a speculum (see Fig. 1-9), provides the magnification and light necessary to enable visualization of the lower vagina and usually the upper vagina and cervix. The child's anxiety will be allayed if she is again shown the otoscope light and efforts are made to gain her full confidence before this part of the examination. A running conversation about school, toys, and siblings often diverts the child's attention and helps her maintain this position for several minutes without moving or objecting. Since the vagina of the prepubertal child is quite short, a foreign body or a lesion is often easily detected. Similarly, a supine position with the child's legs flexed on her abdomen also enhances visualization of the hymen, vagina, and anus.

Vaginoscopy

If vaginal assessment cannot be accomplished in the office for the child with vaginal bleeding or persistent discharge, an examination with sedation or under anesthesia is the next step. An examination with sedation or under anesthesia may also be important if vulvar biopsy is needed for suspected but not clear-cut vulvar dystrophies or for obtaining typing of human papillomavirus (HPV) lesions, or excision of a suspicious nevus or other vulvar lesion. A Killian nasal speculum with a light source can be helpful for direct visualization of the vagina and cervix (Fig. 1-19). The use of a hysteroscope, cystoscope, or flexible narrow-diameter

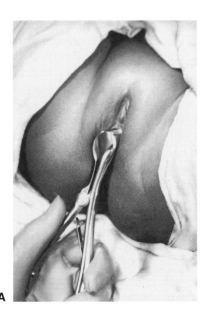

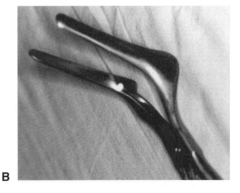

B

FIG. 1-19. (A) Examination of patient under anesthesia, **(B)** using a Killian nasal speculum with fiberoptic light (obtained from Codman and Shurtleff, Inc., Pacella Drive, Randolph, MA).

A

fiberoptic scope with liquid insufflation can be helpful for magnification and identification of vaginal or cervical lesions. As the vagina is filled with the liquid distention media, the labia are "pinched closed" so that the vagina will distend and
facilitate evaluation.

Depending upon the office setting, some clinicians do sometimes use a small
vaginoscope, cystoscope, hysteroscope, or flexible fiberoptic scope with water
insufflation of the vagina for visualization of the upper vagina and cervix in the
cooperative child. The child is examined in a supine position with her knees apart.
A step-by-step method of inserting the vaginoscope in the young child was originally described by Capraro (7). The child is first allowed to touch the instrument
and is told that it feels "slippery, funny, and cool." The instrument is then placed
against her inner thigh and the same words are repeated. Next, the instrument is
placed against her labia, again with the statement, "This feels slippery, funny, and
cool." As the vaginoscope is inserted through the hymen, the examiner repeats the
words and presses the child's buttocks firmly with the other hand to divert her
attention. The application of lidocaine jelly makes insertion easier. Most
vaginoscopy is done under sedation or anesthesia. Very rarely, a narrow vaginal
speculum can be useful in examining the older child if insertion does not cause
pain or trauma.

Vaginal Samples

If a vaginal discharge is present, samples should be obtained for culture and for
saline and potassium hydroxide (KOH) preparations (see section on Wet Preparations, p. 37). Usually, the child prefers to lie on her back with her knees apart and
with her feet together or in the stirrups so that she can watch the procedure without becoming excessively anxious. A nasopharyngeal Calgiswab moistened with
nonbacteriostatic saline, a soft plastic eyedropper, a glass eyedropper with plastic
tubing attached, a small feeding tube with a syringe, or a modified urethral catheter
attached to a syringe (8) can be gently inserted through the hymenal opening to
aspirate secretions or to obtain a vaginal wash sample. The child should be allowed
to feel a cotton-tipped applicator, Calgiswab, feeding tube, or catheter on her skin
before a similar sterile device is inserted into her vagina. For example, a cotton-
tipped applicator can be gently stroked over the back of her hand to allow her to
feel it as "soft" or "ticklish." For the prepubertal child, we usually use a naspha-
ryngeal Calgiswab moistened with nonbacteriostatic saline (such as ampules of
nebulizer saline) (Fig. 1-20A). If a small saline-moistened Calgiswab is used, care
should be taken to place it into the vagina without touching the edges of the hymen.
The child can be asked to cough as the examiner inserts the swab. This action dis-
tracts the child and makes the hymen gape open. The child will be amazed that no
discomfort is felt, and the three samples (one with a Dacron male urethral swab
gently scraping the lateral vaginal wall, if a sample for vaginal *Chlamydia* culture
is desired) can be quickly obtained and directly plated or sent for culture. Pokorny

and Stormer (8) have described a modified syringe and urethral catheter (Fig. 1-20B) in which the proximal 4-in. end of an intravenous butterfly catheter is inserted into the 4-in. end piece of a no. 12 bladder catheter, and a syringe is attached. The catheter is slid into the vagina, similarly to catheterizing the bladder. Sterile saline (0.5 to 1 ml) is injected into the vagina and aspirated. This device is commercially available as the Pediatric Vaginal Aspirator from Cook ObGyn (Spencer, IN). If necessary, a small amount of lidocaine solution can be applied to the hymenal edges to facilitate insertion. For the child who will not allow an intravaginal sampling, Muram has used a technique of squirting saline with an Angiocath (no needle) to fill the vagina followed by holding three swabs perpendicular just outside the vagina with the labia held closed over the swabs by the examiner. The child is asked to cough hard to expel the solution, and the wet swabs are used for the needed tests.

A culture for *Neisseria gonorrhoeae* should be done on modified Thayer–Martin–Jembec medium at the time of the examination. Cultures for other organisms are done by placing the saline moistened Calgiswab into a transport Culturette II with medium. The bacteriology laboratory should plate the swab on the standard genitourinary media, which usually include blood agar, MacConkey, and chocolate media. The laboratory should be notified that the Thayer–Martin–Jembec medium being processed is from the vagina of a *prepubertal* child so that if a *Neisseria* species grows, it is properly and unequivocally identified as *N. gonorrhoeae* for medicolegal purposes. Bacterial isolates initially identified as *N. gonorrhoeae* from children may be other *Neisseria* species such as *N. lactamica, N. meningitidis,* and *N. cinerea* (9,10).

Culture tests for *Chlamydia trachomatis* should be used in the diagnosis of prepubertal infections, since false-positive results can occur with some nonculture

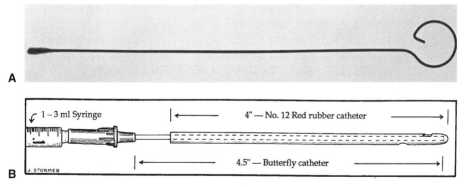

FIG. 1-20. A: Calgiswab for obtaining vaginal specimens in the prepubertal girl. **B:** Assembled catheter-within-a-catheter, for obtaining specimens from a prepubertal child. (From Pokorny SF, Stormer LVN. Atraumatic removal of secretions from the prepubertal vagina. *Am J Obstet Gynecol* 1987;156:581; with permission.)

tests. The association of this organism with sexual abuse necessitates sensitive and specific methods (see Chapters 3, 15, and 24). If culture is not available, some research has indicated that nucleic acid amplification tests (NAATs) are acceptable if another NAAT that targets a different sequence can be performed should the first NAAT test be positive (11,12). For patients who complain of itching or have suspected yeast infection, a Biggy agar culture can be incubated and read in the office.

Completing the Examination

After the vaginal samples have been obtained, a rectoabdominal examination may be indicated for the child with persistent discharge, bleeding, or pelvic/abdominal pain. The bimanual examination is performed with the child in stirrups or supine with her legs apart. The examiner places the index or little finger of one hand into the rectum and the other hand on the abdomen. The child can be reassured that this examination will feel somewhat like having her temperature taken rectally or having a bowel movement. She should be reassured that a finger has a smaller diameter than a bowel movement. Except in the newborn infant, in whom the uterus is enlarged secondary to maternal estrogen, the rectal examination in the prepubertal child reveals only the small "button" or thickening of the cervix and uterus. Since the ovaries are not palpable in the child and are located higher in the pelvis than in the adult, masses should alert the physician to the possibility of a cyst or tumor. At the end of the rectal examination, as the finger is removed from the rectum, the vagina should be gently "milked" to promote the passage of any discharge or extremely rare vaginal (sarcoma botryoides) tumors (Color Plate 8).

After assessing a patient's chief complaint and the results of the examination, the clinician should spend time with the parents and child to discuss the diagnosis, the proposed therapy, and the necessity of follow-up. Praising the young child for her cooperation and bravery helps establish the clinician–patient relationship so important during future examinations.

OFFICE EVALUATION OF THE ADOLESCENT

Evaluation of the adolescent requires different technical skills, including speculum examination of the vagina, bimanual palpation, and an office environment that is welcoming to the adolescent patient. It is most important that the clinician have the interpersonal skills, sensitivity, and time to establish a primary relationship with the adolescent herself. The clinician must be willing to see the teenager alone and listen to her concerns. For example, the patient with oligomenorrhea may ask at each return visit, "Why am I not normal?" Listening to her describe her feelings is just as important as drawing diagrams of the hypothalamic–pituitary–ovarian axis. The statement "Your pelvic exam is normal" answers few of the adolescent's questions.

The office setting should have a welcoming group of administrative assistants and clinical aides. A seating area for teens is optimal, since they may not feel comfortable sitting with babies in the pediatrician's office or with pregnant women older than themselves in the gynecologist's office. Special times can sometimes be reserved in the evening or late afternoon to respond to the needs of teens. In addition, a mechanism to receive telephone calls from teens needs to be arranged by the office staff. In a pediatric, internal medicine, family medicine, or gynecologic practice, examination rooms should be neutral. In a practice limited to adolescents, the office can have posters and pamphlets (see Appendix 1) that are pertinent to their concerns and, for example, give information on birth control, sexually transmitted diseases (STDs), human immunodeficiency virus (HIV), nutrition, and how to say "no" to premature sexual activity. Access to the Internet with appropriate sites bookmarked also aids in patient education.

When a girl reaches the age of 11 or 12 years, the clinician can discuss with her and her family the need for adolescent preventive health care, the opportunities for confidentiality, and the importance of communication among the health care provider, the patient, and her family. The parents should be educated about giving their adolescents the special time they need to discuss concerns with the health care provider about peer relations, school, family, drugs, alcohol, and sexuality. The well teenager should have at least an annual visit; a patient with medical or psychosocial concerns should be seen more frequently. The American Medical Association (AMA) has published a set of 24 recommendations for annual preventive health care for adolescents (Table 1-1), along with questionnaires for patients and families on their Web site (13). A project under the sponsorship of the Maternal Child Health Bureau with representatives from the American Academy of Pediatrics (AAP), Medicaid, Health Care Financing Administration, and other groups provided similar guidelines: *Bright Futures—Guidelines for Health Supervision of Infants, Children, and Adolescents*, first published in 1994 and updated in 2000 (14). Subsequent companion volumes on nutrition, mental health, oral health, and case studies for primary care clinicians (15–17) have also been published for Bright Futures, and updated guidelines will be at www.aap.org.

Parents should be included as much as possible in important medical decisions, but the adolescent's need for medical privacy and confidentiality should be respected. Parents should be encouraged to call in advance of an appointment if they have special concerns, since an adolescent may sometimes be strikingly nonverbal about troubling issues at home or in school. At the same time, parents may need help communicating more effectively with their adolescent. Clinicians should be explicit with both parents and adolescents about the extent of confidentiality. In a survey of high school students, Cheng and colleagues (18) reported that 25% of teens would forgo health care in some situations if their parents found out, and only 57% of teens would go to their regular physician for questions about pregnancy. Thrall and colleagues, in a survey of over 2,000 ninth and twelfth grade students in Massachusetts, found that students who believed that their physicians

TABLE 1-1. *Summary of recommendations of the AMA Guidelines for Adolescent Preventive Services (GAPS)*

General
1. Annual preventive services visit
2. Age and developmentally appropriate preventive services
3. Office policies regarding confidentiality

Health guidance
4. For parents or other adult caregivers at least twice during child's adolescence
5. Physical growth, psychosocial and psychosexual development
6. Reduction of injuries
7. Dietary habits and safe weight management
8. Exercise
9. Responsible sexual behaviors (including abstinence), prevention of STDs, and contraception
10. Avoidance of tobacco, alcohol, other abusable substances, and anabolic steroids.

Screening
11. Hypertension
12. Hyperlipidemia
13. Eating disorders and obesity
14. Use of tobacco products
15. Use of alcohol and other abusable substances
16. Sexual behaviors
17. Screening for STDs
18. Access to confidential HIV testing
19. Pap test
20. Depression and risk of suicide
21. Emotional, physical, or sexual abuse
22. Learning or school problems
23. Tuberculin testing

Immunizations
24. Appropriate immunizations

provided confidential care were much more likely to have discussed sexuality, pregnancy prevention, and alcohol and tobacco use (19). Similarly, Ford and colleagues found that assurances of confidentiality increased the willingness to disclose information of sexuality, substance abuse, mental health, and to return to the physician for care (20,21). Although explicit confidentiality is important, it is essential that teens know the limits of confidentiality and that the clinician needs to involve others in conditions that are life threatening or carry a significant health risk. Letting teens know that the clinician will work with them if there are issues that need to be shared can alleviate many of their concerns.

The transition from childhood to adolescence involves biologic, cognitive, and psychological changes. The prepubertal latency-age girl undergoes major changes in her body as she develops into the sexually mature young woman. The appearance of pubic hair and breast development, over which the girl has no control, can be exciting but also can cause concern. She may view asymmetry of breasts, acne, or normal weight gain as problems. The fact that her pubertal changes occur at the same rate as in her peer group may offer some reassurance; to be early or late can be troubling. A 12-year-old girl who looks 16 may be confronted with sexual demands; a 16-year-old girl who looks 10 may be embarrassed to undress for physical education class or to interact with her peer group. Girls with lesbian attractions may feel uncomfortable in schools and office settings that speak only to the needs and questions of heterosexual girls (22). The young adolescent may not understand the reasons for her pubertal changes and may ask the same questions at each visit. The older teenager is usually more capable of coping intellectually with the physical examination, the diagnosis, and the treatment plan. Young adolescents are concrete thinkers; thus, explanations and directions for medications must take this into account. Even when an older teen, who is more capable of abstraction and orientation to the future, is prescribed oral contraceptives, it is helpful to have the actual pill package in front of her so she can see how the pills look and learn the calendar system of the individual package. The clinician must thus be sensitive to the different needs of each patient and respond to her issues during assessment, physical examination, and treatment plan.

Obtaining the History

The source of the medical history depends on the medical setting and the age of the patient. The older adolescent tends to seek gynecologic care on her own initiative. In a clinic setting, the clinician may see the mother (and/or the father or other caretaker) and the patient together initially to ascertain the nature of the chief complaint and to ask about the girl's medical history, school problems, and psychosocial adjustment. A major portion of the visit should be devoted to seeing the teenager alone, since her presenting complaint is quite often different from her parent's concerns. In other settings, the parent may make the appointment by telephone, and then the teenager may appear alone for the examination.

The history should relate not only to gynecologic issues but to general health concerns, risk behaviors, and a review of systems. The information can be gathered by the clinician, a computer-aided questionnaire, or a health history form. Private space is important if honest answers are expected. Prefacing the questioning with the statement "I ask all my patients these questions" helps patients to feel they have not been singled out or prejudged. Family history and psychosocial history are as important as the medical history. With adolescents, it is best to first ask them why they are in the office for an evaluation that day. Otherwise, the presenting complaint can be lost in the review of systems, attention to birth control needs, and other issues. The clinician should proceed from neutral areas such as review of systems, allergies, headaches, and gastrointestinal problems to menstrual history and then to weight changes and eating patterns, risky behaviors, sexual preference, and sexual activity. Risky behaviors often occur in clusters, and adolescents who begin smoking and using alcohol early are also frequently involved in early sexual activity. It is often helpful to ask the patient first about risky behaviors in the peer group: "Do your friends smoke? Do your friends use drugs? Are your friends having sex? Have any of your friends been pregnant?" An adolescent's sexual and drug-taking behavior frequently is similar to that of her friends. Even if she is not currently involved in such behaviors, she may be influenced by her peers to experiment in the near future. She may also need assistance with ways to resist the pressure and later reassurance that she is making a sound decision: "From what you are telling me, you have made a healthy choice to avoid . . ."

In questioning the patient, the clinician can start with more neutral risk behaviors: "Do you smoke? Do you use a seat belt? Have you ever been in a car with someone drinking? Do you have a sexual partner? Tell me about your partner. Have you ever had sex? Have you ever been forced or pressured into having sex? What would you do if you were feeling pressured to have sex? Have you ever felt threatened, been slapped, or been hit in a relationship? Have you ever had a sexually transmitted infection? Do you need birth control?" It is important that questions be carefully worded so they are not heterosexually biased or do not convey the assumption that all patients are sexually active. The clinician should avoid writing down answers during the interview when asking about risky behaviors such as drug and alcohol use, because the teen may feel reluctant to give honest answers and the dialogue may be interrupted. Similarly, 10–15% of girls may have experienced unwanted sexual intercourse or dating violence (23,24). Other questions might be "If you make a decision to have sexual relations, would you know how to protect yourself from pregnancy? If you had a girl friend who didn't want to get pregnant, could you help her?" If she says, "Yes," ask, "How?" Such discussions require skillful handling, because adolescents who are not sexually active benefit from support in maintaining their choice. Since many adolescents assume that "everyone" is sexually active, they are often reassured when they learn that many teens choose to postpone having sex until they are older or in a permanent relationship. The messages conveyed are important: The clinician may want to encourage the adolescent to postpone sexual intercourse but also wants to be there to help her with sexual decision making and contraceptive choices. The question "Tell me the things you are doing to stay healthy" also assures the teen that she can make healthy decisions for herself.

As clinicians ask these questions, many feel frustrated by the time constraints of the office setting and the slowness of behavioral change in their patients. It is useful to know the content of curricula being taught in the local school system so that messages can be built into community-wide norms. Office interventions can then build upon the framework of the school, faith group, or community initiative. Many clinicians find the *Guidelines for Adolescent Preventive Services (GAPS)* algorithms (Table 1-2) and an understanding of the "stages of change" useful in planning strategies for interventions with adolescents. The clinician gathers initial information using the office interview and/or questionnaires, makes a further

TABLE 1-2. *GAPS algorithm for office interventions for high-risk behaviors*

G = Gather information
A = Assess further
P = Problem identification
S = Solutions

assessment to determine the level of risk, and then identifies problems. The adolescent's goals and perception of risk are sought. It is important to find out whether the teen is interested in change and what she is willing to do. Finally, the clinician works with the adolescent to seek solutions, reinforcing self-efficacy (can the patient make a change?) and solving barriers. Because an adolescent may have more than one health problem, it is essential for the patient and clinician to work together to prioritize health issues and address them over time.

For example, to address the problem of smoking, which is common in teen girls, the clinician Gathers information (does the patient smoke?), Assesses the level of risk (age started, packs per day, efforts to quit), solves the Problem (presents choices, discusses with the teen such problems as impaired athletic performance, stains on fingers and teeth, bad breath, respiratory disease, and cost of cigarettes), and finds Solutions (sets a quit date; supports the teen in avoiding activities associated with smoking; recommends chewing gum, exercise, or nicotine replacement or pharmacological therapy; and arranges follow-up).

Many clinicians have also found an understanding of the stages of change, originally described as a transtheoretical model for substance abusers (Fig. 1-21), to be valuable in conceptualizing interventions for teens (25). In order to move an adolescent toward a particular behavior change, the clinician determines that stage of change for that girl and then assists her to move from one stage to the next over several visits. The clinician helps to personalize the risk for the individual adolescent. *Precontemplators* do not consider the behavior in question to be a problem; it is neither relevant nor a risk to their health. To move an adolescent to the next stage, the provider should give information about the health consequences and promote the benefits of change. *Contemplators* consider that they may indeed have a problem, realize that there are pros and cons to the behavior, and begin to weigh the feasibility of change. The provider needs to address the teen's barriers and concerns about behavior change and to assist with achieving change in steps. "What would happen if you quit smoking? What would happen if you used a condom? How do you imagine your life could improve if you gave up using drugs?"

At the *determination* or *preparation stage,* the adolescent recognizes the need to change (within a month), although the behavior itself remains unchanged. The health care provider assists by emphasizing the importance of the pros and de-emphasizing the value of the cons. In the *action stage*, the adolescent is actively

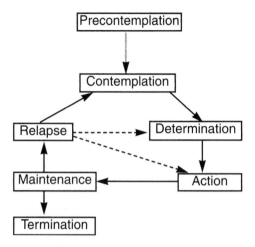

FIG. 1-21. Stages of change. (Adapted from Prochaska JO, DiClemente CC. Transtheoretical therapy: toward a more integrative model of change. *Psychother Theory Res Pract* 1982;19:276.)

changing behavior. The action should be reinforced through visits and telephone calls. In *maintenance,* the adolescent refrains from the risky behavior and is confident in having made a change, which may lead to either a permanent exit (*termination* or *recovery*) from the cycle, or a *relapse* and entry into another cycle. Relapse should be treated as a learning experience, not a failure. This framework provides the clinician with the opportunity to think about a variety of interventions for the risky or unhealthy behaviors noted during the interview.

The clinician providing gynecologic health care to adolescents needs to consider not only the chief complaint for a visit but the more general psychosocial and health needs of the teen. The interventions and recommendations for therapy must be focused on family and life issues beyond those yielding to simple hormonal or antibiotic therapy.

Gynecologic Examination

Once the history has been obtained and the problems have been identified, the patient should be given a thorough explanation of a pelvic examination. The use of diagrams or a plastic model of the pelvis or an Internet module (www.young-womenshealth.org) is helpful. If the teen has ever used tampons or is sexually active, she will find her first examination easier. However, a previous examination that was uncomfortable or a history of sexual assault may make the examination much more challenging. In explaining the first examination, the clinician should acknowledge the feelings of the adolescent. Good communication can be established by a statement such as this: "Some girls I see are worried about pain or embarrassment." It helps to acknowledge that adolescents can be nervous: "A lot of patients I see because of irregular periods are pretty nervous about these exams. It takes only 2 or 3 minutes, and I will explain everything to you now, and then again as I do the exam. I can't do a good exam unless you are relaxed; so it's my job to help you feel comfortable. You are welcome to have someone in the room with you during the exam." Millstein and colleagues (26) noted that messages from friends about pelvic examinations were usually negative and referred to pain, self-consciousness, fear, anxiety, and physical or psychological discomfort. In contrast, messages from mothers and health care providers were primarily descriptions of procedures and their importance. The study underscored the necessity for clinicians to discuss the physical sensations associated with the procedure and to suggest methods of cognitive control. Such a discussion may include the use of imagery, a complete explanation before and during the examination, a mirror, or distraction. Each patient needs individualized attention, and adequate drapes and gowns are important. Allowing the adolescent to control the tempo of the examination is important to alleviate her concerns.

After the explanation, the patient should be asked if she needs to empty her bladder. She should then be given a gown and asked to remove all her clothes, including bra and underpants. If she is covered appropriately and approached in a relaxed manner, she will feel more able to cooperate with the examination. The young adolescent may request that her mother stay with her during a pelvic examination. Most older patients prefer their mothers to stay in the waiting room. The patient's wishes should be respected. It is important for male clinicians to be accompanied by a female chaperone, who can aid in reassuring the patient and helping with samples. A chaperone should always be present if the patient desires one or needs support during the examination, or if medical or legal issues are a factor.

The general physical examination of a teenage girl should always include inspection of the skin, palpation of the thyroid gland, examination of the breasts and abdomen, and a careful notation of the Tanner stages of breast and pubic hair development (see Chapter 4). Demonstrating techniques of self-examination of the breast to the patient during the actual breast examination (see Chapter 19) can be used to put the young woman at ease. However, teaching breast self-examination to the adolescent should not be a goal of preventive clinical services since time in the office is better spent counseling around tobacco, alcohol, and sexual risk prevention than breast self-examination teaching. Breast cancer is not a disease of teenagers, so that teaching breast self-examination to the older teen and young woman should be thought of as part of self-awareness and health promotion, not as an effort to detect cancer. It is essential not to increase the anxiety of the young teen or overload the adolescent with guilt when she does not follow instructions for undertaking breast self-examination.

Inspection of the external genitalia in the adolescent is an important part of the physical examination. Several medical conditions may be detected: folliculitis from shaving or other pubic hair removal methods; *Candida* vulvitis, which can be the first sign of diabetes; vulvar dermatoses; obstructive congenital anomalies such as an imperforate hymen; labial hypertrophy or asymmetry; or clitoromegaly. Similarly, normal sebaceous glands and vulvar papillomatosis may have caused worry. The actual examination frequently elicits questions that the teenager was embarrassed to ask, such as queries about a vaginal discharge, a lump, or irregular periods. Equally important to inspection is reassurance of the adolescent that her perineum is normal. A number of gynecologic conditions including vulvitis and vaginitis can be diagnosed with simple inspection and cotton-tipped applicator samples of vaginal secretions. Screening *Chlamydia trachomatis* and *N. gonorrhoeae* tests can be performed on urine samples in sexually active girls who are not undergoing a speculum examination (see Chapter 15).

Other conditions require varying parts of the complete pelvic examination. For example, in an adolescent girl presenting with primary amenorrhea, the most important objective is to identify whether she has a normally patent hymen and vagina and the presence of a cervix and uterus. Thus a determination of vaginal length using a saline-moistened cotton-tipped applicator, followed by a one-finger vaginal–abdominal examination or rectoabdominal examination, can establish normal or abnormal genital anatomy. If this examination is not possible, external genital examination to establish a patent hymen, exclusion of a transverse vaginal septum by insertion of a cotton-tipped applicator (if tolerated), and ultrasonography of the pelvis can be used similarly to answer the question about genital anatomy. For the non-sexually active teenager with unexplained abdominal or pelvic pain, a bimanual vaginal abdominal or rectoabdominal examination, with the patient in the lithotomy position, will help with the differential diagnosis.

A speculum examination followed by a bimanual examination is usually easily accomplished in the sexually active teen with irregular bleeding, pelvic pain, severe dysmenorrhea, or amenorrhea. Most non-sexually active girls, especially those who have used tampons, can undergo a speculum examination, if needed for similar complaints. The least invasive examination that will answer the question should be performed. On the other hand, examinations should not be omitted solely because of the age of the patient. Contrary to popular belief, rarely is a patient unable to cooperate during a pelvic examination if she has received a careful explanation about the procedure and its importance in evaluating her individual problem. However, it is also important to recognize cultural issues surrounding vaginal examinations. Some families and adolescents are reluctant to permit examination with a speculum because of the misconception that it will alter the hymenal anatomy and virginity. After careful explanation that pelvic examinations have not been shown to be associated with changes in hymens (27), some patients and families are comfortable with a pelvic examination; others are not. Flexibility and respect are the key to good rapport.

As noted above, sexually active patients typically begin routine gynecologic assessments and annual screening for sexually transmitted diseases (STDs) at initiation of vaginal intercourse. It is important that good clinical preventive services for adolescents be unlinked from the prescription of hormonal contraception. The absence of a pelvic examination or Papanicolaou (Pap) test is not a contraindication to the prescription of contraception (28). If a pelvic examination is being performed, cervical (rather than urine) screening for STDs is recommended. Otherwise, urine screening for STDs should be obtained annually. Tests for *N. gonorrhoeae* and *C. trachomatis* should be obtained more frequently when the patient has changed sexual partners, experiences vaginal symptoms, has been exposed to or has a history of STDs, or engages in high-risk behaviors (see Chapter 15 for a discussion of cervical and urine screening tests for STDs). Pap tests should be initiated within 3 years of onset of sexual activity or by age 21 years (29) (see Chapter 17). Girls receiving episodic care, who are immunosuppressed, or who are at increased risk should initiate Pap tests earlier.

An adolescent who is not sexually active can begin routine gynecologic examinations whenever she feels comfortable about the procedure, with the hope that by the age of 18 to 21 years she will have initiated routine care. Using tampons before a first examination is helpful for the virginal patient and increases the ease of the examination for the patient (27). It is important for patients to realize that the pelvic examination and the Pap test are not synonymous, and that a pelvic examination to assure the anatomy is normal does not mandate obtaining a Pap test.

The pelvic examination is done with the patient in the lithotomy position and her feet in stirrups. A mirror can be offered to her. The external genitalia are inspected first; the type of hymenal opening, estrogenization of the vaginal mucosa, the distribution of pubic hair (if not shaved), and the size of the clitoris are assessed. The pubic hair should be inspected for pediculosis pubis if itching is present. Similarly, the mons and inner thighs should be inspected for folliculitis, which can be associated with hair removal methods. The inguinal areas should be palpated for evidence of lymphadenopathy. The estrogenized vagina has a moist or thickened dull pink mucosa in contrast to the thin red mucosa of the prepubertal child. The normal clitoral glans is 2 to 4 mm wide; a width of 10 mm is considered to indicate significant virilization. In a study of 200 consecutive normal women, Verkauf and colleagues (30) reported a mean transverse diameter of the clitoral glans of 3.4 ± 1.0 mm, a longitudinal diameter of 5.1 ± 1.4 mm, and a total clitoral length, including glans and body, of 16.0 ± 4.3 mm. The mean clitoral index (the product of the glans width times glans length) was 18.5 mm^2.

The normal anatomy of the postpubertal external genitalia is illustrated in Figs. 1-22 and 1-23. The hymen in the adolescent girl is estrogenized and thickened. Minor changes due to sexual abuse or minor trauma that might have been easily seen in the thin unestrogenized hymen of the prepubertal child may be difficult to visualize or may have disappeared in the estrogenized vulva and hymen of the adolescent. As the normal hymen is elastic, tampons can be inserted by most adolescents. With very rare exceptions, tampon use does not cause lacerations of the hymen (27). In the virginal adolescent, the hymenal opening is usually large enough to allow the insertion of a small Huffman speculum or a finger for palpation of the cervix, uterus, and ovaries. An adolescent who has been sexually active may have a hymen without any obvious changes or may have transections ("complete clefts" down to the base of the hymen), a narrow rim of hymen, or myrtiform caruncles (small bumps of residual hymen along the lower edge) (Fig. 1-24).

The examination of the sexually abused adolescent should involve a careful assessment of the vulva and hymen. The hymenal edges can be carefully examined by running a saline-moistened cotton swab around the edges (Fig. 1-25). Another method used by some clinicians to facilitate examination of the hymen is the use of a 12- or 14-gauge Foley bladder catheter with a 5- to 10-ml balloon and a 10-ml syringe. The catheter is inserted into the vagina, the balloon filled to capacity, usually to 10 ml, with water and the catheter pulled back gently (avoiding extreme traction) just to the hymenal edge to enhance observation of hymenal disruptions, one side at a time (31). After the examination is completed, the catheter is deflated and removed.

As with the prepubertal child, different configurations of hymens may be seen in adolescents (see Fig. 1-10). A simple hymenotomy is required for the imperforate hy-

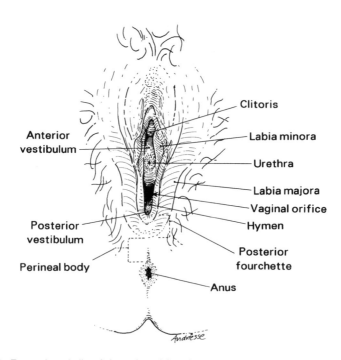

FIG. 1-22. External genitalia of the pubertal female.

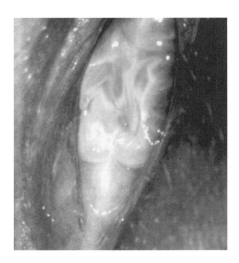

FIG. 1-23. Normal estrogenized hymen. (From Heger A, Muram D, Emans SJ. *Evaluation of the sexually abused child.* 2nd ed. New York: Oxford University Press, 2001; with permission.)

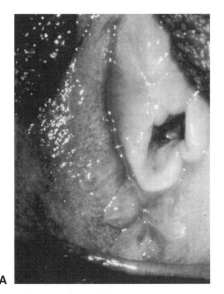

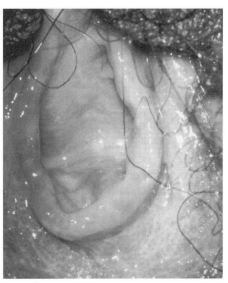

A

B

FIG. 1-24. Adolescent hymens. A: Complete cleft at 4 o'clock from prior sexual abuse. B: Dilated hymenal opening from consensual sexual activity (no clefts on hymen). (From Heger A, Muram D, Emans SJ. *Evaluation of the sexually abused child.* 2nd ed. New York: Oxford University Press, 2001; with permission.)

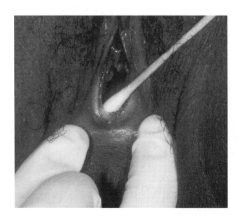

FIG. 1-25. Cotton swab used to examine the edge of the hymen.

men (type B) at the time of diagnosis and for microperforate, cribriform, and septate hymens (types C, D, and E) prior to tampon use or sexual intercourse. The septal band may be excised in the office or in an outpatient operating room with the patient being given intravenous sedation or general anesthesia; it may also break when a tampon is removed or during coitus. It is important for the adolescent with any of the latter three types to be aware of her anatomy so she is not traumatized by difficulty in the use of tampons or in having intercourse. The timing of intervention should be decided by the patient after discussion with her physician.

To avoid surprising the patient during the bimanual or speculum examination, the clinician should precede the examination by a statement such as "I'm now going to touch your bottom" or "I'm now going to place this cool metal speculum first against your thigh and then in your vagina." In the virginal teenager, a slow, one-finger examination will demonstrate the size of the hymenal opening and the location of the cervix, and will allow subsequent easy insertion of the speculum. It is helpful to warm the speculum and then touch it to the patient's thigh to allow her to feel its "cool metal" quality. The speculum should be inserted posteriorly with a downward direction to avoid the urethra. Applying pressure to the inner thigh at the same time the speculum or finger is inserted into the vagina is help-ful. Experts have varying opinions about the value of showing the adolescent the speculum before the examination. In our experience, the adolescent is often much more fearful if she is shown the speculum in advance and does better if she merely feels it initially against her thigh. The patient's wishes should always be respected if she wishes to view or handle a speculum.

If the hymenal opening is small, a Huffman speculum (1/2 × 4 1/4 in.) is used to visualize the cervix. Occasionally, a latex glove with the tip cut off and placed over the narrow speculum or a condom over a longer speculum is needed to keep the vaginal walls from obstructing the view of the cervix. In the sexually active teenager, a Pederson speculum (7/8 × 4 1/2 in.) or occasionally (in the postpar-tum adolescent) a Graves speculum (1 3/8 × 3 3/4 in.) is appropriate. A child's speculum (5/8 × 3 in. or 7/8 × 3 in.) is rarely useful because of its inadequate

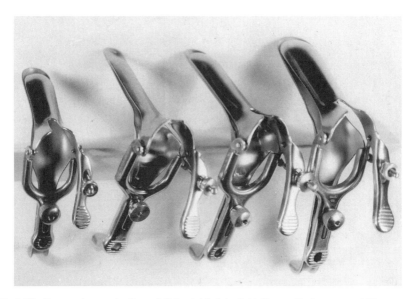

FIG. 1-26. Types of specula *(from left to right):* infant, Huffman, Pederson, and Graves.

length and excessive width (Figs. 1-26 and 1-27). A plastic speculum with an attached light source (Welch Allen) is also useful for facilitating the examination.

The stratified squamous epithelium of the cervix is usually a homogeneous dull pink color; however, in many adolescents an erythematous area surrounding the os is noted. The so-called ectropion is endocervical columnar epithelium on the cervix with the squamocolumnar junction, instead of being inside the endocervical canal, visible on the portio of the cervix. An ectropion does not represent a disease process and may persist throughout the adolescent years, especially if the patient is taking oral contraceptives; it gradually disappears through the process of squamous metaplasia. Mucopurulent cervicitis (MPC) is characterized by purulent discharge from the endocervical canal or on an endocervical swab specimen (and for some specialists, friability of the cervix) (12). MPC may be caused by *N. gonorrhoeae, C. trachomatis,* or other as yet undetermined inflammatory conditions or infections. Small pinpoint hemorrhagic spots on the cervix ("strawberry cervix") can be seen with *Trichomonas* infection. The character of any discharge present should be noted (see Chapter 14). Samples for the Pap test, cultures, pH determination, and saline and KOH preparations are taken with the speculum in place; the techniques are described in the section on diagnostic tests, below. The optimal sequence for endocervical tests is Pap test, followed by tests for *N. gonorrhoeae* and then a test for *C. trachomatis.* After the vagina and cervix have been visualized, the speculum is removed, and the uterus and adnexa are carefully palpated with one or two fingers in the vagina and the other hand on the abdomen: vaginal abdominal bimanual examination (Fig. 1-28). Normal ovaries are usually <3 cm long and are rubbery. The adolescent may complain of mild discomfort with palpation.

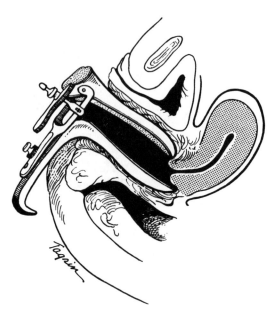

FIG. 1-27. Speculum examination of the cervix. (From Clarke-Pearson D, Dawood M. *Green's gynecology: essentials of clinical practice*, 4th ed. Boston: Little, Brown and Company, 1990; with permission.)

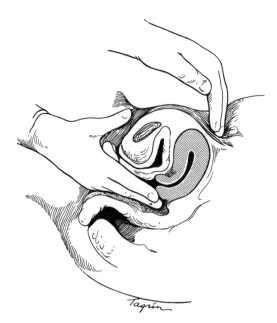

FIG. 1-28. Bimanual abdominal vaginal palpation of the uterus. (From Clarke-Pearson D, Dawood M. *Green's gynecology: essentials of clinical practice,* 4th ed. Boston: Little, Brown, 1990; with permission.)

A rectovaginal abdominal examination, if indicated, is performed with the index finger in the vagina, the middle finger in the rectum, and the other hand on the abdomen, and permits palpation of a retroverted uterus and assessment of the mobility of the adnexa and uterus (Fig. 1-29). The uterosacral ligaments and cul-de-sac should be palpated carefully in patients with pain or dysmenorrhea, since tenderness may be experienced by patients with endometriosis (see Chapter 11). The patient is usually less anxious if she is told in advance that the rectal examination may cause the somewhat uncomfortable sensation that she is "moving her bowels" or "going to the bathroom." Allaying this fear usually elicits better relaxation and cooperation. In patients with a narrow hymenal opening, a simple bimanual rectoabdominal examination with the index finger pushing the cervix upward allows palpation of the uterus and adnexa. In a relaxed patient, an examination revealing no abnormalities rules out the possibility of large ovarian masses or uterine enlargement.

If the adolescent has orthopedic or other disabilities, special attention may be needed for proper positioning during a pelvic examination. The patient's legs may need to be held by one or two assistants rather than supported by her feet in the stirrups. Other positions that may be helpful include the frog-leg position, the

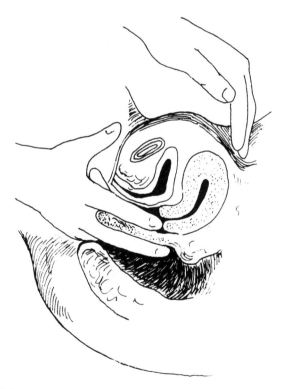

FIG. 1-29. Bidigital rectovaginal examination. (Adapted from Clarke-Pearson D, Dawood M: *Green's gynecology: essentials of clinical practice,* 4th ed. Boston: Little, Brown and Company, 1990; with permission.)

knee–chest position for patients with extreme spasticity, a V position (with the legs abducted and straight or slightly bent), or a side-lying position with an assistant helping to elevate the uppermost leg and the speculum inserted with the handle toward the front or back of the body (see Appendix 1 for videotapes and monographs). An electric examination table that is accessible for adolescents with disabilities is particularly helpful in providing gynecologic care, although with skillful lifting, regular tables can be successfully used. If the adolescent is mentally challenged, the clinician needs to proceed slowly and accomplish as much of the examination as possible to answer the concerns of the patient, family, or caregivers. This may include a bimanual examination, cotton-swab samples of the vaginal secretions, or a Pap test, depending on the age of the patient and her chief complaint. Often an office examination can be accomplished by gaining the confidence of the adolescent with an unhurried, calm approach. Preparation at home before the examination is helpful, and during the examination the adolescent can be encouraged to help with holding the labia or a mirror. It is usually possible to insert a small Huffman speculum. If the young woman will not tolerate a speculum examination, a sample for Pap test can be obtained by inserting a gloved finger moistened with water into the vagina, palpating the cervix, and guiding a cotton-tipped applicator over the finger to the cervical os. However, the percentage of samples with endocervical cells present is much lower than when the standard Pap technique is used. In our experience, the aid of a friendly caretaker who can assist by giving reassurance is preferred to sedation, although other centers have successfully used ketamine and midazolam. Ultrasound examination can help with the differential diagnosis of some conditions. If vaginal examination is imperative and cooperation cannot be elicited, then examination with the patient under anesthesia is necessary (32,33). Most centers use an ambulatory operating room; some have developed specific services within the gynecology clinic (32).

After the examination has been concluded and the patient has dressed, the clinician should sit down and discuss in detail her complaint and the findings from the examination. It is essential that the adolescent be treated as an adult capable of understanding the explanation. If her parent or other caregiver has accompanied her, the patient should be asked whether she would like to tell that person the findings herself or whether she would prefer to have the clinician discuss the diagnosis in her presence. It is extremely important for the patient to know that the clinician and her parent will not have a "secret" about her and that confidential information will not be divulged to her parent.

DIAGNOSTIC TESTS

Papanicolaou Test

The 2002 American Cancer Society Guidelines have recommended that cervical cancer screening using a Papanicolaou (Pap) test begin approximately three years after an adolescent woman begins having vaginal intercourse, but no later than 21 years of age (see Chapter 17) (29). The goal of Pap screening in adolescents is to detect high-grade cervical intraepithelial lesions (HGSIL) to lessen the risk of invasive cervical cancer. If an adolescent or adult woman is immunocompromised or has HIV infection, she should start before 3 years of sexual activity and be screened more frequently. In addition, many favor initiating earlier screening in adolescents receiving episodic gynecologic care and those with a history of high-risk behaviors and STDs. The decision to initiate Pap screening in the non-sexually active woman $\geq$ 21 years old can be individualized by the clinician and the patient if the benefits of screening have been explained and the clinician is comfortable that the patient has never been sexually active or sexually abused (29). The American Cancer Society recommends that cervical screening be done at minimum annually with regular Pap tests or every 2 years using liquid-based tests. ACOG recommends annual Pap test screening for women under 30 years, regardless of the method used. Because the results of Pap test may be falsely negative, the presence of an abnormal growth on the cervix (regardless of Pap test results) should be further assessed with colposcopy and biopsy as indicated.

For accurate cytologic diagnosis, the sample must be collected in such a way as to be representative of normal and abnormal cell populations and must include the squamocolumnar junction and the endocervix. The sample for Pap test should be collected before samples for STD tests, and lubricant should not be used. Ideally, the entire portio of the cervix should be visible. The sample should not be taken during the menses. If vaginal discharge is present in a large amount, it should be gently removed without disturbing the epithelium before the sample is obtained. The laboratory should be given the patient's essential history, such as the date of the last menstrual period, the use of oral or other hormonal contraceptive methods, the presence of an intrauterine device, and a prior abnormal Pap test or treatment.

There are several techniques for obtaining and analyzing cytologic samples. With the regular Pap smear, a spatula is rotated with pressure around the cervix in a circular motion, and the collected material is spread thinly on a slide, both sides of the spatula being applied. In addition, an endocervical specimen should be obtained by using a cytobrush, which is inserted into the os and gently rotated (a cotton-tipped applicator is used by some clinicians for pregnant patients) (34). The sample is rolled onto a second glass slide, or a slide with a line down the middle can be used for both the endocervical and exocervical samples. The slides from the exocervix and endocervix must be fixed immediately with a spray fixative held 10 in. from the slide to prevent dispersal of the cells or by placing the slides in a bottle of Pap fixative (95% ethyl alcohol). Slides with a frosted end are preferred for easy labeling.

Alternatively, a liquid-based technique is used for obtaining cervical cytologic specimens for evaluation. The advantage of liquid based techniques is that the sample examined is more representative of the cells obtained. For Thin Prep, the sample is obtained with a plastic spatula and cytologic brush or with a special broom brush; the technique calls for thorough swishing of the broom or spatula plus brush in the liquid medium to assure adequate transfer of cells. For the AutoCyte PREP System, the broom brush is broken off into the medium. In both methods, the cells are subsequently collected and applied to a glass slide for cytologic reading. Many sites provide reflex HPV testing for ASCUS (atypia of squamous cells of undetermined significance) smears from the cytologic sample (see Chapter 17). Clinicians are encouraged to use the collection and fixation methods that are standard in their communities and to communicate with their cytologists regarding the classification systems used.

Vaginal Smear to Determine Estrogenization

In the absence of inflammation, a vaginal smear is useful for evaluating the patient's estrogen status. The sample for the smear is obtained by inserting a saline moistened cotton-tipped applicator or, in a small child, a moistened Calgiswab through the hymenal opening and scraping the upper lateral sidewall of the vagina. A similar technique can be used while a speculum is in place. The cells obtained are rolled onto a glass slide, and the slide is sprayed with Pap fixative. The cytologist reads the smear by the number of parabasal, intermediate, and superficial cells, and a percentage of each cell type is determined. The greater the estrogen effect, the more superficial cells there are. The patient with little or no estrogen, such as the prepubertal child or the adolescent with amenorrhea due to anorexia nervosa, will have predominantly parabasal cells. The relationship between the percent of superficial cells and the level of estrogenization can be characterized as follows:

<5%	Lack of estrogen effect
5% to 10%	Slight estrogen effect
10% to 30%	Moderate estrogen effect
>30%	Marked estrogen effect

The smear can be correlated with the clinical situation (Table 1-3). The maturation index reports the number of cells as a ratio of parabasal/intermediate/ superficial. In the interpretation, the clinician should remember that the vaginal epithelium is influenced by estrogens, androgens, and progestins and that different patients respond differently to the same level. A preponderance of intermediate cells could be associated with pregnancy, the luteal phase of the cycle, secondary amenorrhea, or long-term administration of a low-dose estrogenic preparation. A scoring system has also proved useful if it is combined with clinical information, especially in the follow-up of girls evaluated and treated for precocious puberty and in those evaluated with secondary amenorrhea. Meisels modified scoring system gives 1 point to superficial cells, 0.5 to intermediate cells, and 0 to parabasal cells (35). The points are multiplied by the per-

TABLE 1-3. *Percentage of parabasal, intermediate, and superficial cells in the vaginal smear*

State	Parabasal	Intermediate	Superficial
Childhood	60–90	10–20	0–3
Early puberty	30	50	20
Stage 5 puberty			
Proliferative phase	0	70	30
Secretory phase	0	80–95	5–20
Pregnancy	0	95	5
Anorexia nervosa (depends on clinical status)	75	25	0
Isosexual precocity	20	50	30
Premature thelarche	60	30	5–10
Premature adrenarche	60–90	10–20	0–3

centage of that type of cell. A score of 90 to 100 is seen in hyperestrogenic patients, 31 to 50 in hypoestrogenic patients, 60 to 70 in newborns, 50 to 60 in pubertal girls, and 0 to 30 in prepubertal girls.

Some clinicians perform the assessment of the vaginal smear at the time of the examination, using a stain formulated by combining 83 ml of light green (5% aqueous solution) with 17 ml of eosin Y (1% aqueous solution). A saline-moistened cotton-tipped applicator is used to obtain the vaginal sample and is then placed in a test tube with 2 ml of saline and three drops of the stain. The tube is gently shaken, and a large drop is applied to a slide and covered with a coverslip for examination under a microscope (36). Since the epithelial cells in urine show the same hormonal changes, the urine of a prepubertal child can be collected for a urocytogram. The first morning urine specimen is centrifuged, and the sediment is spread on a slide. The cytologist records the percentage of superficial, intermediate, and parabasal cells. Two methods of collection and staining have been described (37,38).

Cervical Mucus

An examination of the cervical mucus is another method of evaluating a patient's estrogen status. The cervix is gently swabbed with a large cotton-tipped applicator, and a small sample of cervical mucus is obtained with a saline-moistened cotton-tipped applicator. Profuse, clear, elastic mucus is seen in the preovulatory period and at ovulation. The elastic quality decreases rapidly following ovulation. Thick, sticky mucus is characteristic of the secretory phase of the cycle (see Chapter 4). The mucus is spread on a glass slide and allowed to air dry for 5 minutes. Under the microscope, beautiful ferning patterns will be seen in the smear taken from the late proliferative phase of the cycle (Fig. 1-30). Ferning does not occur in the presence of progesterone.

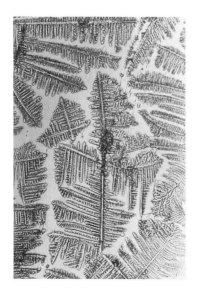

FIG. 1-30. Microscopic evaluation of cervical mucus: ferning during late proliferative phase of the normal menstrual cycle.

Wet Preparations

The so-called wet preparations are useful in defining the etiology of a vaginal discharge. In the prepubertal child, the discharge is usually collected with a saline-moistened Calgiswab or a catheter. In adolescents, a cotton-tipped applicator is inserted directly into the vagina or into the vaginal pool with the speculum in place. The applicator is mixed first with one drop of saline on a glass slide and then with one drop of 10% KOH on another slide. A coverslip is then applied, and the slides are examined under the microscope (low and high dry power) (Fig. 1-31; see also Figs. 14-3 and 14-4 in Chapter 14). On the saline slide, trichomonads appear as lively, flagellated organisms, slightly larger than white blood cells. In bacterial vaginosis, a saline preparation typically shows many refractile bacteria within large epithelial cells (so-called clue cells) and rare leukocytes; mixing this discharge with 10% KOH may liberate an amine-like fishy odor (a positive *"whiff" test* result). In contrast, physiologic discharge is characterized by numerous epithelial cells without evidence of inflammation. On the KOH slide, the presence of budding pseudohyphae and yeast forms is evidence of *Candida* vaginitis.

pH

The pH of the prepubertal vagina is neutral. In contrast, the pH of the vagina of the pubertal adolescent is acid (<4.5). A higher than normal pH (>4.5) occurs with bacterial vaginosis and *Trichomonas* vaginitis. Testing postpubertal vaginal secretions with pH paper can be very helpful in diagnosing the cause of the vaginal discharge (see Chapter 14).

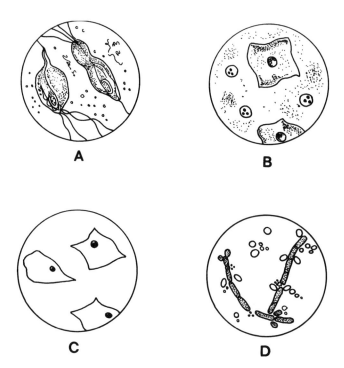

FIG. 1-31. Fresh vaginal smears: **(A)** *Trichomonas*, **(B)** clue cells of bacterial vaginosis, **(C)** normal vaginal discharge, and **(D)** *Candida.* **A, B,** and **C** are saline preparations; **D** is a KOH preparation.

Tests for *N. gonorrhoeae* and *C. trachomatis*

Sexually active teenage girls should have screening tests for sexually transmitted infections, including *N. gonorrhoeae* and *C. trachomatis,* at least annually. These STD tests should be obtained more frequently if the adolescent changes sexual partners, engages in high-risk behaviors, has had an STD or a history of exposure, or has symptoms of cervicitis, breakthrough bleeding on the oral contraceptive pill (or patch or vaginal ring), or lower abdominal pain. In some low-risk suburban and college populations, less frequent or no screening for *N. gonorrhoeae* may be indicated. *C. trachomatis* is common in sexually active adolescents, and thus at least annual screening is important.

In screening for *N. gonorrhoeae*, the optimal test with the best sensitivity and specificity in females is a culture of the endocervix, followed by a nucleic acid amplification test (NAAT) or nucleic acid hybridization test (11). A NAAT performed on urine is an option for patients not undergoing gynecologic examination or screening in nontraditional settings (e.g., schools) (11). For culture, a cotton-tipped applicator is inserted into the cervical os and then streaked directly onto modified Thayer–Martin–Jembec or Thayer–Martin medium. The use of plain Thayer–Martin plates requires immediate transportation of the culture to a bacteriology laboratory and incubation under increased carbon dioxide tension. The Jembec medium, with a small carbon dioxide-generating tablet inserted into a well of the plastic case, is easy to use and reliable; the medium can be transported after an incubation of 24 to 48 hours or processed in the office. The nonculture tests are similarly obtained and sent to the laboratory (see Chapter 15).

For *C. trachomatis,* endocervical samples using a NAAT are preferred if a pelvic examination is being performed. If not, a NAAT can be sent on urine. Alternative tests with less sensitivity and specificity include unamplified nucleic acid hybridization tests, direct immunofluorescent smears, and enzyme immunoassays (see Chapter 15 for sensitivities and specificities of each test). Some methods allow for detection of *Chlamydia* and *N. gonorrhoeae* simultaneously. Culture on endocervical samples in adolescents and vaginal specimens in prepubertal girls remain important for diagnosis of *Chlamydia* in sexually abused girls; culture is less sensitive than the newer methods but 100% specific. The nonculture tests should not be used on rectal or pharyngeal specimens.

Other Cultures

Nickerson-Bismuth Sulfate-Glucose-Glycine-Yeast (Biggy) agar (PML Microbiologicals, Wilsonville, OR) helps confirm a *Candida* vaginitis if the result of the KOH preparation is negative. A sample of the discharge is streaked on the medium, and the tube is incubated at 35°C. The appearance of brown colonies 3 to 7 days later is a positive result for yeast; however, a positive culture suggests but does not prove infection, since *Candida* may be part of the normal flora. Cultures for *Trichomonas* are significantly more sensitive than the "wet prep" but are not widely available (see Chapter 14). PCR tests may be available in the future. Aerobic cultures of the vagina are useful in the diagnosis and treatment of vaginitis in prepubertal girls when respiratory pathogens such as *Streptococcus pyogenes* play a major role, but such cultures are rarely indicated in the diagnosis of vaginal discharge in the adolescent. Normal flora of the adolescent vagina is discussed in Chapter 14.

Progesterone Withdrawal Test

The patient is given medroxyprogesterone, 10 mg orally once a day for 5 or 10 days, micronized progesterone 200 to 300 mg orally for 10 days, or rarely progesterone in oil, 50 to 100 mg intramuscularly once. If the patient has an estrogen-primed endometrium and is not pregnant, she will have a period 3 to 10 days after the last medroxyprogesterone tablet. Progesterone withdrawal is used as a diagnostic test for the evaluation of primary and secondary amenorrhea and typically implies that the estradiol level is >50 pg/ml (see Chapter 7).

Pregnancy Tests

Several highly sensitive, rapid pregnancy tests are available. Qualitative kits used on urine samples are the most practical for office use (39–41). Most kits use specific monoclonal antibodies to human chorionic gonadotropin (HCG) and enzyme-linked immunoassay techniques. For example, the positivity of ICON II HCG (Hybritech) kits is associated with HCG levels of 20 mIU/ml or more; the tests are not affected by blood or protein and have a built-in control (Fig. 1-32). In studies of ectopic pregnancies, 26 of 27 and 95 of 95 ectopic pregnancies were detected by ICON (39,40). Very low levels of HCG (10 to 20 mIU/ml), especially in urine with low specific gravity (<1.015), may be missed. Testpack (Abbott) offers similar advantages. Because of the sensitivity of such tests, the detection of early pregnancies and ectopic pregnancies is significantly enhanced. Pregnancy tests should always be correlated with clinical information and examination (Table 1-4) (see Chapter 21). Positive results may occur in nonpregnant patients because of luteinizing hormone (LH) (ovarian failure), lab error, and HCG-secreting tumors.

Blood tests for measuring HCG can be qualitative or quantitative. For example, Tandem ICON can be used on serum to determine a positive or negative pregnancy test. Quantitative HCG levels are important in the diagnosis of ectopic pregnancy and some spontaneous abortions and threatened abortions and for the follow-up of molar pregnancies and choriocarcinomas. Because not all laboratories use the same units or methods in reporting HCG levels, sequential serum measures in a patient should use the same laboratories (see Chapter 21 for evaluation of disorders of early pregnancy).

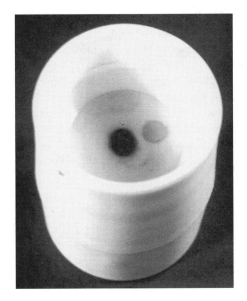

FIG. 1-32. ICON office pregnancy test. The center dot indicates a positive result; the dot on the outer circle is the positive control.

TABLE 1-4. *Mean serum human chorionic gonadotropin levels throughout normal gestation*

Weeks after last menstrual period	Mean (mlU/ml)	SEM (mlU/ml)
3–3.5	22	6
4–4.5	353	9
5–5.5	2270	390
6–6.5	6640	1160
7–7.5	13,610	2740
8–8.5	46,830	4710
9–9.5	44,710	3690
10–10.5	37,750	5420
11–11.5	38,360	8100

SEM = standard error of the mean.
(Adapted from Braunstein GD, Rasor J, Adler D, et al. Serum human chorionic gonadotropin levels throughout normal pregnancy. *Am J Obstet Gynaecol* 1976; 126:678–681.)

Over-the-counter pregnancy tests have improved significantly, and most use monoclonal antibody technology, which yields sensitive and specific results at the time of a missed period or shortly thereafter. However, adolescents may misread the instructions and the results and should therefore be encouraged to use primarily office and laboratory tests and to confirm the results of at-home tests with a medical assessment and a repeat office test.

Bone Age

The bone age is determined by comparing radiographs of the patient's wrist and hand (carpal and phalangeal ossification centers) with the standards in Greulich and Pyle (42) or by applying the Tanner–Whitehouse method (43). A radiograph of the iliac crest can be used in a similar way. At puberty, the epiphysis along the iliac crest undergoes ossification. During adolescence, the ossification progresses from the lateral to the medial part, and fusion occurs at 21 to 23 years of age. Growth hormone and thyroid deficiencies, glucocorticoid excess, delayed puberty, and malnutrition result in delayed maturation; androgens produce an advanced bone age. In the absence of sex steroids (for example, in sexual infantilism associated with Turner syndrome), the bone age will not advance beyond 13 years.

Imaging Techniques

Ultrasonography of the pelvis is useful for evaluating suspected and known gynecologic problems such as ovarian masses, pregnancy, and pelvic anomalies

(44–54). Because an ill-defined adnexal mass in an adolescent may represent a congenital abnormality of the müllerian system, ultrasonography should also include views of the kidneys, as there is a high correlation of müllerian with renal anomalies. Although ultrasonography is an extremely helpful technique, false-positive findings do occur, as when bowel gas is read as an ovarian cyst.

The uterus should be identified in the prepubertal child, with measurements of 2.6 to 3.0 cm in length (50). The uterus is tubular in shape, with the fundus and cervix

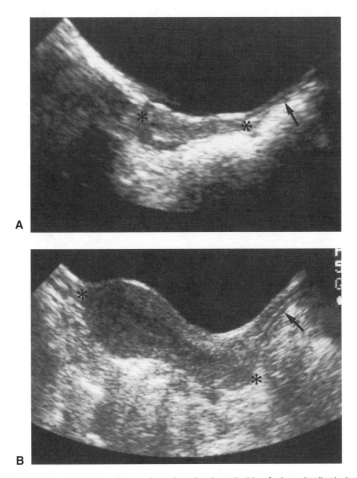

FIG. 1-33. Ultrasound images of prepubertal and pubertal girls. **A:** Longitudinal view of a normal prepubertal uterus, between the *asterisks* (patient's head to the left). The fundus and cervix are approximately the same size. The *arrow* points to the vagina. **(B)** With puberty, the fundus enlarges. This is the longitudinal scan of a normal teenage girl with the fundus shown between the *asterisks*. The *arrow* points to the vagina.

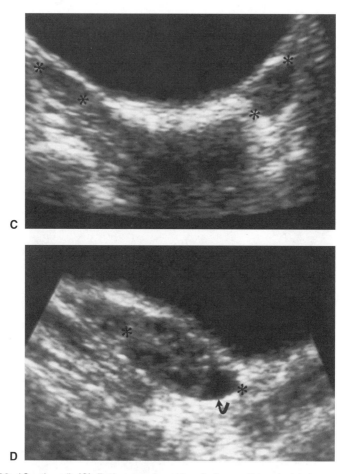

FIG. 1-33. (*Continued*) **(C)** Both normal ovaries (between the asterisks) are seen on the transverse scan of this prepubertal girl. It is not uncommon to see tiny areas of low density in the ovary, presumably representing follicles. **(D)** Longitudinal view of a normal ovary (between the *asterisks*) in a postpubertal girl. The curved *arrow* indicates a normal follicle. (Courtesy of Dr. Jane Share, Children's Hospital Boston.)

equal in size (typically, 1 cm or less in width). With puberty, the fundus increases in size; the postpubertal uterus is 5 to 8 cm in length, and the fundus is up to 4 cm in width. In the prepubertal girl, the ovaries are typically <1 cm³ in volume, although slightly larger ovaries are normal. Follicles are commonly present (51) (Fig. 1-33). In the pubertal girl, the ovaries are 1.8 to 5.7 cm³, with a mean of 4 cm³ (47). The average reproductive ovary varies from 2.5 to 5 cm in length, 1.5 to 3.0 cm in width, and 0.7 to 1.5 cm in thickness; they may normally be slightly asymmetric. A progressive increase in the proportion of normal girls with more than six follicles in each ovary (multicystic ovaries) occurs after the age of 8 1/2 years (48). Follicles of 1 to 3 cm occur normally in adolescent girls, and girls in early and midpuberty may have enlarged ovaries with multiple small "cysts" throughout the ovarian stroma. Small amounts of fluid in the cul-de-sac may be seen in normal girls and with ovulation (52). Cul-de-sac fluid may also occur with bleeding, retrograde menstruation, a ruptured ovarian cyst, endometriosis, or infection.

Ultrasonography is useful when bimanual examination is difficult, when a mass is palpated, and to define the anatomy in patients with probable congenital anomalies. A patient with gonadal dysgenesis should have her renal status assessed by ultrasonography. A patient thought to have uterine agenesis can also be assessed by this technique; the absence of the uterus can be confirmed, the presence of normal ovaries established (in Mayer–Rokitansky–Küster–Hauser syndrome), and the kidneys examined (see Chapter 10). In patients with androgen insensitivity, the testes may sometimes be visualized as soft tissue densities behind the bladder or in the inguinal areas.

Ultrasonography (both 2D and 3D) is also helpful in establishing the presence of uterine, cervical, and vaginal anomalies with or without obstruction. Magnetic resonance imaging (MRI), however, is the definitive test in assessing the complexities of the anatomic abnormalities and planning potential operative approaches. In the assessment of müllerian abnormalities, the kidneys should be scanned for unilateral agenesis, horseshoe kidney, and crossed-fused ectopia. Skeletal anomalies are also common in patients with müllerian anomalies; they include abnormalities of segmentation and rudimentary and wedge vertebrae. Conversely, patients with cervical spine anomalies or congenital scoliosis, or both, should undergo ultrasonography to screen for renal and pelvic anomalies in midpuberty before the menarche. A renal screen can be done much earlier, but pelvic screening is easier in the pubertal child. The girl with unilateral renal agenesis should undergo ultrasonography and gynecologic assessment before menarche. Uterine hypoplasia, as well as ovarian failure, often occurs in patients treated with pelvic radiation therapy for childhood malignancies. Uterine leiomyomas are rare in adolescents; ultrasonography may show uterine enlargement and alterations in the texture and contour. Ultrasound imaging may also be indicated in establishing the gestational age of an intrauterine pregnancy or to sort out abnormalities such as ectopic pregnancy, threatened abortion, and trophoblastic disease (see Chapter 21).

Ovarian enlargement and pelvic pain are often evaluated with ultrasonography (53). The ovaries of patients with polycystic ovaries may be of normal size or enlarged, with multiple cysts and a thickened capsule. Unlike the girl in early adolescence, who may have "multicystic" ovaries, the adolescent with polycystic ovary syndrome may have the small cysts in a "string of pearls" configuration just underneath the cortex (see Chapter 9). Simple ovarian cysts are very common in adolescents. They are usually 3 to 6 cm in diameter, unilocular, and without internal debris, and they often resolve spontaneously. Complex ovarian cysts may be a corpus luteum cyst, a cystadenofibroma, a cystadenoma, a teratoma, a hemorrhagic ovarian cyst, ovarian torsion (see Chapters 11 and 18 for discussion of Doppler ultrasound), ectopic pregnancy, tubo-ovarian abscess, ovarian tumor, or periappendicular abscess. Hemorrhagic ovarian cysts have quite variable findings depending on when they are scanned; most are heterogeneous with mixed solid and cystic areas, which may become more cystic as the clot resorbs. The ultrasound findings in ovarian torsion are also variable; classically, there is a large solid mass with peripheral follicular cysts. Pelvic inflammatory disease (PID) with tubo-ovarian abscess may produce edema and loss of anatomic planes, giving a disorganized pattern and adnexal enlargement, but PID alone cannot be distinguished by ultrasound (44). An ovarian tumor with a cystic component may be easier to visualize than a solid teratoma, which can be obscured by bowel gas. A radiograph of the abdomen may help identify fat, calcifications, or teeth in these tumors (see Chapter 18).

Transvaginal ultrasonography is used frequently in the evaluation of intrauterine and ectopic pregnancy, spontaneous and incomplete abortion (see Chapter 21), pelvic masses, PID, and uterine abnormalities. Signs of abnormal early gestation include irregular decidua, pathologic double ring, subchorionic bleeding, degenerative changes of fetal pole and yolk sac, and absence of fetal heartbeat. Tubo-ovarian disease can also be assessed and the actual tube examined in greater detail in cases of both PID and ectopic pregnancy (54). The vaginal probe can be easily inserted into the vagina of the sexually active adolescent. It can also be used for selected girls who have never been sexually active but who have used tampons and do not experience pain with insertion of the probe.

Computed tomography (CT) and MRI are important additional tests in pathologic conditions of the pelvis when ultrasonography has not yielded sufficient diagnostic information. CT is useful in staging malignancies and in defining abscesses. MRI has become the prime modality for assessing congenital pelvic anomalies. 3D ultrasound is also being evaluated and appears to be very beneficial in the evaluation of uterine and cervical anomalies.

Detection of Ovulation

Several methods have been used to detect ovulation. Most are used primarily in the evaluation and treatment of infertility. Occasionally, in older adolescents with conditions such as oligomenorrhea or Turner syndrome with normal gonadotropin levels, or after exposure to chemotherapy or radiation therapy, the clinician may wish to establish whether ovulatory cycles are occurring. The methods include measurement of basal body temperature charts, determination of serum progesterone levels during the luteal phase, urine or serum testing for LH, ultrasonography, and rarely, endometrial sampling.

In using basal body temperature (BBT) charts, the patient is instructed to take her temperature every morning as soon as she awakens. For accurate recording, a basal thermometer is kept at the bedside, and the patient is told not to go to the

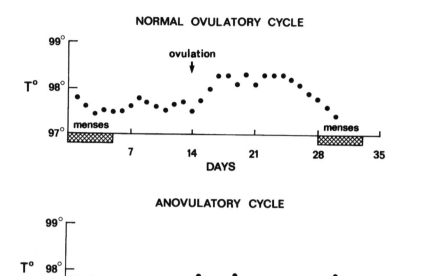

FIG. 1-34. Basal body temperature charts.

bathroom, drink fluids, or have sexual activity before taking her temperature. The temperature is recorded on a special chart. The typical ovulatory and anovulatory cycles are shown in Fig. 1-34. BBT charts are useful if the patient shows a classic pattern, but some ovulatory patients may not have a biphasic chart, may be ill during the recording, or may fail to use the proper method. Owing to the labor intensive nature of BBT testing and its limited appropriate application for adolescents, it is rarely used in this patient population.

Home kits are available for testing the urine to detect the midcycle rise of LH (55). These kits, which use monoclonal antibody technology, are helpful in infertility evaluations, since the time from the detected surge to ovulation is typically about 12 to 24 hours. However, as will be noted in Chapter 4, an LH surge in an adolescent may not be evidence of normal ovulation and a normal luteal phase. Similarly, a random serum progesterone level may be suggestive but not definitive evidence of a normal luteal phase. A luteal progesterone level >10 ng/ml establishes ovulation with normal corpus luteum function. Endometrial sampling, with a small catheter (e.g., Pipelle endometrial suction curette), can be difficult for the physician to perform in the virginal patient. It is uncomfortable for the adolescent and is rarely indicated. Clearly, the use of any of these tests necessitates discussion with the patient of the problems and likely benefits from the results.

REFERENCES

1. Huffman JW, Dewhurst CJ, Capraro VJ. *The gynecology of childhood and adolescence.* Philadelphia: WB Saunders, 1981.
2. Emans SJ, Wood ER, Flagg NT, et al. Genital findings in sexually abused symptomatic and asymptomatic girls. *Pediatrics* 1987;79:778.
3. Pokorny SF. Configuration of the prepubertal hymen. *Am J Obstet Gynecol* 1987;157:950.
4. Jenny C, Kuhns MLD, Arakawa F. Hymens in newborn female infants. *Pediatrics* 1987;80:399.
5. Mor N, Merlob P. Congenital absence of the hymen only a rumor? *Pediatrics* 1988;82:679.
6. Emans SJ, Goldstein DP. The gynecologic examination of the prepubertal child with vulvovaginitis: use of the knee–chest position. *Pediatrics* 1980;65:758.
7. Capraro V. Gynecologic examination in children and adolescents. *Pediatr Clin North Am* 1972; 19:511.
8. Pokorny SF, Stormer J. Atraumatic removal of secretions from the prepubertal vagina. *Am J Obstet Gynecol* 1987;156:581.
9. Alexander ER. Misidentification of sexually transmitted organisms in children: medicolegal implications. *Pediatr Infect Dis J* 1988;7:1.
10. Whittington WL, Rice RJ, Biddle JW, et al. Incorrect identification of *Neisseria gonorrhoeae* from infants and children. *Pediatr Infect Dis J* 1988;7:3.
11. CDC. Screening tests to detect *Chlamydia trachomatis* and *Neisseria gonorrhoeae* infections 2002. MMWR 2002;51 (RR-15):1.
12. CDC. Sexually Transmitted Diseases Treatment Guidelines 2002. MMWR; 2002;51 (RR-6):1.
13. American Medical Association. *Guidelines for Adolescent Preventive Services (GAPS).* Chicago: Department of Adolescent Health, American Medical Association, 1997 (www.ama-assn.org).
14. Green M, Palfrey J, ed. *Bright futures—Guidelines for health supervision of infants, children, and adolescents.* National Center for Education in Maternal and Child Health. Arlington VA, 2000.
15. Knight J, Emans SJ, eds. (and primary authors). *Bright Futures Case Studies for Primary Care Clinicians: A Guide to the Case Teaching Method; and Growth in Children and Adolescents.* Boston, MA: Bright Futures Center for Education in Child Growth and Development, Behavior and Adolescent Health. 2001.
16. Knight J, Frazer C, Emans SJ, eds. (and primary authors). *Bright futures case studies for primary care clinicians: child development and behavior.* Boston, MA: Bright Futures Center for Education in Child Growth and Development, Behavior and Adolescent Health. 2001.
17. Emans SJ, Knight J, eds. (and primary authors). *Bright Futures Case Studies for Primary Care Clinicians: Adolescent Health.* Boston, MA: Bright Futures Center for Education in Child Growth and Development, Behavior and Adolescent Health. 2001.
18. Cheng TL, Savageau JA, Sattler AL, et al. Confidentiality in health care: a survey of knowledge, perceptions, and attitudes among high school students. *JAMA* 1993;269:1404.
19. Thrall JS, McCloskey L, Ettner SL, et al. Confidentiality and adolescents' use of providers for health information and for pelvic examinations. *Arch Pediatr Adolesc Med* 2000;154:885.
20. Ford CA, Millstein SG, Halpern-Feilsher BL, et al. Influence of physician confidentiality assurances on adolescents' willingness to disclose information and seek future health care. *JAMA* 1997;278:1029.
21. Ford CA, Millstein SG. Delivery of confidentiality assurance to adolescents by primary care physicians. *Arch Pediatr Adolesc Med* 1997;151:505.
22. Frankowski BL, and Committee on Adolescence. Sexual Orientation and adolescents. *Pediatrics* 2004; 113; 1827.
23. Wilson KM, Klein JD. Opportunities for appropriate care: health care and contraceptive use among adolescents reporting unwanted sexual intercourse. *Arch Pediatr Adolesc Med* 2002;156(4):341.
24. Youth Risk Behavior Surveillance—United States, 2003. MMWR 2004;53(55-2).

25. Prochaska JO, DiClemente CC. Transtheoretical therapy: toward a more integrative model of change. *Psychother Theory Res Pract* 1982;19:276.
26. Millstein SG, Adler NE, Irwin CE. Sources of anxiety about pelvic examinations among adolescent females. *J Adolesc Health Care* 1984:5:105.
27. Emans SJ, Woods ER, Allred EN, Grace E. Hymenal findings in adolescent women: impact of tampon use and consensual sexual activity. *J Pediatr* 1994;125:153.
28. Stewart FH, Harper CC, Ellertson CE, et al. Clinical breast and pelvic examination requirements for hormonal contraception: Current practice vs evidence. *JAMA* 2001;285(17):2232.
29. Saslow D, Runowicz CD, Solomon D, et al. American Cancer Society guideline for the early detection of cervical neoplasia and cancer. *CA Cancer J Clin* 2002;52:342.
30. Verkauf BS, Von Thron J, O'Brien WE. Clitoral size in normal women. *Obstet Gynecol* 1992;80:41.
31. Starling S, Jenny C. Forensic examination of adolescent female genitalia: the Foley catheter technique. *Arch Pediatr Adolesc Med* 1997;151:102.
32. Rosen DA, Rosen KR, Elkins TE, et al. Outpatient sedation: an essential addition to gynecologic care for persons with mental retardation. *Am J Obstet Gynecol* 1991;164:825.
33. Elkins TE, McNeeley SG, Rosen D, et al. A clinical observation of a program to accomplish pelvic exams in difficult-to-manage patients with mental retardation. *Adolesc Pediatr Gynecol* 1988; 1:195.
34. Germain M, Heaton R, Erickson D, et al. A comparison of the three most common Papanicolaou smear collection techniques. *Obstet Gynecol* 1994;84:168.
35. Meisels A. Computed cytohormonal findings in 3,307 healthy women. *Acta Cytol* 1965;9:328.
36. Rakoff AE. Hormonal cytology in gynecology. *Clin Obstet Gynecol* 1961;4:1045.
37. Lencioni LJ, Staffieri J. Urocytogram diagnosis of sexual precocity. *Acta Cytol (Baltimore)* 1969; 13:302.
38. Preeyasombat C, Kenny E. Urocytogram in normal children and various abnormal conditions. *Pediatrics* 1966;38:436.
39. Cartwright PS, Victory DG, Moore RA, et al. Performance of a new enzyme-linked immunoassay urine pregnancy test for the detection of ectopic gestation. *Ann Emerg Med* 1986;15:1198.
40. Norman RJ, Buck RH, Rom L, et al. Blood or urine measurement of human chorionic gonadotropin for detection of ectopic pregnancy? A comparative study of quantitative and qualitative methods in both fluids. *Obstet Gynecol* 1988;71:315.
41. Klee G. Human chorionic gonadotropin. *Mayo Clin Proc* 1994;69:391.
42. Greulich WW, Pyle S. *Radiographic atlas of skeletal development of the hand and wrist.* Stanford, CA: Stanford University Press, 1959.
43. Tanner JM, Whitehouse RH, Cameron N, et al. *Assessment of skeletal maturity and prediction of adult height (TW2 method).* New York: Academic Press, 1983.
44. Share J, Teele R. Ultrasonography in adolescent gynecology. *Clin Pract Gynecol* 1989;1:72.
45. Sanfilippo JS, Lavery JP. The spectrum of ultrasound: antenatal to adolescent years. *Semin Reprod Endocrinol* 1988;6:45.
46. Salardi S, Orsini IF, Cacciari E, et al. Pelvic ultrasonography in premenarcheal girls: relation to puberty and sex hormone concentration. *Arch Dis Child* 1985;60:120.
47. Lippe BM, Sample WE. Pelvic ultrasonography in pediatric and adolescent endocrine disorders. *J Pediatr* 1978;92:897.
48. Stanhope R, Adams J, Jacobs HS, et al. Ovarian ultrasound assessment in normal children, idiopathic precocious puberty, and during low dose pulsatile gonadotropin releasing hormone treatment of hypogonadotrophic hypogonadism. *Arch Dis Child* 1985;60:116.
49. Wu A, Siegel MJ. Sonography of pelvic masses in children: diagnostic predictability. *AJR* 1987; 148:1199.
50. Cohen HL, Bober SE, Bow SN. Imaging the pediatric pelvis: the normal and abnormal genital tract and simulators of its diseases. *Urol Radiol* 1992;14:273.
51. Cohen HL, Eisenberg P, Mandel F, et al. Ovarian cysts are common in premenarchal girls: a sonographic study of 101 children 2–12 years old. *Am J Roentgenol* 1992;159:89.
52. Rathaus V, Grunebaum M, Konen O, et al. Minimal fluid in asymptomatic children: The value of sonographic finding. *J Ultrasound Med* 2003;22:13.
53. Expert Panel on Pediatric Imaging: Cohen HL, Smith WL, Kushner DC, et al. Imaging evaluation of acute right lower quadrant and pelvic pain in adolescent girls. *Radiology* 2000;215(S):833.

54. Bulas DI, Ahlstrom PA, Sivit CJ, et al. Pelvic inflammatory disease in the adolescent: comparison of transabdominal and transvaginal sonographic evaluation. *Pediatr Radiol* 1992;183(2):435.
55. Rebar RW. Practical appreciations of home diagnostic products: a symposium. *J Reprod Med* 1987; 32(9S):705.

SUGGESTED VIDEOTAPES FOR EXAMINATION

See Appendix 1.

2

Ambiguous Genitalia in the Newborn

Ingrid Holm

Although most clinicians rarely see an infant with ambiguous genitalia at birth, the need to assess the situation as quickly as possible makes this subject essential. Any deviation from the normal appearance of male or female genitalia should prompt investigation, since apparent but incomplete male or female external genitals may be associated with the gonads and genotype of the opposite sex. Even a slight doubt that arises during the initial examination of the newborn should be pursued systematically to prevent the possibility of later confusion. Bilateral cryptorchidism, unilateral cryptorchidism with incomplete scrotal fusion or hypospadias, labial fusion, or clitoromegaly requires evaluation.

DETERMINING SEX ASSIGNMENT

Abnormal sexual differentiation presents medical and psychological issues that need to be addressed in an urgent fashion. Two of these major issues need to be immediately addressed: the relationship of the sexual ambiguity to a possible life-threatening disease and the sex of rearing. In the delivery room, it is critical *not* to make a gender assignment but to postpone that determination until the necessary data have been collected. Clearly, most parents will react with dismay and anxiety. It is important to reassure the parents that they have a healthy baby but that the development of the external genitals is incomplete and tests are necessary to determine the sex. They should be reassured that tests will show the cause of the problem and identify the baby as a girl or a boy and that a definite answer should be possible within a few days, or at most in 1 or 2 weeks. The possibility of an intersex disorder (hermaphroditism) does not need to be raised initially. Speculation about the possible assignment of sex could be psychologically damaging to the parents. The child should be referred to by all caretakers as *the baby* rather than as a boy or girl. Parents should be encouraged to tell other family members and friends, when they ask about the sex of the baby, that the baby is sick, and to delay sending out birth announcements until the gender options have been considered. The physician should examine the baby in the presence of the parents, explain the common genital anlage for boys and girls, and educate the family about normal sexual development. Once the diagnosis is made, the natural history, prognosis, and therapeutic options should be discussed with the parents. Full disclosure and communication is essential. Decisions regarding sex assignment must be made with the parents, taking into account their cultural and religious beliefs and level of understanding. Parents should be made aware of recent controversies in this area of sex assignment and provided with educational information and resources. Once the sex of rearing has been determined, the physician should help the family put aside issues of sexual ambiguity. Parents should be encouraged to use the names previously selected for a boy or girl. Names that are definitely male or female help the family see the child unequivocally as belonging to that sex. As long as parental attitudes toward the child's sex remain unequivocal, the child usually assumes his or her gender role without difficulty, regardless of the genotype.

Although a diagnosis of the patient's condition requires knowledge of the genotype (karyotype), sex assignment is generally based on other criteria as well. The main issues are the potential for an unambiguous appearance, the potential for normal sexual functioning, and fertility. The female pseudohermaphrodite has normal ovaries and uterus, is potentially capable of bearing children, and thus should usually be given a female gender identity. In general, the male pseudohermaphrodite should be raised as a male, unless there is complete androgen resistance, the genitalia are almost completely or completely feminized, or the family makes an informed decision to raise the child as a female. In gonadal disorders in which fertility is not possible, the decision regarding sex assignment is based in part on the potential for reconstructive surgery. In general, surgical techniques are more suited to reduction of the size of the phallus and, later, to the creation of a vagina, than to the construction of a normal male phallus.

In the evaluation of children with ambiguous genitalia, it is critical to provide a multidisciplinary approach. Psychiatrists and social workers should be included as sex assignment is being determined, and in the long-term management. The decision to make a sex assignment must be carefully considered with the knowledge that there are those who advocate making no sex assignment and allowing the child to choose for him/herself, when old enough to do so. This approach is advocated by intersex societies. Thus, the family must be made aware of all options, even as the medical team has come to a consensus as to the best sex assignment. (See Ref. 1 for a review of the psychological ramifications of sex assignment in children with ambiguous genitalia.)

REVIEW OF EMBRYOGENESIS

The bipotential gonads develop prior to the fifth to sixth week of gestation. Steroidogenic factor 1 (SF1) and Wilms tumor 1 (WT1) are critical for the devel-

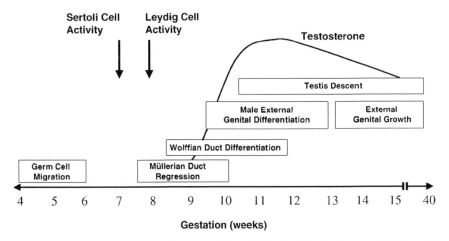

FIG. 2-1. Embryologic events in male sex differentiation depicted in temporal fashion. The *line* depicts the increase in fetal serum testosterone concentrations. The word *activity* refers indirectly to the action of AMH in causing müllerian duct regression and androgens to induce male sex differentiation. (From Hughes IA. Minireview: sex differentiation. *Endocrinology* 2001;142:3282; with permission of The Endocrine Society.)

opment of the genital ridge into the bipotential gonad prior to sexual differentiation (2). Mutations in SF1 and WT1 are associated with abnormal gonadal development, resulting in 46,XY sex-reversal or ambiguous genitalia (3). Other genes proposed to be involved in gonadal development include LIM1 and EMX2, although no mutations responsible for sex reversal have been found in these genes (4) (Fig. 2-1 and Table 2-1). An excellent review of genes involved in sex determination and differentiation, and

TABLE 2-1.

Gene	Localization	Gene Family	Putative Function	Phenotype of Mutations
SRY	Yp11	HMG protein	Transcription factor	XY gonadal dysgenesis
*DAX*1	Xp21.3	Nuclear receptor	Transcription factor	Duplication: XY gonadal dysgenesis Mutation: adrenal hypoplasia congenita
*SOX*9	17q24	HMG protein	Transcription factor	Duplication: XX sex reversal Mutation: campomelic dysplasia with XY gonadal dysenesis
SF-1	9q33	Nuclear receptor	Transcription factor	Gonadal dysgenesis and adrenal insufficiency
WT-1	11p13	Zinc finger protein	Transcription factor	Denys-Drash and Frasier syndromes
*DMRT*1	9p24	DM domain, DNA binding protein	Transcription factor	XY sex reversal?
WNT-4	1p35	Wnt	Signaling molecule	XX sex reversal

From Dewing P, Bernard P, Vilain E. Disorders of gonadal development. *Semin Reprod Med* 2002;20:198; with permission.

of the clinical characteristics resulting from mutations in these genes, is presented by MacLaughlin and Donahoe in their 2004 review article (4).

The bipotential gonads differentiate into either testes or ovaries. In general, maleness is imposed upon the innate tendency of the fetal gonads to develop along female lines. There are three major components to sex determination and differentiation: chromosomal sex, gonadal sex, and phenotypic sex. Chromosomal sex refers to the karyotype, 46,XY or 46,XX, which under normal circumstances determines whether the individual is male or female. More specifically, the chromosomal sex refers to genes important in *sex determination*, i.e., the events that lead to the differentiation of the gonads into either an ovary or testis (4). The first critical gene in the cascade of genes involved in sex determination is the sex-determining region of the Y chromosome (*SRY*), which is located on the short arm of the Y chromosome (Yp) just centromeric to the pseudoautosomal region (the region where the X and Y chromosomes pair during meiosis) (Fig. 2-2). *SRY* is required for differentiation of the gonad into a testis (5,6). If it is absent or abnormal, the gonad differentiates into an ovary. The importance of *SRY* in sex determination is demonstrated by 46,XX males who have *SRY* present (6) and 46,XY females with mutations or deletions in SRY (5,7). The *SRY* protein activates transcription of genes on the sex chromosomes and autosomes that are important in sex determination (5–9). Defects in genes activated by *SRY* are postulated to be responsible for sex reversal in 46,XX males who have no Y sequences detectable (10,11), including no *SRY*, and in 46,XY females with normal *SRY* (12,13).

Sex reversal occurs in patients with abnormalities in *SOX9*, a gene that functions downstream of SRY. *SOX9* encodes a transcription factor related to SRY, and is involved in testicular development. Mutations in *SOX9* disrupt male development and cause 46,XY sex reversal as well as camptomelic dysplasia (14–16). *SF1* and *WT1* interact and are also involved in testicular development. The dosage sensitive sex reversal gene on the X chromosome (*DAX1*) antagonizes this interaction and inhibits the gonad from developing into a testis (2,17) (see Fig. 2-1). In addition, mapping of the Y chromosome has identified regions involved in spermatogenesis (18–20), although the nature of these genes is unclear.

The presence of two X chromosomes appears to be important for development of a normal functioning ovary. 46,XX and 45,X fetuses initially have oocytes. However, in the 45,X fetus, oocyte atresia is accelerated in the second half of intrauterine life and in the prepubertal years. This suggests that two copies of genes on the X chromosome are necessary for oocyte maintenance. Mapping of the X chromosome has identified regions of the X chromosome responsible for short stature, some of the stigmata of Turner syndrome, and ovarian function (Fig. 2-3). Duplications in *DAX1* in 46,XY individuals leads to sex reversal. It now appears that *DAX1* functions by inhibiting the gonad from developing into a testis, and is not an ovary-determining gene (2,21,22). *WNT4* is another gene that may be involved in ovarian development (4). Overall, however, the genes involved in the development and maintenance of the ovary are still largely unknown.

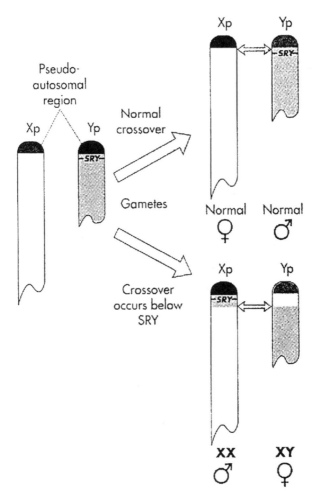

FIG. 2-2. The distal short arms of the X and Y chromosomes exchanging material during meiosis in the male. The region of the Y chromosome in which this crossover occurs is called the *pseudoautosomal* region. The *SRY* gene, which triggers the process leading to male gonadal differentiation, is located just outside the pseudoautosomal region. Occasionally, the crossover occurs on the centromeric side of the *SRY* gene, causing it to lie on an X chromosome instead of the Y chromosome. An offspring receiving this X chromosome will be an XX male, and an offspring receiving the Y chromosome will be an XY female. (From Jorde LB, Carey JC, Bamshad MJ, et al. Clinical cytogenetics: the chromosomal basis of human disease. In: Schmitt W, ed. *Medical genetics.* St. Louis, MO: Mosby, 2000; with permission.)

The gonadal sex is established under the influence of the chromosomal sex. The first sign of gonadal differentiation occurs in the male with the appearance of Sertoli cells at 6 to 7 weeks (23); Leydig cells appear at about 8 weeks (Fig. 2-4). In the female at this stage, the only sign of ovarian differentiation is the absence

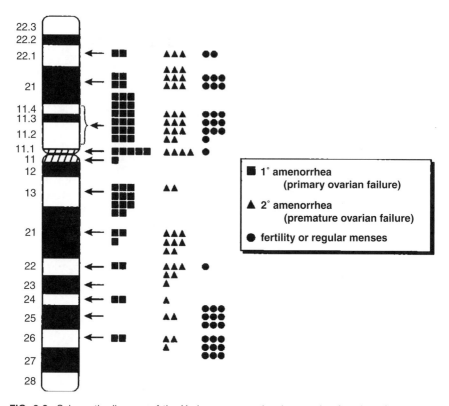

FIG. 2-3. Schematic diagram of the X chromosome showing ovarian function of nonmosaic terminal deletion. Earlier references are provided elsewhere by the author (Simpson, 1987b). Nonmosaic cases described since that report include Naguib et al. (1988). Massa et al. (1992), Veneman et al. (1991), and Schwartz et al. (1987), which is actually a molecular update of Fitch et al. (1982), Tharapel et al. (1993), Zinn et al. (1997), Zinn et al. (1998), Ogata and Matsuo (1995), Marozzi et al. (1998), Davison et al. (1998), James et al. (1998), and Susca et al. (1999). In familial aggregates all affected cases are included because their phenotypes are not always concordant (e.g., Zinn et al.). In some cases, patients are described as having premature ovarian failure, but no information is provided on fertility; in the absence of explicit information it is assumed no pregnancy has occurred. In some younger patients (e.g., ≥14 years but <20 to 25 years), there has been little opportunity to demonstrate pregnancy, nor is there assurance regular menses will continue. Nonetheless, they are designated as having "regular menses/fertility." (From Simpson JL, Rajkovic A. Ovarian differentiation and gonadal failure. *Am J Med Genet* 1999;89:186; with permission of John Wiley & Sons.)

of Sertoli and Leydig cells. The ovarian cortex does not begin to develop until 12 weeks, and primordial follicles appear at 13½ weeks (23). In contrast to the male, in whom testicular cords form in the absence of germ cells, the ovary does not develop if germ cells are not present.

The end result of gonadal differentiation (testis or ovary) determines the hormone that will be secreted to lead to the phenotypic sex. *Sex differentiation* is

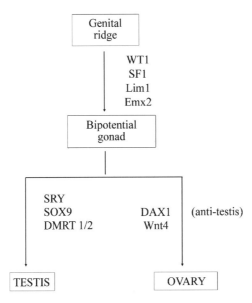

FIG. 2-4. Factors controlling gonad determination. *DAX*-1 may have an indirect role in ovarian development by acting as an antitestis factor. (From Hughes IA. Minireview: sex differentiation. *Endocrinology* 2001;142:3283; with permission of The Endocrine Society.)

the process by which hormone secretion, and the response of end organs to these hormones, results in the phenotypic sex (Fig. 2-5). Testosterone and antimüllerian hormone (AMH), secreted from the Leydig cells and the Sertoli cells of the testes, respectively, induce differentiation of the genital primordia into the male phenotype. In the absence of a functioning testis, whether or not an ovary is present, the genital primordia will differentiate into the female phenotype. However, although the presence of a functioning testis is necessary, it is not sufficient for the development of a male phenotype. Normal androgen metabolism is also required, including normal androgen receptors and 5α-reductase activity.

The internal genitalia are derived from the müllerian ducts in the female and the wolffian ducts in the male (Fig. 2-6). The first phenotypic sign of differentiation of the male internal genitalia is the regression of müllerian ducts at 8 weeks of gestation, mediated by AMH (24). This hormone, a high-molecular-weight glycoprotein secreted from the Sertoli cells, prevents the differentiation of the müllerian duct structures (the fallopian tubes, uterus, and upper vagina); the müllerian duct structures are almost completely absent by 10 weeks. Testosterone secreted from the Leydig cells is responsible for the differentiation of the wolffian ducts (the vas deferens, seminal vesicles, and epididymis). High concentrations of AMH and testosterone are required locally around the müllerian and wolffian ducts, respectively, and androgen receptors must be functional, for differentiation of the male internal genitalia to occur. In the female, or in the absence of testicular tissue secreting

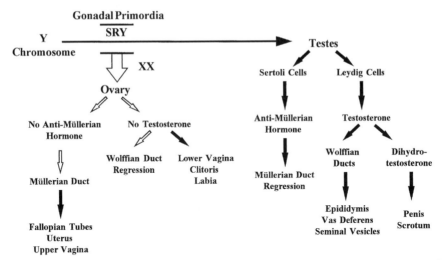

FIG. 2-5. Male and female gonadal differentiation. Gonadal primordia, under the influence of the sex-determining region (*SRY*), become a testis; the presence of antimüllerian hormone (AMH) and testosterone causes the regression of müllerian ducts and the formation of male internal and external genitalia. In the absence of *SRY*, an ovary differentiates, and in the absence of AMH and testosterone, female internal and external genitalia are formed.

AMH and testosterone locally, müllerian duct differentiation and wolffian duct regression occur. This explains why female pseudohermaphrodites, who do not have testes, develop female internal genital structures.

External genital development occurs between the 8th and 12th weeks of gestation (Fig. 2-7) and in the male does not require high local concentrations of testosterone. Normal differentiation of the male external genitalia requires high circulating levels of testosterone, the conversion of testosterone to dihydrotestosterone (DHT) by 5α-reductase in the target organs, and functional androgen receptors. In the male, under the influence of DHT, the urogenital sinus gives rise to the prostate, the genital tubercle forms the glans penis, the labiourethral folds form the urethra and ventral shaft of the penis, and the labioscrotal folds fuse to form the scrotum. In the female, or in the absence of testicular tissue secreting bioactive testosterone, functioning androgen receptors, or 5α-reductase, the genital tubercle forms the clitoris, the labiourethral folds form the labia minora, and the labioscrotal folds form the labia majora.

Thus, from this brief review of embryogenesis, it is clear that a defect in any one of many steps along the pathway of sex determination and differentiation can result in ambiguous genitalia.

ASSESSMENT OF THE NEONATE

The initial evaluation of the newborn with ambiguous genitalia includes a careful history, physical examination, karyotype determination, serum hormone analyses,

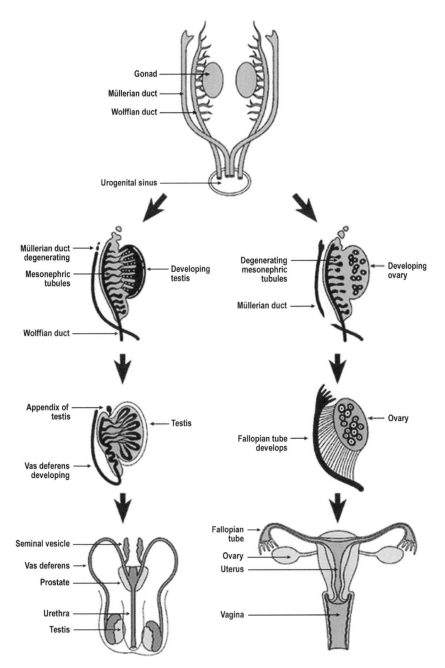

FIG. 2-6. Differentiation of the wolffian and müllerian ducts (From Warne GL, Kanumakala S. Molecular endocrinology of sex differentiation. *Semin Reprod Med* 2002;20:174; with permission of Thieme Medical Publishers.)

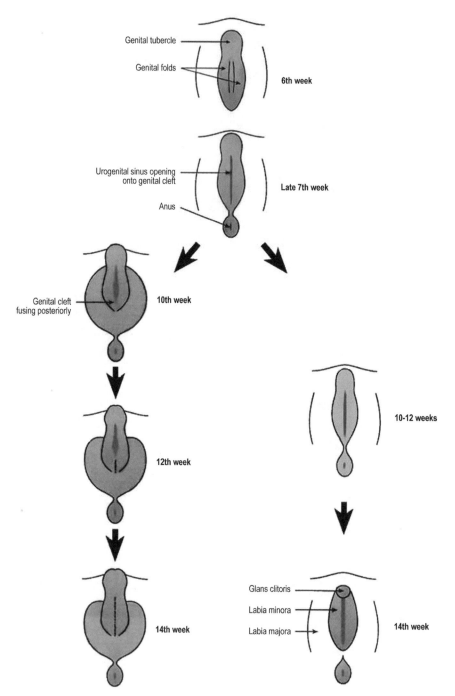

FIG. 2-7. Differentiation of male and female external genitalia. (From Warne GL, Kanumakala S. Molecular endocrinology of sex differentiation. *Semin Reprod Med* 2002;20:175; with permission of Thieme Medical Publishers.)

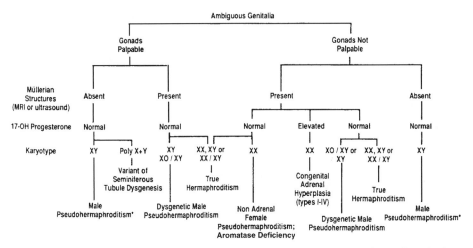

FIG. 2-8. Steps in the diagnosis of intersexuality in infancy and childhood. (From Grumbach MM, Conte FA. Disorders of sex differentiation. In: Wilson JD, Foster DW, Kronenberg HM, et al., eds. *Williams textbook of endocrinology.* Philadelphia: WB Saunders, 1998; with permission of W.B. Saunders Company.)

and radiographic studies (Fig. 2-8). The direction of further studies, including the performance of a human chorionic gonadotropin (HCG) stimulation test, more extensive hormone analyses, DNA studies in a search for *SRY* or mutations in other genes, laparoscopy, or gonadal biopsy, depends on the results of the initial evaluation. Tables 2-2 and 2-3 provide summaries of clinical information regarding gonadal abnormalities and androgen abnormality/insensitivity syndromes.

History

A careful history should be obtained from the parents, particular attention being given to the following points:

TABLE 2-2. *The androgen abnormality/insensitivity syndromes*

Syndrome	5α-reductase	Complete	Incomplete	Reifenstein	Infertile
Inheritance	Autosomal recessive	X-linked recessive	X-linked recessive	X-linked recessive	X-linked recessive
Spermatogenesis	Decreased	Absent	Absent	Absent	Decreased
Müllerian	Absent	Absent	Absent	Absent	Absent
Wolffian	Male	Absent	Male	Male	Male
External	Female	Female	Female clitoromegaly	Male hypospadias	Male
Breasts	Male	Female	Female	Gynecomastia	Gynecomastia

(Adapted from Griffin JE. Androgen resistance—the clinical and molecular spectrum. *N Engl J Med* 1992;326:611–618; and Kim HH, Laufer MR. Developmental abnormalities of the female reproductive tract. *Curr Opin Obstet Gynecol* 1994;6:518–525; with permission.)

TABLE 2-3. *A clarification of the terminology for gonadal abnormalities*

Event	Time of event (days after fertilization)	Nomenclature	Müllerian duct	Wolffian duct	External genitalia
Early embryonic testicular regression	<43	Pure gonadal dysgenesis	Present	Absent	Female
Late embryonic testicular regression	43–59	Swyer syndrome	Present	Absent	Female
Early fetal testicular regression	60–69	Agonadism	Present	Absent	Ambiguous
	70–75	Testicular dysgenesis	Present	Present	Ambiguous
	75–84	Testicular regression	Absent	Present	Ambiguous
Midfetal testicular regression	90–120	Rudimentary testis	Absent	Present	Male infantile
Late fetal testicular regression	>140	Vanishing testis, anorchia	Absent	Present	Male infantile

(Adapted from Speroff L, Glass RH, Kase NG. Normal and abnormal sexual development. In: Mitchell C, ed. *Clinical Gynecologic Endocrinology and Infertility*, 5th ed. Baltimore: Williams & Wilkins, 1994; and Kim HH, Laufer MR. Developmental abnormalities of the female reproductive tract. *Curr Opin Obstet Gynecol* 1994;6:518–525; with permission.)

1. Family history (See Tables 2-1 and 2-4 for a summary of the inheritance of disorders leading to ambiguous genitalia.).
   a. Other family members, especially siblings, with congenital adrenal hyperplasia (CAH).
   b. A history of early neonatal death. The diagnosis of CAH may be missed in males, since there are often no physical signs at birth except, occasionally, increased scrotal rugae, pigmentation, or a large phallus. Thus, a brother may have died in early infancy of vomiting and dehydration, not recognized as secondary to adrenal insufficiency.
   c. Consanguinity, which makes an autosomal recessive disorder, such as CAH or 5α-reductase deficiency, more likely.
   d. Aunts or other relatives with amenorrhea and/or infertility, which may suggest male pseudohermaphroditism.
2. Maternal history
   a. Maternal ingestion of drugs during pregnancy (particularly androgens or progestational agents).

TABLE 2-4. *Patterns of inheritance: ambiguous genitalia*

Disorder	Heredity
Female pseudohermaphroditism	
Congenital adrenal hyperplasia	Autosomal recessive
Male pseudohermaphroditism	
Testosterone biosynthetic defects	Autosomal recessive
Leydig cell hypoplasia	Autosomal recessive
5α-reductase deficiency	Autosomal recessive
Androgen insensitivity syndrome	X-linked recessive
Gonadal disorders	
Gonadal dysgenesis	Sporadic and familial
True hermaphroditism	Sporadic and rarely familial

   b. Maternal exposure to chemical endocrine disrupters in the environment (25)

   c. Maternal history of virilization or CAH.

Physical Examination

The physical examination of the infant starts with a general examination and a search for the stigmata of a malformation syndrome (e.g., intrauterine growth retardation, dysmorphic features, and abnormal body proportions). If a malformation syndrome is identified, further hormonal evaluation may not be necessary (for example, if the suspected diagnosis is trisomy 13). Other signs to look for on the general examination include hypertension, areolar hyperpigmentation, and signs of dehydration, all suggestive of CAH.

The genitalia should be carefully examined. The number of gonads and the size, symmetry, and position are crucial (Table 2-5). A palpable gonad below the inguinal canal is almost always a testis and, if present, generally rules out the diagnosis of female pseudohermaphroditism. An undescended gonad could be a testis, ovary, or ovotestis. Asymmetric labioscrotal folds with a unilateral gonad make mixed gonadal dysgenesis or true hermaphroditism more likely. The infant should be examined for the presence of a hernia, as it may contain a uterus, ovary, or testis. Precise measurements of the phallus should be made, including the stretch penile length (along the dorsum of the stretched phallus from the pubic ramus to the tip of the glans) and the midshaft diameter. The mean stretched penile lengths in normal males are as follows (±1 standard deviation):

2.5 (±0.4) cm for a 30-week newborn
3.0 (±0.4) cm for a 34-week newborn
3.5 (±0.4) cm for a full-term newborn
3.9 (±0.8) cm for a 0- to 5-month old
4.3 (±0.8) cm for a 6- to 12-month old

A good rule of thumb in evaluating the full-term newborn is that the normal male penis should be >2.5 cm (2.5 standard deviations below the mean).

TABLE 2-5. *Patient with intersex state: clinical assessment*

Family history, general examination for dysmorphic features
Examination of external genitalia
  No gonads palpable
    Female pseudohermaphroditism: congenital adrenal hyperplasia (21-hydroxylase
      deficiency)
    Male pseudohermaphroditism
  One gonad palpable = abnormal gonadal differentiation
  Male pseudohermaphroditism
  Mixed gonadal dysgenesis (X0/XY)
  True hermaphroditism
Two gonads palpable = male pseudohermaphroditism
  Impaired testosterone biosynthesis
  Androgen receptor defect
  5α-Reductase deficiency
  True hermaphroditism

From Sultan C, Paris F, Jeandel C, et al. Ambiguous genitalia in the newborn. *Semin Reprod Med* 2002;20:181; with permission.

The thickness and degree of development of the corpora should be assessed. If a clitoris is present, the length and width should be measured. The location of the urethral opening should be noted. In first-degree hypospadias, the urethra opens on the glans of the phallus; in second degree hypospadias, on the shaft; and in third degree, on the perineum. Hypospadias is usually accompanied by chordee, a tethering of the phallus due to incomplete closure of the tissue layers that constitute the covering over the urethra. Any child with hypospadias or a small phallus, bilateral cryptorchism, and a neonatal hernia should be evaluated for the possibility of an intersex disorder. It should be determined whether a vaginal opening or urogenital sinus is present. The labioscrotal folds should be examined for hyperpigmentation, the presence of gonads, and the degree of labial fusion. Labioscrotal folds range in phenotype (from the least to most virilized) from normal labia majora, to labia majora with posterior fusion, to a bifid scrotum, to a fully fused scrotum. Fusion of the labioscrotal folds is an androgen effect and can be assessed by measuring the anogenital ratio: the distance from the anus to the fourchette (AF) divided by the distance from the anus to the base of the clitoris (AC) (i.e., AF/AC). An anogenital ratio greater than 0.5 falls outside the 95% confidence limits (26) and represents fusion of the labioscrotal folds. A rectal examination should always be performed, since if a uterus is present, it is often easily palpable at birth because of uterine stimulation in utero by placental and maternal estrogens.

Laboratory and Radiographic Tests

The most important tests in the initial evaluation include the determination of the blood karyotype, electrolytes, 17-hydroxyprogesterone (17-OHP), dehydroepiandrosterone (DHEA), testosterone, dihydrotestosterone (DHT), luteinizing hormone (LH), and follicle-stimulating hormone (FSH), and performing radiographic studies. The results of the blood karyotype determination are usually available in 2 to 3 days if the laboratory is alerted and processes the blood expediently. Polymerase chain reaction (PCR) analysis of *SRY* on the Y chromosome is performed in some hospitals, as the results can be available in one day. However, an analysis of the karyotype is still mandatory. Buccal smears should not be performed, as they are inaccurate. In primary gonadal defects, and possibly in androgen-resistant states, LH and FSH are elevated. To define the internal structures, an ultrasound examination and a contrast study, either a retrograde genitogram (retrograde injection of contrast material via the urogenital orifice) or a voiding cystourethrogram, should be performed. The location of the gonads and the presence of a uterus and endometrial stripe can be determined by ultrasound examination. The contrast study will delineate the anatomy of the urethra and vagina (if present), the urogenital sinus, and at times, the cervix. Once it has been determined whether the infant is a male or female pseudohermaphrodite, or has a disorder of gonadal differentiation, other studies are usually indicated.

The most common cause of ambiguous genitalia is female pseudohermaphroditism due to CAH, and the majority of patients with this condition have 21-hydroxylase deficiency resulting in a markedly elevated 17-OHP level. If gonads are not palpable, 17-OHP and DHEA determinations should be obtained after 24 hours of life. In the normal infant, 17-OHP is elevated in cord blood but decreases to 100 to 200 ng/dl after 24 hours of life; this decrease may take longer in premature infants. The early-morning 17-OHP is generally greater than 10,000 ng/dl in infants with 21-hydroxylase deficiency. If the 17-OHP is not diagnostic, and CAH is suspected, a repeat level should be obtained a few days later, and fluid and electrolyte balance monitored daily. In infants with 21-hydroxylase deficiency, androstenedione and DHEA are elevated, serum cortisol may be very low or at the lower end of the normal range, and adrenocorticotropic hormone (ACTH) is elevated. Given the frequency of the CAH gene in the population (varying from 1:300 in Alaskan Eskimos to an average of 1:14,500 worldwide), screening of newborns for 21-hydroxylase deficiency has been implemented in most states by measurement of 17-OHP on the neonatal blood filter specimens (27). If the patient is a female pseudohermaphrodite but the etiology is unclear, other steroid precursor levels are measured after ACTH (Cortrosyn) stimulation and may delineate a specific adrenal enzyme defect.

In the male pseudohermaphrodite, testosterone is low in any defect in testosterone production. The testosterone/DHT ratio is elevated in 5α-reductase deficiency. AMH correlates with the degree of müllerian duct development and is a reliable marker for the presence of functional testicular tissue (28–31). AMH is nondetectable in normal females, detectable in normal males, and detectable but low in true hermaphrodites and patients with other disorders of testicular dysgenesis (30,31). In patients with androgen insensitivity syndrome (AIS) and those with defects in testosterone production, AMH is elevated (32). In the persistent müllerian duct syndrome, AMH is nondetectable in patients with defects in AMH, and is detectable in patients with end-organ resistance to AMH (33).

An HCG stimulation test is useful for determining the defect in the male pseudohermaphrodite. Several protocols for intramuscular HCG administration are available, including giving 1,500, 2,000, or 3,000 U/m^2 once a day for 3 to 5 days (34,35) or giving 5,000 U/m^2 for 1 day (36). Testosterone and DHT are measured 24 hours after HCG, and they both increase in the normal male; a sample of serum should be saved for further hormone analyses. In patients with 5α-reductase deficiency, the basal testosterone/DHT ratio may be normal, but the ratio is elevated after HCG stimulation. Failure of testosterone and DHT to rise after HCG stimulation suggests a defect in testosterone biosynthesis, Leydig cell hypoplasia, or gonadal dysgenesis. In this case, steroid hormone precursors should be measured in the serum saved from the test to look for inborn errors of testosterone biosynthesis. Fibroblasts from a scrotal skin biopsy can be assayed for 5α-reductase activity if 5α-reductase deficiency is suspected, or for androgen receptor binding capacity if AIS is suspected. If the patient has a primary gonadal abnormality, a skin biopsy or scrotal skin biopsy may be indicated for a karyotype analysis to rule out mosaicism. A gonadal biopsy may be indicated to determine whether ovarian or testicular tissue is present, or to confirm Leydig cell hypoplasia.

Several genetic studies are now available that may aid in the evaluation of ambiguous genitalia in the infant. A DNA probe for SRY will demonstrate whether SRY is present in the 46,XX male, and it is useful in determining whether Y material is present in a 45,X individual, placing the patient at risk for gonadoblastoma (see section on gonadal abnormalities below, and Chapters 6, 7, and 18). Mutations have been identified in the 21-hydroxylase gene in CAH, the 5α–reductase 2 gene in patients with 5α-reductase deficiency, the androgen receptor gene in AIS, and the AMH gene in persistent müllerian duct syndrome.

Differential Diagnosis of Ambiguous Genitalia in the Newborn

The differential diagnosis of the newborn with ambiguous genitalia can be divided into four broad categories:

1. Female pseudohermaphroditism
2. Male pseudohermaphroditism
3. Disorders of gonadal differentiation
4. Malformation syndromes

The female pseudohermaphrodite has a 46,XX karyotype, ovaries, no wolffian duct structures, well-developed müllerian duct structures, and virilized external genitalia. The male pseudohermaphrodite has a 46,XY karyotype; wolffian duct structures that are normal, hypoplastic, or absent; no müllerian duct structures; and undervirilized external genitalia. Patients with disorders of gonadal differentiation have either both ovarian and testicular tissue (true hermaphrodite) or one dysgenetic testis, one streak gonad, and no ovarian tissue (mixed gonadal dysgenesis [MGD]) (see Table 2-6 for the differential diagnosis of the infant with ambiguous genitalia).

FEMALE PSEUDOHERMAPHRODITISM

Congenital Adrenal Hyperplasia

Congenital adrenal hyperplasia (CAH) is the most common cause of ambiguous genitalia in the 46,XX newborn (see Ref. 37 for a review of CAH). It is caused by a deficiency in one of the adrenal cortical enzymes involved in the synthesis of cortisol (Fig. 2-9) and is inherited in an autosomal recessive manner. The enzyme deficiency results in inadequate cortisol synthesis, inadequate negative feedback to the hypothalamus and pituitary, and increased ACTH secretion. High levels of ACTH leads to adrenal gland hyperplasia, and the block in adrenal cortisol production results in shunting of the adrenal steroid precursors toward adrenal androgen production. The enzyme blocked and the degree of block vary, and ambiguity may range from labial fusion, with or without slight clitoromegaly, to a male-type phallus with labial fusion and rugae on the labioscrotal folds (Fig. 2-10).

More than 95% of CAH is due to 21-hydroxylase deficiency in the adrenal cortex (38). Mutations in the *CYP21* gene on chromosome 6p, which encodes the P450c21 enzyme, leads to the activity of the enzyme being severely reduced or absent. Both alleles of the gene must be affected for classic CAH to occur. Classic 21-hydroxylase deficiency presents in the newborn period, and salt losing is seen in about three-fourths of patients. In salt-losing CAH, the enzyme deficiency is more severe, and aldosterone secretion from the adrenal glomerulosa is decreased as well. Decreased aldosterone secretion decreases renal electrolyte exchange, resulting in hyponatremia, hyperkalemia, and metabolic acidosis. The extent of virilization is not a reliable indicator of the degree of adrenal insufficiency. Thus, the electrolyte status of all infants with 21-hydroxylase deficiency should be monitored.

Congenital adrenal hyperplasia can also be due to 11β-hydroxylase deficiency. Mutations in the *CYP11B1* gene disrupt the activity of the P450C11B1 enzyme. 11-Deoxycortisol and 11-deoxycorticosterone levels are high, and these moderately salt-retaining compounds result in salt retention, volume expansion, and hypertension. Another rare form of CAH, 3β-hydroxysteroid dehydrogenase deficiency (mutations in *HSD3B2* gene), results in severe adrenal insufficiency and increased ACTH. Pregnenolone, 17-hydroxypregnenolone, and DHEA are increased. Virilization is quite mild, since the block occurs in the initial steps of hormone synthesis and thus only the weak androgen DHEA can be produced in excess. Aldosterone deficiency may also occur and lead to salt wasting. Testosterone biosynthesis is decreased; therefore, 3β-hydroxysteroid dehydrogenase deficiency is also a cause of male pseudohermaphroditism.

TABLE 2-6. *Classification of anomalous sexual development*

I. Disorders of gonadal differentiation
   A. Seminiferous tubule dysgenesis (Klinefelter syndrome)
   B. Syndrome of gonadal dysgenesis and its variants (Turner syndrome)
   C. Complete and incomplete forms of XX and XY gonadal dysgenesis
   D. True hermaphroditism
II. Female pseudohermaphroditism
   A. Androgen-induced
      1. Congenital virilizing adrenal hyperplasia
      2. CYP19 (P45$_{arom}$) aromatase deficiency
      3. Androgens and synthetic progestagens transferred from maternal circulation
   B. Other teratologic factors (non-androgen-induced) associated with malformations of intestine and urinary tract
III. Male pseudohermaphroditism
   A. Testicular unresponsiveness to hCG and LH (Leydig cell agenesis or hypoplasia due to hCG/LH receptor defect)
   B. Inborn errors of testosterone biosynthesis
      1. Enzyme deficits affecting synthesis of both corticosteroids and testosterone (variants of congenital adrenal hyperplasia)
         a. StAR deficiency (congenital lipoid adrenal hyperplasia)
         b. 3β-Hydroxysteroid dehydrogenase/Δ^5 isomerase type II (3β-HSD II) deficiency
         c. CYP17 (P450$_{c17}$ [17α-hydroxylase/17,20 lyase]) deficiency
      2. Enzyme defects primarily affecting testosterone biosynthesis by the testes
         a. CYP17 (P450$_{c17}$ [17,20 lyase]) deficiency
         b. 17β-Hydroxysteroid dehydrogenase type 3 (17β-HSD 3) deficiency
   C. Defects in androgen-dependent target tissues
      1. End-organ resistance to androgenic hormones
         a. Syndrome of complete androgen resistance and its variants (testicular feminization and its variant forms)
         b. Syndrome of incomplete androgen resistance and its variants (Reifenstein's syndrome)
         c. Androgen resistance in phenotypically normal males
      2. Defects in testosterone metabolism by peripheral tissues; 5α-reductase-2 (SRD5A2) deficiency (pseudovaginal perineoscrotal hypospadias)
   D. Dysgenetic male pseudohermaphroditism
      1. XY gonadal dysgenesis (incomplete)
      2. XO/XY mosaicism, structurally abnormal Y chromosome, Xp+, 9p−, 10q−
      3. Denys-Drash syndrome (*WT1* mutation)
      4. WAGR syndrome (*WT1* deletion)
      5. Campomelic dysplasia (*SOX9* mutation)
      6. ? *SF1* mutation
      7. Testicular regression syndrome
   E. Defects in synthesis, secretion, or response to antimüllerian hormone: persistent müllerian duct syndrome (female genital ducts in otherwise normal men; herniae uteri inguinale)
   F. Maternal ingestion of progestagens and estrogens
   G. ?Environmental chemicals
IV. Unclassified forms of abnormal sexual development
   A. In males
      1. Hypospadias
      2. Ambiguous external genitalia in XY males with multiple congenital anomalies
   B. In females, absence or anomalous development of the vagina, uterus, and uterine tubes (Rokitansky-Küster syndrome)

(From Grumbach MM, Conte FA. Disorders of sex differentiation. In: Wilson JD, Foster DW, Kronenberg HM, et al., eds. *Williams textbook of endocrinology.* Philadelphia: WB Saunders, 1998:1303; with permission.)

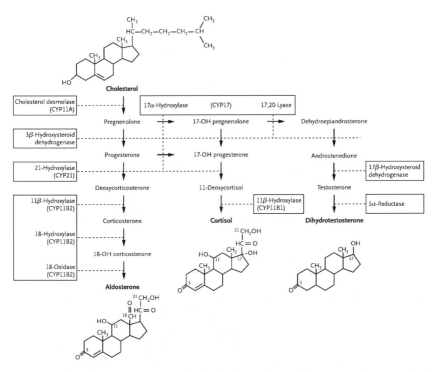

FIG. 2-9. Pathways of steroid biosynthesis in the adrenal cortex. The pathways for the synthesis of progesterone and mineralocorticoids (aldosterone), glucocorticoids (cortisol), and androgens (testosterone) are shown. Enzymes that are encoded by a single gene are shown in *boxes*. For activities mediated by specific P-450 cytochromes (CYP), the systematic name of the enzyme is given in parentheses. CYP11B2 and CYP17 have multiple activities. The planar structures of cholesterol, aldosterone, cortisol, and testosterone are shown. Deficient 21-hydroxylase activity prevents the synthesis of aldosterone and cortisol and shunts precursors such as 17-hydroxypregnenolone into the pathway for androgen biosynthesis. Androstenedione is secreted by the adrenal cortex and then converted to testosterone in the periphery. Testosterone may be aromatized to estradiol or converted by 5α-reductase to dihydrotestosterone (From Speiser PW, White PC. Congenital adrenal hyperplasia. *N Engl J Med* 2003;349:777; with permission.)

Glucocorticoid treatment should be instituted as soon as possible in the female pseudohermaphrodite once the laboratory studies have been obtained. Hydrocortisone, 2.5 mg two or three times daily (10 to 20 mg/m^2 per day), is the usual initial treatment. Since salt losing does not occur until day 6 to day 14 of life, the baby's weight, electrolytes, fluid status, and plasma renin activity (PRA) should be closely monitored. Salt losing is demonstrated by decreased serum sodium, increased serum potassium, decreased aldosterone, and elevated PRA; the elevated PRA is the most sensitive indicator of aldosterone deficiency. If salt losing is documented, salt (2 to 4 g per day) should be added to the formula, and a mineralocorticoid, fludrocortisone acetate (Florinef) 0.05 to 0.1 mg daily, should be given. In some children, the PRA is elevated in the absence of low aldosterone levels and

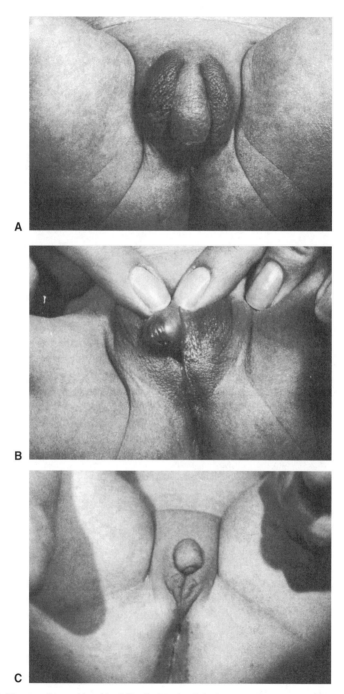

FIG. 2-10. Two newborn girls with virilization and salt-losing congenital adrenocortical hyperplasia: **(A)** and **(B)** patient S.C., **(C)** patient M.T.

salt wasting. In these children, the addition of fludrocortisone acetate normalizes the PRA, improving hormonal control and growth.

The hydrocortisone dose is adjusted on the basis of growth parameters (length, weight, skeletal maturation) and adrenal steroid precursor levels, including serum 17-OHP, Δ^4-androstenedione, DHEA, DHEA sulfate (S), and (except in infants and adolescent boys) testosterone. Therapy should be aimed at keeping the 17-hydroxy-progesterone well below 1000 ng/dl; levels <200 ng/dl in the morning usually indicate oversuppression. In patients in good control, Δ^4-androstenedione is normal, and DHEAS is below the normal range. However, DHEAS is not sensitive for detecting overtreatment. Although not usually used, 24-hour urinary 17-ketosteroid determinations can be used to monitor therapy in older children and should be in the low normal range (for bone age). Overtreatment with glucocorticoids results in growth retardation and delayed skeletal maturation. Undertreatment leads to accelerated skeletal maturation and virilization. The glucocorticoid dosage must be increased at times of stress, such as during illness and in the event of surgery. The adequacy of mineralocorticoid replacement is most accurately determined by measuring the PRA. New approaches include standard therapy plus antiandrogens and aromatase inhibitors (39,40), treatment with growth hormone to improve final adult height (41), and laparoscopic adrenalectomy, which allows for use of lower doses of glucocorticoid replacement (42,43). All of these are considered experimental at this time. (See Chapter 9 for a discussion of late onset congenital adrenal hyperplasia.)

It should be emphasized that female pseudohermaphrodites with CAH are females with ovaries, and are potentially fertile. Thus, regardless of the appearance of the external genitalia, the sex assignment should be female. Surgery, which may include clitoroplasty, labioplasty, and vaginoplasty, is discussed in Chapter 10.

Testing for mutations in *CYP21* and the pseudogene CYP21P are commercially available, and can be useful for prenatal diagnosis in future pregnancies. Prenatal treatment with high doses of glucocorticoids (dexamethasone) given to the mother before the sixth to seventh week of gestation is a somewhat controversial therapy designed to prevent virilization of an affected female (see Refs. 44 and 37 for a review).

Exogenous Androgens

The 46,XX infant with no evidence of CAH may have been exposed to exogenous androgens from either maternal ingestion or production. Androgens, danazol, and synthetic progestins (in doses much higher than in oral contraceptive pills) given before the fourteenth week of gestation can cause labial fusion and clitoromegaly; such therapy after the fourteenth week causes clitoromegaly only. If the maternal drug history is noncontributory, the mother should undergo a careful physical examination and laboratory testing for hyperandrogenism. In the absence of a maternal history of virilization or hormone ingestion, the internal genital anatomy should be evaluated to determine whether there is a primary gonadal abnormality (see below). Placental aromatase deficiency is another rare cause of fetal virilzation, accompanied by virilization of the mother during pregnancy, which resolves postpartum (45).

MALE PSEUDOHERMAPHRODITISM

Understanding the steps involved in the development of normal male genitalia facilitates the diagnosis of the specific defect in the male pseudohermaphrodite (Fig. 2-11). However, it should be noted that in 46,XY individuals, a definitive diagnosis cannot always be made. In one study (46) of 67 patients with ambiguous genitalia and a 46,XY karyotype or testicular tissue, a definitive diagnosis was made in only 48%, and included testicular dysgenesis, true hermaphroditism PAIS, or 17β-hydroxysteroid dehydrogenase.

If the testis is unresponsive to HCG and LH because of absence of LH receptors or abnormal Leydig cell development (Leydig cell hypoplasia or agenesis), wolffian duct structures do not differentiate owing to lack of testosterone (36). Müllerian duct structures regress under the stimulus of AMH, which comes from the Sertoli cells, and testes are present in the abdomen. Testosterone is low, LH is elevated, and testosterone does not rise in response to exogenous HCG. The external genital phenotype is usually female, with a urogenital sinus and a short vaginal pouch. Biopsy of the testicles reveals no distinct Leydig cells, normal Sertoli cells, and spermatogenic arrest in the seminiferous tubules.

Defects in testosterone biosynthesis can be due to deficiencies in one of several enzymes in the pathway toward testosterone synthesis, all of which are inherited in an autosomal recessive manner (see reference 47 for a review). Steroidogenic acute regulatory protein (StAR) regulates the rapid influx of cholesterol in the mitochondria, acutely regulating steroidogenesis (47). Mutations in StAR are responsible for most cases of congenital lipoid adrenal hyperplasia, a rare, often fatal, condition where no steroid hormones are made and severe salt wasting occurs (47,48). Mutations in the cholesterol side chain cleavage enzyme (P45scc or CPY11A) have also been described to cause congenital lipoid adrenal hyperplasia (49). 3β-hydroxysteroid dehydrogenase (HSD3B2) deficiency causes male *pseudohermaphroditism*, as well as female pseudohermaphroditism, since the large amounts of DHEA produced are not able to compensate for the lack of testosterone production. The P45c17 enzyme, encoded by the *CYP17* gene, is now known to be the one enzyme that carries out functions previously thought to be mediated by 17α-hydroxylase and 17,20-lyase, and patients have been described who lack the 17α-hydroxylase activity, 17,20-lyase activity, or both (47). Cortisol levels are decreased, and increased deoxycorticosterone levels can lead to hypertension and hypokalemia. Finally, 17β-hydroxysteroid dehydrogenase, or 17-ketosteroid reductase, deficiency is due to mutations in 17β-HSD-III (HSD17B3), and affected individuals show no signs of CAH. Defects in testosterone production result in absence of wolffian duct structures, regression of müllerian duct structures (AMH is normal), and external genitalia that are either female or ambiguous. Testosterone and DHT are low and do not increase in response to HCG. For all of these enzyme deficiencies, the specific defect can be determined by measuring steroid hormone precursors after HCG stimulation. Enzyme deficiencies that also lead to CAH can be confirmed by an ACTH (Cortrosyn) stimulation test.

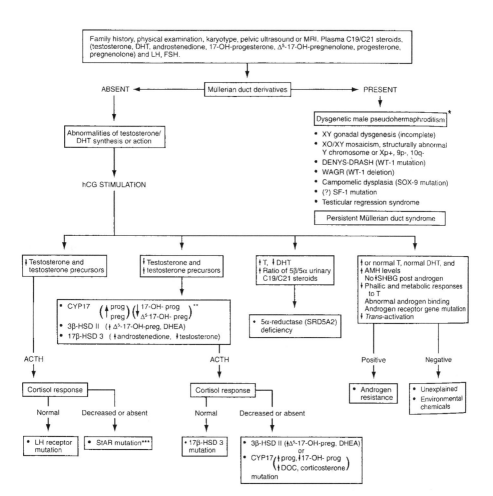

FIG. 2-11. Steps in the differential diagnosis of male pseudohermaphroditism. Patients with dysgenetic male pseudohermaphroditism may manifest varying degrees of testicular dysgenesis with consequent testosterone/DHT and/or AMH deficiency. Therefore, not all patients may manifest either ambiguous genitalia or the presence of müllerian ducts. CYP17 (P450c17) catalyzes the 17-hydroxylation of progesterone and pregnenolone to 17-hydroxyprogesterone and Δ^5-17-hydroxypregnenolone as well as the scission (lyase) of 17-hydroxypregnenolone to DHEA. Patients with 17,20-lyase deficiency have elevated levels of 17-hydroxyprogesterone and Δ^5-17-hydroxypregnenonlone in relation to androstenendione and DHEA either before or after HCG stimulation. The StAR (steroidogenic acute regulatory) protein is involved in the transport of cholesterol from the outer to the inner mitochondrial membrane where the enzyme CYP11A1 (P450scc) resides. Patients with a mutation in the gene for this protein have a markedly diminished ability to convert cholesterol to Δ^5-17-hydroxypregnenolone, although their CYP11A1 enzymatic activity is intact, and they manifest congenital lipoid adrenal hyperplasia. WAGR, Wilms tumor, aniridia, genital anomalies, and mental retardation; SF-1, steroidogenic factor-1; CYP17, 17α-hydroxylase/17, 20-lyase; 3β-HSD II, 3β-hydroxysteroid dehydrogenase/Δ^5-isomerase;17β-HSD 3, 17β-hydroxysteroid dehydrogenase (oxidoreductase); T, testosterone; DHT, dihydrotestosterone; AMH, antimüllerian hormone; SHBG, sex hormone binding globulin; DHEA, dehydroepiandrosterone. (From Grumbach MM, Conte FA. Disorders of sex differentiation. In: Wilson JD, Foster DW, Kronenberg HM, et al., eds. *Williams textbook of endocrinology*. Philadelphia: W.B. Saunders, 1998:1303; with permission.)

Defects in androgen-dependent target tissues include androgen insensitivity syndrome (AIS) and 5α-reductase deficiency, and are the most common causes of male pseudohermaphroditism (see reference 50 for a review). In AIS, binding of testosterone and DHT to the androgen receptor is impaired because of a receptor defect (see Table 2-2 for a summary of findings). Testosterone levels are normal and increase normally after HCG stimulation. Complete AIS (CAIS) gives the classic picture of testicular feminization and is not manifested by ambiguous genitalia at birth, although occasionally testes may be noted in a hernia sac early in life. The phenotypic female infant with a hernia should undergo an evaluation to determine what is in the hernia; 7% of females with a hernia have no cervix by palpation or vaginoscopy, and they are either male pseudohermaphrodites (usually CAIS) or have mixed gonadal dysgenesis. In CAIS, the testes function normally, producing AMH (müllerian ducts regress) and testosterone, which is converted into DHT. However, since androgen-dependent target tissues are unresponsive to testosterone and DHT, wolffian duct structures do not develop, and the external genitalia develop along female lines (Table 2-2). Partial AIS (PAIS), on the other hand, results in a spectrum of ambiguous genitalia syndromes, including the Gilbert–Dreyfus, Reifenstein, Rosewater, and Lubs syndromes. Patients with PAIS have some degree of wolffian development and labioscrotal fusion. The androgen receptor (AR) has been well characterized, and molecular defects in AIS have been described in the AR gene. The AR gene is located on the short arm of the X chromosome, and AIS is inherited in an X-linked recessive manner. Over 250 mutations in the AR gene have been described (51). Of interest, AR mutations are found in 85% to 90% of patients with CAIS or familial PAIS, but in only 10% to 15% of patients with sporadic PAIS (50), suggesting that the diagnosis of PAIS, without the help of a family history of PAIS, is difficult.

5α-Reductase deficiency is an autosomal recessive disorder in which the enzyme that converts testosterone to DHT in androgen-dependent tissues is defective. Testosterone levels are normal, DHT levels are low, and the T/DHT ratio is elevated, especially after HCG stimulation. Since DHT is responsible for the masculinization of the external genitalia, patients with 5α-reductase deficiency have undervirilized external genitalia but develop normal male internal genitalia (wolffian duct structures differentiate, and müllerian duct structures regress). The phenotype is characterized by a bifid scrotum, a clitoris-like phallus, hypospadias, a urogenital sinus that opens onto the perineum, and a blind vaginal pouch. In some families, children with this condition have been initially raised as females, but due to masculinization at puberty (the testes descend, the scrotum enlarges, and the phallus lengthens), take on a male gender identity (52). The disorder is due to mutations in the steroid 5α-reductase 2 gene (SRD5A2)

The persistent müllerian duct syndrome occurs in a 46,XY individual with testes and either defective AMH or end-organ resistance to AMH (33,53,54). Such a patient does not often have ambiguous genitalia but may have cryptorchidism or hernia uteri inguinale (presumably due to the mobilization of müllerian derivatives during testicular descent into the inguinal canal or scrotum). Wolffian duct development varies among individuals. Few males are fertile, and there is a high incidence of postnatal testicular degeneration. Mutations have been found in the AMH and AMH receptor II (AMHR-II) genes and are transmitted in an autosomal recessive manner (55).

As discussed in the section on laboratory and radiographic testing, the evaluation of the 46,XY male with ambiguous genitalia should include an HCG stimulation test. An increased testosterone/DHT ratio is characteristic of 5α-reductase deficiency and can be confirmed by measurement of 5α-reductase activity in cultured genital skin fibroblasts. If the testosterone and DHT are both low, steroid precursors in the testosterone biosynthetic pathway should be measured. If a testosterone biosynthesis defect that also leads to CAH is suspected, an ACTH stimulation test can confirm the diagnosis. If all hormone levels are low, and there is no adrenal insufficiency, Leydig cell hypoplasia is likely and can be verified by testicular biopsy. If hormone levels are normal, the diagnosis of AIS is suggested and can be confirmed by identification of a mutation in the androgen receptor gene or by measurement of androgen receptor binding in scrotal skin.

Sex assignment is usually based on the patient's potential to achieve unambiguous appearance of the external genitalia and normal sexual function after reconstructive surgery and hormonal therapy. Conte and Grumbach (56) have recommended that any child with a 46,XY karyotype be raised as a male, except in the presence of CAIS, completely feminized genitalia, or if there is some other reason, including an informed parental decision, not to do so. In certain rare circumstances, another approach is to use HCG and testosterone, to assure adequate function in puberty and adulthood. In this case, a male gender would be assigned to patient with micropenis or PAIS who respond to a 3- to 5-day HCG stimulation test with adequate penile growth, achieving a length of >2.0 cm (34). Under rare circumstances, sex assignment may be delayed until the patient is given three monthly intramuscular injections of testosterone enanthate, 25mg, which should produce lengthening of the penis by >0.9 cm (56), and in this case, the patient is assigned a male gender. The phallus may not grow well at puberty in patients with PAIS who do not respond to testosterone in the newborn period. In patients with 5α-reductase deficiency, topical DHT cream applied to the external genitalia causes phallic growth (57). If the sex assignment is female, the gonads should be electively removed early, once the diagnosis has been made.

DISORDERS OF GONADAL DIFFERENTIATION

The true hermaphrodite has both testicular and ovarian tissue (with follicles) and represents the rarest intersex disorder. The gonads consist of either one ovary and one testis, two ovotestes, or one ovotestis and one ovary or testis. Over half of patients have a 46,XX karyotype, one-third are chimeric 46,XX/46,XY (two distinct populations of cells with different genetic origins) or mosaic (46,XY/47,XXY or 45,X/46XY), and only a few have a 46,XY karyotype (58). Only a few 46,XX true hermaphrodites have detectable SRY in the blood (59,60), although in some, mosaicism for SRY has been demonstrated in gonadal tissue (58,61). Differentiation of the internal ducts depends on the amount and location of functional testicular tissue; wolffian duct structures differentiate on the side with testicular tissue, and müllerian duct structures on the side with no testicular tissue. A uterus (frequently hypoplastic or abnormal) is present in 90% of patients. Although a few patients have normal female external genitalia or have a penile urethra, the majority have ambiguous genitalia. In the past, most have been reared as males. At puberty, three-quarters of patients develop gynecomastia, and one-half menstruate. Decisions about sex assignment should be based on the internal and external genitalia, and the organs of the opposite sex should be removed. If the patient is to be reared as a male, the phallus must be adequate in size and the testis or testes brought down into the scrotum.

Patients with pure gonadal dysgenesis are phenotypic females, lack the stigmata of Turner syndrome (see Chapter 6), and do not have ambiguous genitalia at birth. The karyotype is either 46,XX or 46,XY; individuals with a 46,XY karyotype are sometimes referred to as having *complete gonadal dysgenesis*. Individuals with pure gonadal dysgenesis have dysgenetic (streak) gonads consisting of ovarian stroma, fibrous tissue, and no primordial follicles. Pure gonadal dysgenesis is usually diagnosed during adolescence when a girl presents with primary amenorrhea and is found to have elevated gonadotropins. In the past, pure gonadal dysgenesis has been referred to as Swyer syndrome. Approximately 15% of 46,XY females with pure gonadal dysgenesis have a mutation in the SRY (62), and in most patients the SRY is intact and the etiology is unknown.

Mixed gonadal dysgenesis (MGD) is characterized by one normal or dysgenetic testis and one streak ovary. All patients have a Y chromosome, and the karyotype is usually 45,X/46,XY mosaic but can be 46,XY (sometimes referred to as *partial gonadal dysgenesis*). The phenotype reflects the level of functioning of the fetal dysgenetic testis. The internal genitalia are usually asymmetric, with müllerian duct differentiation on the side with the streak ovary and variable wolffian duct differentiation on the side with the testis. Approximately one-half of patients with MGD are born with ambiguous external genitalia, which may be asymmetric with an enlarged labioscrotal fold on the side with the testis. The dysgenetic testis is not capable of completely virilizing the external genitalia, but it is capable of producing androgen levels sufficient to virilize an apparent female at puberty (63). Most patients have been raised as females.

The choice of gender in gonadal disorders depends on the external genitalia and the possibility for future coital adequacy. Once the sex assignment has been made, the gonads that conflict with the assignment are electively removed. Any patient with a dysgenetic gonad and a Y-bearing cell line is at high risk for developing a gonadal tumor (64–66). Even if a Y chromosome is not visible cytogenetically,

DNA probes for SRY may detect Y material. Gonadoblastomas occur in 20% to 30% of 46,XY patients with pure gonadal dysgenesis and one-third of patients with MGD, and they may develop into malignant tumors (dysgerminomas or seminomas) in about one-third of patients (65,66) (see Chapter 18 for a further discussion of ovarian masses). True hermaphrodites are also at risk for developing gonadoblastomas, although the risk is lower. All patients with a dysgenetic gonad and a Y-bearing cell line should have the intraabdominal dysgenetic gonads removed in infancy or at the time of diagnosis. Dysgenetic testes may be left in place only in the child with bilateral descended dysgenetic testes given a male sex assignment; in this case, the risk of malignancy is less, and the testes should be routinely examined.

MALFORMATION SYNDROMES

Chromosomal abnormalities that can be associated with ambiguous genitalia include trisomy 13 and 18, triploidy, and 4p- syndrome (67). Monogenic disorders can be associated with ambiguous genitalia, including Smith–Lemli–Opitz and camptomelic dysplasia (67). Associations of defects, such as the CHARGE association (Coloboma, Heart defect, Atresia choanae, Retarded growth and development with or without central nervous system anomalies, Genital anomalies with or without hypogonadism, and Ear anomalies with or without deafness) can include ambiguous genitalia (see Table 2-7 for a summary of malformation syndromes associated with genital ambiguity). Genital abnormalities can be associated with other anomalies, especially those of the urinary tract (see Chapter 10).

HYPOSPADIAS AND CRYPTORCHIDISM

The incidence of hypospadias in newborn males ranges from 1 in 300 to 1 in 800. Familial clustering has been reported, and hypospadias is present in a second individual in 21% of families (68). Variable modes of inheritance suggest that familial hypospadias represents a heterogeneous group of disorders. Defects in the androgen receptor have been described in isolated hypospadias, but are rare (69), and the majority of patients with hypospadias have normal androgen receptors (70). Severe forms of hypospadias, especially if accompanied by unilateral or bilateral cryptorchidism, defects in scrotal fusion, or a cervix palpable by rectal examination, necessitate a complete evaluation.

Cryptorchidism occurs in 2.7% of full-term newborn males and in 21% of premature infants. The incidence decreases to 0.8% by 1 year of age, and descent is unlikely after that time. Malignancy is more common in undescended testes than in scrotal testes (71–73). These two facts have led to the recommendation that evaluation for cryptorchidism occur before 2 years of age (72,74). It should be noted

TABLE 2-7. *Conditions associated with genital ambiguity*

Chromosomal
  Trisomy 13
  Trisomy 18
  Triploidy
  4p-, 13q-
  Aniridia-Wilms
Single gene
  Ellis van Creveld
  Smith-Lemli-Opitz
  Opitz
  Opitz-Frias
  Rieger
  Robinow
  Carpenter
  Meckel-Gruber
  Camptomelic dysplasia
  Androgen insensitivity
  Congenital adrenal hyperplasia
Associations
  CHARGE
  Vater

that both the cryptorchid testis and the contralateral testis have an increased risk of cancer even with surgery. Cryptorchidism can occur in Kallmann syndrome, hormonal deficiencies, dysgenetic or "vanishing" testes, persistent müllerian duct syndrome (33), and congenital syndromes. Thus, disorders of sexual differentiation need to be considered in the infant with cryptorchidism.

If one testis is absent but the genitalia are otherwise completely normal, a rectal examination should be performed to rule out the remote possibility that there is a cervix or large utricle. If a midline structure is not palpated, ultrasonography of the pelvis will rule out the presence of müllerian duct structures. If this is normal, no further evaluation is indicated. If both testes are missing but the genitalia appear to be that of a normal male, karyotype determination and hormone analysis should be performed to rule out female pseudohermaphroditism. If the karyotype is 46,XY and the genitals adequate for male function, the infant should be raised as a male. An HCG stimulation test should be performed to determine whether or not functional testes are present; a lack of rise in testosterone indicates primary testicular failure or an agonadal state. Some of these patients may have congenital anorchia, in which the testes presumably functioned at least until the sixteenth week of gestation and then disappeared. In these patients, serum LH and FSH are elevated, and testosterone and AMH are low. Testosterone therapy at puberty is necessary for the development of secondary sexual characteristics. Testicular implants may be helpful as well. Other patients may have bilateral undescended testes that are capable of function. A 4- to 6-week course of HCG or gonadotropin-releasing hormone can be given to induce descent of the testes. However, this therapy remains controversial; success rates are low with truly cryptorchid testes in contrast to retractile testes, which usually descend with hormonal stimulation (75). Laparoscopy is useful in locating intraabdominal testes or cord structures entering the inguinal canal (76), which suggests a descended but probably atrophic organ. Surgical treatment can be carried out using either open or laparoscopic techniques. There seems to be an inverse correlation between the age of surgery and the degree of fertility; the younger the patient is at surgery, the higher the rate of fertility (72).

REFERENCES

1. Gooren LJ. Psychological consequences. *Semin Reprod Med* 2002;20:285.
2. Koopman P. Sry and Sox9: mammalian testis-determining genes. *Cell Mol Life Sci* 1999;55:839.
3. Cotinot C, Pailhoux E, Jaubert F, et al. Molecular genetics of sex determination. *Semin Reprod Med* 2002;20:157.
4. MacLaughlin DT, Donahoe PK. Sex determination and disease. *N Engl Med* 2004;350:367.
5. Sinclair AH, Berta P, Palmer MS, et al. A gene from the human sex-determining region encodes a protein with homology to a conserved DNA-binding motif. *Nature* 1990;346:240.
6. Berta P, Hawkins JR, Sinclair AH, et al. Genetic evidence equating SRY and the testis-determining factor. *Nature* 1990;348:448.
7. Hawkins JR. Mutational analysis of SRY in XY females. *Hum Mutat* 1993;2:347.
8. Harley VR, Jackson DI, Hextall PJ, et al. DNA binding activity of recombinant SRY from normal males and XY females. *Science* 1992;255:453.
9. Dubin RA, Ostrer H. Sry is a transcriptional activator. *Mol Endocrinol* 1994;8:1182.
10. Fechner PY, Marcantonio SM, Jaswaney V, et al. The role of the sex-determining region Y gene in the etiology of 46,XX maleness. *J Clin Endocrinol Metab* 1993;76:690.
11. Kuhnle U, Schwarz HP, Lohrs U, et al. Familial true hermaphroditism: paternal and maternal transmission of true hermaphroditism (46,XX) and XX maleness in the absence of Y-chromosomal sequences. *Hum Genet* 1993;92:571.
12. Tsutsumi O, Iida T, Nakahori Y, et al. Analysis of the testis-determining gene SRY in patients with XY gonadal dysgenesis. *Horm Res* 1996;46[Suppl 1]:6.
13. Tsutsumi O, Iida T, Taketani Y, et al. Intact sex determining region Y (SRY) in a patient with XY pure gonadal dysgenesis and a twin brother. *Endocr J* 1994;41:281.
14. Wagner T, Wirth J, Meyer J, et al. Autosomal sex reversal and camptomelic dysplasia are caused by mutations in and around the SRY-related gene SOX9. *Cell* 1994;79:1111.
15. Foster JW, Dominguez-Steglich MA, Guioli S, et al. Camptomelic dysplasia and autosomal sex reversal caused by mutations in an SRY-related gene. *Nature* 1994;372:525.
16. Koopman P. Sry, Sox9 and mammalian sex determination. *EXS* 2001:25.
17. Swain A, Narvaez V, Burgoyne P, et al. Dax1 antagonizes Sry action in mammalian sex determination. *Nature* 1998;391:761.
18. Vogt PH, Edelmann A, Hirschmann P, et al. The azoospermia factor (AZF) of the human Y chromosome in Yq11: function and analysis in spermatogenesis. *Reprod Fertil Dev* 1995;7:685.
19. Ferlin A, Moro E, Rossi A, et al. The human Y chromosome's azoospermia factor b (AZFb) region: sequence, structure, and deletion analysis in infertile men. *J Med Genet* 2003;40:18.
20. Foresta C, Moro E, Rossi A, et al. Role of the AZFa candidate genes in male infertility. *J Endocrinol Invest* 2000;23:646.
21. Yu RN, Ito M, Saunders TL, et al. Role of Ahch in gonadal development and gametogenesis. *Nat Genet* 1998;20:353.
22. Parker KL, Schimmer BP. Ahch and the feminine mystique. *Nat Genet* 1998;20:318.
23. Voutilainen R. Differentiation of the fetal gonad. *Horm Res* 1992;38[Suppl 2]:66.
24. Teixeira J, Maheswaran S, Donahoe PK. Müllerian inhibiting substance: an instructive developmental hormone with diagnostic and possible therapeutic applications. *Endocr Rev* 2001;22:657.
25. Toppari J. Environmental endocrine disrupters and disorders of sexual differentiation. *Semin Reprod Med* 2002;20:305.

26. Callegari C, Everett S, Ross M, et al. Anogenital ratio: measure of fetal virilization in premature and full-term newborn infants. *J Pediatr* 1987;111:240.
27. Thompson R, Seargeant L, Winter JS. Screening for congenital adrenal hyperplasia: distribution of 17 alpha-hydroxyprogesterone concentrations in neonatal blood spot specimens. *J Pediatr* 1989;114:400.
28. Gustafson ML, Lee MM, Asmundson L, et al. Müllerian inhibiting substance in the diagnosis and management of intersex and gonadal abnormalities. *J Pediatr Surg* 1993;28:439.
29. Josso N, di Clemente N, Gouedard L. Anti-müllerian hormone and its receptors. *Mol Cell Endocrinol* 2001;179:25.
30. Lee MM, Donahoe PK, Silverman BL, et al. Measurements of serum müllerian inhibiting substance in the evaluation of children with nonpalpable gonads. *N Engl J Med* 1997;336:1480.
31. Lee MM, Donahoe PK, Hasegawa T, et al. Müllerian inhibiting substance in humans: normal levels from infancy to adulthood. *J Clin Endocrinol Metab* 1996;81:571.
32. Rey R, Mebarki F, Forest MG, et al. Anti-müllerian hormone in children with androgen insensitivity. *J Clin Endocrinol Metab* 1994;79:960.
33. Josso N, Picard JY, Imbeaud S, et al. The persistent mullerian duct syndrome: a rare cause of cryptorchidism. *Eur J Pediatr* 1993;152[Suppl 2]:S76.
34. Almaguer MC, Saenger P, Linder BL. Phallic growth after hCG. A clinical index of androgen responsiveness. *Clin Pediatr (Phila)* 1993;32:329.
35. Garg SK, Yopadhyay PK, Ram B. Gonadotrophin stimulation in children with abnormal sexual development. *S Afr Med J* 1989;76:199.
36. Hughes IA, Williams DM, Batch JA, et al. Male pseudohermaphroditism: clinical management, diagnosis and treatment. *Horm Res* 1992;38[Suppl 2]:77.
37. Speiser PW, White PC. Congenital adrenal hyperplasia. *N Engl J Med* 2003;349:776.
38. New MI. Female pseudohermaphroditism. *Semin Perinatol* 1992;16:299.
39. Merke DP, Cutler GB, Jr. New ideas for medical treatment of congenital adrenal hyperplasia. *Endocrinol Metab Clin North Am* 2001;30:121.
40. Merke DP, Bornstein SR, Avila NA, et al. NIH Conference. Future directions in the study and management of congenital adrenal hyperplasia due to 21-hydroxylase deficiency. *Ann Intern Med* 2002;136:320.
41. Quintos JB, Vogiatzi MG, Harbison MD, et al. Growth hormone therapy alone or in combination with gonadotropin-releasing hormone analog therapy to improve the height deficit in children with congenital adrenal hyperplasia. *J Clin Endocrinol Metab* 2001;86:1511.
42. Gmyrek GA, New MI, Sosa RE, et al. Bilateral laparoscopic adrenalectomy as a treatment for classic congenital adrenal hyperplasia attributable to 21-hydroxylase deficiency. *Pediatrics* 2002;109:E28.
43. Meyers RL, Grua JR. Bilateral laparoscopic adrenalectomy: a new treatment for difficult cases of congenital adrenal hyperplasia. *J Pediatr Surg* 2000;35:1586.
44. Consensus statement on 21-hydroxylase deficiency from the Lawson Wilkins Pediatric Endocrine Society and the European Society for Paediatric Endocrinology. *J Clin Endocrinol Metab* 2002;87:4048.
45. Meinhardt U, Mullis PE. The essential role of the aromatase/p450arom. *Semin Reprod Med* 2002;20:277.
46. Morel Y, Rey R, Teinturier C, et al. Aetiological diagnosis of male sex ambiguity: a collaborative study. *Eur J Pediatr* 2002;161:49.
47. Miller WL. Disorders of androgen biosynthesis. *Semin Reprod Med* 2002;20:205.
48. Lin D, Sugawara T, Strauss JF, 3rd, et al. Role of steroidogenic acute regulatory protein in adrenal and gonadal steroidogenesis. *Science* 1995;267:1828.
49. Tajima T, Fujieda K, Kouda N, et al. Heterozygous mutation in the cholesterol side chain cleavage enzyme (p450scc) gene in a patient with 46,XY sex reversal and adrenal insufficiency. *J Clin Endocrinol Metab* 2001;86:3820.
50. Sultan C, Lumbroso S, Paris F, et al. Disorders of androgen action. *Semin Reprod Med* 2002;20:217.
51. Gottlieb B, Beitel LK, Lumbroso R, et al. Update of the androgen receptor gene mutations database. *Hum Mutat* 1999;14:103.
52. Imperato-McGinley J, Peterson RE, Gautier T, et al. Androgens and the evolution of male-gender identity among male pseudohermaphrodites with 5 alpha-reductase deficiency. *N Engl J Med* 1979;300:1233.

53. Josso N, Picard JY, Imbeaud S, et al. Clinical aspects and molecular genetics of the persistent mullerian duct syndrome. *Clin Endocrinol (Oxf)* 1997;47:137.
54. Lang-Muritano M, Biason-Lauber A, Gitzelmann C, et al. A novel mutation in the anti-müllerian hormone gene as cause of persistent müllerian duct syndrome. *Eur J Pediatr* 2001;160:652.
55. Josso N, Belville C, Picard J. Mutations of AMH and its receptors. *Endocrinologist* 2003;13:247.
56. Conte FA, Grumbach MM. Diagnosis and management of ambiguous external genitalia. *Endocrinologist* 2003;13:260.
57. Odame I, Donaldson MD, Wallace AM, et al. Early diagnosis and management of 5 alpha-reductase deficiency. *Arch Dis Child* 1992;67:720.
58. Queipo G, Zenteno JC, Pena R, et al. Molecular analysis in true hermaphroditism: demonstration of low-level hidden mosaicism for Y-derived sequences in 46,XX cases. *Hum Genet* 2002;111:278.
59. McElreavey K, Rappaport R, Vilain E, et al. A minority of 46,XX true hermaphrodites are positive for the Y-DNA sequence including SRY. *Hum Genet* 1992;90:121.
60. Berkovitz GD, Fechner PY, Marcantonio SM, et al. The role of the sex-determining region of the Y chromosome (SRY) in the etiology of 46,XX true hermaphroditism. *Hum Genet* 1992;88:411.
61. Ortenberg J, Oddoux C, Craver R, et al. SRY gene expression in the ovotestes of XX true hermaphrodites. *J Urol* 2002;167:1828.
62. Cameron FJ, Sinclair AH. Mutations in SRY and SOX9: testis-determining genes. *Hum Mutat* 1997;9:388.
63. Mendez JP, Ulloa-Aguirre A, Kofman-Alfaro S, et al. Mixed gonadal dysgenesis: clinical, cytogenetic, endocrinological, and histopathological findings in 16 patients. *Am J Med Genet* 1993;46:263.
64. Gibbons B, Tan SY, Yu CC, et al. Risk of gonadoblastoma in female patients with Y chromosome abnormalities and dysgenetic gonads. *J Paediatr Child Health* 1999;35:210.
65. Savage MO, Lowe DG. Gonadal neoplasia and abnormal sexual differentiation. *Clin Endocrinol (Oxf)* 1990;32:519.
66. Verp MS, Simpson JL. Abnormal sexual differentiation and neoplasia. *Cancer Genet Cytogenet* 1987;25:191.
67. Aarskog D. Syndromes and genital dysmorphology. *Horm Res* 1992;38[Suppl 2]:82.
68. Bauer SB, Retik AB, Colodny AH. Genetic aspects of hypospadias. *Urol Clin North Am* 1981;8:559.
69. Sutherland RW, Wiener JS, Hicks JP, et al. Androgen receptor gene mutations are rarely associated with isolated penile hypospadias. *J Urol* 1996;156:828.
70. Evans BA, Williams DM, Hughes IA. Normal postnatal androgen production and action in isolated micropenis and isolated hypospadias. *Arch Dis Child* 1991;66:1033.
71. Berkmen F, Alagol H. Germinal cell tumors of the testis in cryptorchids. *J Exp Clin Cancer Res* 1998;17:409.
72. Cortes D, Thorup JM, Visfeldt J. Cryptorchidism: aspects of fertility and neoplasms. A study including data of 1,335 consecutive boys who underwent testicular biopsy simultaneously with surgery for cryptorchidism. *Horm Res* 2001;55:21.
73. Herrinton LJ, Zhao W, Husson G. Management of cryptorchism and risk of testicular cancer. *Am J Epidemiol* 2003;157:602.
74. Docimo SG, Silver RI, Cromie W. The undescended testicle: diagnosis and management. *Am Fam Physician* 2000;62:2037.
75. Rajfer J, Handelsman DJ, Swerdloff RS, et al. Hormonal therapy of cryptorchidism. A randomized, double-blind study comparing human chorionic gonadotropin and gonadotropin-releasing hormone. *N Engl J Med* 1986;314:466.
76. Tsujihata M, Miyake O, Yoshimura K, et al. Laparoscopic diagnosis and treatment of nonpalpable testis. *Int J Urol* 2001;8:692.
77. Hughes IA. Minireview: sex differentiation. *Endocrinology* 2001;142:3281.
78. Jorde LB, Carey JC, Bamshad MJ, et al. Clinical Cytogenetics: The Chromosomal Basis of Human Disease. In: Schmitt W, ed. *Medical genetics*. St. Louis: Mosby, 2000:108.
79. Simpson JL, Rajkovic A. Ovarian differentiation and gonadal failure. *Am J Med Genet* 1999;89:186.
80. Warne GL, Kanumakala S. Molecular endocrinology of sex differentiation. *Semin Reprod Med* 2002;20:169.
81. Grumbach MM, Conte FA. Disorders of Sex Differentiation. In: Wilson JD, Foster DW, Kronenberg HM, Larsen PR, eds. *Williams Textbook of Endocrinology*. Philadelphia: WB Saunders, 1998:1303.

82. Dewing P, Bernard P, Vilain E. Disorders of gonadal development. *Semin Reprod Med* 2002;20:189.
83. Sultan C, Paris F, Jeandel C, et al. Ambiguous genitalia in the newborn. *Semin Reprod Med* 2002;20:181.

3

Vulvovaginal Problems in the Prepubertal Child

S. Jean Emans

VULVOVAGINITIS

Vulvovaginitis is a common gynecologic problem in prepubertal girls. Vulvar inflammation, termed *vulvitis*, may occur alone or may be accompanied by a vaginal inflammation, vaginitis. A child may acquire a primary vaginal infection, and the discharge may cause maceration of the vulva and secondary vulvitis. The prepubertal child is particularly susceptible to vulvar and vaginal infections because of the physiology of the genital tract. In the newborn period, the vagina is well estrogenized from maternal hormones. For several months to several years beyond the newborn period, the infant has fluctuating gonadotropin levels, which can result in stimulation of the ovaries to produce low levels of estrogen. As the estrogen levels wane, the hymen becomes thin and the vagina atrophic with a pH of 6.5 to 7.5. The prepubertal child is thus susceptible to both nonspecific and specific vaginal infections and a variety of vulvar skin abnormalities (dermatoses) (Table 3-1) (1–7). Contributing factors are poor hygiene, the proximity of the vagina to the anus, the lack of protective hair and labial fat pads, and the lack of estrogenization. The vulvar skin is susceptible to irritation and is easily traumatized by chemicals, soaps, medications, and clothing. Vulvar itching is a common complaint and frequently does not have a specific etiology (8). Nonabsorbent nylon underpants, nylon tights, nylon bathing suits, close-fitting blue jeans, and ballet leotards may result in maceration and infection, particularly in hot weather. Little girls who are overweight are particularly likely to experience these symptoms. The vulvar irritation of the child with vaginitis may appear similar to the diaper dermatitis seen in infants. Bubble baths and harsh soaps may cause vulvitis and a secondary vaginitis. Girls typically urinate on the toilet with their knees together, increasing the possibility that urine will reflux into the vagina. It has been suggested but not proven that either a high, small hymenal opening that does not allow normal

TABLE 3-1. *Etiology of vulvovaginal symptoms in the prepubertal child*

"Nonspecific" vulvovaginitis
Specific vulvovaginitis
  Respiratory pathogens
    Streptococcus pyogenes (Group A β-streptococcus)
    Staphylococcus aureus
    Haemophilus influenzae
    Streptococcus pneumoniae
    Branhamella catarrhalis
    Neisseria meningitidis
  Enteric
    Shigella
    Yersinia
    Other flora
  Candida
  Sexually transmitted diseases
    Neisseria gonorrhoeae
    Chlamydia trachomatis
    Herpes simplex
    Trichomonas
    Condyloma accuminata (human papillomavirus)
Pinworms, other helminths
Foreign body
Polyps, tumors
Systemic illness: measles, chickenpox, scarlet fever, Stevens-Johnson syndrome,
  mononucleosis, Kawasaki disease, histiocytosis, Crohn disease
Vulvar skin disease: lichen sclerosus, seborrhea, psoriasis, atopic dermatitis, scabies,
  contact dermatitis (nickel allergy), zinc deficiency, bullous pemphigoid
Trauma
Psychosomatic vaginal complaints
Miscellaneous: draining pelvic abscess, prolapsed urethra, ectopic ureter, disposable
  diapers

---

vaginal drainage or a gaping hymenal opening that allows easy contamination of the vagina might predispose a girl to nonspecific vaginitis.

Normal Vaginal Flora

Several studies have provided information on the normal flora of the prepubertal vagina (2, 9–12). Paradise and colleagues (2,12) cultured vaginal specimens from 52 premenarcheal girls without genitourinary signs or symptoms (Table 3-2); 11 of 40 had *Bacteroides* species (*B. bivius, B. fragilis, B. melaninogenicus*) (2). *Bacteroides* species were as commonly found in control subjects as in those with vulvovaginitis. Gardner (10) studied a group of 77 girls, 3 to 10 years of age, who were undergoing minor nongynecological procedures under general anesthesia. She defined normal flora as lactobacilli, *Staphylococcus epidermidis,* enteric organisms (*Streptococcus faecalis, Klebsiella* species, *Proteus* species, *Pseudomonas* species), and viridans species of streptococci other than *Streptococcus milleri.* Additional isolates from the control group included *Escherichia coli* (two girls), *Streptococcus*

TABLE 3-2. *Aerobic bacteria and yeasts recovered from vaginal cultures of 52 girls without genitourinary symptoms or signs*

Microorganisms isolated	n (%)
Normal flora[a]	52 (100)
β-Hemolytic streptococci (not group A or B)	2 (4)
Escherichia coli	4 (8)
Group B streptococcus	1 (2)
Coagulase-positive staphylococcus	1 (2)
Candida tropicalis or "yeast"[b]	2 (4)

(Source: J. Paradise. Unpublished data; with permission.)
[a]Includes diphtheroids, α-hemolytic streptococci, and lactobacilli.
[b]If fewer than one-third of the colonies in a culture are yeasts, the laboratory did not identify their species.

pneumoniae (five), *Staphylococcus aureus* (four), *S. milleri* (one), and *Gardnerella vaginalis* (three). No isolates of *Haemophilus influenzae, Streptococcus pyogenes,* or mycoplasmas were identified. However, since 43% of girls among the 108 controls in all age groups were undergoing ear, nose, and throat procedures and 14% had received antibiotics during the previous month, it is unclear whether the underlying diagnosis or antibiotic therapy given to some girls more than a month previously (percent not specified) may have influenced the flora of the vagina. Another study of vaginal flora in prepubertal girls (mean age 9 years, range 3 months to 16 years) found that the most common aerobic organisms were *S. epidermidis,* enterococci, *E. coli,* lactobacilli, and *Streptococcus viridans* (11). The anaerobes included *Peptococcus* species, *Peptostreptococcus* species, *Veillonella parvula, Eubacterium* species, *Propionibacterium* species, and *Bacteroides* species. Other organisms found in asymptomatic girls included *Proteus mirabilis* (3.2%), *Pseudomonas* species (6.5%), and *Candida albicans* (3.2%).

Etiology of Vulvovaginitis

The spectrum of diagnoses causing vulvovaginal symptoms is quite broad (see Table 3-1). "Nonspecific" vulvovaginitis accounts for 25% to 75% of the cases of vulvovaginitis seen in referral centers (2–7). The pathogenesis and associated alteration in vaginal flora have not been well defined, but the absolute number of colonies of fecal aerobes or an overpopulation with anaerobes may contribute to the symptoms of odor and discharge. Gerstner (11) found *Candida, Peptococcus, Peptostreptococcus,* and *Bacteroides* species more commonly in girls with vaginal discharge and/or vulvovaginitis than in asymptomatic girls. The vaginal culture from girls with vaginitis typically grows normal flora (lactobacilli, diphtheroids, *S. epidermidis,* or α-streptococci) or gram-negative enteric organisms (usually *E. coli*). The significance of *E. coli* and other enteric organisms is unclear. Gerstner and colleagues (11) also found that 23% of asymptomatic girls had *E. coli* in the vagina, compared with 36% of girls with vaginitis. Hammerschlag and co-workers (9) reported that 90% of girls under 3 years of age had vaginal colonization with *E. coli* compared to 15% of 3- to 10-year-old asymptomatic girls. In a study in our program, 47% of 3- to 10-year-old girls with nonspecific vaginitis had *E. coli* on culture (3). Thus, poor hygiene and contamination with bowel flora may play a role in the persistence of symptoms. In addition, pinworms appear to be a major contributor to nonspecific infections in some populations. In a British study, 32% of girls with vulvovaginitis had pinworms detected (6). Children susceptible to recurrent vulvovaginitis may have other factors that promote adherence of bacteria to epithelial cells.

The specific infections that occur in the prepubertal child are typically respiratory, enteric, or sexually transmitted pathogens. The most common respiratory pathogen is *Streptococcus pyogenes* (group A β-hemolytic streptococci), which is isolated from 7% to 20% of girls with vulvovaginitis (6,7,13–18). Vaginal *S. pyogenes* infections may be associated with nasopharyngeal, perianal, or skin infections. Although throat cultures from 28% to 92% of girls with *S. pyogenes* vaginitis are positive, only 25% to 30% have symptoms of pharyngitis (16,18). Specific strains have been identified in some series (18). Scarlet fever and guttate psoriasis can also be associated with streptococcal vaginitis. In New Hampshire, perineal *S. pyogenes* infections peaked in the late winter and early spring (18). Symptoms may include pruritus, dysuria, pain, and vaginal or rectal bleeding. The vulva and perianal areas often have a distinctive bright red ("beefy red") inflamed appearance.

More rarely, vaginal infection may result from *H. influenzae, S. aureus, Branhamella catarrhalis, S. pneumoniae,* and *Neisseria meningitidis* (2,3,6,19). In most series, *H. influenzae* appears to cause infection and not to be part of normal flora (6,20). In the Pierce and Hart study (6), *H. influenzae* was the most commonly isolated organism in girls with vulvovaginitis. *S. aureus* also appears to cause vaginal infections, and associated impetiginous lesions on the vulva and the buttocks are often observed. *Shigella* infection can result in a mucopurulent, sometimes bloody vaginal discharge. In only one-fourth of cases, the discharge occurs in association with an episode of diarrhea (21). Between 70% and 90% of *Shigella* vaginitis is caused by *S. flexneri* (22,23). *Yersinia enterocolitica* has also been reported to be associated with vaginitis (24); whether other enteric pathogens play a role is not known. Although *Candida* vulvovaginitis is common in pubertal, estrogenized girls, it is uncommon in prepubertal children unless the girl has recently finished a course of antibiotics, has diabetes mellitus, is immunosuppressed, is still in diapers, or has other risk factors. *Candida* appears to be present in the normal flora of 3% to 4% of girls.

Sexually acquired vulvovaginal infections occurring in the prepubertal child include *Neisseria gonorrhoeae, Chlamydia trachomatis, Trichomonas,* herpes simplex, and human papillomavirus (condyloma acuminatum) (these infections are also discussed in Chapters 14, 15, and 24) (25–36). Gonococcal infection in the prepubertal child usually causes a green purulent vaginal discharge; occasionally the discharge is mucoid. Confirmatory tests are crucial in prepubertal girls whose vaginal culture appears to be positive for *N. gonorrhoeae.* Gonococcal vaginal infections in prepubertal girls are typically identified by culturing samples from girls presenting with vaginal discharge, *not* by culturing asymptomatic victims of sexual abuse (31) (see Chapter 24). The prevalence of *N. gonorrhoeae* in girls with vaginitis varies from 0% to 26%. Siblings of individuals with known gonococcal infections are also at risk of infection and should be cultured (34). The perpetrator is often a family member who is identified only by culturing samples taken from the entire family. All children with *N. gonorrhoeae* vaginitis should be reported to child protection agencies (25–27,35).

Chlamydia trachomatis may be acquired from sexual contact or from perinatal maternal infant transmission (28,29,37–40). Schachter and associates (37) found that 14% of infants born to *Chlamydia*-positive mothers had vaginal/rectal colonization; none of these infants still had positive cultures at 12 months of age. Bell and colleagues (38) reported that among 120 infants born vaginally to infected women, 22% had positive cultures from the conjunctiva and 25% from the pharynx in the first month of life. Positive rectal and vaginal cultures were obtained during the third and fourth months of life. In a study of 22 infants in Seattle, positive rectal and vaginal cultures were not seen beyond 383 and 372 days, respectively, but positive cultures from the nasopharynx, oropharynx, and conjunctiva persisted up to 866 days (40). Ocular infection may persist for 3 to 6 years (33). However, because the majority of girls will have been treated for other infections by the age of 2 or 3 years with antibiotics to which *Chlamydia* is sensitive (e.g., erythromycin, azithromycin), persistence becomes an unlikely explanation in most girls. Girls over age 2 to 3 are thus likely to have acquired a *Chlamydia* infection from sexual contact. In a study of sexually abused and control girls, Ingram and associates (28) reported that 10 of 124 sexually abused girls and 0 of 90 control girls had a positive introital culture for *C. trachomatis.* In a subsequent study of 1,538 children evaluated for possible sexual abuse, Ingram found *Chlamydia* infections in 1.2% (35). As in adolescents, *C. trachomatis* can occur as a coexisting infection in girls with *N. gonorrhoeae* (41).

How frequently *C. trachomatis* is responsible for signs of vaginitis is a subject of controversy. In a study of 622 girls under 12 years of age who were evaluated for sexual abuse or who had a sexually transmitted disease, six girls had *Chlamydia* without gonorrhea and only one had a discharge on examination (although four gave a history of discharge) (31). Ingram et al. (35) found that only 6 of 17 girls with positive *Chlamydia* cultures had a vaginal discharge at presentation or a history of vaginal discharge in the previous 6 months. Culture tests should be used in the diagnosis of prepubertal infections, since false-positive results can occur with some nonculture tests (42–45). If culture is not available, some research has indicated that nucleic acid amplification tests (NAATS) can be used if another NAAT that targets a different sequence can be performed if the first NAAT test is positive (42,43).

Herpes simplex type 1 (oral-labial herpes) can cause lesions in the mouth and vulva of young girls, with the vulvar infection occurring through self-inoculation. Both types 1 and 2 can be acquired by sexual abuse, although type 2 is more likely to be acquired

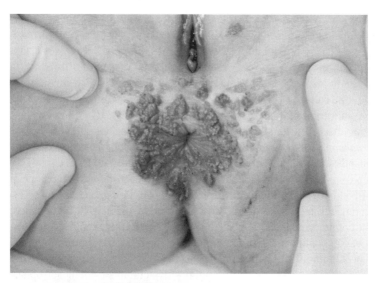

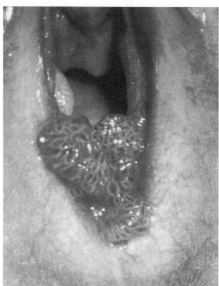

FIG. 3-1. Human papillomavirus infections in prepubertal girls: **(A)** perianal condylomata and **(B)** hymenal condyloma.

by sexual contact. In a study of six cases of genital herpes (five type 1 and one type 2), Kaplan and colleagues (46) reported that infection resulted from sexual abuse in four of six patients. Recurrent lesions may occur with either type of herpes but are more likely with type 2. Varicella-zoster infections in the genital area have been confused with herpes simplex (47). Condylomata acuminata (venereal warts) are caused by human papillomavirus, usually HPV subtypes 6 or type 11, and can occur in the genital and perianal area (Fig. 3-1) (see also Chapters 17 and 24 and Color Plate 14).

Trichomonas vaginalis can be transmitted from the mother to the child at birth and rarely can cause urethritis and vaginitis, which usually resolves spontaneously with the waning of estrogen levels. Occasionally, persistent symptoms require treatment (36). This pathogen is rarely seen in the prepubertal child because the unestrogenized vagina is relatively resistant to infection. It occurs primarily in the sexually active teenager (see Chapter 14). Although *Trichomonas* can theoretically be spread by wet towels and washcloths, it is primarily a sexually transmitted infection.

The role of *G. vaginalis* in causing vaginitis in the child has been controversial (10,48,49). Bartley and co-workers (48) found that the isolation of *G. vaginalis* from the vaginas of prepubertal girls appeared to be more likely in sexually abused girls (14.6%) than in control subjects (4.2%) or in patients with genitourinary complaints (4.2%). However, they did not find any association of this organism with vaginal erythema or discharge. In contrast, Ingram and associates (49) found *G. vaginalis* in the vaginal cultures of 5.3% of 191 sexually abused girls, 4.9% of 144 girls evaluated for possible sexual abuse, and 6.4% of control girls (daughters of friends of the authors). The isolated finding of *G. vaginalis* on vaginal culture should not be confused with a diagnosis of bacterial vaginosis. Bacterial vaginosis is characterized by an alteration of the bacterial flora with the presence of increased concentrations of *G. vaginalis* and anaerobes and in adolescents is characterized by a high vaginal pH and clue cells (see Chapter 14). Bacterial vaginosis has been rarely reported in girls who presented with vaginal odor after an episode of rape; the diagnosis was made by the observation of clue cells on microscopic examination of the discharge and the presence of a characteristic amine (fishy) odor on the "whiff" test (see p. 38).

Other causes of vulvovaginal complaints include vaginal foreign bodies; vaginal and cervical polyps and tumors; cavernous lymphangioma; urethral prolapse; systemic illnesses such as measles, chickenpox (47), scarlet fever, mononucleosis, Crohn disease, Kawasaki disease (50), or histiocytosis; anomalies such as double vagina with a fistula, pelvic abscess or fistula, or ectopic ureter; and vulvar skin diseases such as seborrhea, psoriasis (Fig. 3-2), atopic dermatitis (Fig. 3-3), lichen sclerosus, scabies, contact dermatitis, impetigo, or autoimmune bullous diseases (9) (see Table 3-1, Color Plates, and Chapter 14). Zinc deficiency from insufficient intake (51), urinary loss, or malabsorption (acrodermatitis enteropathica) can result in vulvar dermatitis. Seborrheic dermatitis is associated with seborrhea in other parts of the body; fissures within the folds of the labia can lead to bleeding. Both psoriasis and seborrheic dermatitis can become secondarily infected. Psoriasis in the groin may also be mistaken for diaper dermatitis. Atopic dermatitis usually occurs in other parts of the body as well as the vulva; vulvar lesions are pruritic, dry, papular, scaly patches. Bullous pemphigoid occasionally occurs in young children with recurrent ulcers and erosions; two girls with symmetric ulcers responded to fluocinonide 0.05% cream (52). Chronic bullous disease of childhood is rare and is associated with pruritic and burning vesicles and bullae in the genitals, face, trunk, and extremities. Vesicular lesions

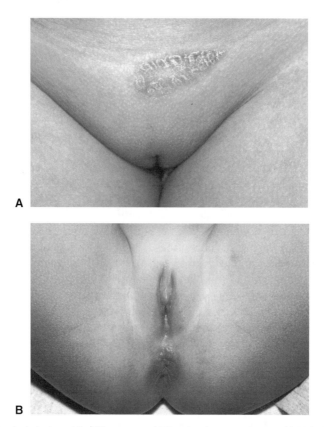

FIG. 3-2. Psoriasis in two girls, **(A)** mons and **(B)** vulva (note erythema of labia). (Photo courtesy of Jonathan Trager, M.D.)

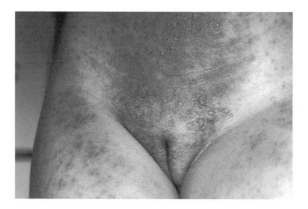

FIG. 3-3. Atopic dermatitis in a 10 year old. (Photo courtesy of Jonathan Trager, M.D.)

in the perineum secondary to nickel allergy from an enuresis alarm has also been reported (53). Histiocytosis can present with firm, yellow, and often purpuric papules in the vulvar area and also has been associated with a persistent 2-cm × 2-cm labial ulcer (54). Epstein-Barr virus infection has been associated with labial ulcers in children (55); we have identified a number of early pubescent girls and adolescents with vulvar ulcers who were found on further evaluation to have mononucleosis (see Color Plate 26). Crohn disease may present with painful asymmetric swelling of the labia, perineal induration (56), and ulcers. Gelatin-like beads from superabsorbent disposable diapers can simulate vaginal discharge (57).

An ectopic ureter may cause daytime wetness, sometimes in quite minimal amounts (see Chapter 13); occasionally ectopic ureters can present in late child-hood or adolescence with purulent discharge and without enuresis (58). If the kidney is infected, purulent perineal discharge will result, and the initial diagnosis may be vaginal discharge. The ectopic ureter usually empties on the perineum adjacent to the normal urethra, but it may also open into the vagina, cervix, uterus, or urethra. The clinician should look for a small drop of urine (or pus) adjacent to the urethra after the child drinks a large amount of a beverage, especially one containing caffeine. Ultrasonography of the kidneys will suggest the anomaly in most cases with obstruction and a purulent discharge. An intravenous pyelogram (IVP) is particularly helpful as an initial test if day-time "dampness" or dribbling (not purulent discharge) is the presenting complaint. Even if the double collecting system cannot be visualized because of poor function in the upper pole, the contour of the kidney is likely to provide the key to diagnosis. It should be noted that there have been at least five cases of clear cell cancer of the vagina in adolescents who have had an ectopic ureter into the vagina from a dysplastic kidney (59,60). We at Children's Hospital Boston thus promote every-other-year exam under anesthesia and Pap tests for children and biyearly vaginal exams and yearly vaginal Pap tests in adolescents with this condition.

Edema of the clitoral hood and labia may occur because of hypoproteinemia, chronic sitting without the ability to move position, inflammation/infection, and obstruction of lymphatic or venous return. Adherence of the clitoral hood, probably secondary to poor hygiene, can cause clitoral pain and itching. Occasionally, children have vaginal or vulvar complaints of itching, tingling, or tickling, sometimes associated with posturing, scissoring, and masturbation. The behavioral changes can precipitate great concern in parents. Psychosomatic complaints may also occur in the absence of any definable signs of vulvovaginal change. In a study of 44 premenarcheal girls presenting with vulvar itching, Paek and colleagues reported that 33 (75%) had no specific cause (negative cultures and no skin disease); five (11%) lichen sclerosus, four (9%) bacterial infection, one (2%) yeast, and one (2%) pinworms (8). At a 2- to 3-year follow-up, symptoms had cleared in 15, were improved in 13, and were unchanged in four.

True vulvovaginitis should not be confused with physiologic pubertal discharge. Newborns and pubescent girls often have copious secretions from the effect of estrogen on the vaginal mucosa. In newborns, maternal estrogen is primarily responsible for the discharge, which typically disappears within a few weeks after birth.

Obtaining the History

In most cases of vulvovaginitis, the parent brings the child to the clinician with a complaint of discharge, dysuria, pruritus, or redness. A complete history is obtained before the examination; a questionnaire may speed the process so that the child does not become fidgety or nervous before the examination. The clinician should elicit information on the quantity, duration, odor, and type of discharge (clear, yellow, green, bloody, etc); perineal hygiene; recent use of medications or bubble baths or harsh soaps; symptoms of anal pruritus (associated with pinworm infection); enuresis; history of atopic dermatitis or allergies; and recent infections in the patient or family. A history of recent infections is important because, for example, group A β-hemolytic streptococcal (*S. pyogenes*) vaginitis, perianal cellulitis, or, rarely, proctocolitis may follow a streptococcal upper respiratory or skin infection in the child or other family members. Girls with recurrent viral URIs also seem to be susceptible to recurrent vaginitis. Overvigorous cleansing of the vulva in a girl with mild vaginal symptoms or odor can lead to significant vulvitis. Questions about caretakers that may give a clue to sexual abuse should be asked. The parent should be asked about behavioral changes, nightmares, fears, abdominal pain, headaches, and enuresis, all of which may suggest the possibility of abuse or other stressors. The vaginal discharge may be copious and purulent, or it may be thin and mucoid.

The child should be included in the history taking by being asked about her symptoms, frequency and amount of discharge, bathing, use of soaps, type of clothing (for example, tights, leotards, blue jeans), and perineal hygiene. She can be asked to demonstrate her motion of wiping and whether she has ever placed anything within her vagina. A child's scratching because of vulvar pruritus may cause conflict between parent and child. Compulsive masturbation may also cause vulvar irritation and erythema and guilty feelings for the child and parents. A cycle of itching and scratching may have started with a vaginal infection and then persisted with resultant chronic vulvitis. The child should be asked about the possibility that someone has touched her in the vaginal area.

The history may give a clue to the diagnosis. For example, a foul-smelling discharge may result from a foreign body (usually toilet paper), a necrotic tumor (rare), or vaginitis. Both *Shigella* and group A β-streptococcal infections can cause bleeding. An odorless, bloody discharge may result from vulvar irritation (from scratching), trauma (from playground equipment, bicycle, or sexual abuse), granulation tissue from prior trauma, precocious puberty, a foreign body, vaginitis, condylomata acuminata, or, rarely, a tumor (adenocarcinoma, sarcoma botryoides) (22,61). A greenish discharge is usually associated with a specific cause of the vaginitis, such as group A β-streptococci, *N. gonorrhoeae, H. influenzae, S. aureus, Shigella,* or a foreign body. Itching and redness are usually nonspecific signs of irritation. However, a history of pruritus and "blood blisters" suggests lichen sclerosus (p.100). In our experience (3), a short duration of symptoms (<1 month) is associated more often with specific diagnoses, perhaps because the parent notices an abrupt change in the vulvovaginal area. Girls with nonspecific vaginitis often have symptoms that have lasted for months or, in some cases, for years before clinical presentation. The discharge on the underwear may appear white or yellow. Nonetheless, even a long history of symptoms calls for a careful assessment and examination.

Physical Examination

For children with symptoms of vulvitis, a brief history and external genital examination in the office and instructions to the parent on improved hygiene, avoidance of irritants, and/or treatment of pinworms are all that are needed. A similar approach is appropriate for many little girls with vulvitis and minimal vaginal discharge. The only findings on external examination are usually a scanty mucoid discharge and an erythematous introitus. Small vulvar papillomatosis should not be mistaken for condylomata acuminata. The cause is usually poor perineal hygiene, which results in infection with mixed bacterial flora. Cultures are unnecessary if the condition responds promptly to improved hygiene.

Any child with persistent, purulent, or recurrent vaginal discharge deserves a thorough gynecologic assessment. The physical examination of the prepubertal child is described in Chapter 1. It is important to ask the child to point to the area of discomfort since it may be clitoral rather than vaginal pain. To diagnose the vaginal complaints, the physician should undertake a stepwise approach: (a) do a general physical examination; (b) inspect the perineum, vulva, and vaginal introitus with the patient supine; (c) visualize the vagina and cervix with the patient in the knee–chest position; (d) obtain specimens for wet preparations and cultures; and (e) if indicated, do a rectoabdominal examination with the patient supine, knees apart, and feet together or in stirrups. Providing a mirror for the child, asking her to assist in the examination, or encouraging the parent to engage in conversation with the child can help her relax. A visible discharge at the time of the examination increases the likelihood that the vaginal culture will be positive for a specific pathogen (2). If the knee–chest position does not allow adequate visualization *and* the symptoms are significant or persistent, an examination with sedation or under anesthesia is usually the next step for complete assessment (see Chapter 1). Some clinicians have experience with using a hysteroscope, cystoscope, or flexible endoscope in the cooperative child in the office. Anesthetic ointment is usually applied to the vulva prior to insertion, after cultures have been obtained. It should be remembered that although visualization of the vagina and cervix is optimal and usually easily performed, this part of the examination can be deferred if mild symptoms of vulvovaginitis improve in 2 to 3 weeks of good perineal hygiene. The rectal examination is usually reserved for girls who have persistent discharge, bleeding, or pelvic/abdominal pain. During a rectal examination, the clinician may be able to express discharge from the vagina not previously seen, palpate hard foreign bodies, or detect an abnormal mass.

Laboratory Tests

If the vaginal discharge is persistent or purulent at the initial office visit, cultures and, if possible, wet preparations should be done. A nasopharyngeal Calgiswab moistened with nonbacteriostatic saline, a soft plastic eyedropper, a glass eyedropper with plastic tubing attached, a small feeding tube, or a small urethral catheter attached to a syringe can be gently inserted through the hymenal opening to aspirate secretions or a vaginal wash sample (see Chapter 1). If a small saline-moistened Calgiswab is used, care should be taken to place it into the vagina without touching the edges of the hymen. The three samples (one with a Dacron male urethral swab if a sample for vaginal *Chlamydia* culture is desired) can be quickly obtained and directly plated or sent for culture. Alternatively, a small amount of saline can be squirted into the vagina with an Angiocath (no needle) and three swabs held right outside the vagina and the child asked to cough hard to expel the solution.

A culture for *N. gonorrhoeae* is typically done on modified Thayer–Martin–Jembec medium at the time of the examination. Cultures for other organisms are done by sending the small Calgiswab, a moistened cotton-tipped applicator (used only if easily inserted without discomfort), or a small amount of aspirated secretions to the bacteriology laboratory for plating on genitourinary media (blood, MacConkey, and chocolate media). The swab can be kept moist in a Culturette II transport tube during transport to the laboratory. Samples for *Chlamydia* culture are generally obtained from girls with persistent symptoms and those with a history of sexual abuse. For suspected *Candida* infection, a sample of the discharge is plated directly onto Biggy agar slant; this culture is incubated in the office and observed for the growth of brown colonies 3 to 7 days later. Patients with vulvar or anal pruritus can be screened for pinworm infestation. Material is obtained in the morning by pressing the sticky side of a piece of cellophane tape against the perineal area. The tape is affixed to a slide and examined under the

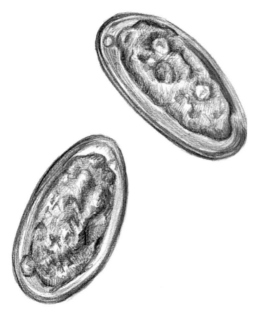

FIG. 3-4. Pinworm eggs *(Enterobius vermicularis).*

microscope for the characteristic eggs (Fig. 3-4). The parent should also check the child's anus late at night (with a flashlight) for adult pinworms. Radiography of the pelvis in a search for foreign bodies should be avoided, since most foreign bodies are not radiopaque, and usually cannot be identified even on ultrasound evaluation.

Treatment

As noted in the section on etiology, no specific cause is found in a substantial portion of prepubertal girls with vulvovaginal symptoms, so-called nonspecific vulvovaginitis. The culture may grow gram-negative enteric organisms such as *E. coli* or normal flora. Treatment of nonspecific vulvovaginitis should focus on improved hygiene (white cotton underpants or cotton crotch, front-to-back wiping, loose-fitting skirts, no nylon tights or tight blue jeans, avoidance of prolonged sitting in nylon bathing suits), hand washing, and sitz baths. The child should be asked to urinate with her knees spread apart so the labia are separated and urinary reflux into the vagina is minimized. The vulvar skin of the prepubertal child is extremely sensitive to drying, chapping, and irritants, including heat, medications, and soaps. The clinician should keep in mind, however, the many causes of vulvar disease noted above.

The child should be instructed to sit in a tub of clear, warm (not hot) water for 10 to 15 minutes once or twice daily. At the end of that time, she should be washed with a bland soap (such as Basis, unscented Dove, Lowila, Oilatum, Aveeno, or Neutrogena), with little or preferably no soap being applied to the vulva. The vulva should not be scrubbed. Hair should be shampooed over a sink or in the shower, rather than in the bathtub while the child is bathing. If neither is possible, the shampooing should occur at the end of the bath and the child rinsed in clear water. A handheld sprayer is helpful. If the child is not afraid of showers, the optimal course is for her to soak for 10 to 15 minutes in several inches of clean water in the tub and then stand up to wash her body in the shower. Some clinicians prefer cleaning the perineum gently with cotton pledgets and Cetaphil cleanser. Bubble bath crystals and solutions should not be used, since the irritant soap may exacerbate the symptoms. After a bath, the child should pat her vulva dry or air dry it with her legs spread apart; a hair dryer on cool setting for 10 to 15 seconds can aid drying. Sleeper pajamas should not be used if possible, since the associated heat and poor air circulation frequently cause maceration of the vulva. Underwear should be washed in a mild detergent (no color, no added scents) and double-rinsed in clear water, and no rinse or dryer additives should be used.

A small amount of A and D ointment, Vaseline, Desitin, or Theraplex emollient can be used to protect the vulvar skin. Loose-fitting clothes such as skirts and knee socks or loose pants or shorts should be worn during the daytime. During the summer, the girl should not spend long periods of time in a wet swimsuit; a change to a pair of shorts or a dry suit should be suggested. Some girls have persistent vaginal discharge despite enhanced hygienic and other measures. Generally, if a discharge persists more than 2 or 3 weeks after such measures have been undertaken, the possibility of pinworms should be excluded or, in the girl with perianal or vulvar itching, empirically treated with mebendazole. A trial of oral antibiotics, such as amoxicillin, amoxicillin/clavulanate, or a cephalosporin, may be given for 10 days. Other clinicians have used topical mupirocin or gentamicin ointment or oral or topical metronidazole or clindamycin. Neomycin containing preparations should be avoided because of the risk of sensitization.

Some children have persistent or frequently recurring symptoms even though a specific cause has been excluded. A variety of measures have been advocated, but none have been studied in clinical trials. We often prescribe a 1-month course of a small dose of an antibiotic at bedtime or even 3 nights a week, similar to the regimen used for suppression of urinary tract infections. Occasionally, estrogen-containing creams (e.g., Premarin cream) can be used to thicken the epithelium, making it more resistant to infection; the cream is applied to the vulva but should be used only briefly (2 to 3 weeks at a time). This cream can also be applied for a brief course to the periclitoral area if erythema and adhesions from a previous inflammation appear to cause sensations of pulling and tingling. The parent should not be given a refillable prescription, since systemic absorption of estrogen does occur. Hygiene needs to be emphasized to all these girls, since the prescription of medication sometimes suggests to parents and child that the other measures can be discontinued. Intravaginal medications are rarely indicated and may be difficult for the parent and child to administer. In some unusually persistent cases, irrigation of the vagina with a 1% povidone–iodine solution, using a syringe and a small infant feeding tube or urethral catheter, may be helpful.

Nonspecific vaginitis often recurs when the child develops an upper respiratory infection or has poor hygiene. Obese girls with inadequate hygiene are particularly prone to recurrences. Other causes of recurrent discharge, though rare, need to be considered, including pelvic abscess and ectopic ureter. Thus, the child with recurrent vaginitis often needs a careful reexamination and a search for a foreign body or an ectopic ureter. Other tests, such as pelvic ultrasonography, IVP, vaginoscopy, or cystoscopy, may be necessary to establish the more unusual diagnosis. Recurrence of vaginitis may become a source of considerable anxiety for the parent, who may express fear that the child's future reproductive capacity will be harmed. In particular, the mother may have concerns about whether her own gynecologic problems of recurrent vaginitis, pelvic infection, or abnormal bleeding are hereditary or are related to the child's symptoms. The clinician can offer important reassurance by performing an adequate physical examination, obtaining vaginal cultures, and outlining a treatment plan.

Some girls without vaginal discharge have recurrent episodes of vulvar irritation, dysuria, and pain (transient vulvitis). Symptoms usually last for 12 to 24 hours and respond to tepid sitz baths and one or two applications of hydrocortisone cream 1% to 2.5% or lidocaine gel, and/or an oral antihistamine at bedtime. These episodes of vaginal pain often occur in the middle of the night and may be triggered by irritants or a long period of time in tights, leotards, or sleeper pajamas.

Specific causes of vulvovaginitis are listed in Table 3-1, and treatment is outlined in Table 3-3. The treatment of group A β-streptococci (*S. pyogenes*) is oral penicillin. Perianal streptococcal infection may occur with a vaginal infection or alone and may require a longer treatment course of 14 to 21 days if symptoms recur. Impetiginous lesions of the buttocks or vulva can be treated topically with mupirocin ointment or systemic oral antibiotics. Recurrences of folliculitis may be prevented by using chlorhexidine (Hibiclens) to wash in the shower, and eradication of nasal carriage of *Staphylococcus* with mupirocin. *H. influenzae* and *S. aureus* can be treated effectively with any of several antibiotics, although symptoms do not always clear up even when the organism has been eradicated. With increasing methicillin resistant *S. aureus* (MRSA) in the community, antibiotic choices may be limited. *S. pneumoniae* is increasingly resistant to penicillin, and alternative therapy may be necessary if the symptoms do not resolve and the organism is resistant. Prolonged symptoms have been reported with *Shigella* vulvovaginitis despite multiple antibiotics; a 14-day course of ciprofloxacin was successful in one case report (62). The finding of *N. gonorrhoeae* should prompt careful evaluation for sexual abuse and mandated reporting. The girl should be examined for *C. trachomatis* as a coinfection and given appropriate treatment to cover both in-

TABLE 3-3. *Treatment of specific vulvovaginal infections in the prepubertal child*

Etiology	Treatment
Streptococcus pyogenes	Penicillin V potassium 250 mg b.i.d—t.i.d. PO × 10 d
Haemophilus influenzae	Amoxicillin 40 mg/kg/d × 7 d Alternate: amoxicillin/clavulanate, cefuroxime axetil, trimethoprim-sulfamethoxazole, erythromycin-sulfamethaxazole
Staphylococcus aureus	Cephalexin 25-50 mg/kg/d PO × 7–10 d Dicloxacillin 25 mg/kg/d PO × 7–10 d Amoxicillin-clavulanate 20–40 mg/kg/d (of the amoxicillin) PO × 7–10 d Cefuroxime axetil suspension 30 mg/kg/d divided b.i.d. (max 1 g) × 10 d (tablets: 250 mg b.i.d.)
Streptococcus pneumoniae	Penicillin, amoxicillin, erythromycin, trimethoprim-sulfamethoxazole, clarithromycin
Shigella	Trimethoprim/sulfamethoxazole or ampicillin × 5 d For resistant organisms: ceftriaxone
Chlamydia trachomatis	≤45 kg Erythromycin 50 mg/kg/d (4×/d) × 14 d ≥45 kg, <8 yr: Azithromycin 1 g PO ≥8 yr Azithromycin 1 g PO OR doxycycline 100 mg b.i.d. PO × 7 d
Neisseria gonorrhoeae	<45 kg Ceftriaxone 125 mg I.M. (alternate: Spectinomycin 40 mg/kg (max 2 g) I.M. once PLUS If *Chlamydia* infection not ruled out Rx for *chlamydia* as above. ≥45 kg: treated with adult regimens
Candida	Topical nystatin, miconazole, clotrimazole, or terconazole cream; fluconazole orally
Trichomonas	Metronidazole 15 mg/kg/d given t.i.d. (max 250 mg t.i.d.) × 7 d
Pinworms (*Enterobius vermicularis*)	Mebendazole (Vermox), 1 chewable 100-mg tablet, repeated in 2 wk

fections (see Chapter 15). Since sexual abuse often involves genital fondling, oral sex, or vulvar coitus rather than vaginal penetration in young girls, normal findings on examination of the girl with *N. gonorrhoeae* or *C. trachomatis* should not be taken as evidence against sexual abuse (see Chapter 24). A history of prior antibiotic therapy that would have been expected to eradicate *Chlamydia* transmitted at birth can help establish the likely timing of acquisition.

In contrast to the frequent occurrence of *Candida* vaginitis in the estrogenized pubertal girl, the presence of this infection in the toilet-trained prepubertal girl who has not recently taken systemic antibiotics should prompt laboratory tests to exclude diabetes mellitus. Topical antifungal creams for the external genitalia are often successful, and if not, oral fluconazole is an effective, easy to administer alternative. For tinea cruris and other dermatophyte infections, topical preparations of terbinafine or naftifine are indicated.

Pinworms (*Enterobius vermicularis*) always need to be kept in mind as a specific cause of recurrent nonspecific vaginitis and are easily treated with oral medication. Mebendazole is not recommended for children under the age of 2 years. Family members may also need to be treated. Occasionally, other helminthic infections require treatment.

A purulent and/or bloody discharge is often the presenting complaint in a girl with a vaginal foreign body, most commonly toilet paper. The child should be questioned alone to determine whether another child or an adult placed the object in her vagina, since sexual abuse may be involved. If the child herself repeatedly places objects in her vagina, a psychosocial assessment is important. Toilet paper in the bathroom can be replaced with witch hazel pads (Tucks) to prevent accidental or purposeful shredding of toilet paper (see page 108 for removal).

Summary of Therapy for Nonspecific Vulvovaginitis

General Measures

1. Good perineal hygiene (including wiping from front to back after bowel movements).
2. Frequent changes of white cotton underpants to absorb discharge.
3. Avoidance of bubble baths, harsh soaps, and shampooing hair in the bathtub.
4. Loose-fitting skirts; no nylon tights or tight blue jeans. Sleep in loose clothing at night.
5. Sitz baths one to three times daily with plain warm water. The vulva should be gently washed (no soap) using soaking alone if possible. If soap is needed, only a mild, nonscented soap (Basis, unscented Dove, Lowila, Oilatum, Aveeno, or Neutrogena) should be applied. The bath should be followed by careful drying (patting, not rubbing). The child should then lie with her legs spread apart for approximately 10 minutes to complete the drying, or a hair dryer used on the cool or low setting for 10 to 15 seconds. Cetaphil Gentle Cleanser can also be used for improving hygiene and removing smegma.
6. Urination with legs spread apart and labia separated (consider having the child sit "backwards"—facing the toilet—which forces her to separate her legs).
7. Even after the discharge clears up, daily sitz baths and other hygiene measures should be continued.

Measures for Nonspecific Pruritus of the Vulva

1. Avoidance of soapy bath water and bubble baths; showers after sitz bath in clear water.
2. Switching to mild or no soap to vulva.

3. Application of a low- to mid-potency topical corticosteroid such as hydrocortisone 2.5% ointment or cream for a short course.
4. A nonsedating antihistamine (such as cetirizine) can be used in the morning and a sedating antihistamine in the evening. Hydroxyzine hydrochloride, 2 mg/kg per day divided into four doses, or diphenhydramine hydrochloride, 5 mg/kg per day divided into four doses are sedating antihistamines.

Therapy for Severe Allergic Contact Dermatitis of the Vulva

1. Elimination of the offending agent.
2. Sitz baths every 4 hours (with plain water or with a small amount of Aveeno colloidal oatmeal or baking soda added). Soap should not be used, and the vulva should be air dried. Powders should be avoided. Petroleum jelly in a lotion (e.g., Theraplex emollient) can be helpful.
3. Prednisone orally in a 14-day tapering course can be prescribed.
4. After the acute phase of 1 to 2 days has passed, if there is no oozing, the sitz baths can be alternated every 4 hours with painting on a bland solution such as calamine lotion.
5. Infection should be treated with an oral antibiotic; a topical antibiotic such as mupirocin ointment may be added for additional antibacterial activity and for a local soothing effect.

Therapy for Persistent Nonspecific Vulvovaginitis

1. Oral antibiotics, such as cephalosporin, amoxicillin, amoxicillin/clavulanate, or clindamycin for 10 to 14 days; a 1- to 2-month low dose of bedtime cephalexin, cefuroxime axetil, amoxicillin/clavulanate, or trimethoprim/sulfamethoxazole may be helpful in the child with many recurrences; or
2. Antibacterial cream or ointment applied locally (mupirocin, gentamicin, metronidazole, clindamycin); or
3. Estrogen-containing cream (e.g., Premarin cream), applied nightly to the vulva for 2 weeks and then every other night for 2 weeks; a repeat course may be necessary.
4. Hygiene must be emphasized. A petrolatum cream can help avoid recurrences of vulvitis.

LICHEN SCLEROSUS

Lichen sclerosus occurs in prepubertal children, and the diagnosis may be delayed (63–73). Patients usually complain of itching, irritation, soreness, bleeding, and dysuria. Less commonly, they may have bowel symptoms and a vaginal discharge. Some girls have painful defecation, constipation, encopresis, or anal stenosis (64). The vulva characteristically has white, atrophic, parchment-like skin and evidence of chronic ulceration, inflammation, and subepithelial hemorrhages. As the disease progresses, there is loss of normal vulvar architecture: loss of the demarcation of the labia, scarring of the clitoral hood, and thickening of the posterior fourchette. Bleeding without a history of trauma has often caused suspicions of sexual abuse. The friction involved with physical and sports activities can produce bleeding. Often, the involvement of the perianal area along with the labia may give the affected area an hourglass (or so-called figure-of-eight) configuration. Secondary infection may occur. The condition should be distinguished from vitiligo, which causes loss of pigmentation but not inflammation or atrophy. The occurrence of vulvar lichen sclerosus in monozygotic twin girls and in other family members suggests that genetic factors play a role (63). In addition, some girls have other autoimmune diseases such as vitiligo, thyroid disease, and alopecia areata as well as autoantibodies.

The diagnosis of lichen sclerosus is made clinically and rarely, if necessary, by examining a biopsy specimen (Fig. 3-5; see also Color Plates 2 to 4). Since the etiology is unknown, the best form of therapy is controversial. A graded approach based on the symptoms and clinical appearance seems best. For mild cases, treatment is aimed at elimination of local irritants and improved hygiene.

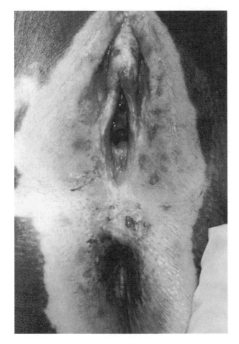

FIG. 3-5. Vulva of girl with lichen sclerosus.

Soaps should be used only minimally in the vulvar area; the child should be encouraged to wear cotton underpants and loose-fitting pants or skirts to minimize local maceration and irritation. A protective ointment such as A and D ointment or petroleum jelly in lotion (e.g., Theraplex emollient) is helpful, and a sedating antihistamine such as oral hydroxyzine hydrochloride is given 1 hour before bedtime to lessen the child's nocturnal scratching. Nails should be trimmed. The child is encouraged to become an active participant by applying the ointment and avoiding scratching. If this therapy is not adequate, a 1- to 3-month course of a topical steroid cream or ointment such as hydrocortisone 2.5% can be used with close followup. If the response is good, the hydrocortisone can be tapered to 1% for several additional months and then discontinued in favor of scrupulous hygiene and emollients. If flare-ups occur or symptoms continue, hydrocortisone cream can be reapplied. Oral antibiotics are prescribed for significant superinfections.

For moderate to severe lichen sclerosus, the use of the potent steroid clobetasol propionate (Temovate) 0.05% cream or ointment or halobetasol propionate (Ultravate) 0.05% ointment has dramatically changed the course and outcome of lichen sclerosus in girls (69,70,72). The high-potency ointment is typically prescribed to be applied sparingly twice a day for 2 weeks; after an assessment of the response, the topical medication is continued for another 2 to 4 weeks or tapered to once a day for 2 weeks, and then once every other day for 2 weeks. Other clinicians have used similar high-potency ointments twice daily for 6 to 10 weeks (treating until the disease is nonvisible and nonsymptomatic), and then tapered or discontinued the medication. A less potent steroid such as hydrocortisone 2.5% is then prescribed and tapered over several months. A burning sensation may be reported by patients using the clobetasol gel (especially with some generic preparations); this side effect seems to be less common with ointments, including halobetasol ointment. Recurrences do occur and can be retreated with short courses of topical steroids (72,73). Secondary infection can be treated with oral antibiotics or topical mupirocin combined with the topical steroid. Close supervision is mandatory to prevent adverse effects from the topical steroids. Recently, tacrolimus 0.1% ointment has been used successfully in a few prepubertal girls (68); more studies are needed.

Occasionally surgical intervention is needed later because of loss of vulvar architecture from the lichen sclerosus and adhesions around the clitoris burying it beneath the scar tissue. If pain occurs from a clitoral entrapment syndrome, a clitoroplasty can be performed to release the scar tissue and permit expansion of the clitoris with excitation. If a lysis of scar tissue is performed, Surgicel can be sewn between the lysed edges to help decrease the chance of re-adherence (74).

In some girls, lichen sclerosus improves with puberty; in many, the symptoms and signs persist (63–66). Among 15 girls (aged 18 months to 9 years) followed up for more than 43 months, seven improved, seven showed no change, and one was worse; there was a trend toward improvement with increasing age (67). Ridley (66) has questioned whether the absence of active lesions really represents disappearance of the condition. The long-term risks of vulvar malignancy in girls with lichen sclerosus have not been well studied (75). A few anecdotal cases have been reported in adolescents (66,67), and in one series of 350 females (mean age 56 years, range 1 to 90 years) with lichen sclerosus, 5% developed squamous cell carcinoma (76).

VAGINAL BLEEDING

Vaginal bleeding in the prepubertal child should always be carefully assessed. In the neonate, vaginal bleeding that can be significant, with clots, sometimes occurs in the first week of life secondary to withdrawal from maternal estrogen. After that, the causes to be considered include vaginitis, lichen sclerosus (Color Plates 2 to 4 and 22), condyloma (Fig. 3-6 and Color Plate 14); trauma (Color Plates 9 to 13, 15 to 18, 25), foreign body (Fig. 3-7), tumor (Color Plate 8), precocious puberty, hypothyroidism, hematological disorders, hemangioma (Fig. 3-8), polyp, and urethral prolapse (Fig. 3-9) (Table 3-4) (77–84). A good history and physical examination are important to the differential diagnosis. Questions should focus on onset and duration of the bleeding, history of trauma, pubertal development and growth, hematuria, rectal bleeding, vaginitis, and sexual abuse. Acceleration of height

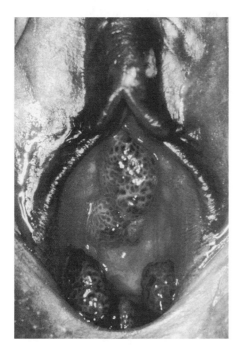

FIG. 3-6. Condyloma acuminatum, presenting as vaginal bleeding.

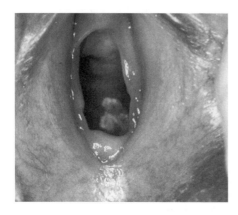

FIG. 3-7. Toilet paper within the vagina, visualized through an irregular hymenal orifice of a prepubertal girl.

and weight or signs of pubertal development before the age of 7 to 8 years suggest precocious puberty (see Chapter 5). A history of foreign bodies in the ears or vagina may implicate another foreign body, which may have been placed by the child or by an abuser. Patients with thrombocytopenia or bleeding disorders typically have other signs of bleeding, such as epistaxis, petechiae, or hematomas.

The physical examination should include a general assessment and a careful gynecologic examination. Trauma, vulvovaginitis, and hemangiomas are usually evident on inspection. Congestion of the vulva with a dark purplish discoloration has been noted in girls with prolonged sitting in wheelchairs with western saddle inserts. A straddle injury typically causes ecchymoses in the vulva and periclitoral folds. A laceration of the labia minora and periurethral tissue may be seen (Color Plates 17 and 18). It is extremely uncommon for a child to have a tear in the hymen without having suffered a penetrating injury (e.g., from a nail, a broom handle, a bedpost). Therefore, in the absence of an appropriate history, sexual abuse should be strongly considered when a hymenal tear is noted

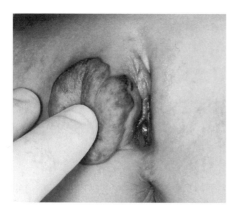

FIG. 3-8. Hemangioma of the vulva.

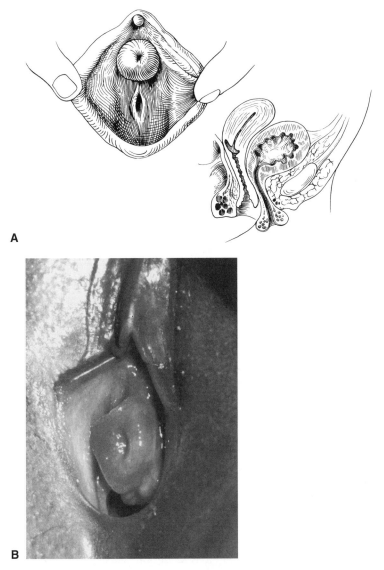

FIG. 3-9. Urethral prolapse. **A:** Schematic drawings (from Nussbaum AR, Lebowitz RL. Interlabial masses in little girls: review and imaging recommendations. AJR 1983; 141:65–71; with permission). **B:** Photograph (courtesy of Dr. Arnold Colodny, Children's Hospital Boston).

(77,78,80). Significant vaginal tears, however, can occur with water skiing, water slides, and other high pressure water injuries with sometimes minor injuries to the hymen (81,82), and this type of injury frequently necessitates an examination under anesthesia to assess to extent of the injury.

TABLE 3-4. Differential diagnosis of vaginal bleeding in the prepubertal girl

---

Trauma
  Accidental
  Sexual abuse
Vulvovaginitis
  Irritation, pinworms
  Nonspecific vulvovaginitis
  S. *pyogenes, Shigella*
Endocrine abnormalities
  Newborn bleeding due to maternal estrogen withdrawal
  Isosexual precocious puberty
  Pseudoprecocious puberty
  Precocious menarche
  Exogenous hormone preparations
  Hypothyroidism
Dermatoses
  Lichen sclerosus
Condyloma acuminatum (HPV)
Foreign body
Urethral prolapse
Bleeding disorders
Hemangioma
Tumor
  Benign
  Malignant

Evaluation and Treatment of Bleeding Resulting from Trauma

Evaluating the girl with active bleeding from the vulva following trauma can be challenging. Some suggestions for examining the child are to wipe 2% lidocaine jelly over the cut, place warm water in a syringe to irrigate the tissue gently, and/or irrigate using IV tubing and solution. The child can also assist by holding cool compresses with strong pressure. As noted in Fig. 3-10, the irrigation allows blood that may have collected in the vagina from a labial laceration to be washed out and the source of bleeding to be identified. If the bleeding is from an abrasion and it is oozing, it can often be treated with ice and compression. If the oozing continues, then Gelfoam or Surgicel can be applied.

If a laceration exists, and sutures are necessary for repair, most emergency wards have a protocol for anesthesia (conscious sedation). Lidocaine 1% to 2% can then be injected locally with a 25-gauge needle and the repair done with no. 4 chromic or Vicryl interrupted sutures. If cooperation is not possible and an intravaginal tear or a periurethral laceration is noted, an examination and repair may need to be performed while the child is under general anesthesia. Straddle injuries may cause deep lacerations in the periurethral tissue; repair may require the placement of a Foley catheter and meticulous suturing. Significant penetrating injuries may have occurred to the upper vagina without obvious symptoms or signs other than a hymenal tear at presentation. Most vulvar injuries heal after repair with little or no residual scarring or other sequelae.

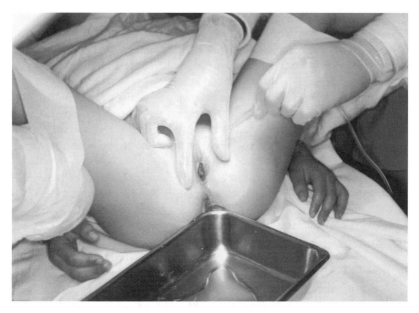

FIG. 3-10. Irrigation of the vulva and vagina with saline to identify the source of bleeding.

Injuries to the vulva can also result in large vulvar hematomas (Color Plate 25). Ice packs should be applied immediately, and if the injury is significant, a Foley catheter for urinary drainage should be inserted before genital anatomy is distorted by the swelling. Patients can be managed as "outpatients" with ice, narcotics, a leg bag for the Foley catheter, and bed rest. Surgical drainage should be avoided in order to prevent the introduction of infection. The swelling and discoloration may take several weeks to resolve. Healing is usually complete without residual defect or long-term adverse effects.

Bleeding Resulting from Nontrauma

Most bleeding in the prepubertal girl occurs not because of major trauma but because of vulvovaginitis, scratching due to pinworm infection, or a vaginal foreign body. Vaginitis caused by group A β-streptococci (*S. pyogenes*) or *Shigella* is especially likely to be accompanied by bleeding. If drops of blood have only recently been seen on the underwear, it is important to visualize the vagina (e.g., with the patient in the knee–chest position) and to obtain specimens for vaginal culture before anesthesia examination is recommended. If excoriations are noted around the anus and vulva, a cellophane tape test should be done to search for pinworms, or the patient should be treated empirically if pinworms are strongly suspected. Intravaginal foreign bodies are usually wads of toilet paper (see Fig. 3-7), but may be pins, paper clips, tampon cartons, beads, marker tips, crayons, or batteries. An irritative vulvitis with sharp demarcation of redness on the vulva may occur secondary to the chronic discharge associated with a foreign body. The upper vaginal mucosa may show a papillary response with small projections of 1 to 2 mm. A study by Paradise and Willis (61) found that 18% of girls under 13 years with vaginal bleeding with or without discharge, and 50% of those with vaginal bleeding and no discharge, had a foreign body. Most girls with a foreign body do not have a foul-smelling discharge with the bleeding. A tumor is a rare cause of bleeding, but the possibility of this diagnosis makes adequate assessment of the vagina important in the child with unexplained bleeding.

Urethral prolapse usually presents with bleeding, often thought by the parent to be vaginal bleeding (see Fig. 3-9 and discussion under Interlabial masses below). Cyclic vaginal bleeding without signs of pubertal development, termed "precocious menarche" (83,84) is rare and usually associated with slightly elevated estradiol levels (see Chapter 5). However, complete examination, with the girl under anesthesia if necessary, is essential before vaginal bleeding can be considered an idiopathic or benign disorder. Bleeding secondary to vulvitis should respond promptly to local measures. Vaginitis due to organisms such as *S. pyogenes* or *Shigella* requires oral antibiotics.

A foreign body may be removed in the outpatient setting if the patient is cooperative. Soft foreign bodies can often be easily removed by twirling a dry cotton-tipped applicator within the vagina with the patient in the lithotomy or knee–chest position. Gentle irrigation of the vagina with saline or water can usually be accomplished with the child supine, using a small urethral catheter or infant feeding tube attached to a 25-ml syringe or an Angiocath attached to a syringe. Lubricant or lidocaine jelly (or liquid) can be applied to the introitus to aid in insertion of the small catheter. It may be possible to remove metallic items such as safety pins with bayonet forceps avoiding the hymenal edges. If the child is frightened or the foreign body cannot be easily removed, general anesthesia is necessary. Sitz baths for a few days after are generally adequate to clear any residual symptoms. Therapy for a tumor depends on the extent of the lesion and requires referral to a tertiary care medical center.

INTERLABIAL MASSES

The causes of interlabial masses include urethral prolapse, paraurethral cyst (Fig. 3-11), hydro(metro)colpos, rhabdomyosarcoma of the vagina (botryoid sarcoma) (Color Plate 8), prolapsed ectopic ureterocele (Fig. 3-12), condyloma acuminatum (see Figs. 3-1 and 3-6 and Chapters 17 and 24), urethral polyp, congenital perineal lipoma, and vaginal or cervical prolapse (85–91).

Urethral prolapse (Fig. 3-9) usually presents with bleeding, and the characteristic friable red–blue (doughnut-like) annular mass is visible in the perineum. The vaginal orifice is sometimes obscured and may be visualized only when the girl is in the

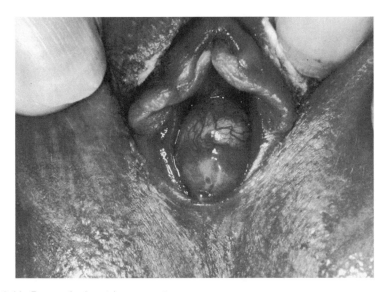

FIG. 3-11. Paraurethral cyst in a neonate.

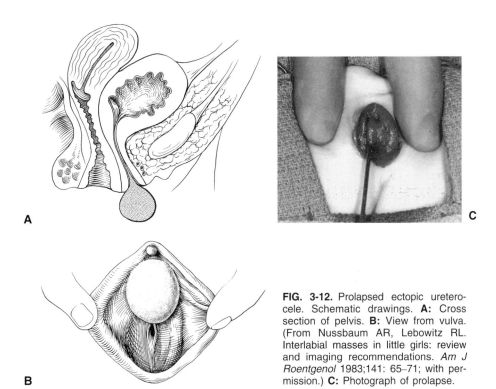

A

B

C

FIG. 3-12. Prolapsed ectopic ureterocele. Schematic drawings. **A:** Cross section of pelvis. **B:** View from vulva. (From Nussbaum AR, Lebowitz RL. Interlabial masses in little girls: review and imaging recommendations. *Am J Roentgenol* 1983;141: 65–71; with permission.) **C:** Photograph of prolapse.

knee–chest position. The patient may complain of dysuria, bleeding, and pain that has occurred after coughing or straining or following trauma. The peak age of prolapse is 5 to 8 years; for unclear reasons the condition has been reported to occur more commonly in black girls in the U.S. The youngest case reported was in a 5-day-old infant (89). Prolapse usually resolves with nonsurgical treatment. Most centers use sitz baths and application of topical estrogen cream. Resolution takes 1 to 4 weeks. Prolapse with tissue necrosis requires surgical resection of the necrotic distal urethra, but surgical intervention is very rarely required.

Paraurethral cysts (Fig. 3-11) may occur in children, especially during the newborn period, and arise from obstruction or cystic degeneration of embryonic remnants of the urogenital sinus: paraurethral glands, Skene duct, mesonephric duct (Gartner duct), or müllerian duct (89). In the newborn, the cysts usually disappear or spontaneously rupture without requiring any treatment. Before surgery is undertaken, the possibility of a urologic or gynecologic problem such as urethral diverticulum, ectopic ureterocele, hymenal or vaginal cyst, or obstructed hemivagina should be excluded by preoperative examination and ultrasonography of the kidneys and bladder. Intraoperatively, radiopaque dye such as Renografin should be injected into the cyst and imaged to enable detection of an anomaly.

A *prolapsed ectopic ureterocele* (Fig. 3-12) is a congenital anomaly that includes cystic dilatation of the terminal (intramural) part of a ureter; 90% are associated with a duplex collecting system (89). *Hydro(metro)colpos* (Fig. 3-13) may present in the nursery with a bulging imperforate hymen or obstruction from a low vaginal septum (a midvaginal or high vaginal septum will not usually present with an interlabial mass). An imperforate hymen is not usually associated with other

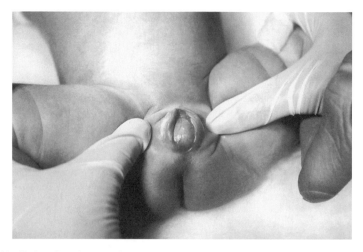

FIG. 3-13. Hydrocolpos in a newborn.

anomalies, but a transverse septum is often associated with genitourinary and gastrointestinal anomalies (89). *Neonatal vaginal prolapse* has been reported in a healthy neonate. The mass was restored to normal position with the examiner's small finger, and the mother was trained to reinsert the vagina subsequently; after 6 months there was no further prolapse (90).

Sarcoma botryoides (Color Plate 8) is a malignant tumor that involves the vagina, uterus, bladder, and urethra of very young girls and is also known as embryonal rhabdomyosarcoma. The symptoms include vaginal discharge, bleeding, abdominal pain or mass, or the passage of grape-like lesions. The peak incidence is in the first 2 years of life, and 90% of cases occur before the child is 5 years old. The tumor usually originates in the lower vagina or urethra in younger girls. In those diagnosed when they are older, the growth usually starts on the anterior vaginal wall near the cervix, and as the tumor grows larger it fills the vagina. On examination, the tumor appears as a prolapse of grapelike masses through the urethra or vagina. Growth of the tumor can be rapid. The prognosis has markedly improved over the past few decades. A combination of chemotherapy and conservative surgery, along with radiation therapy for some patients, can result in a survival rate of 80% to 90% in girls with localized pelvic rhabdomyosarcoma (87,92). In a study of 151 patients with rhabdomyosarcoma of the female genital tract treated with Intergroup Rhabdomyosarcoma Study (IRS) protocols I–IV, Arndt and colleagues reported that noninvasive tumors, being 1 to 9 years old at the time of diagnosis, and the use of IRS-II or IRS-IV treatments were associated with better outcomes (92). The 5-year survival rate for the 1- to 9-year-old girls was 98% (92). In early-stage vulvovaginal rhabdomyosarcoma, systemic vincristine, actinomycin-D, and cyclophosphamide (VAC) have resulted in high cure rates and retention of fertility. The prognosis is poorer in patients with regional or distant spread or recurrences.

CLITORAL LESIONS

The clitoral hood may occasionally develop an infection with intense edema and erythema. An antibiotic such as dicloxacillin or a cephalosporin with antistaphylococcal efficacy should be given orally, and warm soaks should be applied. Surgical incision and drainage are necessary if the abscess becomes fluctuant. In girls with lichen sclerosus, subepithelial hemorrhages may occur around the clitoris and labia minora, and adhesions and scarring may lead to a "buried" clitoris and clitoral pain. Trauma may cause an ecchymotic clitoris and clitoral hood. Edema of the clitoral hood may occur from hypoproteinemia resulting from nephrotic syndrome or gastrointestinal disease. Hypertrophy of the clitoral hood and clitoris can be due to neurofibromatosis (93,94), congenital lipoma (95), congenital hemangiopericytoma (a rare vascular tumor) (96), dermoid cyst (97), or rhabdomyosarcoma (98). A "clitoral tourniquet syndrome" has been described in which a hair had become wrapped around the clitoris, resulting in edema and severe pain (99). After removal of the hair, the clitoris returned to normal size. Recurrent episodes have been reported (100). The syndrome is similar to strangulation by hair of other parts of the body, such as fingers, toes, or the penis. Clitorism, a persistent painful erection of the clitoris, has been reported in one 11-year-old with acute nonlymphocytic leukemia and extremely elevated leukocyte count ($196,000/mm^3$) (101).

LABIAL ADHESIONS

Agglutination of the labia minora, termed labial adhesions or, in the lower half, vulvar adhesions, occurs primarily in young girls aged 3 months to 6 years (Fig. 3-14 and Color Plate 5). Labial adhesions are not seen in newborns because of estrogen effects on the vulva. Occasionally, adhesions occur for the first time after age 6, and adhesions presenting at any age may persist to the time of puberty. Vulvar irritation may play a role in causing the formation of the adhesions or the progression from an initially small posterior adhesion to a near-total fusion. The vaginal orifice may be completely covered, causing poor drainage of vaginal secretions. Parents often become alarmed because the vagina appears "absent." It has

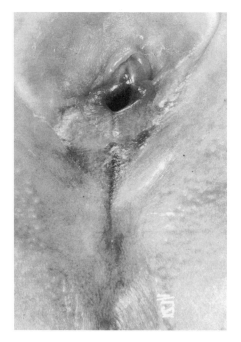

FIG. 3-14. Labial/vulvar adhesions with small opening below the clitoris.

been suggested (although not proved) that fondling and the irritation from sexual abuse may predispose the older girl to labial agglutination (102,103).

The diagnosis of labial adhesions is made by visual inspection of the vulva. The treatment of labial adhesions remains controversial. Spontaneous separation may occur, particularly with small vulvar adhesions at the posterior fourchette and with estrogenization at puberty. If the opening in the agglutination is large enough for good vaginal and urinary drainage, lubrication of the labia with a bland ointment such as A and D ointment, and gentle separation applied by the mother over several weeks, may be helpful. For adhesions that impair vaginal or urinary drainage, the most effective treatment is the application of an estrogen-containing cream (104). We prescribe an estrogen-containing cream (e.g., Premarin) twice daily for 3 weeks and then at bedtime for another 2 to 3 weeks. Approximately half of adhesions will resolve in 2 to 3 weeks (105), and therapy can then be changed to A and D ointment. The other half require a longer course of therapy, as indicated above. The parent must be shown exactly where the labial adhesion is ("a line") and shown how to rub in the cream with gentle separation. The use of a long cotton-tipped applicator may facilitate correct application of the cream and gentle separation (the child may appreciate that the cream is "painted on"). Separating the labia and applying gentle pressure with the applicator in an up and down direction for 10 strokes may improve the chance of success of the treatment. Most failures result when the parent applies the cream over the entire vulva without specific attention to the adhesion or from lack of utilization of enough cream. After separation has occurred, the labia should be maintained apart by daily baths, good hygiene, and the application of a bland ointment (such as A and D ointment) at bedtime for 6 to 12 months. Forceful separation is contraindicated because it is traumatic for the child and may cause the adhesions to form again.

In occasional patients, the extensive, dense labial adhesions fail to respond to estrogen cream, even when proper technique of application of the estrogen cream is used. This is particularly likely if surgical separation has been previously used. In the cooperative patient, separation can be accomplished in the office at the end of the 6-week course of estrogen cream. Approximately 5 minutes after the application of 5% lidocaine ointment, or 30 minutes after EMLA (a eutectic mixture of local anesthetics, lidocaine, and prilocaine) application, the physician can slide a Calgiswab gently along the adhesions thinned by the estrogen cream, teasing them apart in an anterior-to-posterior direction (Fig. 3-15). It is essential that this be atraumatic for the child. If this is not easily accomplished or if the girl has acute urinary retention, separation in an ambulatory surgical setting is recommended. Estrogen cream should be applied for 1 week after the procedure. Rarely, patients in early adolescence who have had labial adhesions since early childhood do not have the usual spontaneous separation, despite their own endogenous estrogen levels and/or topical application of estrogen cream. Our oldest patient with persistent adhesions was 16 years old and required general anesthesia for separation.

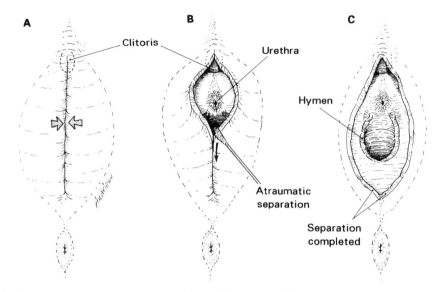

FIG. 3-15. Atraumatic separation of a labial adhesion that failed to separate.

MISCELLANEOUS ENTITIES

Four other entities that should be recognized by the physician are labial abscesses, labial masses, melanoma, and congenital failure of midline fusion. Labial abscesses (Fig. 3-16) in immunocompetent girls are usually caused by infections with *S. aureus* or *S. pyogenes.* The abscesses are treated with antibiotics, sitz baths, and, as indicated, incision and drainage. Immunocompromised and diabetic girls can develop abscesses and life-threatening necrotizing fasciitis. Aggressive shaving of pubic hair in at-risk patients should be discouraged.

Labial masses can also result from a number of conditions, including a hernia, embryonic duct remnants, benign tumors such as a lipoma (Fig. 3-17), fibroma, granular cell tumor, neurofibromatosis, lymphangioma, hamartoma, and hemangioma, and rare malignant tumors (106). Lipomas often present with asymmetry of the labia majora and may initially be mistaken for a hernia. Treatment is observation or excision. Benign granular cell tumors of the labia are of neural origin and may recur locally, and thus close follow-up is important (107). Evaluation and treatment include careful physical examination looking for evidence of hernia or intersex state, ultrasound and occasionally MRI to better define the nature of the enlargement, and observation or excision.

Pigmented lesions of the vulva are fairly common. Since these lesions are difficult for self-monitoring, they often require surgical excision. It is important that the surgeon resect the lesion with adequate margins owing to the possible recurrence of

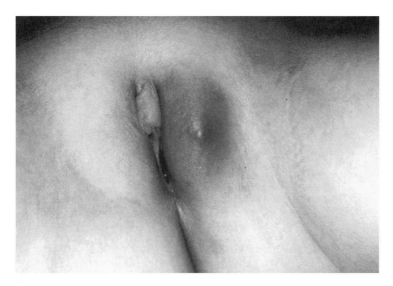

FIG. 3-16. Labial abscess.

atypia. Melanoma is rare in prepubertal girls. However, there have been several case reports on vulvar melanoma in this age group, in two cases in association with lichen sclerosus (108), the significance of which is unknown.

Failure of midline fusion is congenital and may be confused with trauma or sexual abuse; the child in Color Plate 7 underwent excision of the base of the

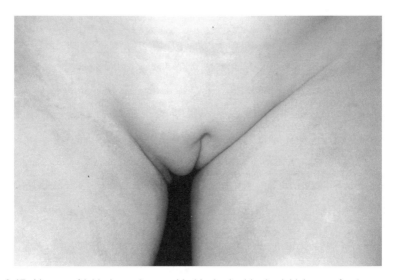

FIG. 3-17. Lipoma of labia in an 8-year-old girl who had had a labial mass for 1 year.

separation, and suturing of the edges to give a normal vulvar appearance, at the age of 4 years.

REFERENCES

1. Fischer G. Rogers M. Vulvar disease in children: a clinical audit of 130 cases. *Pediatr Dermatol* 2000;17:1.
2. Paradise JE, Compos JM, Friedman HM, et al. Vulvovaginitis in premenarchal girls: clinical features and diagnostic evaluation. *Pediatrics* 1982;70:193.
3. Emans SJ, Goldstein DP The gynecologic examination of the prepubertal child with vulvovaginitis: use of the knee-chest position. *Pediatrics* 1980;65:758.
4. Altchek A. Pediatric vulvovaginitis. *J Reprod Med* 1984;29:359.
5. Heller RH, Joseph JH, David HJ. Vulvovaginitis in the premenarchal child. *J Pediatr* 1969;74:370.
6. Pierce AM, Hart CA. Vulvovaginitis: causes and management. *Arch Dis Child* 1992;67:509.
7. Piippo S, Lenko H, Vuento R. Vulvar symptoms in paediatric and adolescent patients. *Acta Paediatr* 2000;89:431.
8. Paek SC, Merritt DF, Mallory SB. Pruritus vulvae in prepubertal children *J Am Acad Dermatol* 2001;44:795
9. Hammerschlag MR, Albert S, Rosner I, et al. Microbiology of the vagina in children: normal and potentially pathogenic organisms. *Pediatrics* 1978;68:57.
10. Gardner JJ. Comparison of the vaginal flora in sexually abused and nonabused girls. *J Pediatr* 1992;120:872.
11. Gerstner GJ, Grunberger W, Boschitsch E, et al. Vaginal organisms in prepubertal children with and without vulvovaginitis. *Arch Gynecol* 1982;231:247.
12. Paradise J. Unpublished data.
13. Figeroa-Colon R, Grunow JE, Torres-Pinedo R, et al. Group A streptococcal proctitis and vulvo-vaginitis in a prepubertal girl. *Pediatr Infect Dis* 1984;3:439.
14. Spear RM, Rithbaum RJ, Keating JP, et al. Perianal streptococcal cellulitis. *J Pediatr* 1985; 107:557.
15. Kokx NP, Comstock JA, Facklam RR. Streptococcal perianal disease in children. *Pediatrics* 1987; 80:659.
16. Straumanis JP, Bocchini JA. Group A beta-hemolytic streptococcal vulvovaginitis in prepubertal girls: a case report and review of the past twenty years. *Pediatr Infect Dis* 1990;9:845.
17. Donald FE, Slack RCB, Colman G. *Streptococcus pyogenes* vulvovaginitis in children in Nottingham. *Epidemiol Infect* 1991;106:459.
18. Mogielnicki NP, Schwartzman JD, Elliott JA. Perineal group A streptococcal disease in a pediatric practice. *Pediatrics* 2000;106:276.
19. Zeiguer NJ, Galvano A, Comparato MR, et al. Vulvar abscesses caused by *Streptococcus pneumoniae. Pediatr Infect Dis J* 1992;11:335.
20. Macfarlane DE, Sharma DE. *Haemophilus influenzae* and genital tract infections in children. *Acta Paediatr Scand* 1987;76:363.
21. Murphy TV, Nelson JD. *Shigella* vaginitis: report of 38 patients and review of the literature. *Pediatrics* 1979;63:511.
22. Yanovski JA, Nelson LM, Willis ED, Cutler GB. Repeated childhood vaginal bleeding is not always precocious puberty. *Pediatrics* 1992;89:149.
23. Gryngarten MG, Turco ML, Ewcobar ME, et al. *Shigella* vulvaginitis in prepubertal girls. *Adolesc Pediatr Gynecol* 1994;7:86.
24. Watkins S, Quan L. Vulvovaginitis caused by *Yersinia enterocolitica. Pediatr Infect Dis* 1984;3:444.
25. Ingram DL. *Neisseria gonorrhoeae* in children. *Pediatr Ann* 1994;23:341.
26. Farrell MK, Billmire ME, Shamroy JA, et al. Prepubertal gonorrhea: a multidisciplinary approach. *Pediatrics* 1981;67:151.
27. Folland DS, Burke RE, Hinman AR, et al. Gonorrhea in preadolescent children: an inquiry into source of infection and mode of transmission. *Pediatrics* 1977;60:153.

28. Ingram DL, White ST, Occhiuti AC, et al. Childhood vaginal infections: association of *Chlamydia trachomatis* with sexual contact. *Pediatr Infect Dis* 1986;5:226.
29. Fuster CD, Neinstein LS. Vaginal *Chlamydia trachomatis* prevalence in sexually abused prepubertal girls. *Pediatrics* 1987;79:235.
30. Shapiro RA, Schubert CJ, Myers PA. Vaginal discharge as an indicator of gonorrhea and *Chlamydia* infection in girls under 12 years old. *Pediatr Emerg Med* 1993;9:341.
31. Sicoli RA, Losek JD, Hudlett JM, et al. Indications for *Neisseria gonorrhoeae* cultures in children with suspected sexual abuse. *Arch Pediatr Adolesc Med* 1995;149:86.
32. Shapiro RA, Schubert CJ, Siegel RM. *Neisseria* gonorrhea infections in girls younger than 12 years of age evaluated for vaginitis. *Pediatrics* 1999;104(6),e72.
33. Goh BT, Forster GE. Sexually transmitted diseases in children: chlamydial oculo-genital infection. *Genitourin Med* 1993;69:213.
34. Desenclos JA, Garrity D, Wroten J. Pediatric gonococcal infection, Florida 1984 to 1988. *Am J Public Health* 1992;82:426.
35. Ingram DL, Everett VD, Lyna PR. Epidemiology of adult sexually transmitted disease agents in children being evaluated for sexual abuse. *Pediatr Infect Dis J* 1992;11:945.
36. Danesh IS, Stephen JM, Gorbach J. Neonatal *Trichomonas vaginalis* infection. *J Emerg Med* 1995; 13:51.
37. Schachter J, Grossman M, Sweet RL, et al. Prospective study of perinatal transmission of *Chlamydia trachomatis*. *JAMA* 1986;255:3374.
38. Bell TA, Stamm WE, Kuo CC, et al. Delayed appearance of *Chlamydia trachomatis* infection acquired at birth. *Pediatr Infect Dis* 1987;6:928.
39. Bell TA. *Chlamydia trachomatis* infections in infants: perinatal or sexual transmission? *Infect Med* 1993;10:32
40. Bell TA, Stamm WE, Wang SP, et al. Chronic *Chlamydia trachomatis* infections in infants. *JAMA* 1992;267:400.
41. Patamasucon P, Rettig PJ, Nelson JD. Cefuroxime therapy of gonorrhea and coinfection with *Chlamydia trachomatis* in children. *Pediatrics* 1981;68:534.
42. Centers For Disease Control and Prevention. Sexually Transmitted Diseases Treatment Guidelines 2002. *MMWR*; 2002;51(RR-6):1.
43. Centers For Disease Control and Prevention. Screening tests to detect *Chlamydia trachomatis* and *Neisseria gonorrhoeae* infections—2002. *MMWR* 2002;51(RR-15):1.
44. Hammerschlag MR, Rettig PJ, Shields ME. False positive result with the use of *Chlamydia* antigen detection tests in the evaluation of suspected sexual abuse in children. *Pediatr Infect Dis J* 1988;7:11.
45. Embree JE, Lindsay D, Williams T, et al. Acceptability and usefulness of vaginal washes in premenarcheal girls as a diagnostic procedure for sexually transmitted diseases. *Pediatr Infect Dis J* 1996;15:662.
46. Kaplan KM, Fleisher GR, Paradise JE, et al. Social relevance of genital herpes simplex in children. *J Pediatr* 1984;104:243.
47. Simon HK, Steele DW. Varicella: pediatric genital/rectal vesicular lesions of unclear origin. *Ann Emerg Med* 1995;25:111.
48. Bartley DL, Morgan L, Rimsza ME. *Gardnerella vaginalis* in prepubertal girls. *Am J Dis Child* 1987;141:1014.
49. Ingram DL, White ST, Lyna PR, et al. *Gardnerella vaginalis* infection and sexual contact in female children. *Child Abuse Neglect* 1992;16:847.
50. Fink CW. A perineal rash in Kawasaki disease. *Pediatr Infect Dis* 1983;2:140.
51. Khoshoo V. Zinc deficiency in a full-term breast-fed infant: unusual presentation. *Pediatrics* 1992; 89:1094.
52. Guenther LC, Shum D. Localized childhood vulvar pemphigoid. *J Am Acad Dermatol* 1990; 22:762.
53. Hanks JW, Venters WJ. Nickel allergy from a bed-wetting alarm confused with herpes genitalis and child abuse. *Pediatrics* 1992;90:458.
54. Otis CN, Fischer RA, Johnson N, et al. Histiocytosis X of the vulva: a case report and review of the literature. *Obstet Gynecol* 1990;75:555.
55. Wilson RW. Genital ulcers and mononucleosis. *Pediatr Infect Dis J* 1993;12:418.
56. Tuffnell D, Buchan PC. Crohn's disease of the vulva in childhood. *Br J Clin Prac* 1991;45:159.

57. Rimsza ME, Chun JJ. Vaginal discharge of "beads" and the new diapers. *Pediatrics* 1988;81:332.
58. See WA, Mayo M. Ectopic ureter: a rare cause of purulent vaginal discharge. *Obstet Gynecol* 1991; 78:552.
59. Ott MM, Rehn M, Muller JG, et al. Vaginal clear cell carcinoma in a young patient with ectopic termination of the left ureter in the vagina. *Virchows Arch* 1994;425:445.
60. Shimao Y, Nabeshima K, Inoue T, et al. Primary vaginal adenocarcinoma arising from the metanephric duct remnant. *Virchows Arch* 2000;436:622.
61. Paradise JE, Willis ED. Probability of vaginal foreign body in girls with genital complaints. *Am J Dis Child* 1985;139:472.
62. Baiulescu M, Hannon PR, Marcinak JF, et al. Chronic vulvovaginitis caused by antibiotic-resistant *Shigella flexneri* in a prepubertal child. *Pediatr Infect Dis J* 2002;21:170.
63. Meyrick Thomas RH, Kennedy CT. The development of lichen sclerosus et atrophicus in monozygotic twin girls. *Br J Dermatol* 1986;114:337.
64. Loening-Bauecke V. Lichen sclerosus et atrophicus in children. *Am J Dis Child* 1991;145:1058.
65. Parks G, Growdon WA, Mason GD, et al. Childhood anogenital lichen sclerosus. *J Reprod Med* 1990;191.
66. Ridley CM. Genital lichen sclerosus in childhood and adolescence. *J R Soc Med* 1993;69.
67. Berth-Jones J, Graham-Brown RA, Burns DA. Lichen sclerosus et atrophicus—a review of 15 cases in young girls. *Clin Exp Dermatol* 1991;16:14.
68. Bohm M, Frieling U, Luger TA, et al. Successful treatment of vulvar lichen sclerosus with topical tacrolimus. Arch Dermatol 2003;139:922.
69. Dalziel KL, Millard PR, Wojnarowska F The treatment of vulval lichen sclerosus with a very potent topical steroid (clobetasol propionate 0.05%) cream. *Br J Dermatol* 1991;124:461.
70. Dalziel KL, Wojnarowska F. Long-term control of vulval lichen sclerosus after treatment with a potent topical steroid cream. *J Reprod Med* 1993;38:25.S.
71. Powell J, Wojnarowska F. Childhood vulvar lichen sclerosus: an increasingly common problem. *J Am Acad Dermatol* 2001;44:803.
72. Garzon MC, Paller AS. Ultrapotent topical corticosteroid treatment of childhood genital lichen sclerosus. *Arch Dermatol* 1999;135:525.
73. Smith YR, Quint EH. Clobetasol propionate in the treatment of premenarchal vulvar lichen sclerosus. *Obstet Gynecol* 2001;98:588.
74. Breech LL, Laufer MR. Surgicel® in the management of labial and clitoral hood adhesions in adolescents with lichen sclerosus. *J Pediatr Adolesc Gynecol* 2000;13:21.
75. ACOG Educational Bulletin. Vulvar nonneoplastic epithelial disorders. *Int J Gynecol Obstet* 1998;60:181.
76. Thomas RH, Ridley CM, McGibbon DH et al. Lichen sclerosus et atrophicus and autoimmunity: a study of 350 women. *Br J Dermatol* 1988;188:41.
77. Pokorny S, Pokorny W, Kramer W. Acute genital injury in the prepubertal girl. *Am J Obstet Gynecol* 1992;166:1461.
78. Bond GR, Dowd MD, Landsman I, et al. Unintentional perineal injury in prepubescent girls: a multicenter, prospective report of 56 girls. *Pediatrics* 1995;95:628.
79. Hostetler BR, Muram D, Jones CE. Capillary hemangiomas of the vulva mistaken for sexual abuse. *J Pediatr Adolesc Gynecol* 1994;7:44.
80. Hostetler BR, Muram D, Jones CE. Sharp penetrating injury to the hymen. *J Adolesc Pediatr Gynecol* 1994;7:94.
81. Perlman SE, Hertweck SP, Wolfe WM. Water-ski douche injury in a premenarcheal female. *Pediatrics* 1995;96:782.
82. Kunkel NC. Vaginal injury from a water slide in a premenarcheal patient. *Pediatr Emerg Care* 1998;14:210.
83. Heller ME, Dewhurst J, Grant DB. Premature menarche without other evidence of precocious puberty. *Arch Dis Child* 1979;54:472.
84. Heller ME, Savage MO, Dewhurst J. Vaginal bleeding in childhood: a review of 51 patients. *Br J Obstet Gynaecol* 1970;85:721.
85. Mercer LJ, Mueller CM, Hajj SN. Medical treatment of urethral prolapse in the premenarchal female. *Adolesc Pediatr Gynecol* 1988;1:181.
86. Fernandes ET, Dekermacher S, Sabadin MA, et al. Urethral prolapse in children. *Urology* 1993; 41:240.

87. Copeland LJ, Gershenson DM, Saul PB, et al. Sarcoma botryoides of the female genital tract. *Obstet Gynecol* 1985;66:262.
88. Klee LW, Rink RC, Gleason PE, et al. Urethral polyp presenting as interlabial mass in young girls. *Urology* 1993;41:132.
89. Nussbaum AR, Lebowitz RL. Interlabial masses in little girls: review and imaging recommendations. *AJR* 1983;141:65.
90. Bayatpour M, McCann J, Harris T, et al. Neonatal genital prolapse. *Pediatrics* 1992;90:465.
91. Chandra MN, Jammieson MA, Poenaru D. Congenital perineal lipoma presenting as "ambiguous genitalia": A case report. *J Pediatr Adolesc Gynecol* 2000;13:71.
92. Arndt CA, Donaldson SS, Anderson JR, et al. What constitutes optimal therapy for patients with rhabdomyosarcoma of the female genital tract. *Cancer* 2001;91:2454.
93. Griebel ML, Redman JF, Kemp SF, et al. Hypertrophy of clitoral hood: presenting sign of neurofibromatosis in female child. *Urology* 1991;37:337.
94. Nonomura K, Kanno T, Tanaka M, et al. A case of neurofibromatosis associated with clitoral enlargement and hypertension. *J Pediatr Surg* 1992;27:110.
95. Van Glabeke E, Audry G, Hervet F, et al. Lipoma of the preputium clitoridis in neonate: an exceptional abnormality different from ambiguous genitalia. *Pediatr Surg Int* 1999;15:147.
96. Brock JW 3rd, Morgan U, Anderson TL. Congenital hemangiopericytoma of the clitoris. *J Urol* 1995;153:468.
97. Abudaia J, Habib Z, Ahmed S. Dermoid cyst: a rare cause of clitorimegaly. *Pediatr Surg* 1999;15:521.
98. Bond SJ, Seibel N, Kapur S, et al. Rhabdomyosarcoma of the clitoris. *Cancer* 1994;73:1984.
99. Press S, Schachner L, Paul P. Clitoris tourniquet syndrome. *Pediatrics* 1980;66:781.
100. Sylwestrzak MS, Fischer BF, Fischer H. Recurrent clitoral tourniquet syndrome. *Pediatrics* 2000; 105:866.
101. Williams DL, Bell BA, Ragab AH. Clitorism at presentation of acute nonlymphocytic leukemia. *J Pediatr* 1985;107:754.
102. Berkowitz CD, Elvik SL, Logan MK. Labial fusion in prepubescent girls: a marker for sexual abuse? *Am J Obstet Gynecol* 1987;156:16.
103. McCann J, Voris J, Simon M. Labial adhesions and posterior fourchette injuries in childhood sexual abuse. *Am J Dis Child* 1988;142:659.
104. Ariberg A. Topical oestrogen therapy for labial adhesions in children. *Br J Obstet Gynaecol* 1975; 82:424.
105. Muram D. Treatment of prepubertal girls with labial adhesions. *J Pediatr Adolesc Gynecol* 1999;12:67.
106. Lowry DLB, Guido RS. The vulvar mass in the prepubertal child. *J Pediatr Adolesc Gynecol* 2000;13:75.
107. Cohen Z, Kapuller V, Maor E, et al . Granular cell tumor (myoblastoma) of the labia majora: a rare benign tumor in childhood. *J Pediatr Adolesc Gynecol* 1999;12:155.
108. Egan CA, Bradley RR, Logsdon VK, et al. Vulvar melanoma in childhood. *Arch Dermatol* 1997;133:345.

FURTHER READING

AAP Report of the Committee on Infections Diseases. Pickering LK, ed. *Red Book 2003*. 26th ed., Elk Grove, IL: AAP, 2003.

Educational Materials for Families and Patients

Labial adhesions: www.naspag.org/labialadhesions

Vaginitis: www.naspag.org/vaginitis

Lichen sclerosus: www.naspag/org/lichensclerosus

www.youngwomenshealth.org/teenlichensclerosus

4

The Physiology of Puberty

Catherine M. Gordon and Marc R. Laufer

Puberty is the natural life transition from childhood to adulthood. Change can be stressful, and puberty is no exception. As a young woman proceeds through this time of change she, her parents, guardians, or teachers may have questions about what is normal or abnormal. In order to gain the needed information, she may approach the family pediatrician, gynecologist, or other health care provider. An understanding of the physiology of puberty and menarche is essential for all health care providers so that they can dispense accurate information and help dispel myths. Once normal development is understood, the foundation is set for the diagnosis and management of precocious puberty (see Chapter 5) and menstrual abnormalities (see Chapters 6 to 9).

HORMONAL CHANGES AT PUBERTY

Normal female pubertal development requires the elaborate orchestration of the hypothalamic–pituitary–gonadal axis. The physical signs of puberty in girls are accelerated growth and the appearance of secondary sex characteristics. Before signs of puberty are visible, hormonal changes result from activation of the hypothalamic pituitary axis and the secretion of ovarian sex steroids. The hypothalamus is responsible for the synthesis and release of gonadotropin-releasing hormone (GnRH), historically referred to as luteinizing hormone–releasing hormone (LHRH) (Fig. 4-1). GnRH is a decapeptide with a serum half-life of 2 to 4 minutes and is released in a pulsatile fashion into the pituitary portal plexus. Higher cortical centers and the limbic system influence the synthesis and secretion of GnRH. In addition, neurotransmitters, sex steroids, and gonadal peptides also affect the synthesis and secretion of GnRH. This hormone binds to surface receptors on anterior pituitary gonadotrophs, which synthesize and store the glycoprotein gonadotropins: follicle-stimulating hormone (FSH) and luteinizing hormone (LH). Pulses of electrical activity have been recorded from the hypothalamus coincident

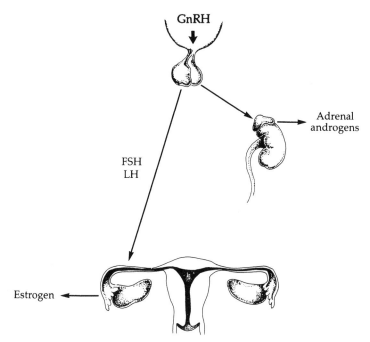

FIG. 4-1. Hormones responsible for the onset of puberty. GnRH, gonadotropin-releasing hormone; FSH, follicle-stimulating hormone; LH, luteinizing hormone. The stimulus for the rise in adrenal androgens is unclear.

with LH pulses (1). The pulsatile GnRH stimulation results in a pulsatile secretion of gonadotropins, as was demonstrated in the classic studies comparing pulsatile versus continuous administration of GnRH to oophorectomized rhesus monkeys (Fig. 4-2) (2). The pulsatile release of gonadotropins is thus responsible for ovarian stimulation and the resultant maturation of the germinal epithelium and synthesis of gonadal steroid hormones.

Sex steroids are produced in the follicles and theca cells of the ovary. In addition, the ovary produces insulin-like growth factor (IGF), inhibin, activin, follistatin, and cytokines. These ovarian products exert a feedback effect upon gonadotropin secretion (Fig. 4-3). The feedback occurs both at the level of the hypothalamus, modulating the frequency and amplitude of GnRH release, and at the level of the pituitary, affecting the amount of LH and FSH released in response to GnRH pulses. Inhibin and activin are structurally similar. Each are disulfide-linked dimers composed of peptide subunits that are encoded by separate genes (3,4). Despite the structural similarity between these factors, they may function as antagonists, with activin stimulating and inhibin inhibiting FSH secretion (3,4). Follistatin is structurally unrelated to inhibin and activin, but acts as a regulator of the activin–inhibin system, decreasing FSH biosynthesis (3,4). Significant changes in these FSH-regulatory

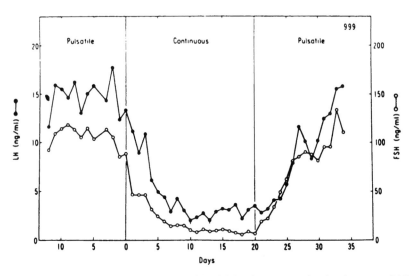

FIG. 4-2. Effect of pulsatile administration of luteinizing hormone–releasing hormone (LHRH) in contrast to continuous infusion of LHRH in adult oophorectomized rhesus monkeys in which gonadotropin secretion has been abolished by lesions that ablated the medial basal hypothalamic LHRH pulse generator. Note the high concentrations of plasma luteinizing hormone (LH) and follicle-stimulating hormone (FSH) in monkeys given one LHRH pulse per hour, the suppression of gonadotropin secretion by continuous infusion of LHRH even though the total dose of LHRH was the same, and the restoration of FSH and LH secretion when the pulsatile mode of LHRH administration was reinitiated. (From Belcheltz PE, Plant TM, Nakai Y, et al. Hypophysial responses to continuous and intermittent delivery of hypothalamic gonadotropin releasing hormone. *Science* 1978;202:631–633; with permission.)

peptides accompany the onset of puberty (4). Serum inhibin A levels increase in midpuberty, while levels of inhibin B peak during midpuberty and decline thereafter (4). Serum inhibin B levels correlate positively with age many years before the clinical onset of puberty, suggesting increasing follicular activity in late prepuberty (4). During the pubertal period, inhibin B levels increase with breast development, suggesting high follicular activity before the onset of ovulatory menses (4). Levels of activin do not appear to vary across pubertal stages or across gender (4,5). Therefore, this factor does not appear to be involved in the endocrine modifications of pubertal development (5). Follistatin levels do not appear to change during puberty but increase with the establishment of regular menses (6). Ultimately, estrogen from the ovary suppresses gonadotropin secretion by negative feedback. Although both FSH and LH are released in pulses, LH pulses are recognizable by minute-to-minute serum measurements, as the half-life of LH is approximately 30 minutes compared with the 300-minute half-life of FSH.

The hypothalamic–pituitary–ovarian system is remarkably well-developed at the time of birth. In fact, the hypothalamic portal system is intact by 14 weeks of gestation. The negative feedback effect of gonadal steroids on the hypothalamus

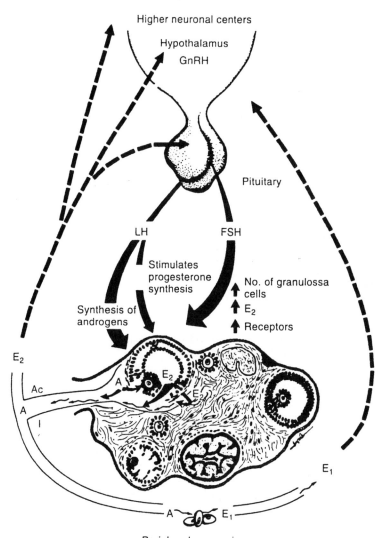

FIG. 4-3. Hypothalamic–pituitary–ovarian axis interaction in the regulation of follicular maturation and steroid biosynthesis. GnRH, gonadotropin-releasing hormone; LH, luteinizing hormone; FSH, follicle-stimulating hormone; E_2, estradiol; A, androstenedione; E_1, estrone; I, inhibin; Ac, activin. The ovary shows the various stages of growth of the follicle and the formation and regression of the corpus luteum.

and pituitary is apparent by midgestation. The production of gonadotropins and ovarian sex steroids is important in the stimulation of germ cell division and follicular development. By 5 to 6 months of gestation, 6 to 7 million oocytes are present, and through the process of atresia, the neonate has approximately 1 to 2 million

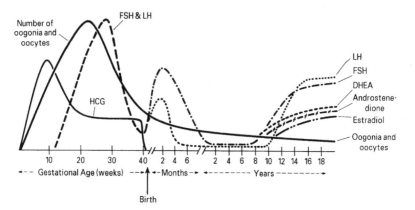

FIG. 4-4. Variations in number of oogonia and oocytes, and fluctuations in levels of hormones throughout gestational, neonatal, childhood, pubertal, adolescent, and adult life. DHEA, dehydroepiandrosterone; FSH, follicle-stimulating hormone; HCG, human chorionic gonadotropin; LH, luteinizing hormone. (Adapted from Speroff L, Glass RH, Kase NG. *Clinical gynecologic endocrinology and infertility,* 5th ed. Baltimore: Lippincott Williams & Wilkins, 1994; with permission.)

oocytes at birth; by puberty only 0.3 to 0.5 million oocytes remain (Fig. 4-4) (3). By 5 days after birth, gonadotropin levels rise sharply to levels considerably higher than those found in the prepubertal child, probably in response to the fall in placental estrogen. Transient rises in plasma FSH and estradiol are apparent in female infants, especially during the first 3 months of life. Thereafter, gonadotropin levels gradually fall to prepubertal levels, although FSH levels may not be maximally suppressed for 1 to 4 years. Girls have an elevated FSH/LH ratio compared with boys (7).

During the prepubertal childhood years, there is a down-regulation of the hypothalamic–pituitary system, with reduction of the amplitude and frequency of GnRH pulses (Fig. 4-5) and a decreased pituitary responsiveness as seen on a GnRH stimulation test (single 2.5-mg/kg IV dose of native GnRH) (8). Table 4-1 shows the method for GnRH stimulation testing (9). Figure 4-6 shows a prepubertal versus a pubertal serum FSH and LH response to GnRH stimulation testing. Prepubertal girls often show little LH response to a single dose of GnRH but a considerable rise in FSH; however, if GnRH is administered in a physiologic manner over the course of time, the pituitary is then "primed" and capable of a pubertal response. This inactivity appears to be in response to a central nervous system signal, with endogenous opiates serving as one of the primary inhibitory influences over GnRH secretion (10). In prepubertal girls, GnRH pulses continue to persist at low levels with enhancement during sleep, and the FSH/LH ratio is higher than in earlier or later stages. Levels of FSH and LH in Turner syndrome, which are markedly elevated in the neonatal period, are suppressed between the ages of 4 and 10 years, although the mean levels are higher than in normal children of similar ages. In some agonadal children between the ages of 5 and 11 years, basal levels

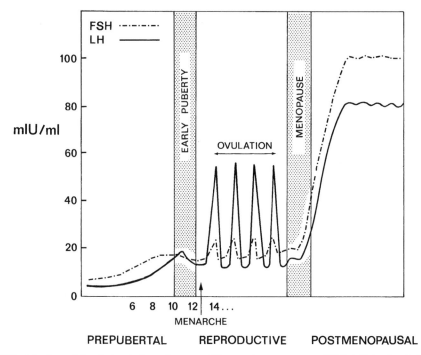

FIG. 4-5. Gonadotropin levels from the age of 6 years to menopause. FSH, follicle-stimulating hormone; LH, luteinizing hormone.

of LH and FSH, and responses to GnRH are comparable to those in normal prepubertal children; this similarity precludes a definitive diagnosis of gonadal failure by hormonal tests alone at this age (11).

The ovary increases in size during the prepubertal years and demonstrates evidence of active follicular growth and atresia. The vagina, which is approximately 4 cm long at birth, grows only 0.5 to 1.0 cm during early childhood but increases in length to 7.0 to 8.5 cm in late childhood. The uterus is about 2.5 cm long in infancy. The corpus/cervix ratio is slightly <1:1; it reaches 1:1 at menarche and the adult ratio of 3:1 postmenarcheally.

An early change associated with pubertal maturation is the secretion of adrenal androgens—dehydroepiandrosterone (DHEA), its sulfate (DHEAS), and androstenedione—between the ages of 6 and 8 years. Termed *adrenarche*, this process involves the regrowth of the zona reticularis (the zone that was large in the fetal adrenal cortex and regressed after birth) of the adrenal cortex with increases in activity of the microsomal enzyme p450c17. Recent data suggest that adrenarche is not the result of sudden rapid changes in adrenal enzymatic activity but rather may be a gradual maturational process that begins in early childhood (12). In a group of preadrenarchal young girls on GnRH agonist therapy to suppress

TABLE 4-1. *Normal responses to luteinizing hormone (LH) in adult women following FACTREL administration in the early follicular phase (days 1–7) of the menstrual cycle*

Subcutaneous administration
    LH peak: mean 67.9 ± 27.5 mIU/ml
        100% ≥ 12.5 mIU/ml
        90% ≥ 39.0 mIU/ml
    Maximum LH increase: mean 52.8 ± 26.4 mIU/ml
        100% ≥ 7.5 mIU/ml
        90% ≥ 23.8 mIU/ml
    LH % response: mean 374 ± 221%, range 108–981%
        90% ≥ 185%
    Time to peak: mean 71.5 ± 49.6 min
Intravenous administration[a]
    LH peak: mean 57.6 ± 36.7 mIU/ml
        100% ≥ 20.0 mIU/ml
        90% ≥ 24.6 mIU/ml
    Maximum LH increase: mean 44.5 ± 31.8 mIU/ml
        100% ≥ 7.5 mIU/ml
        90% ≥ 16.2 mIU/ml
    LH % response: mean 356 ± 282% range: 60–1300%
        90% ≥ 142%
    Time to peak: mean 36 ± 24 min

[a]The results are based on 31 tests in women between the ages of 20 and 35 years, inclusive.
LH peak (mIU/ml)=highest LH value after FACTREL administration.
Maximum increase (mIU/ml)=peak LH value-LH baseline value.
LH % response$=\left(\dfrac{\text{peak LH–baseline LH}}{\text{baseline LH}}\right)\times100\%$
Time to peak (minutes)=time required to reach LH peak value.
(Adapted from Ayerst Laboratories, Inc. FACTREL (Gonadorelin Hydrochloride) Package Insert. New York, 1990.)

precocious puberty, gradual increases in 17,20–lyase activity and decreasing activity of 3β-hydroxysteroid dehydrogenase was seen, even in this young cohort. Adrenal androgens continue to rise through ages 13 to 15 years and are primarily responsible for the appearance of pubic and axillary hair in girls (*pubarche*) (13,14). Acne vulgaris may be an early sign of puberty, resulting from rising levels of DHEAS (15,16). The ovarian androgens androstenedione and testosterone also stimulate growth of pubic and axillary hair.

At approximately 8 years of age or thereafter, although no physical changes are present, GnRH secretion is enhanced, at first during sleep (17). There is a resultant increase in pituitary responsiveness and increased secretion of LH and FSH (18). Baseline luteinizing hormone levels and responsiveness to exogenous GnRH (as seen on GnRH stimulation tests) also increase at this time and allow differentiation between a pubertal and prepubertal pattern (see Fig. 4-6). It also appears that the increase in LH bioactivity at puberty exceeds the changes seen in studies that examine the more commonly used radioimmunoassay. Lucky and associates (19) found that bioactive LH increased 23.1-fold, while immunoreactive LH increased only fourfold during puberty, which suggests a role of the pituitary in controlling the maturational process of puberty.

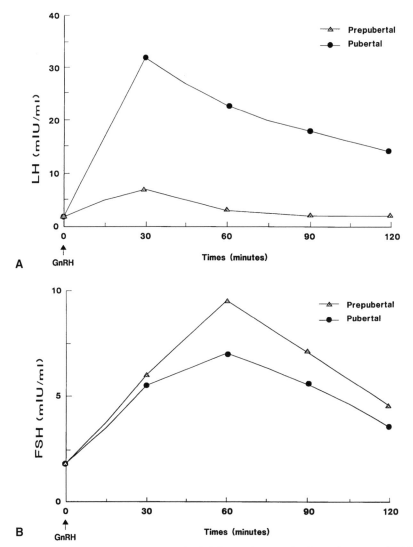

FIG. 4-6. Serum luteinizing hormone (LH) **(A)** and follicle-stimulating hormone (FSH) **(B)** responses as measured following an intravenous bolus of gonadotropin-releasing hormone in prepubertal and pubertal girls. [Adapted from Ayerst Laboratories Inc., Factrel (gonadorelin hydrochloride) package insert. New York: 1990.]

The age-related rise in gonadotropins with an initial sleep enhancement also occurs in patients with Turner syndrome, and menopausal levels of LH and FSH pulses occur at this time (20). It does not appear that ovarian sex steroids play a critical role in the onset of puberty, since patients with Turner syndrome experience adrenarche (the rise of adrenal androgens) and an age-related rise in gonadotropins.

Prepubertal patients with Addison disease can experience normal *gonadarche* (the activation of the hypothalamic–pituitary–ovarian axis) but not adrenarche. Patients in whom precocious puberty begins before age 6 years typically exhibit gonadarche, but not adrenarche. Patients with constitutional delay of puberty frequently have delays in both adrenarche and gonadarche (21). Sex steroids are important for the development of functional feedback mechanisms (18).

During early puberty, there is a gradual augmentation of episodic peaks of LH and FSH during sleep. The onset of puberty is associated initially with a greater increase in LH pulse amplitude compared to frequency (22). There is a gradual increase in daytime pulsatility. LH pulsatility is GnRH dependent at all ages, while there is a decrease in GnRH regulation of FSH pulsatility as there is an increase in ovarian activity (3,23). Luteinizing hormone stimulates the ovarian theca cells to synthesize precursors, and FSH increases the enzyme aromatase, which is responsible for the conversion of androgen precursors to estrogen. Estrogen peaks 10 to 12 hours after gonadotropin secretion (18). In addition, inhibin, activin, and follistatin interact in this complex regulatory system. These peptides are secreted in the highest levels by the gonads. In addition to effect on pituitary FSH secretion, they also act locally in the gonad, affecting steroid biosynthesis and gametogenesis (6,24,25). The ovaries are marked by increased follicular growth and on ultrasonography may appear as "enlarged and multicystic" ovaries. As puberty progresses, the ovaries amplify the gonadotropin message and release greater amounts of sex steroids for a given level of gonadotropins.

Breast budding, estrogenization of the vaginal mucosa, and lengthening and enlargement of the uterus occur with estrogen exposure. The physiologic vaginal discharge of puberty is the result of the desquamation of epithelial cells and mucus from the estrogenized mucosa. The pubertal process is accompanied by a growth spurt; both growth hormone and sex steroids appear to contribute to the growth spurt. The levels of growth hormone and IGF-1 increase during puberty, largely dictated by the rise of serum estrogen (26–29). The effect of estrogen on growth hormone and growth is dose related; low doses of estrogen stimulate growth, growth hormone, and IGF-1, while high doses of estrogen decrease them. This observation has led to the use of large pharmacologic doses of estrogen in an attempt to diminish final adult height in girls who are predicted to have excessively tall stature. In contrast, low doses of estrogen replacement in hypogonadal patients result in increased IGF-1 levels and growth. Since bone age, as determined by the Greulich and Pyle standards (30), correlates best with pubertal age, when an individual with delayed or advanced puberty is evaluated, it is important to obtain a radiograph of the wrist and hand for bone age interpretation. An increase in weight accompanies the growth spurt in normal girls, and body composition changes through late childhood and adolescence with a particularly apparent increase in percentage of body fat.

As puberty progresses, the levels of FSH and LH reached at night are gradually carried over into the waking hours until the sleep augmentation disappears. Even before menarche, circulating estrogen concentrations in pubertal girls have some cyclicity; eventually, these periodic fluctuations are sufficient to result in uterine bleeding. The first 1 to 2 years following menarche are often characterized by anovulatory menses (31–35). This time period coincides with the rapid growth of the uterus, vagina, fallopian tubes, and ovaries. With maturation, a mechanism known as the *biphasic positive feedback system* develops; in this system, a rise in plasma estrogen during the latter part of the follicular phase of the menstrual cycle triggers the surge of LH and FSH, which is responsible for ovulation. Historically, the change in the sensitivity of the feedback system was demonstrated by the use of clomiphene citrate, a nonsteroidal, agonist–antagonist estrogen, which when administered to prepubertal and early pubertal girls caused further suppression of gonadotropin levels (36–38). However, in late pubertal adolescents and adults, clomiphene causes a rise in gonadotropin levels and ovulation, a property that makes it useful as a fertility drug. It is noteworthy that this test is no longer used to determine the normal pubertal status, but the clomiphene challenge test is still used as a predictor of ovarian reserve for women desiring to conceive (37).

Leptin, a hormone secreted by adipose tissue, plays an important role in reproductive physiology. In animal models, it has been shown to stimulate the reproductive system by reversing the sterility of leptin-deficient mice and accelerating the onset of puberty in normal mice (39). In humans, serum leptin concentrations increase during childhood in both sexes and may be involved in the initiation of puberty (40). Serum leptin concentrations show diurnal variation throughout pubertal development in both girls and boys, and these changes follow a gender-specific pattern (41). Ankarberg-Lindgren and colleagues found a positive correlation between both estradiol and testosterone and leptin in girls throughout puberty, while no correlation was noted between estradiol and leptin in boys or between testosterone and leptin in pre- or early pubertal boys (41). To evaluate the relationship between leptin and the onset of puberty, Palmert and colleagues (40) measured serum leptin in children with central precocious puberty and made comparisons with normative data for healthy children and adolescents, adjusted for BMI and pubertal stage. Girls with central precocious puberty were found to have modestly elevated serum leptin concentrations compared to healthy girls, and there was a negative correlation between the leptin standard deviation score and BMI. Therefore, sufficient leptin concentrations appear to be associated with the initiation of puberty in girls.

STAGES OF BREAST AND PUBIC HAIR DEVELOPMENT

In 1969, Marshall and Tanner (42) recorded the rates of progress of pubertal development of 192 English schoolgirls. These stages can be important guidelines in assessing whether an adolescent is developing normally. The Tanner

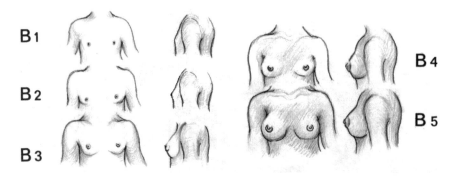

FIG. 4-7. The Tanner stages of human breast development. (Adapted from Grumbach MM, Styne DM. Puberty: Ontogeny, neuroendocrinology, physiology and disorders. In: Wilson JD, Foster DW, eds. *Williams textbook of endocrinology*, 8th ed., Philadelphia: WB Saunders, 1992; and from Marshall WA, Tanner JM. Variations in pattern of pubertal changes in girls. *Arch Dis Child* 1969;44:291.)

stages—also termed *Sexual Maturity Rating* (SMR)—for breast development are as follows (Fig. 4-7) (14, 42):

Stage B1 (preadolescent): elevation of the papilla only

Stage B2 (breast-bud stage): elevation of the breast and papilla as a small mound, enlargement of the areolar diameter

Stage B3: further enlargement of the breast and areola with no separation of their contours

Stage B4: further enlargement with projection of the areola and papilla to form a secondary mound above the level of the breast

Stage B5 (mature stage): projection of the papilla only, resulting from recession of the areola to the general contour of the breast

The pubic hair stages are as follows (Fig. 4-8) (14,42):

Stage PH1 (preadolescent): The vellus over the pubes is not further developed than that over the anterior abdominal wall; no pubic hair.

Stage PH2: Sparse growth of long, slightly pigmented, downy hair, straight or only slightly curled, appearing chiefly along the labia.

Stage PH3: Hair darker, coarser, and curlier spreads to extend sparsely over the junction of the pubes.

Stage PH4: Hair adult in type spreads over the mons pubis but not to the medial surface of the thighs.

Stage PH5 (mature stage): Hair adult in quantity and type spreads to the medial surfaces of the thighs; distribution in an inverse triangle forms the classic feminine pattern.

The mean age of each pubertal stage for British girls is shown in Fig. 4-9. The ages of normal sexual development for American girls are shown in Table 4-2 (43).

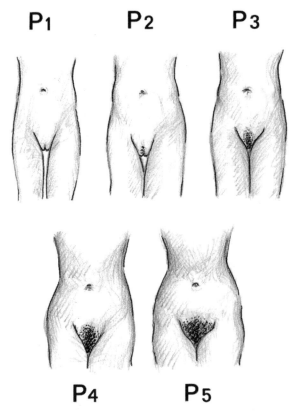

P1　　**P2**　　**P3**

P4　　**P5**

FIG. 4-8. The Tanner stages for the development of female pubic hair. (Adapted from Grumbach MM, Styne DM. Puberty: Ontogeny, neuroendocrinology, physiology and disorders. In: Wilson JD, Foster DW, eds. *Williams textbook of endocrinology*, 8th ed., Philadelphia: WB Saunders, 1992; and from Marshall WA, Tanner JM. Variations in pattern of pubertal changes in girls. *Arch Dis Child* 1969;44:291.)

The first sign of puberty in 85% to 92% of white girls is breast budding, which may initially be unilateral. Some girls pass from stage B3 directly to stage B5, and some remain in stage B4. Developmental stages are assessed most accurately by observation of sequential changes in an individual girl. In the series of Marshall and Tanner (42), the mean interval from stage B2 to stage B5 was 4.2 years. Pubic hair development usually lags by about 6 months and appears at an average age of 11 to 12 years. Pubic hair as the first sign of development may be a normal variant (especially in those of African-American descent), but in some girls, it may reflect an excess of androgens that later may cause hirsutism and menstrual irregularity (see Chapter 9). The mean interval from stages PH2 to stage PH5 is 2.7 years. Generally, pubic hair will not advance beyond stage PH2 or PH3 in the absence of gonadal sex steroids. The beginning of breast development usually corresponds to

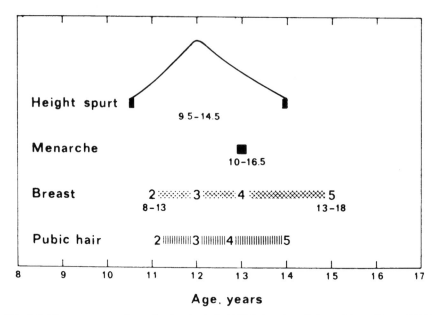

FIG. 4-9. The sequence of events at puberty in British females. (Adapted from Marshall WA, Tanner JM. Variations in pattern of pubertal changes in girls. *Arch Dis Child* 1969;44:291.)

TABLE 4-2. Mean Ages (in Years) at Onset of Pubic Hair, Breast Development, and Menarche for 3 Racial/Ethnic Groups of US Girls: NHANES III, 1988–1994

Puberty Milestone	Non-Hispanic White		Black		Mexican American	
	Mean Age (95% CI)	Mean Age*	Mean Age (95% CI)	Mean Age*	Mean Age (95% CI)	Mean Age*
Pubic Hair**	10.6 (10.4, 10.9)	10.5	9.5 (9.2, 9.8)	9.5	10.3 (10.1, 10.6)	10.3
Breast development***	10.3 (10.0, 10.5)	10.3	9.5 (9.3, 9.8)	9.5	9.7 (9.4, 9.1)	9.8
Menarche**	12.6 (12.4, 12.8)	12.7	12.2 (12.0, 12.4)	12.1	12.2 (12.0, 12.5)	12.2
Menarche***	12.7 (12.5, 12.8)	12.7	12.4 (12.2, 12.5)	12.3	12.5 (12.3, 12.6)	12.5

CI indicates confidence interval.
*Estimated with application of weights from the examination sample of NHANES III.
**Estimated using probit model for the status quo data of the puberty measurements.
***Estimated using failure time model for the recalled age of menarche.
(From Wu T, Mendola P, Buck GM, Ethnic differences in the presence of secondary sex characteristics and menarche among US girls: The Third National Health and Nutrition Examination Survey, 1988–1994, *Pediatrics* 2002;110:752, with permission).

the onset of the growth spurt. The timing of these events is variable, but 98.8% of girls have the first signs of sexual development between the ages of 8 and 13 years.

Data from a large cross-sectional observational study of more than 17,000 girls by community pediatricians noted an even earlier age of pubertal development (44). They noted that among 8- to 9-year-old girls, 7.7% of white girls and 34.3% of African-American girls had Tanner stage 2 or greater pubic hair and that 5% of white girls and 15.4% of African-American girls had Tanner stage 2 or greater breast development. Among girls 12 to 13 years of age, 96% of white girls and 99% of African-American girls had breast development, and 92% of white girls and 99% of African-American girls had pubic hair development. However, it should be noted that Tanner stage 2 breast development may be difficult to identify in obese prepubertal girls, and Biro and colleagues (45) have suggested the utility of the Garn–Falkner system for staging areola. With this system, four areolar stages are identified on the basis of areolar diameter, pigmentation, and contour, with areolar stage 1 being prepubertal. Areolar stage 2 displays palpable subareolar tissue, an increase in size and pigmentation of the areola, and little development of the papilla. Areolar stage 3 has a further increase in size and pigment of the areola, with separation of the areola and papilla from the contour of the breast. Areolar stage 4 has an elevation of the papilla and regression of the areola, with a mature size and color of the areola (not all women develop stage 4). Comparison is made to staging plates. Biro (45) reported that 9 of 15 girls in breast Tanner stage 2 were in areolar stage 1.

Recent data from the Third National Health and Nutrition Examination Survey (NHANES III) showed that black girls entered puberty on average before Mexican-American or white girls (Table 4-2) (43). Using data from 1623 girls from this national survey, black and Mexican-American girls had pubic hair and breast development at younger ages than white girls. In that study, 49.4% of black girls age 9 years had breast development compared with 24.5% of Mexican-American girls and 15.8% of white girls. The mean age of onset of pubic hair, breast development, and menarche for each ethnic group is shown in Table 4-2. The ethnic differences remained even after adjustment for body mass index and specific socioeconomic variables (43). Using this same data set, Sun and colleagues examined racial and ethnic differences in the timing of sexual maturation in both boys and girls (46). Non-Hispanic black girls and boys were found to mature earlier than other ethnic groups, but the children studied in this sample of American youth completed their sexual maturation at approximately the same ages. Kaplowitz and colleagues (47) examined whether nutritional status (i.e., prevalence of obesity) affects timing of puberty. Figure 4-10 is a graphic comparison of white 6- to 9-year old girls with and without breast development. The mean BMI Z-score for each age was markedly greater in girls with compared to without breast development ($p < 0.001$). Their results, also from the NHANES III data set, suggest that obesity is an important contributing factor. However, factors other than obesity are needed to explain the prevalence of earlier puberty in black compared to white girls. These data derived from a large diverse national sample provide meaningful normative reference data regarding the timing of puberty across ethnicity and gender (46).

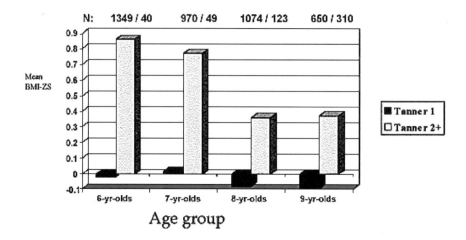

FIG. 4-10. Mean BMI Z-score in 6- to 9-year old white girls with and without breast development from NHANES III sample. The number of girls for each age and Tanner stage is shown above the bars. All of the differences are significant at *p* > 0.001. (From Kaplowitz PB, et al. Earlier onset of puberty in girls: relation to increased body mass index and race. *Pediatrics* 2001; 108:347–353; with permission.)

Breast development before 8 years of age is generally considered precocious and will require further evaluation (see Chapter 5). A girl who has experienced no breast development by the age of 13 is 2 standard deviations from the norm, has delayed development, and should be evaluated to determine the specific cause of the delay (see Chapter 6). It is also extremely unlikely for a young woman to achieve full stage B5 breast development without pubic hair development; this occurrence raises the question of an androgen insensitivity (testicular feminization) syndrome or adrenal insufficiency (see Chapters 2, 7, and 10). The development of pubic hair without any evidence of breast development suggests the presence of androgens alone and raises the possibility of either estrogen deficiency such as Kallmann syndrome or a virilized state such as an intersex disorder. The normal changes in LH, FSH, estradiol, testosterone, DHEA, DHEAS, and androstenedione are shown in Fig. 4-11 (48).

GROWTH PATTERNS

The growth spurt is dependent on the onset of puberty. Growth charts, such as those illustrated in Figs. 4-12 (49) and 4-13 (50) are helpful in evaluating normal development. Special growth charts for Turner syndrome patients (see Chapter 6) can be obtained from Genentech or the Turner Syndrome Society. The inserts (the increment curves) on the charts in Fig. 4-12 (49) represent velocities, that is, the peak is at the maximum rate of linear growth and weight gain. The peak height

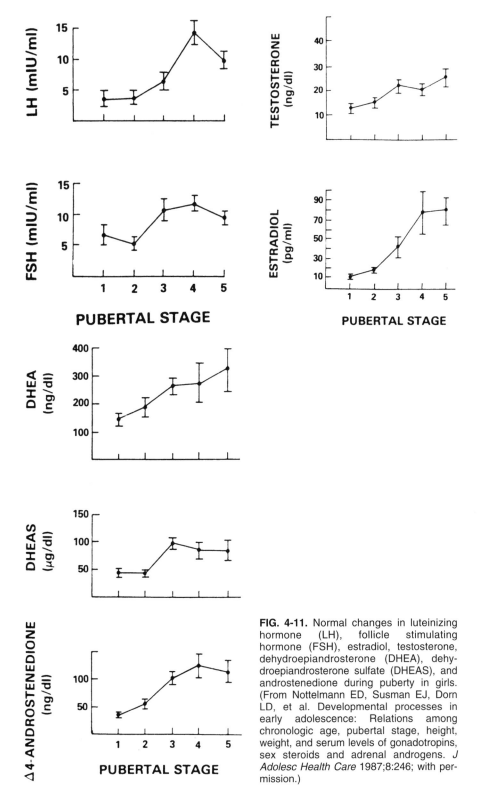

FIG. 4-11. Normal changes in luteinizing hormone (LH), follicle stimulating hormone (FSH), estradiol, testosterone, dehydroepiandrosterone (DHEA), dehydroepiandrosterone sulfate (DHEAS), and androstenedione during puberty in girls. (From Nottelmann ED, Susman EJ, Dorn LD, et al. Developmental processes in early adolescence: Relations among chronologic age, pubertal stage, height, weight, and serum levels of gonadotropins, sex steroids and adrenal androgens. *J Adolesc Health Care* 1987;8:246; with permission.)

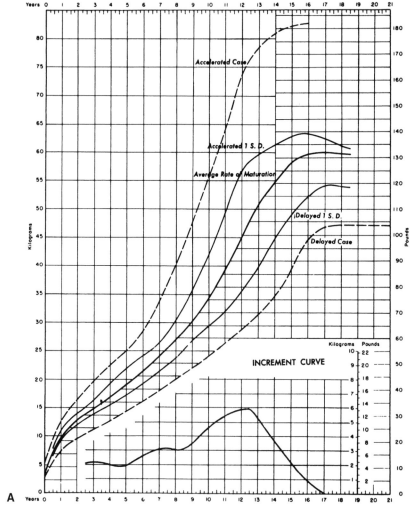

FIG. 4-12. Growth charts. **(A)** Weight.

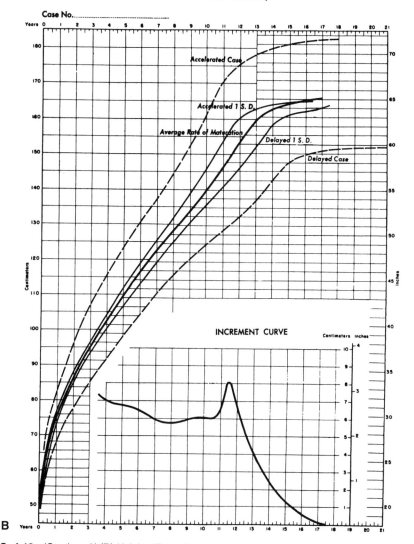

FIG. 4-12. *(Continued.)* **(B)** Height. (From Bayley N. Growth curves of height and weight by age for boys and girls, scaled according to physical maturity. *J Pediatr* 1956;48:187; with permission.)

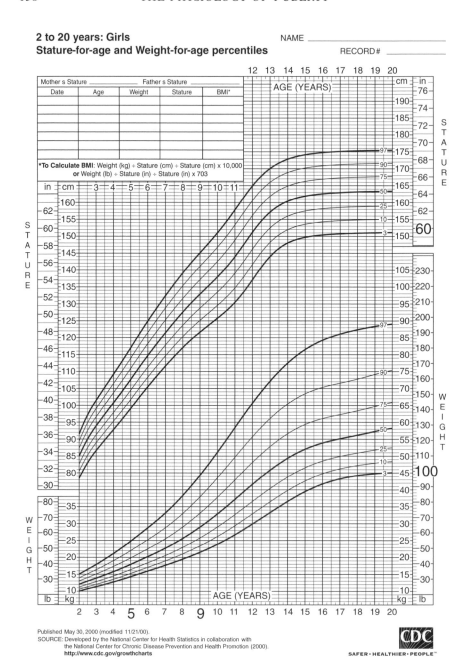

FIG. 4-13. Growth chart. Height and weight percentiles. [Adapted from the National Center for Health Statistics in collaboration with the National Center for Chronic Disease Prevention and Health Promotion (2000).]

velocity is attained in the majority of girls before they reach Tanner stages B3 and PH2. The growth chart in Fig. 4-13 (50) represents data from the National Center for Health Statistics in collaboration with the National Center for Chronic Disease Prevention and Health Promotion (2000). It should be noted that the CDC growth charts are available for download in two formats: (a) charts with the outer limits of the curves (highest and lowest percentiles) of 95% and 5% for routine clinical assessments and (b) charts with the outer limits of 97% and 3% for selective applications such as charting children with growth problems or special health care requirements (most charts in this book use the latter format). Because the data in Fig. 4-13 are cross-sectional rather than longitudinal, as in Fig. 4-12, the pubertal growth spurt is not seen clearly on Fig. 4-13. The average girl grows 2 to 3 in. during the 2 years following menarche. BMI is now being given closer consideration, and normative data are available, especially to determine the significance of weight extremes (obesity or anorexia), and how this index may relate to pubertal development and menarche (http://www.cdc.gov/growthcharts).

Skeletal proportions are determined by the rate of pubertal development. The upper/lower (U/L) body ratio is approximately 1.0 by the age of 10 years, L being the distance from the patient's symphysis pubis to the floor, with the patient standing, and U the height minus L. At puberty, the extremities rapidly increase in length, while the vertebral column lengthens more gradually. Initially, the U/L ratio may dip to 0.9. As the epiphyses of the legs close, the vertebrae continue to add height, and thus the final adult U/L ratio approximates 1.0. In patients with hypogonadism, the lower segment becomes relatively longer because of delayed fusion; thus, the U/L ratio may be approximately 0.8. Span (the distance between the fingertips of outstretched arms) usually reflects the same clinical situation; if the span is more than 2 in. greater than the height, the patient has eunuchoid proportions. A short span suggests skeletal disproportion, as in skeletal dysplasias. Athletes who have undergone intensive training during the prepubertal years may have delayed development and menarche, along with delayed epiphyseal closure, and therefore may have arm spans longer than normal.

BONE DEVELOPMENT AND ACCRETION

The adolescent years are a critical period for the development of peak bone mass (or an adolescent's "bone bank"). During the teenage years, at least half of peak bone mass is achieved, modulated by growth hormone, sex hormones such as estrogen, and adrenal steroids such as dehydroepiandrosterone (DHEA) (51–55). Optimal dietary calcium and vitamin D are also important for efficient deposition of mineralized calcium into the skeleton (55–57). In an adolescent girl, approximately 90% of total body mineral content appears to be accrued by the age of 16.9 years (58–59), and rates of calcium absorption and bone formation decrease significantly with postmenarchal age following onset of menses (59). Exercise, and especially an activity associated with weight-bearing, is another important modifiable determinant of peak

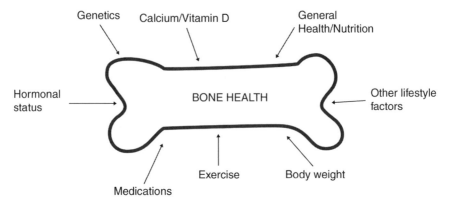

FIG. 4-14. Factors that affect bone development. (Adapted from Gordon CM: Bone density in the adolescent gynecology patients. *J Adolesc Ped Gyn* 2000;13:157–161; with permission.)

bone mass (60–61). However, weight–bearing exercise may have the greatest impact on bone mineral density (BMD) when initiated before the completion of puberty (59). Finally, genetic factors account for 60% to 80% of the variance seen in BMD (62–63) (Fig. 4-14).

Several previous studies have provided evidence to support the conclusion that up to 60% of adult bone mass is acquired during the adolescent growth spurt (51–52,54,58–59,64–67). In addition to the factors mentioned above, bone mass is determined by dietary factors (e.g., vitamin D, calcium, protein), muscle strength, tobacco use, and weight (51–52,54–55,57–61,64–65). Bone density increases in both black and white girls during puberty, but the magnitude of the increase is greater in black girls, who eventually have a higher vertebral bone density at the end of puberty and a higher weight than white girls (66). A recent report found increased calcium absorption in black compared to white teenage girls that may account in part for the higher bone density seen in black adolescents compared to other ethnic groups (68). Bonjour and colleagues (51) and Theintz and colleagues (52) reported marked acceleration of bone mass acquisition during early adolescence (ages 11 to 14 years in girls) (Figs. 4-15 and 4-16). In their study, little bone mass accumulated after 15 years (Tanner stage 5). Rubin and colleagues (67) have similarly noted accelerated bone mass acquisition during puberty, beginning at the age of 10 years in girls, and observed a positive impact of physical activity and calcium intake. Skeletal mineralization at puberty appears to be particularly dependent on the site, with marked gains in areas with a predominance of trabecular bone (e.g., lumbar spine). Weight changes correlate with trabecular mineralization, and height more strongly correlates with cortical bone changes (65).

Although the preponderance of evidence points to the acquisition of most bone mass during early adolescence, Recker and colleagues (69) reported some gains during late adolescence and young adulthood. In a study of 156 college-age women attending professional schools, they observed that 6.8% of lumbar bone mineral density

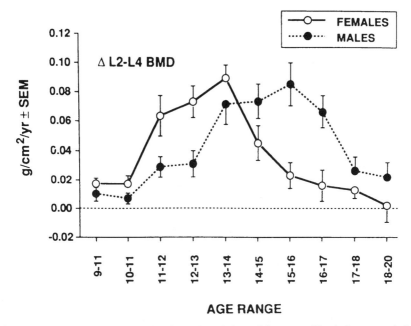

FIG. 4-15. Bone mass gain at the lumbar spine during adolescence. Yearly increases in lumbar bone mineral density (BMD) (L2-L4). (From Theintz G, Buchs B, Rizzoli R, et al. Longitudinal monitoring of bone mass accumulation in a healthy adolescent: evidence for a marked reduction after 16 years of age at the levels of lumbar spine and femoral neck in female subjects. *J Clin Endocrinol Metab* 1992;75:1060–1065; copyright 1992, The Endocrine Society; with permission.)

and 12.5% of total body bone mass was achieved in the third decade of life. The rate of bone density gain correlated positively with calcium/protein intake and physical activity and negatively with age. Oral contraceptive use was associated with a greater gain in total body bone mass.

The specific issue of whether oral contraceptive pills (OCs) have a significant effect on BMD in adolescents and young women is an area of both interest and debate (see Chapter 20). In healthy adult women, OCs have been shown to be beneficial for bone density in some (69–71), but not all studies (72–74). Considering recent studies in healthy adolescents and young adults, there appears to be no significant negative impact of OCs (30 to 40 µg of EE) on BMD (75–77), but whether there are positive effects is less clear. Noteworthy are findings from the prospective 5-year study of Polatti and colleagues in which there was no change seen in BMD in those healthy young women receiving a 20 µg OC compared with a +7.8% increase in the untreated control group (78). The authors speculate that endogenous gonadal steroid production was suppressed by the OC, and the replacement dose administered was inadequate for achievement of peak bone mass. However, other unreported factors may have accounted for the differences observed. Differing doses and prepa-

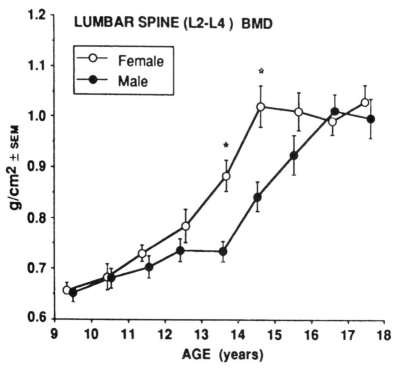

FIG. 4-16. Sex differences in age-related increment in bone mineral density (BMD) at the level of the lumbar spine (L2-L4) by age. (From Bonjour J-P, Theintz G, Buchs B, et al. Critical years and stages of puberty for spinal and femoral bone mass accumulation during adolescence. *J Clin Endocrinol Metab* 1991;73:555–563; copyright 1991, The Endocrine Society; with permission.)

rations of estrogens and progestins, differences in study design, and varying analyses of potential confounders may account for the varying results found among studies.

The management of the young woman with hypothalamic amenorrhea is another area of controversy and research. Gordon and colleagues evaluated the effect of a 1-year course of a 20 µg OC compared to oral DHEA in a cohort of young women with anorexia nervosa. Although no significant gains were seen in either group after controlling for weight gain, maintenance of bone density was seen in this group at high risk for bone loss. In addition, both treatment groups showed significant suppression of bone resorption (79). Recent *in vitro* data complement these clinical findings as both DHEA and estradiol have been shown in human bone marrow cultures to exhibit antiresorptive effects (80). In another study, Warren and colleagues investigated the effect of replacement therapy of conjugated estrogens (0.625 mg daily), in addition to medroxyprogesterone acetate (10 mg daily) for 25 days of the month over 2 years. BMD of the foot, wrist and spine did not change in either treated or placebo group. These findings suggest that mechanisms other than estrogen deficiency are responsible for the bone loss associated with exercise-induced amenorrhea (81). Continued research is needed to delineate the ideal hormonal and nutritional treatment regimen for young women, especially for patients with hypothalamic amenorrhea (see Chapter 7).

MENARCHE

The mean age at menarche in Tanner's classic series of English girls was 13.46 ± 0.46 years, with a range of 9 to 16 years. In a 1969 study by Zacharias and Wurtman (82), the mean age of menarche among student nurses in the United States was 12.65 ± 1.2 years. Recent findings from NHANES III included a median age of menarche of 12.43 years for U.S. girls (32), data similar to that reported for U.S. girls in the National Health Examination Survey of 1973 (83). The similar age of menarche compared to reports from over three decades prior (82,83) suggests that American girls are not progressively gaining earlier reproductive potential. In NHANES III, there were also ethnic differences noted, with the age of menarche of non-Hispanic black girls being significantly earlier than that of non-Hispanic white or Mexican-American girls (32). In a large study, Herman-Giddens reported that by age 12 to 13, 35% of white girls and 62% of African-American girls had initiated menses (44). Table 14-3 (42) shows that most patients in the Tanner study had attained stage 4 breast and pubic hair development at the time of menarche. In Tanner's series, the mean interval from breast development to menarche was 2.3 ± 0.1 years, but the range was 0.5 to 5.75 years. A late onset of pubertal development did not appear to change the intervals between the stages of pubic hair and breast development.

Frisch (84) established a nomogram predicting the age of menarche based on height and weight at the ages of 9 to 13 years, using her observation that menarche was associated with the attainment of a critical body weight (an average of 46 to 47 kg for American and most European girls), the percentage of body fat being the important determinant. According to this theory, a minimum fatness level of about 17% of body weight is necessary for the onset of menstrual cycles, and a minimum of 22% fat is necessary to maintain regular ovulatory cycles (84–85). Early- and late-maturing girls begin their adolescent growth spurt with a weight of about 30 kg. The apparent decline in the age of menarche from the late 1800s to the mid-1900s has been attributed to im-

TABLE 4-3. *Percentage of patients in stages 1 through 5 at time of menarche*

Stage	Breast (% of patients)	Pubic hair (% of patients)
1	0	1
2	1	4
3	26	19
4	62	63
5	11	14

(Adapted from Marshall WA and Tanner JM. Variations in pattern of pubertal changes in girls. *Arch Dis Child* 1969;44:291.)

proved nutrition and in the past two decades, the lack of a further age decline is attributed to the attainment of optimal nutrition (86). Gymnasts, ballet dancers, and long-distance runners with reduced weights and (calculated) percentages of body fat often experience significant delays in development and menarche, especially if their training began in the prepubertal years. Since estrogens are also produced by aromatization of androgen precursors in fat, a low percentage of body fat may contribute less estrogen, which is necessary for hypothalamic–pituitary regulation and the onset of vaginal bleeding. Although helpful in providing an estimate of menarche or resumption of menses, the critical weight hypothesis has been questioned and criticized (87–91). The theory remains controversial primarily because the secretion of GnRH and gonadotropins begins many years before menarche, percentages of body fat are often only calculated figures, and weight at the time of menarche can show tremendous variation in individual girls. Gonzales and Villena (92) reported that the association of body weight, body mass index, or height with menarche is coincidental instead of critical for menarche. Accumulating evidence suggests that maturational timing affects body composition and has a greater long-term effect on fatness than the influence of body fat on the timing of sexual maturation (47,86,92–94).

In a retrospective series, Zacharias and Wurtman (82,95) found that the interval between menarche and regular periods was approximately 14 months, and the interval between menarche and painful (presumably) ovulatory cycles was approximately 24 months. However, ovulatory cycles can begin during the first year following menarche and may be associated with shortened luteal phases. Data from Finland (23) demonstrated that in the first 2 years after menarche, 55% to 82% of cycles were anovulatory (the figure depends on whether only samples drawn <10 days until the next menstrual bleeding or all samples drawn on days 20 to 23 of the menstrual cycle were considered). By 3 years after menarche, the percentage of anovulatory cycles decreased to 50%, and by 5 years, to 10% to 20% (13,23). It appears that the later the age of menarche the longer the interval before 50% of cycles are ovulatory. Apter and Vihko (96) found that this interval was 1 year if menarche occurred before the age of 12 years, 3 years when menarche occurred at 12.0 to 12.9 years, and 4.5 years when menarche was after 13 years of age.

HORMONE LEVELS IN NORMAL OVULATORY CYCLES

The establishment of ovulatory cycles depends on the maturation of a positive feedback mechanism in which rising estrogen levels trigger an LH surge at midcycle. Understanding the hormone changes responsible for ovulation allows the health care provider to understand the pathophysiology of polycystic ovary syndrome (see Chapter 9), amenorrhea, and dysfunctional uterine bleeding (see Chapter 8). Figure 4-3 demonstrates the complex interactions between the changes in the ovary during ovulation and the influence of gonadotropins.

The menstrual cycle is divided into three phases: follicular, ovulatory, and luteal. In the early follicular phase of the menstrual cycle (Fig. 4-17), pulsatile GnRH

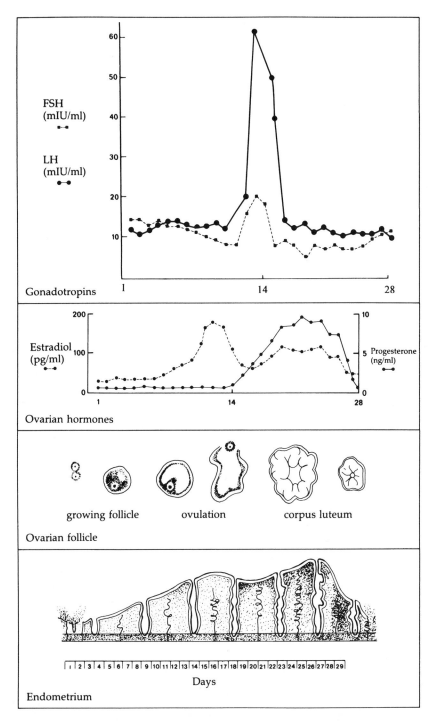

FIG. 4-17. Physiology of the normal ovulatory menstrual cycle: gonadotropin secretion, ovarian hormone production, follicular maturation, and endometrial changes during one cycle. FSH, follicle-stimulating hormone; LH, luteinizing hormone.

145

released from the hypothalamus stimulates the secretion of FSH and LH from the pituitary. In turn, FSH increases the number of granulosa cells in the ovarian follicle, increases the number of receptors for FSH on the granulosa cells, and induces the granulosa cells to acquire an aromatizing enzyme that provides the essential step for the conversion of androgen precursors to estradiol. Estradiol also increases the number of granulosa cells and the number of FSH receptors, which thus leads to further amplification of the effect of FSH. The theca cells, under LH stimulation, secrete androstenedione, testosterone, and estradiol into the bloodstream and also into the follicle as substrate. Usually, a single dominant follicle emerges by day 5 to day 7 of the cycle. The rising estradiol level increases the number of glandular cells and stroma in the endometrium of the uterus. By the midfollicular phase, FSH is beginning to decline, in part because of estrogen-mediated negative feedback. Inhibin, which is secreted by granulosa cells and blocks FSH synthesis and release, rises in the late follicular phase of the cycle, paralleling the rise of estradiol. The highest levels are found during the luteal phase and, together with estradiol and progesterone, appear to play a role in the regulation of FSH in that phase of the cycle as well. Inhibin B reaches a nadir during the midluteal period. Inhibin A reaches a peak during the luteal phase, potentially playing a role in the suppression of FSH secretion to the lowest levels reached during a menstrual cycle (97). Activins, also secreted by the granulosa cells, stimulate FSH secretion. The dominant follicle has the richest blood supply and the most estrogen production and granulosa aromatase. The increased number of FSH receptors on the dominant follicle allows it to continue to respond even as rising estrogen levels lower the FSH. Locally, in the dominant follicle, estradiol levels are greater than androstenedione levels, whereas androstenedione levels are greater than estradiol levels in the atretic follicles.

In a classic group of clinical studies, Crowley's group at the Massachusetts General Hospital (98) has characterized the sleep latency changes in LH that occur during the normal ovulatory menstrual cycle. The LH interpulse interval decreased from a mean of 94 minutes in the early follicular phase to 71 minutes in the late follicular phase, with a change in the mean pulse amplitude from 6.5 mIU/ml in the early follicular phase to 5.1 mIU/ml in the midfollicular phase, to 7.2 mIU/ml in the late follicular phase. In the luteal phase, the LH pulse interval progressively increased from a mean of 103 minutes in the early luteal phase to 216 minutes in the late luteal phase. The mean pulse amplitude was highest in the early luteal phase (14.9 mIU/ml) and decreased to 12.2 mIU/ml in the midluteal phase and to 7.6 mIU/ml by the late luteal phase. FSH was closely correlated to LH secretion.

In the periovulatory phase of the cycle, the dominant follicle is clearly evident; it has increased receptors for LH and secretes increasing levels of estradiol. The rising estrogen levels produce a further proliferation of the endometrium, with increasing length of the glands. The rising LH levels appear to induce a block in steroid pathways, which initiates secretion of 17-hydroxyprogesterone and progesterone and the gradual luteinization of the granulosa cells. The exact mechanism for the positive feedback effect of rising estrogen and progesterone levels on the midcycle release of multiple pulses of LH is unknown. By midpuberty, the hypothalamic–pituitary unit is capable of this positive feedback response. Following the surge of LH, follicular rupture and expulsion of the oocyte occur (ovulation).

The development of the corpus luteum is affected by levels of LH and the rupture of the follicle. As noted, GnRH and thus LH are released in slower pulses. The corpus luteum secretes progesterone and 17-hydroxyprogesterone. Plasma progesterone concentrations are stable over 24-hour studies in the early luteal phase and show no relationship to LH pulses; however, in the middle and late luteal phases, progesterone levels rapidly fluctuate during 24-hour studies from levels as low as 2.3 ng/ml to peaks of 40.1 ng/ml, and they correlate with LH pulses (99). Thus, a single progesterone level in the middle to late luteal phase of the cycle may not always predict the adequacy of the corpus luteum.

Under the influence of rising progesterone and estrogen levels, the endometrium enters the secretory phase, which is characterized by coiling of the endometrial glands, increased vascularity of the stroma, and increased glycogen content of the epithelial cells. Maturation of the endometrium is reached within 8 or 9 days after ovulation, and if fertilization does not occur, regression begins. Exact dating of the endometrium is possible because of the date-specific changes in the structure of the endometrial cells. Evidence for ovulation and the occurrence of a luteal phase may be obtained by endometrial biopsy, basal body temperature charts, and measurement of serum progesterone levels (>10 ng/ml).

Without pregnancy and the concomitant rise in placental human chorionic gonadotropin (HCG) levels, luteolysis begins, and progesterone and estrogen levels begin to decline. Unlike HCG, the luteotropic support of LH cannot extend the life of the corpus luteum beyond 14 days. In contrast to the variable length of the follicular phase, the luteal phase is usually constant at 14 days. Thus, the life span of the corpus luteum is determined by a preset "clock" with time to allow implantation and retention until trophoblastic HCG intervenes. The mechanisms behind the process of luteolysis are unclear, with the demise of the corpus luteum affecting inhibin A secretion as well as steroidogenesis (97). Inhibin A suppresses FSH secretion during this phase of the cycle. The selective action of inhibin on FSH is partly responsible for the rise in FSH seen during the luteal-follicular transition (3,97). With the waning of progesterone and estrogen levels, the endometrium undergoes necrotic changes that result in menstrual bleeding. The stage for the new cycle is in fact set in the late luteal phase when plasma FSH begins to rise to initiate follicular development.

Several researchers have studied adolescent cycles as they pass from anovulatory to ovulatory cycles (33,100). Apter and co-workers (100) reported that in adolescents, follicular development was slower and eventual ovulation took place from a smaller follicle than in older women (ages 25 to 35 years). In adults, the concentration of FSH decreased from day 4 to day 10 of the cycle, whereas in adolescents the FSH level increased. The selection of the dominant follicle seemed disturbed, with seven of eight adolescent patients studied still having several follicles of 8 to 14 mm on days 12 to 15 of the cycle. In the last 3 days before ovulation, the mean increase in the diameter of the dominant follicle was 2.9 mm in the adolescent group and 5.6 mm in the adult group. Ovulation occurred later in the cycle in adolescents than in adults (mean of 5 days longer). Apter and co-workers (33) had previously shown a negative correlation between the FSH concentration on days 3 to 4 of the cycle and the length of the follicular phase. In comparison with adolescents, the adults had slightly but significantly higher mean maximal progesterone levels during the luteal phase.

Apter and co-workers (100) have described several distinct patterns in adolescents with anovulatory cycles. One pattern was characterized by low estradiol levels without LH at midcycle and minor or no follicular growth. A second pattern was characterized by developing follicles, slightly higher estradiol, and minor increases in LH at midcycle. A third pattern was identical to an ovulatory pattern, with an increase in follicular development, increased estradiol levels, and an LH surge but no evidence of ovulation (no rise in progesterone, no cul-de-sac fluid by ultrasound, menses 3 to 4 days after the LH surge). Others have found similar patterns in adolescents and adult women involved in strenuous athletic competition. Bonen and associates (101) found that competitive swimmers may have an LH surge at midcycle but no rise in serum progesterone; abnormal FSH secretion during the first half of the cycle may inadequately prepare the follicle for ovulation. The time from the LH surge to menstruation was 4 or 5 days, resembling the third pattern described by Apter and co-workers. Shangold and associates (102) determined that the luteal phase in a healthy adult runner shortened as she increased her weekly mileage.

In adolescents, the gonadotropin response to a dose of exogenous GnRH appears to change during the follicular phase in the first 2 postmenarcheal years toward that observed in adult women and in the luteal phase from the third to the fifth postmenarcheal year (102, 103). Another pattern that appears to occur early in the adolescent years in association with menstrual irregularity is the overproduction of adrenal and ovarian androgens. Venturoli and associates (104, 105) found that adolescents with persistent anovulatory menses maintained marked hyperandrogenism, increasingly high LH levels, and enlarged multicystic ovaries. Mean testosterone and androstenedione were higher than in ovulatory cycles and in adult controls. The persistence of this pattern sets the stage for classic polycystic ovary syndrome (see Chapter 9) with rapid pulses of GnRH and LH. In contrast, adolescents with anovulatory cycles and normal LH levels were more similar to ovulatory adolescents. Venturoli and associates (104) have suggested that the pulsatile pattern of GnRH and gonadotropin secretion account for the endocrine differences in these groups of postmenarcheal adolescents. In addition, they have suggested that in the postmenarcheal period, progesterone, by modulating LH and FSH pulsatility and thus reducing androgen levels and their action on producing atresia of follicles, may be a regulatory factor in enhancing normal cyclicity.

The term *hypothalamic amenorrhea* has been used to apply to the common problem in which, despite a normal pituitary and ovaries, normal cyclic changes do not occur. The hormonal pattern seen often represents a psychobiologic response to life events (106). In many cases, reduction of metabolic fuel availability below a critical level (e.g., that induced by food restriction) is appropriately accompanied by neuroendocrine-metabolic changes that result in anovulation and amenorrhea (107). Previous work has suggested that abnormalities in pulsatile GnRH are involved and may include a spectrum of changes. The frequency of LH pulses is reduced in most women with hypothalamic amenorrhea (107,108), which suggests that GnRH pulses are too infrequent to stimulate normal follicular maturation. Data from monkeys indicate that corticotropin-releasing hormone (CRH) inhibits gonadotropin secretion, likely by augmenting endogenous opioid secretion (109). Stress likely inhibits reproductive function through this pathway. Women with hypothalamic amenorrhea have reduced secretion of gonadotropins and prolactin, but increased secretion of cortisol (110–112). There is also data suggesting that some patients with hypothalamic amenorrhea have dopaminergic inhibition of GnRH pulse frequency (113). Thus, increases in endogenous opioids and dopamine may account for the suppression of GnRH pulsatile secretion in these patients.

CLINICAL APPLICATIONS

An understanding of the normal cycle is useful in the clinical management of patients with menstrual problems. In patients with anovulatory cycles, the ovary produces continuous levels of estrogen, and thus the endometrium remains in the proliferative phase; menstrual periods may be heavy and irregular. Regulation can often be obtained with medroxyprogesterone (Provera) given 14 days each month to produce a secretory endometrium; 1 to 7 days after taking medroxyprogesterone, the patient then has a menstrual period. In the evaluation of the patient with amenorrhea, a withdrawal flow after intramuscular progesterone or oral medroxyprogesterone has been given implies that the endometrium has been adequately primed with estrogen (see Chapter 7).

Quantification of serum FSH and LH by radioimmunoassay is readily available; laboratories vary both in normal values and in units per milliliter (mIU/ml or ng/ml). Because gonadotropins are released in a pulsatile fashion, a single random serum value of LH and FSH may not be helpful in distinguishing between low and normal levels of these hormones. Variability is common in normal menstrual cycles (114). Using the assay system of Nottelmann et al., FSH or LH levels of 5 to 25 mIU/ml are in the normal range; consistently low values of 2 to 4 mIU/ml may imply hypothalamic or pituitary hypofunction. An FSH level >50 to 60 mIU/ml and an LH level >40 mIU/ml in a prepubertal or poorly estrogenized female imply ovarian failure; such high levels are also found in the postmenopausal woman. Newer assays have reference levels of >30 mIU/ml for the postmenopausal or ovarian failure range (3). In addition, an elevated serum LH with normal FSH in an amenorrheic or oligomenorrheic adolescent may suggest an androgen excess/polycystic ovary syndrome (see Chapter 9). Gonadotropin levels and serum androgen levels should be measured in the oligomenorrheic patient who has hirsutism, acne, or signs of virilization. It is always important to know when the blood samples for FSH and LH levels were drawn in relation to the menstrual cycle, if any. The last menstrual period should be recorded at the time of the office visit, and the patient should be instructed to keep a calendar and call with the date of the next menses. If no menses have occurred by 4 weeks after the visit, the clinician should record this fact to aid in interpreting the levels.

Frequent sampling of the serum for LH and FSH levels over a 24-hour period or over a menstrual cycle has been useful in research settings for investigating normal and abnormal physiology. Clinically, pituitary function can also be studied by the administration of a GnRH stimulation test. A single dose of GnRH is given intravenously or subcutaneously, and serum LH and FSH levels are measured at frequent intervals over a 4-hour period. The LH values should increase 150% *above* baseline in normal pubertal patients (9) (see Table 4-1 for normal responses). Girls with isosexual central precocious puberty will respond with a pubertal LH and FSH response, whereas those with premature thelarche or puberty secondary to an ovarian tumor respond with a prepubertal response. Patients with anorexia nervosa and craniopharyngiomas usually have little response to GnRH, whereas those with prolactin-secreting pituitary microadenomas have a normal pubertal response. Patients with Kallmann syndrome (hypogonadotropic hypogonadism) have heterogeneous responses to GnRH; some may have minimal response to the single dose of GnRH and require longer administration of pulsatile GnRH to cause normal release of LH and FSH.

The observation (2,115–116) that pulsatile GnRH results in secretion of LH and FSH but that the continuous infusion of GnRH results in the suppression of LH and FSH led to GnRH treatment modalities for precocious puberty in children (see Chapter 5). GnRH analogs are also useful for ovarian suppression in the treatment of endometriosis, polycystic ovary syndrome, severe premenstrual syndrome, and, possibly, hormonally dependent malignancies. In addition, the ovarian suppression also results in amenorrhea, which may be helpful in the treatment of some medical diseases (see Chapter 23).

The measurement of serum estrogen, progesterone, and androgen levels is now possible in many laboratories, although variation in quality control and normal levels makes interpretation, especially of androgen levels, problematic at times. In addition, the fact that most of these levels vary during the day and during the menstrual cycle must be kept in mind when one is drawing conclusions from these levels. For example, girls in the early stages of puberty may have low daytime FSH and LH levels and undetectable or very low estradiol levels in spite of normal maturation. As noted, progesterone is secreted in pulses, and thus a single level cannot assess the adequacy of the luteal phase in infertile patients. The importance of the physical examination should not be underestimated, despite the ability to measure many hormone levels. The response of the target organs to these hormones is essential to a correct diagnosis. Pubertal breast development, a pink moist vaginal mucosa, and watery cervical mucus are all signs that suggest functional ovaries and the secretion of estrogen. From the presence of normal axillary and pubic hair, the physician can infer functioning adrenal glands and circulating androgens. Hirsutism and clitoromegaly are signs of androgen excess; a patient with these signs will require an evaluation of her hormone status (see Chapter 9). The assessment of many gynecologic problems depends on a careful physical examination (see Chapter 1) combined with a thorough understanding of normal pubertal development. Primary and secondary amenorrhea, menorrhagia, and virilization can then be evaluated in terms of the hypothalamic–pituitary–ovarian–adrenal axis.

REFERENCES

1. O'Bryne KT, Thalabard J-C, Grosser PM, et al. Radiotelemetry monitoring of hypothalamic gonadotropin releasing hormone pulse generator activity throughout the menstrual cycle of the Rhesus monkey. *Endocrinology* 1991;129:1207.
2. Belchetz PE, Plant TM, Nakai Y, et al. Hypophyseal responses to continuous and intermittent delivery of hypothalamic gonadotropin-releasing hormone. *Science* 1978;202:631.
3. Speroff L, Fritz M. *Clinical gynecologic endocrinology and infertility,* 7th ed. Baltimore: Lippincott Williams & Wilkins, 2004.
4. Foster CM, Phillips DJ, Wyman T, et al. Changes in serum inhibin, activin and follistatin concentrations during puberty in girls. *Hum Reprod* 2000;15:1052.
5. Luisi S, Lombardi I, Florio P, et al. Serum activin A levels in males and females during pubertal development. *Gynecol Endocrinol* 2001;15:1.
6. Kettel LM, Apter D, DePaolo LV, et al. Circulating levels of follistatin from puberty to menopause. *Fertil Steril* 1996;65:472.
7. Burger HG, Famada Y, Bangah ML, et al. Serum gonadotropin, sex steroid, and immunoreactive inhibin levels in the first two years of life. *J Clin Endocrinol Metab* 1991;72:682.
8. Besser GM, McNeilly AS, Anderson DC, et al. Hormonal responses to synthetic luteinizing hormone and follicle stimulating hormone in man. *Br Med J* 1972;3:267.
9. Ayerst Laboratories Inc. Factrel (gonadorelin hydrochloride) package insert. New York: Ayerst, 1990.
10. Goodman RL, Parfitt DB, Evans NP, Dahl GE, Karsch FJ. Endogenous opioid peptides control the amplitude and shape of gonadotropin-releasing hormone pulses in the ewe. *Endocrinology* 1995;136:2412.
11. Conte FA, Grumbach MM, Kaplan SL, et al. Correlation of luteinizing hormone-releasing factor induced luteinizing hormone and follicle stimulating hormone release from infancy to 19 years with the changing pattern of gonadotropin secretion in agonadal patients: relation to the restraint of puberty. *J Clin Endocrinol Metab* 1980;50:163.
12. Palmert MR, Hayden DL, Mansfield MJ, et al. The longitudinal study of adrenal maturation during gonadal suppression: evidence that adrenarche is a gradual process. *J Clin Endocrinol Metab* 2001;86:4381.
13. Apter D, Pakarinen A, Hammond GL, et al. Adrenocortical function in puberty. *Acta Paediatr Scand* 1979;68:599.
14. Neinstein LS, Kaufman FR. Normal physical growth and development. In: Neinstein LS, ed. *Adolescent Health Care.* Philadelphia: Lippincott Williams & Wilkins, 2002.
15. Lucky AW, Biro FM, Huster GA, et al. Acne vulgaris in premenarchal girls. An early sign of puberty associated with rising levels of dehydroepiandrosterone. *Arch Dermatol* 1994;130:308.

16. Leyden JJ. Therapy for acne vulgaris. *N Engl J Med* 1997;336:1156.

17. Landy H, Boepple PA, Mansfield MJ, et al. Sleep modulation of neuroendocrine function: developmental changes in gonadotropin-releasing hormone during sexual maturation. *Pediatr Res* 1990;28:213.

18. Boyar RM Wu RH, Roffwarg H, et al. Human puberty: 24-hour estradiol patterns in pubertal girls. *J Clin Endocrinol Metab* 1976;43:1418.

19. Lucky AW, Rich BI, Rosenfield RL, et al. LH bioactivity increases more than immunoreactivity during puberty. *J Pediatr* 1980;97:205.

20. Conte FA, Kaplan SL, Grumbach MM. A diphasic pattern of gonadotropin secretion in patients with the syndrome of gonadal dysgenesis. *J Clin Endocrinol Metab* 1975;40:670.

21. Sklar CA, Kaplan SL, Grumbach MM. Evidence for dissociation between adrenarche and gonadarche: studies in patients with idiopathic precocious puberty, gonadal dysgenesis, isolated gonadotropin deficiency, and constitutionally delayed growth and adolescence. *J Clin Endocrinol Metab* 1980;51:548.

22. Yen SSC, Apter D, Bhtzow T, Laughlin GA. Gonadotropin releasing hormone pulse generator activity before and during sexual maturation in girls: new insights. *Hum Reprod* 1993;8:66.

23. Apter D, Bhtzow TL, Laughlin GA, Yen SCC. Gonadotropin releasing hormone pulse generator activity during pubertal transition in girls: pulsatile and diurnal patterns of circulating gonadotropins. *J Clin Endocrinol Metab* 1993;76:940.

24. Burger HG, McLachlan RI, Bangah M, et al. Serum inhibin concentrations rise throughout normal male and female puberty. *J Clin Endocrinol Metab* 1988;67:689.

25. Halvorson LM, DeCherney AH. Inhibin, activin, and follistatin in reproductive medicine. *Fertil Steril* 1996;65:459.

26. Rosenfield RL, Frulanetto R. Physiologic testosterone in estradiol induction of puberty increases plasma somatomedin-C. *J Pediatr* 1985;107:415.

27. Moll GW, Rosenfield RL, Fang VS. Administration of low-dose estrogen rapidly and directly stimulates growth hormone production. *Am J Dis Child* 1986;140:124.

28. Zachmann M, Prader A, Sobel EH, et al. Pubertal growth in patients with androgen insensitivity: indirect evidence for the importance of estrogens in pubertal growth of girls. *J Pediatr* 1986; 108:694.

29. Rose SR, Municchi G, Barnes KM, et al. Spontaneous growth hormone secretion increases during puberty in normal girls and boys. *J Clin Endocrinol Metab* 1991;73:428.

30. Greulich WW, Pyle S. *Radiographic atlas of skeletal development of the hand and wrist.* Stanford, CA: Stanford University Press, 1959.

31. Iglesias A, Coupey SM. Menstrual cycle abnormalities: diagnosis and management. *Adolescent Medicine: State of the Art Reviews* 1999;10:255.

32. Chumlea WC, Schubert CM, Roche AF, et al. Age at menarche and racial comparisons in US girls. *Pediatrics* 2003;111:110.

33. Apter D, Viinikka L, Vihko R. Hormonal pattern of adolescent menstrual cycles. *J Clin Endocrinol Metab* 1978;47:944.

34. World Health Organization Task Force on Adolescent Reproductive Health. World Health Organization multicenter study on menstrual and ovulatory patterns in adolescent girls: I. A multicenter cross-sectional study of menarche. *J Adolesc Health Care* 1986;7:229.

35. World Health Organization Task Force on Adolescent Reproductive Health. World Health Organization multicenter study on menstrual and ovulatory patterns in adolescent girls: II. Longitudinal study of menstrual patterns in the early postmenarcheal period, duration of bleeding episodes and menstrual cycles. *J Adolesc Health Care* 1986;7:236.

36. Wentz AC, Schoemaker J, Jones GS, Sapp KC. Studies of pathophysiology in primary amenorrhea. *Obstet Gynecol* 1977;50:129.

37. Wentz AC, Jones GS. Prognosis in primary amenorrhea. *Fertil Steril* 1978;29:614.

38. Scott RT, Hofmann GE. Prognostic assessment of ovarian reserve. *Fertil Steril* 1995;63:1.

39. Chehab FF, Qiu J, Mounzih K, et al. Leptin and reproduction. *Nutr Rev* 2002;60:S39.

40. Palmert MR, Radovick S, Boepple PA. Leptin levels in children with central precocious puberty. *J Clin Endocrinol Metab* 1998;83:2260.

41. Ankarberg-Lindgren C, Dahlgren J, Carlsson B, et al. Leptin levels show diurnal variation throughout puberty in healthy children, and follow a gender-specific pattern. *Eur J Endocrinol* 2001;145:43.

42. Marshall WA, Tanner JM. Variations in pattern of pubertal changes in girls. *Arch Dis Child* 1969;44:291.
43. Wu T, Mendola P, Buck GM. Ethnic differences in the presence of secondary sex characteristics and menarche among US girls: the Third National Health and Nutrition Eamination Survey 1988–1994. *Pediatrics* 2002;110:752.
44. Herman-Giddens ME, Slora EJ, Wasserman RC, et al. Secondary sexual characteristics and menses in young girls seen in office practice: a study from the Pediatric Research in Office Settings Network. *Pediatrics* 1997;99:505.
45. Biro FM. Areolar and breast staging in adolescent girls. *Adolesc Pediatr Gynecol* 1992;5:271.
46. Sun SS, Schubert CM, Chumlea WC, et al. National estimates of the timing of sexual maturation and racial differences among US children. *Pediatrics* 2002;111:911.
47. Kaplowitz PB, Slora EJ, Wasserman RC, et al. Earlier onset of puberty in girls: relation to increased body mass index and race. *Pediatrics* 2001;108:347.
48. Nottelman ED, Susan E, Dorn LD, et al. Developmental processes in early adolescence: relations among chronologic age, pubertal stage, height, weight, and serum levels of gonadotropins, sex steroids, and adrenal androgens. *J Adolesc Health Care* 1987;8:246.
49. Bayley N. Growth curves of height and weight by age for boys and girls, scaled according to physical maturity. *J Pediatr* 1956;48:187.
50. National Center for Health Statistics in collaboration with the National Center for Chronic Disease Prevention and Health Promotion, 2000. http://www.cdc.gov/growthcharts.
51. Bonjour J, Theintz G, Buchs B, et al. Critical years and stages of puberty for spinal and femoral bone mass accumulation during adolescence. *J Clin Endocrinol Metab* 1991;73:555.
52. Theintz G, Buchs B, Rizzoli R, et al. Longitudinal monitoring of bone mass accumulation in healthy adolescent: evidence for a marked reduction after 16 years of age at the levels of lumbar spine and femoral neck in female subjects. *J Clin Endocrinol Metab* 1992;75:1060.
53. Gordon CM, Glowacki J, LeBoff MS. DHEA and the skeleton (through the ages). *Endocrine* 1999;11:1.
54. Gordon CM, Nelson LM. Amenorrhea and bone health in adolescents and young women. *Curr Opin Obstet Gynecol* 2003;15:377.
55. Specker BL. Evidence for an interaction between calcium intake and physical activity on changes in bone mineral density. *J Bone Miner Res* 1996;11:1539.
56. Lloyd T, Andon MB, Rollings N, et al. Calcium supplementation and bone mineral density in adolescent girls. *JAMA* 1993;270:841.
57. Lee WT, Leung SS, Leung DM, et al. A randomized double-blinded controlled calcium supplementation trial, and bone and height acquisition. *Br J Nutr* 1995;74:125.
58. Teegarden D, Proulx WR, Martin BRJ, et al. Peak bone mass in young women. *J Bone Miner Res* 1995;10:711.
59. Weaver CM. Adolescence: the period of dramatic bone growth. *Endocrine* 2002;17:43.
60. Bailey DA, Faulkner RA, McKay HA, et al. Growth, physical activity and bone mineral acquisition. *Exerc Sport Sci Rev* 1996;24:233.
61. Bailey DA, McKay HA, Mirwald RL, et al. A six-year longitudinal study of the relationship of physical activity to bone mineral accrual in growing children: The Univeristy of Saskatchewan Bone Mineral Accrual Study. *J Bone Miner Res* 1999;14:1672
62. Pocock NA, Eisman JA, Hopper JL, et al. Genetic determinants of bone mass in adults. *J Clin Invest* 1987;80:706.
63. Eisman JA. Genetics of osteoporosis. *Endocr Rev* 1999;20:788.
64. Gordon CM. Normal bone accretion and effects of nutritional disorders in childhood. *J Wom Health* 2003;12:137.
65. Slemenda CW, Reister TK, Hui SL, et al. Influences on skeletal mineralization in children and adolescents: evidence for varying effects of sexual maturation and physical activity. *J Pediatr* 1994;125: 210.
66. Gilsanz V, Roe TF, Mora S, et al. Changes in vertebral bone density in black girls and white girls during childhood and puberty. *N Engl J Med* 1991;325:1597.
67. Rubin K, Schirduan V, Gendreau P, et al. Predictors of axial and peripheral bone mineral density in healthy children and adolescents, with special attention to the role of puberty. *J Pediatr* 1993;123:863.
68. Bryant RJ, Wastney ME, Martin BR, et al. Racial differences in bone turnover and calcium metabolism in adolescent females. *J Clin Endocrinol Metab* 2003;88:1043.

69. Recker RR, Davies, Hinders SM, et al. Bone gain in young adult women. *JAMA* 1992;268:2403.
70. Lindsay R, Tohme J, Kanders B. The effect of oral contraceptive use on vertebral bone mass in pre- and postmenopausal women. *Contraception* 1986;34:333.
71. Kleerehoper M, Brienza RS, Schultz LR, Johnson CC. Oral contraceptive use may protect against low bone mass. *Arch Int Med* 1991;151:1971.
72. Hreshchysyn MM, Hopkins A, Zylstra S, Anbar M. Assocations of parity, breast feeding and birth control pills with lumbar spine and femoral neck densities. *Am J Obstet Gynecol* 1988;159:318.
73. Mazess RB, Barden HS. Bone density in premenopasual women: effects of age, dietary intake, physical activity, smoking and birth control pills. *Am J Clin Nutr* 1991;53:132.
74. Cooper C, Hannaford P, Croft P, Kay CR. Oral contraceptive pill use and fractures in women: a prospective study. *Brit J Fam Plan* 1991;16:125.
75. Rodin A, Chapman M, Fogelman I. Bone density users in combined oral contraception; preliminary reports of a pilot study. *Brit J Fam Plan* 1991;16:125.
76. Cromer B, Blair J, Mahan J. et al. A prospective comparison of bone density in adolescent girls receiving depot medroxyprogesterone acetate (Depo-Provera), levonorgestrel (Norplant) or oral contraceptives. *J Pediatr* 1996;129:671.
77. Macdougall J, Daves MC, Overton CE, et al. Bone density in a population of long-term oral contraceptive pill users does not differ from that in menstruating women. *Br J Fam Plan* 1999;25:96.
78. Polatti F, Perotti F, Filippa N, Gallina D, Nappa RE. Bone mass and long-term monophasic oral contrceptive treatment in young women. *Contraception* 1995;51:221.
79. Gordon CM, Grace E, Emans SJ, et al. Effects of oral DHEA on bone density in young women with anorexia nervosa: a randomized trial. *J Clin Endocrinol Metab* 2002;87:4935.
80. Gordon CM, LeBoff MS, Glowacki J. Adrenal and gonadal steroids inhibit IL-6 secretion by human marrow cells. *Cytokine* 2001;16:178.
81. Warren MP, Brooks-Gunn J, Fox RP, et al. Persistent osteopenia in ballet dancers with amenorrhea and delayed menarche despite hormone therapy: a longitudinal study. *Fertil Steril* 2003;80:398.
82. Zacharias L, Wurtman R. Age at menarche: genetic and environmental influences. *N Engl J Med* 1969;280:868.
83. MacMahon B. *National health examination survey: age at menarche.* DHEW Publication 74-1615, Series 11, No. 133, November 1973.
84. Frisch RE. A method of prediction of age and menarche from height and weight at ages nine through thirteen years. *Pediatrics* 1974;53:384.
85. Frisch RE, McArthur JW. Menstrual cycles: fatness as a determinant of minimum weight necessary for their maintenance or onset. *Science* 1974;185:949.
86. Wyshak G, Frisch RE. Evidence for a secular trend in age of menarche. *N Engl J Med* 1982;306:1033.
87. Beunen GP, Malina RM, LeFevre JA, et al. Adiposity and biological maturity in girls 6–16 years of age. *Int J Obes Relat Metab Disord* 1994;18:542.
88. Bronson FH, Manning JM. The energetic regulation of ovultation: a realistic role for body fat. *Biol Reproduc* 1991;44:945.
89. de Ridder CM, Thijssen JH, Bruning JF, et al. Body fat mass, body fat distribution, and pubertal development: a longitudinal study of physical and hormonal sexual maturation of girls. *J Clin Endocrinol Metab* 1997;75:442.
90. Trussell J. Menarche and fatness: reexamination of the critical body composition hypothesis. *Science* 1978;30:506.
91. Trussell J. Statistical flaws in evidence for the Frisch hypothesis that fatness triggers menarche. *Hum Biol* 1980;52:711.
92. Gonzales GF, Villena A. Critical anthropometry for menarche. *J Pediatr Adolesc Gynecol* 1996;9:139.
93. Guo SS, Chumlea WC, Roche AF, Siervogel RM. Age and maturity related changes in body composition during adolescence into adulthood: the Fels longitudinal study. *Appl Radiat Isot* 1998;49:581.
94. Jaruratanasirikul S, Mosuwan L, Lebel L. Growth pattern and age at menarche of obese girls in a transitional society. *J Clin Endocrinol Metab* 1997;10:487.

95. Zacharias L, Wurtman RJ, Schatzoff M. Sexual maturation in contemporary American girls. *Am J Obstet Gynecol* 1970;108:833.
96. Apter D, Vihko R. Serum pregnenolone, progesterone, 17-hydroxyprogesterone, testosterone, and 5α-dihydrotestosterone during female puberty. *J Clin Endocrinol Metab* 1977;45:1039.
97. Welt CK, Martin KM, Taylor AE, et al. Frequency modulation of follicle-stimulating hormone (FSH) during the luteal-follicular transition: evidence for FSH control of inhibin B in normal women. *J Clin Endocrinol Metab* 1997;82:2645.
98. Filicori M, Santoro N, Merriam GR, et al. Characterization of the physiological pattern of episodic gonadotropin secretion throughout the human menstrual cycle. *J Clin Endocrinol Metab* 1986;62:1136.
99. Filicori M, Butler JP, Crowley WE Neuroendocrine regulation of the corpus luteum in the human: evidence for pulsatile progesterone secretion. *J Clin Invest* 1984;73:1638.
100. Apter D, Raisanen I, Ylostalo P, et al. Follicular growth in relation to serum hormonal patterns in adolescent compared with adult menstrual cycles. *Fertil Steril* 1987;47:82.
101. Bonen A, Belcastro AN, Ling WY, et al. Profiles of selected hormones during menstrual cycles of teenage athletes. *J Appl Physiol* 1981;50:545.
102. Shangold M, Freeman R, Thysen B, et al. The relationship between long distance running, plasma progesterone and luteal phase length. *Fertil Steril* 1979;31:130.
103. LeMarchand-Berand T, Zafferey M-M, Reymond M, et al. Maturation of the hypothalamic-pituitary-ovarian axis in adolescent girls. *J Clin Endocrinol Metab* 1982;54:241.
104. Venturoli S, Porcu E, Fabbri R, et al. Postmenarchal evolution of endocrine pattern and ovarian aspects of adolescents in adult menstrual cycles. *Fertil Steril* 1987;48:78.
105. Venturoli S, Porcu E, Gammi L, et al. Different gonadotropin pulsatile fashions in anovulatory cycles of young girls indicate different maturational pathways in adolescence. *J Clin Endocrinol Metab* 1987;65:785.
106. Berga SL. Behaviorally induced reproductive compromise in women and men. *Seminars Reprod Endocrinol* 1997;15:47.
107. Yen SS. Effects of lifestyle and body composition on the ovary. *Endocrinol Metab Clin North Am* 1998;27:915.
108. Marshall JC, Kelch RE. Gonadotropin-releasing hormone: role of pulsatile secretion in the regulation of reproduction. *N Engl J Med* 1986;315:1459.
109. Olster DH, Ferin M. Corticotropin-releasing hormone inhibits gonadotropin secretion in the ovariectomized Rhesus monkey. *J Clin Endocrinol Metab* 1987;65:262.
110. Berga SL, Mortola JF, Suh GB, Laughlin G, Pham P, Yen SSC. Neuroendocrine aberrations in women with functional hypothalamic amenorrhea. *J Clin Endocrinol Metab* 1989;68:301.
111. Biller BMK, Federoff HJ, Koenig JI, Klibanki A. Abnormal cortisol secretion and responses to corticotropin-releasing hormone in women with hypothalamic amenorrhea. *J Clin Endocrinol Metab* 1990;70:311.
112. Berga BL, Daniels TL, Giles DE. Women with functional hypothalamic amenorrhea but not other forms of anovulation display amplified cortisol concentrations. *Fertil Steril* 1997;67:1024.
113. Berga SL, Loucks AB, Rossmanith WG, et al. Acceleration of luteinizing hormone pulse frequency in functional hypothalamic amenorrhea by dopaminergic blockade. *J Clin Endocrinol Metab* 1991;72:151.
114. Nottelmann ED, Susan EJ, Dorn LD, et al. Secondary sex characteristics of girls 12 to 17 years of age: The US Health Examination Survey. *J Pediatr* 1980;96:1074.
115. Knobil E, Plant TM, Wildt L, et al. Control of the rhesus monkey menstrual cycle: permissive role of hypothalamic gonadotropin-releasing hormone. *Science* 1980;207:1371.
116. Crowley WE Jr, Comite F, Vale W, et al. Therapeutic use of pituitary desensitization with a long-acting LHRH agonist: a potential new treatment for idiopathic precocious puberty. *J Clin Endocrinol Metab* 1981;52:370.

Further Reading

Herman-Giddens ME, Bourdony CJ *Assessment of sexual maturity in girls. Pediatric research in office settings,* Elk Grove, IL: American Academy of Pediatrics, 1995.

5

Precocious Puberty

Joan Mansfield

A thorough understanding of the normal progression of puberty (see Chapter 4) is essential in the evaluation of precocious puberty, premature thelarche, and premature adrenarche. In normal adolescence, estrogen is responsible for breast development; for maturation of the external genitalia, vagina, and uterus; and for the initiation of menses. An increase in adrenal androgens is associated with the appearance of pubic and axillary hair. Excess androgens of either ovarian or adrenal origin may cause acne, hirsutism, voice deepening, increased muscle mass, and clitoromegaly. Precocious puberty may be caused by central, gonadotropin dependent puberty, or peripheral, gonadotropin independent precocity. Incomplete forms of puberty include premature thelarche, premature pubarche (adrenarche), and isolated premature menarche without other signs of puberty.

Premature thelarche is defined as the appearance of breast development in the absence of other signs of puberty, growth spurt, or acceleration of skeletal maturation. *Premature pubarche* is the appearance of pubic or axillary hair without signs of estrogenization and is usually associated with increased secretion of adrenal androgens (adrenarche). Although generally self-limited, isolated breast budding or pubic hair development may be the first sign of a true precocious puberty. Isolated premature menarche without breast development may represent precocious puberty or a benign ovarian cyst, but local vaginal lesions as a source of bleeding (trauma, infection, tumor) should be ruled out (see Chapter 3).

The workup of precocious puberty requires fairly sophisticated endocrine studies and management. Thus, referral to a pediatric endocrinologist is advisable. However, the primary care clinician can initiate the investigation and diagnosis.

CENTRAL PRECOCIOUS PUBERTY

Over the past century, the age of onset of pubertal development and menarche has declined in the United States and western Europe, perhaps in part because of improved nutrition (1). Controversy exists as to the definition of precocious puberty in North American girls. Traditionally, breast or pubic hair development in girls under 8 years of age has been defined as precocious. However, in a recent study of 17,000 girls aged 3 to 12 years in the United States, Herman-Giddens and colleagues reported that a group of pediatric practitioners found breast or pubic hair development to be present at age 7 to 8 years in 6.7% of white and 27.2% of African-American girls seen in office practices (2). Mean age of breast development was just under age 10 in white girls and under age 9 in African Americans. Average age of menarche was age 12.8 in whites and 12.1 in African Americans, not different from previous studies. This was the first study to assess puberty in large numbers of girls under age 8. Most earlier studies began at age 9. Thus it is not clear if the percentage of girls with puberty under age 8 has actually increased in the United States. Obesity in children in the United States is increasing, and Herman-Giddens did note an association between obesity and early signs of puberty in her subjects (3). In response to this study, a Lawson Wilkins Pediatric Endocrine Society task force has modified the definition of precocious puberty to be the appearance of secondary sexual characteristics under age 7 in white or under age 6 in African American girls (4). A number of reports have since pointed out that evaluating only those girls with precocious puberty according to this new definition would miss some children who have significant pathology such as central nervous system or hormone secreting tumors presenting only as puberty between the ages of 6 and 8 years (5–7). Girls who have progression to Tanner stage 3 breast development under age 8, girls who have both pubic hair and breast development under age 8, girls who are short with puberty under age 8, those with bone age advancement more than 2 years, and those with any neurological issues suggesting a central process need further assessment. Although the large majority of girls presenting with breast or pubic hair development have idiopathic precocious puberty or its benign variants, premature adrenarche or premature thelarche, some girls do have specific lesions causing their precocity. Specific causes of precocity (Table 5-1), such as tumors, are more common in girls with puberty under the age of 6 years but may occur in girls age 6 to 8 as well.

In true central precocious puberty, the stimulus for development is gonadotropin-releasing hormone (GnRH) secreted in pulses by the hypothalamus. The pituitary gland responds to the GnRH pulsations with the production and release of pituitary gonadotropin [follicle-stimulating hormone (FSH), and luteinizing hormone (LH)] pulses, which in turn stimulate the ovarian follicles to produce estrogen. In response to estrogen, the young girl has a growth spurt, develops breasts, and may begin menstruation. With the establishment of positive estrogen feedback resulting in the cyclic midcycle LH peak, the child may ovulate and thus becomes potentially fertile. Thus, in central precocious puberty, the hormonal process is that of an entirely normal puberty occurring at an early age (8–10).

Precocious puberty is much more common in girls than boys, with a ratio of about 23:1 (11). Although the large majority of cases of central precocious puberty in girls are idiopathic, computed tomography (CT) and magnetic resonance imaging (MRI) of the central nervous system (CNS) have identified CNS abnormalities, such

TABLE 5-1.

Central precocious puberty
    Idiopathic
    Central nervous system lesions
        Space occupying lesions
            Congenital defects
                Hydrocephalus
                Suprasellar/arachnoid cysts
                Hamartoma (GnRH secreting)
                Septo-optic dysplasia
            Tumors
                Optic Glioma
                Ganglioneuroma
                Ependymoma
                Craniopharyngioma
                Dysgerminoma
        Infection/inflammation
            Post encephalitis
            Brain abcess
            Post meningitis
            Granulomas
        Injury
            Post head trauma
            Post irradiation
        Syndromes
            Tuberous sclerosis
            Neurofibromatosis (often with optic glioma)
        Prolonged exposure to sex steroids
            Late/incompletely treated adrenal hyperplasia
            Post exposure to androgens/estrogens (tumors)
    GnRH independent precocity (peripheral)
        Exposure to topical or ingested androgens or estrogens
        Severe hypothyroidism
        Ovarian tumors
            Granulosa/ theca cell
            Germ cell
            Cystadenoma
            Lipoid
            Gonadoblastoma
        Ovarian cysts
            Idiopathic
            McCune–Albright
        Adrenal tumors (feminizing)
Incomplete precocious puberty
    Benign premature thelarche
    Transient/nonprogressive precocious puberty
    Topical/ingested estrogen exposure
    Premature pubarche
        Benign premature adrenarche
        Congenital adrenal hyperplasia
        Adrenal androgen secreting tumors
        Ovarian androgen secreting tumors
            Arrhenoblastoma
            Lipoid tumors
    Isolated vaginal bleeding
        Premature menarche
        Ovarian cyst
        Foreign body
        Vulvovaginitis
        Trauma
        Urethral prolapse
        Tumor
            Rhabdomyosarcoma
            Carcinomas

as hypothalamic hamartomas in some children with sexual precocity. Hamartomas most commonly present with central precocity under age 3 sometimes with gelastic (laughing) seizures (12–15). Although more common in younger children, CNS abnormalities causing precocity may occur at any time during childhood (16).

In gonadotropin independent (peripheral) precocious puberty, an ovarian tumor or cyst or rarely an adrenal adenoma produces estrogen autonomously. These lesions often produce high levels of estrogens, and puberty may progress more rapidly than in a child with central precocity.

Although the etiology of most cases of precocious puberty in girls is idiopathic, the differential diagnosis includes many organic disorders that need to be considered in the evaluation of the girl with early isosexual development (17–26).

CAUSES OF CENTRAL PRECOCIOUS PUBERTY

Idiopathic

Although this is by far the most common cause of precocity in girls, this is a diagnosis of exclusion.

Cerebral Disorders

These disorders include space-occupying lesions such as congenital malformations (hypothalamic hamartomas), brain tumors (e.g., glioma, astrocytoma, ependymoma, neuroblastoma), neurofibromatosis (optic nerve glioma or hypothalamic glioma), brain abscess, hydrocephalus (sometimes secondary to myelomeningocele), tuberous sclerosis, suprasellar cysts, infiltrative lesions such as sarcoid or other granulomatous disease, sequelae of cellular damage from prior infections (meningitis, encephalitis), head trauma, cerebral edema, or cranial radiation.

Secondary Central Precocious Puberty

Prolonged exposure to sex steroids from any source, resulting in the advancement of skeletal maturation to a bone age of 11 to 13 years, can trigger central precocity. Patients with undertreated or late treated congenital adrenocortical hyperplasia (CAH) or androgen-secreting tumors may develop early central puberty (25).

PERIPHERAL (GONADOTROPIN INDEPENDENT) PRECOCIOUS PUBERTY

Ovarian Tumors

Approximately 60% of ovarian tumors that cause sexual precocity are granulosa cell tumors; the rest are cystadenomas, gonadoblastomas, carcinomas, arrhenoblastomas, lipoid cell tumors, thecomas, and benign ovarian cysts. Ovarian tumors can secrete estrogens and androgens, thus resulting in both breast and pubic hair development.

Adrenal Disorders

Adrenal adenomas may secrete estrogen alone and cause sexual precocity. Adrenal carcinomas that secrete estrogen also produce other hormones that cause androgenization/virilization and sometimes Cushing syndrome. Patients with untreated CAH may have virilization as well as some breast development.

Autonomous Follicular Ovarian Cysts

Recurrent ovarian follicular cysts may occur independently but are often associated with McCune–Albright syndrome. Girls with McCune–Albright syndrome have recurrent follicular cysts, polyostotic fibrous dysplasia, and large irregular café au lait spots (26–31). In these girls, ovarian volumes by ultrasonography are often asymmetric and fluctuate in size over time (29). The mechanism of gonadotropin-independent follicular cyst development in McCune–Albright syndrome is now believed to be due to a dominant somatic mutation in certain cell lines, which results in an overactivity of the cyclic adenosine monophosphate pathway owing to a mutation of the Gs alpha gene (30,31). The fluctuating estrogen levels produced by cysts result in sexual development and anovulatory menses.

Gonadotropin-Producing Tumors

Tumors that secrete both LH-like substances, such as human chorionic gonadotropin (HCG) and estrogen (primary ovarian choriocarcinoma), can cause precocious development. The production of LH or HCG alone will cause isosexual precocity in boys but not in girls.

Iatrogenic Disorders

The prolonged use of estrogen-containing creams for labial adhesions may cause transient breast development. Oral estrogen intake (oral contraceptive ingestion) is a rare cause of breast development. It has been speculated that the ingestion of estrogen-like compounds in certain meat or plant foods may play a role in clusters of cases of premature breast development, but this has not been well defined (32,33).

Primary Hypothyroidism

Ovarian cysts may develop in the presence of severe primary hypothyroidism, perhaps because of cross-reaction of high levels of thyroid-stimulating hormone (TSH) with ovarian FSH receptors (20–22). Premature breast development or vaginal bleeding usually regresses following thyroid hormone replacement. Absence of a statural growth spurt and delayed skeletal maturation accompanying breast development may be a clue to hypothyroidism as a cause of premature development.

Patient Assessment

The initial assessment of the patient with precocious development should include a careful history and physical examination. There is often a history of mildly early development in relatives of children with idiopathic central puberty between the ages of 6 and 8 years. Adopted children with a previous history of poor nutrition may have an increased chance of developing precocious puberty (34). A complete family history must include inherited conditions such as neurofibromatosis or CAH.

On reviewing the child's own history, the clinician should look for a history suggestive of CNS damage such as birth trauma, encephalitis, meningitis, CNS irradiation, seizures, headaches, visual symptoms, or other neurologic symptoms. Increased appetite, a growth spurt, and emotional lability suggest a significant estrogen effect. The time course of precocious puberty is similar to that of normal puberty, whereas an abrupt and rapid course of development suggests an estrogen-secreting lesion. Abdominal pain, urinary symptoms, or bowel symptoms may be present in patients with abdominal masses.

Vaginal bleeding may be the first sign of precocity in patients with both true precocity and pseudoprecocity. Some children have no signs of puberty but have recurrent menses. This may be a benign, self-limited condition, although this is a diagnosis of exclusion (35,36).

Growth charts should be accurate and up to date, since the growth spurt often correlates with the onset of development in precocious puberty. The finding of accelerated growth and advanced skeletal maturation is important in distinguishing between true precocious puberty and premature thelarche. The photograph and growth charts of an untreated patient with idiopathic precocious puberty are shown in Fig. 5-1.

The physical examination should include height and weight measurements. A neurologic assessment, including visualization of the optic discs for evidence of papilledema, should be done. The skin should be assessed for acne, apocrine odor, café au lait spots, and pubic or axillary hair. In patients with neurofibromatosis, café au lait spots are multiple brown macules with smooth edges, whereas in those with McCune–Albright syndrome, one or more large macules with irregular borders may be found. The thyroid should be palpated and clinical signs suggestive of severe hypothyroidism (hair and skin changes, low pulse) noted. The breast dimensions and staging of breast development should be recorded. The external genitalia should be examined for evidence of estrogen effect (enlargement of the labia minora, thickening of the vaginal mucosa, and physiological discharge). This is most easily done

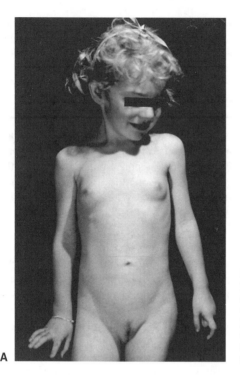

A

FIG. 5-1. Natural history of a girl with idiopathic precocious puberty before the advent of gonadotropin-releasing hormone (GnRH) therapy. She was first seen because of early development at the age of 3²/12 years. Her menarche occurred at 5⁶/12 years of age; she attained adult height at 10 years of age. **A:** At age 3⁶/12 years.

with the child lying on her back in the frog-leg position. Signs of virilization such as clitoromegaly, deepening of the voice, increased muscularity, or hirsutism should alert the examiner to the possibility of contrasexual precocity due to androgen excess. The normal prepubertal clitoral glans is 3 mm in diameter. A clitoral glans width >5 mm, or an index (clitoral length × width) >35 suggests significant androgen exposure (37). If the young child is approached in a relaxed manner, it may be possible to carry out a bimanual rectoabdominal examination. Ovarian masses, when present, are usually easily palpated. A vaginal pelvic exam is not indicated. Ultrasonography of the abdomen is a more sensitive tool for assessment of ovarian masses and is often a better option than a rectoabdominal exam. Girls with true precocity frequently have mildly enlarged ovaries with multiple small follicular cysts similar to the ovaries seen in the adolescent with a normal age of puberty (38). A single large ovarian cyst may occur in isolation or with McCune–Albright syndrome.

The laboratory evaluation of the child depends on the initial clinical assessment. If the examination clearly shows an estrogen effect on the vaginal mucosa and growth charts reveal an acceleration of linear growth, then more extensive testing is needed. If, on the other hand, the clinician suspects premature thelarche, the initial tests would be limited to a radiograph film of the left hand and wrist for

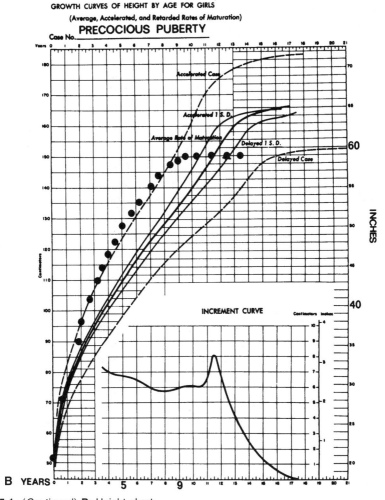

GROWTH CURVES OF HEIGHT BY AGE FOR GIRLS

(Average, Accelerated, and Retarded Rates of Maturation)

PRECOCIOUS PUBERTY

FIG. 5-1. (*Continued*) **B**: Height chart.

bone age. The radiograph for assessment of skeletal maturation is the single most useful test in the evaluation of the child with premature development. The bone age becomes significantly greater than the chronologic age and the height age in patients with true precocious puberty. A vaginal smear (maturational index) can be used to confirm the clinical impression of estrogenization (see Chapter 1). Vaginal smears are often well tolerated in children under age 1, but many older children tend to dislike them. Since it is helpful to visually assess the vaginal introitus for estrogen effect on repeated visits in a child with precocity, it is often preferable to do careful visual inspection instead of a vaginal smear. A typical vaginal smear in a patient with precocious puberty may show 35% superficial, 50% intermediate, and 15% parabasal cells. The findings of estrogen excess (>40% superficial cells) should raise the suspicion of an estrogen-secreting lesion.

If the vagina shows little estrogen effect and growth rate and bone age are normal, the patient can be monitored by her primary care physician at 3-month intervals to observe whether sexual development progresses or acceleration of linear growth occurs. Not uncommonly, a child has one or several transient episodes of breast budding and growth acceleration that resolve without therapy (39,40). Other children have very slow progression of precocity without rapid skeletal maturation. These children represent the "slowly progressive" variant of early puberty (41). They usually reach adult heights in the normal range without intervention.

If the girl has progressive sexual development, advancing bone age, acceleration of growth, or vaginal estrogenization, then consultation with a pediatric endocrinologist is indicated. In addition to determinations of bone age, initial testing for the evaluation of suspected central precocious puberty usually includes serum levels of LH, FSH, estradiol, dehydroepiandrosterone sulfate (DHEAS), TSH, pelvic ultrasound for assessment of ovarian cysts and size and uterine size and configuration, and MRI of the CNS with contrast medium. Girls with precocious puberty between ages 6 and 8 years with height predictions in the normal range do not necessarily require further testing beyond a bone age. They should be followed until at least age 9, however, since height predictions may decline if bone age advances more rapidly than height age.

The interpretation of LH and FSH levels depends on which assay is used. Current commercially available assays include radioimmunoassays (RIA), and the newer and more sensitive immunoradiometric (IRMA), immunochemiluminometric, and immunofluorimetric assays (42–44). Since LH and FSH secretion is associated with sleep in early puberty, the random daytime serum LH and FSH values may not be helpful in differentiating among premature thelarche, pseudoprecocity, and early central precocious puberty. Random LH and FSH levels in the prepubertal range are usually seen in the early stages of true precocity; however, random LH levels in the pubertal range suggest advanced central precocity (Tanner breast stage 3). Thus, random daytime LH levels may be of value in confirming the clinical impression of active central puberty but will probably be in the prepubertal range both in early central puberty and in premature thelarche. Random FSH levels are usually obtained as well but are less useful, since they are generally in the same range in premature thelarche and in precocious puberty. The IRMA and other sensitive assays provide better differentiation between precocious puberty and prepubertal states than the older RIAs.

The GnRH stimulation test (see Chapter 4) can help in the differential diagnosis of premature thelarche, gonadotropin-independent precocity, and true central precocity. Patients with true precocity exhibit nocturnal pulses of LH and FSH and a pubertal, LH-predominant response to the GnRH test, whereas girls with premature thelarche have a prepubertal FSH-predominant response, and those with gonadotropin-independent precocity or ovarian secreting cysts or tumors have a suppressed response to GnRH. The finding of a high estradiol level (100 to 200 pg/ml), low gonadotropin levels, and a suppressed response to GnRH should raise the possibility of an estrogen-secreting tumor or cyst, although this diagnosis should be apparent on ultrasound (see Chapter 18). The GnRH stimulation test is especially useful in tracking the response of the girl to GnRH analog therapy to ensure complete suppression of puberty (42) (Fig. 5-2).

The level of DHEAS is a marker of adrenal androgen production (see Chapter 9). Most girls with precocious puberty have age-appropriate DHEAS levels, although a few have premature adrenarche as well. Patients with precocity between 6 and 8 years of age have mean DHEAS levels similar to those of normal children with the same bone age (45).

In patients with excessive androgen effect, testosterone, DHEAS, early morning 17-hydroxyprogesterone (to detect 21-hydroxylase deficiency) and DHEA may be obtained. An adrenocorticotropic hormone (ACTH) stimulation test may be required to diagnose mild forms of congenital adrenal hyperplasia in the patient with premature pubarche. The child who has clitoromegaly, progressive virilization, or skeletal age advanced by more than 1 year certainly deserves a thorough evaluation.

Treatment and Follow-up

Treatment and follow-up depend on the diagnosis. Ovarian tumors should be managed as outlined in Chapter 18. Successful treatment of a tumor can be monitored by the demonstration of decreasing estrogen effects. Removal of an ovarian cyst will not result in permanent regression of puberty in girls with true precocity or McCune–Albright syndrome; thus, normal follicular cysts accompanying true precocity should not be removed. Severe cases of ovarian hyperstimulation resulting in precocious puberty may require aspiration (22). The ovarian cysts associated with central precocity should be observed because they are likely to regress with suppression of gonadotropins.

Although Depo-Provera and cyproterone acetate were used in the past to treat central precocious puberty, pubertal suppression was incomplete, and therapy did not improve the adult height (46–48). Suppression of puberty with GnRH analog agonists was initially pioneered by Crowley and associates, and these agents have become the treatment of choice for central precocious puberty (49–58). Continuous exposure to GnRH agonist analogs results in desensitization of pituitary gonadotropin-secreting cells. Currently, three GnRH analogs—leuprolide, histrelin, and nafarelin—are approved in the United States for the treatment of precocious puberty. The depot formulation of leuprolide is the most commonly used treatment of precocious puberty in the United States. This is given by intramuscular injection every 28 days. A 3-month depot formulation is now available

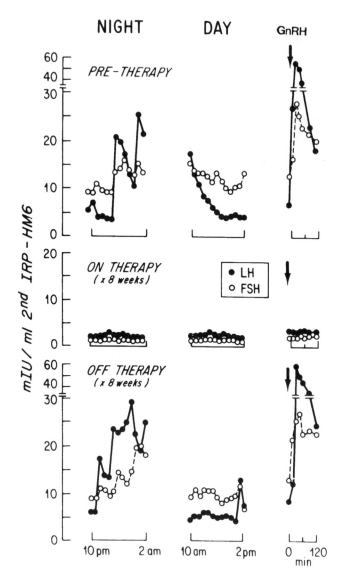

FIG. 5-2. Spontaneous night and daytime gonadotropin secretion and response to exogenous gonadotropin-releasing hormone (GnRH) administration in a 2-year-old with central precocious puberty before, during, and after discontinuation of GnRH analog therapy. LH, luteinizing hormone; FSH, follicle-stimulating hormone. (From Crowley WF, Comite F, Vale W, et al. Therapeutic use for pituitary desensitization with a long-acting LHRH agonist: a potential new treatment for idiopathic precocious puberty. *J Clin Endocrinol Metab* 1981;52:370; Copyright 1981, The Endocrine Society; with permission.)

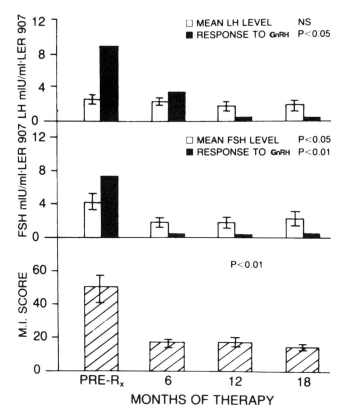

FIG. 5-3. Luteinizing hormone (LH) and follicle-stimulating hormone (FSH) (at baseline and in response to exogenous gonadotropin-releasing hormone [GnRH]), and maturation index (MI) score of vaginal cytology in nine girls with central precocious puberty before and during long-term therapy with GnRH analog. (From Mansfield MJ, Beardsworth DE, Loughlin J, et al. Long-term treatment of central precocious puberty with a long-acting analog of luteinizing hormone-releasing hormone. *N Engl J Med* 1983;309:1286; Copyright, Massachusetts Medical Society; with permission.)

that has been reported to suppress precocious puberty in 95% of children in one study (59). Long-term growth data are not available for this formulation. In girls with central precocity, the advantages of a GnRH agonist analog are the selective and reversible suppression of LH and FSH, the return of estradiol to the prepubertal range, and the regression (or lack of progression) of breast development and the cessation of menses (Figs. 5-2 and 5-3). Growth velocity and skeletal maturation slow during GnRH analog suppression of puberty (Fig. 5-4). Since bone age advancement is slowed more than height age, predicted adult height is increased by this therapy (54,58) (Fig. 5-5). Several series of patients have shown modest to marked improvements in final height with GnRH analog agonist therapy (47,60–62). One randomized trial of girls ages 6 to 8 treated with GnRH analog

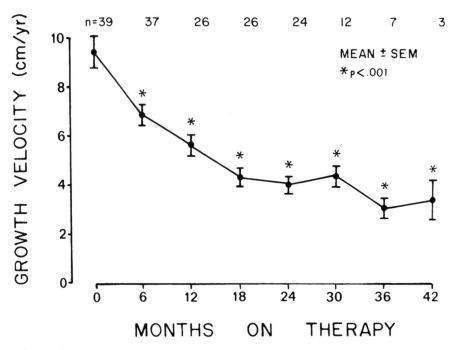

FIG. 5-4. Growth velocity before and during gonadotropin-releasing hormone (GnRH) analog therapy in 32 girls and seven boys treated between 6 and 42 months. (From Boepple PA, Mansfield MJ, Wierman ME, et al. Use of a potent, long-acting agonist of gonadotropin-releasing hormone in the treatment of precocious puberty. *Endocr Rev* 1986;7:24; with permission.)

did not show any increased height in the treated group versus controls without treatment. Final heights were normal in both groups (63). It is important for patients to be closely monitored during GnRH analog therapy to ensure that suppression of puberty is as complete as possible to maximize final height gain. Monitoring is done with physical exams to assess height, weight, breast size, and estrogen effect on the vaginal mucosa. GnRH analog suppression has typically been assessed with GnRH stimulation tests at 3 months, then every 6 to 12 months. A recent study has shown that a single LH and FSH sample 30 to 60 minutes post-depot leuprolide injection is a convenient and less expensive alternative (64).

After GnRH analog therapy, menarche generally occurs within 1 to 2 years in patients with bone ages in the pubertal range, and menstrual cycles are similar to those in normal adolescent girls (65,66). Bone density, initially increased for age in patients with precocious puberty, declines during GnRH analog treatment but remains in the normal range for chronological age, although lower for bone age (67). Calcium supplementation can help to improve bone density during GnRH analog therapy (68). Bone density has been found to be normal in adolescents 2 years post-GnRH analog therapy for precocious puberty (69).

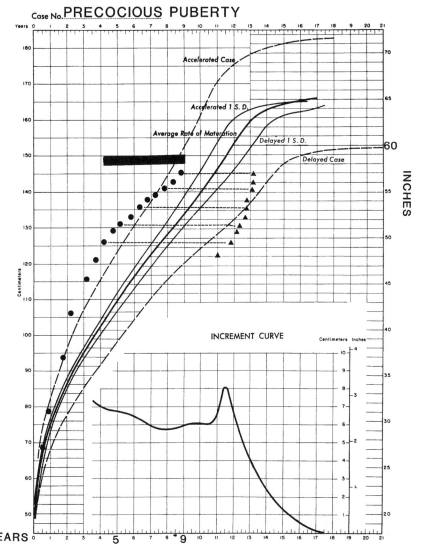

GROWTH CURVES OF HEIGHT BY AGE FOR GIRLS

(Average, Accelerated, and Retarded Rates of Maturation)

Case No. PRECOCIOUS PUBERTY

FIG. 5-5. Growth chart of a girl with true isosexual precocious puberty. Her onset of breast development occurred at 10 months and her menarche at 1¹/₁₂ years. Note the acceleration of growth velocity and bone age. The patient began receiving gonadotropin-releasing hormone (GnRH) analog therapy (*bar*) at 4²/₁₂ years, and her growth decelerated. Bone age, which is shown with ▲ on the horizontal line to the right of the height measurement, was significantly advanced at the beginning of therapy (just under 12 years) but advanced only minimally over the next 4½ years (slightly over 13 years). (Growth chart courtesy of Dr. M.J. Mansfield.)

Therapy with GnRH analogs is expensive and requires monthly injections of depot formulations or daily subcutaneous injections and regular monitoring of indices of pubertal suppression. Nasal analogs generally give less complete suppression. GnRH agonists are also effective in suppressing puberty in girls with precocity secondary to hypothalamic hamartomas and optic nerve gliomas associated with neurofibromatosis (15,19). During treatment with a GnRH analog, normal age-appropriate progression of adrenarche as determined by measurement of DHEAS occurs (45,70). Insulin-like growth factor-1 (also termed *somatomedin-C*) levels and nocturnal growth hormone secretion decrease during GnRH analog therapy, providing one of many lines of evidence that sex steroids augment growth hormone secretion during puberty (71).

Although a girl with precocious puberty may appear tall at the initial evaluation, she may eventually have a short final height because of premature epiphyseal closure. Several series have given final height estimates for girls with precocious puberty at 151 to 155 cm (23,24,46,47); however, recent small series of untreated patients have recorded final heights averaging within 1 standard deviation of normal (47,60). The final heights depended on the age of the children in the study and the rate of progression of their precocity. Children who develop progressive precocious puberty at young ages usually have more height deficit as adults. The majority of children who develop precocious puberty at the age of 6 to 8 years have acceptable final heights. Rosenfield (45) has suggested a useful algorithm for deciding when to initiate treatment for central precocity. If the child is 6 to 8 years old and has an acceptable initial predicted adult height >152 cm, she may be observed. If skeletal maturation progresses rapidly and predicted height declines to <152 cm or declines by ≥5 cm, treatment should be initiated. The psychosocial well-being of the patient and her family needs to be considered as well as the final height. In some patients, suppression of puberty is indicated for psychosocial reasons despite a normal height prediction. Many parents are concerned that menarche will shortly follow the onset of breast development. Overall, the duration of time from thelarche to menarche is longer in younger children (2.8 years with thelarche age 9 versus 1.4 years with thelarche age 12) (72). In patients in whom puberty is slowly progressive or intermittent, the endocrinologist may elect to withhold treatment and monitor the patient closely. Depo-Provera is occasionally used to stop menses when complete suppression of puberty is not required.

Important insights have also been gained on behavioral changes associated with gonadarche. Children with sexual precocity do not automatically manifest intellectual or psychosocial maturity. The degree of psychological maturity of a young girl is more likely to be related to her life experiences and her interactions with her peer group, siblings, and parents. Nevertheless, parents and investigators have noted that girls with sexual precocity sometimes have mood swings and impulsiveness, which resolve with the suppression of puberty during GnRH agonist therapy (73,74). Children with sexual precocity are at special risk for sexual abuse, and one study suggests that they tend to begin sexual relations at a slightly earlier age than their peers. It is important to reassure the young girl with precocious puberty and her parents that her growth and development are "early" but normal and that, if necessary, she can receive medicine to delay her development to a later age. Psychological consultation for the child and family may be indicated to help them with the stress of coping with early development.

Follow-up for the child with precocious puberty depends on the diagnosis and the treatment undertaken. Girls being treated with GnRH analog therapy need to be seen frequently for assessment of compliance with medication, height and weight monitoring, and physical examination. A GnRH stimulation test and determination of estradiol level are usually done within the first 1 to 3 months after the beginning of treatment to establish suppression, and repeated at 6- to 12-month intervals, since the dose may need to be increased. An FSH, LH and estradiol 45 minutes post-depot leuprolide injection may be substituted for a GnRH stimulation test to assess suppression. Bone age is determined at 6-month intervals. Ultrasound can be used to determine regression of uterine size (75). It is important to monitor these patients closely, since incomplete suppression of estrogen by GnRH analog may actually result in a further decrease in final height. The growth chart of a patient treated with an analog is shown in Fig. 5-5.

In girls with McCune–Albright syndrome with gonadotropin-independent puberty and cyclic gonadal steroid production, GnRH agonist therapy does not cause a decrease in estradiol or regression of pubertal changes (26,29). Feuillan and colleagues (27) reported some success with testolactone, an aromatase inhibitor that blocks the synthesis of estrogens, in five girls with McCune-Albright syndrome; however, the effectiveness of this treatment decreases with time in some patients.

CONTRASEXUAL PRECOCIOUS PUBERTY (ANDROGEN EXCESS WITH VIRILIZATION)

Contrasexual precocity arises from excess androgen production from an adrenal or ovarian source, which results in acne, hirsutism, and virilization. The differential diagnosis includes (a) CAH, (b) Cushing syndrome with tumor related androgen excess, (c) adrenal tumors, (d) topical exposure to androgen containing creams or gels and (e) androgen-secreting ovarian tumors such as lipoid cell and arrhenoblastomas.

Patient Assessment

The patient should have a careful physical examination, with emphasis on noting evidence of hirsutism, acne, or clitoral enlargement, and an adequate abdominal and bimanual rectal examination or pelvic ultrasound to exclude an ovarian mass. Ovarian tumors are usually palpable.

Laboratory tests to be considered include serum levels of LH, FSH, estradiol, testosterone, DHEAS, dehydroepiandrosterone (DHEA), 17-hydroxyprogesterone, androstenedione, and 11-deoxycortisol (see Fig. 2-9 in Chapter 2 for pathways of steroid biosynthesis). Blood for the baseline 17-hydroxyprogesterone level is best drawn between 7 and 8 AM, since the diurnal variation of adrenal hormones brings about a normal level in the afternoon in patients with mild deficiencies of 21-hydroxylase. In girls with suspected CAH, a 1-hour ACTH stimulation test (see Chapter 9) is useful in detecting a block in the adrenal pathways. Adrenal tumors are usually associated with elevated serum DHEA, DHEAS, and androstenedione and are not suppressible by dexamethasone. Serum testosterone may be elevated because of direct secretion by the tumor or because of peripheral conversion. Cushing syndrome is usually accompanied by signs of excess cortisol production and poor linear growth. A 24-hour urine collection for determination of free cortisol is useful if Cushing syndrome or cortisol resistance are under consideration. Thus, the diagnosis is made by careful hormone studies with ACTH testing in cases of suspected CAH, abdominal and bimanual rectoabdominal palpation, ultrasonography, CT or MRI scanning for visualizing the adrenals, and resection of identified tumors.

Treatment and Follow-up

Ovarian and adrenal tumors should be surgically excised if possible. Patients with CAH should receive glucocorticoid replacement (e.g., hydrocortisone, 13 to 25 mg/m^2 per day divided in three daily doses) and be monitored every 3 months. If the bone age is not too advanced, breast development may regress when CAH is treated. As noted earlier, some patients may develop secondary central precocity and be candidates for GnRH analog therapy.

PREMATURE THELARCHE

Premature thelarche is defined as breast development without any other signs of puberty and is most commonly seen among young girls under 2 years of age. Occasionally, neonatal breast hypertrophy fails to regress within 10 months after birth; this persistent breast development is also characterized as premature thelarche. The child with typical premature thelarche has bilateral breast buds of 2 to 4 cm with little or no change in the nipple or areola. The breast tissue feels granular and may be slightly tender. In some cases, development is quite asymmetric; one side may develop 6 to 12 months before the other. Growth is not accelerated, and the bone age is normal for height age. No other evidence of puberty appears; the labia often remain prepubertal without obvious evidence of estrogen effect. A vaginal smear for maturation index may show atrophy or may show slight evidence of estrogenization. Similarly, the serum estradiol may be slightly elevated in some patients (76,77).

Occasionally, patients who initially present with premature thelarche eventually develop true central precocious puberty (78). In girls with premature thelarche, basal and post-GnRH serum levels of LH and FSH are generally in the prepubertal range, although Ilicki and colleagues (79) have found that basal levels of FSH and the response to GnRH were higher than in prepubertal control subjects. They have postulated that premature thelarche is due to a derangement in maturation of the hypothalamic-pituitary-gonadal axis, with higher than normal FSH secretion and increased peripheral sensitivity to the sex hormones. This hypothesis would explain the occurrence of this problem principally in 1- to 4-year-old girls. Klein has shown that estradiol is higher in girls with premature thelarche than in controls when measured in an ultrasensitive estradiol assay (79). Premature thelarche is also seen more commonly in very-low-birth-weight infants (80). Thus, evidence points toward the importance of transient ovarian secretion of estrogen under hypothalamic pituitary control. The usual clinical course of regression, or at least lack of progression, of breast development would then correlate with the waning of the estrogen levels as the ovarian follicles become atretic.

Patient Assessment

The assessment of a patient with premature breast development includes a careful review of medications and creams recently used. Occasionally it is discovered that a package of the mother's or sister's oral contraceptive pills has been ingested by the child. Premarin cream applied to the vulva nightly for >2 to 3 weeks may result in breast changes. The physical examination should include notation of the appearance of the vaginal mucosa and of the size of the breasts and, in an infant, a rectoabdominal examination to exclude an ovarian cyst.

A pelvic ultrasound is often used as an alternative to a rectoabdominal exam to assess the uterus and ovaries in infants and older children. The uterus should not be enlarged in patients with premature thelarche. Growth charts should be updated and assessed to see whether the patient is continuing to grow at her previously established percentile of height and weight. Laboratory tests include a radiograph of the left hand and wrist for bone age, a pelvic ultrasound, possibly a vaginal maturational index, and, in some cases, a GnRH stimulation test, and determination of serum estradiol, LH, and FSH levels.

Treatment and Follow-up

Treatment consists mainly of reassurance and careful follow-up to confirm that the breast development does not represent the first sign of precocious puberty (81). A thorough physical examination should be done at each visit. Linear growth and bone age should be monitored. Biopsy of the breast tissue is not indicated, because removal of the breast bud prevents normal development. Although in most cases of premature thelarche breast development regresses or stabilizes, some children do develop central precocious puberty. These patients cannot be distinguished clinically at initial presentation, so that follow-up is appropriate. Parents should be reassured that this is usually a self-limited process and pubertal development will occur at the normal adolescent age.

PREMATURE MENARCHE

Premature menarche most likely represents a similar but less common response than premature thelarche to the transient production of estrogen by the ovary. Prepubertal girls may have uterine bleeding lasting 1 to 5 days, once or in cycles for several months, without other evidence of estrogen effect. Blanco-Garcia and co-workers (35) found estradiol levels to be significantly above the normal prepubertal range and a seasonal increase in isolated menses between September and January. Before the clinician can make this diagnosis, other causes of vaginal bleeding, including infection, trauma, foreign body, and tumors, need to be excluded (see Chapter 3).

PREMATURE ADRENARCHE

Premature adrenarche is defined as the isolated appearance of pubic and occasionally axillary hair before the age of 8 years without evidence of estrogenization or virilization. Patients usually also have axillary odor. The terminology is sometimes confusing, but *premature pubarche* refers to the clinical manifestations of early pubic (and/or axillary) hair and premature adrenarche to the early maturation of adrenal androgen secretion. In common usage, the terms are often interchanged. Most patients have an increase in urinary 17-ketosteroid production and increased plasma levels of DHEA and DHEAS, which suggests that hormone biosynthesis in the adrenal gland undergoes maturation prematurely to a pubertal pattern (82). Although production of these androgens is suppressible by dexamethasone and therefore dependent on ACTH, the mediator for the change at puberty and in premature adrenarche is unknown. Levels of DHEAS are similar to those in girls with stage 2 pubic hair (Fig. 5-6). Bone age is usually normal or 1 year advanced (appropriate for height age).

The cause of premature adrenarche is not yet known. The condition appears to be more common in black and Hispanic girls and obese boys and girls. In some medical centers, including ours, some adolescents with androgen excess and polycystic ovary syndrome have been observed to have a history of premature adrenarche (83,84) (see Chapter 9). Insulin resistance has been documented in children with premature adrenarche even in the absence of obvious acanthosis

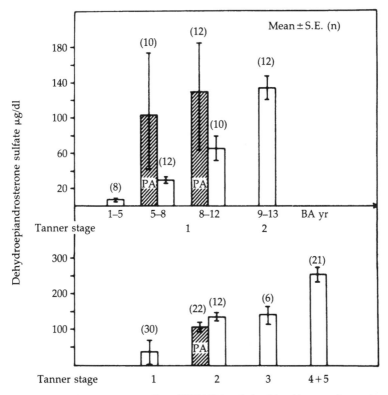

FIG. 5-6. Dehydroepiandrosterone sulfate (DHEAS) levels in girls with precocious adrenarche (PA) compared with normal girls of various bone ages (BA) and stages of pubic hair development (Tanner stages 1 to 4/5). DHEAS levels are appropriate for the Tanner stage of pubic hair but are elevated for the bone age. S.E., standard error; n, number. (From Korth-Schutz S, Levine LS, New MI. Dehydroepiandrosterone sulfate (DS) levels, a rapid test for abnormal adrenal androgen secretion. *J Clin Endocrinol Metab* 1976;42:1005; Copyright 1976, The Endocrine Society, with permission.)

nigricans (85). Ibanez has reported an increased history of low birth weight in girls with premature adrenarche and insulin resistance who had anovulatory cycles as teens (86). Some girls with premature adrenarche do have evidence of a partial deficiency of 21-hydroxylase or are heterozygotes for 21-hydroxylase deficiency (8,87–90). In a referred population with a predominance of ethnic groups known to have a high incidence of nonclassical 21-hydroxylase deficiency (Ashkenazi Jewish, Hispanic, and Italian), Temeck and colleagues (88) found that among girls with premature adrenarche between the ages of 2 and 7 years, 5 of 19 (26%) had 21-hydroxylase deficiency. In a study of 127 Italian children with premature pubarche who underwent ACTH testing, 12% had mild errors in steroidogenesis (90). These studies need to be repeated in ethnic populations with a lower incidence of these disorders, especially among American black children, since premature adrenarche is so common in these girls between the ages of 5 and 8 years (2). Thus, the exact percentage of children with adrenal enzyme deficiencies, the natural history, and the benefits of intervention need to be defined better, since doing a 1-hour ACTH test in all girls with premature adrenarche would add substantially to the expense of the evaluation. A 1-hour ACTH test is indicated in all girls with elevated baseline (7 to 8 AM) 17-hydroxyprogesterone, those whose bone age is advanced >1 year, those with increased linear growth, and those with any signs of clitoromegaly or virilization. Even in the absence of these indications, white girls, especially those from the ethnic groups with an increased risk of nonclassical 21-hydroxylase deficiency, should be screened with a DHEAS level and an early-morning 17-hydroxyprogesterone determination as a minimum.

Patient Assessment

The assessment of the patient with premature adrenarche is similar to that for contrasexual precocious puberty. The important findings on physical examination are the presence of pubic hair and axillary odor and the *absence* of breast development, estrogenization of the labia and vagina, and virilization (clitoromegaly).

The laboratory tests include determination of bone age, serum DHEAS, and early-morning (7 to 8 AM) 17-hydroxyprogesterone. Given the finding of insulin resistance in some of these patients, a fasting blood sugar and insulin level might be added (85,86). As noted earlier, the criteria for ACTH testing need further refinement. However, in many medical centers, this test is performed on all patients to detect enzyme deficiencies and better define the potential causes of this condition. The differential diagnosis must exclude precocious puberty, CAH, and an adrenal or ovarian tumor. Sometimes, the diagnosis of adrenarche is made only in retrospect when further evidence of precocious puberty does not occur. It should be recalled that most patients with precocious puberty have an advanced bone age, growth spurt, and evidence of estrogenization of the external genitalia. Patients with tumors and some patients with CAH have evidence of virilization.

Treatment and Follow-up

The treatment of premature adrenarche is reassurance and follow-up. The child should be examined every 3 to 6 months initially to confirm the original diagnostic impression; evidence of virilization or early estrogen effect points to a different diagnosis. Growth data should be carefully plotted. It is hoped that treatment of late-onset 21-hydroxylase deficiency with corticosteroids will prevent the development of polycystic ovary syndrome in early adolescence. In general, pubertal development at adolescence can be expected to be normal. Some patients will have hirsutism and irregular menses as adolescents (83,91).

REFERENCES

1. Tanner JM. Trend towards earlier menarche in London, Oslo, Copenhagen, the Netherlands, and Hungary. *Nature* 1973;243:95.
2. Herman-Giddens ME, Slora EJ, Wasserman RC, et al. Secondary sexual characteristics and menses in young girls seen in office practice: a study from the Pediatric Research in Office Settings Network. *Pediatrics* 1997;99:505.
3. Kaplowitz PB, Slora EJ, Wasserman RC, et al. Earlier onset of puberty in girls: relation to increased body mass index and race. *Pediatrics* 2001;108:347.
4. Kaplowitz PB, Oberfield SE, et al. Reexamination of the age limit for defining when puberty is precocious in girls in the United States: implications for evaluation and treatment. *Pediatrics* 1999;104:936.
5. Pathomvaanich A, Merke DP, Chrousos GP. Early puberty: a cautionary tale. *Pediatrics* 2000;105:115.
6. Midyett LK, Moore WV, Jacobson JD. Are pubertal changes in girls before age 8 benign? *Pediatrics* 2003;111:47.
7. Haqq AM, Silverberg P, Hanna CE. Precocious puberty caused by an estrogen and androgen secreting adrenal adenoma: a case report and review of the current literature. *The Endocrinologist* 2001;11:9.
8. Rosenfield RL. Normal and almost normal precocious variations in pubertal development. Premature pubarche and premature thelarche revisited. *Horm Res* 1994;41(suppl 2):7.
9. Lee PA. Central precocious puberty: an overview of diagnosis, treatment, and outcome. *Endocrinol Metab Clin North Am* 1999;28:4:901.
10. Fenton C, Tang M, Path M. Review of precocious puberty part 1: gonadotropin-dependent precocious puberty. *The Endocrinologist* 2000;10:107.
11. Bridges NA, Christopher JA, Hindmarsh PC, Brook CGD. Sexual precocity: sex incidence and aetiology. *Arch Dis Child* 1994;70:116.
12. Hochman HI, Judge DM, Reichlin S. Precocious puberty and hypothalamic hamartoma. *Pediatrics* 1981;67:236.
13. Cacciari E, Frejaville E Cicognani A, et al. How many cases of true precocious puberty in girls are idiopathic? *J Pediatr* 1983;102:357.
14. Judge DM, Kulin HE, Pagea R, et al. Hypothalamic hamartoma and luteinizing-hormone release in precocious puberty. *N Engl J Med* 1977;296:7.
15. Mahachoklertwattana P, Kaplan S, Grumbach M. The luteinizing hormone–releasing hormone–secreting hypothalamic hamartoma is a congenital malformation: natural history. *J Clin Endocrinol Metab* 1993;77:118.
16. Chalumeau M, Chemaitilly W, Trivin C et al. Central precocious puberty in girls: an evidence based diagnosis tree to predict central nervous system abnormalities. *Pediatrics* 2002;109:61.
17. Balagura S, Shulman K, Sobel EH. Precocious puberty of cerebral origin. *Surg Neurol* 1979;11:315.
18. Leiper AD, Stanhope R, Kiching P, et al. Precocious and premature puberty associated with treatment of acute lymphoblastic leukemia. *Arch Dis Child* 1987;62:1107.
19. Lane L, Comite F, Hench K et al. Precocious puberty associated with neurofibromatosis and optic gliomas. *Am J Dis Child* 1985;139:1097.
20. Pringle PJ, Stanhope R Hindmarsh P, Brook CG. Abnormal pubertal development in primary hypothyroidism. *Clin Endocrinol* 1988;28(5):479.
21. Anasti JN, Flack MR, Froehlich J, et al. A potential novel mechanism for precocious puberty in juvenile hypothyroidism. *J Clin Endocrinol Metab* 1995;80:276.
22. Gordon CM, Austin DJ, Radovick S, Laufer MR. Primary hypothyroidism presenting as severe vaginal bleeding in a premenarchal girl. *J Pediatr Adolesc Gynecol* 1997;10:35.
23. Sigurjonsdottir TJ, Hayles AB. Precocious puberty: a report of 96 cases. *Am J Dis Child* 1968;115:309.
24. Thamdrup E. Precocious sexual development. *Dan Med Bull* 1961;8:140.
25. Pescovitz OH, Hench K, Green O, et al. Central precocious puberty complicating a virilizing adrenal tumor: treatment with a long-acting LHRH analog. *J Pediatr* 1985;106:612.
26. Wierman ME Beardsworth DE, Mansfield MJ, et al. Puberty with gonadotropins: a unique mechanism of sexual development. *N Engl J Med* 1985;312:65.
27. Feuillan PP, Foster CM, Pescovitz OH, et al. Treatment of precocious puberty in the McCune–Albright syndrome with the aromatase inhibitor testolactone. *N Engl J Med* 1986; 315:1115.
28. Foster CM Feuillan P, Padmanabhan V, et al. Ovarian function in girls with McCune–Albright

syndrome. *Pediatr Res* 1986;20:859.

29. Comite F, Shawker TH, Prescovitz OH, et al. Cyclical ovarian function resistant to treatment with an analogue of luteinizing hormone releasing hormone in McCune–Albright syndrome. *N Engl J Med* 1984;311:1032.

30. Lee PA, VanDop C, Migeon C. McCune–Albright syndrome: long-term follow-up. *JAMA* 1986;256: 2980.

31. Weinstein LS, Shenker A, Gejman PV, et al. Activating mutations of the stimulatory G protein in the McCune–Albright syndrome. *N Engl J Med* 1991;325:1688.

32. Freni-Titulaer LW, Cordero JF, Haddock L, et al. Premature thelarche in Puerto Rico. *Am J Dis Child* 1986;140:1263.

33. Haddad NG, Fuqua JS. Phytoestrogens: effects on the reproductive system. *The Endocrinologist* 2001;11:498.

34. Bourguignon JP, Gerard A, Alvarez Gonzalez ML, et al. Effects of changes in nutritional conditions on timing of puberty: clinical evidence from adopted children and experimental studies in the male rat. *Horm Res* 1992;32(suppl 1):97.

35. Blanco-Garcia M, Evain-Brion D, Roger M, et al. Isolated menses in prepubertal girls. *Pediatrics* 1985;76:43.

36. Saggese G Ghirri P, Del Vecchio A, et al. Gonadotropin pulsatile secretion in girls with premature menarche. *Horm Res* 1990;33:5.

37. Sane K, Pescovitz OH. The clitoral index: a determination of clitoral size in normal girls and in girls with abnormal sexual development. *J Pediatr* 1992;120:264.

38. Stanhope R, Adams J, Jacobs HS, Brook CGD. Ovarian ultrasound assessment in normal children, idiopathic precocious puberty, and during low dose pulsatile gonadotrophin releasing hormone treatment of hypogonadotropic hypogonadism. *Arch Dis Child* 1985;60:116.

39. Palmert MR, Malin HV and Boepple PA. Unsustained or slowly progressive puberty in young girls: initial presentation and long-term follow-up of 20 untreated patients. *J Clin Endocrinol Metab* 1999;84:415.

40. Klein KO. Editorial: precocious puberty: who has it? who should be treated? *J Clin Endocrinol Metab* 1999;84:411.

41. Fontoura M, Brauner R Prevot C et al. Precocious puberty in girls: early diagnosis of a slowly progressing variant. *Arch Dis Child* 1989;64:1170.

42. Lee PA. Laboratory monitoring of children with precocious puberty. *Arch Pediatr Adolesc Med* 1994;148:369.

43. Neely EK, Wilson DM, Lee PA, et al. Spontaneous serum gonadotropin concentrations in the evaluation of precocious puberty. *J Pediatr* 1995;127:47.

44. Garibaldi LR, Picco P, Magier S, et al. Serum luteinizing hormone concentrations, as measured by a sensitive immunoradiometric assay, in children with normal, precocious or delayed pubertal development. *J Clin Endocrinol Metab* 1991;72:888.

45. Rosenfield RL. Selection of children with precocious puberty for treatment with gonadotropin releasing hormone analogs. *J Pediatr* 1993;124:989.

46. Bar A, Linder B, Sobel EH, et al. Bayley-Pinneau method of height prediction in girls with central precocious puberty: correlation with adult height. *J Pediatr* 1995;126:955.

47. Metter GB, Kelch RP Effects of gonadotropin-releasing hormone analog therapy on adult stature in precocious puberty. *J Clin Endocrinol Metab* 1994;79:331.

48. Shoevaart CE, Drop SLS, Otten BJ, et al. Growth analysis up to final height and psychosocial adjustment of treated and untreated patients with precocious puberty. *Horm Res* 1990;34:197.

49. Crowley WF, Comite F, Vale W, et al. Therapeutic use for pituitary desensitization with a long-acting LHRH agonist: a potential new treatment for idiopathic precocious puberty. *J Clin Endocrinol Metab* 1981;52:370.

50. Comite F, Cutler GB, Rivier J, et al. Short-term treatment of idiopathic precocious puberty with a long-acting analogue of luteinizing hormone releasing hormone. *N Engl J Med* 1981;305:1539.

51. Kreiter M, Burstein S. Rosenfield RL, et al. Preserving adult height potential in girls with idiopathic precocious puberty. *J Pediatr* 1990;117:364.

52. Kappy MS, Stuart T, Perelman A. Efficacy of leuprolide therapy in children with central precocious puberty. *Am J Dis Child* 1988;142:1061.

53. Comite F, Cassorla F, Barnes KM, et al. Luteinizing hormone releasing hormone analogue therapy for central precocious puberty. *JAMA* 1986;255:2613.

54. Mansfield MJ, Beardsworth DE, Loughlin JS, et al. Long-term treatment of central precocious puberty with a long-acting analogue of luteinizing hormone–releasing hormone. *N Engl J Med* 1983;309:1286.
55. Manasco PK, Pescovitz OH, Hill SC, et al. Six-year results of luteinizing hormone releasing hormone (LHRH) agonist treatment in children with LHRH-dependent precocious puberty. *J Pediatr* 1989;115:105.
56. Boepple PA, Mansfield MJ, Link K, et al. Impact of sex steroids and their suppression on skeletal growth and maturation. *Am J Physiol* 1988;255:E559.
57. Lee PA, Page JG, Leuprolide Study Group. Effects of leuprolide in the treatment of central precocious puberty. *J Pediatr* 1989;114:321.
58. Boepple PA, Mansfield MJ, Weirman ME, et al. Use of a potent, long-acting agonist of gonadotropin-releasing hormone in the treatment of precocious puberty. *Endocrinol Rev* 1986;7:24.
59. Carel JC, Lahlou N, Jaramillo O, et. al. Treatment of central precocious puberty by subcutaneous injections of leuprorelin 3-month depot (11.25 mg). *J Clin Endocrinol Metab* 2002;87:4111.
60. Brauner R, Adan L, Malandry F, Zantleifer D. Adult height in girls with idiopathic true precocious puberty. *J Clin Endocrinol Metab* 1994;79:415.
61. Oerter KE, Manasco P, Barnes KM, et al. Adult height in precocious puberty after long-term treatment with deslorelin. *J Clin Endocrinol Metab* 1991;73:1235.
62. Carel JC, Roger M, Ispas S, et al. Final height after long-term treatment with triptorelin slow release for central precocious puberty: importance of statural growth after interruption of treatment. *J Clin Endocrinol Metab* 1999;84:1973.
63. Cassio A, Cacciari E, Balsamo A, et al. Randomized trial of LHRH analogue treatment on final height in girls with onset of puberty age 7.5–8.5 years. *Arch Dis Child* 1999;81:329.
64. Bhatia S, Neely EK, Wilson DM. Serum luteinizing hormone rises within minutes after depot leuprolide injection: implications for monitoring therapy. *Pediatrics* 2002;109:30.
65. Jay N, Mansfield MJ, Blizzard RM, et al. Ovulation and menstrual function of adolescent girls with central precocious puberty after therapy with gonadotropin-releasing hormone agonists. *J Clin Endocrinol Metab* 1992;75:890.
66. Manasco PK, Pescovitz OH, Feuillan PP, et al. Resumption of puberty after long term luteinizing hormone–releasing hormone agonist treatment of central precocious puberty. *J Clin Endocrinol Metab* 1988;67:368.
67. Saggese G, Bertelloni S, Baroncelli GI, et al. Reduction of bone density: an effect of gonadotropin releasing hormone analogue treatment in central precocious puberty. *Eur J Pediatr* 1993;152:717.
68. Antoniazzi F, Zamboni G, Bertoldo F, et al. Bone mass at final height in precocious puberty after gonadotropin-releasing hormone agonist with and without calcium supplementation. *J Clin Endocrinol Metab* 2003;88:1096.
69. van der Sluis IM, Boot AM, Krenning EP, et. al. Longitudinal follow-up of bone density and body composition before, during and after cessation of GnRH agonist therapy. *J Clin Endocrinol Metab* 2002;87:506.
70. Weirman ME, Beardsworth DE, Crawford JD, et al. Adrenarche and skeletal maturation during luteinizing hormone releasing hormone analogue suppression of gonadarche. *J Clin Invest* 1986;77:121.
71. Mansfield MJ, Rudlin CR, Crigler JF Jr, et al. Changes in growth and serum growth hormone and plasma somatomedin-C levels during suppression of gonadal sex steroid secretion in girls with central precocious puberty. *J Clin Endocrinol Metab* 1988;66:3.
72. Marti-Henneberg C, Vizmanos B. The duration of puberty in girls is related to the timing of its onset. *J Pediatr* 1997;131:618.
73. Sonis WA, Comite F, Glue J, et al. Behavior problems and social competence in girls with true precocious puberty. *J Pediatr* 1985;106:156.
74. Ehrhart AA, Meyer-Bahlburg HFL, Bell JJ, et al. Idiopathic precocious puberty in girls: psychiatric follow-up in adolescence. *J Am Acad Child Psychiatry* 1984;23:23.
75. Boek-Jensen AM, Brocks V, Holm J, et al. Central precocious puberty in girls: internal genitalia before, during, and after treatment with long-acting gonadotropin-releasing hormone analogues. *J Pediatr* 1998;132:15.
76. Escobar ME, Rivarola MA, Bergada C. Plasma concentration of oestradiol-17β in premature

thelarche and in different types of sexual precocity. *Acta Endocrinol* (Copenh) 1976;81:351.

77. Ilicki A, Lewin RP, Kauli R, et al. Premature thelarche-natural history and sex hormone secretion in 68 girls. *Acta Paediatr Scand* 1984;73:756.

78. Pasquino AM Pucarelli I, Passeri F, et al. Progression of premature thelarche to precocious puberty. *J Pediatr* 1995;126:11.

79. Klein KO, Mericq V, Brown-Dawson JM, et al. Estrogen levels in girls with premature thelache compared with normal prepubertal girls as determined by an ultrasensitive recombinant cell bioassay. *J Pediatr* 1999:134:190.

80. Nelson KG. Premature thelarche in children born prematurely. *J Pediatr* 1983;103:756.

81. Van Winter IT, Noller KL, Zimmerman D, Melton LJ. Natural history of premature thelarche in Olmsted County Minnesota, 1940–1984. *J Pediatr* 1990;116:278.

82. Korth-Schultz S, Levine LS, New M. Dehydroepiandrosterone sulfate (DS) levels, a rapid test for abnormal adrenal androgen secretion. *J Clin Endocrinol Metab* 1976;42:1005.

83. Ibanez L Potau N, Virdis R, et al. Postpubertal outcome in girls diagnosed of premature pubarche during childhood: increased frequency of functional ovarian hyperandrogenism. *J Clin Endocrinol Metab* 1993;76:1599.

84. Miller DP, Emans SJ, Kohane I. A follow-up study of adolescent girls with a history of premature adrenarche. *J Adolesc Health* 1996;18:301.

85. Silfen ME, Manibo AM, McMahon DJ et al. Comparison of simple measures of insulin sensitivity in young girls with premature adrenarche: the fasting glucose to insulin ratio may be a simple and useful measure. *J Clin Endocrinol Metab* 2001;86:2863.

86. Ibanez L, de Zegher F, Potau N. Anovulation after precocious pubarche: early markers and time course in adolescence. *J Clin Endocrinol Metab* 1999;84:2691.

87. Kaplowitz PB, Cockrell JL, Young RB. Premature adrenarche. *Clin Pediatr* 1986;25:28.

88. Temeck JW, Pang S, Nelson C, et al. Genetic defects of steroidogenesis in premature pubarche. *J Clin Endocrinol Metab* 1987;64:609.

89. Granoff AB Chasalow Fl, Blethen SL. 17-Hydroxyprogesterone responses to adrenocorticotropin in children with premature adrenarche. *J Clin Endocrinol Metab* 1985;60:409.

90. Balducci R, Boscherini B, Mangiantini A, et al. Isolated precocious pubarche: an approach. *J Clin Endocrinol Metab* 1994;79:582.

91. Ibanez L, Dimartino-Nardi J, Potau N. and Saenger P. Premature adrenarche—normal variant or forerunner of adult disease? *Endocrine Reviews* 2000;21:671.

6

Delayed Puberty

S. Jean Emans

This chapter presents a practical approach to delayed sexual development, Chapter 7 provides the algorithms for the diagnosis and treatment of amenorrhea, and Chapter 8 reviews dysfunctional uterine bleeding. Chapters 1 and 4 should be mastered before an evaluation of any of these problems is undertaken. Gonadal development and embryogenesis are reviewed in Chapters 2 and 10. The distinction between delayed puberty and amenorrhea can be somewhat artificial because problems that cause pubertal delay can also cause amenorrhea. For example, a patient with 45,X/46,XX (Turner mosaic) or the patient with anorexia nervosa may present to the clinician with no sexual development, primary amenorrhea, or secondary amenorrhea. It is thus helpful for the clinician to think about a general approach to define the source of the hypothalamic–pituitary–ovarian axis abnormality. The differential diagnosis of delayed puberty includes central causes (chronic disease, nutritional deficiency, hypopituitarism, and tumors), hypothyroidism, adrenal disorders, and ovarian failure (Table 6-1). Physiological delay of puberty is a diagnosis of exclusion.

Recent U.S. data from the National Health and Nutrition Examination Survey III (NHANES III) have shown that black girls enter puberty first, followed by Mexican American, and then white girls (1,2). The mean age of initiation of puberty for black, Mexican American, and white girls was 9.5, 9.8, and 10.3 years for breast development, respectively, and 9.5, 10.3, and 10.5 years for pubic hair development (1). Early timing of pubertal maturation in girls is associated with obesity (3,4).

EVALUATION—HISTORY AND PHYSICAL EXAMINATION

A thorough history and physical examination are essential for the evaluation of the adolescent girl with delayed puberty. A girl who has not experienced any pubertal development by the age of 13 years is more than 2 standard deviations beyond the normal age of initiating puberty and thus warrants a medical evaluation. For

TABLE 6-1. *Differential diagnosis of delayed puberty*

Hypogonadotropic hypogonadism

CNS causes
> Chronic disease, especially those associated with malnutrition (cystic fibrosis, Crohn disease, celiac disease, HIV disease, sickle cell disease)
> Physiologic delay
> Weight loss and eating disorders
> Competitive athletics, ballet dancing
> GnRH deficiency (Kallmann syndrome)
> Genetic syndromes: Lawrence-Moon-Biedl, Prader-Willi syndromes
> CNS tumors—e.g., craniopharyngiomas
> Depression
> Drugs, especially associated with hyperprolactinemia
> Pituitary causes—tumor (prolactinoma), infiltrative disease (sarcoid, tuberculosis, histiocytosis X, CNS leukemia), hemochromatosis, head trauma, "empty sella," irradiation, surgery

Thyroid
> Hypothyroidism

Adrenal
> Cushing syndrome
> Addison disease

Hypergonadotropic hypogonadism

Ovaries
> Gonadal dysgenesis (Turner Syndrome)
> Pure gonadal dysgenesis (46,XX or 46,XY)
> Radiation or chemotherapy; oophorectomy
> Autoimmune oophoritis
> Resistant ovary syndrome
> 17α-hydroxylase deficiency
> Aromatase deficiency
> Other—galactosemia, myotonia dystrophica, trisomy 21, fragile X premutation carriers, sarcoidosis, ataxia telangiectasia; ovarian torsion, removal, or destruction; tuberculosis; oophoritis

the exceptional girl who is known to have a debilitating chronic disease (see Chapter 23) or who is involved in ballet or a competitive endurance sport such as track or gymnastics that may be associated with a delay in pubertal development, the full diagnostic workup can be postponed until age 14 years, provided that other parameters of growth and development are compatible with the delay. Each girl should be observed for a steady progression of growth and pubertal development. A halt in maturation also signifies the need to do a thorough endocrine evaluation. Several illustrative case histories are included at the end of this chapter.

The pertinent past history depends in part on the presenting complaint and may include the following:

1. Family history: heights of all family members (if short stature); age of menarche and fertility of sisters, mother, grandmothers, and aunts (familial

disorders include delayed puberty, delayed menarche, androgen insensitivity, congenital adrenal hyperplasia, some forms of gonadal dysgenesis, and fragile X premutation carriers); history of ovarian tumors (e.g., gonadoblastomas in intersex disorders); and history of autoimmune endocrine disorders such as thyroiditis, diabetes, Addison disease, and autoimmune ovarian failure.

2. Neonatal history: Maternal ingestion of androgens can cause clitoromegaly; maternal history of miscarriages; birth weight; congenital anomalies; hernias; lymphedema (Turner syndrome); and neonatal problems such as hypoglycemia that can be suggestive of hypopituitarism.

3. Previous surgery (bilateral oophorectomy), irradiation, or chemotherapy.

4. Review of systems with special emphasis on a history of chronic disease, abdominal pain, diarrhea, headaches, neurologic symptoms, ability to smell, weight changes, disordered eating, caloric intake, sexual activity, galactorrhea, medications, substance abuse, emotional stresses, competitive athletics, acne, and hirsutism.

5. Age of initiation of pubertal development, if any, and rate of development.

6. Growth data plotted on charts, such as those illustrated in Chapter 4, with mid-parental height calculated.

The physical examination involves a general assessment that includes height and weight, blood pressure, palpation of the thyroid gland, and Tanner [Sexual Maturity Rating (SMR)] staging of breast development and pubic hair. The girl may have presented for a complaint of "no development" and yet the physical examination may reveal that her breast development is SMR 2; follow-up over the next 3 to 6 months may establish that the girl is in normal puberty. The presence of congenital anomalies should be assessed, including hernias, renal anomalies, evidence of skeletal disproportion suggestive of chondrodysplasias. If abnormal body proportions are questioned during the visual assessment, measurement of the arm span and upper lower segment (U/L) ratios can be helpful. The arm span is measured from middle fingertip to middle fingertip. The lower segment is measured from the top of the pubic symphysis to the floor (the upper segment is height minus lower segment). In the child with normal proportions, the arm span is approximately the same as the height. The U/L ratio is around 0.95. Midline facial defects may be associated with hypothalamic–pituitary dysfunction. The somatic stigmata of Turner syndrome may be a clue to the diagnosis of delayed development (see page 191). A neurologic examination is important in patients with delayed or interrupted puberty and includes an assessment of the ability to smell, fundoscopic examination, and screening visual field tests by confrontation (formal visual field tests may be indicated if a pituitary tumor is diagnosed). The presence of androgen excess (hirsutism, acne) should also be noted (see Chapter 9).

In the initial examination of the adolescent with no pubertal development, the gynecologic assessment involves simple inspection of the external genitalia to determine if the girl has clitoromegaly and whether there is estrogen effect on the hymen and anterior vagina. The finding of a reddened, thin vaginal mucosa is consistent with lack of estrogen and delayed puberty; this is in contrast to the pink, moist vaginal mucosa consistent with estrogen effect. Because the etiology of pubertal delay likely results from an ovarian problem (e.g., Turner syndrome or ovarian failure) or from a hypothalamic–pituitary problem (e.g., hypogonadotropic hypogonadism), an external examination usually suffices. In contrast, in the girls with normal pubertal development and primary amenorrhea, assessment of internal genital structure is essential to exclude a genital anomaly (see Chapter 7). However, in the nonobese prepubertal teenager, a simple rectoabdominal examination in the dorsal supine position will often allow palpation of the cervix and the uterus. If a pelvic ultrasound is obtained in a prepubertal adolescent girl, the uterus may not be well visualized and thus may be wrongly assumed to be absent. The ultrasound should be repeated in a pediatric center with experience in performing and interpreting ultrasounds in prepubertal girls.

In adolescents, assessment of the pattern of growth can yield valuable information. Accurate measurement using a stadiometer is critical to ascertain changes in growth patterns. Prepubertal growth rate is 2 to 2.5 in. per year with an increase at puberty and then closure of the epiphyses (see Chapter 4). Failure of statural growth for several years in the prepubertal girl may occur with Crohn disease (Chapter 23), a systemic disease, or an acquired endocrine disorder. In conditions associated with poor nutrition, such as anorexia nervosa, celiac disease, and inflammatory bowel disease, weight is typically affected more than height. The patient is usually *underweight for her height.* In contrast, patients with acquired hypothyroidism, cortisol excess (iatrogenic or Cushing syndrome), growth hormone deficiency, and Turner syndrome are typically *overweight for height.*

EVALUATION—LABORATORY TESTING

After completing the history and physical examination and plotting the growth chart, the clinician should obtain laboratory tests including a complete blood count (CBC), urinalysis, and serum levels of follicle-stimulating hormone (FSH), thyroid-stimulating hormone (TSH), and prolactin. Additional thyroid tests (T_4 and TBGI or free T_4) should be obtained initially if a central cause of the delayed puberty or amenorrhea is suspected, since the TSH may be in the normal range despite central hypothyroidism. The differential diagnosis can usually be divided on the basis of FSH levels into categories of hypergonadotropic hypogonadism (high FSH levels, indicating ovarian failure) and hypogonadotropic hypogonadism (low or normal levels of FSH, indicating a hypothalamic problem) (Table 6-1; Fig. 6-1) (5). Unless a high FSH level is suspected because of prior radiation, chemotherapy, or short stature, a single high FSH should be repeated (in 2 weeks) before a definitive statement about ovarian failure is made to the patient and family. Low to normal levels of FSH [and luteinizing hormone

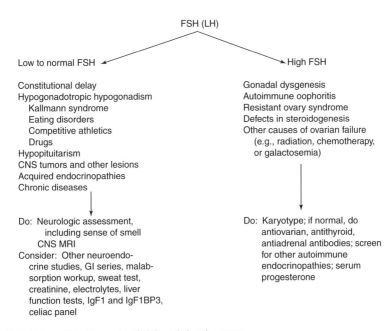

Physical examination
Growth charts
CBC, ESR, TFTs, Prolactin, FSH, Urinalysis
X ray of the hand and wrist for bone age

FSH (LH)

Low to normal FSH   High FSH

Constitutional delay
Hypogonadotropic hypogonadism
    Kallmann syndrome
    Eating disorders
    Competitive athletics
    Drugs
Hypopituitarism
CNS tumors and other lesions
Acquired endocrinopathies
Chronic diseases

Gonadal dysgenesis
Autoimmune oophoritis
Resistant ovary syndrome
Defects in steroidogenesis
Other causes of ovarian failure
    (e.g., radiation, chemotherapy,
    or galactosemia)

Do: Neurologic assessment,
        including sense of smell
        CNS MRI
Consider: Other neuroendo-
    crine studies, GI series, malab-
    sorption workup, sweat test,
    creatinine, electrolytes, liver
    function tests, IgF1 and IgF1BP3,
    celiac panel

Do: Karyotype; if normal, do
        antiovarian, antithyroid,
        antiadrenal antibodies; screen
        for other autoimmune
        endocrinopathies; serum
        progesterone

FIG. 6-1. Differential diagnosis of delayed development.

(LH)] imply a central nervous system (CNS) cause, for example, hypothalamic dysfunction, a pituitary problem, stress, an eating disorder, chronic disease, or, rarely, a CNS tumor. In girls suspected to have Turner syndrome because of significant short stature, determination of the prolactin level can be delayed until the result of the FSH level is known. In girls with unexplained delayed puberty or symptoms of chronic illness, an erythrocyte sedimentation rate (ESR) is obtained in addition to creatinine level, other chemistry determinations, and a celiac panel. For girls with poor linear growth, levels of insulin-like growth factor-1 (IGF-1) and IGF-1 binding protein 3 (IGF-1BP3) can help screen for growth hormone deficiency with the caveat that the levels should be compared to those of similar pubertal status.

A non-dominant hand and wrist x-Ray for *bone age* will help determine how delayed the patient is and allow an estimation of final adult height (Appendix 7). For example, hypothyroidism tends to delay *bone age* more than *height age* (the age at which the patient's height would be on the fiftieth percentile on a growth chart). With constitutional delay, both bone age and height age are similarly delayed (unless the patient is also short genetically). Calculating *mid-parental height* is helpful in determining whether a girl's predicted height is in a target range for her family. For girls, mid-parental height is [(mother's height) + (father's height − 5 in.)] divided by 2; 1 standard deviation (SD) is 2 in. (or 2 SD is 4 in.) (see Case 5). It is extraordinarily helpful as the clinician is taking the history and performing the examination to think of the spectrum of possible diagnoses for delayed puberty or amenorrhea from the hypothalamus to the gonads. A stepwise evaluation using history, growth charts, physical examination, and limited laboratory tests will rule in and rule out the major causes of delayed puberty in adolescent girls.

HYPOGONADOTROPIC HYPOGONADISM

Low to Normal Follicle-Stimulating Hormone (and Luteinizing Hormone) Levels

The majority of girls with delayed puberty will have low or normal FSH levels (hypogonadotropic hypogonadism) from constitutional delay, undernutrition, chronic illness, stress, disordered eating, weight loss, athletic competition, or endocrinopathies such as hypothyroidism. Other less common causes of hypogonadotropic hypogonadism include hypothalamic disorders such as Kallmann syndrome or a tumor, and pituitary problems such as a microadenoma or infiltrative disease. A normal physiologic delay in puberty is a diagnosis of exclusion.

One of the most common causes of delayed puberty is poor nutrition. Caloric counts using food diaries and gastrointestinal evaluation are indicated in those with poor nutrition. Poor intake, malabsorption, and increased caloric requirements commonly occur in chronic diseases such as cystic fibrosis, sickle cell disease, human immunodeficiency virus disease, renal disease, celiac disease, and Crohn disease (6–9). The diagnosis is frequently evident before puberty, but patients with Crohn disease may present with subtle manifestations such as growth failure in the teenage years. On careful history, most, but not all, patients with Crohn disease have a history of intermittent, crampy abdominal pain, diarrhea, or constipation. The ESR is usually, but not invariably, elevated, and mild anemia and hypoalbuminemia may be present as clues. Similarly, celiac disease may present with growth failure and few other suggestive symptoms. If the patient is underweight for height and/or demonstrates poor weight and height gains, further gastrointestinal evaluation and screening tests for celiac disease (celiac panel: transglutaminase, antiendomysial antibodies and IgA) may be indicated before it is assumed that low caloric intake alone is responsible for the problem. If IGF-1 levels are obtained, the binding protein IGF–1BP3 should also be measured because IGF-1 levels may be low in malnutrition and delayed development and do not necessarily indicate growth hormone deficiency. Renal problems associated with impaired growth include renal tubular acidosis, glomerular diseases treated with corticosteroids, and end-stage renal failure.

Self-imposed caloric restriction and intermittent dieting are common among adolescent girls, many of whom view themselves as overweight. Society's preoccupation with a thin physique may lead parents and children to restrict the diet inappropriately, causing weight loss or growth failure. Although anorexia nervosa is typically associated with amenorrhea, fear of obesity can cause significant growth failure in prepubertal children (10). However, it behooves the clinician to exclude a hypothalamic tumor, a malabsorptive state, and chronic disease in the prepubertal child with an apparent eating disorder. Children may also have inadequate access to food because of family psychosocial problems, alcoholism, drug abuse, lack of financial resources, or homelessness.

As noted in the section in Chapter 7 (page 226) on the *female athlete triad* (amenorrhea, disordered eating, and osteopenia), girls who are involved in ballet or competitive endurance sports such as track and gymnastics may have a delay in pubertal development and growth (11–13) (Fig. 6-2). There is debate over whether this delay associated with undernutrition can result in lower final adult height. In a study of gymnasts and swimmers, Theintz and colleagues (13) noted that the growth spurt in gymnasts was suboptimal and associated with short stature (Fig. 6-3). Familial short stature and body type may be contributing factors to the observed results, and other studies have suggested more normal growth curves. However, inadequate nutrition from anorexia nervosa can also impact growth velocity. In addition, delayed puberty and poor linear growth may be caused by endocrinopathies, including hypothyroidism, poorly controlled diabetes mellitus, and Cushing syndrome. Acquired hypothyroidism may have a subtle onset that may be missed except for the slowing of statural growth. The use of pharmacologic doses of corticosteroids to treat many medical diseases frequently causes an iatrogenic picture of Cushing syndrome. Substance abuse and psychological problems such as severe depression can be associated with an interruption of the pubertal process.

Hypothalamic dysfunction may be caused by a number of inherited genetic defects that are increasingly being identified including: X-linked Kallmann syndrome 1 (KAL1 gene) associated with lack of migration of the neurons responsible for gonadotropin-releasing hormone (GnRH) release and the olfactory neurons (and thus anosmia); autosomal dominant Kallmann syndrome (FGFR1 gene); receptor mutations across the hypothalamus, pituitary, and adrenal glands; GnRH receptor mutations (GNRHR gene); mutations in the regulation of GnRH release (GPR54 gene); and leptin mutations (14). Patients with hypothalamic dysfunction may also have midline craniofacial defects. Distinguishing isolated GnRH deficiency from delayed puberty may be difficult if the patient has not begun to show a normal postpubertal response to GnRH or GnRH analogs. Rosenfield (15) has suggested that gonadotropin deficiency is probable in a prepubertal teen girl with normal or low FSH if bone age is >13 years, anosmia or panhypopituitarism is

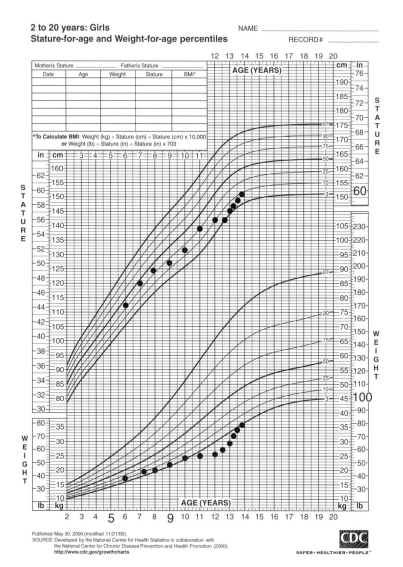

2 to 20 years: Girls
Stature-for-age and Weight-for-age percentiles

NAME _____

RECORD# _____

FIG 6-2. Delayed development and poor growth in a ballet dancer. Medical and nutritional counseling resulted in marked improvement in growth rate. She was still prepubertal at age 13½.

present, there is no sleep-associated increase in LH, and GnRH tests show a flat response (see Chapter 4). Patients with delayed puberty or menarche frequently have other members of the family who have experienced a significant delay. This history alone, however, should not prevent an evaluation of girls with delayed development, since other conditions can be present. Central lesions that need to be

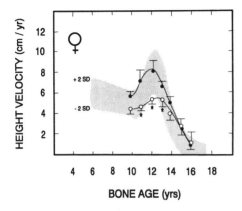

FIG. 6-3. Mean (±SEM) growth velocity as a function of bone age (RUS score) in gymnasts (*clear circles*) and swimmers (*dark circles*); *asterisks* indicate significance (at *p* < 0.05) as a function of chronologic age for normal children. (From Theintz GE, Howald H, Weiss U, Sizonenko PC. Evidence for a reduction of growth potential in adolescent female gymnasts. *J Pediatr* 1993;122:306; with permission.)

considered include tumors, hydrocephalus, brain abscesses, and infiltrative lesions such as tuberculosis, sarcoidosis (16), eosinophilic granuloma, Wegener granulomatosis, lymphocytic hypophysitis, and CNS leukemia. Follow-up is critical to make sure that normal puberty occurs, since one of these conditions may become apparent later.

Craniopharyngiomas typically present between the ages of 6 and 14 years and cause headaches, poor growth, delayed development, and diabetes insipidus. Children who have received cranial radiation for leukemia therapy may have abnormalities of growth hormone secretion and may lack pulsatile GnRH secretion as well (17,18). Iron deposition from hemochromatosis and iron overload associated with transfusion therapy in thalassemia major can result in pubertal delay. Iron deposition in the patient with thalassemia may also cause hypothyroidism, hypoparathyroidism, diabetes, cardiac failure, and/or pituitary dysfunction (19,20). Hypogonadotropic hypogonadism and obesity are also associated with the Laurence-Moon-Biedl and Prader-Willi syndromes. Medications, particularly antipsychotic drugs, can cause hyperprolactinemia (see Chapter 7).

Pituitary causes of interrupted development and irregular menses include hypopituitarism, either congenital or acquired, and tumors. Acquired hypopituitarism can result from head trauma (21), postpartum hemorrhagic shock and pituitary necrosis (Sheehan syndrome), pituitary infarction from conditions such as sickle cell disease, and, rarely, an autoimmune process (22). Empty sella syndrome is rare in children but can be associated with hypothalamic pituitary dysfunction (23) (see Chapter 7). In one series of children with multiple pituitary deficiencies, one-third had an empty sella (24). The most common, but still rare, pituitary tumor in adolescence is a prolactinoma, which most typically causes only primary or secondary amenorrhea rather than complete absence of pubertal development (see section on Hyperprolactinemia in Chapter 7); however, rare tumors have been reported in prepubertal girls (25). Pituitary adenomas that are not prolactinomas are not usually associated with amenorrhea and thus tend to be diagnosed at the time an imaging study is done for some other reason, such as headaches, or because tumor growth causes headaches or visual disturbances. These rare tumors may secrete FSH, LH, or high levels of the α subunit of the glycopeptide hormones (26). Therapy with a GnRH agonist does not cause down-regulation of mildly elevated FSH levels. These patients may have modest elevation of serum prolactin levels. Patients found to have these tumors should have further neuroendocrine evaluation in a search for abnormalities of ACTH production and growth hormone secretion. Consultation with a pediatric endocrinologist and neurosurgeon is important.

Thus, the evaluation of the adolescent with low to normal FSH levels needs to focus on exclusion of a systemic disease, poor nutrition, CNS disorder, or endocrinopathy. Evidence of other chronic diseases such as cystic fibrosis, renal failure, diabetes, or liver disease should be assessed. If a hypothalamic or pituitary tumor is under consideration or if a girl has significantly delayed puberty, then evaluation should include cranial MRI. Further neuroendocrine studies are important in the evaluation of patients with evidence of panhypopituitarism and some patients with tumors. Patients with a history of CNS radiation for leukemia should have their growth monitored carefully and neuroendocrine testing done if linear growth is abnormal. Formal visual field testing should be obtained in patients with pituitary tumors. As noted in Chapter 4 and 7, girls with delayed puberty and especially low weight may not acquire normal bone mass (27), and thus should be counseled about calcium and vitamin D intake, appropriate nutrition, and prescribed hormonal therapy as indicated.

HYPERGONADOTROPIC HYPOGONADISM

High Follicle-Stimulating Hormone (and Luteinizing Hormone) Levels

Adolescents with persistently elevated FSH levels have premature ovarian failure (POF). Patients with POF may have an abnormal karyotype (e.g., Turner syndrome or, rarely, fragile X premutation carriers, or 46,XY gonadal dysgenesis) or a normal karyotype (e.g., autoimmune oophoritis; see Chapter 7, p. 238), idiopathic POF, galactosemia, or ovarian failure associated with radiation or chemotherapy. Patients with Turner syndrome typically present with delayed development, but any of the disorders may also present with primary or secondary amenorrhea after undergoing some, or even complete, pubertal maturation.

Initial evaluation of the adolescent with elevated FSH levels in the absence of a history of radiation or chemotherapy or a known diagnosis such as galactosemia includes a karyotype determination. In patients with 46,XX ovarian failure, further studies include assessment for autoimmune ovarian failure such as antiovarian, antithyroid, and antiadrenal antibodies. In the hypertensive patient with elevated FSH and delayed puberty, serum levels of progesterone (11-deoxycorticosterone and corticosterone) are obtained in a search for the rare case of 17α-hydroxylase deficiency. Laparoscopy or laparotomy with gonadal biopsy is rarely indicated.

Gonadal Dysgenesis

Turner syndrome occurs in approximately 1 of 2,000 live-born girls and in 1 of 15 spontaneous abortions (28). Slightly over one-half of patients with gonadal dysgenesis have the classic 45,X karyotype (Turner syndrome). The stigmata of Turner syndrome include short stature, broad chest, webbed neck, low hairline, short fourth or fifth metacarpals, cubitus valgus, genu valgum, ptosis, low-set ears, narrow high-arched palate, micrognathia, lymphedema, and multiple pigmented nevi. Some anomalies such as the webbed neck, low hairline, rotated auricle, puffy hands and feet, and nail dysplasia appear to be secondary to lymphatic obstruction (29).

The mean final heights of girls with Turner syndrome not treated with growth hormone have been reported to be 142 to 146.8 cm (56 to 58 in.) with an average of 143 cm (30) (Fig. 6-4). A positive correlation has been found between the height standard deviation scores of mosaic patients and the frequency of normal chromosome constitution and a negative correlation of height with the frequency of cells with 45,X (31). Most, but not all studies, have found that the stature of the Turner patients is related to mid-parental height (32,33). Therapy for Turner patients now usually includes treatment with synthetic growth hormone by a pediatric endocrinologist (29,30,34–44). The growth chart of a Turner syndrome patient is shown in Fig. 6-5; the height data are plotted on a special growth chart with percentiles for Turner syndrome (Genentech®). In the

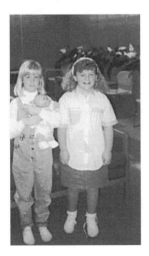

FIG. 6-4. Turner syndrome. A 12-year-old girl with Turner syndrome (*right*) is no taller than her 7-year-old sister. Other signs of the disorder are apparent only on closer inspection. (From Jackson DB, Saunders RB. *Child health nursing: a comprehensive approach to the care of children and their families.* Philadelphia: JB Lippincott Co, 1993; with permission.)

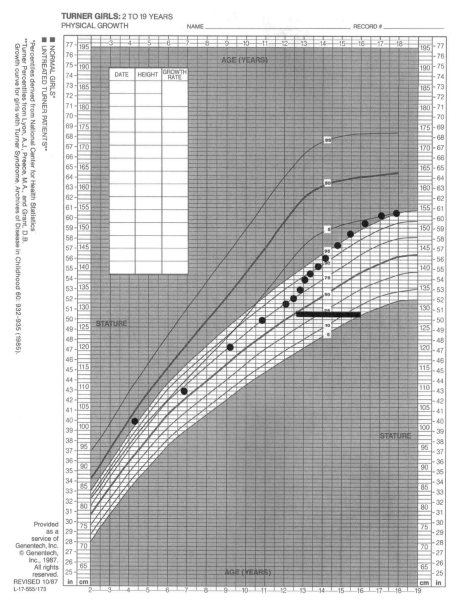

FIG. 6-5. Height chart of a girl with Turner syndrome, treated with growth hormone (*bar*) and subsequently with estrogen–progestin replacement therapy.

first year of therapy of patients with Turner syndrome, Rosenfield and associates (34) found that the mean growth rate for controls was 3.8 cm per year, for human growth hormone (met-HGH) 6.6 cm per year, for oxandrolone 7.9 cm per year, and for combination therapy with human growth hormone and oxandrolone 9.8 cm per year. Although height velocity did decrease after the first year, Rosenfeld and colleagues (35) found sustained increases for at least 6 years in a 3- to 6-year follow-up of girls with Turner syndrome. They reported that 14 of 17 (82%) of girls receiving HGH alone and 41 of 45 (95%) of girls receiving combination therapy with oxandrolone and HGH exceeded their expected adult height. The 30 girls who had completed treatment had a mean height of 151.9 cm, in comparison with a projected mean height of 143.8 cm. The study criteria for cessation of therapy were a bone age ≥14 years and a growth rate <2.5 cm in the past year. (See Fig. 6-5 of a girl with Turner syndrome treated with growth hormone at our hospital.) In a study of 47 girls treated after age 10 years with growth hormone, with or without oxandrolone, Stahnke and colleagues (36) reported that the near final height was 151.7 cm for the GH alone group, 155.1 cm for the GH plus oxandrolone group, and 152.8 cm for the GH plus transient oxandrolone (discontinued because of virilizing side effects). Puberty was induced at a mean of 14.9 years. Ranke and colleagues (37) found an increase of 6 cm with GH treatment. Oxandrolone therapy has not been found beneficial in all studies, and may produce undesired side effects such as virilization and glucose intolerance and should not be used in girls before age 8. Response to GH is dose dependent, with greater gains at higher doses of GH (30,39,41). Patients and parents need to be counseled about the benefits, costs, and potential risks of growth hormone treatment.

A number of recent studies have examined the potential role and timing of estrogen in promoting growth in girls with Turner syndrome. Early treatment with low-dose ethinyl estradiol in addition to GH does not improve final height (30). However, girls who are started on growth hormone early can also start estrogen earlier without compromising adult height (40). In the National Cooperative Growth Study database, Reiter and colleagues (40) found that among the quartile with the earliest age of initiation of growth hormone (mean 8.2 years), estrogen was also initiated at an early age (mean 12.7 ± 1.6 years) with similar heights to the other quartiles. Similarly, a Dutch study (41) found good outcomes for height in girls who received no estrogen for the first 4 years of growth hormone therapy and thereafter were started on estradiol (5 μg/kg per day) when they were 12 years old; their study also found more height gain with higher doses of GH. The advantage of earlier treatment with estrogen would be the development of secondary sexual characteristics more concordant with peers and the opportunity to potentially optimize bone acquisition. However, because the diagnosis of Turner syndrome is often delayed until late childhood or adolescence, estrogen is typically added at a chronologic age of 14 to 15 after the girl has been optimally treated with growth hormone. Estrogen/progestin therapy is further discussed in the Treatment section on page 197.

Other problems associated with Turner syndrome include cardiac anomalies in one-third (bicuspid aortic valve, coarctation of the aorta, mitral valve prolapse, dissecting aneurysms); renal anomalies in 35% to 70% (horseshoe kidneys, unilateral pelvic kidney, rotational abnormalities, duplicated collecting systems, and, rarely, ureteral pelvic obstruction and hydronephrosis); hearing impairment, otitis media, and mastoiditis in one-third; and an increased incidence of hypertension, achlorhydria, glucose intolerance, osteopenia, diabetes mellitus, and Hashimoto thyroiditis (28–30,45–61). Gastrointestinal diagnoses include vascular malformations, which may present with bleeding, and possibly an increased incidence of inflammatory bowel disease. There is conflicting evidence on osteoporosis in patients with Turner syndrome, and studies are needed to control for pubertal status and age and likely examine volumetric bone mineral density as well (49–52,56–61). Benetti-Pinto and co-workers (57) reported that 90% of women with Turner syndrome had osteopenia or osteoporosis; length of estrogen treatment and BMI showed a positive association with bone mineral density. Of interest, girls with normal estrogenization and Turner syndrome have normal bone density (50).

Intelligence appears to be normal in most studies of patients with Turner syndrome, although there can be specific deficits in spatiotemporal processing, visual motor coordination, and specific learning skills (62–64). Similar difficulties have been identified in adult women with Turner syndrome, including deficits of spatial/perceptual skills, visual-motor integration, affect recognition, visual memory, attention, and executive function (28). A high incidence of mental retardation has been reported in girls carrying a small ring chromosome X (28). Girls may be held back in school because of immaturity and short stature, and parents and teachers may expect less of them (30). There is some evidence that girls with Turner syndrome may have more difficulties with social relationships and fewer friends than their peer group (65). Clinicians should ask about potential teasing at school and have counselors address these issues.

A young adolescent with Turner syndrome has prepubertal female genitalia, bilateral streak gonads, and a normal uterus and vagina capable of responding to exogenous hormones; she may have sparse or absent pubic and axillary hair in spite of levels of dehydroepiandrosterone sulfate (DHEAS) that correspond to pubic hair stages 2 to 3. The older teen (15 or 16 years old) with undiagnosed or untreated Turner syndrome usually has pubic and axillary hair, but no breast development or estrogenization of the vaginal mucosa (no ovarian function).

Forty to 50 percent of patients with gonadal dysgenesis have a mosaic karyotype (e.g., 46,XX/45,X) or a structural abnormality of the second X chromosome [e.g., deletion of part of the short arm (p-) or long arm (q-) of the X chromosome, ring chromosome, or isochromosome] (66,67). In a study of 478 patients with Turner syndrome, 52.1% were 45,X; 10.9% were 45,X/46,XX; 4.6% were 45,X/47,XXX or another "superfemale" cell line; 16.1% had isochromosomes; 4% had ring chromosomes; 7.7% had other structural abnormality of the X chromosome; and 4% were mosaic 45,X/46,XY (66). When two tissues are examined (fibroblasts and lymphocytes), mosaicism is more common than would be predicted by just examining blood karyotype results (47). Such patients may show none or all of the classic stigmata of Turner syndrome. "Critical" regions on both the long arm and the short arm of the X chromosome are essential for ovarian function. Deletions in proximal Xq13 and proximal Xq21 are associated with primary amenorrhea, whereas girls with deletions of Xq25-27 develop POF and secondary amenorrhea (29,68). Complete deletion of Xp also results in dysgenetic gonads. Absence or deletion of a portion of Xp correlates with the physical stigmata of Turner syndrome. It is estimated that 5% to 15% of patients with Turner syndrome may have spontaneous pubertal breast development. Girls with mosaic blood karyotypes, especially involving only the loss of the short arm of the X chromosome, are more likely to have pubertal maturation (6% in 45,X; 25% in mosaic patients; and 33% with isolated Xp deletions) (68). Because some of these girls may not have increased FSH, Turner syndrome still should be considered in the adolescent with pubertal development and significantly short stature (in the absence of a family history of short stature). In the majority of girls with Turner syndrome, FSH is usually elevated at birth, is suppressed during childhood, and rises to menopausal levels at the normal pubertal age (9 to 10 years) in those with gonadal failure.

Patients with a 45,X and mosaic karyotypes may have undetected Y DNA, with ranges of 2.5 to 12% (69–72). Cytogenetic examination should include fluorescence *in situ* hybridization, but not routine use of polymerase chain reaction (PCR) techniques unless marker chromosomes of unknown origin are identified or virilization is evident at birth or puberty (47). Gravholt (71) estimated that the occurrence of gonadoblastoma among Y-positive patients to be 7% to 10%, and thus prophylactic gonadectomy is indicated in patients with a Y line to avoid the development of tumors (see Chapter 18) (73).

Rarely, spontaneous pregnancies have been reported among patients with 45,X and mosaics, even among some with elevated gonadotropin levels (74–78). Hreinsson and colleagues reported that follicles could be found in girls up to age 17, raising the question of whether ovarian tissue could be obtained for future reproductive technologies (79). In some studies the outcome of the reported pregnancies has shown an increased risk of abortion, stillbirth, and chromosomally abnormal babies (Turner syndrome and Down syndrome) (76–79). In a recent Danish study (75), 33 women [45,X (n = 1); mosaicism (n = 27); 46,XX and a structural abnormality of the second X (n = 5)], gave birth to 64 children. Two women had become pregnant after in vitro fertilization, including a woman with 45,X after an egg donation. Six of the 25 children who had karyotypes obtained had chromosomal abnormalities (no Down syndrome and only 2 children had malformations). Genetic counseling and prenatal diagnosis should be recommended to all fertile Turner patients. A number of successful pregnancies have been achieved through oocyte donation but the risks of miscarriage and pregnancy related complications are significant (80). Aortic rupture has been reported during oocyte donor pregnancies, with the exact risk unknown (81).

Follow-up of the patient diagnosed with Turner syndrome should include ultrasound examination of the kidneys, cardiac assessment, and monitoring for hypertension, glucose intolerance and diabetes, thyroid dysfunction (those with isochromosome of the long arm of X are especially at risk of Hashimoto thyroiditis), and celiac disease (47,48,82–86). Aggressive treatment of otitis media and audiometry are indicated, and careful attention must be paid to subtle hearing loss and speech defects throughout life (30,53). Patients having surgery should be apprised of their risk of keloid formation (53). Patients who are untreated and who have persistently high gonadotropin levels may show enlarged pituitary fossae, which suggests hyperplasia of the pituitary gland (87). Because of the possibility of increased aortic root diameters (47), patients with Turner syndrome should undergo periodic cardiac evaluation and echocardiography to monitor aortic root diameter and to detect other anomalies. Bicuspid aortic valve, coarctation of the aorta, and hypertension have been noted in 90% of patients with aortic dilatation and dissection (47,54). Monitoring for hypertension, which occurs in up to 40% of girls, is essential and should be aggressively treated (88,89). The optimal periodicity of echocardiograms has not been determined but should depend on baseline assessment and cardiology consultation (53); an interval of 3 to 5 years has been recommended (47). Cardiac MRI has been valuable in the assessment of at-risk patients (47).

Data on long-term follow up of patients with Turner syndrome are providing new information for families. In a study of middle-aged women with Turner syndrome, nearly two-thirds were married, 16% had adopted children, and all were or had been employed (90). Nearly half of the 20 women with 45,X karyotype had had fractures, and many were not taking hormone replacement. Cardiac complications were rare, and hearing loss was reported in 61%. Support groups have been extremely important for providing support and education to patients, their families, and their clinicians. The Turner Syndrome Society of the United States has booklets for families and patients (91) through their website: http://www.turner-syndrome-us.org.

Other Chromosomal Abnormalities Causing Ovarian Failure

The term *pure gonadal dysgenesis* refers to patients with normal or tall stature, streak gonads, and elevated FSH levels. The karyotype is usually 46,XX or 46,XY (Swyer syndrome). In Swyer syndrome, the streak gonads do not produce androgens or antimüllerian hormone (also termed müllerian inhibiting substance) and thus the müllerian system is normal (see Chapters 2 and 10). These 46,XY patients require removal of the gonads. Girls with the 47,XXX karyotype may also have ovarian failure and may have impairment on neuropsychological tests (although preselection bias may play a role in the reported findings) (62).

Patients with 46,XX ovarian failure may have a family history of premature menopause, such as a deletion on the long arm X chromosome in the area responsible for follicular maintenance (92).

Ovarian Failure Secondary to Radiation or Chemotherapy

As more adolescents are surviving their childhood malignancies, the effects of radiation and chemotherapy on gonadal function have become particularly relevant (see

Chapter 23). A teen with delayed puberty or amenorrhea and a history of a malignancy treated with radiation to the pelvis or abdomen and/or chemotherapy suggests a diagnosis of POF. The higher the dose of chemotherapy (particularly alkylating agents) and the older the patient, the greater the possibility of ovarian damage. Children are more resistant to the deleterious effects of chemotherapeutic agents than adults.

17α-Hydroxylase and Aromatase Deficiencies

The extremely rare disorder 17α-hydroxylase deficiency (P450c17) is not true gonadal failure but rather an enzyme deficiency that results in adrenal insufficiency, hypertension, and lack of gonadal sex steroids, including androgens and estrogens. Patients with a 46,XX karyotope have a female phenotype but no secondary sexual characteristics or sexual hair. Patients with a 46,XY karyotype may have a female phenotype, vaginal agenesis, and lack of müllerian structures but, unlike patients with androgen insensitivity (testicular feminization), do not have pubertal breast development. Progesterone levels are elevated. A single case of an adolescent girl with a diagnosis of aromatase deficiency (P450arom), the inability to convert testosterone to estrogen, has been reported (93). The patient had masculinization of the external genitalia at birth but normal female internal genital structures; at the age of 14 years she had absence of breast development, mild virilization (clitoromegaly), multicystic ovaries, elevated testosterone and gonadotropin levels, and delayed bone age.

Other Causes of Premature Ovarian Failure

Premature ovarian failure (POF) also occurs in about 70% to 80% of patients with galactosemia, even those treated from infancy, and may be apparent in late childhood with elevated gonadotropins; it is more likely to occur in those with particular genotypes (94). Other diseases associated with POF are myotonia dystrophica; trisomy 21 (95); fragile X premutation carriers, sarcoidosis; and ataxia telangiectasia. Ovarian destruction has followed mumps oophoritis, gonococcal salpingitis (rarely), and ovarian infiltrative processes (tuberculosis and mucopolysaccharidosis). Autoimmune oophoritis is discussed in Chapter 7 since it is more likely to cause primary or secondary amenorrhea than delayed puberty.

TREATMENT

Treatment is aimed at the cause of the problem, if known; for girls with functional delay in puberty, discussion with the patient and family about risks and benefits of various hormonal therapies is paramount. For conditions such as premature ovarian failure, hormone replacement therapy is the primary therapy. For the teenager with Crohn disease, nutritional rehabilitation and medical and surgical therapies may result in the onset of pubertal growth and development, obviating the need for hormonal interventions.

For many patients with irreversible estrogen deficiency or significant constitutional delay, estrogen replacement therapy is needed to bring about normal secondary sexual characteristics at an age commensurate with the peer group. Although few adolescents with ovarian failure experience vasomotor symptoms such as those seen in postmenopausal women or following oophorectomy, estrogen replacement results in pubertal breast development and menstrual periods, reverses vaginal atrophy, and provides normal levels of estrogen that are important for acquisition of bone mass during adolescence.

For the girl with no secondary sexual characteristics, the approach is relatively straightforward. The clinician should assess readiness for hormone therapy by reviewing growth charts, obtaining a hand and wrist radiograph for estimating bone age and predicted final adult height, and discussing with the girl and her family their view on the optimal age to initiate estrogen replacement. For the girl with Turner syndrome, growth hormone should be offered prior to institution of estrogen replacement therapy to assure optimal linear growth. It is hoped that most of these girls with Turner syndrome would have been diagnosed prenatally or in early childhood and therefore would reach adolescence having been treated with growth hormone, if indicated. However, girls with few stigmata or atypical presentations may not present to the pediatric endocrinologist until the teen years. In girls with Turner syndrome, treatment with estrogen is generally initiated at about the age of 14 or 15 (or after cessation of growth hormone therapy) (see section on Turner Syndrome).

Since many girls with gonadal dysgenesis, premature ovarian failure, or Kallmann syndrome do not come to medical attention until they are 13 to 16 years old, therapy is undertaken at that time. The goals of therapy are to induce normal breast development and menses, increase growth velocity, and promote normal bone mass. In adolescents and young adults, the risk of low bone density appears to be especially related to the lack of spontaneous development, low weight, and exposure to radiation therapy (50). Patients who are known to have undergone chemotherapy and, especially, radiation therapy should have bone age and ovarian status evaluated at a chronologic age of 10 to 12 years and should be considered for replacement therapy when the diagnosis of ovarian failure has been established.

The optimal age for treating patients who have a delay in pubertal development associated with competitive athletic participation or anorexia nervosa is unknown. In general, it seems preferable for patients to make the necessary changes in lifestyle and nutrition to assure normal growth, pubertal development, menses, and bone mass. Delayed menarche is a risk factor for low lumbar bone density (see Chapter 7). Weight, height, growth pattern, and diet should be monitored. Although previously patients were often allowed to remain estrogen deficient for years, which increased their risk of osteopenia, many clinicians do offer estrogen replacement therapy despite the few studies that address efficacy. For example, in girls with no development, we typically offer estrogen therapy when the girl is 14 to 15 years old, taking into account predicted height and the age when breast development and menses are desired by the teen.

Despite the many unknowns in the approach to the adolescent girl with delayed puberty, the clinician needs to undertake therapy for a myriad of conditions, balancing the benefits and risks. In an adolescent girl with an intact uterus, final hormone replacement therapy requires the use of both estrogen and progestin (30,96). The goals of the estrogen component should be considered in three phases: *Phase 1*: induction of breast development; *Phase 2*: establishment of normal menses and, it is hoped, acquisition of normal bone mineralization; and *Phase 3*: long-term maintenance of a normal estrogen state. A patient may need planning for all three phases of estrogen replacement, and the selection of the appropriate doses and the method of cycling depends on her individual needs. The timing of initiating progestin treatment and the appropriate dose are dependent on the amount of breast development and the phase of therapy.

For the induction of breast development in the girl with no secondary sexual characteristics (*Phase 1*), a number of estrogen preparations and dosages have been used. Generally, a low dose of estrogen, such as 0.3 mg of conjugated estrogens (Premarin*), 0.3 mg estrone sulfate (Estratab), or 0.5 mg micronized estradiol (Estrace) is selected to induce initial breast development for 6 to 12 months. Additional options, not commercially available, are 5 to 10 μg of ethinyl estradiol or the sequential administration of estradiol patches of 5, 10, and 25 μg per day over 12 to 24 months (97); the lowest dose of ethinyl estradiol currently available is 20 μg and the lowest dose transdermal patch is 25 μg. The relative potencies of estrogens are summarized in Table 6-2. Oral contraceptives are *not* recommended for initial therapy because they contain progestin throughout the cycle, which is not a physiologic approach to the induction of normal breast development. During normal puberty, there is a long period of unopposed low levels of estrogen until ovulatory cycles begin (see Chapter 4). There has been speculation that particular doses of progestin or estrogen may be more likely to lead to tubular breasts, but a randomized study has not been done.

To further enhance breast development and to induce menses (*Phase 2*), the estrogen dose is increased. For example, the dose might increase to 0.625 mg of conjugated estrogens, 1.0 mg micronized estradiol, 20 μg ethinyl estradiol, or 50 μg transdermal estradiol patch. The timing of this change needs to be adjusted using the bone age determination, the predicted height, and the desire of the patient for rapid breast development. For example, in the girl who is short and initially had no pubertal development, the transition to the higher dose is likely to occur in

---

*The use of brand names is to provide examples, not endorsement of a particular product.

TABLE 6-2. *Comparative effects of estrogen preparations on suppression of follicle-stimulating hormone (FSH) level, liver proteins, and bone density*

Estrogen	FSH levels	Liver proteins	Bone density
Conjugated estrogens	1.0 mg	0.625 mg	0.625 mg
Ethinyl estradiol	5.0 µg	2–10 µg	5–10 µg
Transdermal estradiol	—	—	37.5–50 µg
Piperazine estrone sulfate	1.0 mg	1.25 mg	1.25 mg
Micronized estradiol	1.0 mg	1.0 mg	1.0 mg
Esterified estrogens	—	—	.625 mg
Estradiol valerate	—	—	1.0 mg

(Adapted from Speroff L, Glass RH, Kase NG. *Clinical gynecologic endocrinology and infertility,* 6th ed Philadelphia: Lippincott, Williams & Wilkins, 1999, Chapter 18; with permission. Sources of table: Genant HK, Cann CE, Ettinger B, et al. Quantitative computed tomography of vertebral spongiosa: a sensitive method for detecting early bone loss after oophorectomy. *Ann Intern Med* 1982;97:600. Mashchak CA, Lobo RA, Dozono-Takano R, et al. Comparison of pharmacodynamic properties of various estrogen formulations. *Am J Obstet Gynecol* 1982; 144:511. Horsman A, Jones M, Francis R, et al. The effect of estrogen dose on postmenopausal bone loss. *N Engl J Med* 1983;309:1405. Field CS, Ory SJ, Wahner HW, et al. Preventive effects of transdermal 17β-estradiol on osteoporotic changes after surgical menopause: a two-year placebo controlled trial. *Am J Obstet Gynecol* 1993;168:114. PDR, Vivelle dot.)

12 months. For the girl with ovarian failure who had already started her breast development, has achieved a normal height, and is eager for more breast development, the dose may be increased in 3 to 6 months. The timing of the introduction of progestin varies among centers. Although in the past some girls received unopposed estrogen daily until breakthrough bleeding occurred, we believe that this method should be discouraged because adolescents benefit from a predictable onset of menses, and many girls experience significant dysfunctional bleeding that may require intervention. We suggest the addition of a short course of progestin (5 or 10 mg of medroxyprogesterone) to the continuous estrogen within 2 to 3 months of the *Phase 2* increase in dose: e.g., daily estrogen *plus* medroxyprogesterone 10 mg each day for the first 5 days of each month. This dose of progestin is used only until breast development is completed over the next 6 months and then the dose of progestin is increased to 10 days and ultimately to 12 to 14 days for optimal protection of the endometrium if long-term hormone replacement is planned.

Long-term maintenance (*Phase 3*) includes both an estrogen and a progestin. The estrogen (such as conjugated estrogens 0.625 mg, ethinyl estradiol 20 µg, transdermal estradiol 50 to 100 µg (0.05 to 0.1 mg), esterified estrogens 0.625 mg, or micronized estradiol 1.0 mg is given daily with the progestin for 12 to 14 days each month *or* a cyclic combined estrogen/progestin contraceptive can be prescribed (oral contraceptive, transdermal patch, vaginal ring). Transdermal estradiol patches (such as Vivelle-Dot, Climara, Estraderm) are changed once or twice a week, depending on the preparation. For example, the average estradiol concentration for the Vivelle dot transdermal system is 34 pg/ml for the 0.0375 mg dot,

57 pg/ml for the 0.05 mg dot, 72 pg/ml for the 0.075 mg dot, 89 pg/ml for the 0.1 mg dot, all applied abdominally, and 104 pg/ml for the 0.1 mg dot applied to the buttocks (98). All these doses are superior to placebo for preservation of bone density at the hip and lumbar spine in postmenopausal women with the 0.1 mg superior to the lower doses. Some adolescents tolerate the estradiol patches well and find changing them preferable to daily oral medication (oral or transdermal progestin is still necessary). However, other adolescents complain of the patch falling off, have allergic reactions to the adhesive, or do not like the idea of having a potentially visible acknowledgment of a medical problem. A progestin should be provided for 12 to 14 days each month (e.g., medroxyprogesterone 10 mg or micronized progesterone 200 mg for 12 to 14 days each month) or in a combined oral contraceptive pill, patch, or ring (see Chapter 7). Sequential hormonal regimens are also available prepackaged as dial-paks (e.g., PremPhase has 14 days of conjugated estrogens 0.625 mg and 14 days of conjugated estrogens 0.625 mg and medroxyprogesterone 5 mg). An alternative for teens preferring transdermal estrogen is to give transdermal estrogen/progestin such as Combipatch (estradiol 0.05/0.14 mg norethindrone acetate) for the second 14 days of each month. College students often prefer a combined oral contraceptive pill (or contraceptive patch) in order to be taking a preparation similar to that of many of their friends, avoiding questions about POF or other medical conditions. Of note, elevated gonadotropin levels from POF may only partially suppress, even with what appears to be adequate doses, and the best long-term treatments for individual diagnoses such as Turner syndrome have not been ascertained (99). Monitoring levels of FSH is not generally helpful in determining estrogen dose (100).

Girls with POF need long-term hormonal therapy. The need for hormonal therapy in adolescents should not be confused with the recently changed recommendations about the lack of benefit of hormonal therapy in postmenopausal women. For girls with presumed constitutional delay, therapy can be stopped after the attainment of secondary sexual characteristics and menses to reassess whether the patient has a normal delay or hypothalamic dysfunction. If spontaneous development does not continue, then estrogen can be reinstituted for courses of 6 to 12 months with periodic discontinuation of therapy. Many patients begin to grow pubic hair after receiving estrogen replacement therapy; however, girls who have had CNS tumors and those with panhypopituitarism often have adrenal insufficiency and thus have absent or only scant pubic and axillary hair development.

Adolescent girls, especially those with estrogen deficiency, should be counseled to consume 1300 mg of calcium daily by diet (see Appendix 8 for handout) or supplements (101) and at least 400 IU per day of Vitamin D (daily multivitamin) (100).

The most important part of the therapy undertaken by the physician is the ability to listen to questions and respond in a straightforward fashion. The adolescent needs to know that her parents are not keeping secrets from her about her medical condition. Drawings that underscore how normal she is and that illustrate current and potential technologies are extremely meaningful. The positive aspects of her condition and her ability to function as a normal woman should be emphasized. She may cope better with the issue of infertility if she receives information in response to her own questions. The girl with ovarian failure can be told about the many other young patients with infertility; she may know a couple who has spent years in infertility treatments. The fact that she can make plans that are right for her from early on in relationships can be reassuring. Acceptance of estrogen therapy to promote normal development, menses, and bone mass is the easier part of the counseling, although families and patients often have questions about long-term risks (see Chapter 7). Fertility therapies are discussed in Chapters 7, 10, and 23.

Groups are available in many metropolitan centers for specific diagnoses (e.g., Turner Society groups). Although young adolescents may resist going to meetings, parents, older adolescents, and young adults often find the support and education helpful. Grief and mourning over the lack of function is normal, and frequent visits can help the patient come to terms with the problem. Denial of the diagnosis between visits is common, and the same questions may arise at each visit. The clinician frequently needs to do much of the talking during these appointments, with statements such as "I have other girls in my practice with this problem, and I find they worry about . . ." Sometimes, a young patient will request to be excused from physical education class so that her lack of development will not be the subject of peer discussion; this request should be honored. The empathic health care provider can greatly aid the patient in accepting the medical diagnosis and the treatment plan.

CASES OF DELAYED SEXUAL DEVELOPMENT

Case 1

S. T. was evaluated at the age of 15 years because of "no development." She had always been the shortest member of her class. Physical examination revealed short stature and many of the stigmata of Turner syndrome (low hairline, webbed neck, ptosis, increased carrying angle, and short fourth metacarpals). Her height was 54 in. and her weight 105 lb, her blood pressure was 125/80 mm Hg, and her pulse rate was 78 beats/min. Breast development was stage 1; no pubic or axillary hair was present (stage 1 pubic hair). Pertinent laboratory tests showed an FSH level of 143 mIU/ml, an LH level of 135 mIU/ml, and a karyotype of 45,X (Turner syndrome).

Case 2

C. O. was referred at the age of $15^{10}/_{12}$ because of delayed development. Her developmental milestones were normal; however, she had always been the shortest member of her class. She was an A student in the tenth grade. A review of systems was noncontributory. The family history revealed that one of her father's sisters

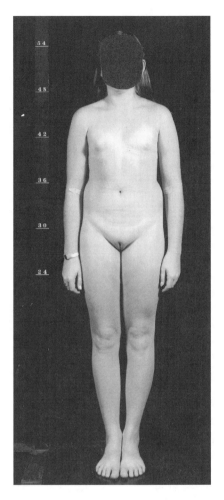

FIG. 6-6. Case 2: Delayed puberty.

had experienced menarche at the age of 20 years. On physical examination (Fig. 6-6), she was short and healthy appearing with a height of 55¾ in. and a weight of 86 lb; her blood pressure was 105/70 mm Hg; and her pulse rate was 66 beats/min. The fundi were normal. Breast development was stage 1, although the areolae were slightly raised with a diameter of 2.4 cm. There was no pubic or axillary hair. The results of CBC, blood urea nitrogen (BUN) determination, thyroid function tests, and urinalysis were normal; the FSH level was low normal. She had an extensive neuroendocrine evaluation, including CNS imaging and neuroendocrine studies, the results of which were normal.

The patient was then given conjugated estrogens 0.3 mg daily, and in a short time her breasts began to develop. Pubic hair appeared gradually. One year later, the estrogen dosage was increased to 0.625 mg given in cycles with 10 mg of medroxyprogesterone. The hormone therapy was discontinued after 18 months, and C. O. continued to have normal cyclic menses.

Case 3

L. C. came to the clinic at the age of $16^6\!/_{12}$ years because of no sexual development. She recalled having been short since the age of 8 or 9 years. With her family, she had moved several times, and two of her grandparents had died when she was between the ages of 8 and 12 years. She had always been in good health and specifically denied having headaches, frequent infections, eating disorders, and gastrointestinal symptoms. Her family members had not experienced any delays in pubertal development. Her father was 65 in. tall; her mother was 62 in. tall and had had menarche at the age of 13.

Physical examination showed her to be healthy with normal blood pressure and pulse rate. Her weight was 105 lb and her height $58\,^1\!/_4$ in. Breast development was Tanner stage 1, and pubic hair was stage 2. No axillary hair was present. The external genitalia were normal but unestrogenized, and a small uterus was palpable on rectoabdominal examination. The results of neurologic examination, including her sense of smell, were normal. Growth charts (Fig. 6-7) showed the patient to be slightly overweight for height; her bone age was $10^9\!/_{12}$ years and her height age $11^6\!/_{12}$ years. The LH level was 0.2 mIU/ml, the FSH level was <2.0 mIU/ml, the estradiol level was <20 pg/ml, the DHEAS level was 109 μg/dl, and the prolactin level was 2.2 ng/ml. The results of thyroid function tests, urinalysis, CBC, and determination of creatinine level and ESR were normal. CNS imaging studies were normal. An overnight study of gonadotropin levels showed no detectable pulsations of LH or FSH (all values <2.0 mIU/ml), and GnRH stimulation testing showed a prepubertal pattern of LH and FSH. Cortisol and growth hormone responses were normal overnight and with insulin testing.

A diagnosis of hypogonadotropic hypogonadism was made, and estrogen therapy was begun: initially 0.3 mg of conjugated estrogens, which was subsequently increased to 0.625 mg with cyclic progestin. With 2 years of therapy, she developed pubertal breasts, with the areola measuring 2.5 cm and glandular tissue 6×6 cm, and pubic hair stage 3. Bone age was 13 years at a chronologic age of 18 years, and she had a significant growth spurt. She currently takes oral contraceptives for estrogen replacement, and becomes estrogen deficient when her therapy is stopped for 2 to 3 months.

Case 4

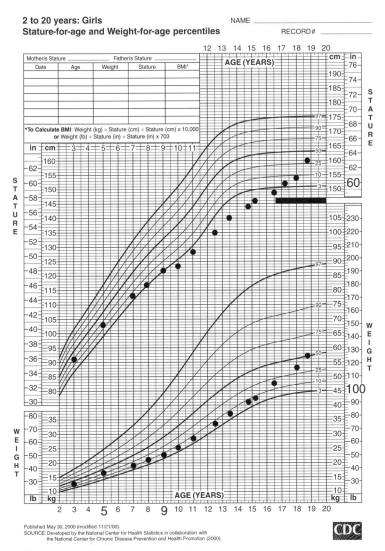

FIG. 6-7. Case 3: Growth chart of patient with delayed development treated with estrogen–progestin therapy (*bar*).

M. C. was referred to the adolescent clinic by the renal clinic at the age of 15 6/12 years because of delayed development. She had been diagnosed with immune complex nephritis at the age of 8 years and had begun dialysis for end-stage renal disease at the age of 11, the time when she recalled having begun to develop pubic hair. She had undergone a successful renal transplant at age 13 years. At the time of her clinic visit, her serum creatinine level was normal, and she was taking prednisone, 15 mg every other day, and azathioprine, 100 mg daily. She was concerned because she had never menstruated and her breasts had not developed.

Physical examination showed her to be short and overweight. Her height was 59½ in. and her weight 131 lb (Fig. 6-8). Her blood pressure and pulse were normal. Breast development was Tanner stage 1, and pubic hair scant stage 2 to 3; no axillary hair was present. The abdominal examination revealed several large

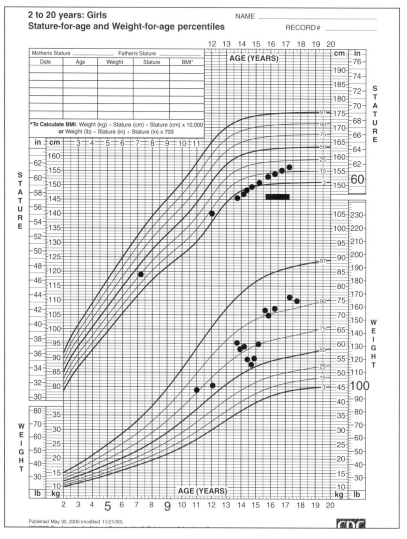

FIG. 6-8. Case 4: Growth chart of patient with delayed development, renal transplant, and 46,XY gonadal dysgenesis, with estrogen progestin therapy *(bar)*.

normal. Breast development was Tanner stage 1, and pubic hair scant stage 2 to 3; no axillary hair was present. The abdominal examination revealed several large scars and a palpable kidney in the right lower quadrant. Pelvic examination revealed a prepubertal unestrogenized hymen; examination with the patient in the knee–chest position showed a normal vagina and cervix. Rectoabdominal examination showed a small, palpable cervix. Although the initial thought was that M.C.'s delay in puberty was likely to have been caused by her chronic illness, the fact that she had started to develop pubic hair at age 11 and not progressed to a normal puberty, in spite of the establishment of normal renal function following the transplant, suggested other diagnoses. Her bone age was 10%12 years. The results of thyroid function tests were normal, but surprisingly, gonadotropin levels were elevated: LH was 216 mIU/ml, and FSH was 297 mIU/ml. Her karyotype was 46,XY. With the diagnosis of 46,XY (Swyer syndrome), M. C. underwent surgery to remove the intraabdominal gonads. The histopathology and staging procedure for ovarian cancer revealed bilateral gonadoblastomas with early invasive dysgerminoma. She has had no recurrence of tumor. M. C. was treated with estrogen replacement therapy and developed only small breasts in spite of the onset of menses. She later underwent an elective breast augmentation with satisfactory results.

Case 5

S. R. is a 13%12 year old seen for slowed growth and delayed pubertal development. She has been in good health with no chronic medical problems and no acute illnesses. She eats a good variety of foods with no restrictions and is active in sports, playing soccer for 2 hours each weekday. She denies abdominal pain, nausea, vomiting, bloating, and diarrhea. Her bowel movements are normal and she has had no skin, joint, or visual complaints. She developed breast buds at age 11 years, followed by development of scant pubic hair but has not changed in the past year. Her mother's height is 64 in. and the father's height is 69 in.; therefore, the parent's mid-parental height is 64 in. (2 SD is 60 in. to 68 in.). Her mother's menarche was at age 13. Her growth chart before and after treatment is shown in Fig. 6-9.

On physical examination, she is a thin, but otherwise well-appearing adolescent girl. Height is 62¼ in. and weight is 84 lb. Her general physical examination is normal. Her breasts and pubic hair are Tanner 2. Her external genitalia are normal. Rectal exam is normal and the stool is negative for occult blood.

Laboratory tests showed a CBC with hematocrit of 34% and MCV of 74 (mild microcytic anemia; other indices within normal limits), normal WBC and platelets, and normal ESR. Liver function tests, electrolytes, BUN, creatinine, glucose, albumin, total protein, Ca, and phosphorus were all normal. Her bone age was 12 years. She had normal thyroid function tests and FSH 2.3 mIU/ml. However, her celiac panel was positive. She was placed on a gluten-free diet, and resumed normal growth and development.

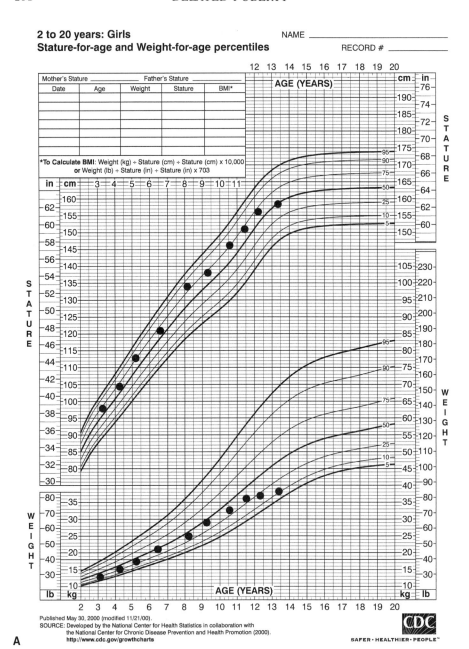

2 to 20 years: Girls
Stature-for-age and Weight-for-age percentiles

NAME _____

RECORD # _____

Published May 30, 2000 (modified 11/21/00).
SOURCE: Developed by the National Center for Health Statistics in collaboration with
the National Center for Chronic Disease Prevention and Health Promotion (2000).
http://www.cdc.gov/growthcharts

A

FIG. 6-9. Case 5: Growth charts of a patient who presented with growth and pubertal delay and was diagnosed with celiac disease **(A)** before, and

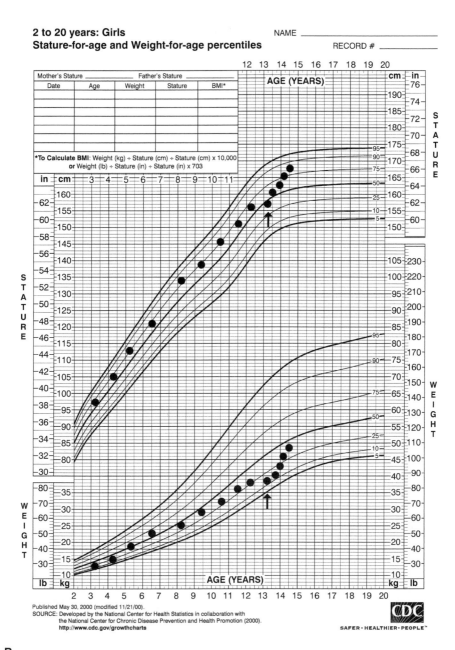

2 to 20 years: Girls
Stature-for-age and Weight-for-age percentiles

NAME _____

RECORD # _____

B

FIG. 6-9. (*Continued*) **(B)** after gluten-free diet (see *arrow*). (From, Knight J, Emans SJ. *A Guide to the Case Teaching Method: and Growth in Children and Adolescents,* Bright Futures Center for Pediatric Education in Growth and Development, Behavior, and Adolescent Health, Children's Hospital, Boston, 2001.)

REFERENCES

1. Wu T, Mendola P, Buck GM. Differences in the presence of secondary sex characteristics and menarche among US girls: the third National Health and Nutrition Examination survey, 1988–1994. *Pediatrics* 2002;110(4):752.
2. Sun SS, Schubert CM, Chumlea WC, et al. National estimates of the timing of sexual maturation and racial differences among US children. *Pediatrics* 2002;110(5):911.
3. Wang, Y. Is obesity associated with early sexual maturation? A comparison of the association in American boys versus girls. *Pediatrics* 2002;110:903.
4. Kaplowitz PB, Slora EJ, Wasserman RC, et al. Earlier onset of puberty in girls: relation to increased body mass index and race. *Pediatrics* 2001;108(2):347.
5. Reindollar RH, Byrd JR, McDonough PG. Delayed sexual development: a study of 252 patients. *Am J Obstet Gynecol* 1981;140:371.
6. Finan AC, Elmer MA, Sasnow SR, et al. Nutritional factors and growth in children with sickle cell disease. *Am J Dis Child* 1988;142:237.
7. Platt OS, Rosenstock W, Espeland MA. Influence of sickle hemoglobinopathies on growth and development. *N Engl J Med* 1984;311:7.
8. Rosenbach Y, Dinari G, Zahavi I, et al. Short stature as the major manifestation of celiac disease in older children. *Clin Pediatr* 1986;25:13.
9. Weizman Z, Hamilton JR, Kopelman HR, et al. Treatment failure in celiac disease due to coexistent exocrine pancreatic insufficiency. *Pediatrics* 1987;80:924.
10. Pugliese MT, Lifshitz F, Grad G, et al. Fear of obesity: a cause of short stature and delayed puberty. *N Engl J Med* 1983;309:513.
11. Frisch RE, Gotz-Welbergen AV, McArthur JW, et al. Delayed menarche and amenorrhea of college athletes in relation to age of onset of training. *JAMA* 1981;246:1559.
12. Warren MP. The effects of exercise on pubertal progression and reproductive function in girls. *J Clin Endocrinol Metab* 1980;51:1150.
13. Theintz GE, Howald H, Weiss U, et al. Evidence for a reduction of growth potential in adolescent female gymnasts. *J Pediatr* 1993;122:306.
14. Beier DR, Dluhy RG. Bench to bedside—The G protein-coupled receptor GPR54 and puberty. *N Engl J Med* 2003;349:1589.
15. Rosenfield RL. Puberty and its disorders in girls. *Endocrinol Metab Clin North Am* 1991;20:15.
16. Murialdo G, Tamagno G. Endocrine aspects of neurosarcoidosis. *J Am Endocrinol Investigation* 2002;25(7):650.
17. Cicognani A, Cacciari E, Vecchi V, et al. Differential effects of 18- and 24-gy cranial irradiation on growth rate and growth hormone release in children with prolonged survival after acute lymphocytic leukemia. *Am J Dis Child* 1988;142:1199.
18. Costin G. Effect of low-dose cranial radiation on growth hormone secretory dynamics and hypothalamic-pituitary function. *Am J Dis Child* 1988;142:847.
19. Maurer HS, Lloyd-Still JD, Ingrisano C, et al. A prospective evaluation of iron chelation therapy in children with severe β-thalassemia. *Am J Dis Child* 1988;142:287.
20. Borgna-Pignatti C, DeStefano P, Zonta L, et al. Growth and sexual maturation in thalassemia major. *J Pediatr* 1985;106:150.
21. Miller WL, Kaplan SL, Grumbach MM. Child abuse as a cause of post-traumatic hypopituitarism. *N Engl J Med* 1980;302:724.
22. Barkan AL, Kelch RP, Marshall JC. Isolated gonadotrope failure in the polyglandular autoimmune syndrome. *N Engl J Med* 1985;312:1535.
23. Shulman DI, Martinez CR, Bercu BB, et al. Hypothalamic-pituitary dysfunction in primary empty sella syndrome in childhood. *J Pediatr* 1986;108:540.
24. Cacciari E, Zucchini S, Ambrosetto P, et al. Empty sella in children and adolescents with possible hypothalamic-pituitary disorders. *J Clin Endocrinol Metab* 1994;78:767.
25. Harris NL, McNeely WF, Shepard JO, et al. Case records of the Massachusetts General Hospital. *N Engl J Med* 2002;347(20):1604.
26. Djerassi A, Coutifaris C, West VA, et al. Gonadotroph adenoma in a premenopausal woman secreting follicle-stimulating hormone and causing ovarian hyperstimulation. *J Clin Endocrinol Metab* 1995;80:591.
27. Csermely T, Halvax L, Schmidt E, et al. Occurrence of osteopenia among adolescent girls with

oligo/amenorrhea. *Gynecol Endocrinol* 2002;16(2):99.

28. Stratakis CA, Rennert OM. Turner's syndrome: molecular and cytogenics, dysmorphology, endocrine, and other clinical manifestations and their management. *Endocrinologist* 1994;4:442.

29. Ogato T, Matsuo N. Turner's syndrome and female sex chromosome aberrations: deduction of the principal factors involved in the development of clinical features. *Hum Genet* 1995;95:607.

30. Rosenfeld RG. Turner's syndrome: a guide for physicians. The Turner's Syndrome Society. Gardiner-Caldwell Synermed, 1992.

31. Partsch CJ, Pankau R, Sippell WG, et al. Normal growth and normalization of hypergonadotropic hypergonadism in atypical Turner syndrome. *Eur J Pediatr* 1994;153:451.

32. Sybert VP. Adult height in Turner syndrome with and without androgen therapy. *J Pediatr* 1984; 104:365.

33. Demetriou E, Emans SJ, Crigler JF, Jr. Final height in estrogen treated patients with Turner syndrome. *Obstet Gynecol* 1984;64:459.

34. Rosenfeld RG, Hintz RL, Johanson AJ, et al. Three year results of a randomized prospective trial of methionyl human growth hormone and oxandrolone in Turner syndrome. *J Pediatr* 1988;113:393.

35. Rosenfeld RG, Franc J, Attie KM, et al. Six-year results of a randomized, prospective trial of human growth hormone and oxandrolone in Turner syndrome. *J Pediatr* 1992;121:49.

36. Stahnke N, Keller E, Landy H, et al. Favorable final height outcome in girls with Ullrich-Turner syndrome treated with low-dose growth hormone together with oxandrolone despite starting treatment after 10 years of age. *J Pediatr Endocrinol Metab* 2002;15(2):129.

37. Ranke MB, Partsch CJ, Lindberg A, et al. Adult height after GH therapy in 188 Ullrich-Turner syndrome patients: results of the German IGLU Follow-up Study 2001. *Eur J Endocrinol* 2002; 147(5):625.

38. Quigley CA, Crowe BJ, Anglin DG, et al. Growth hormone and low dose estrogen in Turner syndrome: results of a United States multi-center trial to near-final height. *J Clin Endocrinol Metab* 2002;87(5):2033.

39. Cacciari E, Mazzanti L. Final height of patients with Turner's syndrome treated with growth hormone (GH): indications for GH therapy alone at high doses and late estrogen therapy. Italian Study Group for Turner Syndrome. *J Clin Endocrinol Metab* 1999;84(12):4510.

40. Reiter EO, Blethen SL, Baptista J, et al. Early initiation of growth hormone treatment allows age-appropriate estrogen use in Turner's syndrome. *J Clin Endocrinol Metab* 2001;86(5):1936.

41. Sas TC, de Muinck Keizer-Schrama SM, Stijnen T, et al. Normalization of height in girls with Turner syndrome after long-term growth hormone treatment: results of a randomized dose-response trial. *J Clin Endocrinol Metab* 1999;84(12):4607.

42. Rosenfield RL, Perovic N, Devine N. Optimizing estrogen replacement in adolescents with Turner syndrome. *Ann NY Acad Sci* 2000;900:213.

43. Elsheikh M, Dunger DB, Conway GS, et al. Turner's syndrome in adulthood. *Endo Rev* 2002;23:120.

44. Hindmarsh PC. What's best for the bones in Turner syndrome? *Clin Endocrinol* 2000;52(5):529.

45. Chernausek SD, Attie KM, Cara JF, et al. Growth hormone therapy of Turner syndrome: the impact of age of estrogen replacement on final height. Genentech, Inc., Collaborative Study Group. *J Clin Endocrinol Metab* 2000;85(7):2439.

46. Allen DB, Hendricks SA, Levy JM. Aortic dilation in Turner's syndrome. *J Pediatr* 1986;109:302.

47. Frias JL, Davenport M. The AAP Committee on Genetics, and the Section on Endocrinology. Health supervision for children with Turner syndrome. *Pediatrics* 2003;111:692.

48. Lippe B, Geffner ME, Dietrich RB, et al. Renal malformations in patients with Turner syndrome: imaging in 141 patients. *Pediatrics* 1988;82:852.

49. Neely EK, Marcus R, Rosenfeld RG, Bachrach LK. Turner syndrome adolescents receiving growth hormone are not osteopenic. *J Clin Endocrinol Metab* 1993;76:861.

50. Emans SJ, Grace E, Hoffer FA, et al. Estrogen deficiency in adolescents and young adults: impact on bone mineral content and effects of estrogen replacement therapy. *Obstet Gynecol* 1990;76:585.

51. Stepan JJ, Musilova J, Pacovsky V. Bone demineralization, biochemical indices of bone remodeling, and estrogen replacement therapy in adults with Turner's syndrome. *J Bone Miner Res* 1989;4:193.

52. Naeraa RW, Brixen K, Hansen RM, et al. Skeletal size and bone mineral content in Turner's syndrome: relation to karyotype, estrogen treatment, physical fitness, and bone turnover. *Calcif Tissue Int* 1991;49:77.

53. Saenger P, Wikland KA, Conway GS, et al. Recommendations for the diagnosis and management of Turner syndrome. *J Clin Endocrinol Metab* 2001;86(7):3061.
54. Rosenfeld RG. Hypertension, aortic dilatation and aortic dissection in Turner syndrome: a potentially lethal triad. *Clin Endocrinol* 2001;54(2):155.
55. Meunier JP, Jazayeri S, David M. Acute type A aortic dissection in an adult patient with Turner's syndrome. *Heart (British Cardiac Society).* 2001;86(5):546.
56. Mora S, Wever G, Guarneri MP, et al. Effect of estrogen replacement therapy on bone mineral content in girls with Turner syndrome. *Obstet Gynecol* 1992;79:747.
57. Benetti-Pinto CL, Bedone A, Magna LA, et al. Factors associated with the reduction of bone density in patients with gonadal dysgenesis. *Fertil Steril* 2002;77(3):571.
58. Sas TC, de Muinck Keizer-Schrama SM, Stijnen T, et al. Bone mineral density assessed by phalangeal radiographic absorptiometry before and during long-term growth hormone treatment in girls with Turner's syndrome participating in a randomized dose-response study. *Pediatr Res* 2001;50(3):417.
59. Sass TC, De Muinck Keizer-Schrama SM, Stijnen T, et al. A longitudinal study on bone mineral density until adulthood in girls with Turner's syndrome participating in a growth hormone injection frequency-response trial. *Clin Endocrinol* 2000;52(5):531.
60. Bertelloni S, Cinquanta L, Baroncelli GI, et al. Volumetric bone mineral density in young women with Turner's syndrome treated with estrogens or estrogens plus growth hormone. *Horm Res* 2000; 53(2):72.
61. Lanes R, Gunczler P, Esaa S, et al. Decreased bone mass despite long-term estrogen replacement therapy in young women with Turner's syndrome and previously normal bone density. *Fertil Steril* 1999;72(5)896.
62. Bender BG, Linden MG, Robinson A. Neuropsychological impairment in 42 adolescents with sex chromosome abnormalities. *Am J Med Genet* 1993;48:169.
63. Ross JL, Roeltgen D, Kushner H, et al. The Turner syndrome-associated neurocognitive phenotype maps to distal Xp. *Am J Hum Genet* 2000;67(3):672.
64. Ross JL, Stefanatos GA, Kushner H, et al. Persistent cognitive deficits in adult women with Turner syndrome. *Neurology* 2002;58(2):218.
65. McCauley E, Feuillan P, Kushner H, et al. Psychosocial development in adolescents with Turner syndrome. *J Dev Behav Pediatr* 2001;22(6):360.
66. Kleczkowska A, Dmoch E, Kubien E, et al. Cytogenetic findings in a consecutive series of 478 patients with Turner syndrome. The Leuven experience 1965–1989. *Genet Couns* 1990;1:227–233; Erratum *Genet Couns* 1991;2:130.
67. Temtamy SA, Ghali I, Salam MA, et al. Karyotype/phenotype correlation in females with short stature. *Clin Genet* 1992;41:147.
68. Heinze HJ. Ovarian function in adolescents with Turner syndrome. *Adolesc Pediatr Gynecol* 1994:7:3.
69. Nishi MY, Domenice S, Medeiros MA, et al. Detection of Y-specific sequences in 122 patients with Turner syndrome: nested PCR is not a reliable method. *Am J Med Genet* 2002;107(4):299.
70. Medlej R, Lobaccaro JM, Berta P, et al. Screening for Y-derived sex determining gene SRY in 40 patients with Turner syndrome. *J Clin Endocrinol Metab* 1992;75:1289.
71. Gravholt CH, Fedder J, Naeraa RW, et al. Occurrence of gonadoblastoma in females with Turner syndrome and Y chromosome material: a population study. *J Clin Endocrinol Metab* 2000;85(9):3199.
72. Alvarez-Nava F, Soto M, Sanchez MA, et al. Molecular analysis in Turner syndrome. *J Pediatr* 2003;142(3):336.
73. Kotzot D, Dufke A, Tzschach A, et al. Molecular breakpoint analysis and relevance of variable mosaicism in a woman with short stature, primary amenorrhea, unilateral gonadoblastoma, and a 46,X,del(Y)(q11)/45,X karyotype. *Am J Med Genet* 2002;112(1):51.
74. Hovatta O. Pregnancies in women with Turner's syndrome. *Ann Med* 1999;31(2):106.
75. Birkebaek NH, Cruger D, Hansen J, et al. Fertility and pregnancy outcome in Danish women with Turner syndrome. *Clin Genet* 2002;61(1):35.
76. Groll M, Cooper M. Menstrual function in Turner's syndrome. *Obstet Gynecol* 1976;47:225.
77. Reyes Fl, Koh KS, Faiman C. Fertility in women with gonadal dysgenesis. *Am J Obstet Gynecol* 1976;126:668.
78. Kaneko N, Kawagoe S, Hizoi M. Turner's syndrome—review of the literature with reference to a successful pregnancy outcome. *Gynecol Obstet Invest* 1990;29:81.

79. Hreinsson JG, Otala M, Fridstrom M, et al. Follicles are found in the ovaries of adolescent girls with Turner's syndrome. *J Clin Endocrinol Metab* 2002;87(8):3618.
80. Foudila T, Soderstrom-Anttila V, Hovatta O. Turner's syndrome and pregnancies after oocyte donation. *Hum Reprod* 1999;14(2):532.
81. Nagel TC, Tesch LG. ART and high risk pregnancies. *Fertil Steril* 1997;68:748.
82. Gruneiro de Papendieck L, Lorcansky S, Coco R, et al. High incidence of thyroid disturbances in 49 children with Turner syndrome. *J Pediatr* 1987;111:258.
83. Miller MJ, Geffner ME, Lippe BM, et al. Echocardiography reveals a high incidence of bicuspid aortic valve in Turner syndrome. *J Pediatr* 1983;102:47.
84. Elsheikh M, Wass JA, Conway GS. Autoimmune thyroid syndrome in women with Turner's syndrome—the association with karyotype. *Clin Endocrinol* 2001;55(2):223.
85. Bonamico M, Pasquino AM, Mariani P, et al. Prevalence and clinical picture of celiac disease in Turner syndrome. *J Clin Endocrinol Metab* 2002;87(12):5495.
86. Gillett PM, Gillett HR, Israel DM, et al. Increased prevalence of celiac disease in girls with Turner syndrome detected using antibodies to endomysium and tissue transglutaminase. *Can J Gastroenterol* 2000;14(11):915.
87. Samaan NA, Stepanas AV, Danziger J, et al. Reactive pituitary abnormalities in patients with Klinefetter's and Turner's syndrome. *Arch Intern Med* 1979;139:198.
88. Nathwani NC, Unwin R, Brook CG, et al. The influence of renal and cardiovascular abnormalities on blood pressure in Turner syndrome. *Clin Endocrin* 2000;52(3):371.
89. Nathwani NC, Unwin R, Brook CG, et al. Blood pressure and Turner syndrome. *Clin Endocrin* 2000;52(3):363.
90. Sylven L, Hagenfeldt K, Brondum-Nielson K, et al. Middle-aged women with Turner's syndrome: medical status, hormonal treatment and social life. *Acta Endocrinol (Copenh)* 1991;125:359.
91. Rieser P, Davenport M. Turner Syndrome: A guide for families. Turner Syndrome Society, 2003.
92. Krauss CM, Turksoy RN, Atkins L, et al. Familial premature ovarian failure due to an interstitial deletion of the long arm of the X-chromosome. *N Engl J Med* 1987;317:125.
93. Conte FA, Grumbach MM, Ito Y, et al. A syndrome of female pseudohermaphrodism, hypergonadotropic hypogonadism, and multicystic ovaries associated with missense mutations in the gene encoding aromatase (P450arom). *J Clin Endocrinol Metab* 1994;78:1287.
94. Guerrero NV, Singh RH, Manatunga A, et al. Risk factors for premature ovarian failure in females with galactosemia. *J Pediatr* 2000;137:833.
95. Hsiang YH, Berkovitz GD, Bland GL, et al. Gonadal function in patients with Down syndrome. *Am J Med Genet* 1987;27:449.
96. Benjamin I, Block RE. Endometrial response to estrogen and progesterone therapy in patients with gonadal dysgenesis. *Obstet Gynecol* 1977;50:136.
97. Lippe B. Turner syndrome. *Endocrinol Metab Clin North Am* 1991;20:121.
98. Vivelle dot transdermal system, www.pdr.net.
99. Guttmann H, Weiner Z, Nikolski E, et al. Choosing an oestrogen replacement therapy in young adult women with Turner syndrome. *Clin Endocrinol* 2001;54(2):159.
100. Yanovski JA, Rose SR, Municchi G, et al. Treatment with a luteinizing hormone-releasing hormone agonist in adolescents with short stature. *N Engl J Med* 2003;348(10):908.
101. Chan GM, Hoffman K, McMurry M. Effects of dairy products on bone and body composition in pubertal girls. *J Pediatr* 1995;126:551.

7

Amenorrhea in the Adolescent

S. Jean Emans

This chapter presents a practical approach to diagnosis and treatment of amenorrhea. Chapter 6 provides the algorithms and differential diagnosis of delayed sexual development, Chapter 8 focuses on dysfunctional uterine bleeding, and Chapter 9 discusses androgen abnormalities and polycystic ovary syndrome (PCOS). As noted in Chapter 6, the distinction between pubertal delay and amenorrhea can be somewhat artificial because many problems that cause pubertal delay can also cause amenorrhea. For example, the patient with 45,X/46,XX (Turner mosaic) or the patient with anorexia nervosa may present to the clinician with no sexual development, primary amenorrhea, or secondary amenorrhea. In the girl with primary amenorrhea, the clinician needs to assess whether there is a hypothalamic–pituitary–ovarian axis abnormality or a genital anomaly present, such as imperforate hymen or vaginal, cervical, and/or uterine agenesis. It is extraordinarily helpful as the clinician is taking the history and performing the examination to think of the spectrum of possible diagnoses for amenorrhea from the hypothalamus to the genital tract (see Fig. 7-1). Diagnoses may range from constitutional delay, eating disorders, stress, and central nervous system (CNS) tumors to thyroid and adrenal disorders to ovarian failure, pregnancy, genital anomalies, and PCOS. A stepwise evaluation using history, growth charts, physical examination, and limited laboratory tests will rule in and rule out the major causes of menstrual disorders in adolescent girls.

The mean age of menarche in the U.S. has decreased significantly over the past 100 years, but little in the past four decades. In the National Health and Nutrition Survey III (NHANES III), the mean age of menarche was 12.1 for black girls, 12.2 for Mexican American girls, and 12.7 for white girls (1). Using this data, Chumlea and colleagues found the mean age was only 0.34 year earlier than 1973 (2). Less than 10% of girls had menarche before age 11, and 90% had begun to menstruate by age 13.75 years. Absence of menarche by age 16 years is termed *primary amenorrhea*. Only three in 1,000 girls will experience

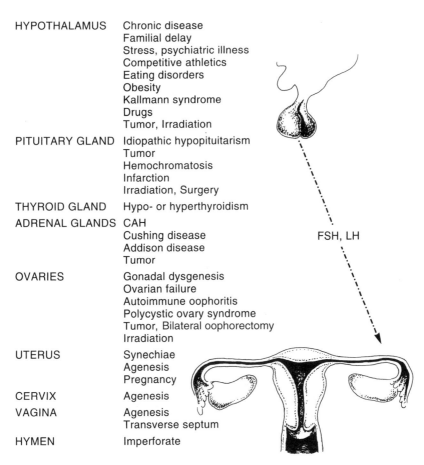

HYPOTHALAMUS	Chronic disease
	Familial delay
	Stress, psychiatric illness
	Competitive athletics
	Eating disorders
	Obesity
	Kallmann syndrome
	Drugs
	Tumor, Irradiation
PITUITARY GLAND	Idiopathic hypopituitarism
	Tumor
	Hemochromatosis
	Infarction
	Irradiation, Surgery
THYROID GLAND	Hypo- or hyperthyroidism
ADRENAL GLANDS	CAH
	Cushing disease
	Addison disease
	Tumor
OVARIES	Gonadal dysgenesis
	Ovarian failure
	Autoimmune oophoritis
	Polycystic ovary syndrome
	Tumor, Bilateral oophorectomy
	Irradiation
UTERUS	Synechiae
	Agenesis
	Pregnancy
CERVIX	Agenesis
VAGINA	Agenesis
	Transverse septum
HYMEN	Imperforate

FSH, LH

FIG. 7-1. Etiology of primary amenorrhea. CAH, congenital adrenocortical hyperplasia; FSH, follicle-stimulating hormone; LH, luteinizing hormone.

menarche after $15\frac{1}{2}$ years. In assessing the individual patient, the clinician needs to keep in mind the normal stages of puberty. Although most girls have the onset of menses within 2 to $2\frac{1}{2}$ years of the beginning of breast development, the range is considerable, and menarche may not occur in an individual girl for 4 years. For example, if the 15-year-old began her pubertal development at the age of 14 years, she can usually be reassured that she can expect her menarche by the age of 16 or 17 years, 2 to 3 years after the onset of secondary sexual characteristics. The patient should be observed for a reassuring steady progression of growth and development. A halt in maturation signifies the need to do a thorough endocrine evaluation. In contrast, the girl who is age 15 years and started her development at age 11 but has not had her menarche warrants an evaluation to determine the cause, including a pelvic examination or ultrasound/MRI to exclude a genital tract anomaly.

The definition of secondary amenorrhea, and thus guidelines for timing of the evaluation, are problematic in the adolescent, since pregnancy is a frequent cause of this complaint. Denial of intercourse is common among teenagers, and young adolescents may not understand their physiology or may have become pregnant by rape or incest. Thus, a pregnancy test should be done whenever an adolescent expresses concern about a menstrual period being late, even if only by 2 or 3 weeks, and as a routine part of evaluation of secondary amenorrhea. Hormone tests and further evaluation of amenorrhea are usually reserved for adolescents who have had 3 to 6 months of amenorrhea without an obvious cause (such as dieting or weight loss) and those with persistent oligomenorrhea, estrogen deficiency, or androgen excess (hirsutism, acne). In a survey of eight high schools [94% of the students white, and ages evenly distributed from 14 to 17 years ($2.5\% \leq 13$, $5.5\% \geq 18$)], Johnson and Whitaker (3) found that abnormal eating patterns were the most important risk factor for missing three consecutive menses in the previous year. The percentage of teens missing three cycles is shown is Table 7-1 by chronologic and gynecologic age (chronologic age minus age of menarche), and the odds ratios for risk factors are shown in Table 7-2. Several illustrative case histories are included in this chapter.

TABLE 7-1. *Percent of adolescent high school girls who reported missing three consecutive menses during the past year (n=2156)*

Chronologic age	%
13	10.8
14	7.8
15	9.4
16	7.9
17	8.1
18	9.8
Gynecologic age	**%**
0	12.5
1	13.5
2	9.7
3	9.6
4	6.1
5	8.5
6	5.3
7	5.4

Gynecologic age is chronologic age minus the age of menarche.
(From Johnson J, Whitaker AH. Adolescent smoking, weight changes, and binge purge behaviors: associations with secondary amenorrhea. *Am J Public Health* 1992;82:47–54; with permission.)

TABLE 7-2. *Risk factors for secondary amenorrhea (3 mos) in 2588 high school girls*

	RR	95% CI
Frequent bingeing and purging	4.17	2.54–6.52
Weight loss and gain	2.59	1.33–4.79
Weight gain ≥4.5 kg	1.71	1.16–2.49
Weight loss ≥4.5 kg	1.45	0.95–2.20
Smoking > 1ppd	1.96	1.21–3.10
First year post menarche	1.74	0.99–1.92

(From Johnson J, Whitaker AH. Adolescent smoking, weight changes, and binge purge behaviors: associations with secondary amenorrhea. *Am J Public Health* 1992;82:47–54; with permission.)

PATIENT ASSESSMENT

A careful history and physical examination are essential for the evaluation of the adolescent girl with amenorrhea. As noted in Chapter 6, the history should include an assessment of familial disorders, including age of menarche and fertility of mother, sisters, and other relatives; neonatal history; previous surgeries; treatments for malignancies, autoimmune disorders, endocrinopathies; review of systems; and rate of pubertal development. The review of systems should focus on headaches, disordered eating, weight changes, athletic participation, medications, acne, and hirsutism.

Assessment of the pattern of growth can yield valuable information. Failure of statural growth for several years may occur with Crohn disease or an acquired endocrine disorder, or it may indicate that the adolescent has reached a bone age of 15 years and her epiphyses have fused. In conditions associated with poor nutrition, such as anorexia nervosa, celiac disease, and inflammatory bowel disease, the patient is typically *underweight for her height.* In contrast, patients with acquired hypothyroidism and cortisol excess (iatrogenic or Cushing syndrome) are typically *overweight for height.* Obtaining a radiograph of the wrist and hand for bone age can be helpful in assessing the amount of growth remaining in patients with primary amenorrhea and short stature [see Appendix 7 for estimates of final height and Chapter 6 (page 186) for discussion of calculation of midparental height]. Menarche is more closely linked to bone age than to chronological age. Girls with classic congenital adrenal hyperplasia (CAH) may have early puberty or may have delayed menarche or secondary amenorrhea with advanced bone age from poor control of elevated androgens.

PHYSICAL EXAMINATION

The physical examination of the girl with primary amenorrhea involves a general assessment including height and weight, blood pressure, palpation of the thyroid gland, and Tanner [Sexual Maturity Rating (SMR)] staging of breast development and pubic hair. The breasts should be compressed gently to assess for the presence of galactorrhea, since patients frequently do not report this finding. Midline facial defects may be associated with hypothalamic–pituitary dysfunction. Renal and vertebral anomalies and hernias may be associated with müllerian malformations. The somatic stigmata of Turner syndrome may be a clue to this diagnosis (p. 191). A brief neurologic examination may include an assessment of the ability to smell, fundoscopic examination, and screening visual field tests by confrontation. The presence of hirsutism, acne, and acanthosis nigricans, which together with amenorrhea are indicative of polycystic ovary syndrome (PCOS), should also be noted (see Chapter 9).

Assessment of the percentage of body fat may also help in explaining to the patient the relationship of amenorrhea to the body composition. A low body mass index (BMI) and low percentage of body fat have been associated with delayed puberty and amenorrhea in athletes and in girls with eating disorders. Although the relationship is an association and not necessarily causative, the determination may aid in setting realistic goals for the future. Methodological issues abound in determining the best way to estimate percentage of body fat, and all office methods have problems (4–7). A clinical *estimate* of percentage of body fat can be obtained by measuring four sites of skinfold thickness (triceps, biceps, subscapular, and suprailiac), using calipers and comparing the results with tables and equations given in Appendix 6 (5,6).

The gynecologic assessment involves first inspection of the external genitalia to determine if the girl has clitoromegaly and a normal hymenal opening and whether there is estrogen effect on the hymen and anterior vagina. Normal breast development and an estrogenized vagina imply that the ovaries are making estrogen. The degree of estrogenization noted at the time of the initial examination can often help the clinician decide the extent of the workup indicated. The finding of a reddened, thin vaginal mucosa is consistent with estrogen deficiency and is more worrisome than the finding of an estrogenized, pink, moist vaginal mucosa.

In the girl with normal pubertal development and primary amenorrhea, assessment of internal genital structures is essential to exclude a genital anomaly. Although an imperforate hymen is typically detected in the newborn nursery or during early childhood, it is sometimes not diagnosed until the patient is an adolescent. A bulging bluish-tinged hymen may be noted in the adolescent with an imperforate hymen and blood-filled vagina (hematocolpos). To assess patency and length of the vagina, a saline-moistened cotton-tipped applicator or urethral catheter can be gently inserted into the hymenal opening (the vaginal sample can also be used for a maturation index to assess estrogenization). The patient with a transverse vaginal septum or vaginal, cervical, and uterine agenesis has normal-appearing external genitalia. Typically in a patient with vaginal agenesis, a cotton-tipped applicator can be inserted only 0.5 to 2 cm. If the vaginal length and width appears normal and the hymenal opening is estrogenized and is adequate for a digital examination, a gentle one-finger examination of the vagina will allow palpation of the cervix and uterus by bimanual vaginal-abdominal examination with the patient in the lithotomy position. If needed, visualization of the cervix is usually possible with a small Huffman speculum. In the nonobese teenager, a simple rectoabdominal examination in the dorsal supine position also can be used to confirm the presence of the cervix and the uterus. In the *unestrogenized* adolescent, the knee–chest position (see Chapter 1) can be used, just as in the prepubertal child, to visualize the vagina and the cervix, although the position is likely to be experienced as embarrassing for most teens.

Pelvic ultrasonography can be obtained for confirmation of the findings or if the patient is not comfortable with a modified pelvic examination. If a pelvic ultrasound is obtained in a poorly estrogenized adolescent girl, the clinician should be cautious in the interpretation because the uterus may be small and difficult to visualize and thus may be assumed to be absent. If questions are raised at the time of the initial evaluation, the ultrasound can be repeated in a pediatric center accustomed to the appearance of the prepubertal uterus or after a course of estrogen therapy. An MRI is important if a congenital anomaly or obstructed genital tract is found; laparoscopy may be needed to better define uterine structures in women with vaginal agenesis (8) (see Chapter 10).

The history and physical examination of the girl with secondary amenorrhea or oligomenorrhea is similar, with the exception that a genital anomaly is unlikely and pregnancy needs to be ruled out early in the assessment. The gynecologic examination may include a speculum examination, a bimanual rectoabdominal examination, or pelvic ultrasound.

The patient's estrogen status can be assessed by vaginal smear, progestin withdrawal, or serum estradiol level. The vaginal smear, obtained during the genital examination, can be sent to the laboratory for maturation index (page 36). The progestin challenge provides an estimate not only of estrogen levels but also confirms the presence of an estrogen-primed normal uterus. After confirming that the patient is not pregnant, the clinician prescribes a progestin challenge with oral medroxyprogesterone (5 or 10 mg once a day for 5 or 10 days) or micronized progesterone (200 to 300 mg once a day for 10 days). The response to progestin challenge tends to correlate with estradiol level. Kletzky and colleagues (9) reported that the mean estradiol concentration was 60 pg/ml in 63 women who had withdrawal bleeding compared to a mean value of 18 pg/ml in 27 women who had no withdrawal response. Among a group of women with a screening estradiol of >50 pg/ml, Shangold and colleagues (10) found that a 10-day course of micronized progesterone, 300 mg, induced withdrawal bleeding in 90%. Bleeding typically occurs 2 to 3 days after the progestin dose but may occur up to 10 days later. The progestin withdrawal test is not indicated in the patient with delayed development or in the patient who clearly appears estrogen deficient on clinical examination (e.g., a girl with anorexia nervosa), as bleeding will not occur. Although a normal menstrual flow in response to progesterone suggests adequate estrogen levels, patients with a variety of pathologic diagnoses such as prolactinomas and those in the early years of ovarian failure may have a normal response. In addition to the vaginal smear and progestin withdrawal test, a serum estradiol level can be obtained but is generally less helpful in assessing estrogenization than the other two tests because it represents a single point in time.

LABORATORY TESTS

Initial laboratory screening tests include a urine or serum human chorionic gonadotropin (HCG) test, a complete blood count (CBC), urinalysis, and serum levels of thyroid-stimulating hormone (TSH), follicle-stimulating hormone (FSH), and prolactin. These should be drawn before any hormones are given, including a progestin challenge, so that levels are not altered. Additional thyroid tests [T_4 and thyroxine-binding globulin index (TBGI) or free T_4] should be obtained initially if a central cause of the amenorrhea is suspected. The HCG result should be obtained early in the workup, since very rarely pregnancy will occur without menarche.

The differential diagnosis can usually be divided on the basis of FSH levels into categories of hypergonadotropic hypogonadism (high FSH levels indicating ovarian failure) and hypogonadotropic hypogonadism (low or normal levels of FSH indicating hypothalamic or pituitary dysfunction) (11) (Fig. 7-2). In girls with amenorrhea and symptoms of chronic illness, an erythrocyte sedimentation rate (ESR) is often obtained in addition to creatinine level, other chemistry determinations, and, as indicated, celiac panel. A luteinizing hormone (LH) level is helpful in girls with suspected PCOS (increased LH to FSH ratio, see Chapter 9). Unless a high FSH level is expected because of prior radiation or chemotherapy, a single high FSH should be repeated in 2 weeks before a definitive statement about ovarian failure is made. Low to normal levels of FSH (and LH) imply CNS cause, for example, hypothalamic dysfunction, which may be primary or secondary to a chronic disease, endocrinopathy, stress, or an eating disorder or, rarely, a CNS tumor. It should be noted that if the LH is drawn during the mid-cycle, ovulatory LH surge, the levels can be three times normal baseline levels. Checking with the oligomenorrheic patient to assure that she did not have menstrual bleeding 2 weeks after the sample was drawn allows correct interpretation of the results. Occasionally, patients with normal FSH levels have subtle disorders of ovarian function, which have been evaluated in adult women with the clomiphene challenge test (12).

In the apparently estrogenized patient with normal gonadotropin levels and failure to have withdrawal bleeding from progesterone, the presence of a normal endometrium can be established by obtaining an ultrasound or by giving estrogen and progestin [e.g., 21 days of an oral contraceptive with 35 μg ethinyl estradiol (EE) *or* conjugated estrogens 0.625 to 1.25 mg on days 1 to 25 and medroxyprogesterone 10 mg on days 16 to 25] for two to three cycles. However, it should be noted that a diagnosis of uterine synechiae (Asherman syndrome) is sufficiently

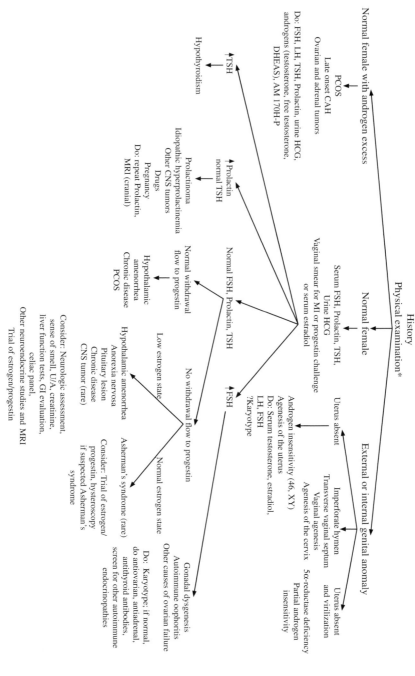

FIG. 7-2. Evaluation of amenorrhea.

rare in the absence of a history of uterine infections, abortion, or dilation and curettage (D&C) that this part of the evaluation can be delayed until the many other possible diagnoses for amenorrhea are considered. Other rare diagnoses resulting in disruption of normal endometrium are tuberculosis and schistosomiasis. Another explanation for the lack of withdrawal flow in the well-estrogenized normal adolescent girl is her failure to take the progestin for the withdrawal challenge.

As noted in Chapter 4, a major concern is whether the patient with amenorrhea is developing normal bone mineral density during her adolescence. Thus assessment of bone density of the lumbar spine and hip is important in girls with more than 6 to 12 months of hypoestrogenic amenorrhea in order to choose appropriate therapies such as observation versus hormonal replacement. The center performing the bone density measurements should have software that can provide age-matched standards for comparison (13). For girls with significant pubertal delay, the results should be corrected for bone age.

A dilemma for the clinician may be whether to obtain radiographic studies of the CNS in the patient with normal serum FSH and prolactin values. There are no absolute guidelines; however, most pituitary tumors associated with primary or secondary amenorrhea in this age group secrete prolactin, interrupt normal prolactin inhibition sufficiently to cause a mild to moderate elevation of prolactin, or are associated with other signs or symptoms. Given the likelihood that most adolescents with hypothalamic amenorrhea have that condition because of stress, athletics, or weight changes, and nonfunctioning tumors that cause amenorrhea are extremely rare, an MRI scan is generally reserved for the evaluation of the patient with interrupted puberty, elevated prolactin level, and/or neurologic signs or symptoms. A MRI may also be indicated in the evaluation of the older adolescent or young adult woman who has persistent amenorrhea with no obvious etiology.

Patients with amenorrhea (primary or secondary) and hirsutism usually have polycystic ovary syndrome (PCOS) or more rarely, late-onset congenital adrenal hyperplasia (CAH) (see Chapter 9). Patients with true virilization are rarer and may have PCOS, late-onset CAH, an ovarian or adrenal tumor, mixed gonadal dysgenesis, an incomplete form of androgen insensitivity, 5α-reductase deficiency, gonadal dysgenesis (with virilization), or true hermaphroditism (see Chapters 2, 9, and 10).

HYPOGONADOTROPIC HYPOGONADISM

The majority of diagnoses in adolescents with primary and secondary amenorrhea fall into this category and include chronic illness (especially those associated with poor nutrition such as Crohn disease, celiac disease, cystic fibrosis, and sickle cell disease), undernutrition, stress, eating disorders, athletic competitions, medications, genetic syndromes, hypothalamic disorders such as Kallmann syndrome and tumors, and pituitary problems such as prolactinomas, non-prolactin-secreting tumors (14), infarction, and infiltrative disease (see Chapter 6). Hydrocephalus due to aqueductal stenosis can present with headaches and amenorrhea during adolescence (15). Acquired hypopituitarism can result from head trauma, postpartum shock and pituitary necrosis (Sheehan syndrome), pituitary infarction from conditions such as sickle cell disease, and, rarely, an autoimmune process (16). An entity known as *empty sella* can occur in children as well as adults and may be associated with hypothalamic pituitary dysfunction; in one series of children with multiple pituitary deficiencies, one-third had an empty sella (17). A normal-sized sella that is empty may be associated with pituitary hypoplasia, an unrecognized pituitary insult, dysfunction of the hypothalamus or higher centers resulting in diminished pituitary growth, or herniation of cerebrospinal fluid through a congenitally incomplete sellar diaphragm (18).

Girls with poorly controlled diabetes mellitus (19,20), depression, psychological problems, and substance abuse may have irregular menses. Self-imposed caloric restriction and intermittent dieting are common among adolescent girls, many of whom view themselves as overweight. Even mild dieting, fat restriction, bingeing and purging are associated with irregular menses and may be initially denied (21–23). Similarly, weight loss even in obese patients who are still significantly overweight for height can result in amenorrhea (24). However, it is important for the clinician to consider the rare hypothalamic tumor, a malabsorptive state, and chronic disease in the adolescent with an apparent eating disorder.

Hypothalamic amenorrhea refers to a spectrum of girls who may have severe estrogen deficiency from anorexia nervosa to those with more minor changes in endocrine function. In a study of 49 adult women with hypothalamic amenorrhea, LH pulses varied from apulsatile (8%) to low frequency/low amplitude (27%), low amplitude/normal frequency (8%), low frequency/normal amplitude (43%), and normal frequency/normal amplitude (14%) (25). The abnormal pattern of gonadotropin-releasing hormone (GnRH) and gonadotropin secretion varies over time in the same woman.

Special sections below review some of the relevant literature on special causes of hypogonadotropic hypogonadism in adolescents: eating disorders, the female athlete triad, and prolactinomas. A normal physiologic delay in menarche is a diagnosis of exclusion and requires a careful medical evaluation before watchful waiting or hormonal therapy is undertaken.

EATING DISORDERS

Eating disorders are prevalent in contemporary society. Some adolescents pursue thinness to the extreme of causing delayed development, delayed menarche, and secondary amenorrhea. Adolescents with bulimia and normal weight for height may have regular or irregular menses. Two peaks of presentation of anorexia nervosa occur, at age 13 years and at 18 years, the first associated with pubertal mat-

TABLE 7-3. *Criteria for diagnosing eating disorders in adolescents*

Anorexia nervosa
Refusal to maintain body weight over a minimal normal weight for age and height (body weight less than 85% of that expected), or failure to make expected weight gain during period of growth.
Intense fear of gaining weight or becoming fat, even though underweight.
Disturbed body image, or denial of the seriousness of the current low body weight.
In postmenarcheal females, amenorrhea of at least three consecutive menstrual cycles.
Types: restricting and binge eating/purging.

Bulimia nervosa
Recurrent episodes of binge eating, characterized by eating, in a discrete period of time, an amount of food that is definitely larger than most people would eat during a similar period of time, AND a sense of lack of control over eating during the episode.
Recurrent inappropriate compensatory behaviors in order to prevent weight gain, such as self-induced vomiting; misuse of laxatives, diuretics, enemas, or fasting; or hyperexercising.
Binge eating or compensatory behaviors at least twice a week for 3 months.
Self-evaluation unduly influenced by body shape and weight.
Disturbance does not occur exclusively during episodes of anorexia nervosa.
Types: purging and nonpurging.

Eating disorders not otherwise specified (EDNOS).
Criteria for anorexia nervosa are met, except the individual has regular menses.
Criteria for anorexia nervosa are met except weight is in the normal range.
Criteria for bulimia nervosa are met, except binges occur <2×/week for <3 months.
Regular use of inappropriate compensatory behavior by an individual of normal body weight after eating a small amount of food.
Repeatedly chewing and spitting out large amounts of food.
Binge eating disorder: recurrent binges without compensatory behaviors.

(Adapted from American Psychiatric Association. *DSM-IV. Diagnostic and Statistical Manual of Mental Disorders, 4th Ed.*, Washington D.C., American Psychiatric Association, 1994, and AAP Committee on Adolescence. Identifying and treating eating disorders. *Pediatrics* 2003;111: 204.)

uration and body image concerns, and the second with separation and choices about jobs and college. Young women with other medical problems such as Turner syndrome or diabetes mellitus may also develop eating disorders. The criteria for the diagnosis of anorexia nervosa are summarized from *The Diagnostic and Statistical Manual of Mental Disorders IV* (DSM-IV) in Table 7-3 (26). Treating patients early in the course of the illness, even before these criteria have been met, may yield a better prognosis. These girls are often preoccupied with thoughts of food; some may restrict intake to several hundred calories per day and may feel inadequate and experience a pervasive lack of control. Other adolescents may binge and then purge by self-induced vomiting or by abuse of laxatives. Since these girls are frequently secretive about their eating patterns, it is useful for the clinician to develop some techniques for eliciting an accurate history, such as saying, "Where would you like your weight to be? How hard do you have to work to keep your weight where you want it to be? Have you ever used vomiting or medicines to control your weight?"

A multitude of medical problems are associated with eating disorders, including dehydration and electrolyte imbalance (27). Vital signs are usually depressed in girls with anorexia nervosa, with low temperature, blood pressure, and pulse rate. Other signs include dry skin, lanugo, bruises, edema (during refeeding), murmurs, abdominal bloating, constipation, cold intolerance, and stress fractures. Substantial deficits in bone density may occur and may be irreversible and associated with low weight, low lean body mass, low fat intake, estrogen deficiency, hypercortisolism, low DHEAS, and insulin-like growth factor-1 (IGF-1) deficiency (28–32). Dual energy x-ray absorptiometry (DEXA) measurements of the spine and hip are significantly related to lean body mass and are lower in women with anorexia nervosa than hypothalamic amenorrhea (28). Leptin levels are low and are associated with amenorrhea. In a study of women with anorexia nervosa, normal cycling women with BMI <18, and normal weighted cycling controls, the low BMI women with menses had higher leptin levels than women with anorexia nervosa but lower levels than normal weighted controls (33). In girls with anorexia nervosa, serum levels of FSH and LH are low (34). Levels of TSH and T_4 are usually normal, but T_3 is often low and the inactive metabolite, reverse T_3, high ("sick euthyroid"). The differential diagnosis of anorexia nervosa includes inflammatory bowel disease, celiac disease, Addison disease, hyperthyroidism, malignancy, diabetes mellitus, depression, and CNS tumors.

Frisch and McArthur (35,36) have proposed a chart for examining the relationships between height/weight and menstrual function (Fig. 7-3). Although the chart can provide some guidance for office counseling, it should be noted that the hypothesis of a critical weight or percentage body fat for establishment of menses has been challenged, and individual patients show variation in the recovery of menstrual function related to weight. The ranges are useful in developing target weights for patients and families and facilitating a discussion of the relationships of height, weight, and menstrual function. For example, a 13-year-old adolescent who is 5 ft 5 in. tall would be expected to weigh a minimum of 44 kg (97 lb) or a *calculated* body fat percentage of 17% at the time of menarche. If instead she lost weight at age 16 to 18 years and developed secondary amenorrhea, she would need to achieve a weight of 49 kg (108 lb) or a *calculated* body fat percentage of 22% to regain her menses. Given the normal weight gain of 10 pounds between the ages of 13 and 18 years, the clinician needs to consider both the patient's age and whether the patient has primary or secondary amenorrhea in utilizing the charts. A weight estimate for a 16- to 18-year-old with primary amenorrhea (and anorexia nervosa) is better determined from the weight for height charts associated with secondary amenorrhea than from the line for primary amenorrhea weights; otherwise, the expected weight will likely be set too low. Statural growth in girls with delayed menarche is often nearly complete because of exposure to low amounts of estrogens and adrenal androgens.

Target ideal body weights (IBW) for height can also be determined using percentiles for weight and height (37) or determinations of normal body mass index (BMI) using the CDC growth charts. Patients benefit from being given a range (92 to 100% IBW or 10th to 25th centile on BMI) of weights, *not a single number*. Patients

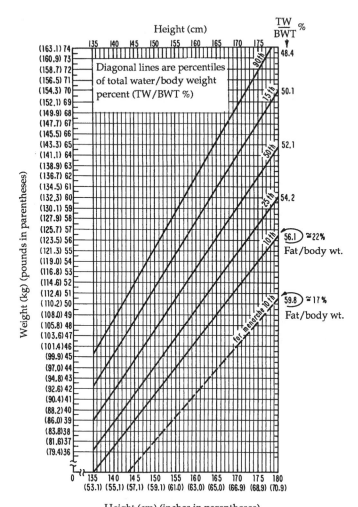

FIG. 7-3. Nomogram indicating the minimal weight a female of a given height should weigh to be likely to have normal menses. The lowest diagonal line is the 10th percentile of total water/body fat for menarche. The second lowest diagonal line is the 10th percentile for 18-year-old adolescents; this diagonal often corresponds to the weight needed for restoration of menses in an adolescent with weight loss and secondary amenorrhea. (From Frisch RE, McArthur JW. Menstrual cycles: fatness as determinant of minimum weight necessary for their maintenance or onset. *Science* 1974;185:949; with permission of the American Association for the Advancement of Science and Dr. Rose Frisch. Figure provided by Dr. Rose Frisch, Center for Population Studies, Cambridge, MA.)

who regain a normal weight for height but persist with amenorrhea frequently continue to have abnormal eating patterns, avoidance of foods containing fat, and preoccupation with food. In a study of girls recovering from anorexia nervosa, Kreipe and colleagues (38,39) found that a mean of 92 ± 7% of ideal body weight (IBW) was associated with the return of menses. In another study, Golden and colleagues (40) noted that menses resumed at a weight 2.05 kg more than the weight at which menses were lost and that the mean percent of IBW was 91.6% ± 9.1%. Eighty six percent of patients resumed menses within 6 months of achieving this weight. Another study found that 79% of 242 girls had return of menses at follow-up (41).

FEMALE ATHLETE TRIAD: DISORDERED EATING, AMENORRHEA, AND OSTEOPOROSIS

Over the past 20 years, more adolescent girls and young women have participated in competitive sports. Exercise clearly has benefits, including improved cardiovascular fitness, socialization, involvement in peer groups, a sense of well-being, weight control, lowering of blood pressure, and improved lipid profile. A lower rate of cancers of the reproductive system and breast cancer has been reported in one study of former athletes (42). However, intense exercise can be associated with amenorrhea. In the early 1990s, clinicians began to recognize the interrelatedness of disordered eating, amenorrhea, and osteoporosis in athletes, and the term *female athlete triad* was coined. The triad is particularly likely to develop in girls who participate in sports in which the theme of achieving or maintaining an ideal body weight or optimal percentage of body fat is a common focus and scoring is partly subjective (42,43). Coaching strategies such as daily weigh-ins and strict weight standards may predispose young women to the triad. A highly structured life, social isolation, lack of a support system, and a family history of disordered eating are also frequently associated with this presentation. Although not all young women athletes with amenorrhea have all elements of the triad, consideration of each is important in evaluation of these patients in the office. Similarly, appropriate counseling of athletes, families, and coaches is essential to lessen long-term morbidity for these active girls.

For the past 20 years, amenorrhea in athletes has received considerable attention (41–53). The incidence of amenorrhea in particular sports has been unclear, in part because of the varying definitions used for secondary amenorrhea (usually 3 to 6 months of amenorrhea). In contrast to an expected incidence of 2% to 5% of amenorrhea in adult women, the incidence in athletes has been reported at 3% to 66%. For example, in a group of 250 premenopausal women runners, the prevalence of amenorrhea increased from 1% in normally active women to 11% in elite runners (47). Irregular menses in athletes have been associated with many factors, shown in Table 7-4. Endurance activities, such as gymnastics, ballet, and running, are particularly likely to be associated with menstrual problems. Even swimmers who have more body fat than runners may experience menstrual dysfunction, most commonly short luteal phases. Surprisingly, a group of competitive synchronized British swimmers with mean body fat of 23% did not experience menstrual disturbance (54). Similarly, adolescents involved in normal after-school sports programs do not appear to be at increased risk of disrupted menstrual cycles (55), although the possibility of more subtle changes in GnRH pulsations or anovulation has not been examined in this population. Lowered salivary progesterone levels have been noted in recreational runners (average 12.5 miles per week) (56). In a study of 20 moderately active women with normal cycle length, 24 of the cycles were ovulatory and 21 of the cycles were deficient in the luteal phase (57). Thus, athletes with seemingly regular menses may in fact have anovulatory cycles or inadequate luteal phases.

Pubertal development and menarche are often delayed in thin athletes, especially ballet dancers, gymnasts, and runners (51,52). Ballet dancers often have delayed thelarche and menarche with a normal age of adrenarche; they may also have irregular menses, a low percentage of body fat, high energy output, and decreased caloric intake with episodes of bingeing (58,59). Malina (60) has proposed that some of the delay in pubertal development in athletes may be attributed to the preselection of girls who have a thin body type and familial late development and who also excel in athletic endeavors. Some of the delay, however, likely also results from the girls' commitment to the sport. Inadequate nutrition from anorexia nervosa can impact growth velocity and final height. Frisch and coworkers (44) found that athletes who began their training premenarcheally experienced a delay in menarche and a higher incidence of amenorrhea than did athletes who began their training postmenarcheally. Each year of training before menarche was associated with a delay of menarche by 5 months.

The intensity of the exercise and the age of the athlete also appear to be contributing factors to amenorrhea. In most studies, a greater number of miles run per week is associated with a higher incidence of amenorrhea. In a survey of college runners,

TABLE 7-4. *Factors associated with irregular menses in athletes*

Low weight and weight loss
Low body fat (?sport related)
Eating disorders
Delayed menarche
Prior menstrual irregularity
Adolescent age group
Nonparous
Stress (associated with exercise)
Type of sport
  Highest in running
  Lower in swimming and cycling
High level of training
Diet (low calorie, vegetarian, high fiber)
Hereditary? metabolic?

the incidence of amenorrhea was 20% for women running 20 miles/week and 43% for those running 60 to 80 miles/week (61). A lower incidence of amenorrhea has been noted in other studies. Runners who are young and nulliparous are more likely to experience irregular cycles than older, multiparous runners.

Diet may be suboptimal in many adolescent athletes. In an attempt to separate weight loss from strenuous exercise as causative factors, Bullen and colleagues (50) carried out a prospective study of menstrual cycles, assigning one group to weight maintenance and the other to weight loss. They found that exercise, especially if accompanied by weight loss, could reversibly disturb menstrual function. Those in the weight loss group experienced more delayed menses, and a higher percentage of patients had loss of the LH surge. Diets low in calories, fat, and red meat and high in carotene have been associated with amenorrhea (49,62–64). Indeed, restriction of fat has emerged as a finding across multiple studies. Weight loss in girls consuming a vegetarian diet appears to be more likely to induce menstrual dysfunction than a nonvegetarian diet (64).

Gadpaille and colleagues (65) reported an association between athletic amenorrhea, eating disorders, and a family history of major affective disorders. Disordered eating including anorexia nervosa, bulimia, purging, bingeing, and fasting has been reported in 15% to 62% of young female athletes (41,43,52). For example, ballet dancers have higher Eating Attitudes Test (EAT) scores, a measure of disordered eating, than nondancers (mean 22.9 vs 4.1) (66); runners with oligomenorrhea also had higher Eating Disorder Inventory scores (53). Similarly, girls with anorexia nervosa may have joined the track team and be exercising compulsively (often beyond the expectation of the coach) to lose additional weight.

The mechanism of exercise-related menstrual changes is unclear, but there are changes in metabolic rate, prolactin, GnRH, gonadotropins, adrenocorticotropic hormone (ACTH), endorphins, catecholamines, thyroid hormone ("sick euthyroid"), insulin levels and sensitivity, leptin, growth hormone, and growth hormone binding protein (23,62,66–71). The low leptin level appears to be particularly related to caloric restriction and low weight (23). A normal LH response to GnRH in most runners suggests that the defect is at the level of the hypothalamus. Stress associated with the athletic endeavor also appears to increase the incidence of amenorrhea. Of interest, a recent report found that not all female athletes have typical hypothalamic amenorrhea, but rather some may have higher levels of free and total testosterone, increased LH:FSH ratios, and lower sex hormone binding globulin (SHBG), suggestive of PCOS (see Chapter 9); these athletes had higher bone mineral density and higher performance values (69).

As noted in Chapter 4, puberty is a critical time period for the acquisition of normal bone mass (72–75). Genetic factors along with normal levels of androgens and estrogens, physical activity, normal weight and BMI, and adequate calcium and vitamin D intake are all important for healthy bones. A number of studies have examined the benefits of athletic participation (which would be expected to enhance bone mass) countered by the occurrence of hypoestrogenic amenorrhea (which may lead to bone loss) (76–83). For example, Marcus and co-workers (76) found that while eumenorrheic runners had better bone density than sedentary eumenorrheic women, amenorrheic runners had decreased bone density by CT. Young runners 17 to 21 years of age who had started training early after menarche were particularly likely to have impressively low bone mineral density (BMD), using quantitative CT (QCT) of the lumbar spine (79). In a study of 67 elite athletes 18 to 31 years old, Wolman and colleagues (80) found that the QCT lumbar spine measurements were substantially lower in the 25 amenorrheic women (≤ 1 menses every 6 months) than the 27 eumenorrheic women and the 15 women taking oral contraceptive pills (168 vs 211 vs 215 mg/cm^3). Weight and height were also lower in the amenorrheic athletes. Increased calcium intake was associated with increased bone density in all groups. In a study of 43 girls 13 to 20 years old, of whom 28 were dancers, girls with low estrogen exposure scores had lower spine bone mineral density by dual photon absorptiometry than girls with moderate or high estrogen scores (59). Spine BMD was also correlated with weight/height and testosterone levels. In a study of 97 female athletes 18 to 38 years old, Drinkwater and colleagues (81) found that women who had always had regular menstrual cycles had higher lumbar densities (measured by DPA) (1.27 g/cm^2) than those with a history of oligomenorrhea interspersed with regular cycles (1.18 g/cm^2) and than those who had never had regular cycles (1.05 g/cm^2). The combination of body weight and menstrual pattern predicted 43% of the total variation in lumbar density. Another study found that body weight combined with months of amenorrhea and age of menarche predicted the bone mineral density at the lumbar spine of amenorrheic athletes ($R^2 = 0.71$) (83). At other sites, BMD was also predicted by duration of amenorrhea and weight. Several studies have raised the question of whether particular sites in the skeleton might be protected because of selective stresses on those bones. The data so far have yielded mixed results (82–89). For examples, Gremion and colleagues found that distance runners with oligomenorrhea had a loss of BMD at the lumbar spine over one year but not the hip (88).

The proposed risk factors for osteoporosis in female athletes include the factors shown in Table 7-5 (41–43,58). Each of these issues needs to be assessed and addressed in the comprehensive evaluation of the adolescent who has amenorrhea and/or who participates in athletics. The consequences of low bone density can be both long-term and short-term. In two surveys of ballet dancers, Warren and associates (52,86) found that the incidence of stress fractures rose with increasing age of menarche and that the incidence of secondary amenorrhea was twice as high among dancers with stress fractures as those without. In a study of 25 athletes with confirmed stress fractures and matched control athletes, Myburgh and colleagues (90) reported that control subjects were more likely to have used oral contraceptive pills, were less likely to have oligomenorrhea or irregular menses, consumed more servings of calcium each day, and had higher BMD of the spine and hip than women with stress fractures. In a study of 2312 women on active duty (mean age

26.1 ± 5.8 years), Friedl (91) reported that a history of stress fracture ranged from 31.6% in nonblack smokers with episodes of amenorrhea and a family history of osteoporosis to 8% for a black nonsmoker with normal menses and a negative family history. The odds ratios of a stress fracture for women ≤25 years old were 2.24 for a history of 6 months of amenorrhea, 1.96 for smokers, 1.78 for white or Asian ethnicity, and 1.66 for a family history of osteoporosis.

The lower bone density appears to be at least partially reversible in girls who begin to menstruate normally (77,81,92,93). Runners who regained their menses after a mean of 40 months of amenorrhea (associated with a decrease in training mileage and increase in body weight) experienced an increase in bone density in the 14-month follow-up; the two runners who remained amenorrheic had further decreases in bone density (92). However, Drinkwater and colleagues (77,81,92) have observed that even though there is an increase in bone density initially in the first 2 years following resumption of menses, the increase ceased over the next 2 years and bone density remained below the average for their age group 4 years after resumption of menses. Among a group of dancers and nondancers with hypothalamic amenorrhea, resumption of menses was associated with increased spinal bone mineral density but not to normal levels (94).

Prevention efforts should involve safe training techniques for adolescents; educational efforts with athletes, parents, and coaches; counseling for healthy nutrition including calcium and vitamin D intake; promotion of positive and realistic images of women; and screening and evaluation of athletes. Adolescent athletes with amenorrhea deserve a medical and gynecologic evaluation, including assessment of estrogenization, appropriate screening laboratory tests, and bone mineral density (using a scanner with appropriate age matched standards). Athletes with amenorrhea, disordered eating and/or at risk for bone loss, deserve early diagnosis, monitoring, and treatment.

TABLE 7-5. *Factors associated with low bone density in athletes*

Low weight
Low percentage of body fat
Low estrogen
Delayed puberty
Duration of amenorrhea (present and past history)
Low use of oral contraceptives and other estrogens
Low androgen levels
Low calcium intake
Low protein intake
High fiber intake
Increased cortisol levels and increased increment during exercise
Eating disorders
Family history of osteoporosis
Lack of mechanical load

HYPERPROLACTINEMIA

The spectrum of prolactin-secreting pituitary tumors, the natural history of prolactinomas, and the outcome of surgically and medically treated patients has become clearer in the past two decades (95–99). The normal serum prolactin level in women ranges from 1 to 20 ng/ml with a mean of 8.9 ng/ml, although laboratories vary in reported values. Hyperprolactinemia results from high levels of monomeric, dimeric or macro forms of prolactin (100–102). The monomeric form is seen in patients with prolactinomas. Patients with macroprolactin (or "big big prolactin," which consists of antigen antibody complex of monomeric prolactin and IgG) has been reported to represent 10% or more of those with elevated prolactin levels; they are often asymptomatic and have normal fertility (101,102). In a study of 113 patients (19 to 67 years old) with hyperprolactinemia, Hauache and colleagues (100) found that 79% of those with "macroprolactinemia" had normal imaging, compared to 25% with monomeric hyperprolactinemia. None of the patients who were asymptomatic and had "macroprolactinemia" had abnormal imaging. The finding of the prolactin complex underscores the importance of drawing prolactin levels in symptomatic patients to avoid false positives. However, the presence of macroprolactin does not exclude a tumor or response to dopamine agonists. If available, assays should be checked for macroprolactin in patients with hyperprolactinemia.

Prolactin is secreted episodically, it has a half-life of about 20 minutes, and peak secretion occurs during sleep. In patients with pituitary tumors, the sleep-related rhythm is often abolished and prolactin levels are elevated night and day. Unlike most pituitary hormones, prolactin is regulated primarily by inhibition from the hypothalamus through secretion of a prolactin-inhibiting factor, dopamine. Dopamine and dopaminergic drugs, such as bromocriptine and cabergoline, lower serum prolactin levels. Drugs such as risperidone (103,104), other antipsychotic drugs (e.g., haloperidol), phenothiazines, reserpine, protease inhibitors (105,106), especially if given with metoclopramide, and α-methyldopa have been reported to raise prolactin levels. Kinon and colleagues reported that 96% of women of reproductive age taking risperidone had hyperprolactinemia and 56% of those experienced menstrual irregularity, often with low estradiol levels (103). Even low doses cause hyperprolactinemia. Drugs such as olanzapine, quetiapine, ziprasidone, and sertindole produce a transient, minimal, or no effect on prolactin levels and appear to be better tolerated without resulting in hyperprolactinemia (103,107). A baseline prolactin level drawn before the initiation of antipsychotic treatment with drugs known to cause hyperprolactinemia is optimal.

Estrogens stimulate prolactin release and result in an increase in the size and number of lactotropes. Prolactin secretion is increased during pregnancy, with prolactin levels peaking at term (100 to 300 ng/ml). Prolactin levels rise with each episode of nursing during the initial postpartum period, but by 4 to 6 months, prolactin levels are normal. Although some patients taking or discontinuing oral contraceptives develop galactorrhea, studies have not shown an association between oral contraceptives and the development of prolactinomas. Hypothyroidism [with elevated thyrotropin-releasing hormone (TRH) and TSH levels] can occasionally be associated with elevated prolactin levels. In a study of 1,003 patients with hypothyroidism, 8% had hyperprolactinemia (108). Antibodies to prolactin can result in elevated prolactin levels, sometimes associated with autoimmune disorders such as lupus (109,110). Other causes of hyperprolactinemia include renal failure (decreased clearance of prolactin), hyperplasia of lactotropes (functional hyperprolactinemia), or a pituitary tumor (Table 7-6). Women with multiple endocrine neoplasia type 1 (MEN1) can also present with prolactinomas (111).

Prolactin secretion is also affected by breast stimulation in some nonpregnant women and can increase following a large high-protein meal or during major stress (such as general anesthesia for surgery), orgasm, hypoglycemia, and marathon running (112,113). Nipple piercing has also been associated with hyperprolactinemia (114). The sample for serum prolactin determination should not be drawn after a large meal, strenuous exercise, or breast examination.

The presenting complaint in the adolescent may be galactorrhea, interrupted pubertal development, or primary or secondary amenorrhea. The absence of galactorrhea is not unusual in the adolescent with hyperprolactinemia, especially in the girl with primary amenorrhea. One-half to two-thirds of adolescents with secondary amenorrhea and hyperprolactinemia have galactorrhea. Patients with galactorrhea, normal menses, and normal serum prolactin virtually never have a tumor, although galactorrhea is unusual in this setting if the patient has never been pregnant (115).

The evaluation of the adolescent with hyperprolactinemia should include a menstrual history and a history of pregnancies and abortions, medications and illicit drugs, hirsutism or acne, symptoms of thyroid dysfunction, visual changes, and headaches. The physical examination should include a neurologic assessment, including fundoscopic examination and screening visual field test by confrontation, palpation of the thyroid gland, notation of vital signs and androgen excess, a breast examination, and evaluation of vaginal estrogenization.

TABLE 7-6. *Differential diagnosis of hyperprolactinemia and/or galactorrhea*

Pregnancy, postpartum, and postabortion
Pituitary tumor
Hypothalamic diseases and tumors: craniopharyngioma, sarcoidosis, eosinophilic
  granuloma, encephalitis, Chiari-Frommel syndrome, pituitary stalk section or compression,
  metastatic disease
Hypothyroidism
Drug-induced: risperidone, phenothiazines, reserpine, prostaglandins, methyldopa,
  amitriptylene, cimetidine, benzodiazepines, haloperidol, cocaine, metoclopramide
Chronic renal failure
Local factors: chest wall surgery, trauma, nipple stimulation, herpes zoster, atopic
  dermatitis, thoracic burns, nipple piercing
Tumors: bronchogenic or renal carcinoma
Other: stress, sleep-induced, hypoglycemia
Idiopathic

Pregnancy, hypothyroidism, renal and hepatic disease, polycystic ovary syndrome, and use of illicit and prescribed drugs should be ruled out in the patient with hyperprolactinemia. In most of these conditions, prolactin values are elevated to only 30 to 150 ng/ml. Repeat serum prolactin values should be measured under optimal conditions: with the patient in the fasting, unexercised state, with no breast stimulation. The TSH level also should be measured. A prolactin level >100 ng/ml is suggestive of a prolactin-secreting tumor and the level usually correlates with the size of the tumor (99), but microadenomas have been identified in women with only mildly elevated prolactin levels. However, patients with craniopharyngiomas, somatotropic tumors causing acromegaly, cysts (suprasellar arachnoid cysts and Rathke cleft cyst), and nonfunctioning tumors may have mildly elevated prolactin values because of stalk compression; levels are usually <150 ng/ml (but occasionally as high as 600 ng/ml) (116). If there are signs of growth hormone excess (acromegaly, large hands and feet), a screening IGF-1 and random growth hormone should be obtained. Similarly, signs of hypercortisolism should prompt measurement of ACTH, cortisol, and 24-hour urinary free cortisol. Prolactinomas are classified as microadenomas (<10 mm) and macroadenomas (>10 mm). Patients classified as having functional hyperprolactinemia represent a spectrum of findings from mild hyperplasia of lactotropes to small pituitary microadenomas not visualized on imaging. Formal visual field testing and neuroendocrine testing are usually reserved for patients with macroadenomas, preoperative evaluation, or patients with clinical signs or symptoms of hypopituitarism.

It is essential to assess estrogen status in these young women with hyperprolactinemia by serum estradiol level, vaginal smear, and/or progestin challenge because of the risk of low bone density associated with hypoestrogenic amenorrhea (117–122). Klibanski and associates (117) have found reduced bone density improved with therapy (118) but did not return to normal in all women. Similarly, Biller and colleagues (119) found that after the restoration of menses, bone density did improve in a subset of women, but a sustained period of amenorrhea may lead to permanent losses. A higher initial percent of ideal body weight and final serum androgen levels [testosterone and dehydroepiandrosterone sulfate (DHEAS)] positively correlated with the slope of the bone density curve. In a study of 40 adolescent and young adult patients, Colao and colleagues found that 80% had osteopenia or osteoporosis, and dopamine agonist therapy did not return bone density to normal (123). Fracture risk appears to be increased in adult patients before diagnosis of prolactinomas (124).

Once a prolactin-secreting pituitary tumor has been diagnosed, the clinician needs to consider the size of the tumor, the estrogen status of the young woman, the presence of troublesome galactorrhea, the need for contraception, and the desire for fertility. For patients who have microadenomas or functional hyperprolactinemia with normal estrogen status and normal menses, and are therefore not at increased risk for osteoporosis, observation is one option. In a study of 59 patients with idiopathic hyperprolactinemia, there was a high tendency to spontaneous cure, and progression to pituitary prolactinoma did not occur (125). In a study of 30 patients (age 16 to 38 years) with hyperprolactinemia followed for 3 to 20 years (mean 5.2 years) with prolactin levels and tomograms or computed tomography (CT) studies, only two patients had evidence of progression at 4 and 6 years (126). Four patients with initially normal radiographs developed signs of a tumor, but in none was there progression to a macroadenoma. Several patients had spontaneous resolution of amenorrhea and galactorrhea, and one-third of those with abnormal CT or tomograms initially had no evidence of tumor at their last follow-up study (126). Other studies of the natural history of these lesions have reported similar findings; many lesions will stay the same size or regress, with lowering of serum prolactin and re-establishment of menses over time (96–98,127,128). If observation is elected, close monitoring with both MRI and serum prolactin determinations is warranted because low prolactin levels alone are not adequate to provide reassurance of a benign course.

Most adolescents with microadenomas are estrogen deficient and therefore in need of therapy. They are at risk of bone loss and, most importantly, of not attaining normal peak bone mass. Treatment with dopamine agonists restores menses, normal levels of bone formation and resorption markers (121), and fertility (ovulation) in most patients. Patients thus need to be counseled to use effective barriers or low-dose oral contraceptives if they become sexually active. The length of treatment is controversial. Some clinicians will give a trial of tapering and discontinuing medication for patients with microprolactinomas after 2 to 3 years of dopamine agonist therapy; some patients will maintain normal prolactin levels and normal menses. Recurrent hyperprolactinemia can occur after even 4 to 8 years of treatment with reductions in dosage or discontinuation. In a study of 131 patients with prolactinomas (27% had had surgery), 25.8% of those with microprolactinomas and 15.9% of those with macroprolactinomas maintained normal prolactin levels 44 months after withdrawal of bromocriptine therapy; the median time of therapy had been 47 months (129). A study of patients with normalized prolactin levels, no evidence of tumor, and had cabergoline withdrawn after 36 months reported a recurrence rate of 31% for microadenomas and 36% for macroadenomas (130). Some patients with idiopathic hyperprolactinemia or nonprogressive microadenomas who are estrogen deficient have also been treated with cyclic conjugated estrogens and medroxyprogesterone for a mean of 4 years, or low-dose (30 to 35 μg) oral contraceptives for a mean of 2.9 years with little if any effect on the long-term prognosis and at lower cost than dopamine agonists (131,132).

Macroadenomas do require therapy because if they are untreated, patients may experience further tumor growth, visual impairment, and hypopituitarism. Medical therapy with a dopamine agonist is the primary approach for the majority of patients, reducing prolactin levels substantially and causing shrinkage of the tumor over weeks to months (see Case 4) (96,130,132). The cytoplasmic volume of cells is decreased. In most patients, therapy will need to be continued indefinitely. Deterioration of visual acuity has been rarely reported, related to presumed chiasmal traction from tumor shrinkage in macroadenomas and improved with reduction in the dose of the dopamine agonist (133). Tumor enlargement may occur in some patients despite medical therapy because of the presence of a nonfunctioning or non-prolactin-secreting tumor (134) or the occurrence of intrapituitary hemorrhage or tumor necrosis. Since prolactin levels may fall with therapy in spite of continued tumor enlargement, successful management must be monitored by prolactin levels, MRI, and clinical assessment and, if indicated, visual field testing, initially every 6 months.

Although a number of series have reported favorable outcomes for microscopic and endoscopic transsphenoidal or transnasal surgery for prolactinomas (135–143), the majority of clinicians favor dopamine agonists as primary therapy. The success rates for surgery have been in the 90% range in the immediate postoperative period, but the recurrence risk for hyperprolactinemia is 20% to 80%, and the patient may become hypogonadotropic. A normal prolactin value less than 10 ng/ml on the first postoperative day suggests a good outcome (144). Some of the patients with initial inadequate response appear to later become normoprolactinemic, even 15 to 20 years later (137). The indications for surgery include an inability to tolerate or adhere to dopamine agonists, unresponsiveness to therapy (which usually indicates a cystic lesion), increasing tumor size despite therapy, persistent visual loss and chiasmal compression despite medical therapy, and pituitary apoplexy (145–147). Radiation therapy has been used for large tumors that are refractory to medical and surgical management in patients who desire definitive therapy, but it may lead to hypopituitarism.

In young women desiring fertility, dopamine agonists (especially bromocriptine) has been used effectively (148–150). Symptomatic enlargement (visual field defects, headaches, and diabetes insipidus) appear to occur in 23% of bromocriptine-induced pregnancies in women with macroprolactinomas but only 1.3% of women with microadenomas (149). Prolactin levels fall after delivery, and there is no contraindication to breast feeding.

Dopamine agonist therapy restores menses and ovulation more rapidly and more reliably than it controls galactorrhea. The two medications used are bromocriptine, which needs to be given two to three times a day, and cabergoline (Dostinex), which is prescribed twice a week (151). Therapy should begin at low doses in order to lessen the nausea and postural hypotension. Other side effects include headache, dizziness, nasal congestion, and fatigue. For bromocriptine, the dose is usually one-half of a 2.5-mg tablet at bedtime, followed a week later by one tablet at bedtime, followed in 1 week by half a tablet in the morning and one tablet at night, followed by one 2.5-mg tablet twice a day. A dosage of 5.0 to 7.5 mg per day is usually adequate in most patients with mild to moderate hyperprolactinemia, although some require a higher dose. The dose of cabergoline typically starts at 0.25 mg and then is increased as needed to 0.5 to 1.5 mg twice a week. The dose may often be decreased after reaching optimal prolactin levels. Cabergoline is more effective and has fewer adverse side effects than bromocriptine (152–154). One study found that response of macroprolactinomas to cabergoline was better if the patient had not been previously treated with bromocriptine (155). In another study (156), cabergoline resulted in normal prolactin levels in 92% with idiopathic hyperprolactinemia or microprolactinemia and 77% of macroprolactinomas; tumor size decreased in 67% of patients. Only 3.9% discontinued therapy because of side effects. Di Sarno and colleagues (154) have defined cabergoline resistance as a dose of >2.0 mg per week for macroprolactinomas and 3.0 mg per week with microprolactinomas; 10% of microadenomas and 20% of macroadenomas were resistant. Quinagolide has also demonstrated efficacy and an improved side effect profile in comparison with bromocriptine, but comparable or less favorable profile than cabergoline (157–159).

HYPERGONADOTROPIC HYPOGONADISM

Premature ovarian failure (POF) can cause primary or secondary amenorrhea (see Chapter 6 for discussion of differential diagnosis). Patients may have an abnormal karyotype such as Turner syndrome or a normal karyotype with autoimmune oophoritis, idiopathic POF, galactosemia, radiation or chemotherapy. POF also occurs in patients with myotonia dystrophica; trisomy 21; fragile X premutation carriers; sarcoidosis; and ataxia telangiectasia. Ovarian destruction has followed mumps oophoritis, gonococcal salpingitis (rarely), and ovarian infiltrative processes (mucopolysaccharidosis and tuberculosis). Cytomegalovirus infection has also been associated with oophoritis in women with HIV infection and with stem cell transplants (160,161).

All patients with elevated FSH, in the absence of a history of chemotherapy or radiation therapy, should have a karyotype obtained. A search for a Y line should be part of the chromosome analysis. Turner syndrome should be particularly considered in the girl with amenorrhea and short stature (under 5 ft). Fragile X premutation carriers should be considered. Oophoritis is often associated with other endocrinopathies and is considered in more detail below.

As more young women are surviving their childhood malignancies and living into adulthood, the effects of radiation and chemotherapy on gonadal function have become particularly relevant (see Chapter 23). A young woman with amenorrhea and a history of a malignancy treated with radiation to the pelvis or abdomen and/or chemotherapy suggests a diagnosis of POF. The likelihood of ovarian failure in relation to chemotheraphy (alkylating agents) and radiation is both dose- and age-related; the higher the dose and the older the patient, the greater the possibility of ovarian damage. Children and adolescents appear to be more resistant to the deleterious effects of chemotherapeutic agents than adults. In addition to POF, an adolescent who received pelvic radiation therapy before puberty often has a very small cervix and uterus despite estrogen therapy. Adolescents may experience amenorrhea, elevated gonadotropins, and bone loss while receiving chemotherapy; subsequently, their menstrual function and hormone levels may return to normal some months to several years after completion of the course (162,163).

Some patients with idiopathic or autoimmune POF may have fluctuating levels of gonadotropins and estradiol for months to years and may recover menstrual function spontaneously with the rare possibility of fertility. Although Alper and co-workers (164) reported that 6 of 80 (7.5%) adult women conceived after the diagnosis of POF, patients with elevated gonadotropins during adolescence are less likely to have a reversal of the POF.

Autoimmune Oophoritis

The possibility of autoimmune oophoritis needs to be considered in any patient with normal karyotype and POF, because she may subsequently develop other endocrinopathies. In studies of adults with premature ovarian failure evaluated in medical centers, 18% to 50% have been reported to have evidence of autoimmune disease (11,164–171). Associated diseases have included thyroid disorders, Addison disease, hypoparathyroidism, myasthenia gravis, diabetes mellitus, pernicious anemia, and vitiligo. Among women with premature ovarian failure, antithyroglobulin and antithyroid microsomal antibodies are commonly present; antibodies to smooth muscle, gastric parietal cells, mitochondria, cell nucleus, pancreatic islet cells, and the adrenals have also been reported (168). Antibodies against theca interna and corpus luteum cells, FSH receptors, and specific enzymes in the adrenals and ovaries have been described (165–170). Localization of staining for the presence of ovarian antibodies has been reported in the primary oocytes and in the granulosa cells of large secondary follicles (166). Patients may not have positive antiovarian antibody tests because the right antigens may not be included in the assay, the antibody may be only transiently present, or the pathogenesis of the ovarian failure may involve primarily lymphocytic infiltration.

Patients with autoimmune oophoritis may have a variable course with spontaneous remissions and the resumption of normal ovarian function (164,171). Amenorrhea and infertility persist in most patients. Whether corticosteroids, combined estrogen–progestin therapy, or other therapies lead to any better prognosis is unclear (172–174), since controlled studies have not been performed. Serious side effects from the steroids can occur (175) and therefore this therapy is not recommended in adolescents. For most patients, assisted reproductive technologies with donor oocytes offer the best possibility for a pregnancy.

At the initial assessment of the patient with suspected autoimmune ovarian failure, baseline thyroid function tests, complete blood count, calcium and phosphorus, and morning cortisol should be obtained. Serum can be sent for antibodies to thyroid, adrenal, ovary, islet cells, and parietal cells, if these tests are available. Patients with autoimmune ovarian failure may develop adrenal insufficiency or other autoimmune endocrinopathies; thus, long-term follow-up is essential. The best way to assess the risk of adrenal insufficiency has not been rigorously evaluated. Some advocate an ACTH test with measurement of cortisol levels at 0 and 30 (or 60) minutes as an appropriate screening test, with repeat measurements done annually to determine adrenal reserve. Others advocate monitoring DHEAS, ACTH, and morning cortisol levels less frequently or doing more extensive testing only in those with antiadrenal antibodies.

RESISTANT OVARY SYNDROME

In resistant ovary syndrome, the ovaries appear normal at laparoscopy and biopsy specimens reveal numerous primordial follicles (176). Ovarian follicular activity can also be identified in some patients with the use of transvaginal ultrasonography. The ovaries may lack a receptor for gonadotropin function. In two reported cases, inhibin levels were normal, suggesting that this may provide a diagnostic test for the disorder. During an infertility evaluation, a trial of exogenous human gonadotropin may be indicated to exclude the remote possibility that the patient has produced biologically inactive FSH and LH. The condition is rare and may not be a unique entity; many hypergonadotropic women have follicles that are intermittently demonstrable by ultrasound.

EXTERNAL OR INTERNAL GENITAL ANOMALIES

Imperforate Hymen and Transverse Vaginal Septum

The diagnosis of imperforate hymen is occasionally made in an adolescent patient who presents with delayed menarche. The patient may have a history of cyclic abdominal pain, often for several months to years, or may be asymptomatic. A bluish, bulging hymen and distention of the vagina with blood are found on genital inspection and rectoabdominal palpation. The repair of imperforate hymen is typically accomplished in infancy or early adolescence or when the diagnosis is made (see Chapter 10 for discussion of genital anomalies).

The rare complete transverse vaginal septum may be low or high in the vagina, but the external genitalia appear normal. The vagina appears short, and a mass is palpable above the examining finger and on rectoabdominal palpation. Obstruction by a high transverse septum results in hematometra and endometriosis. It should be noted that a transverse vaginal septum usually has a central small perforation but still may present with hematocolpos in the adolescent, mucocolpos in the child, or pyohematocolpos because of ascending infection.

Agenesis of the Vagina/Cervix/Uterus

Vaginal agenesis is usually accompanied by cervical and uterine agenesis, although infrequently a patient has a normal but obstructed uterus or rudimentary uterus with functional endometrium. Patients with Mayer-Rokitansky-Küster-Hauser (MRKH) syndrome have a 46,XX karyotype and normal ovaries and hormonal patterns, but the cervix, uterus, and fallopian tubes are absent or rudimentary, and the upper two-thirds of the vagina is absent. The presence of normal breast and pubic hair development and normal female serum testosterone and pubertal estradiol levels makes this syndrome the likely diagnosis. Ultrasonography, which should be done to assess renal status, confirms normal ovaries and the lack of a uterus. Diagnostic and medical and surgical approaches are discussed in Chapter 10. Although chromosome studies are not necessary for girls with classic MRKH syndrome, the finding of an elevated testosterone level, lack of breast development, absent pubic hair, or virilization mandate studies looking for an intersex state.

ANDROGEN INSENSITIVITY

The patient with androgen insensitivity syndrome (AIS) (previously referred to as *testicular feminization*), a form of male pseudohermaphroditism, has normal breast development with pale areola, and very sparse or absent pubic and axillary hair. The vagina is short, and the uterus and cervix are absent. More than 50% of these patients have an inguinal hernia. The karyotype is 46,XY. The gonads, which may be intraabdominal or in the inguinal rings, are testes; thus, the serum testosterone level is in the same range as in the pubertal male and they make müllerian inhibitory substance (MIS) (see Chapter 2). Because of insensitivity to androgens and enhanced estrogen production, the patient develops a female habitus and external genitalia. The lack of pubic and axillary hair is the result of end-organ failure to respond to adrenal and testicular androgens (177–179) (see Chapters 2 and 10). Owing to the presence of MIS, although the external body habitus is female, she lacks an upper vagina, cervix, and uterus. Information and support groups are offered through the international AIS support group web site (www.medhelp.org/www/ais). Patients with incomplete androgen insensitivity have a 46,XY karyotype, agenesis of the uterus, hirsutism, clitoral enlargement, and absence of breast development (178).

AMENORRHEA AND VIRILIZATION

Causes of primary amenorrhea and virilization include mixed gonadal dysgenesis (MGD), 5α-reductase deficiency, incomplete androgen insensitivity syndrome, true hermaphroditism, and ovarian and adrenal tumors (see Chapters 2 and 10). At puberty, patients with MGD show virilization (without evidence of estrogen effect) because the functioning intraabdominal testis produces testosterone. The reported chromosome patterns of patients with MGD have included 46,XY; 45,X/46,XY; 45,X/46,XX/46,XY; and 45,X (some likely have a missed second line). Essential is mosaicism with a 45,X stem and a stem with a Y (fragment) (180) to make the diagnosis of mixed gonadal dysgenesis (MGD). With a uterus present, patients should be given cyclic estrogen–progestin therapy to produce menses and referred to centers for fertility interventions with assisted reproductive technologies and oocyte transfer, if desired. Because a dysgenetic intraabdominal testis has a high incidence of malignant transformation, it should be removed. Patients with 5α-reductase deficiency are 46,XY, lack müllerian structures, and have virilization at puberty. A true hermaphrodite has ovarian and testicular tissue (see Chapter 2). Some appear to be almost normal females who develop mild to moderate virilization at puberty, depending on the balance of ovarian and testicular function. Gonadotropin concentrations may be normal or high (181). Congenital adrenal hyperplasia can cause primary or secondary amenorrhea and virilization, if undertreated. Polycystic ovary syndrome more frequently causes hirsutism and acne but patients can present with clitoromegaly and mild virilization (see Chapter 9).

TREATMENT

Therapy should be directed at the underlying cause of the amenorrhea, if possible, and should target acquisition of normal bone mass. For example, achieving better glucose control in the young diabetic or decreased disease activity in Crohn disease or celiac disease will often bring about menarche. The girl with end-stage renal failure often experiences menarche following a successful renal transplant; in fact, ovulatory cycles may result in an unintended pregnancy for the sexually active adolescent who has not previously used birth control. Girls with anorexia nervosa are typically treated by a multidisciplinary team with medical and nutritional monitoring and mental health counseling; the best treatment for amenorrhea is restoration of normal nutrition and body weight. A reasonable approach for girls with eating disorders is to provide medical treatment and counseling in an attempt to bring about a change in lifestyle for 6 to 12 months before estrogen replacement is considered (182). As noted above, the patient should achieve at minimum 92% of ideal body weight (IBW), and even then the return of menstrual periods is often delayed because of high levels of exercise or preoccupation with diet and weight. Spontaneous recovery of menstrual function may occur in adolescents with hypothalamic amenorrhea, especially with decreased activity, increased weight, and less stress. The findings of Couzinet and colleagues (22) that hypothalamic amenorrhea was often associated with dietary fat restriction suggests that these young women could benefit from nutritional counseling. Some athletic girls will reduce the amount of exercise in order to allow puberty to progress; others may find their training schedule important for optimal performance, or they may be in a compulsive pattern associated with an eating disorder. An assessment of bone density by DEXA or other methodology (compared to bone age standards) can help determine if osteopenia is already a significant problem and provide the girl and her family with information about this potential complication (183). Weight, height, growth pattern, and diet should be monitored. Although previously patients were often allowed to remain estrogen deficient for years, which increased their risk of osteopenia, many clinicians do offer estrogen replacement therapy, extrapolating from bone density studies in postmenopausal women despite the few studies that address efficacy in teens.

In young women, most of the studies of estrogen use have concentrated on oral contraceptives. As noted in Chapter 20, in normal women progestin/estrogen combined pills provide normal menses and reduce the risk of dysmenorrhea, anemia, ovarian cysts (higher dose pills), and ovarian and endometrial cancer. Studies of the impact of oral contraceptive use in normal adolescents and women on bone density have been mixed, with most studies showing an association with higher bone mass, at least for 35-µg ethinyl estradiol (EE) pills (see Chapter 20). Oral contraceptives and other estrogens increase the risk of venous thromboembolism by two- to fourfold over baseline, with a particularly heightened risk in those with Factor V Leiden. The risk of breast cancer appears to be unchanged by oral contraceptive therapy.

The question that arises for families and patients is the extent to which recent data from prospective studies in menopausal women should impact decision making related to hormone replacement therapy in young women, particularly those with premature ovarian failure. Although observational studies of estrogen replacement in postmenopausal women had suggested cardiovascular protection, more recent randomized studies have led to a reanalysis of the risk and benefits for these older women. Published in 2002, the Heart and Estrogen/Progestin Replacement Study (HERS) did not find a reduction in cardiovascular risk for postmenopausal women with coronary heart disease (184). The Women's Health Initiative Study randomized menopausal women age 50 to 79 years to conjugated estrogens 0.625 mg plus medroxyprogesterone acetate 2.5 mg daily versus placebo. The trial was stopped after 5.2 years because of increased risks for coronary heart disease (1.29, 95%CI 1.02 to 1.63), breast cancer (1.26, 95%CI 1.00 to 1.59), stroke (1.41, 95%CI 1.07 to 1.85), and pulmonary embolus (2.13, 95%CI 1.39 to 3.25). Of note, decreased risks were found for colorectal cancer (0.63, 95%CI 0.43 to 0.92), endometrial cancer (0.83, 95%CI 0.47 to 1.47), and hip fracture (0.66, 95%CI 0.45 to 0.98) (185). How this applies to adolescents with premature ovarian failure remains speculative. It is generally agreed that the use of hormonal therapy in adolescents with POF is different from prolonging exposure to hormones for postmenopausal women.

A special group for consideration of hormone therapy are adolescents with anorexia nervosa. Bone density is reduced in both women with anorexia nervosa and women with hypothalamic amenorrhea, but the former are more severely impacted (28). The question that has been debated for some time is whether estrogen replacement therapy, in the absence of weight gain, can bring about normal bone mass acquisition in young women with anorexia nervosa (32,186–189). In a large randomized trial of estrogen therapy in women with anorexia nervosa, Klibanski and colleagues (188) studied 48 amenorrheic women (mean age 24.9; range 16 to 42 years) who had had amenorrhea for a mean of 3.3 years in the estrogen group and 4.6 years in the control group (range 0.5 to 17.3 years). The estrogen replacement therapy used was either conjugated estrogens 0.625 mg on days 1 to 25 and medroxyprogesterone 5 mg on days 16 to 25, or oral contraceptive therapy (35-μg EE pill). The patients were monitored for an average of 1.5 years. Although there was no statistical difference between the treated (+2.8 ±11.0%) and the controls (−5.4 ± 22.6%) in spinal bone density, there was a difference between estrogen-treated patients and controls when patients who regained their menses spontaneously were excluded from the analysis (+2.2 ± 11.1% vs −13.3 ± 17.8%; $p = 0.004$). For those who weighed <70% of their ideal body weight, the difference was particularly striking between the treated patients and the controls (+4.0 ±8.8% vs. −20.1 ±16.2%). In another study of patients with anorexia nervosa treated with oral contraceptive pills, an increase in total body bone mass and lumbar spine bone mineral density was observed (189). A recent randomized study of dancers with amenorrhea (22 ± 4.6 years) comparing conjugated estrogen 0.625 mg for 25 days each month and medroxyprogesterone 10 mg for 10 days each month to placebo found no difference at 2 years in bone density in treated versus control women (187). A randomized study by Gordon found small increases in hip bone density for estrogen replacement therapy and for DHEA (an adrenal androgen), but weight gain was a significant contributor to the improvement (32,186). Similarly, a study of the therapeutic use of intravenous IgF-1 has suggested promising effects on bone turnover in women with anorexia nervosa (190). However, more research is needed on the benefits and risks of drugs such as bisphosphonates, androgens (e.g., DHEA), and growth factors in adolescents with anorexia nervosa before their use is recommended.

For girls with hypothalamic amenorrhea, there are similar considerations. The risk of osteopenia is more variable in this group. Miller and Klibanski (183) recently reviewed the literature related to etiology and treatments. Small retrospective and prospective studies have noted increased bone density at the spine and femoral neck in women treated with hormone replacement therapy (HRT) (45,80,89,191). In a study of 34 elite runners (18 to 35 years old), bone density of the hip (+3.8%) and lumbar spine (+4.8%) increased in the group of women treated with HRT and those with natural return of menses, but decreased in those who remained amenorrheic (89). However, factoring in "intention to treat" analysis found the difference at the lumbar spine to be only 1.5%. Although a variety of doses of estrogen have been shown to provide protection from bone loss in postmenopausal women (192–197), in adolescent girls the optimal dose or type of estrogen for the acquisition of bone mass is unknown (198,199). Our studies of adolescents with estrogen deficiency states treated with conjugated estrogens, 0.625 mg for 21 days of the month, found that a regimen started at a mean age of 16 years prevented further bone loss but did not result in normal bone mass (198), because either the dosage, the duration, or age at initiation was inadequate, or other factors, such as androgen replacement, presently unstudied, played a role. Thus higher doses of estrogens, androgens, or other therapies need to be studied in adolescent girls with panhypopituitarism and hypothalamic amenorrhea.

The optimal progestin type and dosage have not been determined in teens, although several studies suggest that protection of the endometrium from endometrial hyperplasia in postmenopausal women is optimal with 12 to 14 days of medroxyprogesterone (200,201). The most commonly used progestin is medroxyprogesterone, 10 mg; doses as low as 5 mg are sufficient to protect the endometrium from endometrial hyperplasia in the vast majority of patients. In a study of more than 1700 women treated with four different regimens of estrogen and progestin (conjugated estrogens 0.625 mg plus medroxyprogesterone with 2.5 or 5.0 mg daily or 5 or 10 mg for 14 days of a 28-day cycle), endometrial hyperplasia occurred in <1%; there were only five cases among women using the two lower-dose regimens, 2.5 mg continuously and 5 mg sequentially (201). Padwick and colleagues (202) have observed that women given continuous estrogen and cyclic progestin for 12 days have a predominantly proliferative endometrium if bleeding occurs on or before day 10 and a wholly or predominantly secretory endometrium with bleeding on day 11 or later. Several recent studies have shown an increased risk of endometrial cancer with 7 days per month of progestin (203) and <10 days per month (204); 10 or more days a month was protective. Providing 10 mg of medroxyprogesterone for 14 days every 3 months also appears to be effective (203,205). Cyclic medroxyprogesterone alone has also been reported to increase lumbar bone density in 21- to 45-year-old women (206). Micronized progesterone (e.g., Prometrium) appears to be associated with beneficial effects on lipids (207).

If height is normal or skeletal age is mature in the girl with delayed menarche and her breast development is complete, a maintenance dose of estrogen can be prescribed from the onset. Options include estrogens such as conjugated estrogens 0.625 mg, ethinyl estradiol 20 μg, transdermal estradiol patch 50 μg (0.05 mg), esterified estrogens 0.625 mg, or micronized estradiol 1.0 mg given daily *plus* progestin for 12 to 14 days each month *or* a cyclic combined estrogen-progestin contraceptive (oral contraceptive, transdermal patch, vaginal ring). Transdermal estradiol patches (such a Vivelle-Dot, Climara, Estraderm) are changed once or twice a week depending on the preparation (see pp. 200–201 for estradiol levels with doses of transdermal estrogen). Some adolescents tolerate the estradiol patches well and find changing them preferable to daily oral medication (oral progestin is still necessary). However, other adolescents complain of the patch falling off, have allergic reactions to the adhesive, or do not like the idea of having a potentially visible acknowledgment of a medical problem. A progestin should be provided for 12 to 14 days each month (e.g., medroxyprogesterone 10 mg or micronized progesterone 200 mg for 12 to 14 days each month). The combined oral contraceptive pill, patch, or ring provide progestin throughout the cycle. For girls with anorexia nervosa and some athletes, even those that may have had prior menses, starting with a low dose of estrogen (e.g., conjugated estrogens 0.3 mg daily) for 2 to 3 months may lessen estrogen related side effects such as bloating and improve compliance. Increasing doses may also be used in girls who have not completed breast development or develop symptoms from maintenance doses (see Chapter 6, p. 199).

Most adolescents prefer monthly menses, and thus progestin cycles are prescribed monthly. Some adolescents (often athletes and girls with anorexia nervosa), however, may prefer a minimum number of withdrawal menses and can be offered daily estrogen cycled every 60 or 90 days with progestin for 14 days *or* continuous estrogen/progestin. A study of postmenopausal women found that quarterly medroxyprogesterone (10 mg/day for 14 days) resulted in menses that were longer, often heavier, and more often unscheduled than when progestin was used monthly (205). Oral contraceptives (OCs) have been prescribed similarly, with 2, 3, or 4 months of OCs, followed by a 7 day hormone free interval. Sexually active patients should receive oral contraceptives, patch or ring for hormone replacement.

In girls with premature ovarian failure, long term treatment with estrogen/progestin is indicated. In girls with hypogonadotropic hypogonadism in whom contraception is not needed, therapy can be discontinued intermittently (e.g., once a year for 2 to 3 months) to determine whether the hypothalamic–pituitary axis has begun to function more normally.

Adolescent girls, especially those with estrogen deficiency, should be counseled to consume a daily calcium intake of 1300 mg by diet (see Appendix 8 for handout) or supplements. The average adolescent intake is 900 mg/day, below current recommendations. Similarly, adequate intake of Vitamin D is important, and these girls should take a daily multivitamin. Exercise is also important for adolescents with hypoestrogenism to promote normal bone mass and cardiovascular fitness but often needs to be limited in girls with anorexia nervosa who are losing weight.

If the girl is well estrogenized and her examination and laboratory tests are normal, menstrual cycles can be induced by the administration of cyclic progestin therapy every one to three months (e.g., medroxyprogesterone 10 mg or micronized progesterone 200 mg for 12 to 14 days). Patients with chronic anovulatory states, such as those with polycystic ovary syndrome, have an increased risk of endometrial carcinoma and should receive long-term progestin therapy or oral contraceptives (see Chapter 9). Although a withdrawal flow from progesterone is generally reassuring about the continuing presence of normal circulating levels of estrogen and a normal hypothalamic–pituitary axis, persistence of amenorrhea, any signs of headache, visual symptoms, galactorrhea, or an interruption in the tempo of the pubertal process necessitate further tests.

Follow-up studies of adolescent patients with irregular cycles and women with hypothalamic amenorrhea have been few, making it challenging for the clinician to provide the patient and family with definitive information about prognosis. In a 10-year follow-up study of 46 adult women (mean age 24; range 18 to 32 years) with amenorrhea and normal prolactin levels, most women (6 of 9) with hypo-estrogenic amenorrhea (weight loss, exercise) recovered normal cycles, but only 3 of 17 euestrogenic amenorrheic patients progressed to normal cycles (208). None of the patients with polycystic ovary syndrome or premature ovarian failure developed normal ovulatory cycles. In a study of 93 women with hypothalamic amenorrhea followed for 7 to 9 years, 65 (70.5%) recovered (209). Higher BMI, an increase in BMI over the follow-up interval, higher androstenedione levels, and lower cortisol levels were noted to be associated with recovery. Similarly, Kondoh and colleagues (210) found that women with progestin-negative hypothalamic amenorrhea from stress and weight loss had higher levels of cortisol and less response of ACTH and cortisol to human corticotropin releasing hormone (hCRH) than controls. The higher the basal cortisol, the longer the interval for recovery. A retrospective study of 29 women found that those with an identified precipitant such as an eating disorder, weight loss, or stress had a better prognosis for recovery of menstrual function when these factors were reversed than those with no known precipitant (71% vs 29% recovery) (211). LH pulse patterns at presentation did not predict recovery.

Even though considerations of fertility are beyond the scope of this book, it is useful to be able to provide some information to teenagers with estrogen deficiency states. Many patients with irreversible ovarian failure, such as those with Turner syndrome, who desire to have children will choose adoption; however, advances in technology have now shown that oocyte donation and in vitro fertilization are possible in women with premature ovarian failure. Current assisted-reproduction technologies include *in vitro* fertilization (IVF), gamete intrafallopian transfer (GIFT), zygote intrafallopian transfer (ZIFT), ovum donation, and gestational carriers. With these advancements in technologies, there are increased fertility options for women, but there may also be increased risks for some women based on their underlying disease. One example is the risk of oocyte donation for women with Turner syndrome and the risk of death during pregnancy from underlying cardiac disease (212–214).

Rarely, patients with autoimmune oophoritis have been reported to have pregnancies spontaneously (because of the waxing and waning nature of the disorder, or coincident with estrogen treatment). Patients with GnRH deficiency can be induced to ovulate with gonadotropins or pulsatile GnRH. Patients with hypothalamic dysfunction and infertility need to have the issue of weight, exercise, and stress addressed and then, depending on the etiology, may be treated with clomiphene citrate (215), exogenous gonadotropins, or pulsatile GnRH (216). Ovulation can usually be induced in patients with hyperprolactinemia by the use of dopamine agonists.

Groups are available in many metropolitan centers for specific diagnoses (e.g., Turner Society groups). Parents, older adolescents, and young adults often find the support and education helpful. Teens also often discover the benefits of meeting one-on-one with another woman who has the same condition. For example, a girl with vaginal agenesis may find it helpful to meet a young woman who has already used vaginal dilators; similarly, parents often benefit from support from other parents. Denial of the diagnosis between visits is common. The clinician frequently needs to do much of the talking during these appointments, with statements such as "I have other girls in my practice with this problem, and I find they worry about . . ." The health care provider can greatly aid the patient in accepting the medical diagnosis and the treatment plan.

Case 1

E. B. presented with primary amenorrhea at the age of 16 years. Breast and pubic hair development had started when she was 11 or 12 years old. She had noted a slight whitish vaginal discharge for several years. Physical examination showed her to be healthy, with a height of 64 in. and a weight of 125 lb. Breast development was stage 5, and pubic hair development was stage 4. Pelvic examination revealed a well-estrogenized vagina and a normal cervix and uterus. Urine HCG level was negative. A vaginal smear showed 20% superficial and 80% intermediate cells [maturation index = $(80 \times 0.5) + (20 \times 1.0) = 60$]. FSH, TSH, and prolactin levels were normal. Following 10 days of medroxyprogesterone, she had a 4-day menstrual period. She began spontaneous menses 2 months later and continued to have normal menstrual cycles.

Case 2

P. M. presented with primary amenorrhea at the age of 18 years. Breast development had occurred when she was 13 years old, but pubic and axillary hair had not appeared. She had recently gained 70 lb, seemingly because of anxiety over her lack of periods. Her height was 64 in. and her weight was 187 lb. Her blood pressure was 140/80 mm Hg, and her pulse rate was 80 beats/min. Her breasts were stage 5 and pendulous. No axillary or pubic hair was present. Pelvic examination revealed a short vagina and no cervix or uterus. Laboratory tests showed a karyotype of 46,XY. The serum testosterone level was 281 ng/dl (normal female level, <55 ng/dl). A diagnosis of androgen insensitivity syndrome (AIS) was made. After surgery to remove the intraabdominal testes, P M. was given estrogen replacement therapy. She required extensive counseling about the issue of her femininity, sexual function, and her inability to bear children. She subsequently lost 35 lb by dieting.

Case 3

R. L. sought medical attention at the age of 18 years because of "no periods." Her breast and pubic hair development had started at the age of 12 years. She had always been the shortest member of her class, and she had worn bilateral hearing aids since the age of 11. Physical examination (Fig. 7-4) showed her to be short and overweight, with a height of 51 in. and a weight of 105 lb. She had hypertelorism, ptosis, a low hairline, an increased carrying angle, and short fourth metacarpals. Breast development was stage 5; pubic hair was stage 4. Pelvic examination revealed a poorly estrogenized vagina with a small cervix and uterus. Vaginal smear showed no evidence of estrogenization. Laboratory tests revealed a serum FSH level of 258 mIU/ml and an LH level of 173 mIU/ml, indicative of ovarian failure. Her karyotype was 46,X,i(Xq). The patient was given cyclic estrogen/progestin replacement therapy.

Case 4

N. K. was referred at the age of 17 for primary amenorrhea. She was an "A" student in her senior year of high school and was involved in athletics. Her breast and

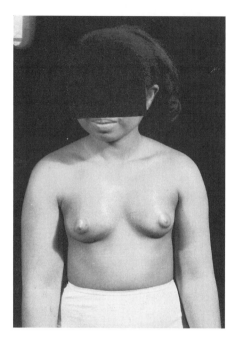

FIG. 7-4. Case 3: gonadal dysgenesis, karyotype 46,X,i(Xq).

pubic hair development had started at the age of 10 but subsequently stopped when she was 12. Her menses had never begun. She had had significant headaches for 4 years, which seemed to increase during the school year. Physical examination showed her to be pleasant and bright, with a height of 64 in. and a weight of 111 lb. Her blood pressure and pulse were normal. The breasts were Tanner stage 3 with small areolae, 1.7 cm on the right and 2.0 cm on the left, and glandular tissue 4 × 4 cm on the right and 5 ×6 cm on the left. No galactorrhea was present. Pubic hair was stage 3 to 4; the vagina was poorly estrogenized. The vagina was normal in length, and rectoabdominal examination revealed a cervix and a uterus. The results of neurologic examination, including fundoscopic examination, visual fields by confrontation, and sense of smell, were normal. The growth chart (Fig. 7-5) showed no increase in height since the age of 12⁶/12 years. The history and examination suggested normal initiation of puberty followed by growth arrest and regression of estrogenization. Laboratory tests showed a bone age of 14 years, normal results of CBC and thyroid function tests, low gonadotropin levels, undetectable estradiol, and markedly elevated prolactin of 13,000 ng/ml (normal <25 ng/ml). Cranial CT (an MRI would be done in this era) demonstrated a large pituitary and suprasellar mass (Fig. 7-6A). The result of formal visual field testing was normal. Neuroendocrine studies revealed prepubertal LH and FSH responses to GnRH, growth hormone deficiency, flat prolactin response to TRH, and normal cortisol levels.

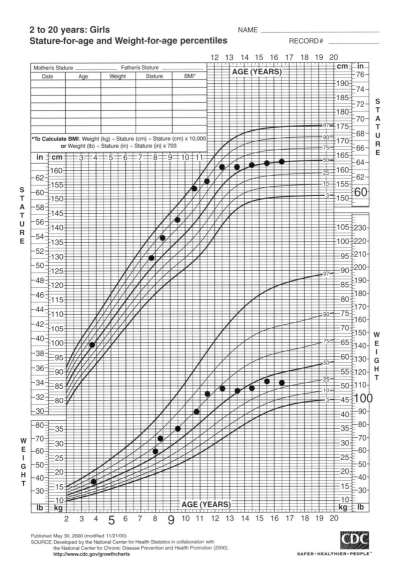

2 to 20 years: Girls
Stature-for-age and Weight-for-age percentiles

NAME _____

RECORD# _____

FIG. 7-5. Case 4: growth chart of patient with primary amenorrhea and a prolactinoma.

After neurosurgical consultation, N. K. was given bromocriptine therapy. The dosage was gradually increased on a weekly basis; the prolactin levels fell progressively, and the tumor showed significant reduction in size (Fig. 7-6B and C). Her headaches disappeared. The estradiol levels ranged between 53 and 283 pg/ml, and breast development and vaginal estrogenization progressed. N. K. had normal

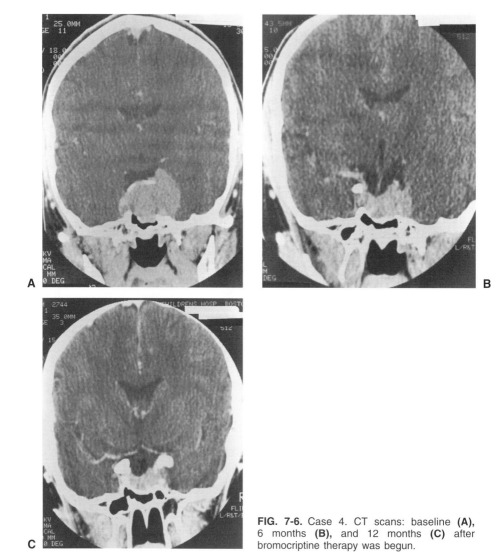

FIG. 7-6. Case 4. CT scans: baseline **(A)**, 6 months **(B)**, and 12 months **(C)** after bromocriptine therapy was begun.

withdrawal flow when medroxyprogesterone was given 1 year after she had started taking bromocriptine. Her first spontaneous menses occurred 2 months later.

Case 5

C. E., a 16⁴/₁₂ year old girl, was referred for primary amenorrhea and tall stature. Her breast and pubic hair development had begun when she was between

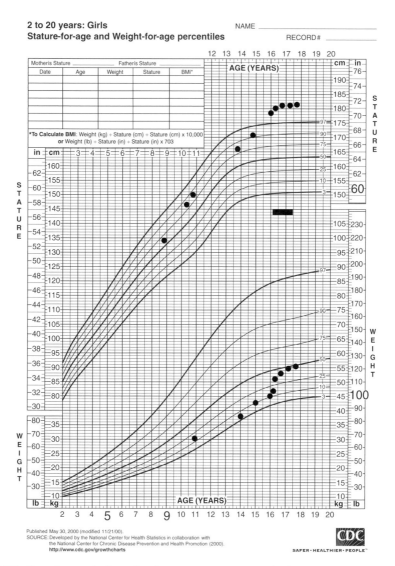

2 to 20 years: Girls
Stature-for-age and Weight-for-age percentiles

NAME _____

RECORD# _____

FIG. 7-7. Case 5: growth chart. *Bar* denotes estrogen–progestin therapy.

the ages of 13 and 14 years. She was active in sports (tennis) and thin. Her father was 6 ft 4 in. and her mother 5 ft 11 in. (mid-parental height, 5 ft 11 in.). She had increasingly become concerned about being too tall and did not wish to be taller than her mother. On physical examination, she was 5 ft 10½ in. (>95%) with a weight of 99 lb (10%) (Fig. 7-7). Her breast development was Tanner stage 3 to 4, and her pubic hair development was Tanner stage 4.

Her external genitalia were normal, and a pelvic examination revealed an estrogenized vagina with a normal cervix and uterus. Her laboratory tests showed a FSH level of 5.4 mIU/ml, a prolactin level of 3.7 ng/ml, and a normal TSH level. Her bone age was between 12 and 12½, giving a predicted height of 6 ft 2 in. to 6 ft 3 in. The benefits and risks of estrogen treatment, including thrombosis and hypertension, were discussed with C. E. and her family, and she elected to take ethinyl estradiol 150 μg per day (increased slowly over a month from 20 μg per day) plus cyclic medroxyprogesterone each month for 1 year to accelerate skeletal maturation. She had normal menses, did not experience nausea or other problems, and was pleased with her final height and weight gain. She has continued to have normal menses while off medication.

It should be noted that the optimal indication or dose of estrogen has not been defined for the treatment of tall stature, but doses of 100 to 250 μg of ethinyl estradiol have been used (217–219) to reduce height by 4 to 6 cm from that predicted. Oral contraceptives (20 to 35 μg EE per day) have not been shown to alter height unless the bone age is 9 to 10 years. Given the potential risks and controversial benefits, we believe high doses of estrogen should be offered only to patients who have a predicted height of over 6 feet, feel strongly about instituting therapy, understand the risks, and are under the care of an experienced physician. Today many more girls are accepting of tall stature.

Case 6

S. Q. is a 16½ year old with primary amenorrhea. She started breast and pubic hair development at 10 to 11 and had some mild vaginal discharge around age 11. She had always been underweight for height and very tall. She eats steak and pasta and avoids vegetables. She denies vomiting or GI symptoms. Her growth chart is in Fig. 7-8. Her mother's menarche was age 16, her grandmother's age 13. Physical examination showed a tall, thin girl: weight 48 kg, height 165 cm, blood pressure 110/60. Her HEENT were benign, and her thyroid was not enlarged. Her breasts were Tanner stage 3, but with only a small amount of glandular tissue. Her lungs were clear. Her heart showed no murmurs. Her abdomen was soft. She has Tanner stage 4 pubic hair and her vagina appeared to be normal in length with a cotton-tipped applicator probe but was unestrogenized.

Pelvic ultrasound showed a small uterus, 4.8 ×1.2 × 2.4 cm, and her ovaries were quite small. Vaginal smear showed 65% parabasal cells, 35% intermediate cells, score 17.5, markedly hypoestrogenic. Laboratory studies: FSH 117 and 121 mIU/ml; prolactin 22 ng/ml; normal thyroid function tests and elevated antithyroid antibodies. Her antiovarian and antiadrenal antibodies were negative. Her karyotype was 46,XX. She was treated initially with estrogen and then estrogen/progestin. Despite an initial impression that she was underweight for her height and that she might have hypothalamic amenorrhea, her laboratory studies revealed premature ovarian failure, possibly autoimmune oophoritis.

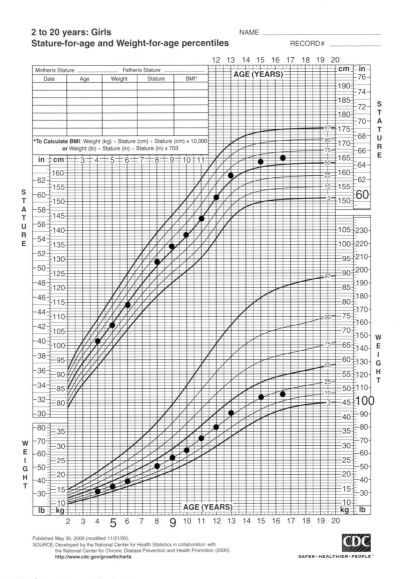

FIG. 7-8. Case 6: growth chart.

SECONDARY AMENORRHEA

Many of the etiologies of delayed menarche are also responsible for secondary amenorrhea, with the most common causes of missed periods being stress, change in environment, weight loss, disordered eating, and pregnancy, as noted on page 222.

If an adolescent presents with a menstrual period that is 2 to 3 weeks overdue, the clinician should obtain a sensitive pregnancy test and never assume that the adolescent is not pregnant simply because she denies a history of sexual intercourse. The magnitude of the weight loss in teens is sometimes evident only after a careful history and weight and height charts have been obtained. A young woman with depression may rapidly gain weight and become amenorrheic, and may then inaccurately view the weight gain as secondary to the loss of periods and retention of blood. Young women also often have irregular menses with changes in environment such as going away to summer camp, boarding school, or college. The involvement of increasing numbers of young adolescents in competitive athletics has been accompanied by increasing reports of menstrual irregularities (see section on the Female Athlete Triad, p. 227). Many older teenagers are still fearful of admitting to having had intercourse; a girl aged 11 or 12 may not understand her own anatomy and cycles well enough to answer the questions accurately or may have been the victim of rape or incest (see Chapter 24).

Given that teenagers may have irregular periods or amenorrhea for 3 to 6 months in the first 1 to 2 years after menarche, the clinician needs to decide which patients to evaluate. Generally, the abrupt cessation of menses for 4 months after regular cycles have begun, or persistent oligomenorrhea 2 years after menarche, should be taken as an indication for an evaluation. Clearly, many patients will not visit the clinician until 2, 3, or 8 months after amenorrhea occurs. Since the evaluation is simple (a physical examination, pregnancy test, progesterone challenge test, and endocrine laboratory studies), there is no need to wait an arbitrary length of time. For patients whose cycles were normal prior to the use of hormonal contraception, a hormonal evaluation (in addition to a physical examination and a pregnancy test) is generally recommended after 6 months in a teen who has discontinued oral contraceptives and 12 months in a teen who has discontinued depot medroxyprogesterone acetate (Depo-Provera). It should also be remembered that adolescents using low-dose birth control pills (which may have been provided confidentially by another clinic) may have scant flow or amenorrhea. As noted in the section on delayed menarche, a progestin challenge provides information on the estrogen status of the adolescent (page 219). Laboratory tests include measurement of serum TSH, FSH, and prolactin levels. Adding an LH level and androgens may help in making a diagnosis if PCOS is a consideration. It should be noted that in some girls, the elevated LH to FSH ratio may be secondary to stress; more generally, it is associated with PCOS. Bone density measurements are helpful in monitoring bone loss in girls with hypoestrogenic amenorrhea.

In most patients who have abundant, watery cervical mucus, a positive vaginal smear for estrogen, or a normal response to progesterone, menses usually return spontaneously without treatment. Medroxyprogesterone, 10 mg orally for 12 to 14 days, is usually prescribed every 6 weeks to 3 months to prevent endometrial hyperplasia resulting from prolonged estrogen stimulation and to reassure the clinician that the patient is continuing to make estrogen. Combined hormonal contraceptives are appropriate to induce menstrual periods in girls who are sexually active and need contraception or in girls who are estrogen deficient.

Case 7

A. N., aged 15, came to the clinic because of fatigue. Further questioning revealed that her last menstrual period had occurred 2 months previously. Her menarche was at the age of 12 years, and she had had regular cycles until the missed period. Although she initially denied the possibility of pregnancy, the urine pregnancy test result was positive, and her uterus was 8-week size.

Case 8

P. A., 14½ years old, was referred for irregular menses. Her breasts and pubic hair had begun to develop when she was 10 to 11 years old, and menarche occurred at 13²⁄₁₂ years. She had had only five menstrual periods over the past 16 months, and her last menstrual period had been 1 month before the visit. She had been short for many years; her father was 5 ft 10 in. and her mother 5 ft ¾ in. (mid-parental height 5 ft 2⅞ in.). Physical examination showed her to have short stature, with a height of 4 ft 9 in. (<5%) and weight of 100 lb (25%) (Fig. 7-9). Her blood pressure was 106/70 mm Hg; her breast development was Tanner stage 5 and her pubic hair Tanner stage 4. The results of external genital examination and pelvic examination were normal. She had no stigmata of Turner syndrome. Her bone age was 14 years; FSH level was 96.5 mIU/ml, and LH level was 34.8 mIU/ml; the TSH level was normal. Her karyotype was 45,X/46,X,i(Xq). She took growth hormone for 4 months at another hospital and then discontinued therapy. She then had several additional spontaneous menses, but had no withdrawal flow in response to medroxyprogesterone at age 15½ years and was given oral contraceptives for estrogen replacement. At age 19, she discontinued the oral contraceptives on her own and continued to have normal regular cycles for 4 months. Her FSH level was 7.7 mIU/ml. She has been counseled about the need to use birth control if she desires to avoid the risk of unintended pregnancy; however, she is at high risk of POF and infertility.

Case 9

B. T., a 17-year-old boarding school student, had had amenorrhea for 3 years. Menarche had occurred when she was 12 years, followed by regular menses for 2 years until she became amenorrheic. The amenorrhea had been attributed to the stress of boarding school. Physical examination showed her to be healthy, with a

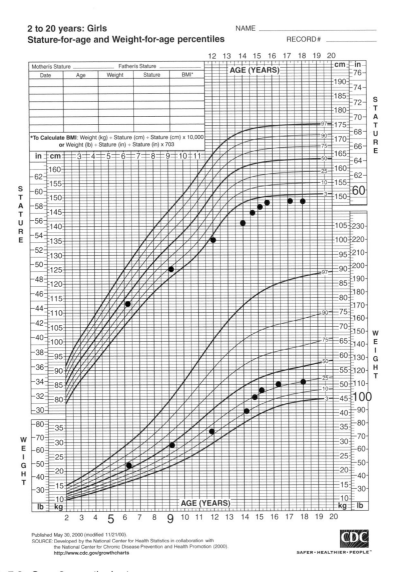

FIG. 7-9. Case 8: growth chart.

height of 63 in. and a weight of 119 lb. Vaginal examination showed poor estrogenization. Laboratory tests showed elevated gonadotropin levels: FSH, 63.9 and >100 mIU/ml; LH, 60.8 and 94.5 mIU/ml. Her karyotype was 46,XX; antiovarian, antithyroid, and antiadrenal antibodies were negative; and thyroid tests were normal. With a diagnosis of premature ovarian failure, she needs to be observed for potential autoimmune endocrinopathies despite negative antibody studies. She initiated estrogen replacement therapy.

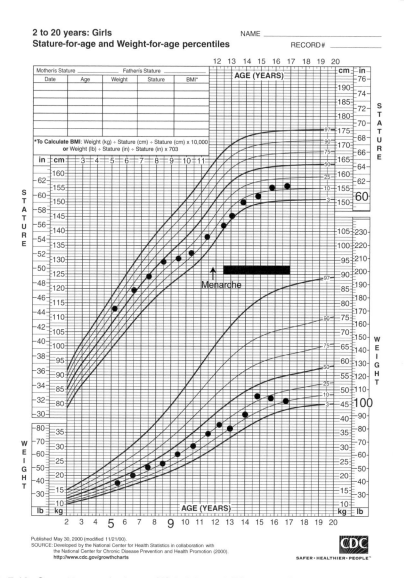

FIG. 7-10. Case 10: growth charts, **(A)** height and **(B)** weight. The *bar* represents therapy with thyroid replacement.

Case 10

K. M. was evaluated at the age of 12⁶/₁₂ years for amenorrhea. She had started her breast and pubic hair development at age 10⁶/₁₂ years and had her menarche at age 11⁹/₁₂ years. She subsequently had two monthly cycles and then amenorrhea for 9 months. She recalled having been short for some time, and had been treated with iron for anemia. She denied constipation, fatigue, intolerance to heat or cold, or school problems. Her mother was 60 in. tall and her father 67½ in. tall; her 17-year-old brother was 69 in. tall. Physical examination showed her height to be 55½ in. and her weight to be 84 lb. Her blood pressure was 112/70 mm Hg, and her pulse was 66 beats/min. Her breast and pubic hair development were both Tanner stage 4. The vagina was well estrogenized, and rectal examination showed a normal-size uterus. Although the history of irregular menses was not particularly unusual in an early adolescent, the growth chart (Fig. 7-10) was a clue to the diagnosis. The patient had had little increase in height between the ages of 8½ and 10½ years but then had experienced the growth spurt of pubertal development. Her bone age was 11 years (delayed for a postmenarcheal adolescent), and indeed, thyroid function tests showed hypothyroidism with a T_4 of 1.8 μg/dl, thyroid-binding globulin index (TBGI) of 0.75, total T_3 of 54 ng/dl, and TSH of 990 μU/ml. Gonadotropin levels were normal (LH, 3.6 mIU/ml; FSH, 9.0 mIU/ml). She was given levothyroxine and experienced some behavioral problems at school as she converted from a placid child to a rebellious adolescent. Her menses resumed after 2 months of thyroid replacement, and she is currently on a dose of 0.125 mg levothyroxine daily. School performance and adolescent adjustment gradually improved over the following years.

Case 11

N. T., 16 years old, was referred for evaluation of amenorrhea that had lasted 2 years. She had normal breast and pubic hair development at the age of 11 and had menarche at the age of 12¹¹/₁₂. Her menses were regular for about 6 months until she lost weight, going from about 125 lb to 104 lb on a "healthy diet" by avoiding sweets, bread, and fats (Fig. 7-11). She subsequently gained weight to 135 lb. She lost weight again, but was gaining again at the time of the visit. She was conscious of trying to maintain a "normal" weight, and she ate no red meat. She was active in after-school sports.

Physical examination showed a healthy appearance, a height of 5 ft 5 in., and a weight of 114 lb. The results of the general physical examination and pelvic examination were normal except for a slightly diminished estrogen effect apparent on the vaginal mucosa. Her estimated percentage of body fat (using calipers) was 21%. The result of a urine pregnancy test was negative. Laboratory tests revealed an FSH level of 6.4 mIU/ml and normal prolactin and TSH levels. A vaginal smear showed 10% parabasal cells, 90% intermediate cells [maturation index (MI) = 45]. She had only a very scant withdrawal flow in response to medroxyprogesterone taken orally for 10 days. The options were discussed with her, and she decided to take estrogen/progestin replacement for one year, to increase her calcium intake, and to stabilize her weight. She subsequently had normal menses.

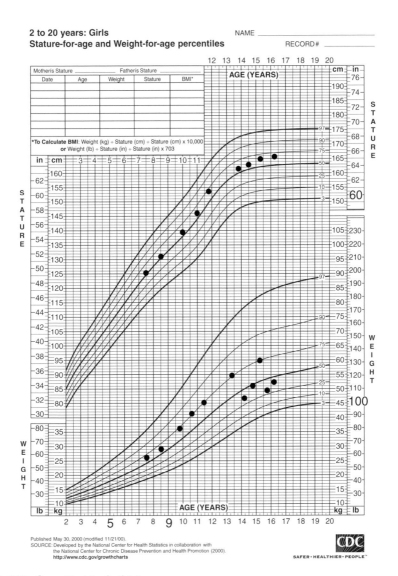

2 to 20 years: Girls
Stature-for-age and Weight-for-age percentiles

NAME _____

RECORD# _____

FIG. 7-11. Case 11: growth chart.

Case 12

Identical twins M. R. and S. R. presented at the age of 20 years with amenorrhea of 2 years' duration. Both had experienced menarche between the ages of 13 and 14 years and had had regular monthly menses until they were 18, when they both increased their level of training in preparation for college athletics. M. R. lost 20 lb and S. R. lost 15 lb. Both had subsequently maintained stable weights between 112 and 120 lb for the past 2 years, and were 66 in. tall. Both continued to be active in competitive sports throughout the year. Physical examination of both patients revealed Tanner stage 5 breast and pubic hair development with markedly diminished estrogenization on vaginal examination. Otherwise, the results of pelvic examination and general assessments were normal. Laboratory values for the two girls were remarkably similar: the LH level was 4.6 mIU/ml for S. R. and 4.7 mIU/ml for M. R.; the FSH level was 10.6 mIU/ml for S. R. and 11.3 mIU/ml for M. R.; the prolactin level was 3.1 ng/ml for S. R. and 3.7 ng/ml for M. R.; the estradiol level was 27 pg/ml for S. R. and 28 pg/ml for M. R. Vaginal smears were slightly different, with S. R., who had lost less weight, having a better maturation index: 15% superficial, 85% intermediate cells (MI = 58) for S. R. versus 16% superficial, 53% intermediate, and 31% parabasal cells (MI = 43) for M. R. The options of weight gain, decreased activity level, improved calcium and vitamin D intake, and estrogen replacement were discussed with the two young women. They both elected to increase dietary calcium and to use transdermal estradiol patches and medroxyprogesterone (14 days per month) for 9 months. Withdrawal flow was normal; however, they discontinued the medication because of concerns about bloating. Six months later they began to decrease their athletic activity in preparation for graduation from college. Spontaneous menses returned.

OLIGOMENORRHEA

Teenagers with menses every 2 to 3 months often consult the clinician. Common diagnoses include PCOS, hypothalamic amenorrhea (usually associated with competitive sports participation, ballet, or weight change), or normal oligoovulatory cycles. Premenstrual symptoms and dysmenorrhea suggest ovulatory cycles, which can be confirmed if needed by demonstrating a shift in the basal body temperature curve (see Chapter 1) and/or by a rise in serum progesterone level in the luteal phase of the cycle. Scant, irregular menses without cramps or heavy, prolonged menses are most likely anovulatory. The presence of signs of acanthosis nigricans, hirsutism, or acne suggest PCOS. In addition, it should be remembered that the sexually active patient with a history of irregular menses who is not using contraception may have an unplanned pregnancy despite any number of negative pregnancy test results in the past.

The importance of evaluating cases of persistent oligomenorrhea was noted in a review at Children's Hospital Boston many years ago. The charts of all adolescents who had been evaluated for oligomenorrhea not associated with weight loss, and who had been assessed over a 2-year period, were reviewed (220). Among the 42 adolescents (mean age 17.3, range 15 to 20 years), 19 had evidence of androgen excess (hirsutism, clitoromegaly, and/or severe acne) consistent with PCOS or adrenal androgen excess, and 23 patients had no evidence of androgen excess.

In the second group, four patients had persistently elevated LH levels that ranged from 34.5 to 41.0 mIU/ml, with normal FSH, DHEAS, and total and free testosterone levels; 15 had hypothalamic amenorrhea (and six of 15 returned to normal menses); one had hyperprolactinemia; and three had ovarian failure. Although the patients were seen in a referral center, the spectrum of potential diagnoses is representative.

Once a diagnosis is made, patients are generally reassured by a careful explanation of menstrual cycles and a discussion of treatment options. The statement "You're normal; don't worry" is not sufficient. Medroxyprogesterone acetate, 10 mg a day for 12 to 14 days each month, can be used to prevent endometrial hyperplasia; it is also especially useful to treat patients with a history of hypermenorrhea associated with irregular periods. Oral contraceptives or other combined estrogen/progestin methods can be prescribed to the adolescent who needs contraception. Patients should be counseled that there is no evidence that hormonal therapy changes the long-term prognosis of patients for irregular cycles (see Chapter 20). However, it is important to make a diagnosis before the institution of hormonal therapy so that the patient realizes that if she has PCOS she is likely to return to oligomenorrhea following the discontinuance of hormonal therapy. No therapy is needed for oligoovulators.

REFERENCES

1. Wu T, Mendola P, Buck GM. Differences in the presence of secondary sex characteristics and menarche among US girls: the third National Health and Nutrition Examination survey, 1988–1994. *Pediatrics* 2002;110(4):752.
2. Chumlea WC, Schubert CM, Roche AF, et al. Age at menarche and racial comparisons in US girls. *Pediatrics* 2003;111:110.
3. Johnson J, Whitaker AH. Adolescent smoking, weight changes, and binge purge behaviors: associations with secondary amenorrhea. *Am J Public Health* 1992;82:47.
4. Frisch RE, Snow RC, Johnson LA, et al. Magnetic resonance imaging of overall and regional body fat, estrogen metabolism, and ovulation of athletes compared to controls. *J Clin Endocrinol Metab* 1993;77:471.
5. Duerenberg P, Pieters JJL, Hautvast JG. The assessment of the body fat percentage by skinfold thickness measurements in childhood and young adolescence. *Br J Nutr* 1990;63:293.
6. Pollock ML, Schmidt DH. Measurement of cardiorespiratory fitness and body composition in the clinical setting. *Compr Ther* 1980;6:12.
7. Oppliger RA, Cassady SL. Body composition assessment in women—special considerations for athletes. *Sports Med* 1994;17:353.
8. Economy KE, Barnewolt C, Laufer MR. A comparison of MRI and laparoscopy in detecting pelvic structures in cases of vaginal agenesis. *J Pediatr Adolesc Gynecol* 2002;15:101.
9. Kletzky OA, Davajan V, Nakamura RM, et al. Clinical categorization of patients with secondary amenorrhea using progesterone-induced uterine bleeding and measurement of serum gonadotropin levels. *Am J Obstet Gynecol* 1975;121:695.
10. Shangold MM, Tomai TP, Cook JD, et al. Factors associated with withdrawal bleeding after administration of oral micronized progesterone in women with secondary amenorrhea. *Fertil Steril* 1991;56:1040.
11. Reindollar RH, Byrd JR, McDonough PG. Delayed sexual development: a study of 252 patients. *Am J Obstet Gynecol* 1981;140:371.

12. Scott RT, Leonardi MR, Hofmann GE, et al. A prospective evaluation of clomiphene citrate challenge test screening of the general infertility population. *Obstet Gynecol* 1993;82:539.
13. Thomas KA, Cook SD, Bennett JT, et al. Femoral neck and lumbar spine bone mineral densities in a normal population 3–20 years of age. *J Pediatr Orthop* 1990;11:48.
14. Djerassi A, Coutifaris C, West VA, et al. Gonadotroph adenoma in a premenopausal woman secreting follicle-stimulating hormone and causing ovarian hyperstimulation. *J Clin Endocrinol Metab* 1995;80:591.
15. Lee JK, Kim JH, Kim JS, et al. Secondary amenorrhea caused by hydrocephalus due to aqueductal stenosis: report of two cases. *J Korean Med Sci* 2001;16:532.
16. Barkan AL, Kelch RP, Marshall JC. Isolated gonadotrope failure in the polyglandular autoimmune syndrome. *N Engl J Med* 1985;312:1535.
17. Cacciari E, Zucchini S, Ambrosetto P, et al. Empty sella in children and adolescents with possible hypothalamic-pituitary disorders. *J Clin Endocrinol Metab* 1994;78:767.
18. Shulman DI, Martinez CR, Bercu BB, et al. Hypothalamic-pituitary dysfunction in primary empty sella syndrome in childhood. *J Pediatr* 1986;108:540.
19. Dorman JS. Steenkiste. AR. Foley TP, et al. Menopause in type 1 diabetes women: is it premature? *Diabetes* 2001;50:1857.
20. Djursing H. Hypothalamic-pituitary-gonadal function in insulin treated diabetic women with and without amenorrhea. *Dan Med Bull* 1987;34:139.
21. Austin SB, Ziyadeh N, Keliher A, et al. Screening high school students for eating disorders: results of a national initiative. *J Adolesc Health* 2001;28:96.
22. Couzinet B, Young J, Brailly S, et al. Functional hypothalamic amenorrhea: a partial and reversible gonadotrophin deficiency of nutritional origin. *Clin Endocrinol* 1999;50:229.
23. Warren MP, Voussoughian F, Geer EB, et al. Functional hypothalamic amenorrhea: hypoleptinemia and disordered eating. *J Clin Endocrinol Metab* 1999;84:873.
24. DiCarlo C, Palomba S. DeFazio M, et al. Hypogonadotropic hypogonadism in obese women after biliopancreatic diversion. *Fertil Steril* 1999;72:905.
25. Perkins RB, Hall JE, Martin KA. Neuroendocrine abnormalities in hypothalamic amenorrhea: spectrum, stability, and response to neurotransmitter modulation. *J Clin Endocrinol Metab* 1999; 84:1905.
26. American Psychiatric Association. *DSM-IV. Diagnostic and statistical manual of mental disorders,* 4th ed. Washington, DC: American Psychiatric Association, 1994.
27. American Academy of Pediatrics, Committee on Adolescence. Identifying and treating eating disorders. *Pediatrics* 2003;111:204.
28. Grinspoon S, Miller K, Coyle C, et al. Severity of osteopenia in estrogen-deficient women with anorexia nervosa and hypothalamic amenorrhea. *J Clin Endocrinol Metab* 1999;84:2049.
29. Rigotti NA, Neer RM, Skates SJ, et al. The clinical course of osteoporosis in anorexia nervosa: a longitudinal study of calcium and bone mass. *JAMA* 1991;265:1133.
30. Bachrach LK, Guido D, Katzman D, et al. Decreased bone density in adolescent girls with anorexia nervosa. *Pediatrics* 1990;86:440.
31. Gordon CM, Goodman E, Emans SJ, et al. Physiologic regulators of bone turnover in young women with anorexia nervosa. *J Pediatr* 2002;141:64.
32. Gordon CM, Grace E, Emans SJ, et al. Effects of oral DHEA on bone density in young women with anorexia nervosa: a randomized trial. *J Clin Endocrinol Metab* 2002;87(11):4935.
33. DiCarlo C, Tommaselli G, DeFillip E et al. Menstrual status and serum leptin levels in anorectic and in menstruating women with low body mass indexes. *Fertil Steril* 2002;78:376.
34. Boyar RM, Katz J, Finkelstein JW et al. Anorexia nervosa: immaturity of the 24-hour luteinizing hormone secretory pattern. *N Engl J Med* 1974;291:861.
35. Frisch RE. Fatness and fertility. *Sci Am* 1988;88.
36. Frisch RE, McArthur JW Menstrual cycles: fatness as a determinant of minimum weight for height necessary for their maintenance or onset. *Science* 1974;185:949.
37. Centers for Disease Control, National Center for Health Statistics. Height and weight of youths 12-17 years, United States. Growth charts at www.cdc.gov/growthcharts/.
38. Kreipe RE, Churchill BH, Strauss J. Long-term outcome of adolescents with anorexia nervosa. *Am J Dis Child* 1989;143:1322.
39. Shomento SH, Kreipe RE. Menstruation and fertility following anorexia nervosa. *Adolesc Pediatr Gynecol* 1994;7:142.

40. Golden NH, Jacobson MS, Schebendach J, et al. Resumption of menses in anorexia nervosa. *Arch Pediatr Adolesc Med* 1997;151:16.

41. Steinhausen HC, Boyadjieva S, Griogoroiu M, et al. The outcome of adolescent eating disorders. *Eur Child Adolesc Psych* 2003;12(S1):91.

42. Wyshak G, Frisch RE, Albright TE, et al. Bone fractures among former college athletes compared with nonathletes in the menopausal and postmenopausal years. *Obstet Gynecol* 1987; 69:121.

43. Yeager KK, Agostini R, Nattiv A, et al. The female athlete triad: disordered eating, amenorrhea, osteoporosis. *Med Sci Sports Exerc* 1993;25:775.

44. Frisch RE, Gotz-Welbergen AV, McArthur JW, et al. Delayed menarche and amenorrhea of college athletes in relation to age of onset of training. *JAMA* 1981;246:1559.

45. White CM, Hergenroeder AC, Klish WJ. Bone mineral density in 15- to 21-year-old eumenorrheic and amenorrheic subjects. *Am J Dis Child* 1992;146:31.

46. Hergenroeder AC. Bone mineralization, hypothalamic amenorrhea, and sex steroid therapy in female adolescents and young adults. *J Pediatr* 1995;126:683.

47. Hetland ML, Haarbo J, Christiansen C. Running induces menstrual disturbances but bone mass is unaffected, except in amenorrheic women. *Am J Med* 1993;95:53.

48. Warren MP Amenorrhea in endurance runners. *J Clin Endocrinol Metab* 1992;75:1393.

49. Baer JT, Taper LJ. Amenorrheic and eumenorrheic adolescent runners: dietary intake and exercise training status. *J Am Diet Assoc* 1992;92:89.

50. Bullen BA, Skrinar GS, Beitins IZ, et al. Induction of menstrual disorders by strenuous exercise in untrained women. *N Engl J Med* 1985;312:1349.

51. Frisch RE, Wyshak G, Vincent L. Delayed menarche and amenorrhea in ballet dancers. *N Engl J Med* 1980;303:17.

52. Warren MP, Brooks Gunn J, Hamilton LH, et al. Scoliosis and fractures in young ballet dancers: relation to delayed menarche and secondary amenorrhea. *N Engl J Med* 1986;314:1348.

53. Cobb KL, Bachrach LK, Greendale G, et al. Disordered eating, menstrual irregularity, and bone mineral density in female runners. *Med Sci Sports Exerc* 2003;35:711.

54. Ramsay R, Wolman R. Are synchronized swimmers at risk for amenorrhea? *Br J Sports Med* 2001; 35:242.

55. Wilson C, Emans SJ, Mansfield MJ, et al. The relationship of calculated percent body fat, sports participation, age, and place of residence on menstrual patterns in healthy adolescent girls at an independent New England high school. *J Adolesc Health Care* 1984;5:248.

56. Ellison PT, Lager C. Moderate recreational running is associated with lowered salivary progesterone profiles in women. *Am J Obstet Gynecol* 1986;154:1000.

57. DeSouza MJ, Van Heest J, Demers LM, et al. Luteal phase deficiency in recreational runners: evidence for a hypometabolic state. *J Clin Endocrinol Metab* 2003;88:337.

58. Warren MP. The effects of exercise on pubertal progression and reproductive function in girls. *J Clin Endocrinol Metab* 1980;51:1150.

59. Dhuper S, Warren MP, Brooks-Gunn J, Fox R. Effects of hormonal status on bone density in adolescent girls. *J Clin Endocrinol Metab* 1990;71:1083.

60. Malina RM. Menarche in athletes: a synthesis and hypothesis. *Ann Hum Biol* 1983;10:1.

61. Feicht CB, Johnson TS, Martin BJ, et al. Secondary amenorrhea in athletes [Letter]. *Lancet* 1978; 2:1145.

62. Laughlin GA, Yen SS. Nutritional and endocrine-metabolic aberrations in amenorrheic athletes. *J Clin Endocrinol Metab* 1996;81:4301.

63. Deuster PA, Kyle SB, Moser PB, et al. Nutritional intakes and status of highly trained amenorrheic and eumenorrheic women runners. *Fertil Steril* 1986;46:636.

64. Pirke KM, Schweiger U, Laessle R, et al. Dieting influences the menstrual cycle: vegetarian versus nonvegetarian diet. *Fertil Steril* 1986;46:1083.

65. Gadpaille WJ, Sanborn CF, Wagner WW. Athletic amenorrhea, major affective disorders, and eating disorders. *Am J Psychiatry* 1987;144:939.

66. Kaufman BA, Warren MP, Dominguez JE, et al. Bone density and amenorrhea in ballet dancers are related to a decreased resting metabolic rate and lower leptin levels. *J Clin Endocrinol Metab* 2002;87:2777.

67. Hale RW, Kosasa T, Krieger J, et al. A marathon: the immediate effect on female runners' luteinizing hormone, follicle-stimulating hormone, prolactin, testosterone, and cortisol levels. *Am J Obstet Gynecol* 1983;146:550.

68. Shangold MM, Gatz ML, Thysen B. Acute effects of exercise on plasma concentration of prolactin and testosterone in recreational women runners. *Fertil Steril* 1981;35:699.

69. Rickenlund A, Carlstrom K, Ekblom B et al. Hyperandrogenicity is an alternative mechanism underlying oligomenorrhea or amenorrhea in female athletes and may improve physical performance. *Fertil Steril* 2003;79:947.

70. Loucks AB, Mortola JF, Girton L, et al. Alterations in the hypothalamic-pituitary-ovarian and the hypothalamic-pituitary-adrenal axes in athletic women. *J Clin Endocrinol Metab* 1989;68:402.

71. Waters DL, Qualls CR, Dorin R, et al. Increased pulsatility, process irregularity, and nocturnal trough concentrations of growth hormone in amenorrheic compared to eumenorrheic athletes. *J Clin Endocrinol Metab* 2001;86:1013.

72. Bonjour J, Theintz G, Buchs B, et al. Critical years and stages of puberty for spinal and femoral bone mass accumulation during adolescence. *J Clin Endocrinol Metab* 1991;73:555.

73. Theintz G, Buchs B, Rizzoli R, et al. Longitudinal monitoring of bone mass accumulation in healthy adolescent: evidence for a marked reduction after 16 years of age at the levels of lumbar spine and femoral neck in female subjects. *J Clin Endocrinol Metab* 1992;75:1060.

74. Slemenda CW, Reister TK, Hui SL, et al. Influences on skeletal mineralization in children and adolescents: evidence for varying effects of sexual maturation and physical activity. *J Pediatr* 1994;125:210.

75. Rubin K, Schirduan V, Gendreau P, et al. Predictors of axial and peripheral bone mineral density in healthy children and adolescents, with special attention to the role of puberty. *J Pediatr* 1993;123:863.

76. Marcus R, Cann C, Madvig P, et al. Menstrual function and bone mass in elite women distance runners: endocrine and metabolic features. *Ann Intern Med* 1985;102:158.

77. Drinkwater BL, Nilson K, Chesnut CH, et al. Bone mineral content of amenorrheic and eumenorrheic athletes. *N Engl J Med* 1984;311:277.

78. Myerson M, Gutin B, Warren MP, et al. Total body bone density in amenorrheic runners. *Obstet Gynecol* 1992;79:973.

79. Louis O, Demeirleir K, Kalender W, et al. Low vertebral bone density values in young non-elite female runners. *Int J Sports Med* 1991;12:214.

80. Wolman RL, Clark P, McNally E, et al. Dietary calcium as a statistical determinant of spinal trabecular bone density in amenorrheic and oestrogen-replete athletes. *Bone Miner* 1992;17:415.

81. Drinkwater BL, Bruemner B, Chesnut CH. Menstrual history as a determinant of current bone density in young athletes. *JAMA* 1990;263:545.

82. Slemenda CW, Johnston CC. High intensity activities in young women: site specific bone mass effects among female figure skaters. *Bone Miner* 1993;20:125.

83. Rencken ML, Chesnut CH, Drinkwater BL. Bone density at multiple skeletal sites in amenorrheic athletes. *JAMA* 1996;276:238.

84. Wolman RL, Clark P, McNally E, et al. Menstrual state and exercise as determinants of spinal trabecular bone density in female athletes. *BMJ* 1990;301:516.

85. Young N, Formica C, Szmukler G, et al. Bone density at weight-bearing and non-weight-bearing sites in ballet dancers: the effects of exercise, hypogonadism, and body weight. *J Clin Endocrinol Metab* 1994;78:449.

86. Warren MP, Gann J, Fox RP, Lancelot C, et al. Lack of bone accretion and amenorrhea: evidence for a relative osteopenia in weight-bearing bones. *J Clin Endocrinol Metab* 1991; 72:847.

87. Myburgh KH, Bachrach LK, Lewis B, et al. Low bone mineral density at axial and appendicular sites in amenorrheic athletes. *Med Sci Sports Exerc* 1993;25:1197.

88. Gremion G, Rizzoli R, Slosman D, et al. Oligo-amenorrheic long-distance runners may lose more bone in spine than in femur. *Med Sci Sports Exerc* 2001;33:818.

89. Gibson JH, Mitchell A, Reeve J, et al. Treatment of reduced bone mineral density in athletic amenorrhea: a pilot study. *Osteoporos Int* 1999;10:284.

90. Myburgh KH, Hutchins J, Fataar AB, et al. Low bone density is an etiologic factor for stress fractures in athletes. *Ann Intern Med* 1990;113:754.

91. Friedl KE, Nuovo JA. Factors associated with stress fractures in young Army women: indications for further research. *Mil Med* 1992;157:334.

92. Drinkwater BL, Nilson K, Ott S, et al. Bone mineral density after resumption of menses in amenorrheic athletes. *JAMA* 1986;256:380.

93. Jonnavithula S, Warren MP, Fox RP, Lazaro MI. Bone density is compromised in amenorrheic women despite return of menses: a 2-year study. *Obstet Gynecol* 1993;81:669.
94. Warren MP, Brooks-Gunn J, Fox RP, et al. Osteopenia in exercise-associated amenorrhea using ballet dancers as a model: a longitudinal study. *J Clin Endocrinol Metab* 2002;87:162.
95. Blackwell RE, Younger JB. Long-term medical therapy and follow-up of pediatric-adolescent patients with prolactin-secreting macroadenomas. *Fertil Steril* 1986;45:713.
96. Schlechte JA. Prolactinoma. *N Engl J Med* 2003;349:2035.
97. Pereira MC, Sobrinho LG, Afonso AM, et al. Is idiopathic hyperprolactinemia a transitional stage toward prolactinoma? *Obstet Gynecol* 1987;70:305.
98. Sisam DA, Sheehan JP, Sheeler LR. The natural history of untreated microprolactinomas. *Fertil Steril* 1987;48:67.
99. Kane LA, Leinung MC, Scheithauer BW, et al. Pituitary adenomas in childhood and adolescence. *J Clin Endocrinol Metab* 1994;79:1135.
100. Hauache OM, Rocha AJ, Maia AC, et al. Screening for macroprolactinoma and pituitary imaging studies. *Clin Endocrinol* 2002;57:327.
101. Vallette-Kasic S, Morange-Ramos I, Selim A, et al. Macroprolactinoma revisited: a study on 106 patients. *J Clin Endocrinol Metab* 2002;87:581.
102. Schlechte JA. The macroprolactin problem. *J Clin Endocrinol Metab* 2002;87:5408.
103. Kinon BJ, Gilmore JA, Liu H, et al. Prevalence of hyperprolactinemia in schizophrenic patients treated with conventional antipsychotic medications or risperidone. *Psychoneuroendocrinology* 2003;28[Suppl 2]:55.
104. Hamner M. The effects of atypical antipsychotics on serum prolactin levels. *Ann Clin Psychiatry* 2002;14:163.
105. Luzzati R, Crosato IM, Mascioli M, et al. Galactorrhea and hyperprolactinemia associated with HIV postexposure chemoprophylaxis. *AIDS* 2002;16:1306.
106. Montero A, Bottasso OA, Luraghi MR, et al. Galactorrhea, hyperprolactinemia, and protease inhibitors. *Lancet* 2001;357:473.
107. Kim KS, Pae CU, Chae JH, et al. Effects of olanzapine on prolactin levels of female patients with schizophrenia treated with risperidone. *J Clin Psychiatry* 2002;63:408.
108. Raber W, Gessl A, Nowotny P et al. Hyperprolactinemia in hypothyroidism: clinical significance and impact of TSH normalization. *Clin Endocrinol* 2003;58:185.
109. Vanbesien J, Schiettecatte J, Anckaert E, et al. Circulating anti-prolactin auto-antibodies must be considered in the differential diagnosis of hyperprolactinemia in adolescents. *Eur J Pediatr* 2002; 161:373.
110. Leanos-Miranda A, Chavez-Rueda KA, Blanco-Favela F. Biologic activity and plasma clearance of prolactin-IgG complex in patients with systematic lupus erythematosus. *Arthritis Rheum* 2001;44:866.
111. Oiwa A, Sakurai A, Sato Y, et al. Pituitary adenomas in adolescent patients with multiple endocrine neoplasia type 1. *Endocr J* 2002;49:635.
112. Dessypris A, Karonen SL, Adlercreutz H. Marathon run effects on plasma prolactin and growth hormone. *Acta Endocrinol (Copenh) (Suppl)* 1979;255:187.
113. Noel GL, Sub HK, Stone JG, et al. Human prolactin and growth hormone release during surgery and other conditions of stress. *J Clin Endocrinol Metab* 1972;35:840.
114. Modest GA, Fangman JJ. Nipple piercing and hyperprolactinemia. *N Engl J Med* 2002;347:1626.
115. Dawajan V, Kletsky O, March CM. The significance of galactorrhea in patients with normal menses, oligomenorrhea, and secondary amenorrhea. *Am J Obstet Gynecol* 1978;130:894.
116. Anonymous. Case record of Massachusetts General Hospital. Weekly clinicopathological exercises. Case 35-2002. A nine-year-old girl with cold intolerance, visual-field defects, and a suprasellar tumor. *N Engl J Med* 2002;347:1604.
117. Klibanski A, Neer RM, Beitins IZ, et al. Decreased bone density in hyperprolactinemic women. *N Engl J Med* 1980;303:1511.
118. Klibanski A, Greenspan SL. Increase in bone mass after treatment of hyperprolactinemia amenorrhea. *N Engl J Med* 1986;315:542.
119. Biller BMK, Baum HBA, Rosenthal DI, et al. Progressive trabecular osteopenia in women with hyperprolactinemic amenorrhea. *J Clin Endocrinol Metab* 1992;75:692.
120. Schlecte J, Walkner L, Kathol M. A longitudinal analysis of premenopausal bone loss in healthy women and women with hyperprolactinemia. *J Clin Endocrinol Metab* 1992;75:698.

121. Shaawary M, El-Dawakhly AS, El-Sadek MM. Biomarkers of bone turnover and bone mineral density in hyperprolactinemic amenorrheic women. *Clin Chem Lab Med* 1999;37:433.
122. Vartej P, Poiana C, Vartej I. Effects of hyperprolactinemia on osteoporotic fracture risk in premenopausal women. *Gynecol Endocrinol* 2001;15:43.
123. Calao A, DiSomma C, Loche S, et al. Prolactinomas in adolescents: persistent bone loss after 2 years of prolactin normalization. *Clin Endocrinol* 2000;52:319.
124. Vestergaard P, Jorgensen JO, Hagen C, et al. Fracture risk is increased in patients with GH deficiency or untreated prolactinomas—a case control study. *Clin Endocrinol* 2002;56:159.
125. Sluijmer AV, Lappohn RE. Clinical history and outcome of 59 patients with idiopathic hyperprolactinemia. *Fertil Steril* 1992;58:72.
126. Schlechte J, Dolan K, Sherman B, et al. The natural history of untreated hyperprolactinemia: a prospective analysis. *J Clin Endocrinol Metab* 1989;68:412.
127. Koppelman MCS, Jaffe MJ, Rieth KG, et al. Hyperprolactinemia, amenorrhea, and galactorrhea: a retrospective assessment of twenty-five cases. *Ann Intern Med* 1984;100:115.
128. Jeffcoate WJ, Pound N, Sturrock ND, et al. Long-term followup of patients with hyperprolactinemia. *Clin Endocrinol* 1996;45:299.
129. Passos VQ, Souza JJ, Musolino NR, et al. Long-term follow-up of prolactinomas: normoprolactinemia after bromocriptine withdrawal. *J Clin Endocrinol Metab* 2002;87:3578.
130. Colao A, DiSarno A, Cappabianca P, et al. Withdrawal of long-term cabergoline therapy for tumoral and nontumoral hyperprolactinemia. *N Eng J Med* 2003;349:2023.
131. Corenblum B, Donovan L. The safety of physiological estrogen plus progestin replacement therapy and with oral contraceptive therapy in women with pathological hyperprolactinemia. *Fertil Steril* 1993;59:671.
132. Tyson D, Reggiardo D, Sklar C, et al. Prolactin-secreting macroadenomas in adolescents. Response to bromocriptine therapy. *Am J Dis Child* 1993;147:1057.
133. Jones SE, James RA, Hall K, et al. Optic chiasmal herniation—an under recognized complication of dopamine agonist therapy for macroprolactinoma. *Clin Endocrinol* 2000;53:529.
134. Horvath E, Kovacs K, Smyth HS, et al. A novel type of pituitary adenoma: morphological features and clinical correlations. *J Clin Endocrinol Metab* 1988;66:1111.
135. Couldwell WT, Rovit RL, Weiss MH. Role of surgery in the treatment of microprolactinomas. *Neurosurg Clin North Am* 2003;14:89.
136. Ciric I. Long-term management and outcome for pituitary tumors. *Neurosurg Clin North Am* 2003; 14:167.
137. Thomson JA, Gray CE, Teasdale GM. Relapse of hyperprolactinemia after transsphenoidal surgery for microprolactinoma: lessons for long-term follow-up. *Neurosurgery* 2002;50:36.
138. Kuroki A, Kayama T. Endoscopic approach to the pituitary lesions: contemporary method and review of the literature. *Biomed Pharmacother* 2002;56[Suppl 1]:158S.
139. Abe T, Ludecke DK. Transnasal surgery for prolactin-secreting pituitary adenomas in childhood and adolescence. *Surg Neurol* 2002;57:369.
140. Nomikos P, Buchfelder M, Fahlbusch R. Current management of prolactinomas. *J Neurooncol* 2001;54(2):139.
141. Duntas LH. Prolactinomas in children and adolescents—consequences in adult life. *J Pediatr Endocrinol Metab* 2001;14[Suppl 5]:1227S.
142. Fideloff HL, Boquete HR, Sequera A, et al. Peripubertal prolactinomas: clinical presentation and long-term outcome with different therapeutic approaches. *J Pediatr Endocrinol Metab* 2000; 13:261.
143. Tyrell JB, Lamborn KR, Hannegan LT, et al. Transsphenoidal microsurgical therapy of prolactinomas: initial outcomes and long-term results. *Neurosurgery* 1999;44:254.
144. Amar AP, Couldwell WT, Chen JC, et al. Predictive value of serum prolactin levels measured immediately after transsphenoidal surgery. *J Neurosurgery* 2002;97:307.
145. Biller BM. Diagnostic evaluation of hyperprolactinemia. *J Reprod Med* 1999;44[Suppl 12]:1095.
146. Mah PM, Webster J. Hyperprolactinemia: etiology, diagnosis, and management. *Sem Reprod Med* 2002;20:365.
147. Acquati S, Pizzocaro A, Tomei G, et al. A comparative evaluation of effectiveness of medical and surgical therapy in patients with macroprolactinoma. *J Neurosurg Sci* 2001;45:65.
148. Mallman ES, Nacul A, Spritzer PM. Pregnancy in hyperprolactinemic women. *Acta Obstet Gynecol Scand* 2002;81:265.

149. Molitch ME. Management of prolactinomas during pregnancy. *J Reprod Med* 1999;44[Suppl 12]:1121.
150. Shewchuk AB, Adamson GD, Lessard P, et al. The effect of pregnancy on suspected pituitary adenomas after conservative management of ovulation defects associated with galactorrhea. *Am J Obstet Gynecol* 1980;136:659.
151. Webster J, Piscitelli G, Polli A, et al. A comparison of cabergoline and bromocriptine in the treatment of hyperprolactinemic amenorrhea. *N Engl J Med* 1994;331:904.
152. Sabuncu T, Arikan E, Tasan E, et al. Comparison of the effects of cabergoline and bromocriptime on prolactin levels in hyperprolactinemic patients. *Internal Med* 2001;40:857.
153. Cannavo S, Curto L, Squadrito S, et al. Cabergoline: a first-choice treatment with previously treated prolactin-secreting pituitary adenoma. *J Endocrinol Invest* 1999;22:354.
154. DiSarno A, Landi ML, Cappabianca P, et al. Resistance to cabergoline as compared with bromocriptine in hyperprolactinemia: prevalence, clinical definition, and therapeutic strategy. *J Clin Endocrinol Metab* 2001;86:5256.
155. Colao A, DiSarno A, Landi ML, et al. Macroprolactinoma shrinkage during cabergoline treatment is greater in naive patients than in patients pretreated with other dopamine agonists: a prospective study in 110 patients. *J Clin Endocrinol Metab* 2000;85:2247.
156. Verhelst J, Abs R, Maiter D, et al. Cabergoline in the treatment of hyperprolactinemia: a study in 455 patients. *J Clin Endocrinol Metab* 1999;84:2518.
157. Schultz PN, Ginsberg L, McCutcheon IE, et al. Quinagolide in the management of prolactinoma. *Pituitary* 2000;3:239.
158. DiSarno A, Landi ML, Marzullo P, et al. The effect of quinagolide and cabergoline, two selective dopamine receptor type 2 agonists, in the treatment of prolactinomas. *Clin Endocrinol* 2000;53:53.
159. DeLuis DA, Becerra A, Lahera M, et al. A randomized cross-over study comparing cabergoline and quinagolide in the treatment of hyperprolactinemic patients. *J Endocrinol Invest* 2000;23:428.
160. Manfredi R, Alampi G, Talo S, et al. Silent oophoritis due to cytomegalovirus in a patient with advanced HIV disease. *Int J STD AIDS* 2000;11(6):410.
161. Nieto Y, Ross M, Gianani R, et al. Post-mortem incidental finding of cytomegalovirus oophoritis after an allogeneic stem cell transplant. *Bone Marrow Transplant* 1999;23(12):1323.
162. Shapiro CL, Manola J, Leboff M. Ovarian failure after adjuvant chemotherapy is associated with rapid bone loss in women with early-stage breast cancer. *J Clin Oncology* 2001;19:3306.
163. Iha T, Kano M, Nakayama M, Nagai, et al. Restoration of menstruation after chemotherapy-induced amenorrhea in a patient with ovarian immature teratoma. *Eur J Obstet Gynecol Reprod Bio* 2001;98:249.
164. Alper MM, Garner MB, Seibel MM. Premature ovarian failure: current concepts. *J Reprod Med* 1986;31:699.
165. Alper MM, Garner PR. Premature ovarian failure: its relationship to autoimmune disease. *Obstet Gynecol* 1985;66:27.
166. Damewood MD, Zacur HA, Hoffman GJ, et al. Circulating antiovarian antibodies in premature ovarian failure. *Obstet Gynecol* 1986;68:850.
167. Ahonen P, Miettinen A, Perheentupa J. Adrenal and steroidal cell antibodies in patients with autoimmune polyglandular disease type I and risk of adrenocortical and ovarian failure. *J Clin Endocrinol Metab* 1987;64:494.
168. Brelvisi L, Bombelli F, Sironi L, Doldi N. Organ-specific autoimmunity in patients with premature ovarian failure. *J Endocrinol Invest* 1993;16:889.
169. Smith BR, Furmaniak J. Adrenal and gonadal autoimmune diseases [Editorial]. *J Clin Endocrinol Metab* 1995;80:1502.
170. Betterle C, Rossi A, Pria SD, et al. Premature ovarian failure: autoimmunity and natural history. *J Clin Endocrinol Metab* 1993;39:35.
171. Rebar RW, Erickson GF, Yen SSC. Idiopathic premature ovarian failure: clinical and endocrine characteristics. *Fertil Steril* 1982;37:35.
172. Alper MM, Jolly EE, Garner PR. Pregnancies after premature ovarian failure. *Obstet Gynecol* 1986;67:595.
173. Kremer D, Droesch K, Navot D, et al. Spontaneous and pharmacologically induced remissions in patients with premature ovarian failure. *Obstet Gynecol* 1988;72:926.

174. Corenblum B, Rowe T, Taylor PJ. High-dose, short-term glucocorticoids for the treatment of infertility resulting from premature ovarian failure. *Fertil Steril* 1993;59:988.
175. Kalantaridou SN, Braddock DT, Patronas NJ, Nelson LM. Treatments of autoimmune premature ovarian failure. *Hum Reprod* 1999;14:1777.
176. Scully RE, ed. Case records of the Massachusetts General Hospital: case 46-1986. *N Engl J Med* 1986;315:1336.
177. Rutgers JL, Scully RE. The androgen insensitivity syndrome (testicular feminization): a clinico-pathologic study of 43 cases. *Int J Gynecol Pathol* 1991;10:126.
178. Griffin JE. Androgen resistance: the clinical and molecular spectrum. *N Engl J Med* 1992;326:611.
179. Siegel SE. Molecular genetics of androgen insensitivity. *Adolesc Pediatr Gynecol* 1995;8:3.
180. Federman D. *Abnormal sexual development.* Philadelphia: WB Saunders, 1968.
181. Hadjiathanasiou CG, Brauner R, Lortat-Jacob S, et al. True hermaphroditism: genetic variants and clinical management. *J Pediatr* 1994;125:738.
182. Shangold M, Rebar RW, Wentz AC, Schiff I. Evaluation and management of menstrual dysfunction in athletes. *JAMA* 1990;263:1665.
183. Miller K, Klibanski A. Amenorrheic bone loss. *J Clin Endocrinol Metab* 1999;84:1775.
184. Grady D, Herrington D, Bittner, et al. Cardiovascular disease outcomes during 6.8 years of hormone therapy: heart and estrogen/progestin replacement study follow-up (HERS II). *JAMA* 2002;288:49.
185. Writing Group for the Women's Health Initiative Investigators. Risks and benefits of estrogen plus progestin in healthy postmenopausal women: principal results from the Women's Health Initiative randomized controlled trial. *JAMA* 2002;288:321.
186. Gordon CM, Grace E, Emans SJ, et al. Changes in bone turnover markers and menstrual function after short-term oral DHEA in young women with anorexia nervosa. *J Bone Miner Res* 1998; 14(1):136.
187. Warren MP, Brooks-Gunn J, Fox RP, et al. Persistent osteopenia in ballet dancers with amenorrhea and delayed menarche despite hormone therapy: a longitudinal study. *Fertil Steril* 2003;80:398.
188. Klibanski A, Biller BM, Schoenfeld DA, et al. The effects of estrogen administration on trabecular bone loss in young women with anorexia nervosa. *J Clin Endocrinol Metab* 1995;80:898.
189. Seeman E, Szmukler GI, Formica C, et al. Osteoporosis in anorexia nervosa: the influence of peak bone density, bone loss, oral contraceptive use, and exercise. *J Bone Miner Res* 1992;7:1467.
190. Grinspoon S, Baum H, Lee K et al. Effects of short-term recombinant human insulin-like growth factor-1 administration on bone turnover in osteopenic women with anorexia nervosa. *J Clin Endocrinol Metab* 1996;81:3864.
191. Cumming D. Exercise-associated amenorrhea, low bone density, and estrogen replacement therapy. *Arch Intern Med* 1996;156:2193.
192. Lindsay R. Estrogen therapy in the prevention and management of osteoporosis. *Am J Obstet Gynecol* 1987;156:1347.
193. Ettinger B, Genant HK, Cann CE. Long-term estrogen replacement therapy prevents bone loss and fractures. *Ann Intern Med* 1985;102:319.
194. The Writing Group for the PEPI Trial. Effect of hormone therapy on bone mineral density. *JAMA* 1996;276:1389.
195. Prestwood KM, Kenny AM, Kleppinger A, et al. Ultralow-dose micronized 17β-estradiol and bone density and bone metabolism in older women. *JAMA* 2003;290:1042.
196. Lindsay R, Hart DM, Clark DM. The minimum effective dose of estrogen for prevention of postmenopausal bone loss. *Obstet Gynecol* 1984;63:759.
197. Ettinger B, Genant HK, Steiger P, Madvig P. Low-dosage micronized 17 β-estradiol prevents bone loss in postmenopausal women. *Am J Obstet Gynecol* 1992;166:479.
198. Emans SJ, Grace E, Hoffer FA, et al. Estrogen deficiency in adolescents and young adults: impact on bone mineral content and effects of estrogen replacement therapy. *Obstet Gynecol* 1990;76:585.
199. Mora S, Wever G, Guarneri MP, et al. Effect of estrogen replacement therapy on bone mineral content in girls with Turner syndrome. *Obstet Gynecol* 1992;79:747.
200. Van Campenhout J, Choquette P, Vauclair R. Endometrial pattern in patients with primary hypo-estrogenic amenorrhea receiving estrogen replacement therapy. *Obstet Gynecol* 1980;56:349.

201. Woodruff JD, Pickar JH. Incidence of endometrial hyperplasia in postmenopausal women taking conjugated estrogens (Premarin) with medroxyprogesterone acetate or conjugated estrogens alone. *Am J Obstet Gynecol* 1994;170:1213.
202. Padwick ML, Pryse-Davies J, Whitehead MI. A simple method for determining the optimal dosage of progestin in postmenopausal women receiving estrogens. *N Engl J Med* 1986;315:930.
203. Pike MC, Ross RK. Progestins and menopause: epidemiological studies of risks of endometrial and breast cancer. *Steroids* 2000;65:659.
204. Archer DF. The effect of the duration of progestin use on the occurrence of endometrial cancer in postmenopausal women. *Menopause* 2001;8:245.
205. Ettinger B, Selby J, Citron JT, et al. Cyclic hormone replacement therapy using quarterly progestin. *Obstet Gynecol* 1994;83:693.
206. Prior JC, Vigna YM, Barr SI, et al. Cyclic medroxyprogesterone treatment increases bone density. *Am J Med* 1994;96:521.
207. The Writing Group for the PEPI Trial. Effects of estrogen or estrogen/progestin regimens on heart disease risk factors in postmenopausal women. The Postmenopausal Estrogen/Progestin Interventions (PEPI) trial. *JAMA* 1995;273:199.
208. Davajan V, Kletzky O, Vermesh M, Anderson DJ. Ten-year follow-up of patients with secondary amenorrhea and normal prolactin. *Am J Obstet Gynecol* 1991;164:1666.
209. Falsetti L, Gambera A, Barbetti L, et al. Long-term follow-up of functional hypothalamic amenorrhea and prognostic factors. *J Clin Endocrinol Metab* 2002;87(2):500.
210. Kondoh Y, Uemura T, Murase M, et al. A longitudinal study of disturbances of the hypothalamic-pituitary-adrenal axis in women with progestin-negative functional hypothalamic amenorrhea. *Fertil Steril* 2001;76(4):748.
211. Perkins RB, Hall JE, Martin KA. Aetiology, previous menstrual function and patterns of neuro-endocrine disturbance as prognostic indicators in hypothalamic amenorrhea. *Human Reprod* 2001;16(10):2198.
212. Karnis M, Zimon A, Lalwant S, et al. Risk of death in pregnancy achieved through oocyte donation in patients with Turner syndrome: a national survey. *Fertil Steril* 2003;80:498.
213. Foudila T, Soderstrom-Anttila V, Hovatta O. Turner's syndrome and pregnancies after oocyte donation. *Hum Reprod* 1999;41:532.
214. Khastgir G, Abdalla H, Thomas A, et al. Oocyte donation in Turner's syndrome: an analysis of the factors affecting outcome. *Hum Reprod* 1997;12:279.
215. Hughes E, Collins J, Vandekerckhove P. Clomiphene citrate for ovulation induction in women with oligo-amenorrhea. *Cochrane Database of Systematic Reviews.* 2000(2):CD000056.
216. Kesrouani A, Abdallah MA, Attieh E, et al. Gonadotropin-releasing hormone for infertility in women with primary hypothalamic amenorrhea. Toward a more-interventional approach. *J Reprod Med* 2001;46(1):23.
217. Normann EK, Trystad O, Larsen S, et al. Height reduction in 539 tall girls treated with three different dosages of ethinylestradiol. *Arch Dis Child* 1991;66:1275.
218. Bailey JD, Park E, Cowell C. Estrogen treatment of girls with constitutional tall stature. *Pediatr Clin North Am* 1981;28:501.
219. Werder EA, Waibel P, Sege D, et al. Severe thrombosis during oestrogen treatment for tall stature. *Eur J Pediatr* 1990;149:389.
220. Emans SJ, Grace E, Goldstein DE. Oligomenorrhea in adolescent girls. *J Pediatr* 1980;97:815.

8

Dysfunctional Uterine Bleeding

S. Jean Emans

One of the most common problems reported by adolescents is irregular, profuse menstruation. Rarely, a teenager with her first period might even show a decrease of 10 to 20 percentage points in her hematocrit. More often, a teenager has irregular menses after menarche. Another teen may have had several years of regular cycles but begins to have periods every 2 weeks or prolonged bleeding for 14 to 20 days after 2 to 3 months of amenorrhea. A young adolescent is prone to anovulatory periods with incomplete shedding of a proliferative endometrium; the older adolescent may develop anovulatory cycles with stress or illness. A study of follicle-stimulating hormone (FSH) and luteinizing hormone (LH) patterns in perimenarcheal girls with anovulatory bleeding suggests the prevalence of a maturation defect (1). The higher-than-normal levels of FSH in relation to LH may result in rapid follicular maturation and increased synthesis of estrogen and absence of the midcycle surge of LH. Although dysfunctional uterine bleeding (DUB) may appear to be simply a defect in positive feedback and the lack of establishment of ovulatory cycles, most adolescents in fact are anovulatory during the first years following menarche and yet do not have DUB. The pathophysiology of DUB is not well understood. Adolescents with DUB appear to have delayed maturation of normal negative feedback cyclicity; rising levels of estrogen do not cause a fall in FSH and subsequent suppression of estrogen secretion, and thus the endometrium becomes excessively thickened. In contrast, normal adolescents have an intact negative feedback mechanism that allows for orderly growth of the endometrium and withdrawal flow before the endometrium is excessively thickened. In addition, the occasional ovulatory cycle stabilizes endometrial growth and allows more complete shedding. Adolescents with conditions that cause sustained anovulation may also be likely to present with abnormal uterine bleeding; such problems include eating disorders, weight changes, athletic competition, chronic illnesses, stress, drug abuse, endocrine disorders, and most importantly, polycystic ovary syndrome (PCOS) (see Chapter 9). Interestingly, Apter and Vihko (2) have observed that adolescents with late menarche have longer intervals until cycles become ovulatory than teens with early menarche.

In deciding whether the pattern of the adolescent is normal or abnormal, the clinician needs to be cognizant of normal variations. The adult menstrual cycle is 21 to 35 days, and an adult tends to have the same interval on a month-to-month basis (3). Although adolescents have a similar range of normal cycles, a given adolescent has more variability within this range than does the adult woman. A normal duration of flow is 3 to 7 days; a flow of >8 to 10 days is considered excessive. Normal blood loss is 30 to 40 mL per menstrual period, which usually translates into 10 to 15 soaked tampons or pads per cycle. Unfortunately, self-reported estimation of blood loss by adolescents (and adult women) is inaccurate, unless the flow is very scant (4). Even counting the number of tampons or pads changed in a day cannot give the clinician an assessment of the likelihood of significant bleeding, defined as a blood loss of >80 mL per menstrual period—an amount that would result in iron deficiency anemia. Thus, the hematocrit should be measured in the girl who reports possible abnormal bleeding to determine the extent of blood loss. *Menorrhagia* (also termed *hypermenorrhea*) is defined as prolonged (>7 days) or excessive (>80 mL) uterine bleeding at regular intervals; *metrorrhagia* is uterine bleeding at irregular, frequent intervals. *Menometrorrhagia* is prolonged uterine bleeding occurring at irregular intervals. *Polymenorrhea* is uterine bleeding occurring at regular intervals of <21 days. *Dysfunctional uterine bleeding* connotes excessive, prolonged, unpatterned bleeding from the endometrium *unrelated to structural or systemic disease,* and thus other diagnoses must be excluded. In adults, 90% of cases of DUB are associated with anovulatory cycles, and 10% have a dysfunctional corpus luteum or atrophic endometrium.

The list of diagnoses to be considered in approaching the problem of abnormal vaginal bleeding in the adolescent is long but necessitates the careful consideration and examination of each patient. The differential diagnosis is shown in Table 8-1. Importantly, disorders of pregnancy and the possibility of pelvic infection must be appraised early in the evaluation. Ectopic pregnancy should be a consideration, especially in the adolescent with a previous history of pelvic inflammatory disease (PID) or sexually transmitted diseases (see Chapter 15). Adolescents with PID and endometritis caused by *Neisseria gonorrhoeae* or *Chlamydia trachomatis* frequently present with heavy or irregular bleeding. The possibility of these infections (especially *C. trachomatis*) needs to be considered in the adolescent taking oral contraceptives who develops new intermenstrual bleeding.

Patients with bleeding disorders usually have other signs of bleeding, such as petechiae, ecchymoses, or epistaxis; however, the teenager with von Willebrand disease may not have a prior history of injuries and thus may be diagnosed only because of profuse menstruation starting with her menarche. Acquired von Willebrand disease can occur in girls with systemic lupus erythematosus with the production of anti-von Willebrand factor antibody (5). Likewise, the teenager with chronic thrombocytopenic purpura, or the cardiac patient on warfarin, may have heavy menstrual bleeding. Patients with significant liver disease or those who have undergone liver transplantation may have coagulopathies.

TABLE 8-1. *Differential diagnosis of abnormal vaginal bleeding in the adolescent girl*

Anovulatory uterine bleeding

Pregnancy-related complications
  Threatened abortion
  Spontaneous, incomplete, or missed
    abortion
  Ectopic pregnancy
  Gestational trophoblastic disease
  Complications of termination
    procedures

Infection
  Pelvic inflammatory disease
  Endometritis
  Cervicitis
  Vaginitis

Bleeding disorders
  Thrombocytopenia
    (e.g., idiopathic thrombocytopenic
    purpura, leukemia, aplastic anemia,
    hypersplenism, chemotherapy)
  Clotting disorders
    (e.g., von Willebrand disease, other
    disorders of platelet function, liver
    dysfunction)

Endocrine disorders
  Hypo- or hyperthyroidism
  Adrenal disease
  Hyperprolactinemia
  Polycystic ovary syndrome
  Ovarian failure

Vaginal abnormalities
  Carcinoma or sarcoma
  Laceration

Cervical problems
  Cervicitis
  Polyp
  Hemangioma
  Carcinoma or sarcoma

Uterine problems
  Submucous myoma
  Congenital anomalies
  Polyp
  Carcinoma
  Use of intrauterine device
  Breakthrough bleeding associated with
    hormonal contraceptives
  Ovulation bleeding

Ovarian problems
  Cyst
  Tumor (benign, malignant)

Endometriosis

Trauma

Foreign body (e.g., retained tampon)

Systemic diseases
  Diabetes mellitus
  Renal disease
  Systemic lupus erythematosus

Medications
  Hormonal contraceptives
  Anticoagulants
  Platelet inhibitors
  Androgens
  Spironolactone
  Antipsychotics

Irregular, heavy menstruation may accompany endocrine disorders that are also associated with secondary amenorrhea and anovulation. Adrenal problems such as late-onset 21-hydroxylase deficiency, Cushing syndrome, and Addison disease can cause anovulation; Addison disease may be associated with ovarian failure. Patients with hyperprolactinemia usually have amenorrhea but may have irregular bleeding from anovulation or a shortened luteal phase. In our experience, adolescents with hypothyroidism and hyperthyroidism may have amenorrhea or less frequently polymenorrhea. Similarly, patients with ovarian failure from Turner syndrome, chemotherapy, or radiation therapy may have irregular bleeding before the onset of amenorrhea. The anovulation of PCOS is present early in adolescence; 20% to 30% of patients with PCOS experience DUB. This diagnosis needs to be considered in adolescents with persistent DUB and those who initially have evidence of androgen excess (hirsutism, acne) or acanthosis nigricans, because these girls are at increased risk of endometrial hyperplasia and the early development of endometrial carcinoma (rarely in the teenage years). Thus, long-term therapy with progestins, oral contraceptives, or other combined hormonal preparations needs to be prescribed in these girls.

Uterine abnormalities manifested by irregular bleeding include submucous myomas, polyps, adenomyomas, congenital anomalies, and intrauterine device (IUD) use. Breakthrough or intermenstrual bleeding from combined hormonal methods (oral contraceptives, patches, rings, and injectables) is common, and patients using progestin-only methods frequently have irregular cycles. Congenital anomalies are sometimes detected by the presence of regular, red menstrual bleeding followed by brown or prune-colored spotting intermenstrually; the bloody fluid may have a foul odor if infected by anaerobes. The normal uterus empties in a cyclic pattern, and the obstructed uterus or vagina empties through a fistula slowly over the month (see Chapter 10). The possibility of breakthrough bleeding in the adolescent taking hormonal contraceptives needs to be kept in mind, since the adolescent may have obtained the method confidentially from a clinic and yet be brought to another clinician by her mother for irregular menses. Unless the girl is seen alone and asked specifically about the use of hormonal methods, the diagnosis may not become apparent. An occasional patient may have slight vaginal bleeding for 1 or 2 days at midcycle because of a fall in estrogen levels at ovulation; we have seen this particularly in athletes who do significant running at midcycle. The bleeding may be more apparent to the adolescent who is exercising vigorously that day because of more rapid emptying of the menstrual blood from the vagina. A carefully kept menstrual calendar helps make the diagnosis.

Carcinoma or sarcoma of the vagina is rare among teenagers. Cervical problems may also cause bleeding, especially with trauma or postcoitally. Sexually transmitted infections such as those caused by *Trichomonas* and *C. trachomatis* can be associated with bleeding from a friable cervix. Young women with cystic fibrosis often have a large cervical ectropion with chronic inflammation; the cervix may bleed easily with coitus or when a speculum is inserted. Hemangiomas rarely occur on the cervix and cause bleeding especially with trauma or coitus. Cervical cancer is extraordinarily rare in adolescence. Endometriosis has been associated with irregular menses from anovulation and also with brown spotting in the premenstrual phase of the cycle (see Chapter 11). Ovarian abnormalities, including tumors and cysts, may cause hypermenorrhea (see Chapter 18).

Systemic diseases (see Chapter 23) may interfere with normal cyclicity because of an impact on ovulation, an interference with normal coagulation, or a local endometrial infection such as tuberculosis (a common cause of bleeding in third-world countries but exceedingly rare in the United States). Patients undergoing renal dialysis frequently have either amenorrhea or excessive menstrual flow; the menorrhagia may increase the transfusion requirement of the patient and thus frequently requires ongoing management with progestins, combined hormonal methods, or GnRH agonists.

Trauma may occur because of acute falls, waterskiing injuries, foreign objects introduced for masturbation, or sexual assault. The most common foreign body is a retained tampon, sometimes left in the vagina for weeks to months. The young adolescent may have tried to use a tampon and not realized the need for removal, or she may have put two tampons in the vagina and forgotten to remove one. The bleeding from a retained tampon is usually accompanied by a foul-smelling discharge.

Medications such as anticoagulants and platelet inhibitors can be associated with excessive bleeding. Adolescent athletes taking anabolic steroids may develop masculinization and anovulatory cycles, with irregular bleeding or amenorrhea. Tricyclic antidepressants, antipsychotic medications such as risperidone, and valproate can also cause irregular menses.

Categorizing bleeding as *cyclic* or *acyclic* may help the clinician focus on the appropriate diagnosis. Adolescents with normal cyclic intervals but very heavy bleeding at the time of each cycle are usually normal but may have a bleeding disorder or a uterine problem (submucous myoma or IUD use). In adults with heavy cyclic bleeding (>80 mL/cycle), the plasma concentrations of LH, FSH, and estradiol and the salivary levels of progesterone are not different from those in women with normal blood loss (6).

An adolescent with normal cycles but superimposed abnormal bleeding at any time throughout the cycle may have a foreign body within the vagina, infection (such as *C. trachomatis* or *N. gonorrhoeae*), uterine polyp, vaginal malignancy, congenital malformation of the uterus with obstruction, cervical abnormality, or endometriosis. Adolescents with no cyclicity apparent, or cycles of <21 days or >40 to 45 days, usually have anovulatory DUB with lack of normal negative feedback. Disorders associated with anovulation include psychosocial problems, eating disorders, athletic competition, PCOS, premature ovarian failure, ovarian tumors, and endocrinopathies.

Several series published in the past 15 years have evaluated adolescents requiring hospitalization for treatment of menorrhagia. The conclusions have varied among studies. In a study of 59 patients hospitalized from 1971 to 1980, Claessens and Cowell (7,8) reported a primary coagulation disorder in 20% of girls: one-fourth of those with hemoglobin <10 g/dL, one-third of those requiring transfusion, and one-half of those presenting at menarche. The diagnoses included idiopathic thrombocytopenia (ITP) (four), von Willebrand disease (three), Glanzmann disease (two), thalassemia major (one), and Fanconi syndrome (one); seven patients had other conditions, and 34% were treated with dilatation and curettage (D&C). A study published in 1994 by Falcone and colleagues (9) reported 61 patients hospitalized between 1981 and 1991. Only 3% had newly diagnosed coagulation disorders: ITP (one), acute promyelocytic leukemia (one). However, 28% had past histories of significant medical problems, including leukemia, ITP, Glanzmann disease, hypothyroidism, mental retardation, and rheumatoid arthritis; 50% had a history of irregular menses (defined as <25 or >35 days apart). The mean hemoglobin was 8.9 g/dL, and 41% required blood transfusions. In contrast to the earlier series, 93% responded to medical management, and only 8% underwent D&C. They reported no difference in the response of patients treated with intravenous conjugated estrogens (Premarin) versus oral estrogen/progestin combinations in the initial hemoglobin, percentage of patients transfused, or days in the hospital (the patients were not randomized). In a study of 71 patients 10 to 19 years old seen for inpatient or outpatient evaluation of menorrhagia at a children's hospital from 1990 to 1998, Bevan and colleagues reported that 9 (13%) has thrombocytopenia (5 ITP, 2 secondary to chemotherapy) and 8 had hereditary coagulation disorders (2 with von Willebrand) (10). One-half had hemoglobin <12 g/dL, and 7 girls in their series had hemoglobin <5.0 g/dL. In contrast, studies of adult women with menorrhagia have found that von Willebrand disease is frequently diagnosed, particularly in white women (11). In our experience at Children's Hospital Boston, most adolescents with severe menorrhagia respond well to oral hormonal therapy, and surgical intervention is very rarely needed. Importantly, those with known coagulopathies and scheduled procedures such as bone marrow transplantation should be managed expectantly.

PATIENT ASSESSMENT

The history, physical examination, and initial laboratory tests are crucial in determining the likely diagnoses as well as the urgency for immediate treatment. Questions should focus on date of menarche; menstrual pattern; duration, quantity, and color of the flow; and the presence of dysmenorrhea. The dates of the last menstrual period and the previous menstrual period should be recorded. A menstrual calendar is invaluable. Information about the use of tampons, condoms, or other foreign objects should be elicited. The patient should be asked whether she is sexually active (realizing that the history must be taken confidentially and the answers may not always be honest), whether the bleeding was postcoital, and whether she is using a hormonal method or an IUD. The patient should also be queried about previous sexually transmitted diseases and recent exposure to a new partner or a partner with urethritis or other infection. A general review of systems, including recent stresses, weight changes, eating disorders, athletic competition, chronic diseases, bleeding disorders, medications, illicit drugs, syncope, visual changes, headaches, gastrointestinal symptoms, acne, hirsutism, and acanthosis nigricans, and a family history of PCOS and bleeding disorders, is essential.

The physical examination should include a general assessment with attention to the height, weight, body type, and fat distribution (to detect Cushing syndrome or Turner syndrome), blood pressure (standing and lying), evidence of androgen excess (acne, hirsutism, clitoromegaly), acanthosis nigricans, thyroid palpation, breast examination to detect galactorrhea, other signs of bleeding such as petechiae or bruises, and if possible, a pelvic examination. In most virginal adolescents (particularly those who have used tampons) and all sexually active adolescents, a one-finger digital examination can be done initially to check for foreign bodies within the vagina and to palpate the cervix. A speculum appropriate for the size of the hymenal opening can then be chosen, usually a Huffman speculum in the virginal patient and a Pederson speculum for the sexually active adolescent. Generally, a virginal patient who has used tampons can cooperate fully if the need for the examination is carefully explained and the examiner obtains her help. Sometimes the application of a small amount of lubricating jelly or lidocaine jelly to the introitus can aid in the insertion of the speculum. In some girls who have never used tampons, the opening is too small to allow a digital or a speculum examination. In these cases, a rectoabdominal examination is an alternative, if acceptable. Sometimes only an external examination can be accomplished, and then ultrasonography of the pelvis can be obtained to exclude an ovarian cyst or other abnormality. Clearly, many adolescents in the early months after menarche may have several closely spaced menses and then revert to a normal pattern, and they can be simply observed without a full pelvic examination. However, a girl with continuous spotting, cyclic bleeding with superimposed bleeding throughout the cycle, bleeding sufficient to cause anemia, or persistent DUB deserves a gynecologic assessment.

During the speculum examination, tests should be obtained for *N. gonorrhoeae* and *C. trachomatis* in any patient who gives a history of being sexually active and in any patient whom the clinician suspects may have had intercourse. In the absence of bleeding at the time of the examination, wet preps are done and a Papanicolaou smear (see Chapter 17 for indications) can also be obtained. A bimanual examination should be done to assess tenderness and enlargement of the uterus and adnexal pain and masses. A soft mass along the anterior-lateral vaginal wall may possibly be an obstruction of the genital tract (see Chapter 10).

Laboratory tests should include a sensitive urine pregnancy test and a complete blood cell count (CBC) with differential and estimate of platelet count. In girls who give an impressive history of bleeding and yet have a normal or only slightly depressed hemoglobin, a reticulocyte count is helpful in assessing the amount of bleeding. In addition, the concentration of hemoglobin in the reticulocyte (CHr) can provide a sensitive indicator of iron sufficiency or deficiency (12,13). An erythrocyte sedimentation rate (ESR) is useful if pelvic infection is a consideration. Coagulation studies (e.g., prothrombin time, partial thromboplastin time, von Willebrand panel) and platelet count are indicated in patients with heavy cyclic bleeding from menarche and those with a significant drop in hemoglobin or a hemoglobin <10 g/dL at presentation. Of importance, the von Willebrand panel should be drawn when the patient is not taking hormones, because the estrogen may elevate the von Willebrand factor into the normal range. Thus the test should be obtained at initial presentation or after the patient has been off hormones for a week (at the end of the pill-free week). It is also important to obtain blood group typing (blood group O is associated with lower von Willebrand levels) and to consult with a hematologist if the levels are low to assure correct interpretation and desmopressin (DDAVP) challenge testing. Blood cross-matching should be done for girls with acute hemorrhage or low hemoglobin when transfusion may be necessary.

Other tests depend on the physical examination and the length of the history of the DUB. The most common additional laboratory test is TSH determination to screen for hypo- or hyperthyroidism. Other potential studies for patients with a long history of DUB include determination of FSH (and LH), prolactin, and serum androgens [total and free testosterone, dehydroepiandrosterone sulfate (DHEAS)], especially in those with hirsutism or acne. Screening tests for diabetes should be individualized. If needed, a progesterone level obtained during the presumed luteal phase of the cycle can aid in the evaluation of ovulatory versus anovulatory menses. Ultrasonography can be helpful when a pelvic mass is felt, a uterine anomaly is suspected, or bimanual examination cannot be accomplished in an adolescent with significant bleeding. If a uterine anomaly is detected, magnetic resonance imaging can help define the anatomy further. A submucous myoma or an endometrial polyp, both rare in adolescents, may require further evaluation with sonohysterogram, hysterosalpingogram, and/or hysteroscopy.

TREATMENT

The goals of the assessment are to determine which adolescent needs medical treatment and which adolescent can be observed in the hope that further maturation of the hypothalamic–pituitary–ovarian axis will result in normal cycles. The objective of hormonal treatment is to give estrogens to heal the endometrial bleeding sites by causing further endometrial proliferation and to give progestins to induce endometrial stability. The evaluation and treatment plan should aim at stopping bleeding; preventing a recurrence; identifying underlying organic disease if present; diagnosing any psychosocial pathology causing and/or exacerbating any menstrual disorders; preventing the progression of acne, hirsutism, and obesity, which can be caused by hormonal imbalances such as PCOS; and preventing long-term pathologic sequelae. Thus, long-term follow-up is essential.

Although opinions clearly vary about the best mode of therapy, various hormonal regimens have been successful (7–10,14–19); most clinicians use monophasic oral contraceptive pills with potent progestin, given cyclically or continuously, to gain control over the irregular menses. Some conditions, such as bone marrow transplantation for malignancies, may be better addressed with prophylactic gonadotropin-releasing hormone (GnRH) agonists (e.g., depot leuprolide) to suppress menses before a problem develops (20–22) (See Chapter 23). Because of the agonist phase of depot leuprolide, it is important to give the first injection (22.5 mg of the 3-month formulation) at least 1 month before the expected bone marrow transplant. Although continuous oral contraceptives have also been used to treat menstrual bleeding in bone marrow transplantation, case reports have indicated that hyperbilirubinemia may be associated with the use of high dose pills (23). Girls with conditions such as von Willebrand disease can be treated with oral contraceptives and/or DDAVP. Girls with bleeding disorders associated with warfarin (e.g., for cardiac conditions) are usually successfully managed with oral contraceptives (patch or ring) cyclically or continuously. However, occasionally because of poor response and a transfusion requirement, depot leuprolide (11.25 mg) is needed every three months with daily add-back therapy prescribed once bleeding is under control; the estrogen/progestin (conjugated estrogens 0.625 mg/medroxyprogesterone 2.5 mg) or norethindrone acetate (5 mg) is given to prevent bone loss with long-term GnRH agonist therapy. In healthy sexually active, monogamous women, the levonorgestrel-releasing intrauterine system (Mirena) is another option for reducing blood loss with heavy menses (24). A few centers have managed heavy menses in patients with severe cognitive challenges and marked difficulty handling menstrual hygiene with hysterectomy or more recently endometrial ablation (25) (with a court order), but erratic bleeding may still occur with the latter.

The following classification and treatment schedules have been helpful in our clinical practices.

Mild Dysfunctional Bleeding

Mild DUB is defined as menses that are longer than normal or in which the cycle is shortened for ≥2 months. The flow is slightly to moderately increased; hemoglobin level is normal. Observation and reassurance are usually adequate. The patient should be encouraged to keep a menstrual calendar so that the need for intervention in the future can be assessed. Iron supplements will help prevent anemia (especially if dietary intake is borderline). Antiprostaglandin medications, such as ibuprofen, naproxen sodium, or mefenamic acid, taken during menstruation have been reported to reduce blood loss in patients with menorrhagia (18).

Moderate Dysfunctional Bleeding

Moderate DUB is defined as menses that are moderately prolonged, or the cycle remains shortened with frequent menses (every 1 to 3 weeks). The flow is moderate to heavy, and hemoglobin level often shows mild anemia. Treatment consists of oral contraceptive pills, oral medroxyprogesterone, or other progestin. Combined oral contraceptive pills are more effective at stopping dysfunctional bleeding that is in progress than medroxyprogesterone. However, if the patient is not bleeding at the time of the visit, the patient or parent dislikes the use of birth control pills, the patient is not sexually active, or there is a medical contraindication to the use of estrogen, medroxyprogesterone can be tried as initial therapy.

For patients with heavy or prolonged dysfunctional bleeding, the initial use of an oral contraceptive with a potent progestin is preferable to progestin-only methods. Although a number of 30- to 35-μg oral contraceptives have been used for this purpose, our program has had the most clinical experience with oral contraceptives

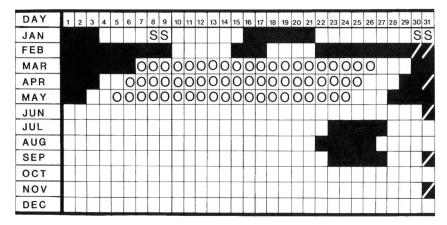

FIG. 8-1. A 14-year-old girl arrives at the emergency ward with profuse vaginal bleeding that followed markedly irregular cycles for the previous 3 months. The results of pelvic examination and clotting studies are normal; hematocrit is 28%. She is given 0.3 mg norgestrel/30 μg ethinyl estradiol three times a day; bleeding ceases the following day. Her dose is decreased to twice a day for the remainder of the cycle; she continues on cyclic pills, one a day, for an additional 2 months. *S,* spotting; *O,* oral contraceptive pill; *solid bars,* bleeding. On the normal menstrual calendar, the months without 30 or 31 days have *slashed bars.*

containing norgestrel (0.3 mg) or levonorgestrel (0.15 mg) (e.g., Lo/Ovral*, Nordette, Levlen). Norgestrel 0.3 mg has essentially the same potency as 0.15 mg of levonorgestrel, the active isomer of norgestrel. For example, for mild bleeding and minimal anemia, the patient can be told to take one tablet of 0.3 mg norgestrel (0.15 mg levonorgestrel)/30 μg ethinyl estradiol (EE) once a day for 21 days. If the bleeding is more significant or there is anemia, the norgestrel/EE can be prescribed twice a day for 3 or 4 days until the bleeding stops and then one a day to finish a 21-day cycle. If bleeding starts again as soon as the dose is decreased from one pill twice a day to one pill once a day, then the dose of twice a day may need to be maintained to complete the 21 day cycle (Fig. 8-1). Other monophasic oral contraceptives containing norethindrone (at least 1.0 mg), desogestrel, and norgestimate have also been used successfully in some patients, given once or twice a day for 21 days. The clinician needs to keep in contact with the patient, since hormonal therapy can cause nausea and noncompliance, and adequate doses must be prescribed to prevent further bleeding. Cyclic pills are typically used in these patients unless there is significant anemia or a bleeding disorder.

The urgency of gaining control of the cycle is related to the amount of bleeding and the hematocrit; thus, in some adolescents with heavy bleeding and anemia, starting with 0.3 mg norgestrel (0.15 mg levonorgestrel)/30 μg ethinyl estradiol four times a day may be necessary to stop bleeding within 24 to 36 hours. A useful

*Brand names are used as examples and do not imply endorsement of a particular product.

regimen is: one pill four times a day for 2 to 4 days, then three times a day for 3 days, then twice a day for 2 weeks. With these doses of estrogen, antiemetics such as meclizine, 25 mg, or chlorpromazine, 5 to 10 mg, may help to prevent nausea if taken by the patient 2 hours before each dose of oral contraceptive (OC). Norethindrone acetate 5 mg may also be used similarly if estrogen is contraindicated. Very occasionally, patients experience excessive nausea with oral contraceptives in spite of using antiemetics; in these cases, the 21-day course of hormone can be shortened to 10 days, and medroxyprogesterone or norethindrone acetate can be given on a cyclic basis. Failure to control bleeding with any of the above regimens should make the clinician consider a diagnosis other than anovulatory uterine bleeding.

A normal withdrawal flow will follow 2 to 4 days after the last hormone tablet has been taken. The oral contraceptive is discontinued for 7 days unless the withdrawal flow is abnormally heavy, in which case the pill-free interval can be shortened to 4 to 5 days. For significant bleeding, the patient usually continues to take oral contraceptives for 3 to 6 months. If a 50-μg EE pill or a twice-daily pill was used for the first cycle, the patient is usually given a lower dose 30- to 35-μg EE OC once a day for the next few cycles. The patient should receive careful instructions on 21-day versus 28-day pills; otherwise, confusion may result, and placebos may be used on hormone days or a 7-day withdrawal time may not be observed. Oral contraceptives should be continued if birth control is needed. Otherwise, the patient can switch to cyclic medroxyprogesterone for an additional 3 to 6 months. A course of oral iron plus folic acid (1 mg daily) should also be prescribed to correct anemia.

As noted above, if oral contraceptives are contraindicated, or the patient or family does not wish the use of oral contraceptives, medroxyprogesterone is an option although less effective. For short-term treatment of mild DUB, medroxyprogesterone 10 mg can be given once a day for 10 to 12 days; for adolescents who require ongoing therapy for persistent DUB (especially associated with PCOS), it is preferable to give 12 to 14 days of progestin each month.

The oral medroxyprogesterone can be prescribed according to the calendar month *or* in cycles based on the first day of menstrual bleeding. If the calendar month is used, the patient is given medroxyprogesterone 10 mg once a day for the first 10 to 14 days of each month; this dosing schedule is simple for most patients to follow. However, some patients begin bleeding before the next dose is to be taken and may then need a start date based on menstrual bleeding or may need to use an oral contraceptive instead. In using the menstrual cycle system, the patient is instructed to start the medroxyprogesterone 10 mg on the 14th day of the menstrual cycle (day 1 is the first day of the last period) or at the time of the visit. After the patient has a withdrawal flow, she starts medroxyprogesterone on day 14 again (Fig. 8-2). The pattern is continued for 3 to 6 months. If the patient starts bleeding even before she gets to day 14 of her cycle, then starting the medroxyprogesterone on day 10 or day 12 of the cycle for several cycles and extending the medroxyprogesterone to 14 days, or preferably switching to an oral contraceptive, will give better control of the cycle. Oral norethindrone acetate

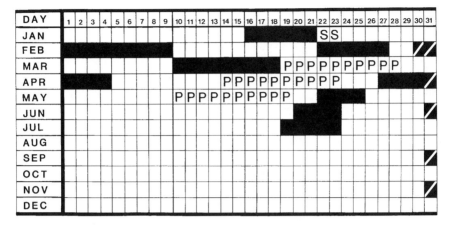

FIG. 8-2. A 14-year-old girl comes to the clinic on March 19 with a history of frequent periods (every 17-22 days). She is not bleeding at the time of her visit. The results of examination and laboratory studies are normal. She is treated with oral medroxyprogesterone, 10 mg daily for 10 days and then for 10 days from the 14th to the 23rd day of the two subsequent cycles. Her menses return to normal in June and July. *S,* spotting; *P,* medroxyprogesterone; *solid bars,* bleeding. On the normal menstrual calendar, the months without 30 or 31 days have *slashed bars.*

(Aygestin), 5 to 10 mg daily for 10 to 14 days, can be given instead of medroxyprogesterone, with 10 to 12 days acceptable for short-term use, and 12 to 14 days preferred for long-term use. Norethindrone acetate may be successful when the cycles have not been regulated successfully with medroxyprogesterone.

Severe Dysfunctional Bleeding

Severe dysfunctional bleeding is defined as bleeding that is prolonged, with normal menstrual cycles disrupted. The flow is very heavy, and the hemoglobin level is reduced, often to <9 g/dL. Clinical signs of blood loss may be present. The patient should be admitted to the hospital if initial hemoglobin is <7 g/dL, or if orthostatic signs are present, or if bleeding is heavy and hemoglobin is <10 g/dL. Clotting studies should be obtained. If the hemoglobin is 8 to 10 g/dL and the patient and family are reliable and can maintain close telephone contact, the patient can be treated at home and monitored daily until bleeding ceases. For most patients with severe bleeding, hospitalization is necessary.

An effective treatment is an oral contraceptive with norgestrel or levonorgestrel (see above) with 30 or 50 μg ethinyl estradiol every 4 hours until bleeding slows or stops (usually 4 to 8 tablets), then every 6 hours for 24 hours, every 8 hours for 48 hours, and then twice a day to complete a 21-day course of hormones. Alternatively, the same dose can be started every 4 hours until bleeding is controlled and then can be tapered to one tablet four times a day for 2 to 4 days, three times a day for 3 days, and twice a day for 2 weeks; this schedule may be especially easy for emergency medicine personnel to administer. Other monophasic oral contraceptives have been used in similar doses, although the clinical experience has not been as vast. In acute severe hemorrhage, some physicians use conjugated estrogens (Premarin), 25 mg IV every 4 hours for two to three doses, whereas others use only combined oral contraceptives because of concern about possible thromboembolism and questionable efficacy of intravenous estrogens (19). We have generally used intravenous conjugated estrogens only when the patient may not be given anything by mouth or is unstable and may require critical care measures. Intravenous estrogen appears to increase clotting at the capillary level. If intravenous estrogen is used, oral contraceptives must be started within 24 to 48 hours to provide a progestin to stabilize the endometrium. Antiemetics are usually needed with any of the high-dose estrogen therapies. Transfusion needs are individualized on the basis of hemoglobin, blood loss, orthostatic symptoms, and the ability to rapidly gain control of the bleeding.

If there is a contraindication to the use of estrogen, a trial of progestin such as norethindrone acetate, 5 to 10 mg, or medroxyprogesterone, 10 mg, can be given every 4 hours and then tapered to the regimen of four times a day for 4 days, three times a day for 3 days, and then twice a day for 2 weeks. Norethindrone acetate appears to be more effective than medroxyprogesterone.

Rarely, only very high doses of progestin (medroxyprogesterone, 40 to 80 mg per day; megestrol acetate, 80 mg twice a day; or depot medroxyprogesterone acetate (Depo-Provera), 100 mg intramuscular daily for up to a week and then weekly to monthly) are effective to cause endometrial atrophy. Breakthrough bleeding can be avoided by using a several-day course of estrogen (conjugated estrogens, 2.5 mg for 5 to 7 days, or a transdermal estradiol patch). Patients may become cushingoid with these high doses of progestin, and injections are usually avoided, if possible, in patients with bleeding disorders. More recently, long-acting GnRH analogs have provided another option. Because of the initial agonist phase and bleeding that can be expected at 2 to 3 weeks, planning is important in advance of a girl becoming thrombocytopenic with bone marrow transplantation (see p. 278 and Chapter 23).

If the various regimens of hormones fail to control bleeding within 24 to 36 hours in an ill patient, the possibility of pelvic pathology should be excluded by ultrasound, anesthesia examination, and D&C. Dilatation and curettage may be needed earlier to treat a patient who cannot be given estrogen. Although this procedure can be both diagnostic and curative, the overwhelming majority of adolescents can be treated successfully with hormones alone. In addition, the adolescent with a long history of anovulation still needs follow-up care to prevent a recurrence of heavy bleeding.

In patients with significant anemia, the placebo (off-pill) interval should be avoided, and the oral contraceptive given continuously until the hematocrit returns toward normal. Once the hematocrit has increased, the patient can be cycled for

3 to 6 months (or longer) with an oral contraceptive. If necessary, the pill-free interval can be shortened to 4 to 5 days. Iron and folic acid therapy should be given along with hormone therapy as soon as the situation has stabilized (1 to 2 days).

FOLLOW-UP

Patients with a long history of anovulatory cycles and dysfunctional uterine bleeding, especially those with PCOS, have an increased risk of later infertility and endometrial carcinoma (26). Thus, regular withdrawal with progestins (such as medroxyprogesterone, 12 to 14 days per month) or oral contraceptives is needed on a long-term basis in these high-risk girls. Careful follow-up is essential.

Case 1

O. N., 15 years old, was evaluated for irregular frequent menses every 14 to 62 days. She was first seen in the clinic at the age of $13\frac{2}{12}$ because of short stature. Breast and pubic hair development had begun when she was 11, and her menarche occurred when she was $12\frac{11}{12}$. Her father was 5 ft 11 in., and her mother was 5 ft 3 in. At the initial evaluation, she had a height of 135 cm and a weight of 37 kg (Fig. 8-3). She had Tanner stage 3 to 4 breast development and Tanner stage 4 pubic hair development. Her external genitalia were normal and estrogenized. Her bone age was 12 years. Because of the short stature, she had determinations of FSH (92.8 mIU/mL and 53.8 mIU/mL), thyroid function tests (normal results), and karyotype: 46,X,i(Xq). Despite her elevated gonadotropins, her ovaries appeared normal on ultrasound, and a 1-cm follicle was evident. She was treated with growth hormone until she had reached a bone age of $14\frac{1}{2}$ years. Her menses were irregular the first year of treatment, and then she began to have frequent menses every 16 to 20 days. She was initially treated with medroxyprogesterone, which did not result in normal cycles, and was then given norethindrone acetate 5 mg for 14 days each calendar month. She was subsequently prescribed oral contraceptives at age 16 to provide menstrual regulation, estrogen replacement, and contraception.

Case 2

A. J., 17 years old, presented for evaluation of heavy bleeding and pain. Her menarche had occurred when she was 13, and she had always had regular menses lasting 4 to 6 days, with mild dysmenorrhea. Her last menstrual period had begun 7 days before, and instead of decreasing by the sixth day, the flow had increased and was accompanied by moderately severe cramps. She denied ever having been sexually active. Physical examination showed her to be afebrile and cooperative.

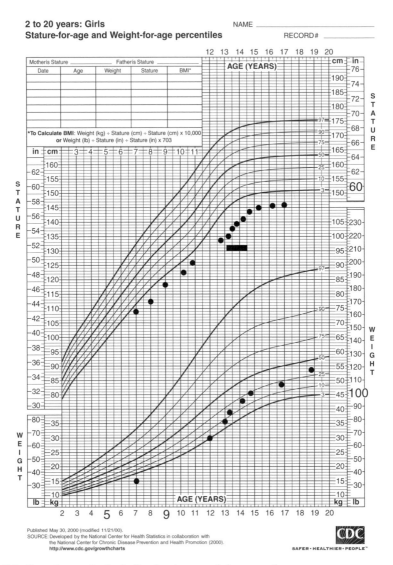

2 to 20 years: Girls
Stature-for-age and Weight-for-age percentiles

NAME _____

RECORD# _____

Published May 30, 2000 (modified 11/21/00).
SOURCE: Developed by the National Center for Health Statistics in collaboration with
the National Center for Chronic Disease Prevention and Health Promotion (2000).
http://www.cdc.gov/growthcharts

FIG. 8-3. Case 1: growth chart. *Bar* denotes growth hormone therapy.

Abdominal examination showed bilateral lower abdominal tenderness; pelvic examination showed a 2-cm hymenal opening, moderate vaginal bleeding, and cervical motion and adnexal tenderness. Samples were taken from the endocervix for *C. trachomatis* and *N. gonorrhoeae* tests. Urine human chorionic gonadotropin (HCG) was negative. Since the clinical impression was PID in spite of a negative history of sexual activity, a CBC and sedimentation rate were obtained, and the patient was treated for PID. In 2 days, she was markedly improved. Initial laboratory tests showed a hematocrit of 36%, white blood cell count (WBC) of 13,600/mm^3, and a sedimentation rate of 26 mm per hour. Endocervical tests were positive for both *N. gonorrhoeae* and *C. trachomatis*. The patient finally admitted to having been sexually active, and her boyfriend was also treated. Oral contraceptives were prescribed for birth control. Even if a patient initially denies sexual activity, the clinician seeing adolescents needs to consider the possibility of PID in the evaluation of pelvic or abdominal pain or irregular bleeding.

Case 3

N. T., 19 years old, presented with a complaint of irregular menses and abdominal pain. Her menarche was at age 13 years, and she had a long history of irregular menses occurring every 3 to 8 weeks. She had previously been treated with oral contraceptives for dysfunctional uterine bleeding and had discontinued her pills 2 months prior to the appointment. Her last menstrual period had started 5 days before the visit, and she had experienced increasing bleeding and cramps. Her previous menstrual period had been 6 weeks earlier. Physical examination revealed bilateral lower abdominal tenderness and rebound. Pelvic examination revealed moderate bleeding and cervical motion and adnexal tenderness. Cultures were taken from the endocervix for *N. gonorrhoeae* and *C. trachomatis*. The result of urine HCG was positive, and quantitative HCG was 340 mIU/mL. Hematocrit was 35%, WBC 9000/mm^3, and sedimentation rate 36 mm/hr. The repeat HCG was unchanged, and the *Chlamydia* culture was positive. Laparoscopy revealed PID and an ectopic pregnancy. These two diagnoses are important considerations for the clinician seeing adolescents with vaginal bleeding.

Case 4

P H., a 13-year-old asthmatic, was brought to the emergency ward because of a 1-week history of vomiting and headache and a 1-day history of bizarre behavior and hallucinations. She had been taking theophylline for many years, and the initial impression was that she might have taken a drug overdose. Her menarche had occurred at the age of 11, and she had had regular menses until 16 days before the visit, when heavy bleeding had begun. Physical examination showed pallor, disorientation, and heavy vaginal bleeding. The hymenal opening was small, and bimanual examination showed a normal uterus and adnexa. The hematocrit was 8.5%, WBC 6,000/mm^3, and platelet count 14,000/mm^3. She was transfused with 6 units of blood, given 25 mg of conjugated estrogens intravenously, and given oral contraceptive therapy every 4 hours. After the bleeding had slowed, the oral contraceptives were tapered to one tablet every 6 hours for 2 days, then every 8 hours for 2 days, then twice daily for 2½ months as maintenance until her platelet count was sufficient to allow menstrual flow. Bone marrow evaluation showed aplastic anemia. After her platelet count improved, her medication was switched to cyclic oral contraceptives.

REFERENCES

1. Ansel S, Jones G. Etiology and treatment of dysfunctional uterine bleeding. *Obstet Gynecol* 1974;44:1.
2. Apter D, Vihko R. Early menarche, a risk factor for breast cancer, indicated early onset of ovulatory cycles. *J Clin Endocrinol Metab* 1983;57:82.
3. Treloar AE, Boynton RE, Behn BG, et al. Variation of the human menstrual cycle through reproductive life. *Int J Fertil* 1967;12:77.
4. Fraser IS, McCarron G, Markham R. A preliminary study of factors influencing perception of menstrual blood loss volume. *Am J Obstet Gynecol* 1984;149:788.
5. Soff GA, Green D. Autoantibody to von Willebrand factor in systemic lupus erythematosus. *J Lab Clin Med* 1993;121:424.
6. Eldred JM, Thomas EJ. Pituitary and ovarian hormone levels in unexplained menorrhagia. *Obstet Gynecol* 1994;84:774.
7. Claessens EA, Cowell CA. Acute adolescent menorrhagia. *Am J Obstet Gynecol* 1981;139:277.
8. Claessens EA, Cowell CA. Dysfunctional uterine bleeding in the adolescent. *Pediatr Clin North Am* 1981;28:369.
9. Falcone T, Desjardins C, Bourque J, et al. Dysfunctional uterine bleeding in adolescent. *J Reprod Med* 1994;39:761.
10. Bevan JA, Maloney KW, Hillery CA, et al. Bleeding disorders: a common cause of menorrhagia in adolescents. *J Pediatr* 2001;138:856.
11. Dilley A, Drews C, Miller C, et al. von Willebrand disease and other inherited bleeding disorders in women with diagnosed menorrhagia. *Obstet Gynecol* 2001;97:630.
12. Stoffman N, Brugnara C, Woods ER. Use of reticulocyte hemoglobin content measurement in screening for iron deficiency. Society for Adolescent Medicine, Seattle, WA, March 21, 2003.
13. Brugnara C, Zurakowski D, DiCanzio J, et al. Reticulocyte hemoglobin content to diagnose iron deficiency in children. *JAMA* 1999;281:2225.
14. Bayer SR, DeCherney AH. Clinical manifestations and treatment of dysfunctional uterine bleeding. *JAMA* 1993;269:1823.
15. Hillard PA. Abnormal uterine bleeding in adolescents. *Contemp Pediatr* 1995;12:79.
16. Athen PI, Henderson MC, Witz CA. Abnormal uterine bleeding. *Med Clin North Am* 1995;79:329.
17. Cowan BD, Morrison JC. Management of abnormal genital bleeding in girls and women. *N Engl J Med* 1991;324:1710.
18. Fraser IS, Pearse C, Shearman RP, et al. Efficacy of mefenamic acid in patients with a complaint of menorrhagia. *Obstet Gynecol* 1981;58:543.
19. Devore GR, Owens O, Kase N. Use of intravenous Premarin in the treatment of dysfunctional uterine bleeding—a double-blind randomized control study. *Obstet Gynecol* 1982;59:285.
20. Laufer MR, Rein MS. Treatment of abnormal uterine bleeding with gonadotropin-releasing hormone analogues. *Clin Obstet Gynecol* 1993;36:668.
21. Laufer MR, Townsend NL, Parsons KE, et al. The use of leuprolide acetate for the induction of amenorrhea in women undergoing bone marrow transplantation (BMT): a pilot study. *J Reprod Med* 1997;42:537.
22. Ghalie R, Porter C, Radwanska E, et al. Prevention of hypermenorrhea with leuprolide in premenopausal women undergoing bone marrow transplantation. *Am J Hematol* 1993;42:350.
23. Kline RM, Fennewald L, Vore M, et al. Oral contraceptives: a cause of hyperbilirubinemia in stem cell transplant patients [Comment]. *J Pediatr Hematol Oncol* 1999;21:436.
24. Hidalgo M, Bahamondes L, Perrotti M. Bleeding patterns and clinical performance of the levonorgestrel-releasing intrauterine system (Mirena) up to 2 years. *Contraception* 2002;65:129.
25. Wingfield M, McClure N, Mamers PM, et al. Endometrial ablation: an option for the management of menstrual problems in the intellectually disabled. *Med J Aust* 1994;160:533.
26. Southam AL, Richart RM. The prognosis for adolescents with menstrual abnormalities. *Am J Obstet Gynecol* 1966;94:637.

9

Androgen Abnormalities in the Adolescent Girl

S. Jean Emans

Signs of androgen excess, especially hirsutism and acne, can be troubling problems for the adolescent girl. Oligomenorrhea or anovulatory dysfunctional uterine bleeding accompanying the signs of androgen excess should especially alert the clinician to the possibility of polycystic ovary syndrome (PCOS). Although the degree of hirsutism may be related to familial, racial, or ethnic factors that determine the capacity of the hair follicle to respond to androgens, in most cases excess androgen production from the ovaries and/or adrenal glands is responsible for the clinical problem of hirsutism. Whatever the cause of the hirsutism, the patient will benefit from a careful explanation of the etiology, diagnosis, and therapy, since acne and hirsutism may have a negative impact on the self-image of the maturing adolescent.

POLYCYSTIC OVARY SYNDROME

Polycystic ovary syndrome (PCOS), sometimes termed *functional ovarian hyperandrogenism*, is found in 4% to 6% of adolescent girls and young women and is the leading cause of oligomenorrhea, hirsutism, and infertility. PCOS is the most common endocrinopathy in premenopausal women, and yet the clinical criteria, the pathophysiology, and the treatment are still debated. At an NIH consensus conference, experts identified the key features needed to diagnose PCOS. Of the 58 experts who responded, definite or probable criteria included hyperandrogenism (64%), menstrual dysfunction (52%), clinical hyperandrogenism (48%), and exclusion of congenital adrenal hyperplasia (CAH) (59%). Possible criteria included insulin resistance (IR) (69%), perimenarcheal onset (62%), elevated luteinizing hormone (LH)/follicle-stimulating hormone (FSH) ratio (55%) and PCOS by sonography (52%) (1). Menstrual irregularity (oligoovulation) and hyperandrogenism (clinical or biochemical) were thus early defined as the key features of PCOS. Over the past decade, hyperandrogenism has remained a key criterion for diagnosis with recognition that some women may be ovulatory and that ultrasound criteria may have assumed more importance in the diagnosis than previously (see p. 295) (2).

Of importance to those caring for adolescents, PCOS begins in the perimenarcheal period. PCOS has been characterized as an abnormal and exaggerated transition to puberty in four key physiological processes:

1. The increase in LH secretion
2. The increase in adrenal androgen production
3. The increase in body mass
4. The onset of adult patterns of insulin resistance (IR).

The contribution of each of these processes is subject to debate (3). Even before puberty, however, an early sign of PCOS may be the appearance of early pubic hair (premature pubarche) and IR (4–7). Some normal girls pass through a hyperandrogenic phase in the first 3 years after menarche and yet have ovulatory cycles 5 years later; however, other girls with hyperandrogenism noted in early puberty will persist with classic PCOS (8,9). Making this distinction can sometimes be challenging, and the clinician needs to follow these girls closely throughout adolescence. PCOS has lifelong implications of increased risk of diabetes mellitus, obesity, insulin resistance, infertility, and impaired quality of life (Fig. 9-1).

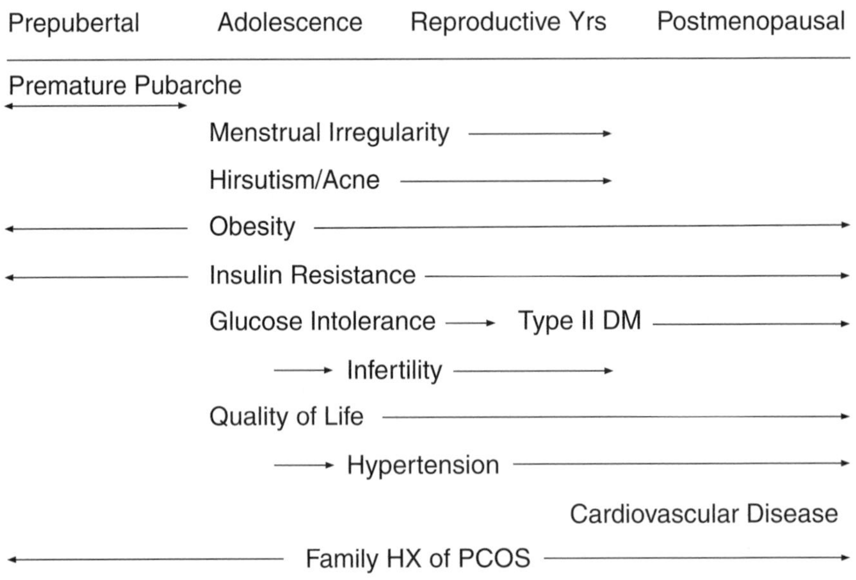

FIG. 9-1. PCOS over the lifespan.

Polycystic ovary syndrome is a spectrum of clinical disorders associated with increased androgen production from the ovaries and frequently the adrenal glands as well, often with abnormal gonadotropin secretion and insulin resistance. Clinical presentations vary and include hirsutism, acne, obesity, oligomenorrhea, dysfunctional uterine bleeding, and infertility. Adolescents with PCOS usually have a normal age of menarche, although occasionally menarche may be delayed and associated with hirsutism or virilization. Most adolescents with PCOS are overweight for height. The majority of patients have irregular menses from the time of menarche; in addition, they often have hirsutism and/or acne beginning either before or around the time of menarche. The abnormal gonadotropin secretory patterns seen in many, but not all, patients with PCOS are also apparent very early in adolescence (10,11). There is exaggerated pulsatile release of LH with increased pulse frequency and amplitude (12), which may be a primary defect or secondary to the hormonal milieu from ovarian enzyme dysregulation (11). The LH levels are often tonically elevated, and the LH/FSH ratio may be elevated. The high LH levels stimulate the ovary to secrete increased amounts of androgen from the stromal tissue; the androgens are converted peripherally to estrone and estradiol. Estrogens, which are secreted tonically rather than cyclically, have been hypothesized to augment pituitary sensitivity to gonadotropin-releasing hormone (GnRH) (12–14). Under long-term LH stimulation, the polycystic ovaries secrete excess androstenedione and testosterone. Body mass index (BMI) inversely correlates with LH levels, but not frequency (15), so that obese patients (BMI > 30) may not have an elevated LH:FSH ratio (16).

In contrast to the high LH levels in many patients with PCOS, FSH levels are low to normal. The low levels may result from (a) the inhibitory feedback of estrogen on FSH, (b) the relative insensitivity of FSH secretion to GnRH, and (c) the production of inhibin from the polycystic ovaries that could in turn stimulate androgen production and inhibit the release of FSH. In the ovary, a relative aromatase defect secondary to FSH deficiency and high intraovarian androgen levels impairs follicular maturation and cyclic production of estradiol and induces follicular atresia. The action of testosterone is further augmented because androgens decrease sex hormone-binding globulin (SHBG), which is produced in the liver, and thereby increase the level of free testosterone. In contrast, estrogen increases SHBG. Thus, sex steroids tend to amplify their own effects. In hirsute women, the low SHBG level facilitates the rapid uptake of free androgens and their peripheral conversion to estrogen. Peripheral conversion of androgens to estrogens takes place in muscle and adipose tissue, the latter being increased in many PCOS patients. With low levels of SHBG, PCOS patients have free estrogen levels that are higher than in normal women in the midfollicular phase of the cycle (12). The constant, acyclic levels of estradiol result in unopposed stimulation of the endometrium, placing the woman with PCOS at a higher risk of developing endometrial uterine cancer (17,18).

Recent evidence, however, has suggested that the hypothesis linking LH levels to changes in androgens and estrogens does not account for all the changes noted in patients with PCOS and may not be the primary defect (13). Studies have increasingly focused on the role of insulin in the pathogenesis of PCOS. Barbieri and associates (19) have noted that approximately 50% of women with significant ovarian androgen excess (serum testosterone >100 ng/dl) have IR and compensatory hyperinsulinemia. A positive correlation has been noted between fasting insulin levels and circulating testosterone and androstenedione levels (20). Caribbean Hispanic women have twice the prevalence of PCOS of other ethnic groups and have an increased prevalence of IR (21). Of note, women can have IR without PCOS. Indeed, IR is also an early marker of PCOS in adolescents with a 50% reduction in insulin sensitivity in adolescents with PCOS compared to obese controls (22). Some women have a severe form of insulin resistance, inherited in an autosomal recessive pattern.

Insulin and insulin-like growth factor-1 (IGF-1) work with LH to directly increase androgen production from the ovaries, even in nonobese women. *In vitro* studies have shown that insulin and insulin-like growth factors (IGFs) can stimulate androgen accumulation in incubations of ovarian stroma obtained from hyperandrogenic women (23) and can regulate thecal and stromal responsiveness to gonadotropins (24). IGFs are associated with binding proteins (BP), which modulate their bioavailability (25). High levels of insulin increase IGF-1, decrease the binding protein IGFBP1, and stimulate activity of the ovarian enzyme P-450c17α CYP 17 (17α-hydroxylase/C17,20 lyase), which is pivotal to the production of androgens by the ovary (Fig. 9-2). Women with PCOS appear to have dysregulation of this enzyme. It has been suggested that for some patients with PCOS serine phosphory-

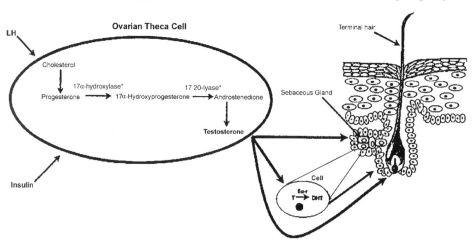

FIG. 9-2. Within the theca cell of the ovary, insulin and LH may stimulate cytochrome P450c17α activity, resulting in increased 17-α-hydroxylase and 17,20-lyase activity, as denoted by *asterisks*. These two enzymes comprise the P450c17α complex. Ovarian testosterone, along with DHT from 5α-reductase(5α-r) activity within the pilosebaceous unit, subsequently stimulates the androgen receptors at the hair follicle and sebaceous glands. Hirsutism and acne can result. (From Gordon CN. Menstrual disorders in adolescents: excess androgens and the polycystic ovary syndrome. *Pediatr Clin North Am* 1999;46:519; with permission.)

lation inhibits activity of the insulin receptor, resulting in insulin resistance, and also up-regulates C17,20-lyase activity (26,27).

In a randomized controlled trial (28), metformin, an insulin-sensitizing agent that decreases hyperinsulinemia, was shown to reduce levels of LH, androstenedione, and testosterone (decreased ovarian cytochrome P-450c17α activity) when administered to women with PCOS for 4 to 8 weeks. Similar effects have been observed by other investigators (29) and with troglitazone (30) and other insulin-sensitizing agents. Nutritional factors and insulin play important roles in determining the production of SHBG; insulin decreases hepatic SHBG production, thereby increasing free testosterone levels (31–33). There is, however, conflicting evidence on whether decreasing insulin levels leads to decreased LH sensitivity of granulosa cells or whether the primary action is increasing SHBG. Of interest in PCOS, IR is *selective in vivo*, affecting glucose transport and metabolic pathways in peripheral tissues such as muscle, at the same time that ovarian metabolic pathways and response are preserved (34,35) (Fig. 9-3).

The presence of acanthosis nigricans (velvety, verrucous, hyperpigmented skin often over the nape of the neck, in the axillae, beneath the breasts, and in the vulva, inguinal area, and other body folds) (Fig. 9-4) is a nonspecific skin marker that has been associated with IR (36,37), although it can occur in non-insulin-resistant obese girls. AN consists of hyperkeratosis, epidermal papillomatosis, and hyperpigmentation. Growth factors thought to be responsible for the appearance of AN include insulin, IGF-1, epidermal growth factor, and

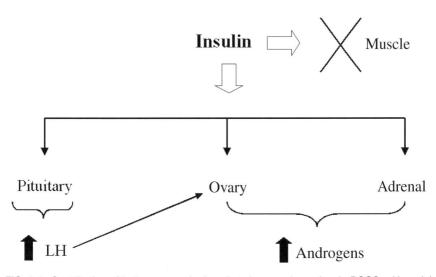

FIG. 9-3. Contribution of both ovary and adrenals to hyperandrogenism in PCOS, with peripheral insulin resistance and excessive levels of LH and insulin, each stimulating androgen production. (Adapted from Dunaif A. Insulin resistance and the polycystic ovary syndrome: mechanism and implications for pathogenesis. *Endocr Rev* 1997;18:774.)

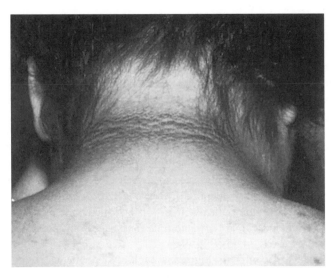

FIG. 9-4. Acanthosis nigricans. (From Chang RJ. Polycystic ovary syndrome and hyperandrogenic states. In: Strauss JF, Barbieri RL, eds. *Reproductive endocrinology: physiology, pathophysiology, and clinical management*, 5th ed. Philadelphia: Elsevier Saunders, 2004:602; with permission.)

testosterone. The combination of hyperandrogenism (HA), IR, and AN has been termed the HAIR-AN syndrome.

The finding of IR in women with PCOS is of particular importance because of the elevated risk of non-insulin-dependent diabetes mellitus (NIDDM) among these women. In a study of 254 women with PCOS, given a 75-g glucose challenge and glucose levels determined at 0 and 2 hours, 31.1% had impaired glucose tolerance (IGT) and 7.5% diabetes. In nonobese women with PCOS, the percentages were smaller but still significant with 10.3% having IGT and 1.5% diabetes (38). In a study of 122 women with PCOS, Ehrmann and colleagues found that 35% had IGT and 10% NIDDM. Women at greatest risk were those with a first degree relative with NIDDM and obese. Fasting glucose was found to be a poor predictor of the 2-hour glucose level (39). There was a significant worsening of glucose tolerance over a two-year follow-up. Similar data have been reported in other ethnic groups. For example, a study of Asian women with PCOS found that 20.3% had IGT and 17.7% NIDDM (40); fasting glucose levels alone would have identified a much lower prevalence of DM (6.3%). Palmert and colleagues at Children's Hospital Boston reported similar results in adolescents with PCOS: 8 of 27 had IGT and 1 of 27 NIDDM (41). Abnormal fasting glucose level was a poor predictor of IGT (2 of 8). Similarly, a glucose:insulin ratio of <4.5, which has been associated with IR in adults, would have detected all of the abnormal patients but would have also predicted that 15 of 18 with normal glucose tolerance tests (GTT) would be abnormal. Follow-up data on adults with PCOS suggests significant deterioration of glucose tolerance over time even in those with initially normal GTT results. In a follow-up study (average 6.2 years) of women with PCOS and normal GTT at baseline, Norman and colleagues found that 5 of 54 (9%) developed IGT and 4 of 54 (8%) developed DM (42). Of those with IGT at baseline, 7 of 13 (54%) developed DM. As expected, BMI at baseline was a significant predictor of adverse glucose tolerance at follow-up. Similarly, women with type II diabetes mellitus have an increased risk of having PCOS (43–45). Obese women with PCOS develop a greater degree of IR as body mass increases than do eumenorrheic controls. Of note, there is no single test for insulin resistance, making the diagnosis imprecise. However, studies of glucose tolerance are an important part of the follow-up of adolescents diagnosed with PCOS and IR (46).

Of interest, a short-term glucose load can produce a large rise in insulin and increases in circulating androgens (androstenedione, testosterone, and dihydrotestosterone) in women with PCOS and IR but not in control subjects or non-insulin-resistant women with PCOS (47). However, the transient physiologic hyperinsulinemia produced by an oral glucose load (such as might occur after a normal meal) appears to be insufficient to produce hyperandrogenism (32). Lowering androgen levels to the normal range in women with PCOS using long-acting GnRH analogs, cyproterone acetate, or bilateral oophorectomy does not improve the insulin resistance, and thus the IR can be considered an essential part of the syndrome (48). Hyperinsulinemia and PCOS are associated with an increased risk of having factors associated with cardiovascular disease (49–52). Wild found that women with PCOS appear to have an increased risk of hypertension (OR 1.4, 95% CI 0.9 to 2.0), diabetes mellitus (2.2, 0.9 to 5.2), hypercholesterolemia (3.2, 1.7 to 6.0) and cerebrovascular disease (2.8, 1.1 to 7.1), but not coronary artery disease (1.5, 0.7 to 2.9) (49). In adolescent girls with PCOS and IGT, the normal nocturnal decline in blood pressure does not occur, suggesting that this could be an early marker of cardiovascular risk (53). However, studies of risk are often confounded by obesity, and prospective studies are lacking to confirm cardiovascular risk attributable solely to PCOS (51).

Since the percent conversion of androstenedione to estrone is related to body weight, obesity at the time of puberty and during adolescence and the normal IR that occurs with puberty could be additive factors in producing the abnormalities of PCOS. Obesity is also associated with lower levels of SHBG and higher levels of unbound testosterone (52). Recent studies have also focused on the potential role of leptin in PCOS. Veldhuis suggested that there may be disruption of coordinated release of leptin with androgens and more variation in leptin levels in adolescents with PCOS compared to controls (54). However, Telli found similar mean leptin levels in PCOS and obese women (55), suggesting that leptin abnormalities may be secondary to obesity and not a primary factor in pathogenesis of the disorder.

The role of the adrenal glands in the pathogenesis of PCOS is controversial. Although many patients (up to 60%) with PCOS have mildly to moderately elevated DHEAS levels (300 to 600 μg/dL) and evidence of hyperresponsive adrenal glands on adrenocorticotropic hormone (ACTH) testing and adrenal scintiscans (56), most adolescents with androgen excess do not have specific adrenal enzyme deficiencies. Although some patients may have an "exaggerated adrenarche"(57), recent studies have suggested that the adrenal hyperandrogenism is due to dysregulation of adrenal steroidogenesis, similar to what is seen with dysregulation of the enzyme P-450c17α CYP 17 (17 α-hydroxylase/C17,20-lyase) in the ovary and may be increased by hyperinsulinemia. It is possible that adrenal hyperandrogenism is an inherited risk factor for PCOS (58). Emotional stress at puberty could perhaps also cause increased ACTH production, adrenal sensitivity, or both (13,59,60). Patients with PCOS and elevated DHEAS produced more androgens in response to ACTH stimulation than did control women before, but not after, 2 months of ovarian suppression with GnRH agonists. Carmina and colleagues (60) also documented a blunted response to ACTH with 6 months of ovarian suppression. The relative hyperestrogenic state of PCOS may be an important factor in enhancing adrenal sensitivity. Insulin may also modulate adrenal androgen production.

Recent interest has also focused on the possible relationship between premature pubarche and the later development of PCOS in some adolescents. Patients with premature pubarche may have adrenal hyperresponsiveness (dysregulation of adrenal steroidogenesis), elevated insulin and IGF-1 levels, and decreased levels of SHBG and IGFBP-1. Girls with premature pubarche, especially those who are insulin resistant, appear to be more likely to progress to PCOS in adolescence than other girls (5–7,61–63). An association between premature pubarche, hyperinsulinemia, and low birth weight has suggested that PCOS is a part of the *Syndrome X metabolic syndrome* (4).

There is a familial incidence of PCOS, and a number of investigators are exploring potential genetic linkages (64). In a study of 115 sisters of 80 probands with PCOS (diagnosed by having elevated serum androgens and less than six menses per year), Legro and colleagues found that 22% of sisters fulfilled criteria for PCOS and another 24% had hyperandrogenemia and regular menses (65). The probands, sisters with PCOS, and sisters with hyperandrogenemia had elevated serum LH levels compared to controls. PCOS appears to be autosomal dominant with variable presentation, including oligomenorrhea, PCOS on ultrasound, hirsutism and enlarged ovaries, premature balding, insulin resistance, and hyperandrogenism. Interestingly, brothers of women with PCOS have higher DHEAS levels than control men (66).

Genetic and endocrinologic factors also play a role in whether signs of hyperandrogenism are clinically evident. Patients have variable end-organ sensitivity of the pilosebaceous unit to the same level of hormones. Differing sensitivities are seen with different ethnicities. For example, Asian women with PCOS uncommonly present with clinical signs of hirsutism and acne. In a study of women with PCOS from the United States, Italy, and Japan, similar levels of LH, testosterone, and estradiol were found, but levels of 3α-androstanediol (a reflection of utilization of androgens by target tissues) were high in women from Italy and the United States and normal in Japanese women, who had much less hirsutism (21).

Ultrasound

Ovarian morphology in PCOS is variable and ranges from normal-appearing ovaries to enlarged ovaries with a thickened glistening capsule ("oyster shell"), multiple small peripheral cysts, and increased stroma or hyperthecosis. The number of growing and atretic follicles is doubled in patients with PCOS to 20 to 100 cystic follicles. The spectrum of ovarian pathology in PCOS is mirrored in the ultrasound findings (67–77). The ovaries may appear normal on ultrasound, although more commonly the ovaries appear enlarged, with multiple ($\geq$10 follicular cysts 2 to 8 mm in diameter) tiny cysts in a peripheral pattern underneath the cortex of the ovary, giving a "string of pearls" configuration (69,75) (Fig. 9-5). Ovarian stromal hyperechogenicity and increased cross-sectional area are common, but not uniformly found, in PCOS. The degree of total ovarian enlargement or stromal volume does not appear to be correlated with the testosterone levels (76). Fulghesu and colleagues (71) have suggested that with transvaginal ultrasound the finding of a stroma/total area (S/A) of the ovary of >0.34 is sensitive in diagnosing

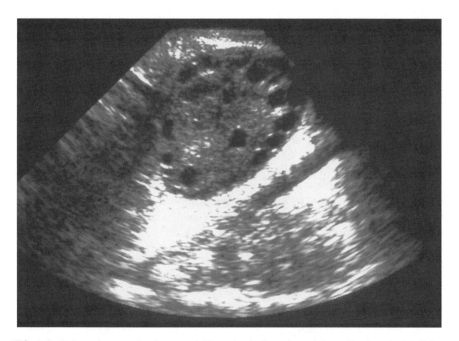

FIG. 9-5. Polycystic ovary in ultrasound. Note the "string of pearls" small subcortical follicles.

PCOS. Atiomo and colleagues (77) found the most sensitive features to be ≥ 10 follicles and peripheral distribution; stromal brightness (increased stromal to total area) was felt to be most specific. In contrast, multicystic or multifollicular ovaries with the small cysts distributed throughout the ovary without increased stroma are more typical of early pubertal or perimenarcheal anovulatory adolescents. However, the distinction can be difficult and may represent a spectrum, and Stanhope et al. (70) have documented the progression from multicystic to polycystic ovaries in one adolescent with delayed menarche. Women with hirsutism and regular menses (idiopathic hirsutism) frequently have "polycystic ovaries" demonstrated by ultrasound (71). "PCO-like" ovaries can occur in patients who have other sources of androgen excess, such as untreated or undiagnosed congenital adrenocortical hyperplasia (CAH) and adrenal adenomas or carcinomas, or in women who have conditions associated with chronic anovulation (including Cushing disease, acromegaly, hypothyroidism, and hyperprolactinemia). Ultrasound can help in defining the likely pathogenesis in some patients and in excluding some ovarian lesions, but it cannot be used to definitely rule out or in the diagnosis of PCOS. In a research study, Silfen and colleagues found that 100% of nonobese adolescents with PCOS had "polycystic-appearing ovaries" compared to 75% of obese patients with PCOS and 31% of obese controls (72). Up to 25% of normal cycling adult women may have "polycystic ovaries" by ultrasound (74). Pelvic ultrasound may not be as helpful in suggesting a diagnosis of PCOS in adolescents as in adults (26).

Quality of Life

PCOS has a profound impact on the quality of life for adolescent and adult women. Cronin and colleagues developed a specific *Health-Related Quality of Life Questionnaire in Adults* with 5 domains: emotions, body hair, weight, infertility, and menstrual problems (78). Trent and colleagues studied the quality of life of adolescents with PCOS and controls at Children's Hospital Boston and found significant disruption in general health perceptions, physical functioning, and family activities (79). The patient's *perceived* severity of PCOS, not the clinical severity assessed by the health care provider, was associated with quality of life. In addition, Trent and colleagues also found that similar to adults, adolescent girls with PCOS are concerned about their fertility (80) (Fig. 9-6).

DEFINITION OF HIRSUTISM

Two types of hair are found on the human body: terminal hair (>0.5 cm long, coarse, and usually pigmented) and vellus or lanugo hair (downy, fine, and light colored). Terminal hairs undergo several phases, including a growing phase (anagen),

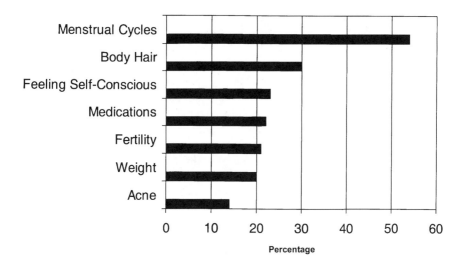

FIG. 9-6. Concerns of adolescent girls with PCOS (percentage). (Data from Trent ME, Rich M, Austin SB, Gordon CM. Quality of life in adolescent girls with polycystic ovary syndrome. *Arch Pediatr Adolesc Med* 2002;156:556.)

an involutional phase (catagen), and a resting phase (telogen). The initiation of anagen is influenced by hormonal factors. The distribution and density of the pilosebaceous units (sebaceous gland and hair follicle) are largely determined by genetic and racial/ethnic factors but are influenced by endocrinologic factors such as the rate and amount of androgen secretion, the concentration of sex hormone-binding globulin (SHBG), the peripheral conversion of weak androgens to potent androgens, and the sensitivity of the pilosebaceous unit to androgens (81).

An increase in the distribution and quantity of *terminal hair* may bring the patient to the health care provider with the complaint of hirsutism. The appreciation of the degree of hirsutism is partially subjective and related to a comparison of the degree of hirsutism in the patient to that noted in other female family members. Hirsutism may also be noted by the physician during a routine physical examination or during an evaluation of irregular menses. Excessive downy hair (*lanugo*) is usually referred to as *hypertrichosis* and occurs, for example, in adolescents with anorexia nervosa.

The clinician may encounter difficulty in establishing whether the amount of hair is excessive, since the spectrum of "normal" is at best ill-defined. In a study of 400 young women in Wales, McKnight (82) reported that 84% of women had terminal hair on the lower arm and leg, 70% also had terminal hair on the upper arm and leg, and 26% had terminal hair on the face, usually on the upper lip. In 10% of the women, the facial hair was noticeable, and in 4%, it was characterized as a true disfigurement. Seventeen percent of women had hair on the chest or breast, usually periareolar; 35% had hair on the abdomen, usually along the linea alba up to the umbilicus; 16% had hair in the lumbosacral area; and 3% had hair on the upper back. Nine percent had considerable hair on most or all of these areas. The Ferriman and Gallwey scoring system (83) has been used by many clinicians to define hirsutism (see p. 305). In a study of 430 women aged 15 to 74 years, a score above 7 was found in 4.3% of women and a score above 10 in 1.2%.

Testosterone induces the production of enzymes in the hair follicle, and thus once a terminal hair begins to grow, less androgen is required to stimulate its continued growth. This factor probably accounts, in part, for the fact that a less than optimal response is frequently achieved by hormone suppression therapy, which by biochemical parameters (lowering of free testosterone) should be successful.

ETIOLOGY OF HIRSUTISM

The differential diagnosis of hirsutism is listed in Table 9-1. As noted above, most cases of significant hirsutism result from the overproduction of androgens or their precursors from an ovarian and/or adrenal source, with PCOS the most common diagnosis. Most women with hirsutism have increased testosterone production rates, and increased levels of free testosterone are detectable in 80% to 85% of hirsute women. In cases in which hyperandrogenism is not detected,

TABLE 9-1. *Causes of hirsutism in adolescents*

Ovarian disorders
  Polycystic ovary syndrome (PCOS)
  Hyperthecosis
  Tumors
  Enzyme deficiency
Adrenal disorders
  Congenital adrenal hyperplasia (21-hydroxylase, 11β-hydroxylase, 3β-hydroxysteroid
    dehydrogenase deficiencies)
  Cushing disease
  Tumors
Idiopathic hirsutism
Drugs (phenytoin, danazol, diazoxide, minoxidil, glucocorticoid excess, androgens, valproate)
Pregnancy
Hypothyroidism
Central nervous system injury
Hyperprolactinemia
Stress
Anorexia nervosa, malnutrition
Peripheral tissue sensitivity
Male pseudohermaphroditism, mixed gonadal dysgenesis

hirsutism may be due to an increased sensitivity of the follicle to low levels of androgen, increased conversion of testosterone to dihydrotestosterone (DHT), an androgen other than testosterone and androstenedione, an elevated level not detected because of the normal fluctuation of secretion, or the presence of more numerous hair follicles. In some women with hirsutism, normal menses, and normal testosterone levels, the cause may be related to increased 5α-reductase activity in the skin. However, a recent study has suggested that many of the women diagnosed with "idiopathic hirsutism" have mild PCOS (84). Among 62 hirsute ovulatory women, 8 (13%) had normal androgen levels (idiopathic hirsutism); 24 (39%) had characteristic polycystic ovaries on ultrasound and/or an exaggerated response of 17-OH progesterone to leuprolide; and 30 (48%) had unspecified hyperandrogenism. Compared to the women with idiopathic hirsutism, the women with mild PCOS had higher fasting insulin levels, lower glucose/insulin ratios, and higher low-density lipoprotein cholesterol (LDL-C).

Drugs such as phenytoin, corticosteroids, danazol, diazoxide, minoxidil, anabolic steroids, and androgens cause hirsutism. Studies on the association of valproate and PCOS have been conflicting. An early study found that 80% of women treated with valproate before the age of 20 years had PCOS or hyperandrogenism (85). In a small study of adult women with focal epilepsy, Bauer and colleagues found similar percentages of women diagnosed with PCOS for those treated with valproate (11%) compared to those treated with carbamazepine or not treated with antiepileptic drugs (86). Among a sample of 43 women in another study, PCOS was found in three (two of the 22 treated with valproate) (87). Further research is needed but close observation of adolescents treated with valproate is indicated. Pregnancy, hypothyroidism, anorexia nervosa, malnutrition, and chronic central nervous system disorders (e.g., mental and motor retardation) can be accompanied by excess hair growth.

Occasionally, stress may precipitate excess secretion of LH and increased production of androgens from the theca cells; the abnormal hormone production reverses when the acute stress is over. With her immature hypothalamic–pituitary–ovarian axis, an adolescent may be particularly prone to this type of disorder. As noted earlier, adolescents may have transient oligomenorrhea and mild hyperandrogenemia in the first few years after menarche and then establish normal ovulatory menses (88). Many others may have persistent anovulatory cycles and typical PCOS. In a small study of 4 groups of adolescents with menstrual irregularity (< or >3 years following menarche), with PCOS, and normal controls, Avvad and colleagues found that the girls with menstrual irregularity and with PCOS had similar androgen levels and ovarian volumes by ultrasound (89). Similarly, in an unselected population of adolescent girls 14 to 16 years old, girls with oligomenorrhea has higher mean LH, testosterone, and DHEAS levels that those with regular cycles; 57% of oligomenorrheic girls had LH levels above the 95th percentile (90). In a study of 13 adolescents with mild to moderate hyperandrogenism, Apter and colleagues found that hyperinsulinemia, elevated LH, and reduced SHBG contributed to PCOS (91). In a 15-year follow-up, Apter found that age-adjusted high concentrations of LH, testosterone, and androstenedione during adolescence were associated with subsequent low fertility rates as adult women (9).

Hyperprolactinemia may be accompanied by increased secretion of adrenal androgens, especially dehydroepiandrosterone sulfate (DHEAS), because of prolactin receptors in the adrenal glands, and may also be associated with PCOS. Hirsutism is mild, as the peripheral action of the androgens is limited because prolactin has a blocking action on the conversion of testosterone to DHT (81). A rare cause of hyperandrogenism is glucocorticoid resistance, caused by mutations in the receptor gene. Diagnostic criteria include elevated cortisol levels (in the absence of symptoms of Cushing syndrome), normal diurnal cortisol variation, lack of dexamethasone suppression, and elevation of adrenal androgens. Treatment is not usually needed (92).

Ovarian and adrenal tumors can present with rapid onset of hirsutism and usually virilization as well. Male pseudohermaphroditism or mixed gonadal dysgenesis may present with virilization at puberty. Any signs of rapid progression of hirsutism or the presence of virilization (clitoromegaly, temporal hair recession, deepening of the voice, changes in muscle pattern) should prompt an immediate assessment of hormone status to exclude the possibility of an androgen-producing tumor or male gonad.

Production of Androgens

The rate of testosterone production in adult women correlates most closely with the degree of hirsutism/virilization, with stepwise increases in testosterone production corresponding to increasing hirsutism and clitoromegaly (93). Free (or unbound) testosterone levels correlate better with the clinical signs of hirsutism and testosterone production rate than total testosterone levels. All but a small fraction of serum testosterone is bound tightly to SHBG, and more weakly bound to albumin. Free and albumin-bound testosterone are the biologically active forms. Although normal adult women have twice the SHBG concentration of normal men, hirsute women with elevated androgen levels have SHBG levels lower than those of normal women.

The sources of androgens are noted in Fig. 9-7. The relative contributions vary during the menstrual cycle and with the time of day. The major adrenal androgens are dehydroepiandrosterone (DHEA) and its sulfate, DHEAS; androstenedione; and testosterone. The stroma and theca interna of the ovaries secrete primarily testosterone and androstenedione. In normal women, approximately 80% to 90% of DHEA is secreted by the adrenal glands and 10% to 20% by the ovaries. More than 90% of DHEAS is secreted by the adrenal glands. The diurnal variation of DHEA is similar to that of cortisol, with peak levels in the early morning. DHEAS

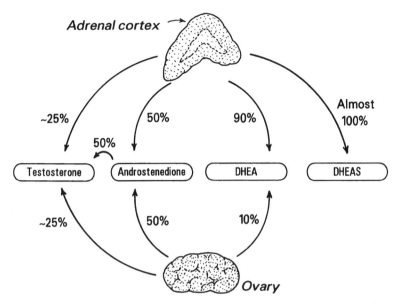

FIG. 9-7. Source of androgens in adult women. DHEA, dehydroepiandrosterone; DHEAS, DHEA sulfate.

has a long half-life, with less fluctuation in levels, and thus, measurement of DHEAS is more easily interpreted in the evaluation of hirsute patients. Androstenedione is secreted equally by the adrenal glands and the ovaries in normal women and has about 10% of the androgenic potency of testosterone.

The source of testosterone is variable: 0% to 30% comes from the adrenal glands, 5% to 25% from the ovaries, and 50% to 60% is produced by the peripheral conversion of precursors, such as DHEA and androstenedione. In hirsute women with PCOS, the ovaries are responsible for a much greater percentage of the testosterone production. Ovarian theca cells from patients with PCOS appear to convert androgen precursors to testosterone more efficiently than cells from normal women (94). Virtually all DHT comes from peripheral conversion of testosterone through the enzymatic action of 5α-reductase; DHT is the biologically active and potent androgen at the level of the hair follicle. The DHT from the pilosebaceous unit does not reenter the circulation as DHT but rather as 3α-androstanediol glucuronide.

Adrenal Enzyme Deficiencies

Depending on the population studied (ethnic origin and referral versus primary care practice), late-onset 21-hydroxylase deficiency, also termed *nonclassic*

CAH, is found in 1% to 10% of adult women with hirsutism (6,95–103). Overall, the severe form of congenital adrenal hyperplasia with 21-hydroxylase deficiency is found in 1 of 12,000 and the mild or nonclassic form in approximately 1 of 1,000 non-Jewish white women. In other populations nonclassic CAH is more common: 3% among Ashkenazi Jews, 1% to 2% among Hispanics (102,103). In a referral population of adolescents with significant hirsutism, we found 21-hydroxylase deficiency in two of 22 patients (99). Ibanez found this deficiency in one of 42 (6). In 100 consecutive women with the classic features of PCOS, Benjamin and colleagues (100) reported that 4% of women had homozygous CAH and 15% had heterozygous CAH. Thus the utility of screening all girls with irregular menses and hirsutism for late onset CAH depends in part on the ethnicity of the patients and the expected prevalence in the patient population. Lower prevalences of late onset CAH would be expected in non-referred, primary care populations.

New and colleagues (104,105) have studied many family pedigrees of patients with nonclassic 21-hydroxylase CAH. The enzyme 21-hydroxylase is a specific microsomal cytochrome P-450 (cytochrome P450c21). Nonclassic CAH is an autosomal recessive disorder with a gene located on chromosome 6, in proximity to the HLA locus. More than 40 mutations of the *CYP21* gene have been associated with CAH (92,106). Patients with nonclassic CAH have a spectrum of clinical presentations: some have severe hirsutism and menstrual irregularity; others are asymptomatic. Asymptomatic patients with nonclassic CAH and abnormal hormone levels have been termed "cryptic." Speiser and New (104) have also identified a group of patients termed compound heterozygotes with one severe (classic) and one mild (nonclassic) 21-hydroxylase allele; these patients have a higher 17-hydroxyprogesterone response to ACTH than do homozygous nonclassic patients but were not found to be more likely to have signs of androgen excess. Moran and colleagues found that ACTH-stimulated 17-OHP levels, but not baseline levels, were higher in patients with clitoromegaly than those without (107).

ACTH testing with measurement of 17-hydroxyprogesterone levels at baseline and 60 minutes later has been the cornerstone of diagnosis of 21-hydroxylase deficiency (99,108), although overlap between heterozygotes and normal subjects and heterozygotes and homozygotes for nonclassic CAH does occur (see p. 311). The use of early morning levels (7 to 8 A.M.) of serum (or salivary) 17-hydroxyprogesterone is a helpful screening test for this disorder (109,110) (see section on Laboratory Studies). Although some have argued that diagnosis is not essential since treatment of adult women with nonclassic 21-hydroxylase deficiency is adequate without the use of corticosteroids, we believe that an adolescent with 21-hydroxylase deficiency should be appropriately diagnosed and treated with corticosteroids with the hope that the long-term androgenic sequelae and PCOS can be prevented with early intervention.

There has been a long controversy about whether there is a partial form of 3β-hydroxysteroid dehydrogenase (3β-HSD) deficiency that can cause hirsutism and oligomenorrhea in the general population (111,112). Increasing evidence suggests that almost all patients previously diagnosed with this disorder have partial defects in enzyme action that result from the hyperandrogenic milieu, not a primary genetic disorder. The elevated levels of DHEA and 17-hydroxypreg-nenolone are often reversible with suppression of androgens. Azziz and col-leagues (111) have argued that responses of DHEA and 17-hydroxypregnenolone fall in a continuum and that patients diagnosed with 3β-HSD deficiency were merely above the 95th percentile but not clearly a distinct population. Using the stringent criteria of requiring patients to have responses that are three times the upper control limit for either steroid response, they found that no patients among 86 women with hirsutism and hyperandrogenic oligomenorrhea met this standard. Three women (2.3%) were diagnosed with 21-hydroxylase deficiency. The women with exaggerated DHEA and 17-OH pregnenolone responses had higher DHEAS values than their less responsive counterparts, but similar total and free T, SHBG, LH, FSH, DHEA/androstenedione, and 17-OH pregnenolone/17-OH progesterone levels. In addition, most girls with premature pubarche and those with hirsutism tested for the 3β-HSD genes have an inherited deficiency (113).

Deficiencies of 11α-hydroxylase and 17-ketosteroid reductase are quite rare (114,115). The 11-hydroxylase deficiency is not HLA linked (105); the structural gene for cytochrome P-450c11 enzyme (for 11-hydroxylation, 18-hydroxylation, and 18-oxidation) is located on chromosome 8. Lee and colleagues (116) have reported a familial hypersecretion of adrenal androgens transmitted as a dominant non-HLA-linked trait; the affected family members had premature adrenarche, hirsutism, and amenorrhea.

Other Diagnoses

Other rare diagnoses to be considered in the patient with oligomenorrhea and androgen excess are Cushing disease, ovarian or adrenal tumors, and intersex states. Cushing disease should be considered in the hypertensive obese adolescent with irregular menses and hirsutism, particularly if other stigmata of Cushing syndrome are present (weakness, spontaneous ecchymoses, purple striae larger than 1 cm, hypokalemia, osteoporosis).

Androgen-producing ovarian and adrenal tumors should be considered in patients with virilization, rapid onset of hirsutism, or markedly elevated baseline androgen levels (117, 118). Adrenal carcinomas are usually palpable at the time of diagnosis; these lesions typically secrete DHEA and androstenedione, which are converted to testosterone in the periphery. Some secrete testosterone directly. Since some lesions lack the ability to convert DHEA to DHEAS, both these hormones need to be measured in the patient suspected of having a tumor. Adrenal adenomas can be quite small at presentation in spite of high levels of androgens. Ovarian tumors may cause hirsutism (see Chapter 18) and, with the exception of luteomas, are usually palpable on bimanual examination or detectable by ultrasound. Occasionally, small ovarian tumors are suppressible by estrogen/progestin therapy.

PATIENT EVALUATION

The initial history should focus on (a) menstrual pattern (age of onset and regularity); (b) history of premature pubarche; (c) weight changes, especially related to puberty; (d) timing, location, rate of progression, and recent changes in the amount of hair; (e) acne; (f) drug intake (including anabolic steroid use in athletes); (g) stress; (h) changes in voice pitch and scalp hair distribution (including evidence of balding); (i) skin changes suggestive of AN (see Fig. 9-4); (j) family history of hirsutism, PCOS, adrenal enzyme deficiencies, diabetes, hyperinsulinism, or infertility; and (k) ethnic background. Increased terminal hair over the face (especially the chin), sternum, upper abdomen, or back is usually a sign of significant hirsutism. The combination of slowly progressive hirsutism, obesity, acanthosis nigricans, and menstrual irregularity suggests PCOS. Patients who have acne that had a very early or late age of onset, is persistent or recalcitrant, or relapses after oral isotretinoin (Accutane) should also have a hormonal evaluation for PCOS whether or not hirsutism is also present (119). Obese patients with PCOS may also have also complications of obesity including obstructive sleep apnea (120) and steatohepatitis. A history of virilization or an abrupt onset of hirsutism should raise the suspicion of a tumor or intersex state.

The physical examination should include a search for signs of thyroid disorders, galactorrhea, acne, AN, stigmata of Cushing disease, and abdominal and pelvic masses. The distribution and quantity of the hair should be noted. Hirsutism should be scored to enable assessment of the degree of the problem and to provide baseline data for followup. Bardin and Lipsett (121) have suggested a criteria of 1+ for each portion of the face involved (upper lip, chin, sideburns) and 4+ for the entire chin, neck, and face. A more time-consuming but preferable method is the use of the Ferriman and Gallwey scoring system (83) (Fig. 9-8). The appearance of the patient can be circled on a flow sheet in the chart and the total score recorded. A score ≥ 8, using the first nine areas, is considered hirsutism. Mild temporal or vertex alopecia may occur in hyperandrogenic states. Similarly, acne can be graded using a clinical scoring system (122,123) (Fig. 9-9).

A lower skinfold dimension has been observed for the dorsum of the hand at the midpoint of the second and third proximal phalanges in adult women with Cushing disease (1.5 $\pm$ 0.2 mm, range 1.0 to 1.8 mm) compared with adult women with either PCOS (2.8 $\pm$ 0.5, range 2.0 to 4.0 mm) or HAIR-AN (mean

(Grade 0 at all sites indicates absence of terminal hair.)

Site	Grade	Definition
1. Upper Lip	1	A few hairs at outer margin.
	2	A small moustache at outer margin.
	3	A moustache extending halfway from outer margin.
	4	A moustache extending to mid-line.
2. Chin	1	A few scattered hairs.
	2	Scattered hairs with small concentrations.
	3 & 4	Complete cover, light and heavy.
3. Chest	1	Circumareolar hairs.
	2	With mid-line hair in addition.
	3	Fusion of these areas, with three-quarter cover.
	4	Complete cover.
4. Upper back	1	A few scattered hairs.
	2	Rather more, still scattered.
	3 & 4	Complete cover, light and heavy.
5. Lower back	1	A sacral tuft of hair.
	2	With some lateral extension.
	3	Three-quarter cover.
	4	Complete cover.
6. Upper abdomen	1	A few mid-line hairs.
	2	Rather more, still mid-line.
	3 & 4	Half and full cover.
7. Lower abdomen	1	A few mid-line hairs.
	2	A mid-line streak of hair.
	3	A mid-line band of hair.
	4	An inverted V-shaped growth.
8. Arm	1	Sparse growth affecting not more than a quarter of the limb surface.
	2	More than this; cover still incomplete.
	3 & 4	Complete cover, light and heavy.
9. Forearm	1, 2, 3, 4	Complete cover of dorsal surface; 2 grades of light and 2 of heavy growth.
10. Thigh	1, 2, 3, 4	As for arm.
11. Leg	1, 2, 3, 4	As for arm.

A

FIG. 9-8. **A** and **B**: Hirsutism scoring sheet. The Ferriman and Gallwey system for scoring hirsutism. A score of 8 or more indicates hirsutism. (From Hatch R, Rosenfield RL, Kim MH, et al. Hirsutism: implications, etiology, and management. *Am J Obstet Gynecol* 1981;149:815. Adapted from Ferriman D, Gallwey JD. Clinical assessment of body hair growth in women. *J Clin Endocrinol Metab* 1961;21:1440; with permission.)

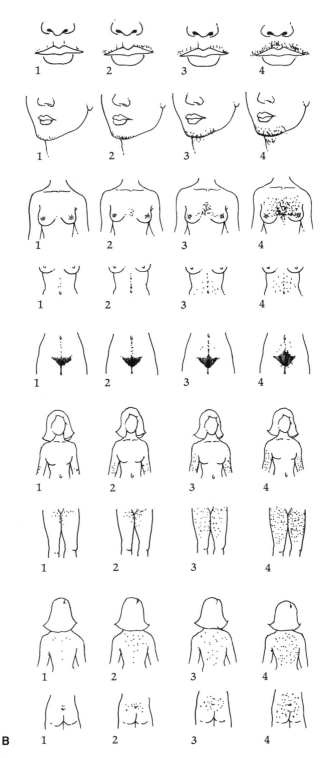

FIG. 9-8. (*Continued*)

Fig. 9-9 A. Clinical Scoring System for Acne Vulgaris*		
Score	Class	Lesions
	Microcomedones	Comedones, <2mm diameter
1	Minor	Comedones, 2 mm or greater (<10)
2	Mild	Comedones (10-20; pustular or nonpustular)
3	Moderate	Comedones (>20) or pustules (<20)
4	Severe	Pustules (>20)
5	Cystic	Inflammatory lesions >5 mm
*Face and trunk may be graded separately		

A

Fig. 9-9 B. The Global Acne Grading System (GAGS)		
Location	Factor x Grade (0-4)* = Local score	
I Forehead	2	
II Right cheek	2	
III Left cheek	2	
IV Nose	1	
V Chin	1	
VI Chest and upper back	3	
	Global Score =	
	*Grade	Global score
	0, No lesions	0 None
	1, ≥ one comedone	1-18 Mild
	2, ≥ one papule	19-30 Moderate
	3, ≥ one pustule	31-38 Severe
	4, ≥ one nodule	>39 Very Severe

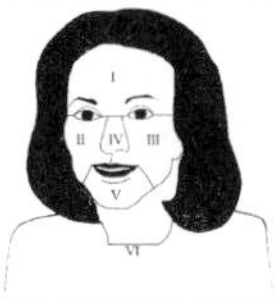

B

FIG. 9-9. Two acne scoring systems. **A**: Clinical scoring system for acne vulgaris. (From Rosenfeld RL. Hyperandrogenism in peripubertal girls. *Pediatr Clin North Am* 1990;37:1333; with permission.) **B**: The six locations (I to VI) of the global acne grading system (GAGS). (From Doshi A, Zaheer A, Stiller M. A comparison of current acne grading systems and proposal of a novel system. *Intl J Dermatol* 1997;36:417; with permission.)

4.4 ± 0.5, range 4.0 to 5.0 mm) (124). This finding needs to be validated in adolescents. Any signs of virilization—significant temporal balding, deepening of the voice, clitoral enlargement (Fig. 9-10), or changes in body fat or muscle distribution—should prompt an assessment to exclude hyperthecosis, an adrenal or ovarian tumor, adrenal enzyme deficiency, or intersex disorder. The width of the clitoral glans should be measured; a normal width is considered to be <5 mm (see Chapter 1, p. 27). If the patient has hirsutism, signs of virilization, and/or irregular menses, a vaginal or rectal bimanual examination or pelvic ultrasound is generally part of the evaluation.

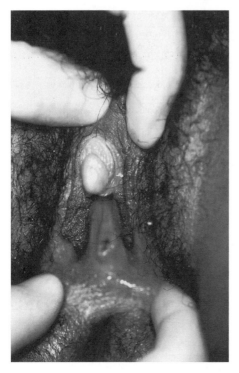

FIG. 9-10. Clitoral enlargement.

LABORATORY STUDIES

The aim of laboratory tests is to assist in determining the cause of the patient's irregular menses and androgen excess (Table 9-2). In most cases, PCOS is the cause of the symptom complex, and thus, laboratory tests should be based on the clinical presentation and the need to exclude other potential diagnoses. If the evolution of symptoms such as progressive hirsutism has occurred over 6 to 12 months, or if virilization is present, more extensive studies are necessary to rule out a possible androgen-producing tumor.

Levels of serum androgens should be determined at a qualified laboratory, which needs to report normal ranges of each hormone. Since hormonal levels vary throughout the day, morning sampling is preferred. Because hormone tests are expensive, some endocrinologists prefer to draw two samples (30 minutes apart), pool equal aliquots of serum from each sample, and then obtain a single determination. Others use a single blood sample initially, and if androgen levels are all normal on the random sample in a hirsute patient and further diagnostic information is needed, the determinations are repeated or several aliquots are pooled. In the adult patient, the clinician has the advantage of evaluating patients with 10 or

TABLE 9-2. *Laboratory evaluation of adolescent girl with suspected PCOS*

At time of clinic visit,
    FSH, LH, prolactin, TSH
    Testosterone, free testosterone [sex hormone binding globulin (SHBG)]
    DHEAS
    Cholesterol, HDL-C (or fasted lipid profile with cholesterol, HDL-C, LDL-C, triglycerides)
    Random blood glucose
If patient is obese and/or has acanthosis nigricans *or* all girls with PCOS,
    Fasting glucose and insulin level; 2-h glucose level after 75-g oral glucose
    American Diabetes Association criteria

Fasting glucose (mg/dl)	Glucose 2 h 75-g OGT (mg/dl)
Normal: <100	Normal: <140
Impaired: 100 to 125	Impaired: 140 to 199
Diabetes: ≥126	Diabetes: ≥200

If suspicious of late-onset CAH (high DHEAS, clitoromegaly, premature pubarche, early onset)
    or all patients in some protocols,
    17-hydroxyprogesterone (17-OHP) in follicular phase drawn between 7 and 8 AM

    If 17-OHP <200 ng/dl, unlikely to have 21-hydroxylase deficiency.
        200 to 1000 ng/dl—Perform 1-h ACTH stimulation test
        >1000 ng/dl—21-hydroxylase deficiency
If pelvic examination is inadequate, testosterone level is high, or evaluation of ovarian
    morphology is desired,
    Pelvic ultrasound
High suspicion of adrenal tumor:
    CT/MRI

---

more years of menstrual history, which increases the likelihood that the hirsute, oligomenorrheic woman indeed has PCOS, which can be diagnosed with a minimum of laboratory tests. In dealing with the adolescent patient, the clinician is often in much more of a quandary about the differential diagnosis because menstrual cycles may be irregular for several years in normal adolescents, hirsutism is often much less striking in the young teen with PCOS, and transient hyperandrogenism can occur during the normal pubertal process. Additionally, in patients with mild hirsutism, apparent skin sensitivity to androgens and the level of serum free testosterone seem to contribute equally; thus, about half of patients with mild hirsutism may have normal free testosterone levels (125). Even women with moderate to severe hirsutism, normal ovarian function, and normal menses can have normal screening serum androgen levels (see p. 296).

Although recommendations vary depending on the clinical presentation, the initial laboratory evaluation of a patient with significant or progressive hirsutism usually includes serum levels of testosterone, free testosterone, and DHEAS. If amenorrhea, oligomenorrhea, or chronic anovulation is present, LH, FSH, and prolactin are measured. The TSH level is also usually determined, because the subtle signs and symptoms of hypothyroidism in adolescents are easy to miss, and treatment is simple. Serum levels of FSH are important to exclude gonadal failure in the amenorrheic adolescent; LH levels, if elevated, may help suggest the clinical diagnosis of PCOS in the young adolescent (72). In the adult woman, LH levels may be less frequently determined because the clinical history is usually more conclusive. Because the samples are drawn at one point in time, elevated LH levels may be found in normal adolescents at ovulation, those under stress, and those with PCOS. Adolescents with PCOS may have normal or elevated LH levels, with elevated levels more likely to be found in those with a BMI <30. LH-to-FSH ratios are 2.5:1 to 3:1 in some, but not all, patients with PCOS. Samples for serum hormone levels should not be drawn immediately following the withdrawal flow to a progestin challenge or while the patient is taking oral contraceptive levels, since hormone levels are decreased (126). Waiting 3 months after oral contraceptives are discontinued is preferred for those already taking hormones.

Although at some centers only the total testosterone level is determined in hirsute adult women with the aim of using the test primarily to exclude a tumor, we have found that adding a *free* testosterone level is helpful because adolescents may have only mild hirsutism and irregular menses at the initial presentation of PCOS. However, the free testosterone level should be included in the testing only if the laboratory assays are of high quality and meaningful. The presence of an abnormal free testosterone level is useful in establishing a likely diagnosis and outlining therapy and follow-up for the adolescent and her family. If virilization is present or a tumor is under consideration, serum levels of DHEA and androstenedione are added. Turhan and colleagues reported that the LH/FSH ratio, insulin, and testosterone levels were the most predictive tests in diagnosing PCOS in adults with oligomenorrhea (127). In epidemiological studies, Escobar and colleagues found that decreased SHBG, increased free androgen index, free testosterone, and DHEAS levels were highly effective in detecting women with PCOS (128).

A testosterone level above 150 to 200 ng/dl (depending on the laboratory normal values), DHEAS above 600 to 700 μg/dl, or androstenedione above 500 ng/dl should raise the suspicion of a tumor or intersex disorder. Testosterone levels between 100 and 200 ng/dl have rarely been associated with tumors. Testosterone levels may be quite elevated (150 to 220 ng/dl) in girls with hyperthecosis. Because of the need for extensive and expensive tests to exclude a tumor, it is critical that a markedly elevated testosterone be verified in a specialized endocrine laboratory; commercial laboratories may use less specific assays that include cross-reacting substances and thus falsely elevate the total testosterone value. Derksen and colleagues (129) have reported that benign ovarian and adrenal disorders can be differentiated from adrenal carcinoma by a dexamethasone test (3 mg/day for 5 days with DHEAS normally suppressed and cortisol <3.3 μg/dl in patients without tumor); however, the clinical presentation of the patients diagnosed with tumors was suggestive of the need for further evaluation. Determination of the karyotype is reserved for adolescents with significant virilization especially if associated with vaginal/uterine agenesis, a serum testosterone level in the male range, or elevated FSH and is helpful in detecting mixed gonadal dysgenesis or male pseudohermaphroditism.

The need to do ACTH testing in patients with hirsutism is controversial. Since testing is expensive, our current approach is to suggest that ACTH testing for 21-hydroxylase deficiency be done on girls with clitoromegaly, markedly elevated DHEAS, a history of premature adrenarche, a family history of CAH, an ethnic origin from a group with a high prevalence of CAH, and, most importantly, a high baseline early-morning level of 17-OHP (Fig. 9-11). Girls with what appears to be "typical PCOS" can have 17-OHP measured between 7 and 8 A.M. in the follicular phase of the menstrual cycle. Girls with PCOS may have minor elevations of 17-OHP. If the 17-OHP level is <200 ng/dL and the history is not suggestive, no further testing is needed. If the baseline level 17-OHP is >1000 ng/dl, the diagnosis of 21-hydroxylase deficiency can be made without further testing. For a 17-OHP level between 200 and 1000 ng/dl, a simple ACTH test is recommended: 17-OHP is measured at baseline and then 60 minutes after giving 0.25 mg of ACTH (cosyntropin). Azziz and Zacur (110) found that a basal 17-OHP level >200 ng/dl had a positive predictive value of 80% (95% CI: 28% to 99%) and a negative predictive value of 100% (95% CI: 97% to 100%). Moran and colleagues reported that at most 10% of patients with late-onset CAH will be missed using an AM 17-OHP of <200 ng/dl to exclude the diagnosis (107). The likelihood of a 21-hydroxylase deficiency is increased if the baseline level of 17-OHP is >400 ng/dl. Some clinicians prefer to perform a modified ACTH test on all patients with significant hirsutism, but most use a first AM 17-OHP as a screening test. The rise seen with late-onset CAH is typically >6.5 ng/dl/min with levels >1000 ng/dl (usually >1500 ng/dl) at 60 minutes. Pang and colleagues (130) reported that women with nonclassic CAH had 60-minute stimulated levels of 17-OHP of 5404 ± 3234 ng/dl (normal, 334 ± 194 ng/dl) with a markedly abnormal ratio of 17-OH pregnenolone to 17-OHP of 0.4 ± 0.2 (normal, 3.4 ± 1.5). In heterozygotes for nonclassic CAH, the rise in 17-OHP may be in the normal range or intermediate between the normal range and the homozygous response (500 to 1000 ng/dl) (Fig. 9-12).

Because of the metabolic abnormalities commonly associated with PCOS, clinicians should assess the lipid profile (cholesterol, HDL-C, LDL-C, and triglycerides) and the presence of hyperinsulinemia and impaired glucose tolerance. Elevated levels of LDL-C are an important lipid abnormality in women with PCOS, independent of obesity (131,132). Triglyceride levels are also typically elevated and HDL-C levels reduced. Fasting glucose and insulin levels may provide an imperfect estimate of insulin resistance. Fasted glucose/insulin ratios of <4.5 has been associated with IR in obese women with PCOS; a ratio of <7.0 has been proposed as a better cutoff in girls with premature pubarche, but further studies to define "insulin resistance" are needed (133,134). In addition, many girls with obesity and IR do not have PCOS (72). As part of the periodic evaluation of adolescents with PCOS, especially those with obesity and AN, we suggest a modified glucose tolerance test using 75 g glucose—obtaining a baseline fasted glucose level followed by a 2-hour glucose level—to assess for IGT and DM. A random glucose drawn at the time of the clinic visit does not exclude DM or

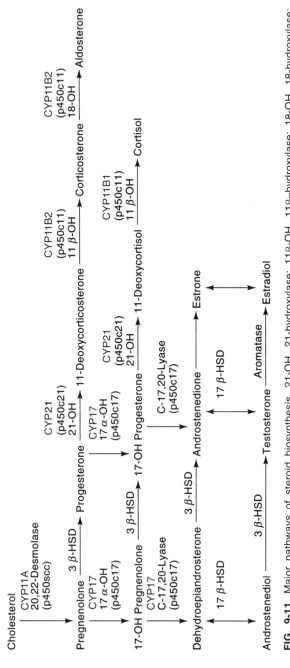

FIG. 9-11. Major pathways of steroid biosynthesis. 21-OH, 21-hydroxylase; 11β-OH, 11β–hydroxylase; 18-OH, 18-hydroxylase; 3–hydroxysteroid dehydrogenase; 17β–HSD, 17β-hydroxysteroid dehydrogenase (17-ketosteroid reductase); 17β–OH, 17–β hydroxylase; C-17,20 lyase also termed 17,20 desmolase.

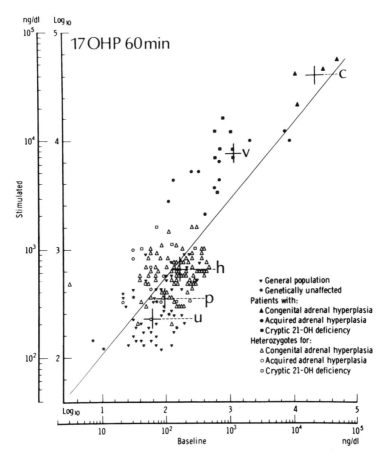

FIG. 9-12. Nomogram relating baseline to ACTH-stimulated serum concentrations of 17-hydroxyprogesterone. The scales are logarithmic. A regression line for all data points is shown. The mean for each group is indicated by a large *cross* and adjacent letter; c, classic 21-hydroxylase deficiency; v, variant or nonclassic 21-hydroxylase deficiency (combined mean of all values in patients with cryptic and late-onset disease); h, heterozygotes for all forms of 21-hydroxylase deficiency; p, general population; u, persons known to be unaffected (e.g., siblings of patients with 21-hydroxylase deficiency who carry neither affected parental haplotype as determined by HLS typing); OH, hydroxyl. (From White PC, New MI, Du Pont B. Congenital adrenal hyperplasia. Parts I and II. *N Engl J Med* 1987;316:1519, 1580; Copyright 1987, Massachusetts Medical Society with permission.)

IGT, but a level of >200 ng/dl should suggest the need for rapid testing of the patient for DM.

Imaging is obtained selectively; for example, if the pelvic exam is inadequate or not possible, the testosterone level is high, or evaluation of ovarian morphology is desired. Ultrasonography can be helpful in assessing the ovaries of obese and poorly relaxed adolescents. Although transvaginal ultrasonography provides better detail of ovarian morphology, most teens prefer transabdominal ultrasound. Ultra-sonography can also be used to evaluate the endometrium. Computed tomography or magnetic resonance imaging is obtained, as indicated, for evaluation of an adrenal or ovarian tumor.

If the stigmata of Cushing disease are present, a 24-hour urine sample should be collected for determination of urinary free cortisol and creatinine. The urinary creatinine should be 16 to 22 mg/kg body weight to assure an adequate collection was accomplished. If urinary free cortisol cannot be obtained or is elevated, an 8 a.m. cortisol level after a bedtime (11 p.m.) dose of 1 mg of dexamethasone is measured. If the serum level of cortisol is not well suppressed (<5 μg/dl), or if the level of urinary free cortisol is abnormal, formal dexamethasone suppression testing is done. A pituitary adenoma should be excluded in hyperandrogenic adolescents with hyperprolactinemia.

Five- and 7-day dexamethasone testing is rarely used for the evaluation of girls who have hirsutism, but are not being evaluated for Cushing disease or a tumor. In our clinic, we use dexamethasone tests occasionally in patients with markedly elevated DHEA and DHEAS to ensure that suppression is normal. Typically, we will give a 5-day dexamethasone test (0.5 mg four times a day) following an ACTH stimulation test. Testosterone, free testosterone, DHEA, DHEAS, androstenedione, and cortisol are measured at baseline and on the morning of the fifth day of dexamethasone. In patients with PCOS, DHEA and DHEAS typically suppress to $<80\%$ and 50%, respectively, with a dexamethasone test. However, even if the free testosterone level falls into the normal range in a patient with PCOS, the level rises on typical doses of dexamethasone (0.1 to 0.5 mg/day), clinical improvement is unlikely, side effects are common, and oral contraceptives or insulin sensitizing agents remained the preferred treatment approach (see Treatment section).

A few centers have reported that androstanediol glucuronide levels are helpful in examining the etiology of hirsutism in adult women, since an increased level reflects utilization of androgens by target tissue (135,136). Androstanediol glucuronide, although not an androgen itself, is a metabolite of the pathway of testosterone to dihydrotestosterone, which is an important step in androgen expression. However, it may arise from hepatic as well as skin sources. Levels of this metabolite appear to correlate with the clinical response to spironolactone therapy in patients with idiopathic hirsutism (136).

The diagnosis of PCOS in adolescents can be made by the typical clinical history, the exclusion of other clinical entities, and the finding of elevated free testosterone in the setting of anovulatory cycles and androgen excess (hirsutism, acne). The total testosterone level is also often elevated. The LH levels may be elevated (may be >15 mIU/ml) and/or the ratio of LH/FSH is >2.5. It should be remembered that an increased LH/FSH ratio may be associated with andro-gen excess per se, as with ovarian tumors or CAH. An increased LH/FSH ratio in the absence of elevated free testosterone does not make a diagnosis of PCOS, although the patient may later develop the more evident clinical and laboratory signs. In some clinical research centers, further confirmatory studies of PCOS are done, such as looking for an exaggerated LH response with normal FSH response to GnRH and increased androstenedione and/or testosterone response to human chorionic gonadotropin (HCG) stimulation. Suppression-stimulation testing, however, cannot be used to exclude a neoplasm definitively in the patient with markedly elevated testosterone.

TREATMENT

Treatment of androgen excess should target the cause. The vast majority of patients with progressive hirsutism and menstrual irregularities have PCOS. Other patients may need surgery for resection of a tumor (See Chapter 18) or steroids for treatment of late onset CAH (see below). As noted earlier, it is important not to underdiagnose or overdiagnose PCOS. Transient hyperandrogenism can occur and may need watchful waiting. However, if the diagnosis of PCOS is delayed, then hirsutism may progress. For example, girls with a family history of PCOS, a history of premature pubarche, or taking medications such as valproate should be followed closely for development of PCOS and treated early if signs or symptoms occur. The potential aims of therapy for PCOS should be discussed with each patient and a therapeutic decision made. The aims of treatment may include:

1. Protection of the endometrium from continuous stimulation with estrogen (and dysfunctional uterine bleeding) and the later development of endometrial cancer
2. Management of irregular menses
3. Decrease in hirsutism and acne, or at least prevention of further new hair growth
4. Decrease risk of developing diabetes mellitus
5. Improvement of quality of life
6. Address infertility

A critical part of all therapies for patients with PCOS and obesity is a lifestyle change that includes weight loss, cessation of smoking, and exercise. Weight loss reduces peripheral production, reduces insulin resistance, suppresses ovarian androgen production, and reduces cardiovascular risks (137–141). Fat cells appear to be responsible for some of the peripheral conversion of the prehormone androstenedione. Obesity per se is associated with increases in total and free testosterone and DHEAS in adults as well as adolescent girls. Guzick and colleagues (141) reported that an average weight loss of 16.2 kg in 12 hyperandrogenic, anovulatory women resulted in an increase of SHBG, a decline in free testosterone, and a decline in fasting insulin levels. Four of six women resumed ovulation. Prevention of diabetes mellitus is an important goal. A randomized trial of diabetes prevention in adults (>25 years old) with IGT at 2 hours and fasting glucose 95 to 125 mg/dl included three arms: lifestyle change with 7% weight loss and 150 minutes of exercise per week, metformin, and placebo. During follow-up (average 2.8 years), 4.8 cases of diabetes/100 person-years developed in the lifestyle group, 7.8 cases/100 person-years in the metformin group, and 11.0 cases/100 person-years in the placebo group (142). Diets that are high in fiber and complex carbohydrates may lower insulin secretion. Low-glycemic-index diets lower insulin secretion, enhance satiety, and lead to weight loss (143). However, randomized studies are needed to determine whether any specific diets beyond one for weight loss are helpful in PCOS. Cessation of smoking is important to lessen cardiovascular risk.

Pharmacologic therapies include progestins, estrogen/progestins, metformin, corticosteroids, and GnRH analogues. In the adolescent who is not sexually active and does not have significant or progressive hirsutism or acne, management of menstrual irregularity can be addressed by the use of progestin withdrawal (12 to 14 days of 10 mg medroxyprogesterone every 4 to 8 weeks). While oral medroxyprogesterone therapy did decrease LH and testosterone and increase insulin sensitivity in a short-term (10 days) study (144), the patient should understand that much of the abnormal physiology is not altered by this therapy.

Estrogen/Progestin Therapy

For most adolescents with PCOS, and especially those with significant hirsutism or acne or in need of contraception, a combined estrogen/progestin hormonal method (oral contraceptives, patch, injectable, or ring) is a first-line therapy. Combined estrogen/progestin therapy such as oral contraceptives (OC) suppresses the hypothalamic–pituitary–ovarian axis, lowers ovarian secretion of steroids, usually lowers adrenal androgen secretion (decreases DHEAS), and provides protection to the endometrium (24,145–149). The estrogen in the OC increases SHBG and thereby decreases free testosterone. However, insulin sensitivity is not changed with OC use, including newer progestins such as norgestimate (150,151). Although few comparative studies have been done for different OC pill formulations, most clinician prescribe OCs with 30- to 35-μg of ethinyl estradiol (EE) (see Chapter 20). Very rarely, a pill with 50 μg EE is needed for a few cycles, especially in patients with markedly elevated free testosterone and hyperthecosis; the dosage can be lowered in several months to a 30- to 35-μg EE pill once the free testosterone levels decrease. Continuous pills (or patches or rings) for 3 to 4 months (followed by 7 days off) also may help to lessen the increase in LH and testosterone during the time for taking placebo pills in patients with very high levels of these hormones (145) or inadequate response; total testosterone was lower is nonobese women with PCOS treated with continuous OCs (28 ng/dl) than cyclic OCs (50 ng/dl) at 3 months.

In patients who develop hypertension or nausea on the pill, even an OC with 20 μg of EE can effectively decrease free testosterone levels. As noted in Chapter 20, body weight may play a role in increasing the risk of OC failure (152) although the absolute risk of a pregnancy is very small. A recent study of lean and obese women with PCOS suggested that obese patients had less response of clinical androgenic symptoms to OCs than lean women (153).

In adolescents with typical PCOS, mildly elevated testosterone, and clinical response to therapy, serum androgen levels do not need to be repeated. However, in adolescents who initially have high levels of testosterone, the testosterone level should be measured in the second or third week of the second cycle of hormones to make sure that adequate suppression has occurred. However, it is important to consider the possibility of the rare tumor in adolescents with a pretreatment serum testosterone >150 to 200 ng/dl (done in a reliable laboratory) even if suppression occurs, because tumors can be suppressed by oral contraceptives, norethindrone, and GnRH analogs. For adolescents with poor response to treatment or if questions arise about adequate suppression or compliance, total and free testosterone levels can be checked at follow-up and continuous pills (patches or rings) prescribed. Hirsutism improves in 50% to 70% of hirsute women treated with OC suppression. The adolescent girl needs to understand that the goal is to prevent the growth of new hairs while she uses cosmetic measures such as electrolysis or laser to treat preexisting hair follicles.

Antiandrogens

Spironolactone has been used successfully in adult women and adolescents for the treatment of hirsutism, generally in addition to OC therapy. Spironolactone is an aldosterone antagonist with antiandrogenic effects; this drug competes at the androgen receptor level and inhibits 5α-reductase activity to decrease conversion of testosterone to DHT, thus lessening hair growth, midshaft diameter, and sebum production (Fig. 9-13). This drug is particularly useful with idiopathic hirsutism (154–157). The drug has been administered in several regimens, usually at 100 to 200 mg per day in two divided doses (154,155). In patients not also taking oral contraceptives, the cyclic administration on days 4 to 22 of the cycle may reduce the occurrence of irregular menses. The dosage of 100 mg per day (given as 50 mg twice daily) is less likely to be associated with metrorrhagia than the higher 200 mg/day (156). Side effects (which include polyuria, polydipsia, dizziness, lethargy, nausea, hyperkalemia, breast pain, and headache) are usually transient and disappear without any intervention. The possible long-term problems have not been fully defined. Adolescents should not use this drug if they are at risk of pregnancy because the drug can potentially prevent normal masculinization of the male fetus. Thus, for most adolescents with moderate to severe hirsutism, spironolactone should be given along with oral contraceptives for therapy. Some clinicians prefer to give oral contraceptives for 1 to 3 months alone first, and then the spironolactone is added so that side effects

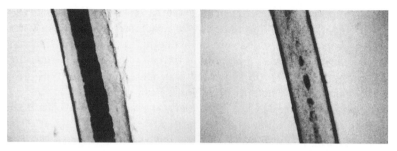

FIG. 9-13. Hair plucked from the facial area of a woman with hirsutism before *(left panel)* and after *(right panel)* treatment for 6 months with spironolactone plus oral contraceptives. Notice the decrease in the medullary diameter of the hair. (From O'Brien RC, Cooper ME, Murray RM, et al. Comparison of the sequential cyproterone acetate/estrogen versus spironolactone/oral contraceptive in the treatment of hirsutism. *J Clin Endocrinol Metab* 1991;72:1008; Copyright 1991, The Endocrine Society; with permission.)

related to either drug are not confused. Others begin both medications at the same time. It must be stressed to the adolescent that a noticeable difference may not be appreciated for 6 to 9 months and the existing hair will not disappear.

Cyproterone acetate along with low-dose estrogen replacement, available in Europe, has yielded comparable or better results than spironolactone plus oral contraceptives in reducing total hair diameter and medullary diameter (the part with the pigment) (158). It is a competitive inhibitor of DHT, binding to its specific receptors; it reduces 5α-reductase in the skin and lowers ovarian androgen secretion by inhibiting gonadotropin release. Finasteride, a specific competitive inhibitor of 5α-reductase, not approved for women in the United States, appears to have a clinical effect similar to spironolactone; both treatments result in a decrease in anagen hair diameters and in Ferriman–Gallwey scores (159), but is not recommended in adolescents. Flutamide, an antiandrogen, both alone and in combination with oral contraceptives, appears efficacious in reducing hirsutism score, hair diameter, and acne with an efficacy similar to that of spironolactone (160,161), but the potential for unexpected hepatotoxicity during treatment with the drug has limited its use and it is not approved in the United States (162). A recent study suggested that spironolactone was more effective than cyproterone or finasteride at 12 months of use (157). Several other antiandrogens, such as ketoconazole, which is an inhibitor for P-450 steroidogenic enzymes and blocks synthesis of androgens, have also been tried but can also be associated with adverse side effects and are not recommended.

Metformin and Insulin-Sensitizing Agents

Metformin, a biguanide that improves hyperinsulinemia, has not only been useful in elucidating the pathophysiology of PCOS but has provided new therapies for women with PCOS (28,29,163–170). In study protocols, metformin (500 mg t.i.d.,

850 mg b.i.d. to t.i.d. or 1000 mg b.i.d.) suppresses hepatic glucose production, increases peripheral insulin sensitivity, increases SHBG levels, decreases androgen levels, and results in resumption of menses in 68% to 96% of patients. A reduction in insulin levels is associated with a reduction in testosterone levels (164). Doses, however, have been empiric and vary with protocols. Metformin treatment induces ovulation in 30% to 55% of patients. The effect on hirsutism has been variable (134,169). There was less response in one study of women with increased DHEAS (170). Overweight patients with PCOS have tended to select metformin because of the belief that it will result in dramatic weight loss. Although metformin may induce slight weight loss, which may then encourage the patient to adhere to a lifestyle program, decreased weight has been observed in only some studies (163,169). Gastrointestinal side effects such as flatulence, diarrhea, nausea, and vomiting can occur in up to 30% to 40% of patients but are lessened by starting with a low dose and gradually increasing the dose over several weeks. Typically metformin 500 mg is given with the evening meal and then one week later the dose is increased to 500 mg b.i.d. (with meals). The dose is increased every 1 to 2 weeks until a dose of 1500 to 2500 mg a day is reached; if side effects occur, the dose can be decreased to a level tolerated. A single long-acting (sustained release SR) form of metformin (750 mg SR) given with dinner also may lessen side effects and improve compliance; the maximum SR dose is 2000 mg per day. Prior to therapy, renal and liver function should be assessed; metformin should not be prescribed if creatinine is elevated. Patients should have annual creatinine and CBC drawn to detect changes in renal function and rare B_{12} deficiency. Patients should be counseled about avoiding significant or binge alcohol use, and metformin should be discontinued before major surgery or radiologic procedures (especially those using contrast agents) that require the patient to not take a usual amount of fluid. Similarly, metformin should be discontinued if the patient has a gastrointestinal illness or vomiting with potential dehydration owing to rare risk of lactic acidosis. Metformin plus an oral contraceptive lowers androstenedione and increases SHBG more than OCs alone (168). Rosiglitazone, an insulin-sensitizing agent, is being studied in trials for adults but is category C for pregnancy. Other drugs that improve insulin sensitivity that have been evaluated in small studies include *N*-acetylcysteine (171), acarbose, an alphaglucosidase inhibitor (172), and D-chiro-inositol (173). Troglitazone was previously used in trials of PCOS with promising outcomes (30,174), but the drug was removed from the market because of liver toxicity.

Several studies of metformin have specifically looked at adolescents. In obese male and female adolescents without clinical PCOS but with hyperinsulinemia and a family history of type 2 diabetes mellitus (14 treated with metformin and 15 controls), metformin therapy resulted in decrease of 0.5 kg/m^2 in BMI (–1.3%) and 5.5% decrease in leptin (175). In a study of nonobese girls (BMI 21.4 kg/m^2) with increased androgens, anovulation, and a history of premature pubarche, Ibanez and colleagues reported that treatment with metformin (1275 mg per day) resulted in regular menses in all 18 girls in 6 months, with ovulation documented in 14 girls

(Fig. 9-14) (176). Therapy was associated with decreased hirsutism scores, decreased fasting insulin and total T levels, and increased SHBG levels. No change occurred in fasting blood sugar levels or BMI. However, once the metformin was stopped after the trial, oligomenorrhea and hyperandrogenism recurred. In a small study of 11 adolescents with PCOS treated with metformin (1500 to 2550 mg per day) and diet for 10.5 (4.5 to 26.5) months, Glueck and colleagues found that 10 of 11 (91%) resumed normal menses and nine (82%) lost weight (5 to >11 lb) (177). A study of 15 obese adolescents with PCOS and IGT found that metformin therapy not only improved glucose tolerance and insulin sensitivity and decreased serum androgens but also attenuated the adrenal steroidogenic response to ACTH (suggesting that the drug impacts on adrenal P-450c17α activity) (178). Similar results have been noted in adult women (179).

The clinical trials in adults and in adolescents have not yet defined which adolescents should be offered metformin therapy. Vrbikova observed that the best predictor of improvement in menstrual cyclicity in adults was a combination of higher basal levels of 17-OH progesterone, SHBG, and testosterone, and lower levels of androstenedione (180). Kolodziejczyk and colleagues (170) found that women with high DHEAS had less response to metformin with less improvement in menstrual cyclicity and hirsutism. Another study found that higher plasma insulin, lower serum androstenedione, and less severe menstrual abnormality were the best

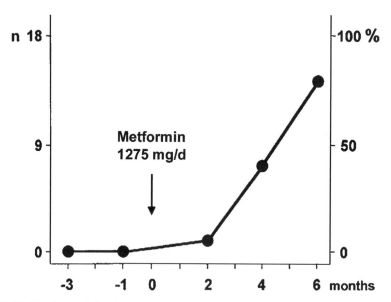

FIG. 9-14. Number and fraction of ovulatory adolescents before and after metformin treatment. (From Ibanez L, Valls C, Ferrer A, et al. Sensitization to insulin induces ovulation in nonobese adolescent with anovulatory hyperandrogenism. *J Clin Endocrinol Metab* 2001; 86:3595; Copyright 2001, The Endocrine Society; with permission.)

predictors of response to metformin (181). To date, studies of metformin have been short-term, and good results generally require both lifestyle change and medication. PCOS recurs when therapy is stopped. Ovulatory cycles may be seen as a benefit or a risk for an adolescent, who may then experience an unintended pregnancy. Adolescents with PCOS and type II diabetes mellitus or IGT are clearly candidates for therapy with metformin. Metformin, as noted above, can reduce the risk of diabetes in patients with IGT. Metformin may also be helpful in those with significant acanthosis nigricans. Other patients who may benefit from metformin include those with IR with or without obesity. Whether teens without IR will also benefit is unclear. It is also unknown whether treatment in early adolescence might prevent some of the progression to PCOS in girls with premature pubarche and insulin resistance. Studies are needed to evaluate whether metformin will lessen the risk of endometrial hyperplasia/cancer (3). Long-term studies are needed to see if outcomes are improved by early treatment with metformin and to delineate the best candidates. Metformin can be used in addition to OCs and spironolactone, if needed.

Other Therapies

Eflornithine hydrochloride 13.9% cream (Vaniqa), a topical antiandrogen, is an inhibitor of ornithine decarboxylase, an enzyme that mediates cell division and growth in hair follicles. The cream is applied to the face twice a day; the primary side effects are burning and folliculitis, which is more likely if the cream is applied to shaved skin. The cream must be used long term because it is needed for ongoing effect. Results have been variable.

GnRH analogs have been helpful for lessening the hirsutism score and the hair shaft diameter in patients with PCOS in most, but not all, studies (182–188). Therapy is generally reserved for severe cases not responding to oral contraceptives, spironolactone, and metformin. Szilagyi found that although androgens decreased with GnRH therapy, hirsutism did not improve at 6 months (187). Add-back estrogen/progestin therapy needs to be administered with the GnRH analogs to prevent the long-term consequences of estrogen deficiency (see Chapter 11 for discussion of add-back therapy). Combined therapy with GnRH analogs and an OC may be more effective in treating hirsutism and decreasing ovarian volume (188). Leuprolide acetate plus oral contraceptives and spironolactone can also lead to clinical improvement in women when previous therapy has failed. In a small study, Rittmaster and Thompson (189) reported that GnRH analogs appeared to be marginally more efficacious in women with PCOS than in those with idiopathic hirsutism. Bromocriptine has been prescribed in women with both hyperprolactinemic PCOS and normoprolactinemic PCOS (190–192); the studies have reported variable results.

Although some studies in adult women initially suggested short-term and long-term benefits of dexamethasone in the reduction of high androgen levels and the establishment of normal menses, our experience in treating adolescents with PCOS and hirsutism with corticosteroids and the experience of other investigators treating adults have not found this to be efficacious for patients (146,193,194). Many patients with PCOS do have elevated adrenal androgen levels (without an adrenal enzyme deficiency) and will experience lowering of serum androgen levels during a dexamethasone test, but few adolescents have clinical improvement in hirsutism or regularity of menses with long-term corticosteroid suppression and are at risk of overtreatment, weight gain, and osteoporosis. Very rare patients with both PCOS and late-onset CAH have benefited from a course of both oral contraceptives and low dose corticosteroids to lessen androgen excess.

Patients with late-onset 21-hydroxylase deficiency CAH have traditionally been treated with glucocorticoid therapy, such as low-dose dexamethasone or prednisone. As overtreatment is more common with dexamethasone, we prefer to prescribe prednisone 5 mg at bedtime (or 2.5 mg twice a day). These girls should wear MediAlert bracelets. Some investigators have argued that other forms of treatment without glucocorticoids are as efficacious as corticosteroids, or more so, in these women. Carmina and Lobo (195) found that suppression of the ovary with a GnRH analog was beneficial for patients with demonstrated late-onset 21-hydroxylase deficiency and that the decrease in hirsutism was greater than during the previous 6-month treatment with dexamethasone. Spritzer and colleagues (196) also reported that cyproterone acetate therapy was more effective in reducing the hirsutism score (but not the serum testosterone or androstenedione levels) than hydrocortisone (20 mg per day) therapy for women with late-onset CAH. Because we generally diagnose patients with late-onset CAH in early to mid-adolescence at our center, we have been prescribing corticosteroid therapy to try to avoid the long-term consequences of the development of PCOS. Whether this approach will be successful in the prevention of hirsutism and PCOS is unknown at present.

Regardless of the therapy chosen, the patient also needs help in achieving good cosmetic results including mechanical treatments such as electrolysis, laser, depilatories, plucking, waxing, shaving, and bleaching. Bleaching of the fine hair, especially on the face, can be accomplished with 6% hydrogen peroxide or commercial preparations of facial bleaches. The addition of 10 drops of ammonia per 30 ml of peroxide just before use will activate the peroxide and increase bleaching. Depilatories, shaving, and wax epilation remove hair temporarily. Electrolysis, if done by an experienced person, permanently destroys the hair bulb and, in most cases, avoids pitlike scars and regrowth of incompletely destroyed hairs. A patient should have her own individual electrolysis needle and should also be given the option of using EMLA cream (lidocaine 2.5% and prilocaine 2.5%) for 1 hour before the electrolysis to lessen the discomfort (197). Laser epilation appears to be promising in selected patients and works best in growing, high melanin hair with light skin. Regrowth of hair is common. The field of laser therapy is rapidly evolving. Side effects include hyper- and hypopigmentation and pitting of the skin surface, which usually improves. Acanthosis nigricans (AN) may improve with weight loss and/or metformin therapy. Topical therapy with lac-hydrin 12% or tretinoin cream have also been used with variable success to lessen AN. Similarly, acne should be treated with topical retinoic acid, topical and systemic antibiotics, OCs (patch or ring) and, if needed, spironolactone. Often systemic antibiotics can be discontinued after 3 months of OC use.

The induction of ovulation in infertile patients with PCOS is beyond the scope of this book, but patients and families often ask questions at the time of the visit. Approximately 80% of patients will have anovulatory infertility. Spontaneous pregnancies do occur, and adolescents may have an unintended pregnancy because they mistakenly believe that they are infertile. Because of oligomenorrhea, teens may present quite late in pregnancy. The most successful treatment for PCOS-related anovulatory infertility is weight loss. Medical therapies for anovulation and infertility have included clomiphene citrate, metformin alone, clomiphene plus metformin, exogenous gonadotropins and HCG, isolated FSH, adrenal suppression, pulsatile GnRH, and GnRH analogs followed by exogenous gonadotropins, (167,198,199). Women with PCOS are at risk of hyperstimulation syndrome and multiple pregnancy from gonadotropin therapy (3). Metformin given through pregnancy appears to decrease the risk of gestational diabetes 10-fold (31% to 3%) (200). However, utilization of metformin during pregnancy is controversial at this time and it is not approved for pregnancy; some obstetricians thus choose to continue the drug and others discontinue it at the time of documentation of pregnancy.

Surgical approaches to PCOS include laparoscopic diathermy or laser "drilling" to decrease the stromal ovarian component that is producing the androgens; however, the increased stroma will return. The disadvantages have included intraabdominal adhesions, the need for surgery and general anesthesia, and in one case ovarian atrophy (201–205) and thus is offered to women with infertility who have failed conservative approaches. Farquhar reported cumulative pregnancy rates to be similar comparing 6 to 12 months post drilling and 3 to 6 cycles of ovulation induction with gonadotropins, with lower multiple pregnancy rates (204).

Just as important as the pharmacologic and lifestyle approaches to adolescents with PCOS is attention to their quality of life. Counseling, support groups, and health information for girls are essential. Adult-oriented PCOS web sites often focus on infertility and personal issues. Teen sites need to address the questions of this age group (see www.youngwomenshealth.org). Similarly, school nurses and other professionals should learn about this common endocrine disorder so they can address the myriad of questions and challenges for these girls. Workplace and school no-harassment policies are essential to improve their environment and self-esteem. A continuing challenge for girls with PCOS and their families is the lack of insurance coverage for the needed therapies including hormonal therapies, laser, electrolysis, etc., that are scarcely viewed as "cosmetic" by the girls with PCOS. The next decade of research and clinical care should bring enhanced knowledge of pathogenesis, therapies, and holistic approaches to PCOS.

Case 1

K. T. presented at the age of 15 years with a history of irregular menses and increasing hirsutism. She had started her pubic hair development at age 11 and her breast development at age 12. Her menarche occurred at age 13 ¹⁰⁄₁₂ years, and she had a second menstrual period 7 months later. She was otherwise in good health, and her increments in height and weight had been normal. On physical examination, she appeared to be healthy and to have moderate facial hirsutism and mild acne. Her height was 156.5 cm (10th percentile) and her weight 46 kg (10th percentile). She had increased hirsutism on the upper lip, chin, and sideburns, and the Ferriman–Gallwey score was 25. Otherwise, the results of her general examination and pelvic examination were normal. Initial laboratory tests revealed an elevated LH to FSH ratio, normal DHEAS of 198 μg/dl, testosterone of 63 ng/dl (normal <55 ng/dl), and free testosterone of 8.8 pg/ml (normal <6.3 pg/ml). An ACTH stimulation test showed that her 17-OHP increased from 1,352 ng/dl at baseline to 7,849 ng/dl at 60 minutes, consistent with late-onset 21-hydroxylase deficiency. She was given prednisone 5 mg at bedtime. As she remained amenorrheic with significant hirsutism, oral contraceptives were begun, initially norethindrone 0.5 mg/ethinyl estradiol 35 μg and then changed to norethindrone 1 mg/ethinyl estradiol 20 μg because of nausea. Her acne resolved, and she underwent electrolysis. She had good cosmetic results and has chosen to continue taking oral contraceptives. Her younger sister had a rise in 17-OHP from 68 ng/dl at baseline to 1,349 ng/dl at 60 minutes in response to ACTH and has no hirsutism; this sister has been shown to be a heterozygote (97).

The ACTH test was performed on K. T. because of her early and progressive hirsutism in spite of an increased LH/FSH ratio and normal DHEAS; however, the diagnosis could have been made by determination of a single early-morning 17-OHP.

Case 2

L. K., 15 years old, presented because of irregular menses. Her menarche occurred at the age of 11, and she had had irregular menses every 2 to 4 months. Her LMP had been 4 months earlier. She had been overweight since childhood and had gained 60 pounds in the past 2 years. She had been sexually active once, 2 years before the office visit. She had a family history of obesity and diabetes mellitus. On physical examination she was obese with a height of 164.7 cm (60%) and weight 116.2 kg (>95%). Her blood pressure was 112/74 mm Hg. She had moderate acne on her face and back with hyperpigmented velvety skin on the back of her neck and in her axilla (acanthosis nigricans). She had mild striae on her abdomen. Her breast and pubic hair development was Tanner stage 5. Her Ferriman–Gallwey score was 15. Her pelvic examination was normal, and she did not have clitoromegaly. Laboratory evaluation revealed negative urine HCG, LH 11.3 mIU/ml, FSH 4.9 mIU/ml, testosterone 62 ng/dl (normal <55 ng/dl), free testosterone 12.0 pg/ml (normal <6.3 pg/ml), normal DHEAS 251 μg/dl, normal TSH and prolactin levels, elevated fasting insulin of 40 μU/ml, normal fasting glucose of 83 mg/dl, and elevated cholesterol of 239 mg/dl. She was diagnosed with hyperandrogenism, insulin resistance, and acanthosis nigricans (HAIR-AN). She was treated with medroxyprogesterone to give normal withdrawal flow and started on oral contraceptives. She made several visits to the nutritionist and managed to lose some weight. She is considering initiating metformin therapy.

REFERENCES

1. Zawadski JK, Dunaif A. Diagnostic criteria for polycystic ovary syndrome: towards a rational approach. In: Dunaif A, Givens JR, Haseltine F, et al., eds. *Polycystic ovary syndrome*. Boston: Blackwell Science, 1992:377.
2. Lobo RA. What are the key features of importance in polycystic ovary syndrome? *Fertil Steril* 2003;80(2):259.
3. Legro RS. Polycystic ovary syndrome: the new millennium. *Mol Cell Endocrinol* 2002;186:219.
4. Ibanez L, Valls C, Potau N, et al. Polycystic ovary syndrome after precocious pubarche: ontogeny of the low-birth-weight effect. *Clin Endocrinol* 2001;55(5):667.
5. Temeck J, Pang S, Nelson C, et al. Genetic defect of steroidogenesis in premature pubarche. *J Clin Endocrinol Metab* 1987;64:609.
6. Ibanez L, Potau N, Zampolli M, et al. Source localization of androgen excess in adolescent girls. *J Clin Endocrinol Metab* 1994;79:1778.
7. Miller D, Emans SJ, Kohane I. A follow-up study of adolescent girls with a history of premature pubarche. *J Adolesc Health* 1996;18:301.
8. Venturoli S, Porcu E, Fabbri R, et al. Postmenarcheal evolution of endocrine pattern and ovarian aspects of adolescents with menstrual irregularities. *Fertil Steril* 1987;48:78.
9. Apter D, Vihko R. Endocrine determinants of fertility: serum androgen concentrations during follow-up of adolescents into the third decade of life. *J Clin Endocrinol Metab* 1990;71:970.
10. Zumoff B, Freeman R, Coupey S, et al. A chronobiologic abnormality in luteinizing hormone secretion in teenage girls with the polycystic-ovary syndrome. *N Engl J Med* 1983;309:1206.
11. Apter D, Butzow T, Laughlin GA, et al. Accelerated 24 h luteinizing hormone pulsatile activity in adolescent girls with ovarian hyperandrogenism: relevance to the developmental phase polycystic ovarian disease. *J Clin Endocrinol Metab* 1994;79:119.
12. Waldstreicher J, Santoro NF, Hall JE, et al. Hyperfunction of the hypothalamic–pituitary axis in women with polycystic ovarian disease: indirect evidence for partial gonadotrophic desensitization. *J Clin Endocrinol Metab* 1988;66:165.
13. Rosenfield RL, Cara JF. Androgens and the adolescent girl. In: Sanfilippo JS, Muram D, Dewhurst J, Lee PA. *Pediatric and adolescent gynecology*. 2nd ed.. Philadelphia: WB Saunders, 2001:269.
14. Rebar R, Judd HL, Yen SSC, et al. Characterization of the inappropriate gonadotropin secretion in polycystic ovary syndrome. *J Clin Invest* 1976;57:1320.
15. Taylor AE. Determinants of abnormal gonadotropin secretion in clinically defined women with polycystic ovary syndrome. *J Clin Endocrinol Metab* 1997;82(7):2248.
16. Yen SSC. Polycystic ovary syndrome. In: Yen SSC, Jaffe RB, Barbieri RL. *Reproductive Endocrinology*, 4th ed. Philadelphia, PA: WB Saunders; 1999:436.
17. Farhi DC, Nosanchuk J, Silverberg SG. Endometrial adenocarcinoma in women under 25 years of age. *Obstet Gynecol* 1986;68:741.
18. Coulam CB, Annegers JF, Kranz JS. Chronic anovulation syndrome and associated neoplasia. *Obstet Gynecol* 1983;61:403.
19. Barbieri RL, Smith S, Ryan KJ. The role of hyperinsulinemia in the pathogenesis of ovarian hyperandrogenism. *Fertil Steril* 1988;50:197.
20. Burghen GA, Givens JR, Kitabchi AE. Correlation of hyperandrogenism with hyperinsulinism in polycystic ovary disease. *J Clin Endocrinol Metab* 1980;50:113.

21. Carmina E, Koyama T, Chang L, et al. Does ethnicity influence the prevalence of adrenal hyperandrogenism and insulin resistance in polycystic ovary syndrome? *Am J Obstet Gynecol* 1992;167:1807.
22. Lewy VD, Danadian K, Witchel SF, et al. Early metabolic abnormalities in adolescent girls with polycystic ovarian syndrome. *J Pediatr* 2001;138(1):38.
23. Barbieri RL, Makris A, Randall RW, et al. Insulin stimulates androgen accumulation in incubations of ovarian stroma obtained from women with hyperandrogenism. *J Clin Endocrinol Metab* 1986; 62:905.
24. Barbieri RE. Hyperandrogenism, insulin resistance and acanthosis nigricans. 10 years of progress. *J Reprod Med* 1994;39:327.
25. Morales AJ, Laughlin GA, Butzow T, et al. Insulin, somatotropic, and luteinizing hormone axes in lean and obese women with polycystic ovary syndrome: common and distinct features. *J Clin Endocrinol Metab* 1996;81:2854.
26. Rosenfield RL, Ghai K, Ehrmann DA, et al. Diagnosis of the polycystic ovary syndrome in adolescence: comparison of adolescent and adult hyperandrogenism. *J Pediatr Endocrinol* 2000; 13[Suppl 5]:1285.
27. Gordon CN. Menstrual disorders in adolescents: excess androgens and the polycystic ovary syndrome. *Pediatr Clin North Am* 1999;46:519.
28. Nestler JE, Jakubowicz DJ. Decreases in ovarian cytochrome P450$c17\alpha$ activity and serum free testosterone after reduction of insulin secretion in polycystic ovary syndrome. *N Engl J Med* 1996;335:617.
29. Loverro G, Lorusso F, De Pergola G, et al. Clinical and endocrinological effects of 6 months of metformin treatment in young hyperinsulinemic patients affected by polycystic ovary syndrome. *Gynecol Endocrinol* 2002;16(3):217.
30. Dunaif A, Scott D, Finegood D, et al. The insulin sensitizing agent troglitazone: a novel therapy for polycystic ovary syndrome. *J Clin Endocrinol Metab* 1996;81:3299.
31. Poretsky L, Piper B. Insulin resistance, hypersecretion of LH, and a dual-defect hypothesis for the pathogenesis of polycystic ovary syndrome. *Obstet Gynecol* 1994;84:613.
32. Fox JH, Licholai T, Green G, et al. Differential effects of oral glucose-mediated versus intravenous hyperinsulinemia on circulating androgen levels in women. *Fertil Steril* 1993;60:994.
33. Buyalos RP, Geffner ME, Watanabe RM, et al. The influence of luteinizing hormone and insulin on sex steroids and sex hormone-binding globulin in the polycystic ovarian syndrome. *Fertil Steril* 1993;60:626.
34. Dunaif A. Insulin resistance and the polycystic ovary syndrome: mechanism and implications for pathogenesis. *Endocr Rev* 1997;18:774.
35. Venkatesan AM, Dunaif A, Corbould A. Insulin resistance in polycystic ovary syndrome: progress and paradoxes. *Recent Prog Horm Res* 2001;56:295.
36. Grasinger CC, Wild RA, Parker IJ. Vulvar acanthosis nigricans: a marker for insulin resistance in hirsute women. *Fertil Steril* 1993;59:583.
37. Barbieri RL, Ryan KJ. Hyperandrogenism, insulin resistance, acanthosis nigricans: a common endocrinopathy with unique pathophysiologic features. *Am J Obstet Gynecol* 1983;147:90.
38. Legro RS, Kunselman AR, Dodson WC, et al. Prevalence and predictors of risk for type 2 diabetes mellitus and impaired glucose tolerance in polycystic ovary syndrome: a prospective controlled study in 254 affected women. *J Clin Endocrinol Metab* 1999;84:165.
39. Ehrmann DA, Barnes RB, Rosenfield RL. Prevalence of impaired glucose tolerance and diabetes in women with polycystic ovary syndrome. *Diabetes Care* 1999;222:141.
40. Weerakiet S, Srisombut C, Bunnag P, et al. Prevalence of type 2 diabetes mellitus and impaired glucose tolerance in Asian women with polycystic ovary syndrome. *Intl J Gynaecol Obstet* 2001; 75:177.
41. Palmert MR, Gordon CM, Kartashov AI, Legro RS, Emans SJ, Dunaif A. Screening for abnormal glucose tolerance in adolescents with polycystic ovary syndrome. *J Clin Endocrinol Metab* 2002;87:1017.
42. Norman RJ, Masters L, Milner CR, et al. Relative risk of conversion from normoglycaemia to impaired glucose tolerance or non-insulin-dependent diabetes mellitus in polycystic ovarian syndrome. *Hum Reprod* 2001;16:1995.
43. Peppard HR, MarforiIuorno MJ, et al. Prevalence of polycystic ovary syndrome among premenopausal women with type 2 diabetes. *Diabetes Care* 2001;24(6):1050.

44. Escobar-Morreale HF, Roldan B, Barrio R, et al. High prevalence of the polycystic ovary syndrome and hirsutism in women with type 1 diabetes mellitus. *J Clin Endocrinol Metab* 2000;85(11):4182.
45. Conn JJ, Jacobs HS, Conway GS. The prevalence of polycystic ovaries in women with type 2 diabetes mellitus. *Clin Endocrinol* 2000;52(1):81.
46. Legro RS. Diabetes prevalence and risk factors in polycystic ovary syndrome. *Obstet Gynecol Clin North Am* 2001;28(1):99.
47. Smith S, Ravnikar VA, Barbieri RL. Androgen and insulin response to an oral glucose challenge in hyperandrogenic women. *Fertil Steril* 1987;48:72.
48. Geffner ME, Kaplan SA, Bersch N, et al. Persistence of insulin resistance in polycystic ovarian disease after inhibition of ovarian steroid secretion. *Fertil Steril* 1986;45:327.
49. Wild S, Pierpoint T, McKeigue P, et al. Cardiovascular disease in women with polycystic ovary syndrome at long-term follow-up: a retrospective cohort study. *Clin Endocrinol* 2000; 52(5):595.
50. Wild RA. Polycystic ovary syndrome: a risk for coronary artery disease? *Am J Obstet Gynecol* 2002;186(1):35.
51. Solomon CG. The epidemiology of polycystic ovary syndrome. Prevalence and associated disease risks. *Endocrinol Metab Clin North Am* 1999;28(2):247.
52. Wild RA, Alaupovic P, Givens JR, et al. Lipoprotein abnormalities in hirsute women. *Am J Obstet Gynecol* 1992;167:1813.
53. Arslanian SA, Lewy VD, Danadian K. Glucose intolerance in obese adolescents with polycystic ovary syndrome: roles of insulin resistance and beta-cell dysfunction and risk of cardiovascular disease. *J Clin Endocrinol Metab* 2001;86(1):66.
54. Veldhuis JD, Pincus SM, Garcia-Rudaz MC, et al. Disruption of the synchronous secretion of leptin, LH, and ovarian androgens in nonobese adolescents with the polycystic ovary syndrome. *J Clin Endocrinol Metab* 2001;86:3772.
55. Telli MH, Yildirim M, Noyan V. Serum leptin levels in patients with polycystic ovary syndrome. *Fertil Steril* 2002;77(5):932.
56. Gross MD, Wortsman J, Shapiro B, et al. Scintigraphic evidence of adrenal cortical dysfunction in polycystic ovary syndrome. *J Clin Endocrinol Metab* 1986;62:197.
57. Lucky AN, Rosenfield RL, McGuire J, et al. Adrenal androgen hyperresponsiveness to adreno-corticotropin in women with acne and/or hirsutism: adrenal enzyme defects and exaggerated adrenarche. *J Clin Endocrinol Metab* 1986;62:840.
58. Moran C, Azziz R. The role of the adrenal cortex in polycystic ovary syndrome. *Obstet Gynecol* 2001;28:63.
59. Ditkoff EC, Fruzzetti F, Chang L, et al. The impact of estrogen on adrenal androgen sensitivity and secretion in polycystic ovary syndrome. *J Clin Endocrinol Metab* 1995;80:603.
60. Carmina E, Gonzalez F, Chang L, et al. Reassessment of adrenal androgen secretion in women with polycystic ovary syndrome. *Obstet Gynecol* 1995;85:971.
61. Ibanez L, Potau N, Zampolli M, et al. Hyperinsulinemia and decreased insulin-like growth factor-binding protein-1 are common features in prepubertal girls with a history of premature pubarche. *J Clin Endocrinol Metab* 1997;82(7):2283.
62. Silfen ME, Manibo AM, Ferin M, et al. Elevated free IGF-I levels in prepubertal Hispanic girls with premature adrenarche: relationship with hyperandrogenism and insulin sensitivity. *J Clin Endocrinol Metab* 2002;87:398.
63. Battaglia C, Regnani G, Mancini F, et al. Isolated premature pubarche: ultrasonographic and color Doppler analysis—a longitudinal study. *J Clin Endocrinol Metab* 2002;87(7):3148.
64. Seminara SB, Crowley WF Jr. Genetic approaches to unraveling reproductive disorders: examples of bedside to bench research in the genomic era. *Endocr Rev* 2002;23(3):382.
65. Legro RS, Driscoll D, Strauss JF, et al. Evidence for a genetic basis for hyperandrogenemia in polycystic ovary syndrome. *Proc Natl Acad Sci* 1998;95:14956.
66. Legro RS, Kunselman AR, Demers L, et al. Elevated dehydroepiandrosterone sulfate levels as the reproductive phenotype in the brothers of women with polycystic ovary syndrome. *J Clin Endocrinol Metabol* 2002;87:2134.
67. Franks S. Polycystic ovary syndrome. *N Engl J Med* 1995;333:853.
68. Adams J, Polson DW, Franks S. Prevalence of polycystic ovaries in women with anovulation and idiopathic hirsutism. *Br Med J* 1986;293;355.
69. Brook C, Jacob H, Stanhope R. Polycystic ovaries in childhood. *Br Med J* 1988;296:878.

70. Stanhope R, Adams J, Brook C. Evolution of polycystic ovaries in a girl with delayed menarche. *J Reprod Med* 1988;33:482.
71. Fulghesu AM, Ciampelli M, Belosi C, et al. A new ultrasound criterion for the diagnosis of polycystic ovary syndrome: the ovarian stroma/total area ratio. *Fertil Steril* 2001;76(2):326.
72. Silfen M, Denburg MR, Manibo AM, et al. Early endocrine, metabolic, and sonographic characteristics of polycystic ovary syndrome (PCOS): comparison between nonobese and obese adolescents. *J Clin Endocrinol Metab* 2003;88:4682.
73. Conway GS, Honour JW, Jacobs HS. Heterogeneity of the polycystic ovary syndrome: clinical, endocrine, and ultrasound features in 556 patients. *Clin Endocrinol (Oxf)* 1989;30:459.
74. Michelmore KF, Balen AH, Dunger DB, et al. Polycystic ovaries and associated clinical and biochemical features in young women. *Clin Endocrinol* 1999;51(6):779.
75. Kaltsas GA, Korbonits M, Isidori AM, et al. Ultrasound criteria in the diagnosis of polycystic ovary syndrome (PCOS). *Ultrasound Med Biol* 2000;26(6):977.
76. Nardo LG, Buckett WM, White D, et al. Three-dimensional assessment of ultrasound features in women with clomiphene citrate-resistant polycystic ovarian syndrome (PCOS): ovarian stromal volume does not correlate with biochemical indices. *Hum Reprod* 2002;17(4):1052.
77. Atiomo WU, Pearson S, Shaw S, et al. Ultrasound criteria in the diagnosis of polycystic ovary syndrome (PCOS). *Ultrasound Med Biol* 2000;26(6):977.
78. Cronin L, Guyatt G, Griffith L, et al. Development of a health-related quality-of-life questionnaire (PCOSQ) for women with polycystic ovary syndrome (PCOS) *J Clin Endocrinol Metab* 1998;83:1976.
79. Trent ME, Rich M, Austin SB, et al. Quality of life in adolescent girls with polycystic ovary syndrome. *Arch Pediatr Adolesc Med* 2002;156:556.
80. Trent M, Rich M, Austin SB, et al. Fertility concerns and sexual behavior in adolescent girls with polycystic ovary syndrome: implications for quality of life. *J Pediatr Adolesc Gynecol* 2003;16:33.
81. ACOG. Evaluation and treatment of hirsute women. *Tech Bull* 1995;203:1.
82. McKnight E. The prevalence of "hirsutism" in young women. *Lancet* 1964;1:410.
83. Ferriman D, Gallwey JD. Clinical assessment of body hair growth in women. *J Clin Endocrinol Metab* 1961;21:1440.
84. Carmina E, Lobo RA. Polycystic ovaries in hirsute women with normal menses. *Am J Med* 2001;111(8):602.
85. Isojarvi JIT, Laatikainen TJ, Pakarinen AJ, et al. Polycystic ovaries and hyperandrogenism in women taking valproate for epilepsy. *N Engl J Med* 1993;329:1383.
86. Bauer J, Jarre A, Klingmuller D, et al. Polycystic ovary syndrome in patients with focal epilepsy: a study in 93 women. *Epilepsy Res* 2000;41(2):163.
87. Luef G, Abraham I, Trinka E, et al. Hyperandrogenism, postprandial hyperinsulinism and the risk of PCOS in a cross sectional study of women with epilepsy treated with valproate. *Epilepsy Res* 2002;48(1,2):91.
88. Siegberg R, Nilsson CG, Stenman UH, et al. Endocrinologic features of oligomenorrheic adolescent girls. *Fertil Steril* 1986;46:852.
89. Avvad CK, Holeuwerger R, Silva VC, et al. Menstrual irregularity in the first postmenarcheal years: an early clinical sign of polycystic ovary syndrome in adolescence. *Gynecol Endocrinol* 2001;15(3):170.
90. van Hooff MH, Voorhorst FJ, Kaptein MB, et al. Endocrine features of polycystic ovary syndrome in a random population sample of 14–16 year old adolescents. *Hum Reprod* 1999;14(9):2223.
91. Apter D, Bützow T, Laughlin GA, et al. Metabolic features of polycystic ovary syndrome are found in adolescent girls with hyperandrogenism. *J Clin Endocrinol Metab* 1995;80(10):2966.
92. Witchel SF. Hyperandrogenism in adolescents. *Adolescent Med: STARS* 2002;13:89.
93. Rosenfield RL. Studies of the relation of plasma androgen levels to androgen action in women. *J Steroid Biochem* 1975;6:695.
94. Nelson VL, Qin K, Rosenfield RL, et al. The biochemical basis for increased testosterone production in theca cells propagated from patients with polycystic ovary syndrome. *J Clin Endocrinol Metab* 2001;86:5925.
95. Blankenstein J, Faiman C, Reyes F, et al. Adult onset familial adrenal hyperplasia due to incomplete 21-hydroxylase deficiency. *Am J Med* 1980;68:441.

96. Lobo RA, Goeblesmann U. Adult manifestation of congenital adrenal hyperplasia due to incomplete 21-hydroxylase deficiency mimicking polycystic ovary disease. *Am J Obstet Gynecol* 1980;138:720.

97. Migeon CJ, Rosewaks Z, Lee P, et al. The attenuated form of 21-hydroxylase deficiency as an allelic form of 21-hydroxylase deficiency. *J Clin Endocrinol Metab* 1980;51:647.

98. Kohn B, Levine LS, Pollack MS, et al. Late-onset steroid 21-hydroxylase deficiency: a variant of classical congenital adrenal hyperplasia. *J Clin Endocrinol Metab* 1982;55:817.

99. Emans SJ, Grace E, Fleischnick E, et al. Detection of late-onset 21-hydroxylase deficiency congenital adrenal hyperplasia in adolescents. *Pediatrics* 1983;72:690.

100. Benjamin F, Deutsch S, Saperstein H, et al. Prevalence of and markers for the attenuated form of congenital adrenal hyperplasia and hyperprolactinemia masquerading as polycystic ovarian disease. *Fertil Steril* 1986;46:215.

101. Eldar-Geva T, Hurwitz A, Vecsei P, et al. Secondary biosynthetic defects in women with late-onset congenital adrenal hyperplasia. *N Engl J Med* 1990;323:855.

102. Speiser PW, White PC. Congenital adrenal hyperplasia. *N Engl J Med* 2003;349:776.

103. Miller WL. Genetics, diagnosis, and management of 21-hydroxylase deficiency. *J Clin Endocrinol Metab* 1994;78:241.

104. Speiser PW, New MI. Genotype and hormonal phenotype in nonclassical 21-hydroxylase deficiency. *J Clin Endocrinol Metab* 1987;64:86.

105. Speiser PW, New MI, White PC. Molecular genetic analysis of nonclassic steroid 21-hydroxylase deficiency associated with HLA-B14, DR1. *N Engl J Med* 1988;319:19.

106. Siegel SF, Lee PA, Rudert WA, et al. Phenotype/genotype correlation in 21-hydroxylase deficiency. *Adolesc Pediatr Gynecol* 1995;8:9.

107. Moran C, Azziz R, Carmina E, et al. 21-Hydroxylase-deficient nonclassic adrenal hyperplasia is a progressive disorder: a multicenter study. *Am J Obstet Gynecol* 2000;183:1468.

108. New MI, Franzieska L, Lerner AJ, et al. Genotyping steroid 21-hydroxylase deficiency: hormonal reference data. *J Clin Endocrinol Metab* 1983;57:320.

109. Zerah M, Pang S, New MI. Morning salivary 17-hydroxyprogesterone is useful screening test for nonclassical 21-hydroxylase deficiency. *J Clin Endocrinol Metab* 1987;65:227.

110. Azziz R, Zacur HA. 21-Hydroxylase deficiency in female hyperandrogenism: screening and diagnosis. *J Clin Endocrinol Metab* 1989;69:577.

111. Azziz R, Bradley EL Jr, Potter HD, et al. 3β-hydroxysteroid dehydrogenase deficiency in hyperandrogenism. *Am J Obstet Gynecol* 1993;168:889.

112. Mathieson J, Couzinet B, Wekstein-Noel S, et al. The incidence of late-onset congenital adrenal hyperplasia due to 3β-hydroxysteroid dehydrogenase deficiency among hirsute women. *Clin Endocrinol* 1992;36:383.

113. Carbunaru G, Prasad P, Scoccio B, et al. The hormonal phenotype of nonclassic 3β-hydroxysteroid dehydrogenase (HSD3β) deficiency in hyperandrogenic female is associated with insulin-resistant polycystic ovary syndrome and is not a variant of inherited HSD3B2 deficiency. *J Clin Endocrinol Metab* 2004;89:783.

114. Pang S, Softness B, Sweeney WJ, et al. Hirsutism, polycystic ovarian disease, and ovarian 17-ketosteroid reductase deficiency. *N Engl J Med* 1987;316:1295.

115. Cathelineau G, Brerault JL, Fier J, et al. Adrenocortical 11α-hydroxylation defect in adult women with postmenarchial onset of symptoms. *J Clin Endocrinol Metab* 1980;51:345.

116. Lee PA, Migeon CJ, Bias WB, et al. Familial hypersecretion of adrenal androgens transmitted as a dominant, non-HLA-linked trait. *Obstet Gynecol* 1987;69:259.

117. Lee PDK, Winter RJ, Green OC. Virilizing adrenocortical tumors in childhood: eight cases and a review of the literature. *Pediatrics* 1985;76:437.

118. Chetkowski RJ, Judd HL, Jagger PI, et al. Autonomous cortisol secretion by a lipoid cell tumor of the ovary. *JAMA* 1985;254:2628.

119. Lucky AW, Biro FM, Simbarti LA, et al. Predictors of severity of acne vulgaris in young adolescent girls: results of a five year longitudinal study. *J Pediatr* 1997;130:30.

120. Fogel RB, Malhotra A, Pillar G et al. Increased prevalence of obstructive sleep apnea syndrome in obese women with polycystic ovary syndrome. *J Clin Endocrinol Metab* 2001;86:1175.

121. Bardin CW, Lipsett MB. Testosterone and androstenedione blood production rates in normal women and women with idiopathic hirsutism or PCOS. *J Clin Invest* 1967;46:891.

122. Doshi A, Zaheer A, Stiller M. A comparison of current acne grading systems and proposal of a novel system. *Intl J Derm* 1997;36:416.
123. Rosenfield RL. Hyperandrogenism in peripubertal girls. *Pediatr Clin North Am* 1990;37:1333.
124. Corenblum B, Kwan T, Gee S, et al. Bedside assessment of skin-fold thickness: a useful measurement for distinguishing Cushing's disease from other causes of hirsutism and oligomenorrhea. *Arch Intern Med* 1994;154:777.
125. Reingold SB, Rosenfield RL. The relationship of mild hirsutism or acne in women to androgens. *Arch Dermatol* 1987;123:209.
126. Anttila L, Koskinen P, Kaihola H-L, et al. Serum androgen and gonadotropin levels decline after progestogen-induced withdrawal bleeding in oligomenorrheic women with or without polycystic ovaries. *Fertil Steril* 1992;58:697.
127. Turhan NO, Toppare MF, Seckin NC, et al. The predictive power of endocrine tests for the diagnosis of polycystic ovaries in women with oligomenorrhea. *Gynecol Obstet Invest* 1999; 48(3):183.
128. Escobar-Morreale HF, Asuncion M, Calvo RM, et al. Receiver operating characteristic analysis of the performance of basal serum hormone profiles for the diagnosis of polycystic ovary syndrome in epidemiological studies. *Eur J Endocrinol* 2001;145(5):619.
129. Derksen J, Nagesser SK, Meinders AE, et al. Identification of virilizing adrenal tumors in hirsute women. *N Engl J Med* 1994;331:968.
130. Pang S, Lerner A, Stoner E, et al. Late-onset adrenal steroid 3β-hydroxysteroid dehydrogenase deficiency. I. A cause of hirsutism in pubertal and postpubertal women. *J Clin Endocrinol Metab* 1985;60:428.
131. Legro RS, Kunselman AR, Dunaif A. Prevalence and predictors of dyslipidemia in women with polycystic ovary syndrome. *Am J Med* 2001;111(8):607.
132. Mather KJ, Kwan F, Corenblum B. Hyperinsulinemia in polycystic ovary syndrome correlates with increased cardiovascular risk independent of obesity. *Fertil Steril* 2000;73(1):150.
133. Silfen ME, Manibo AM, McMahon DJ, et al. Comparison of simple measure of insulin sensitivity in young girls with premature adrenarche: the fasting glucose to insulin ratio may be a simple and useful measure. *J Clin Endocrinol Metab* 2001;86:2863.
134. Kent SC, Legro RS. Polycystic ovary syndrome in adolescents. *Adolescent Med: STARS* 2002; 13(1):73.
135. Paulson RJ, Serafini PC, Catalino JA, et al. Measurements of 3α, 17β-androstanediol glucuronide in serum and urine and the correlation with skin 5α-reductase activity. *Fertil Steril* 1986;46:222.
136. Kirschner MA, Samojlik E, Szmal E. Clinical usefulness of plasma androstanediol glucuronide measurements in women with idiopathic hirsutism. *J Clin Endocrinol Metab* 1987;65:597.
137. Glass AR, Dahms WT, Abraham GE. Secondary amenorrhea in obesity: etiologic role of weight related androgen excess. *Fertil Steril* 1978;30:243.
138. Harlass FE, Plymate SR, Fariss BL. Weight loss is associated with correction of gonadotropin and sex steroid abnormalities in the obese anovulatory female. *Fertil Steril* 1984;42:649.
139. Hosseinian AH, Kim MH, Rosenfield C. Obesity and oligomenorrhea are associated with hyperandrogenism independent of hirsutism. *J Clin Endocrinol Metab* 1976;42:765.
140. Pasquali R, Antenucci D, Casimirri F, et al. Clinical and hormonal characteristics of obese and amenorrheic hyperandrogenic women before and after weight loss. *J Clin Endocrinol Metab* 1989; 68:173.
141. Guzick DS, Wing R, Smith D, et al. Endocrine consequences of weight loss in obese, hyperandrogenic, anovulatory women. *Fertil Steril* 1994;61:598.
142. Diabetes Prevention Program Research Group. Reduction in the incidence of type 2 diabetes with lifestyle intervention or metformin. *N Engl J Med* 2002;346:393.
143. Ludwig, DS. The glycemic index: Physiological mechanisms relating to obesity, diabetes, and cardiovascular disease. *JAMA* 2002;287(18):2414.
144. Bagis T, Gokcel A, Zeyneloglu HB, et al. The effects of short-term medroxyprogesterone acetate and micronized progesterone on glucose metabolism and lipid profiles in patients with polycystic ovary syndrome: a prospective randomized study. *J Clin Endocrinol Metab* 2002;87(10):4536.
145. Ruchhoft EA, Elkind-Hirsch KE, Malinak R. Pituitary function is altered during the same cycle in women with polycystic ovary syndrome treated with continuous or cyclic oral contraceptives or a gonadotropin-releasing hormone agonist. *Fertil Steril* 1996;66:54.
146. Emans SJ, Grace E, Woods ER, et al. Treatment with dexamethasone of androgen excess in adolescent patients. *J Pediatr* 1988;112:821.

147. Nappi C, Farace MJ, Leone F, et al. Effect of a combination of ethinyl estradiol and desogestrel in adolescent with oligomenorrhea and ovarian hyperandrogenism. *Eur J Obstet Gynecol Reprod Biol* 1987;25:209.

148. Jung-Hoffmann C, Kuhl H. Divergent effects of two low-dose oral contraceptives on sex hormone binding globulin and free testosterone. *Am J Obstet Gynecol* 1987;156:199.

149. Wiebe RH, Morris CV Effect of an oral contraceptive on adrenal and ovarian androgenic steroids. *Obstet Gynecol* 1984;63:12.

150. Cibula D, Sindelka G, Hill M, et al. Insulin sensitivity in non-obese women with polycystic ovary syndrome during treatment with oral contraceptives containing low-androgenic progestin. *Hum Reprod* 2002;17(1):76.

151. Armstrong VL, Wiggam MI, Ennis CN, et al. Insulin action and insulin secretion in polycystic ovary syndrome treated with ethinyl oestradiol/cyproterone acetate. *QJM* 2001;94(1):31.

152. Holt VL, Cushing-Haugen KL, Daling JR. Body weight and risk of oral contraceptive failure. *Obstet Gynecol* 2002;99(5):820.

153. Cibula D, Hill M, Fanta M, et al. Does obesity diminish the positive effect of oral contraceptive treatment on hyperandrogenism in women with polycystic ovarian syndrome? *Hum Reprod* 2001; 16(5):940.

154. Shapiro G, Evron S. A novel use of spironolactone: treatment of hirsutism. *J Clin Endocrinol Metab* 1980;51:429.

155. Cumming DC, Yang JC, Rebar RW, et al. Treatment of hirsutism with spironolactone. *JAMA* 1982;247:1295.

156. Helfer EL, Miller JL, Rose LI. Side-effects of spironolactone therapy in the hirsute woman. *J Clin Endocrinol Metab* 1988;66:208.

157. Lumachi F, Rondinone R. Use of cyproterone acetate, finasteride, and spironolactone to treat idiopathic hirsutism. *Fertil Steril* 2003;79:942.

158. O'Brien RC, Cooper ME, Murray RM, et al. Comparison of sequential cyproterone acetate/estrogen versus spironolactone/oral contraceptive in the treatment of hirsutism. *J Clin Endocrinol Metab* 1991;72:1008.

159. Wong IL, Morris RS, Ghang L, et al. A prospective randomized trial comparing finasteride to spironolactone in the treatment of hirsute women. *J Clin Endocrinol Metab* 1995;80:233.

160. Erenus M, Gurbuz O, Durmusoglu F, et al. Comparison of the efficacy of spironolactone versus flutamide in the treatment of hirsutism. *Fertil Steril* 1994;61:613.

161. Cusan L, Dupont A, Gomez JL, et al. Comparison of flutamide and spironolactone in the treatment of hirsutism: A randomized controlled trial. *Fertil Steril* 1994;61:281.

162. Wysowski DK, Fireman, Tourtelot JB, et al. Fatal and nonfatal hepatotoxicity associated with flutamide. *Ann Intern Med* 1993;118:860.

163. Lord JM, Flight IH, Norman RJ. Metformin in polycystic ovary syndrome: systematic review and meta-analysis. *BMJ* 2003;327:951.

164. Taylor AE. Insulin-lowering medications in polycystic ovary syndrome. *Obstet Gynecol Clin North Am* 2000;27(3):583.

165. Pasquali R, Gambineri A, Biscotti D, et al. Effect of long-term treatment with metformin added to hypocaloric diet on body composition, fat distribution, and androgen and insulin levels in abdominally obese women with and without the polycystic ovary syndrome. *J Clin Endocrinol Metabol* 2000;85(8):2767.

166. Glueck CJ, Wang P, Fontaine R, et al. Metformin-induced resumption of normal menses in 39 of 43 (91%) previously amenorrheic women with the polycystic ovary syndrome. *Metabolism* 1999; 48(4):511.

167. Nestler JE, Stovall D, Akhter N, et al. Strategies for the use of insulin-sensitizing drugs to treat infertility in women with polycystic ovary syndrome. *Fertil Steril* 2002;77(2):209.

168. Elter K, Imir G, Durmusoglu F. Clinical, endocrine and metabolic effects of metformin added to ethinyl estradiol-cyproterone acetate in non-obese women with polycystic ovarian syndrome: a randomized controlled study. *Human Reprod* 2002;17:1729.

169. Awartani KA, Cheung AP. Metformin and polycystic ovary syndrome: a literature review. *J Obstet Gynaecol Canada* 2002;24(5):393.

170. Kolodziejczyk B, Duleba AJ, Spaczynski RZ, et al. Metformin therapy decreases hyperandrogenism and hyperinsulinemia in women with polycystic ovary syndrome. *Fertil Steril* 2000;73(6):1149.

171. Fulghesu AM, Ciampelli M, Muzj, et al. *N*-acetyl-cysteine treatment improves insulin sensitivity in women with polycystic ovary syndrome. *Fertil Steril* 2002;77(6):1128.

172. Ciotta L, Calogero AE, Farina M, et al. Clinical, endocrine and metabolic effects of acarbose, an alpha-glucosidase inhibitor, in PCOS patients with increased insulin response and normal glucose tolerance. *Hum Reprod* 2001;16(10):2066.

173. Nestler JE, Jukubowicz DJ, Reamer P, et al. Ovulatory and metabolic effects of D-chiro-inositol in the polycystic ovary syndrome. *N Engl J Med* 1999;340:1314.

174. Azziz R, Ehrmann D, Legro RS, et al. PCOS/Troglitazone Study Group. Troglitazone improves ovulation and hirsutism in the polycystic ovary syndrome: a multicenter, double blind, placebo-controlled trial. *J Clin Endocrinol Metab* 2001;86(4):1626.

175. Freemark M, Bursey D. The effects of metformin on body mass index and glucose tolerance in obese adolescents with fasting hyperinsulinemia and a family history of type 2 diabetes. *Pediatrics* 2001;107:E55.

176. Ibanez L, Valls C, Ferrer A, et al. Sensitization to insulin induces ovulation in nonobese adolescent with anovulatory hyperandrogenism. *J Clin Endocrinol Metab* 2001;86:3595.

177. Glueck CJ, Wang P, Fontaine R, et al. Metformin to restore normal menses in oligo-amenorrheic teenage girls with polycystic ovary syndrome (PCOS). *J Adolesc Health* 2001;29(3):160.

178. Arslanian SA, Lewy V, Danadian K, et al. Metformin therapy in obese adolescents with polycystic ovary syndrome and impaired glucose tolerance: amelioration of exaggerated adrenal response to adrenocorticotropin with reduction of insulinemia/insulin resistance. *J Clin Endocrinol Metab* 2002;87(4):1555.

179. la Marca A, Morgante G, Paglia T, et al. Effects of metformin on adrenal steroidogenesis in women with polycystic ovary syndrome. *Fertil Steril* 1999;72(6):985.

180. Vrbikova J, Hill M, Starka L, et al. Prediction of the effect of metformin treatment in patients with polycystic ovary syndrome. *Gynecol Obstet Invest* 2002;53(2):100.

181. Moghetti P, Castello R, Negri C, et al. Metformin effects on clinical features, endocrine and metabolic profiles, and insulin sensitivity in polycystic ovary syndrome: a randomized, double blind, placebo controlled 6-month trial, followed by open, long-term clinical evaluation. *J Clin Endocrinol Metab* 2000;85:139.

182. Carr BR, Breslau NA, Givens C, et al. Oral contraceptive pills, gonadotropin-releasing hormone agonists, or use in combination for treatment of hirsutism: a clinical research center study. *J Clin Endocrinol Metab* 1995;80:1169.

183. Falsetti L, Pasinetti E. Treatment of moderate and severe hirsutism by gonadotropin-releasing hormone agonists in women with polycystic ovary syndrome and idiopathic hirsutism. *Fertil Steril* 1994;61:817.

184. Morcos RN, Abdul-Malak ME, Shikora E. Treatment of hirsutism with a gonadotropin-releasing hormone agonist and estrogen replacement therapy. *Fertil Steril* 1994;61:427.

185. Carmina E, Janni A, Lobo RA. Physiological estrogen replacement may enhance the effectiveness of the gonadotropin-releasing hormone agonist in the treatment of hirsutism. *J Clin Endocrinol Metab* 1994;78:126.

186. Elkind-Hirsch KE, Anania C, Mack M, et al. Combination gonadotropin-releasing hormone agonist and oral contraceptive therapy improves treatment of hirsute women with ovarian hyperandrogenism. *Fertil Steril* 1995;63:970.

187. Szilagyi A, Homoki J, Bellyei S, et al. Hormonal and clinical effects of chronic gonadotropin-releasing hormone agonist treatment in polycystic ovary syndrome. *Gynecol Endocrinol* 2000; 14(5):337.

188. Genazzani AD, Battaglia C, Gamba O, et al. The use of a combined regimen of GnRH agonist plus a low-dose oral contraceptive improves the spontaneous pulsatile LH secretory characteristics in patients with polycystic ovary disease after discontinuation of treatment. *J Assisted Reprod Genet* 2000;17(5):269.

189. Rittmaster RS, Thompson DL. Effect of leuprolide and dexamethasone on hair growth and hormone levels in hirsute women: the relative importance of the ovary and the adrenal in the pathogenesis of hirsutism. *J Clin Endocrinol Metab* 1990;70:1096.

190. El Tabbakh GH, Loutfi IA, Azab I, et al. Bromocriptine in polycystic ovarian disease: a controlled clinical trial. *Obstet Gynecol* 1988;71:301.

191. Steingold KA, Lobo RA, Judd HL, et al. The effect of bromocriptine on gonadotropin and steroid secretion in polycystic ovarian disease. *J Clin Endocrinol Metab* 1986;62:1048.

192. Hagag P, Hertzianu I, Ben-Shlomo A, et al. Androgen suppression and clinical improvement with dopamine agonists in hyperandrogenic-hyperprolactinemic women. *J Repro Med* 2001;45:678.

193. Loughlin T, Cunningham S, Moore A, et al. Adrenal abnormalities in polycystic ovary syndrome. *J Clin Endocrinol Metab* 1986;62:142.
194. Azziz R, Black VY, Knochenhauer ES, et al. Ovulation after glucocorticoid suppression of adrenal androgens in the polycystic ovary syndrome is not predicted by the basal dehydroepiandrosterone sulfate level. *J Clin Endocrinol Metab* 1999;84(3):946.
195. Carmina E, Lobo RA. Ovarian suppression reduces clinical and endocrine expression of late-onset congenital adrenal hyperplasia due to 21-hydroxylase deficiency. *Fertil Steril* 1994;62:738.
196. Spritzer P, Billaud L, Thalabard J-C, et al. Cyproterone acetate versus hydrocortisone treatment in late-onset adrenal hyperplasia. *J Clin Endocrinol Metab* 1990;70:642.
197. Wagner RF Jr, Flores CA, Argo LE. A double blind placebo controlled study of a 5% lidocaine/prilocaine cream (EMLA) for topical anesthesia during thermolysis. *J Dermatol Surg Oncol* 1994;20:148.
198. Vandermolen DT, Ratts VS, Evans WS, et al. Metformin increases the ovulatory rate and pregnancy rate from clomiphene citrate in patients with polycystic ovary syndrome who are resistant to clomiphene citrate alone. *Fertil Steril* 2001;75(2):310.
199. Iuorno MJ, Nestler JE. Insulin-lowering drugs in polycystic ovary syndrome. *Obstet Gynecol Clin North Am* 2001;28(1):153.
200. Glueck CJ, Wang P, Kobayashi S, et al. Metformin therapy throughout pregnancy reduces the development of gestational diabetes in women with polycystic ovary syndrome. *Fertil Steril* 2002; 77(3):520.
201. Donesky BW, Adashi EY. Surgically induced ovulation in the polycystic ovary syndrome: wedge resection revisited in the age of laparoscopy. *Fertil Steril* 1995;63:439.
202. Heylen SM, Puttermans PJ, Brosens IA. Polycystic ovarian disease treated by laparoscopic organ laser capsule drilling: comparison of vaporization versus perforation technique. *Hum Report* 1994: 9:1038.
203. Balen AH, Jacobs HS. A prospective study comparing unilateral and bilateral laparoscopic ovarian diathermy in women with polycystic ovary syndrome. *Fertil Steril* 1994;62:921.
204. Farquhar C, Vandekerckhove P, Lilford R. Laparoscopic "drilling" by diathermy or laser for ovulation induction in anovulatory polycystic ovary syndrome. *Cochrane Database of Systematic Reviews* 2001;(4):CD001122.
205. Pirwany I, Tulandi T. Laparoscopic treatment of polycystic ovaries: is it time to relinquish the procedure? *Fertil Steril* 2003;80:241.

Additional Reading

The Rotterdam ESHRE/ASRM-sponsored PCOS consensus workshop group. Revised 2003 consensus on diagnostic criteria and long-term health risks related to polycystic ovary syndrome. *Fertil Steril* 2004;81:19.

10

Structural Abnormalities of the Female Reproductive Tract

Marc R. Laufer, Donald P. Goldstein, and W. Hardy Hendren

The development of the female reproductive tract is a complex process that involves cellular differentiation, migration, fusion, and canalization with probable apoptosis (programmed cell death). This integrated series of events creates numerous possibilities for abnormal development and anomalies. Structural anomalies of the female reproductive tract become apparent at varying chronologic times during life, and the diagnosis and treatment may not be straightforward. Most anomalies involving the external genitalia are apparent at birth (see Chapter 2), while obstructive and nonobstructive anomalies of the reproductive tract can be apparent at birth, during childhood, puberty, menarche, adolescence, or later in adult life.

In this chapter, the normal embryologic development of the female reproductive tract will be presented, followed by anatomic and clinical descriptions of developmental anomalies. Anomalies of the reproductive tract can be remembered with the assistance of the pneumonic: C.A.F.E., which stands for canalization, agenesis, fusion, and embryonic rests. These congenital anomalies result from defects of lateral and vertical fusion of the urogenital sinus and müllerian duct systems. In addition, the diagnosis, management, and treatment of developmental and acquired structural disorders of the labia and vulva, such as labial hypertrophy, clitoral hood scarring/clitoral entrapment, and ritual female "circumcision"/mutilation, will be discussed.

The diagnosis, management, and surgical treatments of all female reproductive tract anomalies have changed with improvements in diagnostic imaging techniques, surgical and nonsurgical techniques and instrumentation, and the rapidly expanding field of reproductive medicine and assisted reproductive technologies. Long-term follow-up of the differing structural anomalies will be presented in relation to body image, patient satisfaction, and sexual and reproductive function.

NORMAL DEVELOPMENTAL EMBRYOLOGY OF THE REPRODUCTIVE TRACT

The development of the female genital tract begins at 3 weeks of embryogenesis and continues into the second trimester of pregnancy. During the first 3 months of embryonic life, the primordia of both the male and the female reproductive tracts are present and develop together. Gonadal development results from the migration of primordial germ cells to the genital ridge (see Chapter 2), whereas the genital tract itself results from the formation and reshaping of the müllerian ducts (paramesonephric ducts), urogenital sinus, and vaginal plate.

The cell layers involved in the formation of the female reproductive tract are the mesoderm, the endoderm, and the ectoderm.

The *mesoderm* is divided into (a) paraxial mesoderm, which breaks up into segmental blocks (somites), forming the sclerotome (spinal cord, bone), dermatome (dermis), and myotome (musculature); (b) the intermediate mesoderm, which connects the paraxial and lateral plate as it differentiates into nephrogenic cord, forming the three kidney systems (pronephros [degenerates], mesonephros [only the wolffian system remains], metanephros [develops into the true kidney]); and (c) the lateral plate, which forms mesothelial or serous membranes of the peritoneal and pericardial cavities. In the peritoneum, the mesoderm provides primordium for the müllerian system and gonads. A defect or insult at any given somite or its contiguous mesoderm may give rise to congenital defects of multiple systems, such as the kidneys, the gonads, and corresponding ducts.

The *endoderm* is the epithelial lining of the primitive gut, the intraembryonic portions of the allantois and vitelline duct, respiratory tract, tympanic cavity and eustachian tube, tonsils, thyroid, parathyroid, thymus, liver, pancreas, urinary bladder, and urethra. The urogenital sinus forms the urinary bladder, allantois, and the prostatic, membranous, and penile urethra in males. It forms the urethra and vestibule in females. Both the prostate in males and the urethral/paraurethral glands in females are outbuddings of the urethra.

The *ectoderm* forms the central nervous system, the peripheral nervous system, and the sensory epithelium of sense organs. Of note, the fusion of endoderm and ectoderm contributes to patency (opening) and canalization, and defects result in fusion failures or imperforate/obstruction defects.

During the "indifferent" stage of development, two pairs of genital ducts develop in both sexes: the mesonephric ducts and the paramesonephric ducts. Paired mesonephric or wolffian ducts connect the mesonephric kidney to the cloaca (Fig. 10-1A). The ureteric bud arises from the mesonephric duct at approximately the fifth week and induces differentiation of the metanephros, which later becomes the functional kidney; the mesonephric kidney degenerates at 10 weeks (Fig. 10-1B). The müllerian (paramesonephric) ducts are first identified in embryos of both sexes at the 10-mm stage (sixth week) by the thickening of the anterior lateral coelomic

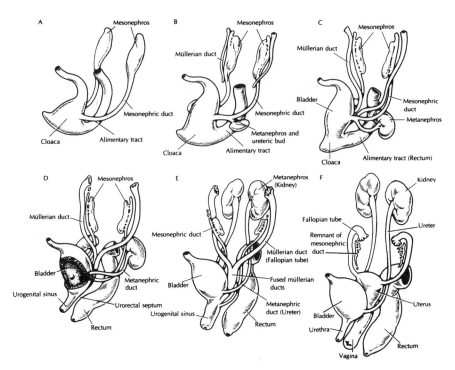

FIG. 10-1. Embryonic development of the female genitourinary tract. **A:** Paired mesonephric or wolffian ducts connect the mesonephric kidneys to the cloaca. **B:** The utereric bud arises from the mesonephric duct at approximately the fifth week and induces differentiation of the metanephros, which later becomes the functional kidney with degeneration of the mesonephric kidney at 10 weeks. **C:** Paired müllerian ducts develop from invagination of the coelomic epithelium at approximately 6 weeks and grow alongside the mesonephric ducts to end near the cloaca. **D:** The urorectal septum forms by the seventh week to separate the rectum from the urogenital sinus. **E:** Adjacent sections of the distal müllerian ducts fuse to form the uterovaginal canal, which inserts into the urogenital sinus at Müller tubercle. **F:** The vaginal plate forms at Müller tubercle and canalizes to form the vagina by the fifth month. (From Shatzkes DR, Haller JO, Velcek FT. Imaging of uterovaginal anomalies in the pediatric population. *Urol Radiol* 1991;13:58; and Markham SM, Waterhouse TB. Structural anomalies of the reproductive tract. *Curr Opin Obstet Gynecol* 1992;4:867; with permission.)

epithelium covering the wolffian body; a slight groove lined with distinct epithelial cells is present, and a tube is subsequently formed by fusion of the lips of the groove. The elongating müllerian ducts lie lateral to the wolffian ducts until they reach the caudal end of the mesonephros, at which point they direct medially to nearly touch in the midline near the cloaca (Fig. 10-1C). The urorectal septum forms by the seventh week to separate the rectum from the urogenital sinus (Fig. 10-1D). By the 30-mm stage (ninth week), the müllerian ducts progress caudally and reach the urogenital sinus to form the uterovaginal canal, which inserts into the urogenital sinus at Müller's tubercle (Figs. 10-1E, 10-2A, and 10-3A). By the 48-mm stage (twelfth week), the two ducts have completely fused into a single tube, the primitive uterovaginal canal, and two solid evaginations grow from the distal aspects of the müllerian tubercle: the sinovaginal bulbs (Figs. 10-1F and 10-2B). The sinovaginal bulbs are of urogenital sinus origin. Proximal to the sinovaginal bulbs, outgrowths from the müllerian ducts at müller tubercle result in the formation of the vaginal plate (Figs. 10-1F and 10-2B). The first and second portions of the müllerian ducts eventually form the fimbria and the fallopian tubes (Figs. 10-1F and 10-3B), while the distal segment forms the uterus and the upper vagina (Figs. 10-2C and 10-3B).

It is the growth of the vaginal plate in conjunction with the sinovaginal bulbs that results in the restructuring of the urogenital sinus from a long, narrow tube to a broad, flat vestibule. These changes result in the positioning of the female urethra down to the future perineum. Canalization of the vaginal plate begins caudally and continues in a cephalad direction, creating the lower vagina (Fig. 10-2B and C). Canalization is complete by the fifth month of gestation. The distal-most portions of the sinovaginal bulbs proliferate to form the hymenal tissue (Fig. 10-2C). The hymen becomes perforate before birth.

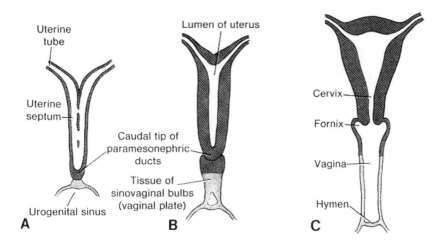

FIG. 10-2. Schematic drawing showing the formation of the uterus and vagina. **A:** At 9 weeks. Notice the disappearance of the uterine septum. **B:** At the end of the third month. Notice the tissue of the sinovaginal bulbs. **C:** Newborn. The upper portion of the vagina and the fornices are formed by vacuolization of the paramesonephric tissue and the lower portion by vacuolization of the sinovaginal bulbs. Prior to birth the hymen becomes perforate. (From Sadler TW. *Langman's medical embryology,* 6th ed. Baltimore: Williams & Wilkins, 1990; with permission.)

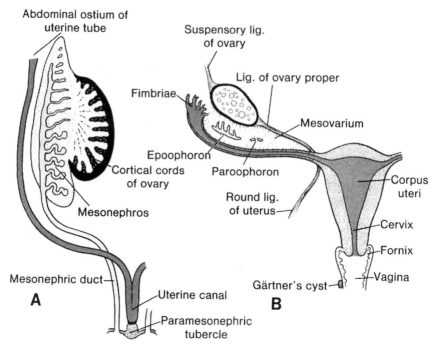

FIG. 10-3. A: Schematic drawing of the female genital ducts at the end of the second month of development. Notice the paramesonephric or müllerian tubercle and the formation of the uterine canal. **B:** The genital ducts after descent of the ovary. The only parts remaining of the mesonephric system are the epoophoron, the paroophoron, and Gärtner cyst. Notice the suspensory ligament of the ovary, the ligament of the ovary proper, and the round ligament of the uterus. (From Sadler TW. *Langman's medical embryology,* 6th ed. Baltimore: Williams & Wilkins, 1990; with permission.)

ABNORMALITIES OF THE FEMALE REPRODUCTIVE TRACT

External Genitalia

Ambiguous Genitalia

The diagnosis, evaluation, and medical management of ambiguous genitalia are presented in Chapter 2. The surgical management of these conditions is presented here by diagnosis.

Female Pseudohermaphrodites/Adrenogential Syndromes   It should be emphasized that female pseudohermaphrodites are females with ovaries and are potentially fertile. Thus, regardless of the appearance of the external genitalia, the sex assignment should be female. The majority of these individuals have masculinized external genitalia from congenital adrenal hyperplasia, but this can also result from maternal ingestion of exogenous androgens or from a maternal androgen-producing tumor. The type and extent of surgery depends on the degree of masculinization and the defined anatomy (1–5). In addition to the variations in the external genitalia, there are variations in the degree of masculinization of the lower urinary tract. Thick midline fusion with a single orifice may be appreciated with a urogenital sinus into which the vagina and urethra open separately, termed a *low vagina* (see Figs. 10-4A, 10-6, and 10-7), or the vagina can enter the urethra high between the external urethral sphincter and the bladder neck, termed a *high vagina* (see Fig. 10-4B) (6). For a low vagina, a cutback (see Figs. 10-5 to 10-9) or flap (see Fig. 10-10) vaginoplasty will create an adequate vaginal introitus. In cases of a high vagina, a pull-through procedure is necessary (see Fig. 10-11). Clitoral recession is usually accompanied by partial corporectomy, preserving the neurovascular bundle, and reanastomosis and preservation of the glans (see Figs. 10-12 and 10-13).

Historically, surgeons (pediatric general surgeons, urologists, and gynecologists) have performed the entire procedure (clitoroplasty, labioplasty, and vaginoplasty) in one, or at the most two, operations at 6 to 12 months of life (see Figs. 10-14 and 10-15). This technique usually requires an additional operation for revision of the vagina due to vaginal stenosis during adolescence (7). Alternatively, clitoroplasty can be

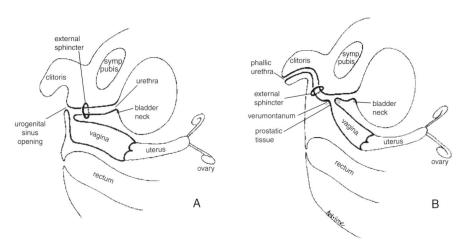

FIG. 10-4. Variable anatomy of the lower urinary tract in females with adrenogenital syndrome. **A:** Urogenital sinus into which the vagina and urethra open separately, below the urethral sphincter. **B:** Very masculinized configuration of the lower urinary tract, with entry of the vagina into the proximal urethra at a pseudoverumontanum, between the sphincter and the bladder neck. For a low vagina, a cutback or flap vaginoplasty is adequate. For a high vagina, a pull-through procedure is necessary. (Hendren WH. Surgical approach to intersex problems. *Semin Pedi Surg* 1998;7:8–18; with permission.)

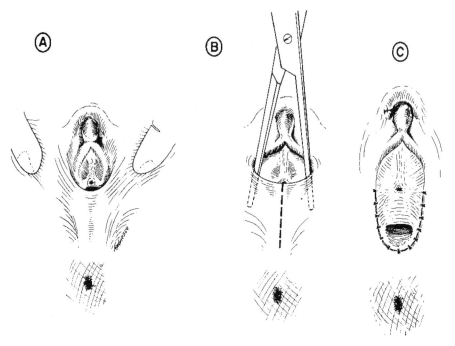

FIG. 10-5. Cutback vaginoplasty is suitable only in cases with minimal labial fusion. **A:** Labial fusion covering back half of vaginal introitus. **B:** Vertical incision. **C:** Transverse closure. This Heineke–Mikulicz procedure is useful to enlarge a well-defined area of narrowing in many surgical circumstances. (Hendren WH. Surgical approach to intersex problems. *Semin Pedi Surg* 1998;7:8–18; with permission.)

performed at a young age and then a flap vaginoplasty and labioplasty delayed until later in adolescence (see Figs. 10-16 to 10-18). The labioscrotal tissue is advanced inferiorly so that the labia are positioned in appropriate proximity to the vaginal orifice; a monsplasty can also be performed to create a normal "flat" mons as opposed to the grooved indentation seen in Fig. 10-16. There is evidence that girls undergoing vaginoplasty in adolescence report a higher level of satisfaction (8,9), whereas those undergoing vaginoplasty early in life have a low rate of compliance with dilators and less satisfaction with the long-term outcome (7,10). In addition, waiting to perform the vaginoplasty during adolescence will avoid the need for parents to insert vaginal dilators in the postoperative child, which can be emotionally challenging to the child and parent. Many pediatric surgeons, pediatric urologists, and gynecologists support the concept that it is best to recess the phallus in childhood and wait until adolescence for the creation of a functional vagina when the young woman can direct the time line and be compliant with the needed utilization of vaginal dilators (11).

Classically the goals of sex assignment and reconstructive surgical procedures have been based on the patient's potential to achieve an unambiguous appearance to the exter-

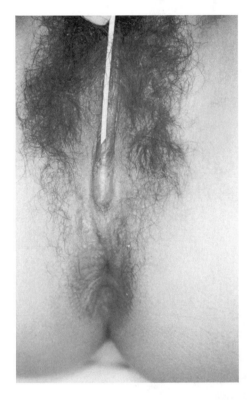

FIG. 10-6. Low urogenital sinus.

nal genitalia and achieve normal sexual function. A discussion of the determination of sex assignment is addressed in Chapter 2. As also discussed in Chapter 2, debate regarding the appropriate timing of "sex assignment" has gained additional attention by adult individuals with genital abnormalities. The Intersex Society provides information and detailed options for patients and their families at www.isna.org.

Androgen Abnormality/Insensitivity   Androgen abnormality/insensitivity, a form of male pseudohermaphroditism, may result from a wide variety of syndromes as outlined in Table 2-2 (9,10,12,13). With *complete androgen insensitivity* (CAIS) (previously referred to as *testicular feminization*), the individual has normal breast development but has pale areola, absent or very sparse pubic and axillary hair, a short vaginal pouch, and absence of the uterus and cervix (see Chapters 2 and 7). The gonads may be intraabdominal or in the inguinal rings; the serum testosterone level is in the range of the normal male. Because of insensitivity to androgens and enhanced estrogen production, the patient develops a normal female habitus and external genitalia. These patients have elevated levels of antimüllerian hormone, also called *müllerian inhibitory substance (MIS)*, during the first year of life; normal values from age 1 to puberty; and elevated levels again after pubertal development begins (14).

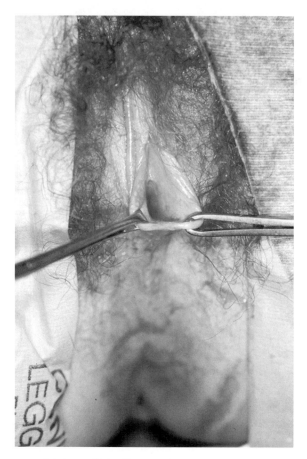

FIG. 10-7. Low urogenital sinus with traction.

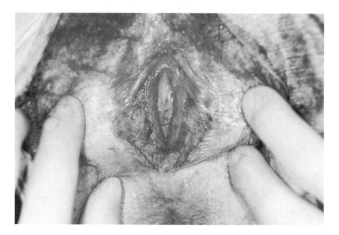

FIG. 10-8. Post incision of the low urogenital sinus. Note the presence of a normal urethra and vaginal orifice.

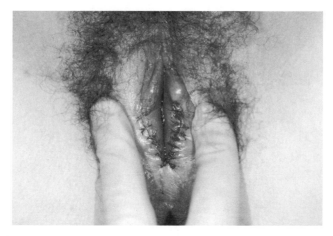

FIG. 10-9. Suture closure of the low urogenital sinus seen in Figs. 10-6 to 10-8.

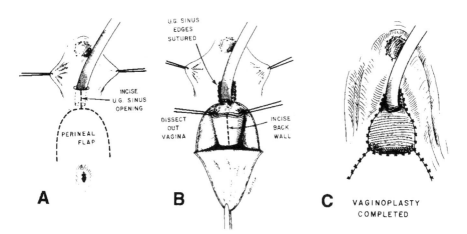

FIG. 10-10. Flap vaginoplasty. This is suitable only for cases with low confluence of the urethra and vagina, distal to urethral sphincter. **A:** Marking flap. **B:** The urogenital sinus is opened a short distance, if appropriate. The flap is raised. The back wall of the vagina is opened to receive the perineal flap. It is safest to perform the vaginal dissection with a finger in the rectum. Bowel should be prepared in all such cases to avert fecal soiling. Also, a Betadine-soaked gauze is placed in the rectum for added protection. **C:** Completed cutback vaginoplasty. (Hendren WH. Surgical approach to intersex problems. *Semin Pedi Surg* 1998;7:8–18; with permission.)

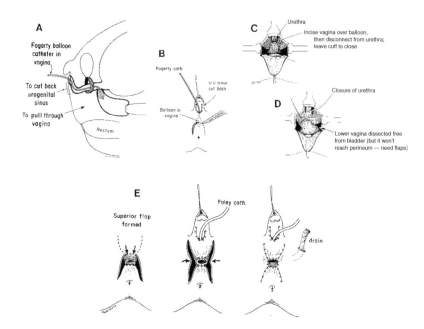

FIG. 10-11. Operative technique for pull-through vaginoplasty. **A:** With the patient in the lithotomy position, a Fogarty balloon catheter is placed in the vagina; the balloon is inflated and is pulled back gently to the entry of the vagina and into the urogenital sinus. The balloon catheter is clamped securely so that it does not deflate, and the endoscope is removed. **B:** The urogenital sinus is cut back to an appropriate length. Through an inverted U incision anterior to the anus, exposure is obtained. The bowel is always prepared, and a Betadine pack is placed in the rectum for further protection against contamination from the colon. The dissection anterior to the rectum is facilitated by placement of a finger in the rectum, until the dissection reaches the vagina. Gloves are changed before the perineal wound is reentered. **C:** By tugging gently on the Fogarty catheter, the precise junction of the vagina with the urethra can be identified. A transverse incision across the lower vagina will disclose the balloon, which is removed, and the opening into the urogenital sinus is visualized. There is no need to encircle the vagina with tape, which can lead to injury of the urethra. Accurate separation of the vagina is facilitated by being able to view it from within the lumen. **D:** The urethra is closed after a Foley catheter is passed from the urethral meatus into the bladder. Care is taken not to narrow the lumen. Usually there is immature prostatic tissue at this closure site. A second layer of tissue is closed over this to avert possible fistula formation between the urethra and the vagina. For this second layer, we have used the adjacent prostatic tissue or a labial fat flap. The vagina is dissected free to gain maximum length. **E:** Creation of flaps of perineum to reach the vagina. (Hendren WH. Surgical approach to intersex problems. *Semin Pedi Surg* 1998;7:8–18; with permission.)

Because the gonads in such patients have a high rate of malignant degeneration with formation of dysgerminoma, they should be prophylactically removed after the patient has completed pubertal development and attained full height and breast development (see Chapter 18). Rarely, children have had malignant degeneration of 46,XY gonads during childhood; therefore, it is suggested that patients in whom the diagnosis is made before puberty be monitored with ultrasound imaging to assess for

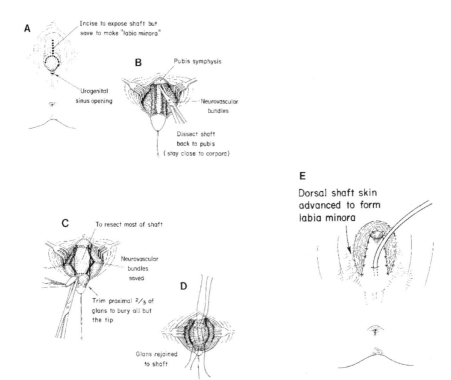

FIG. 10-12. Clitoroplasty by subtotal resection of the shaft and epithelium of the proximal glands to recess the tip of the phallus as "clitoris." Note use of the shaft skin to fashion the labia minora. (Hendren WH. Surgical approach to intersex problems. *Semin Pedi Surg* 1998;7:8–18; with permission.)

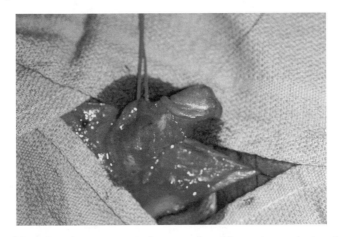

FIG. 10-13. Clitoroplasty in progess, note the separation of the neurovascular bundles from the shaft, and the preservation of the glans. The majority of the shaft will then be resected and the glans attached to the base of the shaft.

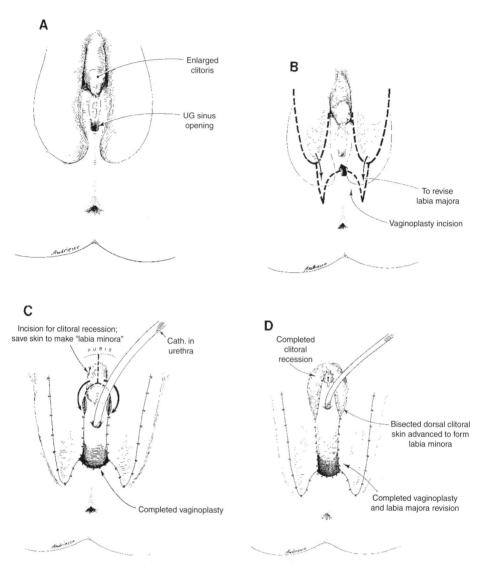

FIG. 10-14. Illustration shows posterior advancement of labioscrotal tissue, which is often inappropriately too forward in position. This is also common in cloacal cases. This type of advancement can be as a separate procedure, or simultaneously with clitoroplasty and vaginoplasty as shown here. **A:** Enlarged clitoris and forward labioscrotal tissue. **B:** The labia are mobilized to advance them posteriorly toward the anus. (Flap vaginoplasty also was performed in this case). **C:** Labia in position. **D:** Shaft skin is inserted, as labia minora, if clitoral recession is performed simultaneously. (Hendren WH. Surgical approach to intersex problems. *Semin Pedi Surg* 1998;7:8–18; with permission.)

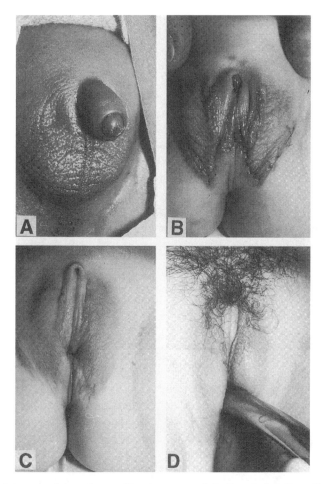

FIG. 10-15. Adrenogenital syndrome with severe masculinization. **A:** Age 5 months. There is a well-formed "penis" with a urethra at the tip. The scotum is empty. The infant was believed to be a male until a salt-losing crisis occurred at age 1 week, and the female gender was discovered. **B:** after phallic reduction, phallic recession, and labioplasty (age 5 months). **C:** At age 3 years, soon after pull-through vaginoplasty. **D:** At age 13 years there was a satisfactory female appearance. With a Hegar dilator in place, the satisfactory position and depth of the vagina were confirmed. (Hendren WH. Surgical approach to intersex problems. *Semin Pedi Surg* 1998;7:8; with permission.)

the development of a pelvic mass (15,16). Breast development is usually better in patients who have their gonads in place during adolescent development than in those who have undergone gonadectomy in childhood. The gonads can be removed by a laparoscopic technique. After gonadectomy, the patient should receive estrogen replacement.

Before surgery is undertaken, the patient needs to understand her anatomy. The physician should stress the patient's femininity and her ability to have normal sexual relations; she must, however, ultimately accept the fact that she cannot have menses

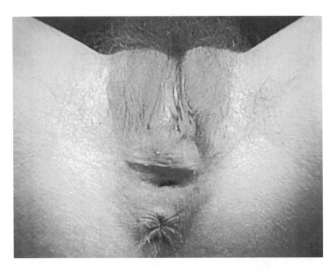

FIG. 10-16. 18 year old with adrenal genital syndrome. Note lack of flat mons, lack of a clitoral hood, narrow vaginal opening, and abnormal superior location of the labia.

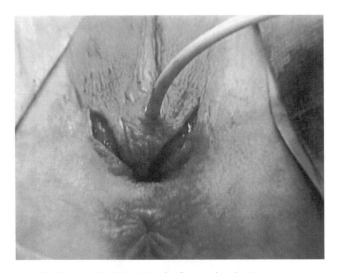

FIG. 10-17. Patient in Fig. 10-16 with incision for flap vaginoplasty.

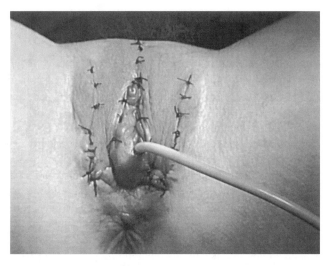

FIG. 10-18. Patient in Figs. 10-16 and 10-17 status post flap vaginoplasty, monsplasty, creation of a clitoral hood, and inferior mobilization of the labia.

or bear children. Relating the patient's condition to genes or chromosomes can be helpful. Because of the openness of medical records to patients and families, the patient deserves a careful explanation about genetic patterns and assurance that although most people think that an XY individual is a male, in fact, there are women with this genetic pattern because of changes at the level of the DNA. The health care provider needs to answer questions honestly and at the same time emphasize that the patient's phenotype is that of a normal female. The necessary surgery can be explained as removal of gonads, rather than testes; gonads can be viewed as organs that did not develop into either testes or ovaries because of the chromosomal problem. The risk of tumor should be openly discussed. Patients with androgen insensitivity syndromes usually have a blind vaginal pouch that, if needed, can be elongated with the use of vaginal dilators as described later (see Vaginal Agenesis). A multidisciplinary approach with involvement of a mental health provider is helpful, as studies have shown that individuals with intersex disorders have a high rate of dissatisfaction regarding physical and psychological health (17).

Partial or *incomplete androgen insensitivity* has also been reported but is less frequent than complete androgen insensitivity (see Table 2-2) (10,12). A typical reported patient may have a 46,XY karyotype, labial fusion, a blind vas deferens, and testes located in the labioscrotal folds. At puberty, the patient develops breasts and pubic and axillary hair. Because of the absence of the uterus (due to the fact that production of MIS occurs normally), the patient usually seeks medical care for the evaluation of primary amenorrhea (see Fig. 7-2). Gonadal removal should not be delayed in adolescents with incomplete androgen insensitivity because of the potential for further virilization once the diagnosis has been made. In one series of 11 patients with incomplete androgen insensitivity, of whom five were prepubertal, eight showed evidence of germ cell neoplasia (15).

Patients with androgen abnormality/insensitivity syndromes or other gonadal abnormalities may present with ambiguous genitalia or infantile male genitalia. It may be determined that these individuals should be reared as female (see Chapter 2); thus, feminizing genital reconstruction will need to be performed (3,18). An inadequate phallus for urination in a standing position and sexual function has historically been the basis for the decision to proceed with feminizing reconstruction. The procedure is performed with the goals of maintaining clitoral sensation, clitoral recession and decreasing the length of the clitoral shaft, properly positioned and creation of a clitoral hood, mobilization of the labia in appropriate proximity to the vaginal orifice, and creation of an adequate vagina (size, location, and consistency). The surgery should result in the girl's ability to void in a seated position and to have a normal-appearing vulva (3,18). Clitoral recession, relocation of the labia with labioplasty and vaginoplasty in an adolescent, is demonstrated in Figs. 10-13, and 10-15 to 10-18.

Labial Hypertrophy

Enlargement of one or both labia minora (Fig. 10-19A B) can result in irritation, chronic infection, and pain or can interfere with sexual activity or activity involving vulvar compression, such as horseback riding. In addition, the cosmetic deformity may result in psychosocial distress. Nonsymptomatic patients should be reassured that asymmetry or hypertrophy is not a serious developmental abnormality. Symptomatic labial hypertrophy can be addressed with counseling about hygiene and the avoidance of tight clothes; these measures are usually sufficient to relieve the discomfort. If symptoms persist, or if the appearance is troublesome to the young woman, then a surgical procedure for labioplasty can be recommended. The labioplasty can be accomplished by resection of the hypertrophic excess labial tissue and the creation of symmetrically reduced labia (Fig. 10-20A); an alternative technique has been described with wedge resection and reanastomosis in an attempt to decrease the exposed scar and improve outcome (Fig. 10-20B) (9,19,20). During the postoperative period, patients should protect the vulvar area from friction by the thighs when walking and strive to keep the area clean and dry to improve healing. Protection of the vulvar area during the postoperative healing period can be aided by a plastic athletic support cup worn inside the patient's underwear; this allows for normal activity without the risk of friction from the thighs against the suture area (19).

Female Circumcision/Female Genital Mutilation

Female circumcision/female genital mutilation (FC/FGM) refers to the alteration of the external genitalia for nonmedical reasons (21) and is practiced in approximately 28 African countries, in the Middle East, and in Indonesia and Malaysia

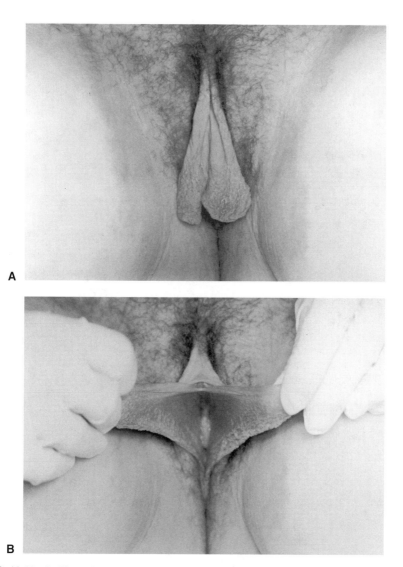

FIG. 10-19. A: Bilateral labial hypertrophy. **B:** Bilateral labial hypertrophy fully extended.

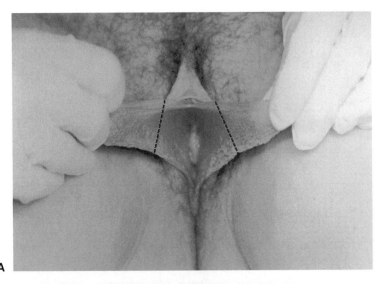

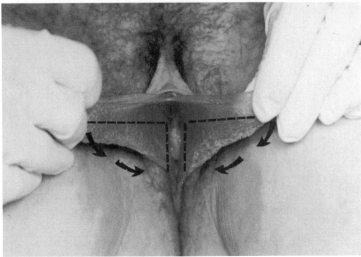

FIG. 10-20. A: Resection of the excess labial tissue in a case of labial hypertrophy. **B:** An alternative method for labioplasty. (From Laufer MR, Galvin WJ. Labial hypertrophy: a new surgical approach. *Adolesc Pediatr Gynecol* 1995;8:39; with permission.)

(22,23). This custom is practiced by Muslims, Christians, and Ethiopian Jews. In these countries, the prevalence rates range from 5% to 99% (22); it is estimated that 80 to 110 million women worldwide are affected (23). Female mutilation procedures present a health hazard and have short- and long-term physical, psychological, sexual, and reproductive effects.

The procedure is usually performed between the ages of 4 and 10 years, most commonly at the age of 7 years (22,23). The procedure varies according to ritual and has been classified by the World Health Organization (WHO) (24) according to the degree of tissue removal/destruction as follows:

Type I ("sunna" circumcision or removal of clitoris). Removal of a part of the clitoris or the whole organ.

Type II (excision). Excision of the clitoris and part or all of the labia minora.

Type III ("pharonic" circumcision or infibulation). Removal of the clitoris and the labia minora, with incision of the labia majora to create raw surfaces. The lateral raw surfaces are approximated, creating a hood of skin covering the urethra and introitus, leaving an opening inferiorly for the passage of urine and menstrual blood.

Type IV (unclassified). Pricking, piercing or incision of the clitoris and/or labia. Cauterization by burning of the clitoris and surrounding tissues. Introduction of corrosive substances or herbs into the vagina to cause bleeding or scarring/narrowing of the vagina.

The procedure is usually performed without anesthesia by a midwife or village woman and usually involves ritual and ceremony as a rite of passage into the adult village society (23,25). The reapproximation of the raw labial surfaces described in type III is accomplished with sutures of silk or catgut or by thorns or twigs (23). The legs of the girl are then bound from the hip to the ankles for up to 40 days so that scar tissue will form (23).

In 1993, WHO condemned FC/FGM and has attempted to educate and politically pressure African nations to discourage this practice (26). Even with the education and political pressure, the prevalence remains at 98% in some parts of Africa (27).

The immediate risks from the procedure include pain, hemorrhage, damage to the urethra and/or anus, local infection, shock, sepsis, and death (22,23). The long-term risks include transmission of blood-borne pathogens from unsterilized instruments (hepatitis, human immunodeficiency virus [HIV]), chronic pain, keloid/scar formation, recurrent urinary tract infections, chronic vaginitis and/or endometritis, dysuria, dysmenorrhea, dyspareunia, apareunia, the need for "surgical" revision prior to intercourse, and possible further revision prior to vaginal delivery (22,23,28).

Health care providers must be cognizant of the existence of ritual female "circumcision," its long-term side effects, and the physical appearance of the perineum after the procedure has been done (see Color Plate 27). A woman may request a revision or a deinfibulation procedure. Extreme sensitivity is essential so that the woman can identify exactly what area of the genital region she wants revised. We usually have the patient demonstrate with a hand-held mirror the exact areas that she wants revised, and we also use drawings to specifically illustrate the appearance of the external genitalia before and after the procedure. With this level of detailed informed consent, the patient's cultural, sexual, and reproductive wishes can be respected. In addition, with the patient dictating the final result, she is retaking control of the genital area that was mutilated by the direction of adults at a time when she was not in control.

Defibulation is performed under local or general anesthesia. The fused labial tissue is incised with care to avoid damage to the underlying clitoral tissue at the superior aspect of the dissection. The labia edges are sutured for hemostasis and to avoid reagglutination of the labia. Postoperative care of ice packs and Sitz baths are prescribed. Figure 10-21 shows a schematic drawing of the revision procedure, and Color Plate 28 shows the result of the revision in the patient shown in Color Plate 27.

At the Brigham and Women's Hospital in Boston, Massachusetts, Nawal Nour, MD, MPH, has established the first African Women's Health Center in the United States; the Female Genital Cutting Education and Networking Project also provides updated information. Additional information for health care providers and affected girls and young women from these and other resources can be found at: *http://www.brighamandwomens.org/africanwomenscenter/default.asp* or *http://www.fgmnetwork.org/*; *http://www.acog.org*; *www.rainbo.org*

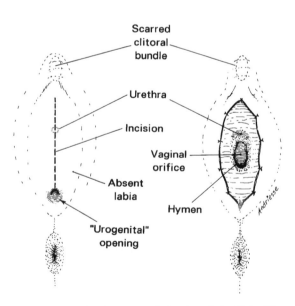

FIG. 10-21. Schematic diagram after female mutilation (see Color Plate 27), and re-creation of the introitus (see Color Plate 28).

Disorders of Mesonephric Remnants

Persistent wolffian duct derivatives are commonly found in normal females (29,30). These remnants can result in pain or pelvic masses as follows:

A *hydatid of Morgagni cyst* itself does not usually cause pain (Fig. 10-22), although torsion of the cyst can result in colicky, lower abdominal/pelvic pain with or without nausea and vomiting. Once torsion has occurred, the cyst may become gangrenous. Intermittent torsion of the cyst can also occur, resulting in intermittent symptoms. These cysts can be removed laparoscopically; the fallopian tube can be salvaged and not compromised.

Cysts of the broad ligament can result in large simple cystic pelvic masses (Fig. 10-23). Patients may present with pain and/or abdominal distention, or the cysts may be identified on routine examination. The cysts are usually simple in appearance on ultrasound. Surgery may be indicated if there is pain or abdominal distention; resection is not mandatory for small asymptomatic broad ligament cysts, as they are benign embryologic remnants. If surgery is undertaken, care must be taken to identify the cyst as arising from the broad ligament, with appropriate identification of the fallopian tube (Fig. 10-24), as the fallopian tube may be distended and stretched over the surface of the cyst (Fig. 10-23). After removal of the cyst, the distended fallopian tube and redundant peritoneum are left to regress to normal size (Fig. 10-25).

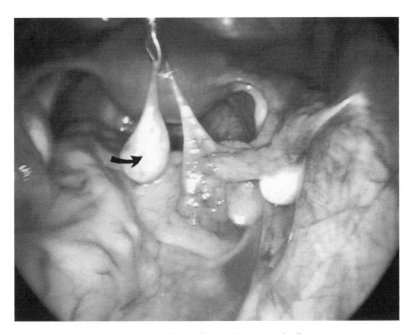

FIG. 10-22. A hydatid of Morgagni cyst (*arrow*) seen laparoscopically.

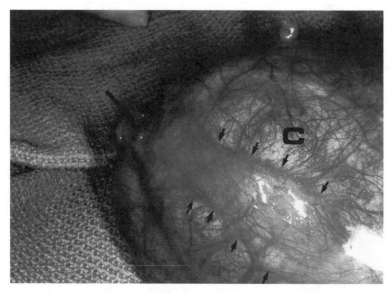

FIG. 10-23. Distorted, stretched left fallopian tube over the left broad ligament cyst. C, cyst, small arrows pointing to edges of stretched fallopian tube, large arrow pointing to fimbriated end of tube.

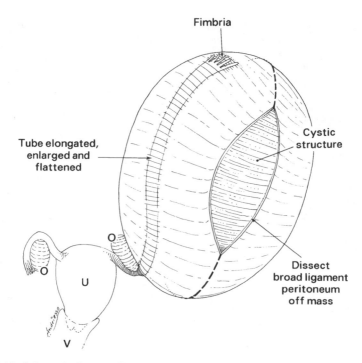

FIG. 10-24. Schematic diagram of broad ligament cyst with demonstration of incision for preservation of fallopian tube. O, ovary; U, uterus; V, vagina.

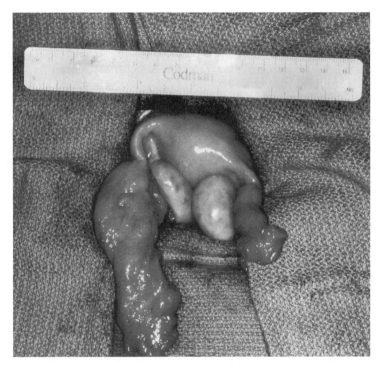

FIG. 10-25. Fallopian tubes, ovaries, and uterus seen after resection of the broad ligament cyst seen in Fig 10-23. Notice distorted enlarged left fallopian tube which will involute and return to a normal size.

Gärtner's canal (duct) may retain a ureteral connection and form an ectopic ureter, which may communicate with the perineum. In addition, remnants of Gärtner's ducts can result in cystic formations of the cervix or vaginal walls (see Fig 13-11). These embryologic remnants do not need to be resected unless they cause pain or interfere with sexual activity or the use of tampons.

Introital Abnormalities

Masses

Introital masses are common in the neonate and young child and include developmental and nondevelopmental abnormalities (see Chapters 1, 3 and 13). The differential diagnosis includes urethral prolapse (see Figs. 3-9 and 13-8), ectopic ureter, prolapsed ureterocele (see Fig. 3-12), hymenal skin tag (see Fig. 1-17), rhabdomyosarcoma (see Color Plate 8), condyloma (see Color Plate 14 and Figs. 3-3 and 3-6), paraurethral cyst (see Fig. 3-11), vaginal cyst (see Fig. 13-11), obstructed hemivagina (Fig. 10-26), or imperforate hymen (see Figs. 1-10, 1-14, and 3-13). The patient should be examined in order to determine the origin of the mass. In a neonate or child, the "pull-down" traction maneuver for visualizing the introitus should be utilized (see Fig. 1-6) to visualize the entire vestibule and distal vagina.

Bartholin's Duct Cyst/Abscess   In the adolescent, the above-mentioned abnormalities may exist, and in addition Bartholin duct cysts or abscesses may occur. Bartholin duct cysts do not need to be drained or removed unless the patient is symptomatic. If the Bartholin duct becomes infected and an abscess forms, it may need to be drained when it is "pointing." A Ward catheter should be placed to maintain a drainage tract. If the abscess recurs, a marsupialization or resection procedure should be considered (see Chapter 15).

Ectopic Ureter

An ectopic ureter (see Chapter 13) that communicates with the perineum can cause chronic vaginal irritation, vulvar/vaginal "wetness," or pain (see Chapter 3) (31). Ultrasound may be utilized to assist in the diagnosis, and an intravenous pyelogram is confirmatory. According to the Weigert–Meyer rule, the ectopic ureter communi-

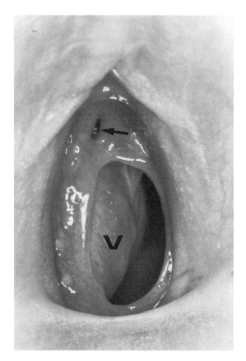

FIG. 10-26. Obstructed left hemivagina with mucocolpos in a 6-year-old. *Arrow* shows urethra; V, wall of obstructed hemivagina seen as a lateral sidewall bulge.

cates with the upper pole of the duplex kidney; the greater the distance of the ectopic location from the orthotopic ureteral orifice, the more dysplastic is the upper pole of the duplex kidney (32). A pediatric urologist should be consulted for corrective surgery to appropriately ligate/implant the ectopic ureter and/or to perform an upper pole nephrectomy. (See Chapter 13).

It should be noted that there have been at least five cases of clear cell cancer of the vagina in adolescent women who have had an ectopic ureter into the vagina from a dysplastic kidney (33,34). We thus promote every-other-year exam under anesthesia and Pap tests for children and biyearly vaginal exams and yearly vaginal Pap tests in adolescents with this condition.

Prolapsed Ureterocele

When the duplex collecting system has a ureter that ends in a ureterocele, the ectopic ureter with ureterocele also arises from the upper collecting system in the duplex kidney. The ureterocele may present as an introital mass if it prolapses through the urethra (see Fig. 3-12 and Chapter 13). The prolapsed ureterocele is managed by marsupialization of the obstructed end to relieve the obstruction, and then the nonobstructed duplex ureter prolapse is reduced into the bladder; additional urologic procedures of the ectopic ureter, bladder, or upper pole of the kidney may be required (35,36).

Introital Cysts

Hymenal, periurethral, and vaginal cysts are usually of the epidermal inclusion variety. Most of these cysts will resolve spontaneously within 3 months. If the cyst does not resolve and is symptomatic, then the cyst should be marsupialized. Prior to surgical intervention, a transperineal ultrasound is helpful to confirm the diagnosis. In addition, cystoscopy should be performed at the time of marsupialization to rule out a urethral diverticulum.

Hymenal Skin Tags

Hymenal skin tags (see Fig. 1-17) are common findings. They usually regress, but if a lesion is symptomatic with inflammation or bleeding, it should be excised to make sure that there is no malignancy, and to relieve the symptoms.

Congenital Hymenal Abnormalities

Congenital variations of the hymen are demonstrated in Fig. 1-10. An adolescent's abnormal hymen that results in a small orifice should be corrected surgically if she is unable to use tampons, insert vaginal cream or suppositories, or have vaginal intercourse. The cribriform, septate, or microperforate hymen can be revised with resection of the "excess" hymenal tissue to create a functional hymenal ring. It should be

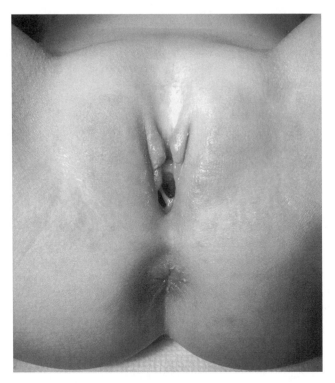

FIG. 10-27. Subsymphyseal epispadias.

noted that there have been reports of familial occurrence of hymenal abnormalities, and thus women should be aware that their daughters may have a similar abnormality. Patient handouts addressing abnormal hymenal abnormalities are available at *http://www.youngwomenshealth.org/hymen.html*

Subsymphyseal Epispadias   Subsymphyseal epispadias is a rare urologic condition (see Chapter 13) that can be seen in Fig. 10-27. The vagina and upper reproductive tract are normal although the hymen may be septate, as seen in this image.

Bladder Exstrosphy

Exstrophy of the urinary bladder is an uncommon anomaly that requires timed reconstruction in a series of stages (see Chapter 13). The anal orifice is usually close to the vagina. Years after repair, adolescents may complain of introital stenosis or of the structural abnormality of the mons and/or clitoris. The upper reproductive tract is usually normal. Individuals with this condition have a bifid clitoris (Fig. 10-28). It is not uncommon for women with a history of bladder exstrophy to develop cervical/uterine prolapse. Surgery can alleviate the prolapse and its associated symp-

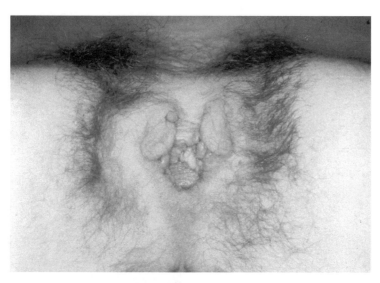

FIG. 10-28. Gynecologic features in an adolescent with a history of bladder exstrophy following successful bladder repair; notice bifid clitoris and pubic hair.

toms of pain, irritation, vaginal discharge/bleeding, or difficulty with sexual activity. The repair usually requires a monsplasty, a Williams vulvovaginoplasty, and a Manchester–Fothergill procedure in a one-stage operation. The result is usually excellent, and patients have full sexual and reproductive function. Pregnancy can occur without complication; delivery can be achieved by either a vaginal or an abdominal route (37).

Cloacal Anomalies

A cloaca is a common canal involving the gastrointestinal, urinary, and genital tracts. A wide range of anatomic variation can occur with the interruption of the normal differentiation of these three organ systems (38–39). The abnormality usually results in a failure of the normal fusion of the müllerian ducts with subsequent duplication of the uterus and proximal vagina (Fig. 10-29A). The sinovaginal bulbs do not form, and the vaginal plate does not develop normally. The urogenital sinus persists, and the urethra enters high on the anterior wall; the hymen and lower vagina do not form appropriately. The examination reveals a "blank" perineum (Fig. 10-29B). Before corrective surgery is performed, the patient needs to have the existing anatomy clearly defined with radiologic and endoscopic evaluations (38,40). According to W. Hardy Hendren's reports of extensive experience with over 195 patients, surgical repair for a primary cloaca is usually done when the patient is between the ages of 9 and 18 months (38,41). Surgical construction for individuals with a cloacal abnormality is performed by a pediatric surgeon or by a team consisting of a pediatric sur-

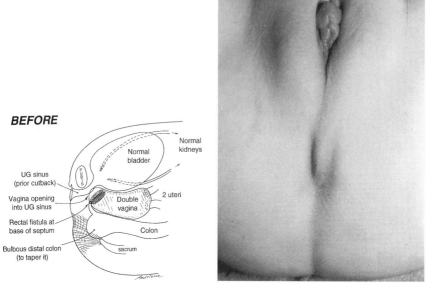

BEFORE

A
B

FIG. 10-29. **A:** Cloacal anomaly before reconstruction. UG, urogenital. (From Hendren WH. Urogenital sinus and cloacal malformations. *Semin Pediatr Surg* 1996;5:72; with permission.) **B:** The "blank" perineum of the cloacal anomaly. (From Hendren WH. Urogenital sinus and cloacal malformations. *J Pelvic Surg* 1995;1:149; with permission.)

geon, a pediatric urologist, and a pediatric gynecologist. Through extensive procedures, separate functional urinary, gastrointestinal, and reproductive tracts are created (Fig. 10-30A). As shown in Fig. 10-30B, there is a perineal body between the new anus and the pull-through vagina. The new urethra lies just beneath the somewhat enlarged clitoris. When the patient is older, the labial tissue can be moved more posteriorly to surround the vaginal opening, as demonstrated in Figs. 10-16 to 10-18 (6,38,39). Multiple revisions of the surgery may be required to create a satisfactory result for all affected functional systems. Full sexual and reproductive function is possible for genetic female individuals with the cloacal anomaly; pregnancy has been reported with both abdominal and vaginal deliveries (38,42). Discordant sexual identity has been reported in some genetic males with cloacal exstrophy assigned to female sex at birth (43).

Anomalies of the Uterus, Cervix, and Vagina

In general, anomalies of the female reproductive tract result from abnormalities of agenesis/hypoplasia, vertical fusion (canalization abnormalities resulting from abnormal contact with the urogenital sinus), lateral fusion (duplication), or resorption (septum). Each of these abnormalities is associated with specific symptoms, physical

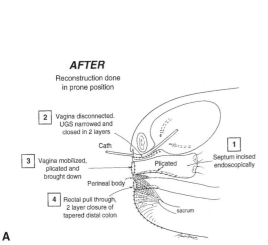

AFTER

Reconstruction done
in prone position

2 Vagina disconnected.
UGS narrowed and
closed in 2 layers

Cath

3 Vagina mobilized,
plicated and
brought down

Plicated

1 Septum incised
endoscopically

Perineal body

4 Rectal pull through,
2 layer closure of
tapered distal colon

sacrum

A

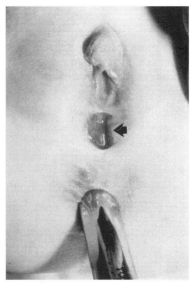

B

FIG. 10-30. **A:** Cloacal anomaly after reconstruction. **B:** Three months after reconstruction of patient in Fig. 10-29 with arrow at constructed vaginal orifice, and a dilator in the anorectal canal. UGS, urogenital sinus. (From Hendren WH. Urogenital sinus and cloacal malformations. *Semin Pediatr Surg* 1996;5:72; with permission.)

findings, evaluation, and therapy. Uterine and vaginal malformations may be identified by the clinician when a patient experiences primary amenorrhea, acute and/or chronic pelvic pain, abnormal vaginal bleeding, or a foul-smelling vaginal discharge (often worse at the time of menses), or incidentally on physical examination. Patients with anomalies that result in obstruction of a functional reproductive tract usually have complaints that differ from those without an obstructive anomaly. Combined uterine and vaginal obstructions may be difficult to diagnose and treat. Although rare, these entities are challenging and are frequently missed in the early adolescent years because the pelvic pain, irregular bleeding, or vaginal discharge may be attributed to functional disturbances. Ultrasonography, magnetic resonance imaging (MRI), laparoscopy, examination with the patient under anesthesia, and/or intraoperative hysterosalpingograms may be useful in defining the anatomy in these patients so that the appropriate management options can be presented and reconstruction, if needed, can be performed. Obstructive anomalies may require immediate intervention to relieve an obstruction, whereas nonobstructive anomalies do not require surgical intervention unless the patient has reached reproductive age and has been shown to be adversely affected by the anomaly.

Classification Systems

The basic classification of anomalies of the müllerian tract include agenesis/hypoplasia, vertical fusion (canalization) defects, and lateral fusion (duplication) defects. The American Society for Reproductive Medicine (ASRM) (formerly the American Fertility Society [AFS]) has adopted a classification system of müllerian anomalies, which is shown in Table 10-1 (44,45).

The ASRM system is based on the degree of failure of normal development and separates the anomalies into groups with similar clinical manifestations and prognoses for fetal salvage upon treatment. These different subtypes of anomalies based on reproductive function were proposed to allow for long-term studies of the reproductive outcomes of each type of anomaly in order to provide better information for health care providers who counsel affected individuals.

The ASRM classification system does not include vaginal anomalies but allows for the inclusion of a description of associated vaginal, tubal, or urinary anomalies. Others have suggested classification systems for vaginal anomalies as demonstrated in Table 10-2 (46,47).

Figure 10-31 shows a schematic drawing of a normal reproductive tract, and Figs. 10-32 to 10-62 demonstrate schematic diagrams of variations of defects of the female genital tract that include and demonstrate uterine, cervical, tubal, vaginal, and renal abnormalities.

TABLE 10-1. *Classification of müllerian anomalies according to the ASRM Classification System*

Type I:	"Müllerian" agenesis or hypoplasia
	A. Vaginal (uterus may be normal or exhibit a variety of malformations)
	B. Cervical
	C. Fundal
	D. Tubal
	E. Combined
Type II:	Unicornuate uterus
	A. Communicating (endometrial cavity present)
	B. Noncommunicating (endometrial cavity present)
	C. Horn without endometrial cavity
	D. No rudimentary horn
Type III:	Uterus didelphys
Type IV:	Uterus bicornuate
	A. Complete (division down to internal os)
	B. Partial
Type V:	Septate uterus
	A. Complete (septum to internal os)
	B. Partial
Type VI:	Arcuate
Type VII:	DES-related anomalies
	A. T-shaped uterus
	B. T-shaped with dilated horns
	C. T-shaped

Adapted from Buttram VC, Jr. Müllerian anomalies and their management. *Fertil Steril* 1983;40:159; Buttram VC Jr, Gibbons WE. Müllerian anomalies: a proposed classification (an analysis of 144 cases). *Fertil Steril* 1979;32:40; The American Fertility Society. The American Fertility Society classifications of adnexal adhesions, distal tubal occlusion, tubal occlusion secondary to tubal ligation, tubal pregnancies, müllerian anomalies, and intrauterine adhesions. *Fertil Steril* 1988;49:944; with permission.)

TABLE 10-2. *Vaginal classification*

Classification	Features
Class I	Transverse
	a. Obstructing
	b. Nonobstructing
Class II	Longitudinal
	a. Obstructing
	b. Nonobstructing
Class III	Stenosis/iatrogenic

From Gidwani G, Falcone T. Congenital malformations of the female genital tract. *Diagnosis and Management*. Philadelphia: Lippincott Williams & Wilkins, 1999:146.

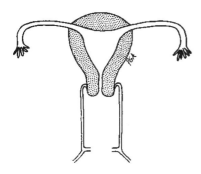

FIG. 10-31. Normal anatomy.

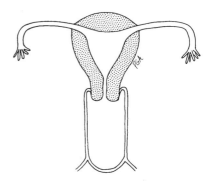

FIG. 10-32. Imperforate hymen.

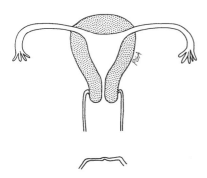

FIG. 10-33. Agenesis (atresia) of the lower vagina.

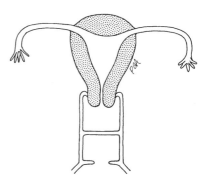

FIG. 10-34. Transverse vaginal septum.

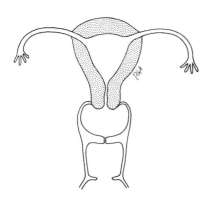

FIG. 10-35. Transverse vaginal septum with microperforation.

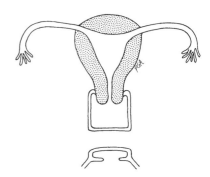

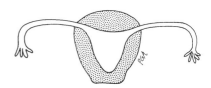

FIG. 10-36. Agenesis (atresia) of the lower vagina, or thick transverse vaginal septum.

FIG. 10-37. Vaginal agenesis with rudimentary uterine horns (of note, in cases of vaginal agenesis the uterus may be normal or exhibit a variety of malformations).

FIG. 10-38. Vaginal agenesis with agenesis of the cervix.

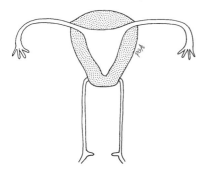

FIG. 10-39. Cervical agenesis with the presence of a vagina.

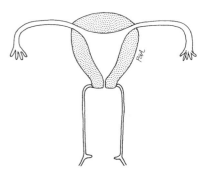

FIG. 10-40. Cervical hypoplasia with the presence of a vagina.

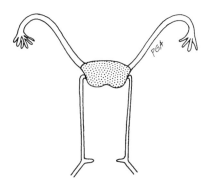

FIG. 10-41. Uterine/cervical hypoplasia.

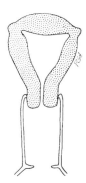

FIG. 10-42. Fallopian tube agenesis.

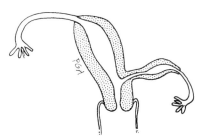

FIG. 10-43. Unicornuate uterus with communicating uterine horn.

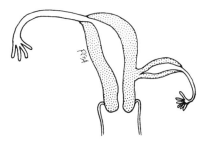

FIG. 10-44. Unicornuate uterus with non-communicating uterine horn (containing an endometrial cavity) fused to unicornuate uterus.

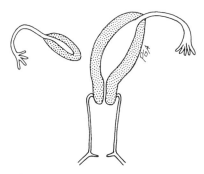

FIG. 10-45. Unicornuate uterus with non-communicating uterine horn (containing an endometrial cavity) not fused to unicornuate uterus.

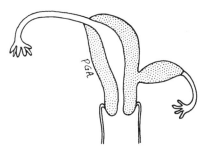

FIG. 10-46. Unicornuate uterus with uterine horn (not containing an endometrial cavity) fused to unicornuate uterus.

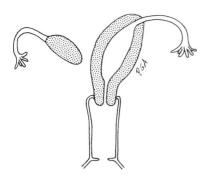

FIG. 10-47. Unicornuate uterus with uterine horn (not containing an endometrial cavity) not fused to unicornuate uterus.

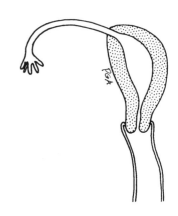

FIG. 10-48. Unicornuate uterus.

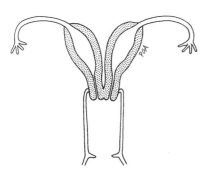

FIG. 10-49. Uterus didelphys, bicollis, with normal vagina.

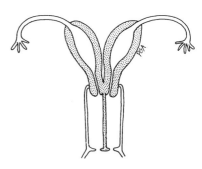

FIG. 10-50. Uterus didelphys, bicollis, with complete vaginal septum.

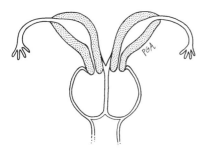

FIG. 10-51. Uterus didelphys, bicollis, with complete upper vaginal septum with bilateral obstruction.

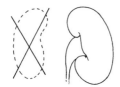

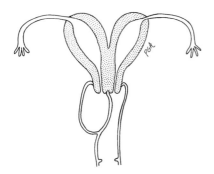

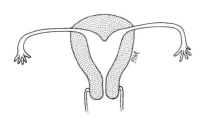

FIG. 10-52. Uterus didelphys with obstructed hemivagina and ipsilateral renal agenesis.

FIG. 10-53. Uterus bicornuate: complete (division down to internal os).

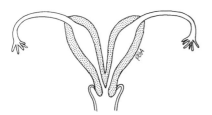

FIG. 10-54. Uterus bicornuate: partial.

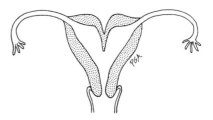

FIG. 10-55. Arcuate uterus.

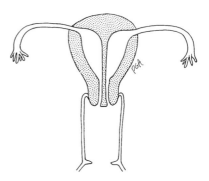

FIG. 10-56. Septate uterus: complete (septum to external os).

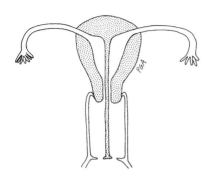

FIG. 10-57. Septate uterus: complete with associated vaginal septum.

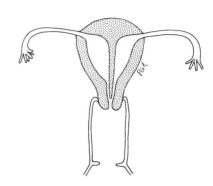

FIG. 10-58. Septate uterus: complete (septum to internal os).

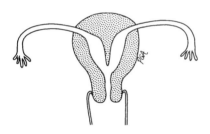

FIG. 10-59. Septate uterus: partial.

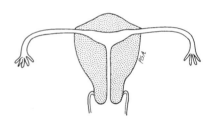

FIG. 10-60. Diethylstilbestrol-related anomalies: T-shaped uterus.

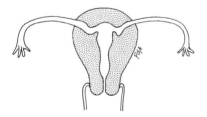

FIG. 10-61. Diethylstilbestrol-related anomalies: T-shaped with dilated horns.

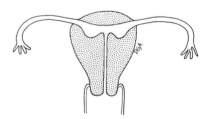

FIG. 10-62. Diethylstilbestrol-related anomalies: T-shaped variation.

TABLE 10-3. *Syndromes associated with vaginal agenesis*

Syndromes	Reproductive anomaly	Etiology/gene
Antley-Bixler	Vaginal atresia: "hypoplastic uterus, atresia of the lower third of the vagina"; urogenital sinus, hypoplastic labia majora, fusion of labia minora, hypertrophy clitoris.	Autosomal recessive
Apert	Vaginal atresia	Autosomal dominant
Bardet-Biedl	Vaginal atresia	Autosomal recessive
Del (1)(q12)	Vaginal stenosis	Chromosomal
Ellis Van Creveld	Vaginal atresia	Autosomal recessive
Fraser	Vaginal atresia	Autosomal recessive
Laurence-Moon syndrome	Vaginal atresia	Autosomal recessive
McKusick-Kaufman	Vaginal atresia uncommonly, transverse vaginal septum more common cause of obstruction	
Pallister Hall	Vaginal atresia	Autosomal dominant
Prune belly	Vaginal atresia	Unknown (?polygenic/ multifactorial)
Robinow	Vaginal atresia and hematocolpos	Autosomal dominant or autosomal recessive

(Adapted from Simpson J. Genetics of the female reproductive ducts. *Am J Med Genet* 1999;89:224.)

Genetics

The etiology of anatomic defects of the female genital tract is not fully understood. Most forms of isolated müllerian duct and urogenital sinus malformations are inherited in a polygenic/multifactorial fashion. Mendelian forms of inheritance with a single gene mutation have been described to explain the McKusick–Laufman syndrome (MKS), and the hand–foot–genital syndrome involves the HOXA13 gene (48). Table 10-3 lists syndromes associated with vaginal atresia, Table 10-4 lists syndromes associated with longitudinal vaginal septum, and Table 10-5 lists syndromes associated with müllerian aplasia.

Incidence

The true incidence of müllerian duct anomalies is not known. Different reports have described a wide range of incidence, depending on whether a general population is evaluated at the time of obstetric delivery, or one with a history of infertility or habitual miscarriage (49–52). In a study of fertile women who were evaluated for müllerian duct anomalies at the time of tubal ligation, an incidence of 3.2% was iden-

TABLE 10-4. *Syndromes associated with longitudinal vaginal septum*

Syndrome	Anomaly	Etiology/gene
Camptobrachydactyly	Longitudinal vaginal septum	Autosomal dominant
Johanson-Blizzard syndrome	Longitudinal vaginal septum	Autosomal recessive

(Adapted from Simpson J. Genetics of the female reproductive ducts. *Am J Med Genet* 1999;89:224.)

TABLE 10-5. *Syndromes associated with müllerian aplasia**

Wolf-Hirschhorn syndrome	Absent uterus	Chromosomal [del (4)(p16.3)]
Goldenhar syndrome	"Rokitansky sequence"	Unknown; autosomal dominant or polygenic/ multifactorial
Al-Awadi syndrome	"Müllerian aplasia"	Autosomal recessive
Klippel-Feil anomaly	Müllerian aplasia	Unknown
MURCS association	Müllerian aplasia	Unknown
Mosaic trisomy 7	Absence of uterus	Chromosomal
Urogenital dysplasia	Absence of uterus	Polygenic/multifactorial; possibly autosomal dominant
Acro-renal mandibular	Uterus didelphys	Autosomal recessive
Apert	"Bicornuate uterus"	Autosomal dominant
Bardet-Biedl	"Uterus duplex, vaginal septa"	Autosomal recessive
Beckwith-Wiedemann	Incomplete müllerian fusion	Autosomal dominant; some cases trisomy 11p
Caudal duplication	"Duplication" of cervix and uterus	Unknown
Caudal regression (dysplasia)	"Duplication of the uterus and vagina"	Unknown
Cloacal exstrophy	Incomplete müllerian fusion	Unknown
de Lange	Incomplete müllerian fusion	Duplication 3q some cases
Leprechaunism (Donahue syndrome)	Incomplete müllerian fusion	Autosomal recessive
Fraser (cryptophalamos)	Bicornuate uterus, gonadoblastoma	Autosomal recessive
Fryns	"Bicornuate uterus"	Autosomal recessive
Halal	"Uterus didelphys with septate vagina"	Autosomal dominant
Hydrolethalus	"Uterus duplex"	Autosomal recessive
Laryngeal atresia	"Bicornuate uterus"	Unknown
Meckel	"Bicornuate with a thin septum down to the upper end of the vagina"	Autosomal recessive
Prune belly	"Bicornuate uterus", XX genital ambiguity	Unknown
Pterygium	Incomplete müllerian fusion	Autosomal dominant
Roberts	"Bicornuate uterus" with "complete longitudinal septum," hypertrophy of uterine cervix, "Agenesis of the uterus and agenesis or atresia of the vagina"	Autosomal recessive
Rüdiger	"Bicornuate uterus"	Autosomal recessive
Triploidy	Septate vagina	Chromosomal
Trisomy 13	Incomplete müllerian fusion	Chromosomal
Trisomy 18	Incomplete müllerian fusion	Chromosomal
Urogenital dysplasia	"Unicornuate" or "bicornuate" uteri	Unknown; probably polygenic/multifactorial or autosomal dominant

(Adapted from Simpson J. Genetics of the female reproductive ducts. *Am J Med Genet* 1999;89:224.)

tified (51). Many women may have an underlying asymptomatic müllerian duct anomaly; since they have no pain, pelvic mass, infertility, or reproductive compromise, they may not come to diagnosis. Because familial occurrences of anomalies of the female reproductive tract have been reported, families should be screened by history for the possibility that female relatives have also been affected (53).

Most uterine abnormalities are asymptomatic but may be diagnosed after habitual abortions, menstrual abnormalities, or infertility. Patients with segmental agenesis/hypoplasia usually present with primary amenorrhea if there is no functioning endometrium in a remnant/rudimentary obstructed uterus, or with cyclic or chronic pelvic pain if there is a vaginal, cervical, or uterine obstruction but a normally functioning endometrium. As the ovaries form from the genital ridge they usually have normal structure and function. In cases of vaginal agenesis, cervical and/or uterine structures may or may not be present. If the cervix and uterus are absent, the ovaries and distal fallopian tubes are present, as they are not of müllerian origin. Patients with a totally obstructed genital tract usually have a mucocolpos at birth (see Fig 3-13) or a hematocolpos at the time of menarche (see Fig 10-63).

Diagnosis

The diagnosis of a structural defect of the female genital tract is usually based on symptoms, history, and physical examination. The genital exam may reveal an im-

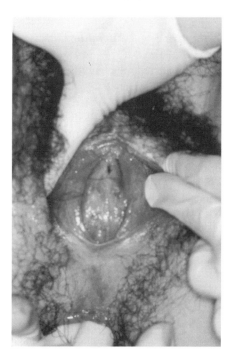

FIG. 10-63. Imperforate hymen with hematocolpos.

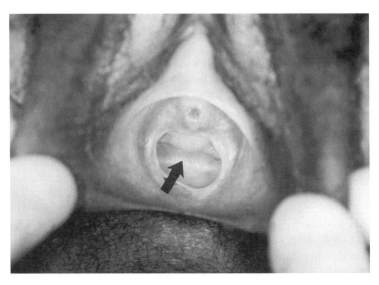

FIG. 10-64. "Blind" vaginal pouch, with transverse vaginal septum at arrow.

perforate hymen (see Figs. 1-10, 1-14,and 10-63), or a vaginal dimple with vaginal agenesis (see Color Plate 29). Alternatively, the exam may reveal a "blind" vaginal pouch with only the lower vagina present (Fig. 10-64).

Imaging Studies for Reproductive Tract Anomalies

Diagnostic imaging of abnormalities of the female reproductive tract can assist in determining the correct diagnosis with delineation of the anatomy and guidance in the formation of a surgical plan for correction of the anomaly. As a result of the obstructive anomaly, patients may have a grossly enlarged blood-filled vagina (hematocolpos) (Fig. 10-65), uterus (hematometra), and/or fallopian tubes (hematosalpinix). Ultrasound is helpful in identifying the anatomy in all cases of reproductive tract anomalies and can be used in a transabdominal, transvaginal, or transperineal approach (54–59). MRI can be helpful in determining the anatomy in cases of complicated obstructive anomalies, and many consider it the "gold standard" for imaging of anomalies of the reproductive tract (60–63). It should be noted that an unestrogenized normally small prepubertal uterus may be difficult to image even with MRI. MRI is especially useful in determining the presence or absence of the cervix in complex anomalies, or the presence of functioning endometrium in cases of a noncommunicating obstructed rudimentary uterine horn. It should be noted, however, that MRI may not be able to identify a rudimentary uterine horn if it is located laterally along the psoas muscle and pelvic sidewall (64). A hysterosalpingogram, performed on an outpatient basis with the use of fluoroscopy, can be helpful in determining the patency and possible complex communications in cases of genital tract anomalies

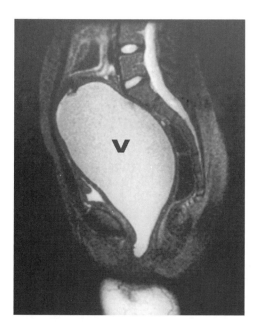

FIG. 10-65. Magnetic resonance imaging of atresia of the lower vagina resulting in a large hematocolpos. V, obstructed blood-filled vagina. (Courtesy of Carol Barnewolt, M.D., Children's Hospital Boston.)

(62). Sonohysterography and 3-D ultrasound have also been shown to be helpful (65,66). In cases of complicated müllerian anomalies, additional information may also be obtained by examination with the patient under anesthesia, vaginoscopy, laparoscopy, and/or hysteroscopy, although with radiologic advances these procedures are now required less frequently (62,67).

Renal and Other Anomalies

Urinary tract anomalies (see Chapter 13) are the most common abnormality associated with congenital anomalies of the female reproductive tract, as the development of a normal müllerian duct is unlikely without the normal development of the mesonephric duct (54,68). Urinary tract abnormalities in patients with müllerian duct anomalies include ipsilateral renal agenesis, duplex collecting systems, renal duplication, and horseshoe-shaped kidneys. In the general population, the incidence of unilateral renal agenesis has been estimated to be between 1 in 600 and 1 in 1,200, on the basis of autopsy studies (69,70). The incidence of associated genital abnormalities in female patients with renal anomalies is estimated to be between 25% and 89% (70,71).

Other extragenital malformations include congenital scoliosis, limb bud deformity, lacrimal duct stenosis, external auditory canal stenosis and resulting hearing loss, congenital heart disease, inguinal hernia, imperforate anus, and malposition of the ovary (see MURC section on page 386) (72,73). Patients with obstructive and nonobstructive anomalies have an increased incidence of endometriosis (see Chapter 11) and resultant extensive adhesions (74–76).

DIAGNOSIS AND TREATMENT OF SPECIFIC ANOMALIES OF THE FEMALE GENITAL TRACT

Imperforate Hymen

Imperforate hymen (Fig. 10-32) is probably the most common obstructive anomaly of the female reproductive tract. Familial occurrences of imperforate hymen have been reported; although most cases are isolated events, families should be screened by history for possibly affected female relatives (53). The diagnosis of imperforate hymen should be made at birth, as obstetricians and pediatricians should determine whether there is a patent hymen during the newborn period; many young women with an imperforate hymen may reach menarche before the diagnosis is made. At birth a bulge from the mucocolpos (see Fig. 3-13) may be evident, as there is an increase in vaginal secretions during the newborn period because of maternal estradiol stimulation. If the imperforate hymen is not diagnosed, the mucus will most likely resorb and the bulge will no longer be present. The thin membrane of the imperforate hymen can be visualized within the hymenal ring.

The adolescent patient with an imperforate hymen may have a history of cyclic abdominal pelvic pain, often for several years, or she may be asymptomatic. A bluish, bulging hymen (Fig. 10-63) and a vagina distended with blood may be found on genital inspection and rectoabdominal palpation. In some cases, the vagina may be extremely large, and the condition may result in back pain, pain with defecation, nausea and vomiting, and/or difficulty with urination. In extreme cases, hydronephrosis due to mechanical obstruction of the ureters from the grossly enlarged vagina can occur.

Surgical Repair

The repair of an imperforate hymen can be accomplished in infancy, childhood, or adolescence, although the repair is facilitated when estrogen stimulation is present (early infancy or postpubertal). In the unestrogenized state of childhood it may be difficult to differentiate vaginal agenesis and an imperforate hymen.

Bupivacaine hydrochloride 0.5% is injected into the area before the incision is made. One method utilizes a Bovie device (with the plastic shield cut back and placed on three-fourths of the tip to help prevent inadvertent injury to the surrounding tissues) to incise the membrane of the imperforate hymen close to the hymenal ring (Fig. 10-66). An elliptical incision is made, and the mucus, secretion (Fig. 10-67), or old blood (Fig. 10-68) is evacuated. Care must be taken, as the fluid within the obstructed vagina may be under considerable pressure; in addition, the "old blood" is usually very thick and may clog the suction tubing. We find it helpful to have more

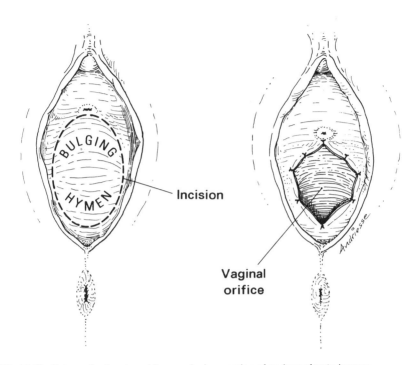

FIG. 10-66. Schematic drawing of the surgical correction of an imperforate hymen.

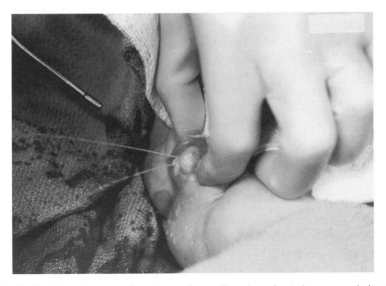

FIG. 10-67. Draining of a mucocolpos in a newborn with an imperforate hymen; predrainage image is shown in Fig. 3-13.

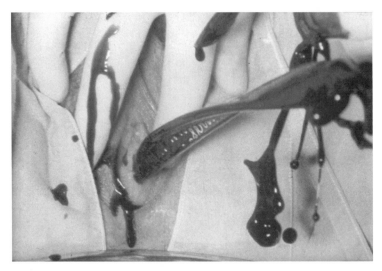

FIG. 10-68. Draining of a hematocolpos in an adolescent with an imperforate hymen.

than one wall suction setup available. Once an initial incision has been made and the obstructed fluid drained, the hymenal area is opened further to create an orifice of "normal" size and remove the excess hymenal tissue. The vaginal mucosa is then sutured to the hymenal ring so that the area does not adhere and result in a recurrence of the obstruction (Fig. 10-66). Additional bupivacaine hydrochloride 0.5% is injected into the repair area, or topical 2% lidocaine jelly can be placed at the conclusion of the procedure for additional postoperative analgesia.

In treatment of the imperforate hymen, puncture of a mucocolpos or hematocolpos without definitive surgical repair should be avoided, since the viscous fluid may not drain adequately and the small perforations will allow ascension of bacteria and the possibility of infection, such as pelvic inflammatory disease or tuboovarian abscess. Patient information regarding types of hymens is available at *http://www.young-womenshealth.org/hymen.html*

Transverse Vaginal Septum

Transverse vaginal septa (Fig. 10-34) are believed to arise from a failure in fusion and/or canalization of the urogenital sinus and müllerian ducts. The complete transverse vaginal septum may be located at various levels (low, middle, or high) in the vagina (Fig. 10-69); the external genitalia appear normal. Approximately 46% of vaginal septa occur in the upper vagina, 40% in the middle vagina, and 14% in the lower vagina (77). The vagina is short or appears as a "blind pouch" (Fig. 10-64). The

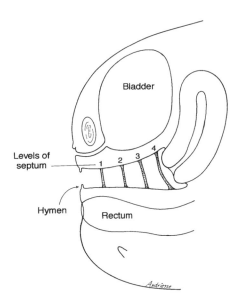

FIG. 10-69. Schematic drawing of locations of transverse septum

septa are usually less than 1 cm thick and may completely or incompletely extend from one vaginal sidewall to the other. Transverse vaginal septa commonly have a small central (Figs. 10-35 and 10-70) or eccentric perforation (78) but still may present with hematocolpos in the adolescent, mucocolpos in the child, and/or pyohematocolpos caused by ascending infection through the small perforation. If there is no

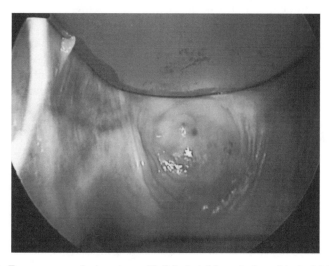

FIG. 10-70. Transverse vaginal septum with "pin hole" fenestration, (black dot in center of bulge).

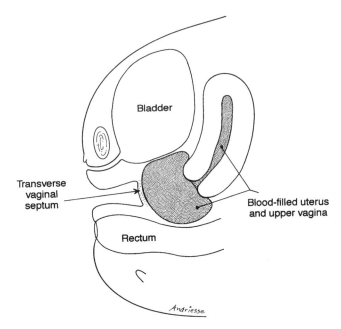

FIG. 10-71. Drawing of non-fenestrated transverse vaginal septum with resulting hematocolpos and hematometra.

perforation in the transverse septum, there is a resultant obstruction with hematocolpos during menses; a mass is palpable above the examining finger and on rectoabdominal palpation (Fig. 10-71). An obstruction with a transverse septum resulting in hematometra may lead to endometriosis (79).

Ultrasound or MRI may help define the septum and its thickness preoperatively (Fig. 10-72). Knowing the thickness of the septum can be helpful at the time of surgery. It is also extremely important to identify a cervix on ultrasound or MRI in order to differentiate between a high septum and congenital absence of the cervix (see Cervical Atresia/Hypogenesis on page 398).

Surgical approaches depend on the septal thickness and the possible need for vaginoplasty to create a patent tract. The surgical procedure involves incision of thin septa with resection of the septal tissue and end-to-end anastomosis of the upper and lower vaginal mucosa (Fig. 10-73). Preoperative dilatation of the transverse septum with hard vaginal dilators may decrease the thickness of the vaginal septum and facilitate the reanastomosis of the upper and lower vaginal mucosa. We find that it is best to perform this procedure when the patient has an upper vagina distended with menstrual blood products, as this acts as a natural tissue expander to increase the amount of upper vaginal tissue available to be reanastomosed to the lower vagina, and may also thin the septal tissue. A Z-plasty technique may help prevent circum-

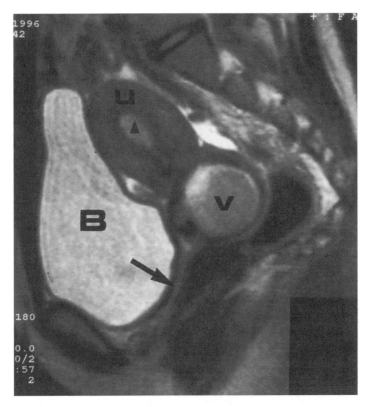

FIG. 10-72. Magnetic resonance imaging of transverse vaginal septum with resulting blood-filled upper vagina (V) and uterus (U) with hematometra (▲). B: bladder, *arrow* at lower vagina. (Courtesy of Carol Barnewolt, M.D., Children's Hospital Boston.)

ferential scar formation (resulting in an "hour-glass" vagina) perpendicular to the vaginal axis in a case of thicker septum (Fig. 10-74) (80,81). To prevent injuries to the urethra or rectum, a urinary bladder catheter and a finger in the rectum can guide surgery. For difficult cases, a probe can be passed transfundally through the uterus, down through the endocervical canal, and into the upper vagina so as to tent up the septum and aid in the resection. If the suture line is under tension, a large (no. 24 French) Malecot catheter or a flexible dilator should be left in place to avoid stricture and reobstruction of the vaginal tract. If there is not enough vaginal mucosa to accomplish a pull-through procedure and reanastomosis of the vaginal mucosa, a skin graft may be necessary to create a patent vaginal tract.

It is very important to attempt to differentiate between a high transverse vaginal septum and cervical agenesis, as the management varies and attempts of surgical correction of the latter have been associated with death (82). MRI can be helpful in this determination. The management of cervical agenesis is discussed below.

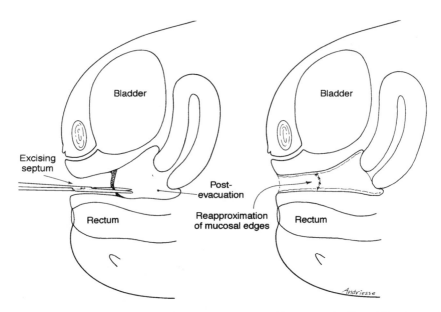

FIG. 10-73. Drawing of resection of transverse septum with reapproximation of the mucosal edges.

Vaginal Atresia/Agenesis of the Lower Vagina/Segmental Vaginal Agenesis

Vaginal atresia (Figs. 10-33 and 10-36) occurs when the urogenital sinus fails to contribute to the lower portion of the vagina. The uterus, cervix, and upper vagina are normal, and the absent section of the vagina is replaced by fibrous tissue. These patients usually present with primary amenorrhea, and with menarche they may develop cyclic or chronic pain and a pelvic or abdominal mass as the upper vagina fills with obstructed blood and secretions (Fig. 10-75).

Physical examination reveals normal secondary sexual characteristics; the introital examination reveals a vaginal dimple, as seen in Color Plate 29. A rectoabdominal exam is helpful to palpate possible midline structures (upper vagina, cervix, and/or uterus) in order to differentiate this condition from vaginal agenesis (see Vaginal Agenesis on page 386).

Ultrasonography, which should be done to assess renal status, can confirm normal ovaries, the presence of an obstructed upper vagina, and the presence of a normal cervix and uterus (56). Also, MRI (Fig. 10-65) may be helpful in the evaluation of these patients, especially to determine whether a cervix is present and to exclude the diagnosis of cervical agenesis (see below) and if functional endometrium is present in a normal uterus or rudimentary uterine horn.

In individuals with agenesis or atresia of the lower vagina, an obstruction with a hematocolpos of the upper vagina will result at the time of menarche and requires a

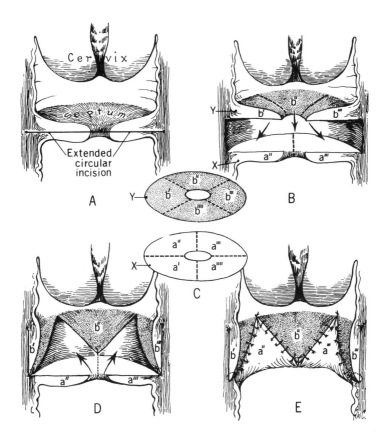

FIG. 10-74. Z-plasty technique for thick vaginal septum. (From Garcia RE. Z-plasty correction for congenital transverse vaginal septum. *Am J Obstet Gynecol* 1967;99:1164–1165; with permission.)

surgical procedure to relieve the obstruction when the hematocolpos is diagnosed. The surgery is best performed when a large hematocolpos is present (Fig. 10-75). A transverse incision is made in the area where the hymenal ring should be located (Fig. 10-76). Dissection is carried out through the fibrous area of the absent lower vagina, until the bulging upper vagina is reached. The obstruction is then drained and the vaginal mucosa identified. It is then possible to do a pull-through procedure to bring the distended upper vaginal tissue down to the introitus (Fig. 10-77). The upper vaginal tissue is held in place and sutured (with interrupted sutures) to the hymenal ring, as shown in Fig. 10-78. After the pull-through procedure has been performed, patients must use a vaginal dilator to avoid stenosis, but will subsequently have normal sexual and reproductive function.

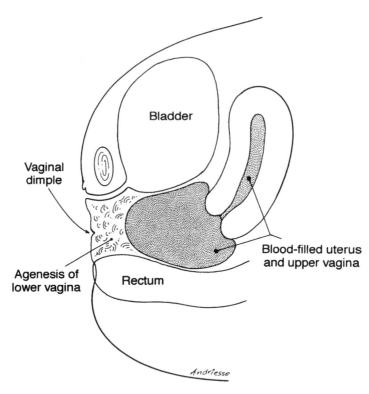

FIG. 10-75. Diagram of agenesis of the lower vagina with normal uterus and cervix, and resulting blood-filled upper vagina.

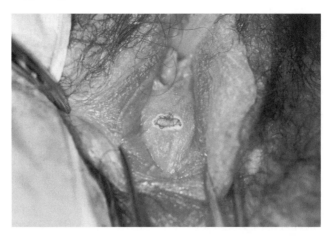

FIG. 10-76. Transverse incision made to create a vaginal orifice. The incision is made and the noted fibrous tissue is dissected to reach the obstructed upper vagina.

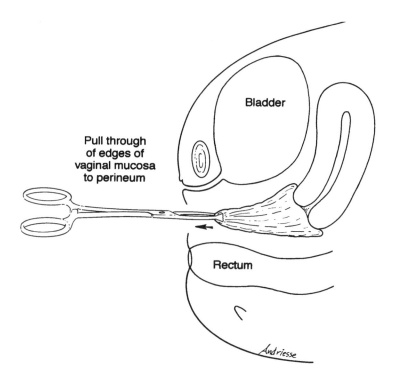

FIG. 10-77. After drainage of obstructed lower vagina (as seen in Fig 10-75), the normal upper vaginal tissue is pulled through to the perineum to create a normal vagina.

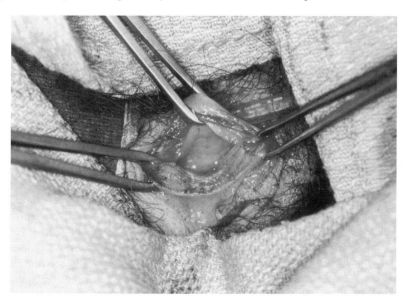

FIG. 10-78. After drainage of obstructed lower vagina (from patent in Fig 10-76), the normal upper vaginal tissue is pulled down to the perineum; the upper vaginal mucosa is stitched to the created introitus with interrupted sutures to create a normal patent vagina. (Notice that the clamps are approximating the upper and lower tissue to be stitched together.)

Vaginal Agenesis (Müllerian Aplasia)

Vaginal agenesis, müllerian aplasia, Mayer-von Rokitansky–Küster–Hauser (MRKH) syndrome, is the congenital absence of the vagina with variable müllerian duct and possible associated renal, skeletal, and auditory abnormalities (83–86). Vaginal agenesis is usually accompanied by cervical and uterine agenesis, although approximately 7% to 10% of affected individuals have a normal but obstructed uterus or a rudimentary uterus with functional endometrium (87–92) (Figs. 10-37 and 10-38 and Color Plates 29, 34, and 35). Vaginal agenesis must be differentiated from vaginal atresia (Figs. 10-33 and 10-36). Another variant is the presence of a uterus but agenesis of the vagina and cervix (Fig. 10-38).

Müllerian aplasia is estimated to occur in about 1 in 1,000 to 1 in 83,000 female births, but the most widely cited incidence is approximately 1 in 5,000 female births (93). MRKH is second only to gonadal dysgenesis as a pathologic cause of primary amenorrhea in a tertiary referral center (94).

Individuals with MRKH have a normal female 46, XX karyotype and normal ovarian hormonal/oocyte function. Ovarian sex steroid production is normal in these women, and thus puberty and the development of secondary sexual characteristics progress normally except that menstrual flow is absent. The presence of normal breast and pubic hair development, and normal female serum testosterone and pubertal estradiol levels, make this syndrome the likely diagnosis. Although chromosomal studies are not necessary for all of these individuals, an elevated testosterone level, lack of breast development, absent pubic hair, or virilization mandate further studies for an intersex state (see Chapters 2 and 7). The average age at the time of diagnosis has been reported to be between 15 and 18 years. Müllerian aplasia has also been associated with maternal deficiency of galactose-I-phosphate uridyl transferase (95).

A high percentage of individuals with müllerian aplasia exhibit renal and skeletal abnormalities. An association has been demonstrated between MRKH and Klippel–Feil (congenital fusion of the cervical spine, short neck, low posterior hairline, and painless limitations of cervical movement) syndromes (96). In addition the *MURCS* association has been described, which includes: MU: Müllerian duct aplasia, R: renal agenesis/ectopia, and CS: cervicothoracic somite dysplasia (97).

Physical examination reveals normal secondary sexual development, normal perineum, and a vaginal dimple/small pouch (see Color Plate 29). The hymenal fringe is usually present along with the small vaginal pouch, as they are both derived embryologically from the urogenital sinus. A rectoabdominal exam is helpful to determine whether the midline structures (upper vagina, cervix, and/or uterus) are present.

Ultrasonography, which should be done to assess renal status, can confirm normal ovaries and the lack of a uterus. Remnants of uterine structures may be present (see Fig 10-37 and Color Plates 34 and 35) and may cause cyclic or chronic abdominal/pelvic pain and require surgical excision if endometrium is present in a noncommunicating rudimentary horn. MRI may be helpful in the evaluation of vaginal agenesis, especially to determine whether functional endometrium is present in a normal uterus or rudimentary uterine horn (98). It is possible that MRI may not be able to identify uterine horns that are laterally displaced and resting on the psoas muscles (64).

Laparotomy is almost never indicated in the diagnostic evaluation, and laparoscopy for cases of vaginal agenesis without pelvic pain is not necessary unless the anatomy cannot be defined by other modalities. Alternatively, if cyclic or chronic pelvic pain develops, then an assessment and treatment of the pelvis for an obstructed uterine horn and possible endometriosis are indicated.

Counseling

This diagnosis can be quite upsetting to a girl, young adolescent, or adult woman, and her family. Counseling by experienced nurses, social workers, psychologists and/or psychiatrists is strongly recommended, and should be encouraged by the treating health care provider (99,100). It is important to stress to the young woman and her family that she has normal ovarian function, normal production of sex steroids, that a functional vagina can be created, and fertility is possible utilizing her own oocytes through assisted reproductive technologies and a gestational carrier (101,102).

Treatment

The treatment of müllerian aplasia should be preceded by counseling of the young woman and her parents. Attention must be given to the psychosocial issues as well as to the correction of the anatomic abnormality. The patient's cooperation and positive attitude are vital to the ultimate success of the creation of a functional vagina (103). The timing for the nonsurgical or surgical creation of a vagina for those individuals with agenesis of the vagina, cervix, and uterus is elective and not a surgical emergency. Since this is not a surgical emergency, pediatric surgeons, pediatric urologists and gynecologists should refrain from creating a vagina for girls with MRKH during childhood, and instead should wait until the young woman opts to move ahead with a self-selected specific treatment (104). It is challenging for children and their parents to be asked to utilize vaginal dilators after surgical creation of a vagina during childhood. Parents commonly complain that they are not comfortable inserting a dilator into their daughter's vagina. Treatment should thus wait until the affected individual is able to determine the treatment and timing of the treatment. Parents of girls with MRKH may seek consultation for surgical correction during childhood to "resolve" the anomaly. It is recommended to delay any technique for creation of a functional vagina until the mid-to-late teens, when the young woman (and not her parents) opts for treatment and is comfortable with and is willing to participate in the process. Some women may elect never to create a vagina. It is important to provide patients and their families with resource information presenting all options such as that available at *www.youngwomenshealth.org* or *www.MRKH.org*

Creation of a Functional Vagina

The creation of a vagina may be accomplished both nonoperatively and operatively (104,105). The goal of any method is to create a vaginal canal of adequate diameter and length and appropriate axis to accommodate sexual intercourse. In addition the vagina should have a "normal" amount of secretion and lubrication and require minimal care for maintenance. No procedure achieves all of these goals and thus there are many options, each with associated advantages and disadvantages.

Nonoperative Techniques for Creation of a Vagina   The nonoperative approaches attempt to use progressive invagination of the vaginal dimple to create a vagina of adequate diameter and length. It has been noted that a functional vagina can be created with repetitive coitus (106), but care must be taken not to dilate the urethra, which can lead to urinary incontinence. The nonoperative method of creating a functional vagina involves the use of pressure against the vaginal dimple in order to create a progressive invagination of the mucosa. The Frank (107) nonsurgical approach for creation of a vagina involves the use of graduated hard dilators. The use of vaginal dilators is the first line of therapy offered to our patients with MRKH. The rationale for this approach is based on the fact that this technique requires no surgical intervention or anesthesia, leaves no scars, results in "normal vaginal lubrication," and is completely in the control of the young woman. Recent studies have shown that the utilization of dilators is greater than 85% to 90% successful for the creation of a functional vagina (108,109), and we have had a similar experience in our patient population.

The young woman is instructed on how to use a hard dilator for constant pressure to create a vagina. This technique works best if she has a vaginal dimple, but can be utilized in all cases of MRKH. It may take 2 months to 2 years to create a functional vagina depending on patient motivation and the frequency of dilation. The smallest dilator (or a small pediatric blood drawing tube) is pressed firmly (until she feels mild discomfort, not pain) against the vaginal dimple (Fig. 10-79) daily for at least half an hour after a warm bath. The young woman is instructed to insert the tube downward and inward in the line of the normal vaginal axis. We begin the dilatation process with the use of a pediatric blood drawing tube, and once an adequate vaginal dimple has been established we currently utilize Syracuse Medical Vaginal Dilators (Fig. 10-80). The Ingram modification of the Frank method utilizes a bicycle seat mounted on a stool to facilitate vaginal dilatation (110). Although this modification is an interesting concept and adaptation of the Frank method, many young women initially find this technique very awkward, but as the vagina gains length it can be helpful. We have found that the greatest success can be achieved through education, nursing support, mental health counseling, and a "big sister" program (see Chapter 12). Patient educational materials regarding the creation of a functional vaginal with the use of vaginal dilators is available at *www.youngwomenshealth.org/dilators* and at *www.MRKH.org*.

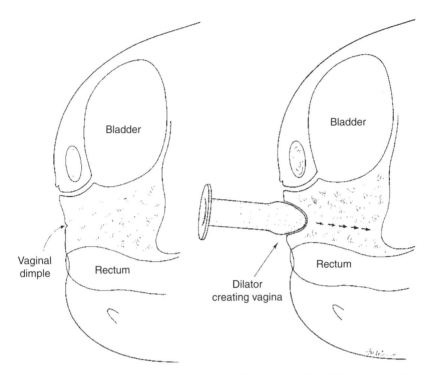

FIG. 10-79. Graduated hard dilator pressed against the perineum in the Frank nonsurgical approach for creation of a vagina; note that the dilator is aimed towards the sacrum and not straight.

Surgical Techniques for Creation of a Functional Vagina   Surgical procedures should be considered only if the young woman has been unable to create a functional vagina with the utilization of dilators. Surgery should not be used as a first option; standard guidelines addressing when to proceed to a surgical procedure need to be developed. Some young women are interested in a "quick fix" and think that surgery will be able to achieve this goal. It is important that the health care provider and mental health provider help the young women understand the short and long term issues related to surgery, and the fact that most surgical interventions require the postoperative utilization of dilators.

If the use of dilators has been unsuccessful, or if the mature patient elects surgery after a thorough discussion of the advantages and disadvantages, surgical creation of a vagina can be accomplished by one of several techniques (111–114). The McIndoe procedure (112,113), used commonly by gynecologists, utilizes a split-thickness skin graft (0.018 to 0.022 in.) taken from the buttocks. To make sure that the graft is aesthetic, the patient can use a magic marker to outline her bathing suit borders so that the graft site is not visible when she wears a bathing suit. The skin graft is placed over a stent, dermal side out (Counsellor technique) (Fig. 10-81). With the patient in the

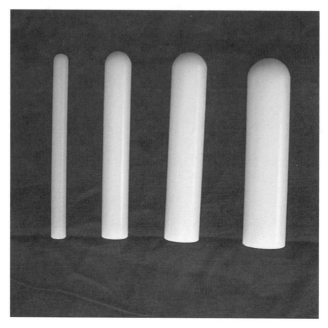

FIG. 10-80. Syracuse Medical Dilators.

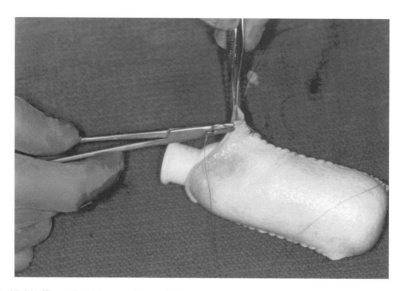

FIG. 10-81. The split thickness skin grafts are sewn around a mold.

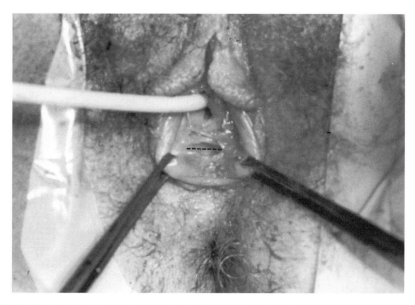

FIG. 10-82. Incision of the perineum (*dashed line*) followed by dissection of the fibrous tissue below the urethra and bladder, above the anus and rectum, and to the level of the peritoneal reflection for creation of a neovagina.

lithotomy position, a transverse incision is made at the vaginal dimple (see Color Plate 29 and Fig. 10-82), and a cavity is dissected to the level of the peritoneum (Fig. 10-83), meticulous hemostasis and asepsis being observed. The mold and skin graft are inserted, and the labia minora are secured around the stent to prevent expulsion. The Foley catheter inserted earlier is removed, and suprapubic bladder drainage is accomplished. After 7 days of strict bed rest and a low-residue diet, the stent is removed (Fig. 10-84) and the graft site revised. A dilator is needed to prevent contraction of the vaginal graft, and the patient is instructed to wear the dilator continually for 3 months, removing it only during urination, defecation, showering, or sexual activity (which can be initiated 3 weeks postoperatively if the patient desires). The patient is seen for frequent follow-up visits to check the graft (Fig. 10-85). After the initial 3 months, the patient is instructed to wear the dilator at night for 6 months unless she has regular intercourse. Since failure to comply with follow-up treatment can lead to vaginal stenosis, surgery should not be contemplated until the patient understands the procedure and her involvement. Talking with another patient who has already had successful surgery is very helpful for many adolescents.

Long-term follow-up of patients who have had a McIndoe vaginoplasty has shown excellent function and patient satisfaction (7,8,115,116). A patient with a neovagina requires yearly examinations, as there have been cases of carcinoma involving the skin grafts (117,118).

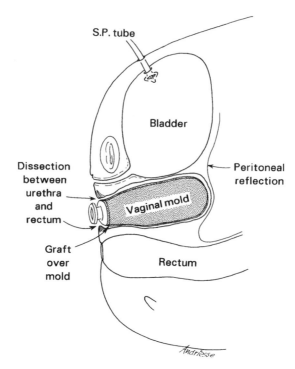

FIG. 10-83. Vaginal mold with skin graft in place; notice that the mold with the skin graft reaches the level of the peritoneal reflection. S.P, suprapubic.

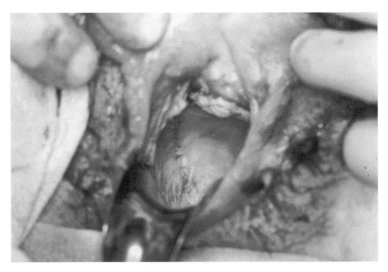

FIG. 10-84. After 7 days of strict bed rest and a low-residue diet, the stent is removed. Notice the suture line of the skin graft of the newly created vagina.

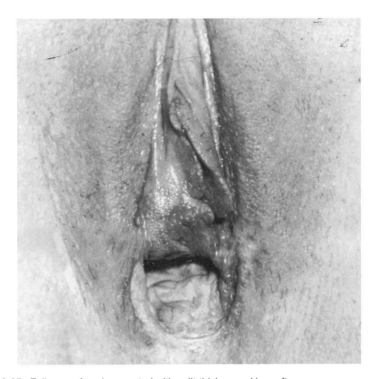

FIG. 10-85. Followup of vagina created with split-thickness skin graft.

Patient information regarding the McIndoe procedure is available at *www.young-womenshealth.org/McIndoe*

The use of full-thickness skin grafts for the creation of a vagina has been described (119–121). Its proponents report that there is less graft stricture or stenosis than in the split-thickness technique.

The Williams vulvovaginoplasty (122) (Fig. 10-86) involves the creation of a vaginal pouch. A U-shaped incision is made, and full-thickness skin flaps from the labia majora are used to create a kangaroo-like pouch, horizontal to the perineum (Fig. 10-87A). A dilator is used daily for 3 to 4 weeks but is not necessary after that. The axis of the vagina is different for coitus, but difficulties can be overcome. Coitus and the use of a dilator assist in the creation of a functional vagina (Fig. 10-87B). The pelvic structures are not entered in this operation, and thus the risk of fistula formation is low. It is particularly useful in patients with a previously failed vaginoplasty and those who have had radical pelvic surgery or irradiation. This procedure has not been popular in the USA as it is felt to create an awkward angle for sexual intercourse and a poor cosmetic appearance. This is not the feeling in other parts of the world, as Creatsas and colleagues have reported greater than 90% success with their modified technique (123).

The use of bowel for the creation of a vagina is an option advocated primarily by pediatric surgeons (124–127). The procedure is accomplished via a laparotomy with the creation of a loop of bowel and preservation of its vascular pedicle (Fig. 10-88A). The bowel loop is them positioned so that one end is pulled down to the introitus for creation of a neovagina, and the distal end is closed to create the blind pouch (Fig. 10-88B). An end-to-end reanastomosis is then performed to recreate a patent

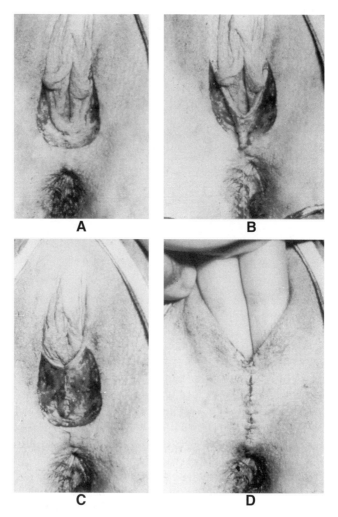

FIG. 10-86. Williams vulvovaginoplasty. **A:** Initial incision. **B:** The edges of the inner skin layer are brought together and sutured. **C:** The edges of the inner layer are almost completely brought together. **D:** The outer layer is sutured over the inner layer. Two fingers are inserted into the introitus of the new "vagina." (From Edmonds DK. *Dewhurst's practical paediatric and adolescent gynecology,* 2nd ed. London: Butterworth-Heinmann, 1989; with permission.)

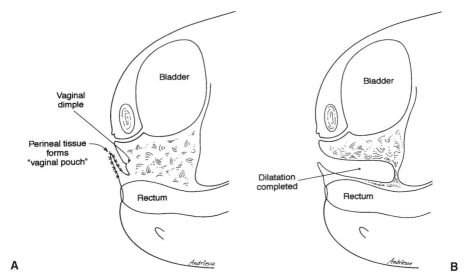

FIG. 10-87. A: Schematic drawing at completion of Williams procedure. **B:** Schematic drawing months after completion of Williams procedure with creation of a vagina with the use of dilators and vaginal intercourse.

gastrointestinal tract (Fig. 10-88C). The final result is shown in Fig. 10-89. Stenosis is believed to be more common when ileum is used than when colon is used (125), and thus, procedures have been proposed to reconfigure the small bowel to increase the diameter (126). This procedure has the advantage over a McIndoe procedure in that the patient is not required to remain at bed rest for 7 days, as with the McIndoe procedure. Disadvantages have been reported. Patients complain of the need to wear a pad daily because of the chronic vaginal discharge from the bowel mucosa. In addition, some patients find that they need to douche daily to avoid a foul odor. Adenocarcinomas have developed in the large or small bowel intestinal grafts for the vaginal reconstruction (128). With the increasing risk of HIV transmission during adolescence and young adulthood (see Chapter 16) and the poor barrier effect of gastrointestinal mucosa compared with skin, we prefer the McIndoe procedure for the surgical creation of a vagina in cases of vaginal agenesis. This technique is best reserved for cases where there is no adequate space between the urethra and the rectum for alternative options of vaginal creation.

Other methods for creation of a functional vagina that use the pelvic peritoneum (129–131), Interceed (Johnson & Johnson Patient Care Inc., New Brunswick, NJ) (132,133), or human amnion have been reported (134). The use of human amnion is not practical because of the risk of HIV transmission. In addition, the use of muscle and skin flaps for the creation of a vagina has been described (135–137).

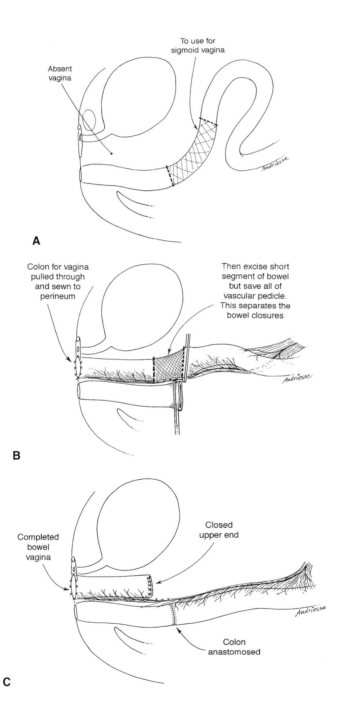

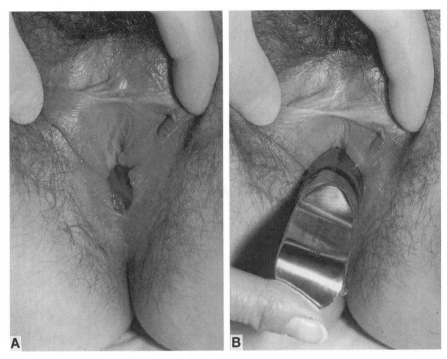

FIG. 10-89. A: Postoperative view of the perineum with the sigmoid vagina anastomosed to vaginal introitus. **B:** No. 26 Hegar dilator (6 in. long) reveals normal vaginal caliber and depth. Patients are advised to pass the dilator periodically to ensure continuation of adequate caliber. This procedure is not as important as it would be for a skin graft vagina, which will contract if not periodically dilated in this fashion or by coitus. (From Hendren WH, Atala A. Use of bowel for vaginal reconstruction. *J Urol* 1994;152:752; with permission.)

Some procedures modify the Frank technique of perineal pressure for the creation of a vagina. The Vecchietti procedure utilizes a laparoscopic approach for the placement of a plexiglass "olive" placed against the vaginal dimple. The "olive" has sutures attached to it, which are laparoscopically guided through the vesicorectal space into the peritoneal cavity and out through the abdominal wall (138–142). Tension is

FIG. 10-88. Technique for sigmoid vaginoplasty. **A:** Identification of distal sigmoid with blood supply that will reach to the perineum. The bowel segment should not be isolated and divided at both ends at this point, lest length of mesentery be misjudged. **B:** Distal end of bowel segment is divided and pulled through to perineum and sewn there, which ensures that the bowel comes down with adequate slack and no tension on its mesentery. Only then is the upper end of the bowel segment divided, care being taken to preserve its adjacent blood supply. Removing the short segment of bowel above that will separate the rectosigmoid anastomosis from the closure of the upper end of the bowel used for the vagina to protect against fistula formation. **C:** Completed sigmoid vagina. (From Hendren WH, Atala A. Use of bowel for vaginal reconstruction. *J Urol* 1994;152:752; with permission.)

increasingly applied to the abdominal wall sutures that pull the "olive," resulting in the creation of a dilated vagina. After sufficient length of the new vagina has been achieved with serially increased tension the mold and sutures are removed. The patient continues to use hard vaginal dilators to create a functional length of the vagina.

Cervical Atresia/Hypogenesis

Cervical agenesis (Figs. 10-37 to 10-41 and Figs. 10-90 and 10-91) and dysgenesis (Fig. 10-92) are rare (143–146) but are extremely important to diagnose correctly. The true diagnosis of cervical atresia requires the absence of the upper vagina, as embryologically the upper vagina does not develop in the absence of the cervix. Patients may present with primary amenorrhea, cyclic or chronic abdominal or pelvic pain, and/or a distended uterus. Ultrasonography and MRI can aid in defining anatomy (60).

If cervical agenesis is diagnosed, hysterectomy with removal of the obstructed uterus has usually been recommended, as this condition has not yet been particularly amenable to surgical attempts at reconstruction (145–148). However, the creation of an epithelialized "endocervical" tract and vagina, utilizing a specially created vaginal/cervical mold and both skin and mucosal grafts, has been reported (143,149,150). The creation of a "vaginal–uterine fistula tract" places the patient at risk of an ascending infection, recurrent obstruction, sepsis, and possible septic death (82,144,151,152). However, successful pregnancies have followed these procedures (89,153,154), and a zygote intrafallopian tube transfer (ZIFT) in a patient with congenital cervical atresia following a fistulous drainage procedure has been reported (155). Based on the options available and the risk of sepsis and death, it is our practice to offer a young woman with cervical agenesis hormonally suppressive therapy

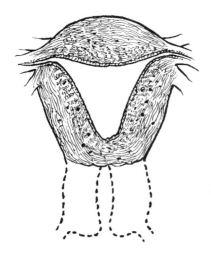

FIG. 10-90. Congenital cervical agenesis. The fundus of the uterus is present without the body of the cervix. (Rock JA, Carpenter SE, Wheeless CR, et al. The clinical management of maldevelopment of the uterine cervix. *J Pelvic Surg* 1995;1:129; with permission.)

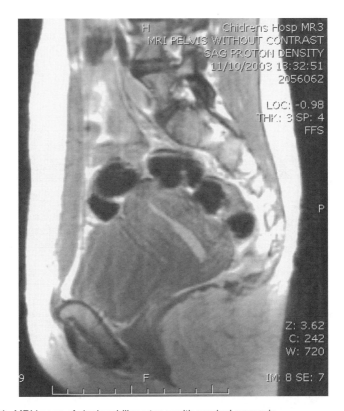

FIG. 10-91. MRI image of single midline uterus with cervical agenesis.

with either combination hormonal therapy or GnRH agonist with add-back therapy (see Chapter 11). With long term hormonal suppression she can maintain her uterus with the plan for assisted reproductive technologies in the future with a planned abdominal delivery of the child.

Variations of cervical agenesis can occur with a single midline uterus, or with hemiuteri, as shown in Color Plates 34 and 35. If a patient has a hemiuterus with an endometrial stripe, then suppressive hormonal therapy can be used to maintain the uterine horns for future ART, or the uterine horns can be removed laparoscopically with the intent to utilize a gestational carrier for future pregnancy.

Obstructed Uterine Rudimentary Horns

In women with müllerian aplasia and cyclic or chronic abdominal or pelvic pain, a noncommunicating uterine horn with functional endometrium should be suspected (Figs. 10-44 and 10-45). Ultrasound and/or MRI may be useful in identifying the noncommunicating uterine horn and determining whether an endometrial stripe is present. Laparoscopy may be needed to diagnose and remove the obstructed rudimentary noncommunicating uterine horn (see Color Plate 36). Figures 10-93 to 10-95 demonstrate the laparoscopic approach to the removal of the obstructed uterine horn seen in Color Plate 36 (156). Patients with an obstructed uterine horn are at in-

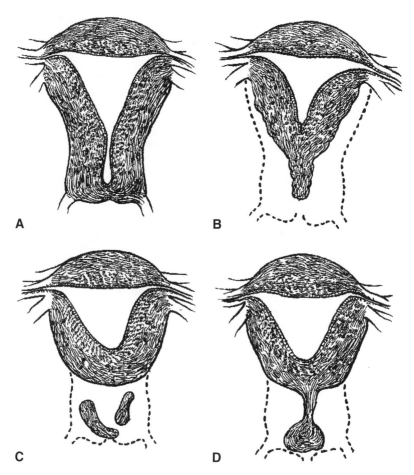

FIG. 10-92. Congenital cervical dysgenesis. The cervical body is intact **(A)** with obstruction of the cervical os. Variable portions of the cervical lumen are obliterated. The cervical body **(B)** consists of fibrous bands of variable diameter that may contain endocervical glands. Fragmented portions of the cervix are noted **(C)** with no connection to the uterine body. Hypoplasia of the uterine cavity may be associated with cervical cords or fragmentation. The midportion of the cervix **(D)** is hypoplastic with a bulbous tip. No cervical lumen is identified. (Rock JA, Carpenter S, Wheeless C, *et al.* The clinical management of maldevelopment of the uterine cervix. *J Pelvic Surg* 1995;1:129–133; with permission.)

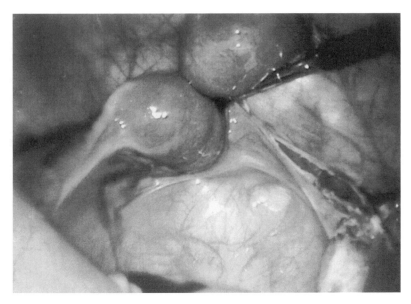

FIG. 10-93. Laparoscopic approach to removal of the obstructed right uterine horn shown in Color Plate 36.

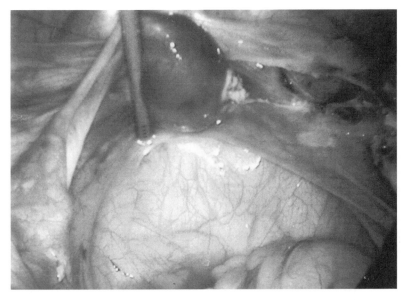

FIG. 10-94. Completion of laparoscopic resection of obstructed right uterine horn in Color Plate 36 and Fig 10-93.

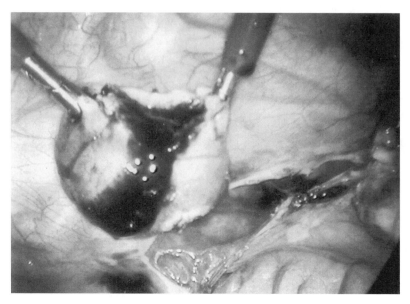

FIG. 10-95. Right uterine horn from Color Plate 36 and Figs 10-93 and 10-94 being morcellated to facilitate laparoscopic removal. Notice the dark old blood of the hematometra.

creased risk of endometriosis, but the endometriosis usually resolves after the correction of the obstruction (see Chapter 11). Excision of the obstructed rudimentary blind horn will prevent endometriosis by eliminating reflux. Spontaneous pregnancies in obstructed uterine horns have been reported (157).

True Duplication and Incomplete Fusion of the Müllerian Ducts

A true duplication of the uterus is rare (Figs. 10-49 to 10-52). This abnormality results from unilateral or bilateral duplication of the müllerian ducts and subsequent doubling of reproductive structures on one or both sides. These are not hemiuteri. True duplication may also result in the very rare occurrence of complete duplication of the vulva, bladder, urethra, vagina, and anus (Fig. 10-96).

Septate uteri (Fig. 10-57) with a septate vagina can be associated with duplication of the colon, anus, urethra, bladder, vagina, and vulva. A uterus didelphys with bicollis has separate uterine cavities and two cervices (Fig. 10-49); in 75% of cases the vagina is septate (see Longitudinal Vaginal Septum below) (Figs. 10-50 to 10-52). Patients with a didelphic uterus usually have adequate reproductive outcomes, and thus metroplasty is contraindicated.

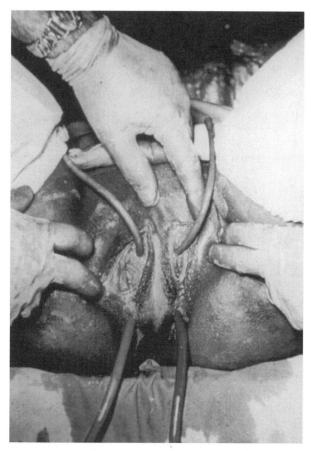

FIG. 10-96. Complete duplication of the vulva, bladder, urethra, vagina, and anus. (Courtesy of James L. Breen, M.D., Saint Barnabas Medical Center, Livingston, New Jersey.)

Longitudinal Vaginal Septum

The fusion of the two müllerian ducts results in a single vagina, but a duplex system with a longitudinal vaginal septum may be created if the fusion is incomplete. Disorders of longitudinal fusion may result in a septate vagina (Figs. 10-50 and 10-97) which may be bilaterally (Fig. 10-51) or unilaterally (Fig. 10-52) imperforate (see Obstructed Hemivagina). Women with a longitudinal vaginal septum may experience difficulties such as a need to use two tampons (one in each hemivagina), difficulty with sexual intercourse, or difficulty with vaginal delivery at childbirth. Resection of the vaginal septum, if needed, can be accomplished in an outpatient surgical setting. The vaginal septum is removed by "wedging" out the complete septum, and

then the normal remaining vaginal mucosa is reapproximated. This technique re-
moves all of the thickened septum so that no "ridge" remains. Care must be taken to
avoid compromise to the cervix, or more commonly the two cervixes at the apex of
the vaginas.

Obstructed Hemivagina (Usually with Ipsilateral Renal Agenesis)

A variation of this abnormality is the obstructed hemivagina with ipsilateral renal
agenesis (158–160) (Figs. 10-52 and 10-98). Patients with this condition have regular periods, as they have a nonobstructed hemivagina with associated cervix and

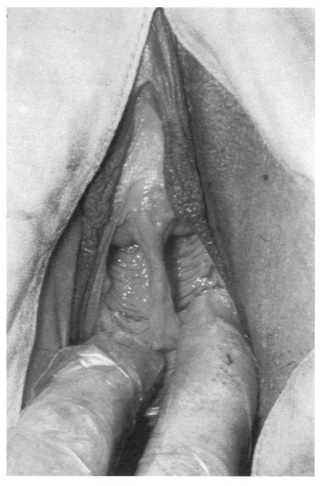

FIG. 10-97. Longitudinal vaginal septum.

hemiuterus. On physical exam, a mass is felt to bulge from the lateral wall of the vagina toward the midline. Ultrasound is helpful in making the diagnosis. In addition, if unilateral renal agenesis is known to exist, the possibility of an obstructed hemivagina must be entertained. In cases of an obstructed hemivagina, the wall of the obstructed vagina must be resected to relieve the obstruction (Figs. 10-98 and 10-99).

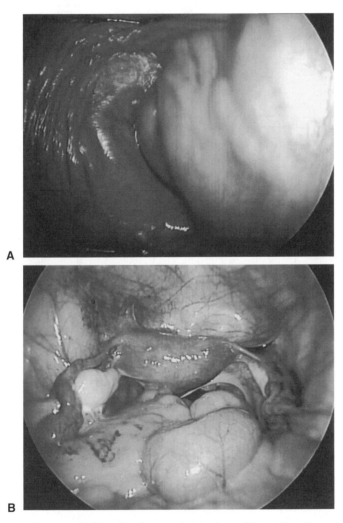

FIG. 10-98. A: Obstructed left hemivagina seen bulging toward the midline. The cervix that communicates with the right vagina and right uterus can be partially seen. **B:** The same patient laparoscopically. Note that the dye injected into the single visible cervix in **(A)** flows out of the right fallopian tube.

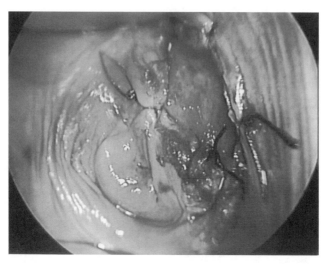

FIG. 10-99. Post resection of the obstruction in patient shown in Fig. 10-98. The second cervix is present in the left hemivagina.

Initially, a wide incision is made in the wall of the obstructed hemivagina to allow adequate drainage of the obstructed fluid. The remainder of the septal wall is then resected to create a single vaginal vault. If there is distorted anatomy from the marked dilatation of the obstructed hemivagina, then a second procedure to resect the remaining septal wall may be necessary. After resection of the septal wall of the obstructed hemivagina, the patient has normal function with a single vagina, two cervices, and two hemiuteri.

Disorders of the Uterus

Complete Uterine Septum

In cases of uterine septum, the external surface of the uterus appears to have a normal configuration, but there are two endometrial cavities (Figs. 10-56 to 10-59, 10-100, and 10-101). Most uterine fusion/duplication abnormalities do not require surgical intervention; if patients experience pain, recurrent miscarriage, infertility, or premature labor, the abnormality should be repaired by hysteroscopic resection (Figs. 10-102 to 10-105) (161–167). In a recent study all women who presented with a divided uterine cavity and first trimester pregnancy loss had a uterine septum and not a bicornuate uterus (168).

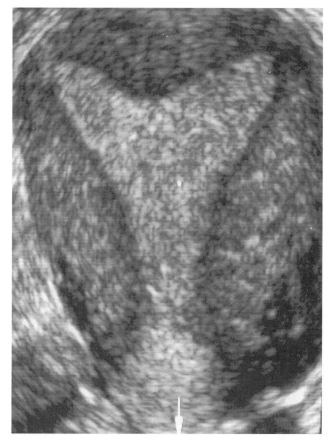

FIG. 10-100. Ultrasound image of two endometrial cavities. Laparoscopy confirmed that this was a septate uterus due to a single uterine myometrial structure as seen in Fig 10-101.

Bicornuate Uterus

In the patient with a bicornuate uterus, the uterine fundus is deeply indented. The level of the indentation can be complete (Fig. 10-53), partial (Fig. 10-54) or arcuate (Fig. 10-55); the vagina is usually normal.

Unicornuate Uterus

A unicornuate uterus (Fig. 10-48) is a single horned uterus that has a single round ligament and fallopian tube. The other hemiuterus, round ligament, and fallopian tube are usually absent. Variations of hemiuteri can occur with the existence of non-communicating uterine horns with or without active endometrium (see Color Plate

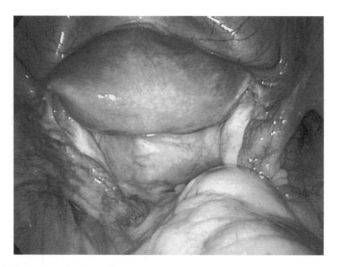

FIG. 10-101. Laparoscopic view of septate uterus. Note broad fundus.

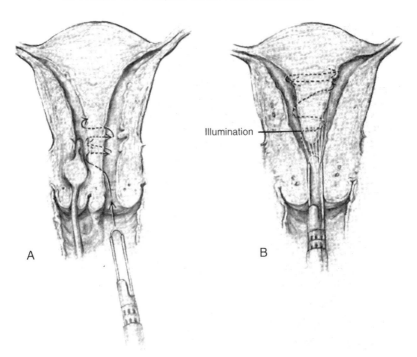

FIG. 10-102. Resectoscopic metroplasty. **A:** A Foley catheter is placed in one cavity of a complete septate uterus (AFS class VA uterus). The resectoscope is inserted in the opposite cavity, and the septum is incised until the Foley is visualized. The septum can be easily incised with the resectoscope until both internal ossa are visible. **B:** A septate uterus with a single cervix. The septum can be incised with the straight loupe of the resectoscope.

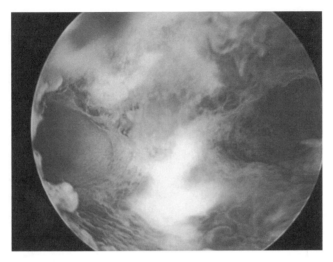

FIG. 10-103. Hysteroscopic view of uterine septum.

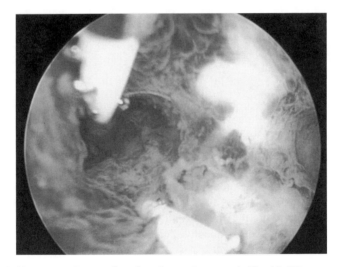

FIG. 10-104. Hysteroscopic resection of uterine septum seen in Fig. 10-103.

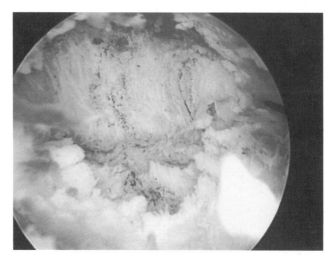

FIG. 10-105. Hysteroscopic view after completed resection of septum seen in Figs. 10-103 and 10-104.

36; Figs. 10-43 to 10-48). The single asymmetric uterus communicates with a single cervix and a normal vagina. Associated renal anomalies are common. Patients with a unicornuate uterus are at increased risk of infertility, endometriosis, premature labor, and breech presentation (52,169).

Pregnancy Outcome in Women with Müllerian Duct Anomalies

Several studies have examined the outcomes of pregnancies in women with müllerian duct abnormalities (170–173). In general, there is an increased rate of unexplained infertility, endometriosis, spontaneous abortion, breech presentation, and premature delivery (52). Women who have had lower vaginal agenesis corrected by the creation of a neovagina are able to conceive and to maintain a pregnancy if a normal cervix and uterus are present. The wider use of assisted reproductive technologies will also enhance the reproductive function of women with congenital abnormalities of the reproductive tract.

REFERENCES

1. Engert J. Surgical correction of virilized female external genitalia. *Prog Pediatr Surg* 1989;23:151–164.
2. Bailez MM, Gearhart JP, Migeon C, et al. Vaginal reconstruction after initial construction of the external genitalia in girls with salt-wasting adrenal hyperplasia. *J Urol* 1992;148:680.

3. Duckett JW, Baskin LS. Genitoplasty for intersex anomalies. *Eur J Pediatr* 1993;152:S80.
4. Donahoe PK, Gustafson ML. Early one-stage surgical reconstruction of the extremely high vagina in patients with congenital adrenal hyperplasia. *J Pediatr Surg* 1994;29:352.
5. Hendren WH, Atala A. Repair of the high vagina in girls with severely masculinized anatomy from the adrogenital syndromes. *J Pediatr Surg* 1995;20:91.
6. Hendren WH. Surgical approach to intersex problems. *Sem Ped Surg* 1998;7:8.
7. Goerzen JL, Gidwani GP. Outcome of surgical reconstructive procedures for the treatment of vaginal anomalies. *Adolesc Pediatr Gynecol* 1994;7:76.
8. Strickland JL, Cameron WJ, Krantz KE. Long-term satisfaction of adults undergoing McIndoe vaginoplasty as adolescents. *Adolesc Pediatr Gynecol* 1993;6:135.
9. Costa EMF, Mendonca BB, Inácío M, et al. Management of ambiguous gentalia in pseudo-hermaphrodites: new perspectives on vaginal dilation. *Fertil Steril* 1997;67:229.
10. Kim HH, Laufer MR. Developmental abnormalities of the female reproductive tract. *Curr Opin Obstet Gynecol* 1994;6:518.
11. Costa E, Arnhold I, Mendonca B, et al. Management of ambiguous genitalia in pseudo-hermaphrodites: new perspectives on vaginal dilation. *Fertil Steril* 1997;67:229.
12. Griffin JE. Androgen resistance: The clinical and molecular spectrum. *N Engl J Med* 1992;326:611.
13. Speroff L, Glass RH, Kase NG. Normal and abnormal sexual development. In: *Clinical gynecologic endocrinology and infertility,* Speroff L, Glass RH, Kase NG, eds., 6th ed. Baltimore: Lippincott Williams & Wilkins, 1999.
14. Rey R, Mebarki F, Forest MG, et al. Anti-müllerian hormone in children with androgen insensitivity. *J Clin Endocrinol Metab* 1994;79:960.
15. Cassio A, Cacciari E, E'Errico A, et al. Incidence of intratubular germ cell neoplasia in androgen insensitivity syndrome. *Acta Endocrinol (Copenh)* 1990;123:416.
16. Rutgers JL, Scully RE. The androgen insensitivity syndrome (testicular feminization): a clinico-pathologic study of 43 cases. *Int J Gynecol Pathol* 1991;10:126.
17. Minto C, Liao K, Conway G, et al. Sexual function in women with complete androgen insensitivity syndrome. *Fertil Steril* 2003;80:157.
18. Kogan S. Feminizing genital reconstruction for male pseudohermaphroditism. *Eur J Pediatr* 1993;152:585.
19. Laufer MR, Galvin WJ. Labial hypertrophy: a new surgical approach. *Adolesc Pediatr Gynecol* 1995;8:39.
20. Rouzier R, Louis-Sylvestre C, Bernard-Jean P, et al. Hypertrophy of labia minora: experience with 163 reductions. *Am J Obstet Gynecol* 2000;182:35.
21. World Health Organization. Female genital mutilation: A Joint WHO/UNICEF/UNFPA statement. Geneva, WHO, 1997.
22. Toubia N. Female circumcision as a public health issue. *N Engl J Med* 1994;331:712.
23. Council on Scientific Affairs, American Medical Association. Female genital mutilation. *JAMA* 1995;274:1714.
24. World Health Organization,. Female genital mutilation: report of a WHO Technical Working Group, July 17–19, 1995. Geneva, WHO, 1995
25. Strickland J. Female circumcision/female genital mutilation. *J Pediatr Adolesc Gynecol* 2001;14:109.
26. World Health Organization. WHO leads action against female genital mutilation. World Health Forum 1994;15:416.
27. ACOG Task Force on Female Circumcision/Female Genital Mutilation. Female circumcision/female genital mutilation: clinical management of circumcised women.1999.
28. Aziz FA. Gynecologic and obstetric complications of female circumcision. *Int J Gynecol Obstet* 1980;17:560.
29. Gardner GH, Greene RR, Peckham BM. Normal and cystic structures of the broad ligament. *Am J Obstet Gynecol* 1948;55:917.
30. Bransilver BR, Ferenczy A, Richart RM. Female genital tract remnants. An ultrastructural comparison of hydatid of Morgagni and mesonephric ducts and tubules. *Arch Pathol* 1973;96:255.
31. See WA, Mayo M. Ectopic ureter: a rare cause of purulent vaginal discharge. *Obstet Gynecol* 1991;78:552.
32. Meyer R. Normal and abnormal development of the ureter in the human embryo—a mechanistic consideration. *Anat Rec* 1946;96:355.
33. Ott M, Rehn M, Müller J, et al. Vaginal clear cell carcinoma in a young patient with ectopic termination of the left ureter in the vagina. *Virchows Arch* 1994;425:445.

34. Shimao Y, Nabeshima K, Inoue T, et al. Primary vaginal adenocarcinoma arising from the metanephric duct remnant. *Virchows Arch* 2000;436:622.
35. Hendren WH, Monfort GJ. Surgical correction of ureteroceles in childhood. *J Pediatr Surg* 1971;6: 235.
36. Hendren WH, Mitchell ME. Surgical correction of ureteroceles. *J Urol* 1979;121:590.
37. Krisiloff M, Puchner PJ, Tretter W, et al. Pregnancy in women with bladder exstrophy. *J Urol* 1978;119:478.
38. Hendren WH. Urogenital sinus and cloacal malformations. *J Pelvic Surg* 1995;1:149.
39. Hendren WH. Urogenital sinus and cloacal malformations. *Semin Pediatr Surg* 1996;5:72.
40. Jaramillo D, Lebowitz RL, Hendren WH. The cloacal malformation radiologic findings and imaging recommendations. *Radiology* 1990;177:441.
41. Hendren WH. Cloaca, the most severe degree of imperforate anus. *Ann Surg* 1998;228:331.
42. Greenberg J, Hendren WH. Vaginal delivery after cloacal malformation repair. *Obstet Gynecol* 1997;90:666.
43. Reiner WG, Gearhart JP. Discordant sexual identity in some genetic males with cloacal exstrophy assigned to female sex at birth. *N Engl J Med* 2004;350:333.
44. Buttram VC Jr, Gibbons WE. Müllerian anomalies: a proposed classification (an analysis of 144 cases). *Fertil Steril* 1979;32:40.
45. The American Fertility Society. The American Fertility Society classifications of adnexal adhesions, distal tubal occlusion, tubal occlusion secondary to tubal ligation, tubal pregnancies, müllerian anomalies, and intrauterine adhesions. *Fertil Steril* 1988;49:944.
46. Powell DM, Newman KD, Randolph J. A proposed classification of vaginal anomalies and their surgical correction. *J Ped Surg* 1995;30:271.
47. Gidwani G, Falcone T. *Congenital malformations of the female genital tract: Diagnosis and management.* Philadelphia: Lippincott Williams & Wilkins;1999.
48. Simpson J. Genetics of the female reproductive ducts. *Am J Med Genet* 1999;89:224.
49. Bennett MJ, Berry JVJ. Preterm labour and congenital malformations of the uterus. *Ultrasound Med Biol* 1979;5:83.
50. Stray-Petersen B, Stray-Petersen S. Etiologic factors and subsequent reproductive performance in 195 couples with a prior history of habitual abortion. *Am J Obstet Gynecol* 1984;148:140.
51. Simón C, Tortajada M, Martinez L, et al. Müllerian defects in women with normal reproductive outcome. *Fertil Steril* 1991;56:1192.
52. Lin P, Bhatnagar K, Nettleton S, et al. Female genital anomalies affecting reproduction. *Fertil Steril* 2002;78:899.
53. Usta IM, Awwad IT, Usta JA, et al. Imperforate hymen: report of an unusual familial occurrence. *Obstet Gynecol* 1993;82:655.
54. Shatzkes DR, Haller JO, Velcek FT. Imaging of uterovaginal anomalies in the pediatric population. *Urol Radiol* 1991;13:58.
55. Valdes C, Malini S, Malinak LR. Ultrasound evaluation of female genital tract anomalies: a review of 64 cases. *Am J Obstet Gynecol* 1984;149:285.
56. Scanlan KA, Pozniak MA, Fagerholm M, et al. Value of transperineal sonography in the assessment of vaginal atresia. *AJR* 1990;154:545.
57. Nussbaum Blask AR, Sanders RC, Gearhart JP. Obstructed uterovaginal anomalies: demonstration with sonography. Part I: neonates and infants. *Pediatr Radiol* 1991;179:79.
58. Nussbaum Blask AR, Sanders RC, Rock JA. Obstructed uterovaginal anomalies: demonstration with sonography. Part II: teenagers. *Pediatr Radial* 1991;179:84.
59. Raga F, Bonilla-Musoles F, Blanes J, et al. Congenital müllerian anomalies: diagnostic accuracy of three-dimensional ultrasound. *Fertil Steril* 1996;65:523.
60. Markham SM, Parmley TH, Murph AA, et al. Cervical agenesis combined with vaginal agenesis diagnosed by magnetic resonance imaging. *Fertil Steril* 1987;48:143.
61. Fedele L, Dorta M, Brioschi D, et al. Magnetic resonance imaging in Mayer-Rokitansky-Kuster-Hauser syndrome. *Obstet Gynecol* 1990;76:593.
62. Pellerito JS, McCarthy SM, Doyle MB, et al. Diagnosis of uterine anomalies: relative accuracy of MR imaging, endovaginal sonography and hysterosalpingography. *Radiology* 1992;183:795.
63. Bakri YN, Al-Sugair A, Hugosson C. Bicornuate nonfused rudimentary uterine horns with functioning endometria and complete cervical vaginal agenesis: magnetic resonance diagnosis. *Fertil Steril* 1992; 58:620.
64. Economy KE, Barnewolt C, Laufer MR. A comparison of MRI and laparoscopy in detecting pelvic structures in cases of vaginal agenesis. *J Pediatr Adolesc Gynecol* 2002;15:101.

65. Soares SR, Barbosa dos Reis MMB, Camargos AF. Diagnostic accuracy of sonohysterography, transvaginal sonography, and hysterosalpingography in patients with uterine cavity diseases. *Fertil Steril* 2000;73:406.
66. Alborzi S, Dehbashi S, Parsanezhad M. Differential diagnosis of septate and bicornuate uterus by sonohysterography eliminates the need for laparoscopy. *Fertil Steril* 2002;78:176.
67. Markham SM, Waterhouse TB. Structural anomalies of the reproductive tract. *Curr Opin Obstet Gynecol* 1992;4:867.
68. Sadler TW. *Langman's medical embryology,* 6th ed. Philadelphia: Williams & Williams, 1990.
69. Fielding C. Obstetric studies in women with congenital solitary kidneys. *Acta Obstet Gynecol Scand* 1965;44:555.
70. Thompson DP, Lynn HB. Genital anomalies associated with solitary kidney. *Mayo Clin Proc* 1966;41:538.
71. Erdogan E, Okan G, Daragenli O. Uterus didelphys with unilateral obstructed hemivagina and renal agenesis on the same side. *Acta Obstet Gynecol Scand* 1992;71:76.
72. Tran ATB, Arensman RM, Falterman KW. Diagnosis and management of hydrohematometrocolpos syndrome. *Am J Dis Child* 1987;141:632.
73. Golan A, Langer R, Bukovsky I, et al. Congenital anomalies of the müllerian system. *Fertil Steril* 1989;51:747.
74. Sanfilippo JS, Wakim NG, Schikler KN, et al. Endometriosis in association with uterine anomaly. *Am J Obstet Gynecol* 1986;154:39.
75. Olive DL, Henderson DY. Endometriosis and müllerian anomalies. *Obstet Gynecol* 1987;69:412.
76. Fedele L, Bianchi S, DiNola G, et al. Endometriosis and nonobstructive müllerian anomalies. *Obstet Gynecol* 1992;79:515.
77. Lodi A. Contributo clinico statistico sulle malformazioni della vagina osservate nella clinica ostetrica e ginecologica di Milano dal 1906 al 1950. *Ann Obstet Ginecol* 1951;73:1246.
78. Suidan FG, Azoury RS. The transverse vaginal septum: a clinicopathologic evaluation. *Obstet Gynecol* 1979;54:278.
79. Rock JA, Zacur HA, Dlugi AM, et al. Pregnancy success following surgical correction of imperforate hymen and complete transverse vaginal septum. *Obstet Gynecol* 1982;59:448.
80. Garcia RE. Z-plasty correction for congenital transverse vaginal septum. *Am J Obstet Gynecol* 1967;99:1164.
81. Wierrani F, Bodner K, Spangler B, et al. "Z"-plasty of the transverse vaginal septum using Garcia's procedure and the Grünberger modification. *Fertil Steril* 2003;79:608.
82. Casey AC, Laufer MR. Cervical agenesis: septic death after surgery. *Obstet Gynecol* 1997;90:706.
83. Mayer CAJ. Über Verdoppelungen des Uterus and ihre Arten, nebst Bemerkungen über Hasenscharte und Wolfsrachen. *J Chir Auger* 1829;13:525.
84. von Rokitansky KE. Über die sogenannten Verdoppelungen des Uterus. *Med Jb Öst Stoat* 1938;26:39.
85. Küster H. Uterus bipartitus solidus rudimentarius cum vagina solida. *Z Geb Gyn* 1910;67:692.
86. Hauser GA, Schreiner WE. Das Mayer-Rokitansky-Küster syndrome. *Schweiz Med Wochenschr* 1961;91:381.
87. Solomons E. Conception and delivery following construction of an artificial vagina: a report of a case. *Obstet Gynecol* 1956;7:329.
88. Murray J, Gambrell RD. Complete and partial vaginal agenesis. *J Reprod Med* 1979;22:101.
89. Singh J, Devi YL. Pregnancy following surgical correction of nonfused müllerian bulbs and absent vagina. *Obstet* Gynecol 1983;61:267.
90. Bates WG, Wiser WL. A technique for uterine conservation in adolescents with vaginal agenesis and a functional uterus. *Obstet Gynecol* 1985;66:290.
91. Ludwig KS. The Mayer-Rokitansky-Küster syndrome: an analysis of its morphology and embryology. Part I: morphology. *Arch Gynecol Obstet* 1998;262:1.
92. Ludwig KS. The Mayer-Rokitansky-Küster syndrome: an analysis of its morphology and embryology. Part II: embryology. *Arch Gynecol Obstet* 1998;262:27.
93. Evans TN, Poland ML, Boving RE. Vaginal malformations. *Am J Obstet Gynecol* 1981;141:910.
94. Reindollar RH, Byrd JR, McDonough PG. Delayed sexual development: a study of 252 patients. *Am J Obstet Gynecol* 1981;140:371.
95. Cramer DW, Ravnikar VA, Craighill M, et al. Müllerian aplasia associated with maternal deficiency of galactose-1-phosphate uridyl transferase. *Fertil Steril* 1987;47:930.

96. Willemson WNP. Combination of Mayer-Rokitansky-Küster and Klippel-Feil syndromes. a case report and review of the literature. *Eur J Obstet Gynecol Reprod Biol* 1982;13:229.

97. Duncan PA, Shapiro LR, Strangel JJ, et al. The MURCS association of müllerian duct aplasia, renal aplasia, and cervicothoracic somite dysplasia. *J Pediatr* 1979;95:399.

98. Fedele L, Dorta M, Brioschi D. Magnetic resonance imaging in Mayer-Rokitansky-Küster-Hauser syndrome. *Obstet Gynecol* 1990;76:593.

99. Foley S, Morley GW. Care and counseling of the patient with vaginal agenesis. The Female Patient 1992;17:73.

100. Weijenborg P, Kuile M. The effect of a group programme on women with the Mayer-Rokitansky-Küster-Hauser Syndrome. *Br J Obstet Gynaecol* 2000;107:365.

101. Batzer FR, Corson SL, Gocial B, et al. Genetic offspring in paitents with vaginal agenesis: Specific medical and legal issues. *Am J Obstet Gynecol* 1992;167:1288.

102. Petrozza JC, Gray MR, Davis AJ, et al. Congenital absence of the uterus and vagina is not commonly transmitted as a dominant genetic trait: outcomes of surrogate pregnancies. *Fertil Steril* 1997;67:387.

103. Coney PJ. Effects of vaginal agenesis on the adolescent: prognosis for normal sexual and psychological adjustment. *Adolesc Pediatr Gynecol* 1992;5:8.

104. Laufer, MR. Congenital absence of the vagina: in search of the perfect solution. When, and by what technique, should a vagina be created? *Curr Opin Obstet Gynecol* 2002;14:441.

105. Croak A, Gebhart J, Klingele C, et al. Therapeutic strategies for vaginal müllerian agensis. *J Reprod Med* 2003;48:395.

106. Moen M. Creation of a vagina by repeated coital dilatation in four teenagers with vaginal agenesis. *Acta Obstet Gynecol Scand* 2000;79:149.

107. Frank RT. The formation of an artificial vagina without operation. *Am J Obstet Gynecol* 1938;35:1053.

108. Edmonds DK. Vaginal and uterine anomalies in the paediatric and adolescent patient. *Curr Opin Obstet Gynecol* 2001;13:463.

109. Roberts CP, Haber MJ, Rock JA. Vaginal creation for mullerian agenesis. *Am J Obstet Gynecol* 2001;185:1349.

110. Ingram JM. The bicycle seat stool in the treatment of vaginal agenesis and stenosis: a preliminary report. *Am J Obstet Gynecol* 1981;140:867.

111. Abbé R. New method of creating a vagina in a case of congenital absence. *Med Rec* 1898;54:836.

112. McIndoe AIL, Banister JB. An operation for the cure of congenital absence of the vagina. *J Obstet Gynaecol Br Commonw* 1938;45:490.

113. Counsellor VS. Congenital absence and traumatic obliteration of vagina and its treatment with inlaying Thiersch grafts. *Am J Obstet Gynecol* 1938;36:632.

114. McIndoe A. Treatment of congenital absence and obliterative conditions of the vagina. *Br J Plast Surg* 1950;2:254.

115. Buss JG, Lee RA. McIndoe procedure for vaginal agenesis: results and complications. *Mayo Clin Proc* 1989;64:758.

116. Martintez-Mora J, Isnard R, Castellvi A, et al. Neovagina in vaginal agenesis: surgical methods and long-term results. *J Pediatr Surg* 1992;27:10.

117. Duckler L. Squamous cell carcinoma developing in an artificial vagina. *Obstet Gynecol* 1972;40:35.

118. Rotmensch J, Rosenshein N, Dillon M, et al. Carcinoma arising in the neovagina: case report and review of the literature. *Obstet Gynecol* 1983;61:534.

119. Sadove RC, Horton CE. Utilizing full-thickness skin grafts for vaginal reconstruction. *Clin Plast Surg* 1988;15:443.

120. Chen YB, Cheng JJ, Lin HH, et al. Spatial W-plasty full-thickness skin graft for neovaginal reconstruction. *Plast Reconstr Surg* 1994;94:727.

121. Selvaggi G, Monstrey S, Depypere H, et al. Creation of a neovagina with use of a pudendal thigh fasciocutaneous flap and restoration of uterovaginal continuity. *Fertil Steril* 2003;80:607.

122. Williams EA. Congenital absence of the vagina—a simple operation for its relief. *J Obstet Gynaecol Br Commonw* 1964;71:511.

123. Creatsas G, Deligeoroglou E, Makrakis E, et al. Creation of a neovagina following Williams vaginopasty and the Creatsas modification in 111 patients with Mayer-Rokitansky-Küster-Hauser syndrome. *Fertil Steril* 2001;76:1036.

124. Wesley JR, Coran AG. Intestinal vaginoplasty for congenital absence of the vagina. *J Pediatr Surg* 1992;27:885.

125. Hensle T, Dean G. Vaginal replacement in children. *J Urol* 1992;148:677.
126. Hendren WH, Atala A. Use of bowel for vaginal reconstruction. *J Urol* 1994;152:752.
127. Communal PH, Chevret-Measson M, Golfier F, et al. Sexuality after sigmoid colpopoiesis in patients with Mayer-Rokitansky-Kuster-Hauser syndrome. *Fertil Steril* 2003;80:600.
128. Andryjowicz E, Qizilbash MB, DePetrillo AD, et al. Adenocarcinoma in a cecal neovagina—complication of irradiation: Report of a case and review of the literature. *Gynecol Oncol* 1985;21:235.
129. Davydov SN, Zhvitiashvili OD. Formation of vagina from peritoneum of Douglas pouch. *Acta Chir Plast* 1974;16:35.
130. Tamaya T, Imai A. The use of peritoneum for vaginoplasty in 24 patients with congenital absence of the vagina. *Arch Gynecol Obstet* 1991;249:15.
131. Templeman CL, Hertweck SP, Levine RL, et al. Use of laparoscopically mobilized peritoneum in the creation of a neovagina. *Fertil Steril* 2000; 74:589.
132. Jackson ND, Rosenblatt PL. Use of Interceed Absorbable Adhesion Barrier for vaginoplasty. *Obstet Gynecol* 1994;84:1048.
133. Estrada Portilla A, Vital Reyes VS, Tellez Velasco S, et al. Flexible vaginal cast covered with oxidated cullulose. Surgical option in neovagina for patients with Rokitansky-Küster-Hauser syndrome. *Ginecol Obstet Mex* 2000;68:301.
134. Morton KE, Dewhurst CJ. Human amnion in the treatment of vaginal malformations. *Br J Obstet Gynaecol* 1986;93:50.
135. McGraw JB, Massey FM, Shanklin KD, et al. Vaginal reconstruction with gracilis myocutaneous flaps. *Plast Reconstr Surg* 1976;58:176.
136. Wang TN, Whetzel T, Mathes SJ, et al. A fasciocutaneous flap for vaginal and perineal reconstruction. *Plast Reconstr Surg* 1987;80:95.
137. Tobin GR, Day TG. Vaginal and pelvic reconstruction with distally based rectus abdominis myocutaneous flaps. *Plast Reconstr Surg* 1988;81:62.
138. Vecchietti G. Le neo-vagin dans le syndrome de Rokitansky-Küster-Hauser. *Rev Med Suisse Romande* 1979;99:593.
139. Gauwerky JFH, Wallwiener D, Bastert G. An endoscopically assisted technique for construction of a neovagina. *Arch Gynecol Obstet* 1992;252:59.
140. Ghirardini G, Popp LW. New approach to the Mayer-von-Rokitansky-Küster-Hauser syndrome. *Adolesc Pediatr Gynecol* 1994;7:41.
141. Fedele L, Busacca M, Candiani M, et al. Laparoscopic creation of a neovagina in Mayer-Rokitansky-Küster-Hauser syndrome by modification of Vecchietti operation. *Am J Obstet Gynecol* 1994;171:268.
142. Fedele L, Bianchi S, Zanconato G, et al. Laparoscopic creation of a neovagina in patients with Rokitansky syndrome: analysis of 52 cases. *Fertil Steril* 2000;74:384.
143. Farber M. Congenital atresia of the uterine cervix. *Semin Reprod Endocrinol* 1986;4:33.
144. Niver DH, Barrette G, Jewelewicz R. Congenital atresia of the uterine cervix and vagina: three cases. *Fertil Steril* 1980;33:25.
145. Dillon WP, Mudalier N, Wingate M. Congenital atresia of the cervix. *Obstet Gynecol* 1979;54:126.
146. Rock JA, Carpenter SE, Wheeless CR, et al. The clinical management of maldevelopment of the uterine cervix. *J Pelvic Surg* 1995;1:129.
147. Rock JA, Schlaff WD, Zacur, HA, et al. The clinical management of congenital absence of the uterine cervix. *Int J Gynaecol Obstet* 1984;22:231.
148. Regan L, Dewhurst J. Atresia of the cervix. *Pediatr Adolesc Gynecol* 1985;3:83.
149. Farber M, Marchant DJ. Reconstructive surgery for congenital atresia of the uterine cervix. *Fertil Steril* 1976;27:1277.
150. Culkier J, Batzofin JH, Connors JS, et al. Genital tract reconstruction in a patient with congenital absence of the vagina and hypoplasia of the cervix. *Obstet Gynecol* 1986;68:32S.
151. Geary LW, Weed JC. Congenital atresia of the uterine cervix. *Obstet Gynecol* 1973;42:213.
152. Baker ER, Horger EO, Williamson HO. Congenital atresia of the uterine cervix: two cases. *J Reprod Med* 1982;27;39.
153. Zarou GS, Espesito JM, Zarou DM. Pregnancy following surgical correction of congenital atresia of the cervix. *Int J Obstet Gynecol* 1973;11:143.
154. Hampton HL, Meeks GR, Bates GW, et al. Pregnancy after successful vaginoplasty and cervical stenting for partial atresia of the cervix. *Obstet Gynecol* 1990;76:900.
155. Thijssen RFA, Hollanders JMG, Willemsen WN, et al. Successful pregnancy after ZIFT in a patient with congenital cervical atresia. *Obstet Gynecol* 1990;76:902–904.

156. Laufer MR. Laparoscopic resection of obstructed hemi-uteri in a series of adolescents. *J Pediatr Adolesc Gynecol* 1997;10:163.
157. Kirschner R, Löfstrand T, Mark J. Pregnancy in a non-communicating, rudimentary uterine horn. *Acta Obstet Gynecol Scand* 1979;58:499–501.
158. Constantian HM. Ureteral ectopia, hydrocolpos, and uterus didelphys. *JAMA* 1966;197:54.
159. Stassart JP, Nagel TC, Prem K, et al. Uterus didelphys, obstructed hemivagina, and ipsilateral renal agenesis: the University of Minnesota experience. *Fertil Steril* 1992;57:756.
160. Zurawin RK, Dietrich JE, Heard MJ, Edwards CL. Didelphic uterus and obstructed hemivagina with renal agenesis: case report and review of the literature. J Pediatr Adolesc Gynecol 2004;17:137.
161. Jones HW, Rock JA. Reproductive impairment and the malformed uterus. *Fertil Steril* 1981;36:137.
162. Rock J, Schlaff W. The obstetric consequences of uterovaginal anomalies. *Fertil Steril* 1985;43:681.
163. Sanfilippo JS. Strassman procedure for correction of a class II müllerian anomaly in an adolescent. *J Adolesc Health* 1991;12:63.
164. Daly DC, Walter CA, Soto-Albors CE, et al. Hysteroscopic metroplasty: surgical technique and obstetric outcome. *Fertil Steril* 1983;39:623.
165. DeCherney AH Russell JB, Graebe RA, et al. Resectoscope management of müllerian fusion defects. *Fertil Steril* 1986;45:726.
166. Rock J, Roberts C, Hesla J. Hysteroscopic metroplasty of the Class Va uterus with preservation of the cervical septum. *Fertil Steril* 1999;72:942.
167. Homer H, Li T, Cooke I. The septate uterus: a review of management and reproductive outcome. *Fertil Steril* 2000;73:1.
168. Proctor JA, Haney AF. Recurrent first trimester pregnancy loss is associated with uterine septum but not bicornuate uterus. *Fertil Steril* 2003;80:1212.
169. Fedele L, Zamberletti D, Vercellini P, et al. Reproductive performance of women with unicornuate uterus. *Fertil Steril* 1987;47:416.
170. Michalas SP. Outcome of pregnancy in women with uterine malformations: evaluation of 62 cases. *Int J Gynecol Obstet* 1991;35:215.
171. Makino T, Umeuchi M, Nakada K, et al. Incidence of congenital uterine anomalies in repeated reproductive wastage and prognosis for pregnancy after metroplasty. *Int J Fertil* 1992;37:167.
172. Kirk EP, Chuong CJ, Coulam CB, et al. Pregnancy after metroplasty for uterine anomalies. *Fertil Steril* 1993;59:1164.
173. Lin PC, Bhatnagar KP, Nettleton GS, Nakajima ST. Female genital anomalies affecting reproduction. Fertil Steril 2002;78:899.

11

Gynecologic Pain: Dysmenorrhea, Acute and Chronic Pelvic Pain, Endometriosis, and Premenstrual Syndrome

Marc R. Laufer and Donald P. Goldstein

A vast array of gynecologic entities and conditions exist that can result in pain for adolescent girls and young women. Pain is the physiologic response to many pathophysiologic conditions such as distension, stretching, compression, irritation (chemical or infectious), ischemia, neuritis, and necrosis. Pelvic pain can also be referred from another anatomic site. Pelvic pain can arise from numerous causes, including diseases or conditions affecting the gastrointestinal (GI) tract, the urogenital tract, the reproductive tract, and the musculoskeletal system. Stress and psychosocial issues may increase the intensity of the symptoms and affect the individual's response to pain and the ability to cope with it. This chapter discusses the approach, diagnosis, and treatment of the adolescent with dysmenorrhea, acute and/or chronic pelvic pain, endometriosis, and premenstrual syndrome.

DYSMENORRHEA

Dysmenorrhea, or pain with menses, is very common in adolescents. Dysmenorrhea is highly prevalent in adolescent women, as 20 to 90% of adolescent women report dysmenorrhea. Fifteen percent of adolescent women describe their dysmenorrhea as severe. Analyzing data from the National Health Examination Survey for 12- to 17-year-old girls, Klein and Litt (1) found that 59.7% of 2699 reported dysmenorrhea, and of those with dysmenorrhea, 14% frequently missed school because of cramps. In a survey of private school girls (mean age 15.5 ± 1.1 years) done by our faculty, dysmenorrhea was reported as mild by 32%, moderate by 15%, and severe by 6% (2). Most dysmenorrhea in adolescents is primary (or functional), but it may also be secondary to endometriosis (see later), obstructing müllerian anomalies (see Chapter 10), or other pelvic pathology.

Typically, the 14- or 15-year-old teenager, 1 to 3 years after menarche, begins to experience crampy lower abdominal pain with each menstrual period. Usually, the pains start within 1 to 4 hours of the onset of the menses and last for 24 to 48 hours. In some cases, the pain may start 1 to 2 days before the menses and continue for 2 to 4 days into the menses. Nausea and/or vomiting, diarrhea, lower backache, thigh pain, headache, fatigue, nervousness, dizziness, or rarely syncope may accompany the cramps.

Etiology

Historically, the etiology of primary dysmenorrhea was poorly understood, and many myths and hypotheses were promoted. Pickles (3) was the first to suggest that dysmenorrhea might be related to a "menstrual stimulant" found in human menstrual fluid that induced smooth muscle contractions. In later studies, he found that the substance was a mixture of prostaglandins $F_{2\alpha}$ ($PGF_{2\alpha}$) and E_2 (PGE_2) (4,5). Menstrual fluid prostaglandin levels were several times higher in ovulatory than in anovulatory cycles. Uterine jet washing, endometrial sampling, and collection of menstrual fluid have generally confirmed higher endometrial prostaglandin levels in women with primary dysmenorrhea than in those without symptoms (5,6).

In the uterus, phospholipids from the dead cell membranes are converted to arachidonic acid, which can be metabolized by at least two enzymes: lipoxygenase, which begins the production of leukotrienes, and cyclooxygenase (COX), which leads to cyclic endoperoxides (PGG_2 and PGH_2). The cyclic endoperoxides are then converted by specific enzymes to prostacyclin, thromboxanes, and the prostaglandins PGD_2, PGE_2, and $PGF_{2\alpha}$. Prostaglandin $PGF_{2\alpha}$ mediates pain sensation and stimulates smooth muscle contraction, whereas PGE_2 potentiates platelet disaggregation and vasodilatation (7). Exogenously administered PGE_2 and $PGF_{2\alpha}$ can produce uterine contractions as well as systemic symptoms such as vomiting, diarrhea, and dizziness, and are commonly used by obstetricians for the induction of labor. Although plasma levels of prostaglandins are normal in dysmenorrheic women, increased sensitivity or generalized overproduction of prostaglandins may occur.

Nonsteroidal antiinflammatory drugs (NSAIDs) have both analgesic and antiinflammatory properties. The principal action of NSAIDs is inhibition of the COX enzyme. This enzyme is responsible for the production of prostaglandins. Two isoforms of the COX enzyme have been identified, COX-1 and COX-2. Prostaglandins produced by COX-1 are mainly involved in maintaining the GI mucosal barrier, renal hemodynamics, platelet function, vascular homeostasis, and play some role in inflammation (8–11). The COX-2 enzyme is induced in inflammation, resulting in prostaglandin production (9,10). Nonselective NSAIDs (ibuprofen and naproxen) inhibit both COX-1 and COX-2, whereas selective COX-2 inhibitors (celecoxib, rofecoxib, valdecoxib) exert their actions more specifically on inflammatory processes (11).

The prostaglandin hypothesis has been further strengthened by the observation that drugs that inhibit prostaglandin synthesis can relieve dysmenorrhea and the associated symptoms (7,12–16). Several clinical studies have found that nonsteroidal anti-inflammatory drugs are effective in the relief of pain. NSAID agents (see Appendix 9) are divided into different groups: salicylate group [aspirin (Ecotrin, Ascriptin), choline magnesium trisalicylate (Trilisate)]; benzenesulfonamide group [celecoxib (Celebrex), valdecoxib (BEXTRA)]; acetic acid group [diclofenac (Voltaren), etodolac (Lodine), indomethacin (Indocin), nabumetone (Relafen), sulindac (Clinoril), tolmetin (Tolectin)]; propionic acid group [fenoprofen (Nalfon Pulvules), flurbiprofen (Ansaid), ibuprofen (Motrin), ketoprofen (Orudis, Oruvail), naproxen (Naprosyn, Naprelan), oxaprozin (Daypro)]; fenamates [mefenamic acid (Ponstel), meclofenamate]; oxicam group [meloxicam (Mobic), piroxicam (Feldene)]; and the furanose group [rofecoxib (Vioxx)] (7,17,18).

The salicylate, acetic acid, propionic acid, and fenamate groups are most frequently used in the treatment of dysmenorrhea. The salicylic acids appear to inhibit cyclooxygenase; but aspirin has little potency compared with some of the other NSAIDs in reducing prostaglandin synthesis, and it may increase menstrual flow (19). Thus, aspirin is used less often in the treatment of dysmenorrhea. Indomethacin is the best known drug of the acetic acid group for treating dysmenorrhea, but its side effects have prevented its use by most, if not all, patients. Thus the clinician selects chiefly from the two last groups, propionic acids and fenamates, for clinical treatment of dysmenorrhea.

Ibuprofen and naproxen have been most widely studied for the relief of pain in dysmenorrhea. For example, Chan and associates (13) correlated the relief of dysmenorrhea by ibuprofen with the reduction in menstrual prostaglandin release as measured by a method that can detect menstrual prostaglandin activity in tampon specimens. Total menstrual prostaglandin release per cycle fell from a control level of 59.8 ± 7.2 to 16.8 ± 2.3 (gram $PGF_{2\alpha}$ equivalents) with the use of ibuprofen (13). Numerous clinical studies have found these agents to be effective in both adult and adolescent women, giving pain relief in 67% to 86% of patients. The sodium salt of naproxen has a more rapid absorption than naproxen and can give very rapid relief of symptoms. The prostaglandin inhibitor flurbiprofen also appears to be very effective in the relief of dysmenorrhea (20).

The fenamates are potent inhibitors of prostaglandin synthesis and in addition can antagonize the action of already formed prostaglandins (16). This increased activity may give this class of drug a theoretic advantage in treatment. Clinical studies of meclofenamate have shown effectiveness (21,22); this drug also inhibits the activity of 5-lipoxygenase, but the clinical importance of the inhibition of leukotrienes is unknown. These medications are useful when less expensive NSAIDs, have not been beneficial.

Combination hormonal therapy (CHT), such as oral contraceptive pills, combination hormonal patch, or vaginal ring, lessen dysmenorrhea. This therapy is effective in part owing to their antiovulatory actions as well as their ability to produce endometrial hypoplasia, less menstrual flow, and subsequently less prostaglandins (13,23).

With the advent of the research on prostaglandins as the cause of dysmenorrhea, the potential influence of psychological issues on dysmenorrhea has received little attention. However, in a study of adolescents treated for dysmenorrhea with naproxen sodium, DuRant and colleagues (24) made the interesting observation that girls with increased life crisis events experienced greater severity of symptoms in the first month of therapy than did other girls. It is possible that prostaglandins may increase in response to physical and psychological stress or that the patient may be more keenly aware of pain when distressed by other problems in her life. As therapy was continued, life stress ceased to have a significant influence on the severity of dysmenorrhea. Those with persistent symptoms, however, did have lower self-concept at follow-up, perhaps because of their initial high expectation of receiving relief.

Patient Assessment

In assessing the adolescent with dysmenorrhea, the physician needs to know her menstrual history and the timing of her cramps, pain, and/or premenstrual symptoms, as well as her response to them. The key questions are these: Is she missing school? If so, how many days? Does she miss other activities? Social events? Does she have nausea and vomiting, diarrhea, or dizziness? What medications has she used to treat the symptoms? What makes the pain better? Worse? What is the nature of the mother–daughter interaction? Does or did her mother or sister have cramps? Is there a family history of endometriosis? Young women whose cramps are disabling out of proportion to the apparent severity may have confounding factors contributing to their symptoms, such as a reluctance to attend school, a history of physical or sexual abuse, or significant psychosocial problems. The questions about previous medications are particularly crucial, because with the availability of over-the-counter NSAIDs, many adolescents have tried these medications in subtherapeutic doses and have subsequently discarded the concept of their usefulness.

For the virginal adolescent who has mild symptoms, a normal physical examination, including inspection of the genitalia to exclude an abnormality of the hymen, is reassuring. Adolescents with moderate or severe dysmenorrhea who are sexually active should have a speculum and bimanual pelvic examination. In the majority of adolescents who are carefully prepared, a vaginal examination is atraumatic. A rectoabdominal examination with the patient in the lithotomy position is all that is possible for some non–sexually active girls, and this exam will exclude adnexal tenderness and masses. A speculum examination is not necessary if it is not easily tolerated.

For the non-sexually active adolescent, a Q-tip can be inserted into the vagina to help determine the presence or absence of a hymenal abnormality and/or a transverse vaginal or longitudinal vaginal septum. The Q-tip is inserted to document the length of the vagina and can be moved from side to side to rule out a fenestrated transverse vaginal septum (see Chapter 10). If the pelvic anatomy needs to be further evaluated, and a rectoabdominal exam is noncontributory or not an option, ultrasonography may be necessary. Ultrasonography is useful in defining suspected uterine and vaginal anomalies with obstruction but will not detect abnormalities such as intraabdominal or pelvic adhesions or endometriosis.

Treatment

Treatment includes a careful explanation to the patient of the nature of the problem and a chance for her to ask questions regarding her anatomy. If the results of examination are normal, treatment should be directed at symptomatic relief. The most common approach is to prescribe one of the NSAID compounds (see Appendix 9 for compounds, available dose, and dosing intervals).

Most patients can obtain effective relief by starting the antiprostaglandin medicine at the onset of the menses and continuing for the first 1 to 2 days of the cycle, or for the usual duration of cramps. The patient should be told to begin taking the medicine as soon as she knows her menses are coming: "at the first sign of cramps or bleeding." A loading dose is important in patients with symptoms that are severe and occur rapidly. For such patients, a rapidly absorbed drug such as naproxen sodium would be preferable. Generally, giving the medicine at the onset of the menses prevents the inadvertent administration of the drug to a pregnant woman. However, a patient who is not sexually active and has severe cramps accompanied by early vomiting, and thus is unable to take medication, may often benefit from starting the drug 1 or 2 days before the onset of her menses. A patient may respond to a higher dose or to another NSAID. Since life stresses may lessen the pain relief in the first cycle, the determination of effectiveness in an individual patient should be based on the response in more than one cycle. Usually, medication is prescribed for two to three cycles before it is changed. In addition, a patient may have previously taken inadequate doses of a medicine, particularly ibuprofen, to obtain relief. There is variability in response to NSAIDs with 70% to 80% of individuals responding to a particular NSAID; lack of response to one NSAID does not preclude a response to another (25,26).

The NSAID compounds should be avoided in preoperative patients and patients with known or suspected ulcer disease, GI bleeding, clotting disorders, renal disease, allergies to aspirin or NSAIDs, or aspirin-induced asthma. All of the NSAIDs should be taken with food, even though some patients prefer only liquids on the first day of the cycle. The side effects of these drugs appear minimal in short-term use, but the possibility of allergy and GI irritation and bleeding should be explained to the patient. Some patients complain of fluid retention or fatigue with the use of these agents.

In some patients, NSAID drugs are contraindicated or produce undesirable side effects. In these adolescents, an alternative is tramadol hydrochloride tablets. Tramadol is a centrally acting analgesic that acts by binding to μ-opioid receptors and inhibiting the reuptake of norepinephrine and serotonin; it is not a member of either the NSAID or narcotic drug groups. It is indicated for moderate to severe pain, and it appears to be nonaddictive. Its efficacy is comparable to that of codeine (30 mg) and oxycodone (5 mg). It is prescribed as 50-mg pills that are taken as 50 to 100 mg every 6 hours; an individual should not take more than eight pills in 24 hours.

In addition to traditional Western medical therapies, patients should be encouraged to exercise, eat a well-balanced diet, and work to reduce stress in their lives. Some girls can continue to exercise or participate in competitive sports during their menses; others may find the discomfort to be too great. Some herbal teas, fruits, and vegetables have been reported to be beneficial to women with dysmenorrhea (27). Magnesium functions in controlling muscle tone and has been studied in the treatment of dysmenorrhea. A decrease in magnesium in women in the luteal phase of the cycle has been demonstrated (28). Some studies have shown a benefit from treating dysmenorrhea with magnesium therapy (see Chapter 25) (29).

The adolescent should be seen initially every 3 or 4 months to evaluate the effectiveness of the therapies. Such visits also facilitate the rapport between health care provider and patient that is essential in the treatment of this problem. Only a few adolescents use their symptoms for secondary gains, such as an excuse to stay out of school or to gain sympathy from their parents. The vast majority of adolescents need to be encouraged to discuss their symptoms and should not be made to feel emotionally unstable because they complain of pain.

If the patient fails to respond to antiprostaglandin drugs and continues to have severe pain or vomiting, or if at the initial evaluation she needs birth control, a course of CHT (see Chapter 20 and Appendix 3) should be initiated. Cramps are usually substantially, if not completely, relieved with the anovulatory cycles and scantier flow. If severe cramps persist despite three cycles of ovulation suppression therapy, laparoscopy is indicated to exclude endometriosis or other organic causes (30,31).

If dysmenorrhea is relieved by CHT, medication is usually prescribed for 3 to 6 months and then discontinued (frequently during the summer, when school attendance will not be disrupted). Often, the patient will continue to have relief from cramps for several additional (commonly anovulatory) cycles before the more severe dysmenorrhea recurs. When the cramps recur, a trial of other antiprostaglandin drugs may again be attempted as the sole therapy before CHT is reinstituted. The adolescent with severe dysmenorrhea usually prefers to continue with long-term CHT. The return of increasingly severe dysmenorrhea in spite of continued use of CHT again raises the possibility of organic disease such as endometriosis and calls for a reevaluation and consideration of laparoscopy for definitive diagnosis.

PELVIC PAIN

Pelvic pain is common in adolescent women and can be characterized as acute or chronic. Pelvic pain can result from gynecologic and nongynecologic etiologies. An extensive listing of nongynecologic and gynecologic causes of acute and chronic pelvic pain is given in Table 11-1 (32,33). Some adolescents may suffer from acute or chronic pelvic pain and not seek attention due to embarrassment or fear.

Acute Pelvic Pain

The adolescent girl with acute pelvic pain should receive aggressive evaluation and management, as the differential diagnosis includes life-threatening conditions. The gynecologic causes of acute pain include infections, ovarian cysts (see Color Plate 37), endometriosis (see Color Plates 44 to 46), ectopic pregnancy (see Color Plate 39), and adnexal torsion (see Color Plates 40 and 41). A genital tract obstruction (see Chapter 10) may cause acute symptoms at the time of menarche, although these anomalies can also result in chronic or cyclic pelvic pain. Symptoms associated with infection usually occur over several days. Pelvic inflammatory disease (PID) (see Chapter 15) is extremely important to consider in the differential diagnosis of acute pelvic pain in the sexually active adolescent; it has been identified as the most common gynecologic disorder leading to the hospitalization of reproductive-age women in the United States (34). The onset of pain associated with adnexal torsion, rupture of an ovarian cyst (see Color Plate 38) (see Chapter 18), or an ectopic pregnancy (see Chapter 21) can be abrupt, sharp, and severe. Nausea and/or vomiting may occur with severe pain and is commonly seen with adnexal torsion. However, intermittent or partial adnexal torsion, or an unruptured ectopic pregnancy, may produce crampy pain for several days to weeks prior to an acute episode of complete torsion with infarction of the fallopian tube and/or ovary, or rupture of the ectopic pregnancy.

In deciding whether the pain is gynecologic in origin, the health care provider must consider GI causes, such as appendicitis, intestinal obstruction or perforation, volvulus, inflammatory bowel disease, infections (e.g., *Giardia, Shigella, Salmonella*), lactose intolerance, irritable bowel syndrome, or constipation (see Table 11-1). Urinary tract infections and calculi may result in acute pain. Orthopedic causes of pain are frequently forgotten and can be missed initially; the evaluation should include a complete history, an examination of the range of motion of the hips and spine, and tests of the sacroiliac joints.

A complete pain history must include its location, nature, intensity, and radiation; factors that relieve and exacerbate the pain such as walking, exercise, eating, urination, or bowel movements; the date of the last menstrual period; contraceptive and sexual history; associated symptoms such as fever, chills, diarrhea, vomiting, or dysuria; and previous pelvic pain and/or surgery. Infants and prepubertal girls (and

TABLE 11-1. *Differential diagnosis of pelvic pain in adolescents*

Nongynecologic
  Gastrointestinal
    Appendicitis
    Intestinal obstruction
    Perforation
    Gastric ulcer
    Gastritis
    Abdominal angina
    Cholecystitis/cholangitis
    Diverticular disease
    Gastroenteritis (bacterial, parasitic)
    Irritable bowel disease
    Ulcerative colitis
    Crohn's disease (granulomatous colitis)
    Meckel's diverticulum
    Mesenteric adenitis
    Pancreatitis
    Hepatitis
    Metabolic disease (steatorrhea, sprue,
      intermittent acute porphyria, lactase
      deficiency)
    Obstruction (adhesions, hernias,
      irradiation, tumors, volvulus)
    Psychogenic (anxiety)
    Constipation
  Genitourinary
    Pyelonephritis/abscess
    Cystourethritis
    Interstitial cystitis
    Calculi
    Ureteral obstruction
    Ureteral diverticulum/polyp
  Musculoskeletal
    Congenital anomalies
    Bone and joint inflammations/infections
      (spine, sacrum, ilium, femoral head)
    Trauma
    Tumors
  Neurologic
    Nerve entrapment
    Neuroma
  Psychologic
    History of physical/sexual abuse
    History of trauma
    Psychosomatic
  Systemic
    Systemic lupus erythematosus
    Neurofibromatosis
    Lymphoma

Gynecologic
  Acute
    Pregnancy-related
      Ectopic pregnancy (with/without
        rupture)
      Threatened/spontaneous abortion

    Ovarian
      Cyst/mass (benign/malignant)
      Mumps oophoritis
      Torsion
    Fallopian tube
      Hydrosalpinx
      Torsion
    Infection
      Endometritis (post therapeutic
        abortion, postpartum)
      Pelvic inflammatory disease/
        tubo-ovarian abscess
      Septic pelvic thrombophlebitis
    Vaginitis/vulvitis
      Contact dermatitis
      Inflammatory/infection
      Lichen sclerosis
      Bartholin's cyst/abscess
  Cyclic
    Mittelschmerz
    Dysmenorrhea
    Endometriosis/adenomyosis
    Leiomyomata (fibroids)
    Obstructive müllerian anomalies
    Premenstrual syndrome
    Ovarian
      Cyst/mass (benign/malignant)
      Torsion
    Fallopian tube
      Hydrosalpinx
      Torsion
    Dyspareunia (pain with sexual intercourse)
      Vaginismus
      Inflammatory/infection
  Chronic
    Endometriosis/adenomyosis
    Pelvic adhesions
    Leiomyomata (fibroids)
    Chronic infection
      Endometritis (post therapeutic
        abortion, postpartum)
      Pelvic inflammatory disease/
        tubo-ovarian abscess
      Septic pelvic thrombophlebitis
    Obstructive müllerian anomalies
    Premenstrual syndrome
    Ovarian
      Cyst/mass (benign/malignant)
      Torsion
    Fallopian tube
      Hydrosalpinx
      Torsion
    Vaginitis/vulvitis
      Chronic dermatitis
      Inflammatory/infection
      Lichen sclerosis
      Bartholin's cyst/abscess

(Adapted from Rapkin AJ, Reading AE. Chronic pelvic pain. *Curr Probl Obstet Gynecol Fertil* 1991;14:101; and Laufer MR. Endometriosis in adolescents. *Curr Opin Pediatr* 1992;4:582; with permission.)

adolescents less commonly) may have torsion of a normal adnexa (ovary and/or tube) (Figs. 11-1 and 11-2) (see Chapter 18). Several weeks to years later, these same individuals may experience torsion of the other adnexa, and if the second torsed ovary is not salvageable the individual is sterile (34–37). Prophylactic oophoropexy (of the contralateral normal ovary) should be considered at the time of the surgery for detorsion of the torsed adnexa. The psychosocial history should be elicited to assess whether stress, substance use, or sexual abuse might be contributing factors to any case of pelvic pain.

A complete physical examination should be undertaken, special attention being given to palpation of the abdomen, in a search for evidence of masses, tenderness, organomegaly, or peritoneal irritation (peritonitis). Depending on the age of the patient and the size of the hymenal opening, a bimanual vaginal-abdominal, rectoabdominal, or rectovaginal-abdominal examination should be done to assess the size of the uterus, the presence or absence of cervical motion tenderness, and/or ovarian/adnexal tenderness. A speculum examination to assess the vagina and cervix should be done in all sexually active patients and should be considered in virginal patients if the examination can be accomplished without trauma. Tests for *Chlamydia trachomatis* and *Neisseria gonorrhoeae* should be obtained in all patients who have ever had consensual or nonconsensual sexual activity, but these tests can be obtained without the need for a speculum exam with the utilization of urinary PCR testing (see Chapter

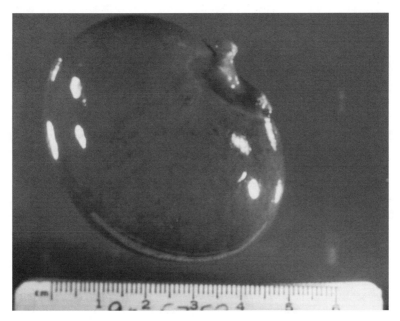

FIG. 11-1. Torsion of an ovary in a 6-week-old infant.

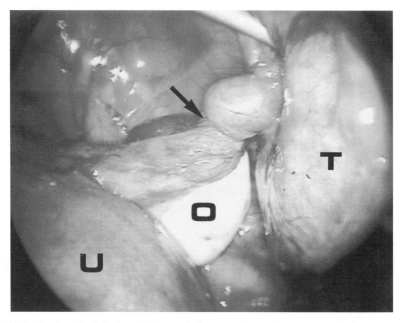

FIG. 11-2. Torsion of a fallopian tube (*arrow*). O, ovary; U, uterus; T, distal fallopian tube.

15). Lubricant should not be used for the digital vaginal or speculum examination unless cervical specimens have already been obtained.

Laboratory tests depend on the initial assessment and may include complete blood count (CBC) with differential, erythrocyte sedimentation rate (ESR), C-reactive protein (CRP), urinalysis, urine culture, cervical or urinary PCR testing for chlamydia and gonorrhea, sensitive urine or serum pregnancy test, and stool specimen for occult blood. A high leukocyte count (WBC) usually indicates infection or inflammation; the WBC may be slightly elevated or high in cases of ischemia, as may occur secondary to adnexal torsion or bowel obstruction. In acute hemorrhage, the hematocrit may not reflect the extent of blood loss, as there may not have been time for intravascular equilibration to have occurred.

In children or adolescents in whom a pelvic or adnexal mass is palpated or an adequate pelvic examination is not possible, ultrasonography (transabdominal and/or vaginal probe) can be used to aid in the evaluation. It is important to remember that adolescents normally have 1- to 2-cm ovarian follicles, which, though often termed *simple cysts* on ultrasound evaluation, are normal findings. In addition, children can have numerous small simple ovarian cysts, which usually measure 1 to 5 mm. Endometriosis and PID cannot be excluded by a normal ultrasound. Ultrasound is not ideal for identifying vaginal congenital anomalies (transverse vaginal septum) and thus a single Q-tip insertion and documentation of a normal vaginal length is important to document in addition to the ultrasound.

Cul-de-sac free fluid can be present with ruptured simple or hemorrhagic ovarian cysts (see Color Plates 37 and 38), leaking or ruptured ectopic pregnancies (see Color Plate 39), or with endometriosis (see Color Plates 44 to 46). The free fluid can be serous clear fluid or blood. The type of free fluid may be determined by the ultrasonic appearance, or it can be definitively determined by culdocentesis. Culdocentesis can be performed in an ambulatory setting but can be painful. In culdocentesis, a speculum is placed into the vaginal vault, povidone-iodine is used to prep the vaginal vault, local anesthetic can be infiltrated with a spinal needle into the anterior lip of the cervix, a tenaculum is used to grasp the anterior lip of the cervix, and a spinal needle is used to aspirate fluid from the posterior cul-de-sac. Cul-de-sac free fluid from a ruptured simple cyst or endometriosis is clear or straw colored, whereas that from a ruptured hemorrhagic cyst or ectopic pregnancy demonstrates free blood. If the blood does not clot, it most likely originates from an intraperitoneal process, whereas if it does clot, it is most likely the result of a misdirected intravascular aspiration. The utility of culdocentesis in the clinical setting of a sensitive and rapid pregnancy test and ultrasound has been questioned (38). At our institution we find this procedure rarely useful because of the availability of a sensitive pregnancy test and ultrasound, and also because of the severity of pain during the procedure.

A patient experiencing "waves" of acute pelvic pain with or without nausea may be experiencing complete or intermittent torsion of an ovary or fallopian tube (Figs. 11-1 and 11-2). Ultrasonography in a case of ovarian torsion may reveal an echogenic mass within the ovary, or an enlarged ovary without a discrete mass with a "string of pearls " appearance of peripheral follicles (Fig. 11-3). Ultrasound Doppler flow studies may be helpful in the assessment of ovarian torsion but are controversial since it is frequently difficult to determine the presence of Doppler flow in normal ovaries (35–42). The theory of the usefulness of Doppler flow is that at the site of the torsion, the diameter of the vessel proximal to the occlusion is increased, and thus the disruption of flow can be identified. Cost-benefit studies are still under investigation, and thus the value of color Doppler for screening for ovarian torsion is as yet unproved (43). Ovarian torsion is more common on the right side and may mimic acute appendicitis, with right lower quadrant pain, vomiting, rebound tenderness, and leukocytosis. For unclear reasons, girls in the 7- to 11-year-old range are especially prone to this problem. Reports have demonstrated that torsed ovaries can be surgically "detorsed" with salvage of the ovary, even if the ovary appears discolored (see Color Plate 40) (44–47) (see Chapter 18). Whether oophoropexy of the contralateral ovary can be helpful in preventing a second asynchronous episode of ovarian torsion of a normal ovary needs evaluation (37). If oophoropexy is elected, it can be safely accomplished by an operative laparoscopic approach (48).

When evaluating pelvic pain, gastrointestinal and skeletal radiographs, bone scans, and other radiologic studies should be ordered as clinically indicated by the history and physical examination.

Depending on clinical and laboratory assessment, patients with pelvic pain will fall into one of several categories requiring further surgical evaluation, nonsurgical

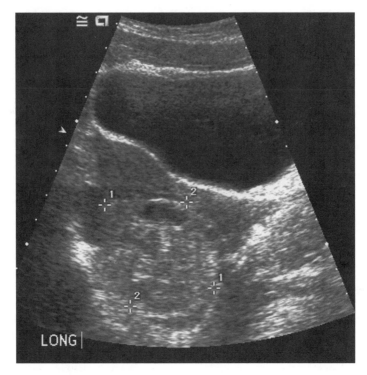

FIG. 11-3. "String of Pearls " appearance of ovarian follicles with torsion and stromal edema. (Courtesy of Carol Barnewolt, M.D., Children's Hospital Boston.)

evaluation, or discharge with follow-up (49). Some conditions such as acute hemoperitoneum, ruptured tubo-ovarian abscess, appendicitis, and other GI surgical emergencies require definitive surgery. Some conditions such as gastroenteritis, urinary tract infection, and PID require medical management; others (e.g., urinary calculi) require further investigation.

Not infrequently, the diagnosis remains in doubt, and diagnostic and/or operative laparoscopy may be invaluable for a definitive assessment. Laparoscopy is a safe means of evaluating the pelvis in adolescents and young adults and is also increasingly used in the management of general surgical, cardiovascular, and thoracic neurosurgical conditions in infants and children. At the time of laparoscopy, the appendix should be visualized to confirm that it is normal. Laparoscopy has been shown to be useful in the diagnosis of salpingitis (50–53), although its use for this diagnosis is not the current standard of care in the United States because of the risks of general anesthesia. When PID or appendicitis may exist, laparoscopy may help to define the underlying disease process. Microlaparoscopy with the utilization of conscious sedation has been shown to be a feasible option for the evaluation of presumed PID for adolescents in an emergency room setting (54). Visualization of a "normal pelvis"

TABLE 11-2. *Principal laparoscopic diagnoses in 121 adolescent patients 11 to 17 years old with acute pelvic pain (Children's Hospital Boston, 1980–1986)*

Diagnosis	No.	(%)
Ovarian cyst	47	(39)
Acute pelvic inflammatory disease	21	(17)
Adnexal torsion	9	(8)
Endometriosis	6	(5)
Ectopic pregnancy	4	(3)
Appendicitis	13	(11)
No pathologic condition	21	(17)

(Color Plates 31 to 33) rules out the need for further surgical intervention and can help direct the subsequent evaluation and therapy. Often, in cases of ruptured ovarian cysts or hemorrhagic corpus luteum, free blood and clots (see Color Plate 38) can be aspirated and hemostasis ensured by fulguration of areas of bleeding via laparoscopy. Hemoperitoneum is not a contraindication to laparoscopy as long as the patient is not hypotensive. Laparoscopy can be implemented in a standard operating room fashion utilizing a 5-, 7-, or 11-mm laparoscope and general anesthesia, or with one of the newer 1.6-, 1.8-, or 2-mm laparoscopes and local anesthesia (55). As mentioned above, we have shown that it is feasible to evaluate adolescent women with suspected PID with a 2-mm laparoscope utilizing conscious sedation (54). Others have explored the use of laparoscopy as an office or outpatient procedure in evaluating pelvic pain in adult women (56,57).

The principal findings in 121 adolescent girls (11 to 17 years old) who underwent laparoscopy by the Gynecology Service of Children's Hospital Boston, for acute pelvic pain between 1980 and 1986 are shown in Table 11-2. The most common diagnosis was a complication of an ovarian cyst. Interestingly, the causes of acute pelvic pain did not appear to be age related (Table 11-3). This data is now over 20 years old and with the improvement and availability of ultrasound and

TABLE 11-3. *Age-related prevalence of principal laparoscopic findings in 121 adolescent patients 11 to 17 years old with acute pelvic pain (Children's Hospital Boston, 1980–1986)*

Diagnosis	No. of patients (%)		
	Age 11–13	Age 14–15	Age 16–17
Ovarian cyst	12 (50)	16 (35)	19 (37)
Acute pelvic inflammatory disease	4 (17)	7 (16)	10 (19)
Adnexal torsion	0 (0)	7 (16)	2 (4)
Endometriosis	0 (0)	2 (4)	4 (7)
Ectopic pregnancy	0 (0)	3 (7)	1 (2)
Appendicitis	3 (13)	4 (9)	6 (12)
No pathologic condition	5 (20)	6 (13)	10 (19)
Total	24 (20)	45 (37)	52 (43)

rapid HCG testing laparoscopy has become less needed in the evaluation of acute pelvic pain. Emergent surgery is now reserved for cases of adnexal torsion, hemorrhagic ruptured ovarian cysts with hemodynamic compromise, and management of appendicitis.

Acute pain in the adolescent may also occur at menarche if there is an obstructive müllerian anomaly. This can result in hematometra or hematocolpos. The presentation, diagnosis, evaluation, and treatment of anomalies of the reproductive tract are discussed in Chapter 10.

Mittelschmerz

Mittelschmerz is the term applied to ovulatory pain. The patient typically experiences dull pain at the time of ovulation in one lower quadrant, lasting from a few minutes to 6 to 8 hours. In rare instances, the pain is severe and crampy and persists for 2 to 3 days. The cause of this pain is unknown, but the spillage of normal follicular fluid as the follicle cyst ruptures and expels the oocyte may irritate the peritoneum. Ultrasonography studies have detected small quantities of fluid at midcycle in 40% of normal women's cycles (58).

In most cases, the diagnosis of mittelschmerz is evident from the recurrent nature of the mild discomfort. Documentation of the midcycle occurrence of the pain by menstrual charts is helpful, but many adolescents do not have regular periods and thus the pain may not be able to be documented as "midcycle." If the patient is being examined for the first episode or for an exceptionally severe episode, other diagnoses must be excluded, including appendicitis, ovarian torsion, rupture of an ovarian cyst, and ectopic pregnancy.

Therapy for mittelschmerz should aim first at a careful explanation to the young woman and her family of the benign nature of the pain and its cause. A heating pad and analgesics such as prostaglandin inhibitors (ibuprofen, naproxen sodium) are helpful. If the pain becomes repetitive in an expected cyclic fashion, CHT can be used to inhibit ovulation.

Chronic Pelvic Pain

Chronic pelvic pain (CPP) is a common and serious health issue for women, and is usually defined as 3 to 6 months of pain. CPP is estimated to have a prevalence of 3.8% in women aged 15 to 73, which is higher than that of migraines (2.1%), and similar to that of asthma (3.7%) and back pain (4.1%) (59,60). One study found that although CPP occurred in one of seven women in the United States between the ages of 18 and 50, only 49% of those with pain reported that the cause was known (61). For adolescents, CPP can lead to suffering, inability to participate in social interactions, and frequent or prolonged school absence.

The diagnosis of CPP in an adolescent is similar to that for acute pelvic pain except that the tempo of the investigation is usually not urgent. An accurate assessment of psychosocial issues and the impact of the pain on the life of the child or adolescent is essential. Chronic pain can be a significant source of frustration for the patient and her parents, and it is not unusual for them to search for multiple opinions from the medical community. Many of these teenagers will have missed many days of school and will be far behind in their schoolwork. If, for example, bowel spasm resulted in the initial symptoms of pain, reluctance to return to school may intensify the pain, causing further absences. Although short-term tutoring may be essential, the clinician should work with the adolescent and her family to encourage her to return to normal social interaction and to school. Granting a request for long-term home tutoring is rarely in her best interests. On the other hand, a definitive diagnosis is extremely important because parents and patients are often concerned that cancer or some other life-threatening condition is present. The girl/young woman's complaints should be assessed thoroughly so that she feels that her symptoms are taken seriously by the health care provider. A recommendation "to see a counselor" may be interpreted by the adolescent as meaning "the pain is in your head." In addition, important diagnoses such as PID or endometriosis may be missed unless a complete assessment is undertaken in the patient with persistent pelvic pain. The health care provider needs to reassure the patient that efforts will be made to sort out her problem and that she will not be abandoned even if no diagnosis can be established.

The evaluation of the child or adolescent with CPP requires a history and physical examination similar to that just described for acute pelvic pain. The common problems included in the differential diagnosis are shown in Table 11-1. The history and assessment should take into account the possible gynecologic, GI, urologic, musculoskeletal, and psychosomatic causes. The patient can be asked to grade the pain on a scale of 1 to 10. This can be helpful in deciding on the long-term management of the chronic pain. A complete history must include questions relating to past or present sexual abuse, as sexual abuse and physical abuse have both been noted to be associated with CPP (62–65). The International Pelvic Pain Society (66) has developed an adult pelvic pain questionnaire that can be adapted to an adolescent practice. A complete physical examination including abdominal palpation, musculoskeletal evaluation, assessment for hernias, and pelvic examination should be performed. It is helpful to ask the patient during the examination to point with one finger to the location of the pain and then to ask her what factors (e.g., exercise, sexual activity, food, urination, bowel movement) relieve or exacerbate the pain. For example, girls with endometriosis may have a constellation of symptoms that include cyclic severe dysmenorrhea, rectal pressure and other bowel problems, and dyspareunia. Activity may increase the symptoms in patients with adhesions and with many of the musculoskeletal problems. Since constipation and other GI disorders (irritable bowel syndrome, lactose intolerance) are such common causes of pelvic discomfort in adolescents, a careful bowel history, dietary history (including information about gum chewing and carbonated beverages), and rectal examination are important. A trial of stool softeners, high-fiber diet, and increased fluid intake is often essential before other diagnoses are considered.

The practitioner performing the musculoskeletal examination should assess the range of motion of the hips and spine, straight-leg raising test, symptoms with pelvic compression, and bone tenderness. Neoplasms of the pelvis and lower spine may be missed on plain radiographs and may require a bone scan for detection. Stress fractures of the pubic ramus and ischium can occur in runners, who may present with hip or groin pain, exacerbated by activity, and bone tenderness.

As noted previously, the pelvic examination should be performed with the patient in the lithotomy position so that the reproductive structures can be adequately assessed. A vaginal assessment is important to identify genital tract obstruction and anomalies. This can be accomplished with a visual inspection and a Q-tip insertion into the vagina to document vaginal tract patency, or with a speculum examination. In addition, samples should be obtained for *C. trachomatis* and *N. gonorrhoeae* tests, if the patient was ever or is possibly sexually active. The bimanual palpation (rectoabdominal or rectovaginal-abdominal) should attempt to localize tender areas, and the posterior cul-de-sac should be assessed for pain.

The laboratory evaluation usually includes a CBC with differential, ESR or CRP, urinalysis and urine culture, cervical tests, and a sensitive test for pregnancy. As described above, pelvic ultrasonography can be used to assess a mass or a suspected genital tract malformation and to screen patients in whom a satisfactory pelvic examination is not possible. It is advisable to ask the radiologist to screen the kidneys by ultrasound to look for unilateral renal agenesis or other renal anomalies if a genital tract anomaly is suspected.

In our practice, we have evaluated several young adolescents in the earliest stages of pubertal development who have persistent pelvic discomfort and large tender multifollicular ovaries (Fig. 11-4); we have treated them symptomatically with analgesics and low doses of NSAIDs, and the symptoms have resolved with further pubertal development. As noted above, some investigators have suggested that transabdominal color Doppler ultrasound can be useful in the evaluation of a painful ovary in adolescents. When prepubertal ovaries are found to be enlarged and multicystic, an evaluation for thyroid disease is indicated. In many young girls or adolescents, multicystic ovaries are asymptomatic and are noted when ultrasonography is done for other indications. Operative evaluation should be avoided unless ovarian torsion or tumor is suspected. A full presentation of the diagnosis and management of ovarian masses is presented in Chapter 18. Gastrointestinal series, urologic studies, bone scans, and consultations by specialists should be obtained as needed, not routinely in all adolescents with CPP.

When working with adolescents, the clinician should understand that 3 to 6 months of debilitating pain may interfere with school and social activities. For undiagnosed CPP in adolescents, laparoscopy has become an invaluable aid to diagnosis and therapy (30,49,67–69). It may be necessary to proceed with a surgical laparoscopic evaluation prior to the full 3 to 6 months. Laparoscopy allows the physician to make or confirm a specific diagnosis, obtain samples for biopsy, lyse adhesions, and perform operative therapeutic procedures. Before the procedure, the gynecologist should dis-

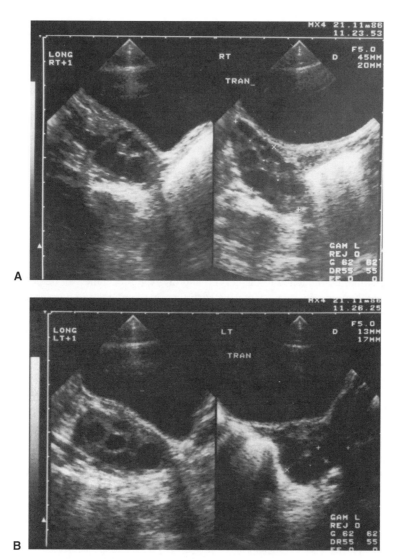

FIG. 11-4. Longitudinal and transverse ultrasound views of enlarged multicystic ovaries in an 11-year-old girl with chronic pelvic pain: **(A)** right ovary. **(B)** left ovary. Such ovaries are often asymptomatic in early pubertal girls.

cuss with the patient and her family the possibilities and limitations of operative surgery during the laparoscopy, and determine whether the patient desires a laparotomy if the needed procedure cannot safely be performed by laparoscopy. This preoperative counseling can avoid the need for a later second anesthetic for a lapa–

rotomy. Negative findings (see Color Plates 31–33) at laparoscopy can be equally valuable in reassuring the patient and her family and in helping her accept the fact that she has a functional problem that is likely to respond to medical and psychological therapy (49,67–69).

At our institution, laparoscopy in the evaluation of the adolescent or young adult with CPP is indicated if the patient's pain is unresponsive to prostaglandin inhibitors and CHT over a 3- to 6-month interval. As previously noted, laparoscopy is useful for the confirmation or exclusion of clinically suspected endometriosis, chronic PID, ovarian cysts, or pelvic adhesions.

Laparoscopy for Chronic Pelvic Pain

At Children's Hospital Boston, laparoscopy is performed with the patient under general endotracheal anesthesia, in the ambulatory surgery unit. A 2-, 5-, 7-, or 10-mm laparoscope is used through an umbilical vertical incision, and a secondary trocar site is established in the suprapubic area. We generally do not use a uterine mobilizer/manipulator attached to the cervix, and thus the procedure can be performed in the dorsal supine position. A uterine mobilizer/manipulator can be placed in the cervix of a sexually active patient, but it is usually not necessary in the majority of patients. If a uterine manipulator is used, the patient is placed in the dorsal lithotomy position. A Foley catheter is placed in all patients, as it is unclear how long the surgical procedure will take, and if a catheter is used to empty the bladder and is then removed the bladder may refill to a point of obstructing the surgeon's view. An orogastric tube is helpful in emptying the stomach, and the patient's respirations are temporarily ceased during the moments of insertion of the insufflation needle and trocar. We prefer to utilize the radially expanding trocar dilation technique as there is no cutting of the fascia with this method and thus decreased risk of postoperative hernias (70). In addition the surgeon should be aware of adolescent specific issues that increase the risks of laparoscopy such as low BMI (increased risk of injury with the insufflation needle insertion) (71).

The results of laparoscopy in the diagnosis of CPP at Children's Hospital Boston, between July 1974 and December 1983 are shown in Table 11-4. It should be noted

TABLE 11-4. *Postoperative diagnosis in 282 adolescent patients with chronic pelvic pain (Children's Hospital Boston, 1974–1983)*

Diagnosis	No. of patients	(%)
Endometriosis	126	(45)
Postoperative adhesions	37	(13)
Serositis	15	(5)
Ovarian cyst	14	(5)
Uterine malformation	15	(5)
Other*	4	(2)
No pathologic condition	71	(25)

*Ileitis, infarcted hydatid of Morgagni, pelvic congestion.

TABLE 11-5. *Age-related incidence of laparoscopic findings in 129 adolescent patients with chronic pelvic pain (Children's Hospital Boston, 1980–1983)*

Diagnosis	No. of patients (%)				
	Age 11–13	Age 14–15	Age 16–17	Age 18–19	Age 20–21
Endometriosis	2 (12)	9 (28)	21 (40)	17 (45)	7 (54)
Postoperative adhesions	1 (6)	4 (13)	7 (13)	5 (13)	2 (15)
Serositis	5 (29)	4 (13)	0 (0)	2 (5)	0 (0)
Ovarian cyst	2 (12)	2 (6)	3 (5)	2 (5)	0 (8)
Uterine malformation	1 (6)	0 (0)	1 (2)	0 (0)	1 (0)
Other	0 (0)	1 (3)	2 (4)	1 (3)	0 (0)
No pathologic condition	6 (35)	12 (37)	19 (36)	11 (29)	3 (23)

that patients suspected of having PID on the basis of history and elevated sedimentation rate were not included in this series, since the laparoscopy in these patients was performed largely to confirm the diagnosis and evaluate the severity of PID rather than to establish the diagnosis of CPP.

As noted in Table 11-4, three-fourths of the adolescents who underwent laparoscopy at Children's Hospital Boston, for CPP had intrapelvic pathologic conditions; endometriosis was diagnosed most frequently. The age-related incidence of findings is shown in Table 11-5. As expected, the finding of endometriosis increases with age. The next most common finding was postoperative adhesions, usually associated with a history of appendectomy or ovarian cystectomy. In most of these adolescents, the pain was acyclic, was often aggravated by physical activity or coitus, and was relieved by rest. Preoperative treatment was variable; predominantly, suppression of ovulation with CHT or antiprostaglandins was used. Because of the small number of patients, the natural history is unknown except that a few have subsequently developed endometriosis.

Other findings included PID (see Chapter 15), ovarian cysts (see Chapter 18), genital tract malformations with obstruction (see Chapter 10), and cases of ileitis, infarcted hydatid of Morgagni, inguinal defects (Fig. 11-5), and adhesions (Fig. 11-6). The pain in the patients with chronic PID was generally acyclic and not related to physical activity; pelvic examination revealed tender or nontender adnexal thickening in most of these girls.

No apparent gynecologic cause of the chronic pain was found in one-fourth of the patients; of those with negative findings, 74% felt that their symptoms were improved at follow-up. Whether the knowledge of normal anatomy contributed to the positive outcome is unknown, although several patients with a history of PID were considerably reassured. At other centers, a larger percentage of normal laparoscopic examination results has been reported. The much higher number of patients with early endometriosis in the Children's Hospital Boston series may reflect the difficulty of identifying very early endometriosis (see later: Clinical Presentation and Diagnosis of Endometriosis), thus underscoring the need for a gynecologic surgeon familiar

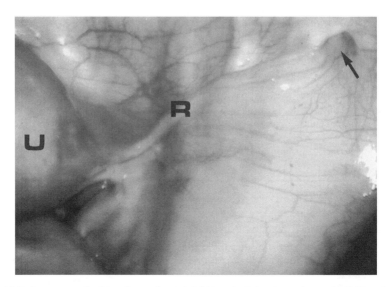

FIG. 11-5. Laparoscopic view of an enlarged right inguinal ring (*arrow*), a potential hernia site. R, round ligament; U, uterus.

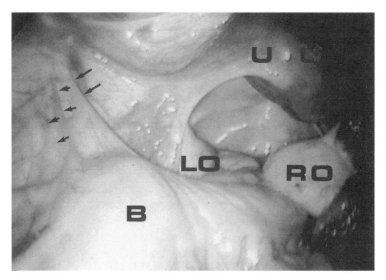

FIG. 11-6. Bowel adhesions (*arrows*) to sidewall. B, bowel; LO, left ovary; RO, right ovary; U, uterus.

TABLE 11-6. *Results of initial treatment in 140 adolescent patients with chronic pelvic pain*

Condition	No. of patients	Improved (%)	Recurrence (%)
Endometriosis alone	66	47 (71)	19 (29)
Postoperative adhesions	18	16 (89)	2 (11)
Uterine anomalies			
With endometriosis	8	8 (100)	0 (0)
Without endometriosis	4	4 (100)	0 (0)
Pelvic inflammatory disease	10	5 (50)	5 (50)
Hemoperitoneum	6	5 (83)	1 (17)
Functional ovarian cysts	5	4 (80)	1 (20)
Serositis	4	3 (75)	1 (25)
No pathologic condition	19	14 (74)	5 (26)
Total	140	106 (76)	34 (24)

(From Goldstein DP, deCholnoky C, Emans SJ, et al. Laparoscopy in the diagnosis and management of pelvic pain in adolescents. *J. Reprod Med* 1980;24:254; with permission.)

with the appearance of adolescent endometriosis. The results of treatment of the first 140 patients in our earlier series are shown in Table 11-6.

In a more recent study at Children's Hospital Boston, adolescent women aged 13 to 21 were evaluated when their pelvic pain had lasted longer than 3 months and had not responded to NSAIDs and CHT (30). Approximately 70% had endometriosis; the laparoscopic findings are shown in Table 11-7. The presenting symptoms of the

TABLE 11-7. *Laparoscopic findings in adolescent patients with chronic pelvic pain not responding to oral contraceptives and nonsteroidal antiinflammatory drugs*

Laparoscopic findings	Number (%)
Visible endometriosis	31/46 (67.4)
Adhesions	11/46 (23.9)
prior surgery	8
with endometriosis	3
without endometriosis	5
no prior surgery	3
with endometriosis	3
without endometriosis	0
Grossly normal pelvis	5/46 (10.9)
Functional cysts	4/46 (8.7)
Paratubal cysts	4/46 (8.7)
Müllerian anomalies	3/46 (6.5)
with endometriosis	1
without endometriosis	2

(From Laufer MR, Goitein L, Bush M, Cramer DW, Emans SJ. Prevalence of endometriosis in adolescent women with chronic pelvic pain not responding to conventional therapy. *J Pediatr Adolesc Gynecol* 1997;10:199.)

TABLE 11-8. *Characteristics of subjects with and without endometriosis*

Characteristics	Patients with endometriosis (n = 32) Number (%)	Patients without endometriosis (n = 14) Number (%)
Age (years)		
≤14	7 (21.8)	1 (7.2)
15–17	20 (62.5)	10 (71.4)
≥18	5 (15.6)	3 (21.4)
Mean age (years) at menarche	12.3	12.3
Mean time (months) at menarche	3.7	3.9
Duration of oral contraceptives (months)		
≤3	17 (53.1)	5 (35.7)
4–11	9 (28.1)	6 (42.9)
≥12	6 (18.8)	3 (21.4)
Prior surgery	3 (9.4)	5 (35.7)
Presenting symptoms		
Acyclic and cyclic pain	20 (62.5)	8 (57.1)
Acyclic pain	9 (28.1)	3 (21.4)
Cyclic pain	3 (9.4)	3 (21.4)
Gastrointestinal pain	11 (34.3)	6 (42.9)
Urinary symptoms	4 (12.5)	4 (33.3)
Irregular menses	3 (9.4)	6 (42.9)*
Vaginal discharge	2 (6.3)	2 (14.3)

*$p < 0.05$.
(From Laufer MR, Goitein L, Bush M, Cramer DW, Emans SJ. Prevalence of endometriosis in adolescent women with chronic abdominal/pelvic pain not responding to conventional therapy. *J Pediatr Adolesc Gynecol* 1997;10:199.)

patients with and without endometriosis are shown in Table 11-8. A study by Rock and colleagues showed a similar rate of endometriosis in their adolescent patient population with chronic pelvic pain (72).

An association between CPP and bowel-to-pelvic sidewall adhesions (Fig. 11-6) has been debated. The cause of adhesions is unknown, but it is believed to be the result of infection, previous surgery, or endometriosis. In women with CPP, a recent study found a higher rate of colon-to-sidewall adhesions than in controls (93.3% vs. 13.3%) (73). These authors also found that adhesions may occur with or without the presence of endometriosis, but that those patients with CPP had a higher rate of endometriosis than controls (46.7% vs. 6.7%). Others have suggested that a causal relationship between adhesions and pelvic pain is unproved (74). At our institution, when bowel adhesions are identified in adolescents with CPP, a laparoscopic lysis of adhesions is undertaken, and then a random posterior cul-de-sac biopsy specimen is obtained for microscopic evaluation to rule out microscopic endometriosis (see below). Our studies have shown a correlation of adhesions with endometriosis in patients with pelvic pain; as shown in Table 11-7, no cases of adhesions were identified in patients without a history of previous surgery or the existence of endometriosis (30). Patients who have undergone prior surgery may have adhesions as a result, or may have a herniation of bowel or omentum at the site of a previous laparoscopy incision.

The data collected at our institution and others reinforce the need to take the symptoms of CPP seriously. A careful history, pelvic examination, appropriate laboratory tests, and laparoscopy as indicated should be done in the pursuit of a diagnosis and treatment.

ENDOMETRIOSIS

Background

Endometriosis is defined as the presence of endometrial glands and stroma outside the normal anatomic location of the lining of the uterus (see Color Plates 44 to 46). In 1948, Meigs (75) reported that the incidence of endometriosis in all adolescents was 6%. Others have also attempted to estimate the prevalence (76,77). It is estimated that 4 to 17% of postmenarchal females have endometriosis (78). Studies have shown that 25% to 38.3% of adolescents with chronic pelvic pain have endometriosis (79,80), and 50% to 70% of adolescents undergoing laparoscopy for CPP who did not have control of pelvic pain with CHT and NSAIDs are found to have endometriosis (30,68,72,81–82).

Historically, endometriosis was considered a disease of women in the reproductive years, with onset only after many years of menstruation. However, studies have described endometriosis prior to menarche (83) and 1 (67) and 5 (84) months after menarche. An accurate determination of the prevalence in the adolescent population is difficult because the definitive diagnosis requires a laparoscopic evaluation, which only occurs with a specific indication; a selection bias thus exists for determining the prevalence in the overall adolescent population.

Treatment of CPP with NSAIDs and CHT are the first line approach as noted above; however, many adolescents continue to experience symptoms of pelvic pain despite these medications. For these young women, it is important to evaluate for endometriosis. Endometriosis in adult women is commonly associated with pain with menses; however, the symptoms in adolescents are typically acyclic and cyclic pain (30). Most adult patients with endometriosis present with pain, a pelvic mass, or infertility. Adolescents usually present with pelvic pain, as endometriomas and infertility are rare in this patient population.

Etiology of Endometriosis

There are many proposed theories to explain the origin of endometriosis, and no one theory accounts for all presentations of endometriosis.

Proposed theories about the causes of endometriosis include the following:

1. Sampson's (85,86) theory of retrograde menstruation proposes that there is retrograde transport of viable fragments of endometrium through the fallopian

tubes at the time of menstruation that leads to seeding of the peritoneal cavity. Studies of women undergoing laparoscopy (87,88) or peritoneal dialysis (89) have shown that retrograde menstruation occurs in 76% to 90% of all menstruating women. The extent of the reflux may be different or immunologic responses may be variable in women with endometriosis than in those free of the disease. Factors such as shorter cycle lengths, longer duration of flow, and possibly heavier flow in women with endometriosis than in control women lend credence to the hypothesis that retrograde menstruation is primarily responsible for endometriosis (90). This theory is supported by the observation that endometriosis occurs most commonly in the dependent portion of the pelvis. Furthermore, obstructive anomalies of the female genital tract that enhance retrograde flow have been associated with endometriosis in the adolescent population (67,91–92). Schifrin and colleagues identified six adolescents with müllerian anomalies associated with endometriosis, the youngest being a 12 year old with vaginal atresia and bicornuate uterus leading to a hematocolpos (91). Furthermore, repair of this type of obstructive anomaly has been associated with resolution of endometriosis (92).

2. Meyer's (93) theory of embryologically totipotent cells postulates that these cells undergo metaplastic transformation into functioning endometrium.

3. Halban's (94) theory hypothesizes of metastases of endometrial cells though vascular or lymphatic spread; this theory serves to explain the occurrences of endometriosis in anatomic locations remote from the pelvic such as the lung (95) or brain (96).

4. The theory of deficient cell-mediated immunity, promotes the concept that there is impaired "clearing" of endometriotic cells from aberrant locations (97,98). This theory suggest that a deficiency in cellular immunity allows the ectopic endometrial tissue to proliferate (98–100). This theory has also been supported by the high rates of autoimmune disorders in women with endometriosis (101).

5. A theory of environmental exposures has also been implicated as the etiology of endometriosis or as a confounding factor to the development of endometriosis in women with a genetic predisposition (102).

All these theories help explain some aspects of endometriosis. No single theory explains all cases of endometriosis, especially when relating to adolescents. One very challenging scenario is that of postpubertal/premenarcheal endometriosis (83). Most likely the cause of endometriosis is multifactorial, and all proposed mechanisms may contribute to the etiology of this disease process.

Genetic Predisposition

There may be a genetic predisposition to, or etiology of, endometriosis. Ranney (103) first reported the familial occurrence of endometriosis in a retrospective study of 53 families. Simpson and associates (104) reported a 6.9% rate of endometriosis in first-degree relatives of women with the disease, compared with only 1% of control relatives, the most probable mode of inheritance being polygenic and multifactorial. As the general population and health care providers have become increasingly educated about the existence and prevalence of endometriosis, there is an increase in referrals for young women to undergo definitive diagnosis for chronic pelvic pain. It is our observation that this is especially true of mothers who suffered from chronic pelvic pain as adolescents but received diagnosis and treatment for endometriosis only as adults.

Clinical Presentation and Diagnosis of Endometriosis

Endometriosis is the most common pathologic condition of the pelvis in adolescents with chronic pelvic pain (Tables 11-4 to–11-7). As noted in Table 11-5, endometriosis as a cause of chronic pelvic pain increases with age, from 12% in the 11- to 13-year old group to 54% in the 20- to 21-year-old group. The history usually reveals cyclic and/or acyclic pelvic pain. In one study from our institution, 64% of adolescents with endometriosis had cyclic pain and 36% acyclic pain (81). Our more recent study of adolescents with chronic pain not responding to NSAIDs and CHT showed that approximately 90% of the patients with endometriosis had some acyclic pain (Table 11-8). Some patients experience an increase in symptoms at midcycle and again with menses. The pain tends to increase in severity over time and may occur throughout the month. A pain diary documenting frequency and character of pain will help the adolescent and her caregiver to determine the timing of the pain, and if it is related to bowel or bladder function. Complaints of difficulty participating in normal activities, missing school, or avoiding extracurricular activities secondary to pain suggests that more aggressive intervention is appropriate. As mentioned above, a family history of endometriosis is correlated with a higher likelihood of endometriosis in the patient (104). A history of sexual abuse or physical abuse may also be associated with chronic pelvic pain (65) but should not preclude further evaluation.

Although CHT and antiprostaglandin medications may give some initial relief from dysmenorrhea, the pain of endometriosis usually persists, leading to laparoscopy for a definitive diagnosis and therapy as shown in Fig. 11-7 (31,105). Other presenting symptoms of adolescents with chronic pelvic pain not responding to NSAIDs and CHT are shown in Table 11-8, categorized according to those with and without endometriosis (30). Most adolescents with diagnosed endometriosis present with symptoms of pain, although adult women may be asymptomatic and the disease detected during an evaluation for infertility. The cause of the pain may be related to prostaglandin release or swelling and bleeding within the endometriotic implants. In addition, pain may be related to the type of lesion as studies have suggested that the clear and red lesions of endometriosis, which are most common in adolescents, are the most painful (see Table 11-9) (106). Endometriosis pain may be incapacitating in patients with both minimal and extensive disease; no clear correlation has been es-

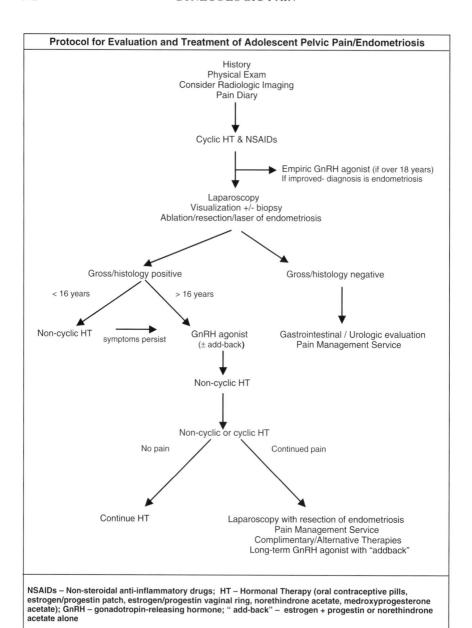

FIG. 11-7. Protocol for evaluation and treatment of pelvic pain/endometriosis (From Laufer MR, Sanfilippo J, Rose G. Adolescent endometriosis: diagnosis and treatment approaches. *J Pediatr Adolesc Gynecol* 2003;16:S3 and Propst AM, Laufer MR. Endometriosis in adolescents: incidence, diagnosis, and treatment. *J Reprod Med* 1999;44:751; with permission.)

TABLE 11-9. *Type of lesion and pain.*

Type of lesion	Association with pain
Clear	76%
Red	84%
White	44%
Black	22%

Pain perception 1 to 27 mm from lesion

(From Demco L. Mapping the source and character of pain due to endometriosis by patient-assisted laparoscopy. *J Am Assoc Gynecol Laparosc* 1998;5:241; with permission.)

tablished between the extent of disease and severity of pain (see Table 11-10) (107–110). Cornillie and colleagues (107) found that it is the deeply infiltrating endometriotic lesions that are most active and strongly correlate with pelvic pain, while Fedele and colleagues (108) found no relation between the severity of pain and stage of the disease or site of the endometriosis lesions (see Table 11-10).

Pelvic examination in the adult woman with endometriosis classically reveals tender nodules in the posterior vaginal fornix (cul-de-sac) and along the uterosacral ligaments. The ovary may be involved, with an endometrioma or dense periovarian adhesions, and the uterus may be fixed and retroverted. In contrast, the pelvic examination of adolescents with endometriosis often reveals mild to moderate tenderness rather than nodules or masses. As mentioned above, a pelvic exam should not be viewed as a necessity prior to proceeding with an evaluation of pelvic pain; most adolescents will have minimal disease and no specific findings on exam.

There is no imaging study that can identify endometriosis in the absence of an endometrioma. MRI, CT, and ultrasound are unable to detect the small lesions of endometriosis. In addition there is no specific blood test to identify endometriosis. CA-125 is a nonspecific marker of peritoneal inflammation and is elevated in women with endometriosis; it is not a useful screening test due to its high rate of false positives (111).

Empiric Gonadotropin-Releasing Hormone-agonist for a Diagnosis of Endometriosis

Empiric gonadotropin-releasing hormone-agonist (GnRH-a) (depot leuprolide) has been utilized in adult women with chronic pelvic pain and clinically suspected

TABLE 11-10. *Staging and pain are unrelated.*

Stage of disease	Percent of patients with pain
Stage I	40%
Stage II	24%
Stage III	24%
Stage IV	12%

(From Fedele L, Parazzini F, Bianchi S, et al. Stage and localization of pelvic endometriosis and pain. *Fertil Steril* 1990;53:155; with permission.)

endometriosis (112,113). If a woman with CPP responds to a 3 month injection of GnRH-a and her pain is relieved, then she is given a diagnosis of endometriosis without the need for a surgical procedure. Although controversial, the utilization of empiric GnRH-a therapy alleviates the need for a surgical procedure and the disease is treated medically. If the patient's symptoms persist then she is offered a laparoscopic evaluation and treatment. We, however, do not routinely utilize GnRH-a for women 16 years or younger due to concerns of adverse effects on final bone density acquisition (105). Additionally some parents are not interested in utilizing empiric therapy due to concerns of using a medication with adverse side effects without a definitive diagnosis. We thus do not routinely recommend empiric GnRH-a therapy for treatment of presumed endometriosis for young women under age 18, but it is an option for consenting women over age 18.

Surgical Diagnosis of Endometriosis

Operative laparoscopy can be undertaken to make a definitive diagnosis of endometriosis. If a gynecologist is going to perform the surgical procedure, he or she must feel comfortable operating on patients in this age range and be able to perform the required surgery. A diagnostic laparoscopy with subsequent referral to a "specialist" for definitive surgery places the patient at undue risk from two anesthesias. The gynecologist operating on an adolescent with pelvic pain must be familiar with the appearance of endometriosis implants in this age group. A diagnosis of endometriosis can be made by the visual appearance of the lesions or by taking a specimen for pathologic evaluation. Some authors have suggested that there is poor correlation between visually diagnosed endometriosis and pathology specimens and have thus recommended that all diagnoses be made with pathologic specimens (114). We currently utilize pathologic specimens for lesions that are difficult to classify or have an atypical appearance. If the surgeon is not familiar with the appearance of endometriosis in adolescents, then liberal use of biopsies for pathologic diagnosis may be helpful.

Appearance and Staging of Endometriosis

Endometriosis is staged according to the criteria of the American Society for Reproductive Medicine, which are based on a point system (Fig. 11-8) (115). Classic endometriosis has been described as blue/brown/gray "powder burns." Classic and "atypical" implants have been categorized on an expanded basis of morphologic appearance: white lesions; red, "flame," or petechial lesions (Color Plate 44); clear vesicular lesions (Color Plate 45); reddish-brown implants; and blue/brown/gray powder burn implants (115–119). The implants seen in adolescents are not typical of the lesions seen in adult women; adolescents predominantly have clear vesicles, pearly granular punctations (white implants), and/or small hemorrhagic or petechial

AMERICAN SOCIETY FOR REPRODUCTIVE MEDICINE
REVISED CLASSIFICATION OF ENDOMETRIOSIS

Patient's Name _____ Date_____

Stage I (Minimal) - 1-5
Stage II (Mild) - 6-15
Stage III (Moderate) - 16-40
Stage IV (Severe) - >40
Total_____

Laparoscopy_____ Laparotomy_____ Photography_____
Recommended Treatment_____
_____
Prognosis_____

PERITONEUM	**ENDOMETRIOSIS**	<1cm	1-3cm	>3cm
	Superficial	1	2	4
	Deep	2	4	6
OVARY	R Superficial	1	2	4
	Deep	4	16	20
	L Superficial	1	2	4
	Deep	4	16	20

	POSTERIOR CULDESAC OBLITERATION	Partial	Complete
		4	40

	ADHESIONS	<1/3 Enclosure	1/3-2/3 Enclosure	>2/3 Enclosure
OVARY	R Filmy	1	2	4
	Dense	4	8	16
	L Filmy	1	2	4
	Dense	4	8	16
TUBE	R Filmy	1	2	4
	Dense	4*	8*	16
	L Filmy	1	2	4
	Dense	4*	8*	16

*If the fimbriated end of the fallopian tube is completely enclosed, change the point assignment to 16.

Denote appearance of superficial implant types as red [(R), red, red-pink, flamelike, vesicular blobs, clear vesicles], white [(W), opacifications, peritoneal defects, yellow-brown], or black [(B) black, hemosiderin deposits, blue]. Denote percent of total described as R___%, W___% and B___%. Total should equal 100%.

Additional Endometriosis: _____ | Associated Pathology: _____

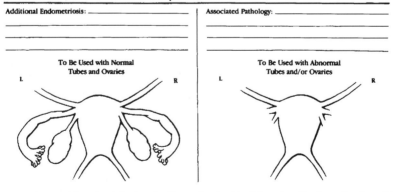

To Be Used with Normal Tubes and Ovaries

To Be Used with Abnormal Tubes and/or Ovaries

A

FIG. 11-8. Revised American Society for Reproductive Medicine classification of endometriosis: 1996. (From American Society for Reproductive Medicine. Revised American Society for Reproductive Medicine Classification of Endometriosis: 1996. *Fertil Steril* 1997;67:817; with permission.)

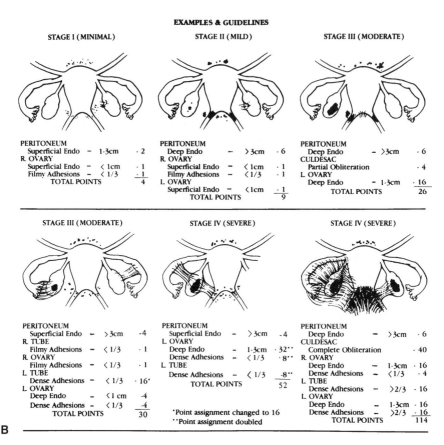

EXAMPLES & GUIDELINES

STAGE I (MINIMAL)	STAGE II (MILD)	STAGE III (MODERATE)

PERITONEUM
　Superficial Endo – 1-3cm · 2
R. OVARY
　Superficial Endo – < 1cm · 1
　Filmy Adhesions – < 1/3 · 1
　　　　TOTAL POINTS　　　4

PERITONEUM
　Deep Endo – > 3cm · 6
R. OVARY
　Superficial Endo – < 1cm · 1
　Filmy Adhesions – < 1/3 · 1
L. OVARY
　Superficial Endo – < 1cm · 1
　　　　TOTAL POINTS　　　9

PERITONEUM
　Deep Endo – > 3cm · 6
CULDESAC
　Partial Obliteration · 4
L. OVARY
　Deep Endo – 1-3cm · 16
　　　　TOTAL POINTS　　26

STAGE III (MODERATE)	STAGE IV (SEVERE)	STAGE IV (SEVERE)

PERITONEUM
　Superficial Endo – > 3cm -4
R. TUBE
　Filmy Adhesions – < 1/3 · 1
R. OVARY
　Filmy Adhesions – < 1/3 · 1
L. TUBE
　Dense Adhesions – < 1/3 · 16*
L. OVARY
　Deep Endo – < 1 cm -4
　Dense Adhesions – < 1/3 -4
　　　　TOTAL POINTS　　30

PERITONEUM
　Superficial Endo – > 3cm · 4
L. OVARY
　Deep Endo – 1-3cm · 32**
　Dense Adhesions – < 1/3 · 8**
L. TUBE
　Dense Adhesions – < 1/3 · 8**
　　　　TOTAL POINTS　　52

*Point assignment changed to 16
**Point assignment doubled

PERITONEUM
　Deep Endo – > 3cm · 6
CULDESAC
　Complete Obliteration · 40
R. OVARY
　Deep Endo – 1-3cm · 16
　Dense Adhesions – < 1/3 · 4
L. TUBE
　Dense Adhesions – > 2/3 · 16
L. OVARY
　Deep Endo – 1-3cm · 16
　Dense Adhesions – > 2/3 · 16
　　　　TOTAL POINTS　　114

B

FIG. 11-8. (*Continued*)

spots of the pelvic peritoneum. We have recently described a new technique of filling the pelvis with liquid to aid in the visualization of clear lesions of endometriosis (120). Peritoneal defects, Alan-Masters windows, are also common in adolescents and should be recognized by the operating gynecologist (see Color Plate 46).

In earlier reports from our institution, adolescents with chronic pelvic pain were found to have a rate of endometriosis of 45% and a rate of serositis of 5% (Table 11-4). The cases of serositis may be what is now referred to as atypical clear lesions of endometriosis, thus giving an overall prevalence of 50% of adolescents with chronic pelvic pain having endometriosis. If endometriosis is suspected but difficult to identify, or if the gross appearance of the pelvis is normal in a patient with chronic pelvic pain, a biopsy from the particular lesion or a random pelvic peritoneal biopsy specimen from the posterior cul-de-sac may help confirm a diagnosis of endometriosis (121,122). Nisolle and colleagues (121) found microscopic endometriosis in 6% of patients with a grossly visible pelvis. In our series, one of five patients (20%) with a visibly normal pelvis was found to have biopsy-proven endometriosis (30). In the ovary, large endometrial cysts can develop: so-called endometriomas or chocolate cysts, which are much less common in adolescents and are usually found with more advanced disease. In our experience, endometriomas are not commonly identified in women under age 20.

There may be a natural progression of endometriosis, evolving from the subtle lesions in adolescents to the classic lesions in adult women. Adolescent endometriosis usually presents with clear or red lesions of the cul-de-sac and no other definable disease. Martin and colleagues (123) reported a pattern of evolution of subtle lesions in adolescence and more classic disease a decade later. Redwine demonstrated that "clear" and "red" lesions occur at a mean age 10 years earlier than do "black" lesions (77). In our recent series, 77.4% of adolescents were found to present with stage I disease and 22.6% with stage II disease; no patients presented with stage III or IV disease (30). This finding is in contrast to those in adults showing a higher stage of endometriosis at the time of presentation (124), and it also argues for the possibility that the disease progresses with age.

Endometriosis and Obstructive Anomalies of the Reproductive Tract

As mentioned above, the incidence of endometriosis is found to be greatly increased in patients with obstructive anomalies of the reproductive tract (see Chapter 10) (125). Schifrin and co-workers (91) concluded that müllerian tract anomalies predispose adolescents to endometriosis. Adolescents with congenital obstructing müllerian malformations often have severe endometriosis classified as stage III or IV, even in early adolescence. Endometriosis associated with obstructive anomalies has been reported to completely resolve after correction of the obstruction (92). Congenital anomalies associated with endometriosis include imperforate hymen, vaginal septum, hematocolpos, hematometra, and uterine anomalies.

Endometriosis and Future Fertility

The importance of finding endometriosis early lies not only in the relief of symptoms but also, it is hoped, in the preservation of reproductive potential and suppression of possible natural disease progression (109,126). Infertility commonly results when endometriosis causes anatomic distortion of the pelvic organs and/or the fallopian tubes. In addition, stage I disease has been shown to be associated with infertility (127). Data from animal studies show a clear cause-and-effect relationship between endometriosis and infertility (128–130). The causes of infertility as they relate to endometriosis are beyond the scope of this book, but it is important for the health care provider to refer patients with chronic pain or diagnosed endometriosis to gynecologists who provide state-of-the-art therapies to treat the pelvic pain and, it is hoped, avoid the progression of the disease and its sequelae. Since endometriosis is known to be a progressive disease, it is thus our philosophy that pelvic pain should be evaluated in an expedient fashion and if endometriosis is diagnosed it should be treated aggressively until the patient has completed child bearing.

Endometriosis and Cancer

Very rarely endometriomas can contain an endometrioid adenocarcinoma. Since endometriomas are rare in the adolescent, this condition is extremely rare. Endometriosis has been associated with dysplastic nevi and melanoma (131).

Treatment of Endometriosis

The optimal therapy for adolescents and adult women with endometriosis is still being debated. The patient needs to understand the pros and cons of each surgical and medical option and that there is no cure for the disease. Recurrence of symptoms from endometriosis is common. The patient and the health care provider should follow success or failure of the varied treatments. Adolescents should be asked to rate their pain on a scale of 0 to 10 at the time of each visit. Therapy should be utilized to decrease pain and permit the adolescent to function. The patient should be aware that she may not be pain free but her treatments should be adjusted to maximize pain relief and promote school and social function and participation.

Surgical Treatment Options of Endometriosis

Treatment of endometriosis in adolescents usually begins with surgical resection/destruction of visible lesions at the time of diagnosis (Fig. 11-9). A laparoscopy should never be performed only to diagnose endometriosis without advantage being taken of the opportunity for surgical therapy. Surgical therapy utilizes several techniques to maximally remove or destroy visible lesions of endometriosis; these techniques include gross resection, laser vaporization, endocoagulation, and electrocoagulation (unipolar or bipolar) (132). Advances in operative laparoscopic techniques and instrumentation have increased the extent and degree of difficult surgical procedures that can be approached via laparoscopy. Whatever the surgical approach, the goal is removal and destruction of all visible endometriosis, lysis or resection of adhesions, restoration of normal pelvic anatomy, and maintenance of all reproductive organs. Resection or lysis of adhesions can be achieved with laparoscopic scissors, with or without cautery. In our institution, we favor the gross resection of endometriotic lesions, electrocautery, and/or carbon dioxide (CO_2) laser vaporization. Regardless of the surgical approach to treating the endometriosis and/or adhesions,

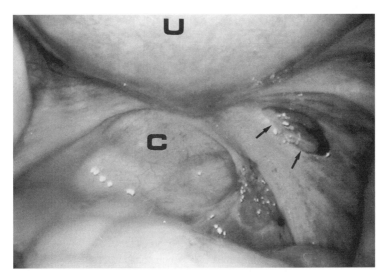

FIG. 11-9. Peritoneal "defects" (*arrows*) created by resection of endometriosis. U, uterus; C, cul-de-sac.

care must be taken to avoid damage to the bowel, bladder, ureters, and major blood vessels; the patient must be informed that these complications are a known risk of all operative laparoscopic procedures, and if an injury occurs it will be repaired by laparoscopy or laparotomy when that injury is identified.

The use of laparotomy to treat endometriosis has decreased as laparoscopic surgeons have become more experienced. Although rare in adolescents, advanced staged endometriosis can be surgically managed via laparoscopy; laparotomy is rarely indicated. Historically, it has been argued that laparotomy provides better depth perception and has the added advantage of allowing direct palpation of the diseased tissue. The relevance of these points is minimized with the improved skill of the laparoscopist and with improved instrumentation. Laparoscopy has the advantages of magnification. Laparotomy may be needed if there are extensive adhesions, or endometriotic implants that are not safely resectable via pelviscopy.

The success rate of surgery in resecting/ablating endometriotic lesions causing pain is variable (132,133). Surgery alone is not adequate treatment for endometriosis as there can be microscopic residual disease that must be suppressed with medical therapy (113). With surgery alone, studies have shown that symptoms will return in approximately 50% of adult women within 1 year (113,134–136).

Endometriosis and Adhesions

Endometriosis can be associated with pelvic adhesions. A lysis of these adhesions can be undertaken laparoscopically to try to improve pelvic pain. Adhesions can recur. Tubal scarring should be addressed if it is felt to be an etiology for pain; tubal surgery to improve fertility is best undertaken at the time that the individual is trying to conceive.

Endometriomas in Adolescents

Endometriomas do not usually present until the mid-20s. When they do occur, we manage the endometrioma with surgical drainage and excision of the endometrioma cyst wall. If the cyst wall is not removed, then there is a higher rate of recurrence (137,138). When the cyst wall is being removed, great care should be taken not to remove normal ovarian tissue, as this could potentially have an adverse effect on future fertility (139,140).

Medical Treatment Options of Endometriosis

Since endometriosis is a chronic disease, following the initial optimal surgical resection/vaporization of all visible lesions of endometriosis, medical therapy should be initiated (Fig. 11-7). Medical management can achieve two goals: pain control and hormonal suppression of the disease to avoid progression. In the selection of a medical therapy, it is important to consider the patient's age, the severity of symptoms, the duration of symptoms, and the extent of disease.

Endometrium and endometriotic implants contain receptors for estrogen, progesterone, and androgens (141–143). Estrogens stimulate the growth of endometriotic tissue, whereas androgens result in atrophy. Progesterone stimulates endometrial growth, while synthetic progestins inhibit endometrial growth through their androgenic properties. Thus, the basis of medical therapy for pain from endometriosis is to take advantage of the reliance of endometrial tissue on steroid hormones for growth and function. A complete listing of possible hormonal therapies and their side effects is given in Table 11-11.

Combination Estrogen and Progestin Therapy

Oral contraceptives (OCs), contraceptive patch, and the vaginal ring, all contain both estrogen and progestin. Continuous low-dose CHT diminishes pain from endometriosis by creating a hormonal "pseudopregnancy" state in which endometrial implants become relatively inactive (144). This term is used because of the amenorrhea and decidualization of the endometrial tissue induced by the combined estrogen and progestin. The adolescent should be instructed that she may have irregular bleeding for up to 3 months before amenorrhea is induced. This form of treatment has been reported to relieve the pelvic pain associated with endometriosis (145). A progestin-

TABLE 11.11. *Comparison of hormonal therapies for endometriosis and possible side effects*

Therapy	Resultant hormone state			Side effects
	Acyclic	Hypoestrogenic	Hyperandrogenic	
NSAIDs	–	–	–	Inadequate pain control, gastrointestinal irritation
Noncyclic OCs	+	–	–	Nausea, breakthrough bleeding, other side effects listed for OCs
Progestins	+	+	–	Breakthrough bleeding, depression, bloating, decreased libido
Methyltestosterone	±	–	++	Virilization, masculinization of a female fetus
Danazol	+	+	++	Weight gain, acne, hirsutism, voice changes
GnRH agonist	+	++	–	Vasomotor symptoms (hot flushes), bone loss, vaginal dryness
GnRH agonist plus steroid add back (Premarin and Provera or Aygestin)	+ +	? ?	– –	Possible decreased vasomotor symptoms, bone loss, vaginal dryness
Mifepristone (RU 486)	+	±	–	Anorexia, nausea, dizziness, sommolence
Bilateral oophorectomy	++	++	–	Vasomotor symptoms, bone loss, vaginal dryness

NSAIDs, nonsteroidal antiinflammatory drugs; OC, oral contraceptive; GnRH, gonadotropin-releasing hormone; ++, extremely effective; +, effective; ±, sporadically effective; –, not effective; ?, questionably effective.
(From Laufer MR. Endometriosis in adolescents. *Curr Opin Pediatr* 1992;4:582; with permission.)

dominant monophasic pill, the combination hormonal contraceptive patch, or the hormonal vaginal ring should be initiated. If breakthrough bleeding occurs, it is often due to the lack of compliance with taking the pill or changing the patch or ring at the appropriate time. With the utilization of a combination hormonal pill continuously, it is very important that the pill be taken at the exact same time daily, or else there is an increased risk of irregular bleeding. A patient handout with information regarding continuous CHT is provided in Appendix 3. Low dose monophasic OCs may be used continuously; triphasic agents are not effective because of the change/fluctuation in hormonal dose. The principal problems with the "pseudopregnancy" therapy are headaches, fluid retention, nausea, weight gain, emotional lability, and hypertension. There is a lack of data on the long-term utilization of continuous CHT although this has been a widely utilized treatment modality. There has been a recent small study showing benefits of long term hormonal therapy (146). In a similar fashion to the continuous pills, the contraceptive patch (Ortho Evra Transdermal System) or the vaginal ring (Nuvaring) can be used in a continuous fashion without breaks to attempt to suppress menses, pain, and endometriosis.

Progestins have been found to have varying effectiveness in the treatment of endometriosis (147,148). Commonly used regimens include norethindrone acetate 15 mg daily by mouth, medroxyprogesterone acetate (MPA) 30 to 50 mg orally per day, or depot MPA 150 mg intramuscularly every 1 to 3 months (147–149). High dosages are required for benefit, and side effects are not well tolerated (150). The principal complaints in adolescents are weight gain, bloating, acne, headaches, fluid retention, emotional lability, and irregular menses. This treatment modality is usually reserved for those individuals who cannot tolerate continuous CHT or have a contraindication to their use. Oral progestin therapy should be considered prior to long-term intramuscular injections so that side effects can be identified and addressed or the medication discontinued. The long-term utilization of depo medroxyprogesterone acetate has been shown to result in loss of bone density in some patients and therefore monitoring of serum estradiol and/or bone density is advised (151,152). In at-risk patients, low dose estrogen therapy can be used. The cardiovascular effects of long-term therapy remain unknown and warrant investigation.

Testosterone and Danazol

The creation of a high androgen state with exogenous androgens has been shown to produce atrophy of endometriotic implants and improve pelvic pain (153). Methyltestosterone can improve pelvic pain associated with endometriosis; its usual dosage is 5 to 10 mg given buccally every day (153). When this dosage is used, pain will be improved but ovulation is not usually inhibited. This therapy can result in the undesirable side effect of masculinization, and if ovulation is not inhibited and a conception results while the patient is receiving this therapy, a masculinized female fetus may result. In our institution, we do not utilize this therapy for adolescents with endometriosis because of the severe adverse effects such as weight gain, bloating, acne, headaches, fluid retention, emotional lability, irregular menses, and virilization.

Danazol, an isoxazole derivative of 17α-ethinyl testosterone, is effective in the treatment of pain associated with endometriosis, as it results in an acyclic hypoestrogenic-hyperandrogenic state by interrupting ovarian follicular development and thereby inhibiting the growth and function of the endometriotic tissue (154,155). Although danazol appears to be very effective in the treatment of pelvic pain associated with endometriosis, we do not prescribe it for adolescents because of its unacceptable side effects, which include weight gain, edema, irregular menses, acne, oily skin, hirsutism, and a deep voice change. Some side effects, such as hirsutism and voice deepening, are not always reversible with discontinuation of the medication. The standard dosage is 800 mg per day in divided dosages. Danazol offers effective contraception at doses of 400 to 800 mg per day (154); sexually active patients treated with <400 mg per day require additional methods of contraception. Pain from endometriosis treated with danazol has been reported to be relieved in 85% to 90% of patients (156). In the same study, pain returned to the majority of treated patients within 1 year after they stopped therapy. In another study, the recurrence rate of symptoms and physical findings in patients treated with danazol was approximately 5% to 20% per year (154). A prospective randomized study in adult women has failed to show that danazol was superior to placebo in improving pregnancy rates in women with minimal endometriosis (157), in agreement with a previous study (158). Other problems with this medication include decreased high-density lipoprotein cholesterol, a mild increase in insulin resistance, an alteration in liver proteins, and androgenic effects on the developing fetus if the adolescent becomes pregnant while taking the drug. The drug should therefore be avoided in patients with hepatic dysfunction, severe hypertension, congestive heart failure, and borderline renal function. Because of these side effects, other treatment modalities have replaced this therapy, and as mentioned above, we do not currently prescribe danazol to adolescents.

Gonadotropin-Releasing Hormone Agonists

Currently, the first-line and most widely used therapy for endometriosis is the creation of an acyclic, low-estrogen environment to prevent bleeding in the implants and to prevent additional seeding of the pelvis during retrograde menstruation (31). This goal has been pursued by the use of gonadotropin-releasing hormone agonists (GnRH-a), such as nafarelin and leuprolide. Continuous GnRH stimulation results in down regulation of the pituitary and resultant hypoestrogenism. This reversible medical return to a prepubertal (hypoestrogenic, hypogonadotropic) state is very effective in creating a hypoestrogenic environment for the suppression of endometriosis. Gonadotropin-releasing hormone agonists are available in many formulations: nasal spray, subcutaneous injection, and intramuscular injection. In the adolescent population, compliance is a major issue, and thus the decision whether to use a twice-daily nasal spray or an intramuscular injection every 3 months is important. The nasal spray, if selected, is given as one puff twice daily in alternating nostrils (159). If depot-leuprolide (Lupron) is used, a dosage of 3.75 mg every 4 weeks will induce amenorrhea and hypoestrogenism in over 90% of women (126). Lupron is also available in an 11.25 mg dosage given every 3 months. If irregular bleeding occurs and the induction of amenorrhea is not achieved with these dosages, then an estradiol level should be checked and if not suppressed (less than assay), the dosage can be increased to 7.5 mg every 4 weeks, or 22.5 mg every 3 months.

It is important to make sure that patients understand that since this is a GnRH-agonist (GnRH-a), there will be a stimulatory phase prior to the down regulation. Thus patients will experience a final withdrawal bleed 21 to 28 days after the initiation of the GnRH-a. They will most likely experience a worsening of symptoms with the initial withdrawal bleed (160) prior to the suppression of pain and bleeding. Henzl and colleagues (161) examined the comparative effects of nafarelin and danazol in the treatment of endometriosis. They showed that GnRH-a was as effective as danazol in reducing endometriosis as demonstrated on second-look laparoscopy, and it was better tolerated. Other authors have reported similar results (159,162). Dlugi and colleagues (163) found that 3.75 mg of depot leuprolide given intramuscularly every 4 weeks for six doses was effective in improving pelvic pain in 85% of patients, compared with improvement in 43% of patients receiving placebo.

The side effects of GnRH-a therapy include hypoestrogenic symptoms such as hot flashes, vaginal dryness, and decreased libido (155,161). The most worrisome long-term side effect of GnRH-a therapy is decreased bone density, and thus the United States Food and Drug Administration (FDA) has not approved its prescription for courses of therapy lasting longer than 6 consecutive months (164–166). The prolonged hypoestrogenic state places the patient at risk for trabecular bone loss. Dawood and colleagues (164) showed a 7% trabecular bone loss in individuals when GnRH-as were used for 6 months. Reports differ about the reversibility of this bone loss, and its clinical significance is questionable (165). The use of GnRH-a therapy in adolescents, however, may present the added risk of long-term effects on bone because of the importance of the adolescent years to acquisition of normal bone density (166,167). Once again, the risks, benefits, and alternatives of various therapies need to be openly discussed with all adolescents and their parents.

Numerous studies have been undertaken in an attempt to alleviate the long-term side effects of the GnRH-as. The goal of GnRH-a therapy with "add-back" hormonal therapy is to reduce the deleterious side effects on bone and lipid metabolism. Studies of add-back regimens have examined the use of differing combinations of hormonal replacement. Surrey and others (168) reported on the effects of combining norethindrone with a GnRH-a in the treatment of symptomatic endometriosis, while Cedars and colleagues (169) studied the use of GnRH-a with medroxyprogesterone. Other studies have shown beneficial effects of the long-term use of GnRH-a in combination with the use of progestin therapy in maintaining bone density (168–172). Barbieri (170) has proposed an "estrogen threshold hypothesis" in the treatment of women with endometriosis. This theory proposes that there is an estrogen threshold for the reduction of endometriosis that is of a lesser degree of hypoestrogenism than the degree of hypoestrogenism resulting in bone resorption (Fig. 11-10). Sex steroid "add-back therapy" can be given with either norethindrone acetate 5 mg daily or conjugated estrogens (0.625) and MPA (5 mg) daily, or tibolone (2.5 mg) daily which is not currently available in the United States (173–176). Studies have shown greater patient satisfaction with the utilization of norethindrone as compared to conjugated estrogens and MPA for add-back therapy (173). Studies are needed to determine if long-term GnRH-a with sex steroid add-back therapy is safe for adolescents (166). When prescribing add-back therapy in adolescents, we currently use norethindrone acetate 5 mg per day in a continuous fashion. Oral contraceptive pills should not be used as add-back therapy, as the dosage of hormones is too high and the patient will have the same response as if she is on CHT alone. Calcium and vitamin D supplementation is prescribed with either add-back regimen. In addition to evaluating add-back with steroid hormones, others have studied the sole use or additional use of bisphosphonates or parathyroid hormone to preserve bone density (177,178). We do not currently utilize bisphosphonates in women who have not yet completed childbearing due to concerns that a fetus could "leach" the bisphosphonate from the mother's bones.

We utilize add-back therapy once amenorrhea has been induced with the initial course of GnRH-a therapy. There is no reason to avoid the utilization of add-back therapy, as studies have not shown increased return of pain with the initiation of add-back therapy (173).

It is our current practice to offer all adolescents over age 16 with endometriosis a 6-month course of GnRH-a therapy with norethindrone acetate add-back therapy

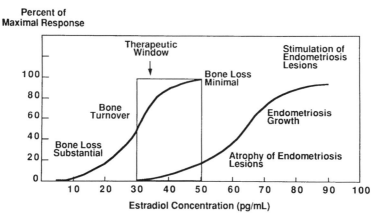

FIG. 11-10. Estradiol therapeutic window in the treatment of endometriosis. The concentration of estradiol required to cause growth of the lesions of endometriosis may be greater than the concentration required to stabilize bone mineral density. (From Barbieri RL. Hormone treatment of endometriosis: the estrogen threshold hypothesis. *Am J Obstet Gynecol* 1992;166:740; with permission.)

following surgical diagnosis and resection/vaporization. At the conclusion of this initial GnRH-a therapy, continuous CHT (see earlier) are prescribed. If patients do well with this therapy, they continue to take continuous CHT until they desire fertility. If they have pain with the continuous hormonal therapy and irregular bleeding, a different monophasic combined hormonal pill should be used to try to induce amenorrhea and suppress pain. If there is pain without bleeding, then resuming GnRH-a therapy with add-back should be utilized on a long-term basis.

For adolescents less than 16 years of age, we utilize continuous CHT as first-line medical therapy so as to avoid possible adverse effects of GnRH-a on bone formation. If these therapies do not succeed, then patients are offered additional surgery and/or GnRH-a therapy. It is important for the clinician to keep in mind other diagnoses in addition to the endometriosis, such as irritable bowel syndrome, lactose intolerance, or psychological issues in the adolescent with persistent pain.

Pain Management

NSAIDs are effective in the treatment of some cases of pain from endometriosis (17,18) (see Appendix 9), but many patients do not respond to this management. Naproxen sodium was proved to be significantly better than placebo in relieving the symptoms of dysmenorrhea in patients with endometriosis (179). Long-term narcotic use should be avoided, and if the patient is in such significant pain, further evaluation and treatment of the disease process are indicated. It is important to stress that hormonal therapy is suppressive and not curative, and there is no cure for the disease.

A multidisciplinary approach to the management of the chronic pain of endometriosis is very beneficial. A pain management service should be utilized (180). In addition, alternative and complementary medicines including herbal therapy and acupuncture should be encouraged (see Chapter 25).

Management of Refractory Pain from Endometriosis

Other Surgical Procedures (Laser Uterosacral Nerve Ablation and Presacral Neurectomy)

Additional surgical options for patients with persistent pelvic pain include pelvic denervation procedures such as laser uterosacral nerve ablation (LUNA) (181,182) and presacral neurectomy (183–186). These procedures come in and out of vogue, as the data are limited and difficult to interpret.

LUNA can safely be achieved with the use of a CO_2 laser through a laparoscope, but recent studies have not supported the efficacy of this procedure. It is important to know the surgical landmarks; we ablate the medial two-thirds of the uterosacral ligaments (which contain the uterosacral nerves) within 1 cm of the uterus so as to avoid damage to the ureters (Figs. 11-11 and 11-12). In a randomized trial comparing LUNA with sham surgery for dysmenorrhea, ablation was found to be more effective in relieving pain for the first 3 months after surgery; <50% of women continued to have relief 1 year later (181). A later study showed that LUNA benefited women with dysmenorrhea who had not responded to NSAIDs (182). Presacral neurectomy procedures have been performed for many years, with successful relief of dysmenorrhea and dyspareunia as great as 73% to 77% (183,187). Another evaluation of presacral neurectomy showed a high rate of relief of dysmenorrhea and central pelvic pain, but no improvement in lateral pain, back pain, or dyspareunia (184). Additional reports have shown that this procedure can be performed safely and effectively by either laparotomy or laparoscopy (185,186,188).

Although it is not appropriate treatment for adolescents and young adults, hysterectomy with bilateral salpingo-oophorectomy is believed to be the definitive surgical procedure for the treatment of endometriosis, with approximately 90% elimination of symptoms postoperatively (133). If one or both ovaries remain in situ, there is believed to be a 7% rate of recurrence of symptoms (189). If the disease is severe, as many as 33% of women experience recurrence of symptoms if bilateral oophorectomy is not performed (133). For adolescent women with endometriosis and a contraindication for future fertility (severe cognitive or medical disease) then laparoscopic bilateral oophorectomy is an alternative to long-term GnRH-a therapy if continuous combination hormonal therapy has not been effective.

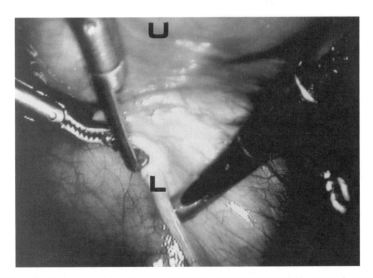

FIG. 11-11. Right laser uterosacral nerve ablation (LUNA) in progress. U, uterus; L, uterosacral ligament.

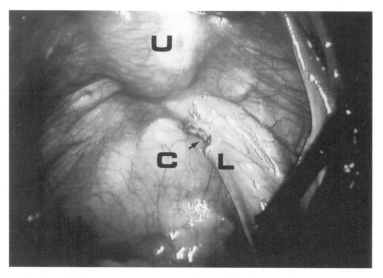

FIG. 11-12. Result of right laser uterosacral nerve ablation (LUNA) (*arrow*) in Fig. 11-11. U, uterus; L, uterosacral ligament; C, cul-de-sac.

Prolonged GnRH-a Therapy

Following additional surgery, or after initial medical therapy has failed, then prolonged utilization of GnRH-a with add-back therapy can be initiated. We have had patients with surgically diagnosed disease refractory to other medications on this prolonged GnRH-a with add-back for over 10 years. Prior to the initiation of "re-treatment" with a GnRH-a or if therapy is to be prolonged greater than 9 months, a baseline bone density evaluation should be obtained, and then repeated 6 months later and if stable repeated every 2 years. As noted above, the long-term utilization of GnRH-a with add-back therapy has not been studied in the adolescent population (166).

Other Medical Therapies (GnRH Antagonists and RU-486)

Theoretically, GnRH antagonists should be advantageous over GnRH-as, as there is no initial stimulatory phase and they thus result in faster gonadal suppression. The many side effects of the antagonists have limited their approval by the FDA, including histamine release and anaphylaxis. Further studies and improvement of these drugs are needed before they can be widely tested for the treatment of endometriosis.

RU 486 (mifepristone) is a synthetic steroid with both antiprogesterone and antiglucocorticoid activity. Numerous studies have shown that long-term treatment results in anovulation. Kettel and colleagues (190) showed a decrease in pelvic pain in patients with endometriosis treated with 100 mg per day of RU-486, but no improvement in gross disease as seen at follow-up laparoscopy. Further double-blind studies are needed.

Future developments in the treatment of endometriosis may be able to take advantage of the protein growth factors that regulate the epithelial and stromal elements of the endometrium. Modulation of the immune system, which may possibly play a critical role in pain, scarring, and infertility, may offer another method of treating endometriosis. Women with endometriosis may have elevated levels of serum CA-125, and this marker may provide a potential means for monitoring treatment (125,155,191). Studies have not been done in adolescents, and we prefer to rely on pain symptoms as a predictor of recurrence or progression of disease.

Therapy for adolescent pelvic pain associated with endometriosis clearly needs to be individualized because adolescents are very conscious of side effects and will become noncompliant. Frequent appointments, support, and careful listening and response to concerns and questions are an important part of the medical care. Diet and exercise are extremely important in assisting adolescents with endometriosis to cope with this chronic disease.

Support and Education Relating to Endometriosis

In addition, adolescents with endometriosis find a support network with meetings, a newsletter, phone conversations, and "big sisters with endometriosis" helpful. We have collaborated to establish such a group, the Teen Endometriosis Education Network (TEEN) in Boston within the structure of the Endometriosis Association's Boston chapter (192). The adolescents reported that the support group was beneficial in providing educational material and support to themselves, their families, and school systems. In addition, the Boston chapter of the Endometriosis Association and the Division of Gynecology at the Children's Hospital Boston, have collaborated in the creation of an educational video on adolescent endometriosis for schools, health care providers, patients, and their families. Educational information is available for patients and families at *www.endometriosisassn.org* and *www.youngwomenshealth.org*.

Issues in Adolescent Endometriosis for Future Consideration

Early diagnosis of endometriosis and treatment will hopefully suppress progression and advancement of disease; this is an area that needs future investigation (31). Additionally there are some areas that are particularly challenging. For instance, how should we treat the adolescent daughter of a woman who had no pelvic pain but who had stage IV endometriosis and infertility. Should she have an evaluation and treatment with continuous OCs, even though she has no pelvic pain in an attempt to avert the silent development of stage IV endometriosis and future infertility? These areas should be addressed in future investigations.

With education of young women, their families, pediatricians, nurse practitioners, family practitioners, gynecologists, and pediatric surgeons, we may be able to decrease the length of time from the onset of symptoms to presentation, and from the time of presentation to diagnosis of endometriosis. In addition, with early diagnosis of endometriosis it may be possible to decrease the long-term effects of the disease (pain, endometriomas, and infertility), and thus improve an affected adolescent's quality of life.

Endosalpingiosis

Endosalpingiosis is a pathologic condition that differs from endometriosis in that glands without stroma are present. Little is known of the clinical correlation with this pathologic entity. Only one published report describes a correlation with pelvic pain in three patients with endosalpingiosis (193). In a recent study, we reviewed the pathologic reports from women younger than 22 who had undergone peritoneal biopsy identified with endosalpingiosis; those with a pathologic diagnosis of endometriosis were excluded (194). The presenting symptoms included pelvic pain (100%), acyclic pain (36%), cyclic pain (9%), cyclic and acyclic pain (55%), irregular menses (45%), GI symptoms (55%), urinary symptoms (36%), and vaginal discharge (9%). Initial postoperative therapy included cyclic OCs (55%), continuous OCs (36%), and progestin-only pills (9%). Long-term follow-up was obtained for an average of 12.6 months. Subjects had pain when not taking medications, and all were maintained by medical management for endometriosis (OCs, danazol, or GnRH-a). Thirty-three percent of the subjects required additional surgery 6, 10, or 12 months after the initial surgery, at which time all were found to have endometriosis. It is thus our conclusion that the clinical presentation of endosalpingiosis is one of pelvic pain, operative findings are varied, and the clinical course and response may be similar to that of endometriosis. Additional studies are required to better define the clinical disease of endosalpingiosis so that surgeons and patients confronted with this pathologic entity have a better understanding of its clinical course and possible treatment options.

Uterine and Vaginal Malformations with Obstruction

Obstructive müllerian anomalies can result in both acute or chronic pelvic pain. In addition, as mentioned above, there is a high rate of endometriosis in cases of obstructive müllerian anomalies (91). A complete description of the presentation, diagnosis, and treatment of these conditions is given in Chapter 10.

PREMENSTRUAL SYNDROME AND
MENSTRUAL DYSPHORIC DISORDER

Premenstrual syndrome (PMS) includes a cluster of symptoms that occur in a cyclic fashion beginning 1 to 2 weeks prior to menses and disappearing within a few days of the onset of menses. These symptoms have been reported to affect as many as 75% of women of reproductive age women during their lives (195). PMS includes mild to moderate emotional and physical symptoms without impacting the individual's level of functioning. Premenstrual dysphoric disorder (PMDD) is a severe form of PMS and is included in *Diagnostic and Statistical Manual of Mental Disorders,* 4th ed, text revision (DSM-IV-TR) to allow better diagnostic criteria and enhanced therapeutic approaches (196) (see Table 11-12) (197). PMDD is reported to affect 3% to 8% of women of reproductive age (197).

TABLE 11-12. *Criteria for premenstrual dysphoric disorder.[a]*

In most menstrual cycles during the past year, presence of greater than or equal to five of the following symptoms for most of the last week of the luteal phase[b], with remission beginning within a few days after the onset of the follicular phase, and absence of symptoms during the week after menses; inclusion of more than or equal to one of the first four symptoms:
Markedly depressed mood, feelings of hopelessness, or self-deprecating thoughts
Marked anxiety, tension, feelings of being "keyed up" or "on edge"
Marked affective lability (e.g., feeling suddenly sad or tearful or having increased (sensitivity to rejection)
Persistent and marked anger or irritability or increased interpersonal conflicts
Decreased interest in usual activities (e.g., work, school, friends, and hobbies)
Subjective sense of difficulty in concentrating
Lethargy, easy fatigability, or marked lack of energy
Marked change in appetite, overeating, or specific food cravings
Hypersomnia or insomnia
Subjective sense of being overwhelmed or out of control
Other physical symptoms, such as breast tenderness or swelling, headache, joint or muscle pain, a sensation of "bloating," weight gain
Marked interference with work or school or with usual social activities and relationships with others (e.g., avoidance of social activities or decreased productivity and efficiency at work or school)
Disturbance not a mere exacerbation of the symptoms of another disorder, such as major depressive disorder, panic disorder, dysthymic disorder, or a personality disorder (although possibly superimposed on any of these disorders)
Confirmation of three criteria above by prospective daily ratings during at least two consecutive symptomatic menstrual cycles. (Diagnosis may be made provisionally before such confirmation.)

[a]The criteria are from the *Diagnostic and Statistical Manual of Mental Disorders,* 4th ed., text revision (DSM-IV-TR). (From Grady-Weliky, TA. Premenstrual dysphoric disorder. *N Engl J Med* 2003;348:433; with permission.)
[b]In menstruating women, the luteal phase corresponds to the period between ovulation and the onset of menses, and the follicular phase begins with menses. In nonmenstruating women (e.g., women who have had a hysterectomy), determination of the timing of the luteal and follicular phases may require measurement of circulating reproductive hormones.

The PMS constellation of symptoms commonly reported by adolescents and adult women includes bloating, weight gain, breast soreness, hunger, thirst, fatigue, acne, constipation, hot flashes, chills, difficulty concentrating, and mood change (irritability or depression) (198–200). Adolescents and adults with migraine headaches may suffer an increase in headaches premenstrually and with menses; similarly, those with epilepsy may note an increase in the severity and/or frequency of seizures in the luteal phase of the cycle, premenstrually, or with the onset of menses. Cognitively challenged individuals may have behavioral outbursts that are difficult for their caretakers to cope with, and psychotic patients may exhibit more uncontrollable actions in a cyclic fashion in the luteal phase of the cycle. Premenstrual exacerbation may occur in some rare medical conditions, such as hepatic porphyria (201). In addition, recent case reports have indicated that rare patients develop sensitivity to naturally produced progesterone and may have hives or even life-threatening allergic reactions during the luteal phase; these manifestations are reversed by GnRH-a or oophorectomy (202,203).

Most adolescent girls are aware of some premenstrual symptoms, and active listening, reassurance, and improvement in diet and exercise are usually sufficient to manage them. Adolescents who experience severe symptoms often are under stress and have other psychosocial issues that need to be addressed, not just by medical evaluation of the PMS but also by psychological counseling. About 20% to 40% of adult women of reproductive age have symptoms sufficiently bothersome to cause a temporary deterioration in interpersonal relationships or job effectiveness; fewer than 5% of adult women have severe symptoms (198,204).

The cause of PMS has been variously attributed to estrogen and progesterone because of the occurrence of these symptoms in the luteal phase of the cycle and the disappearance when ovulation (and the resultant rise in progesterone levels) is inhibited by GnRH-a (205,206). Although several forms of progesterone have been prescribed for treatment, double-blind studies have not demonstrated the efficacy of this approach (207). In fact, it has been suggested that higher adverse premenstrual scores occur in menstrual cycles with high luteal-phase plasma progesterone and estradiol concentrations (208). Other studies have not detected a difference in hormone levels between women with a mood disorder of PMS and those without symptoms (209). In addition, one study has demonstrated that neither the timing nor the severity of PMS symptoms was altered by mifepristone-induced menses or luteolysis, which suggests that the endocrine events of the late luteal phase do not directly generate the symptoms of PMS (210).

Women with PMS appear to have symptoms consistent with exaggerated neurotransmitter responses to estrogen and progesterone fluctuations. The changes occur in the opioidergic system, the γ-aminobutyric system (GABA), and the serotonergic system. In 1981, Reid and Yen (211) proposed a hypothesis that endogenous opiates triggered the premenstrual symptoms. In an assessment of the pattern of symptoms, Reid (212) attributed the changes in the 2 weeks before menses—breast swelling and tenderness, lower abdominal bloating, and constipation—to the production of endogenous central, and perhaps peripheral, opiates. Since actual body weight may not increase in spite of bloating, changes that the patient notes may occur because of local fluid shifts and bowel wall edema. The release of the opiates may also increase the appetite and result in unusual food cravings as well as fatigue, depression, and emotional lability. Later in the cycle, the shift toward anxiety and irritability, vague abdominal cramps with loose bowel movements or diarrhea, headaches, chills, and sweats may result from withdrawal of endogenous opiates as hormone levels fall. In sensitive women, cyclic exposure to the neuropeptides, and subsequent withdrawal from their central effects, may result in a cascade of neuroendocrine changes that cause clinical symptoms. Support for this hypothesis has come from animal experiments, the observation of the effects of opiates on nonaddicts and the consequences of withdrawal in addicts, and the improvement in symptoms with the administration of the opiate antagonist (naltrexone) and with exercise (213). Support for the involvement of the GABA and serotonergic system in the pathogenesis of PMS comes from the positive therapeutic responses to alprazolam and the selective serotonin-reuptake inhibitors (SSRIs) including fluoxetine, sertraline, and fluvoxamine (214–218). In addition administration of metergoline, a serotonin antagonist, to fluoxetine treated women with PMDD causes a return of mood symptoms (219).

Therapeutic Options for PMS/PMDD Treatment

Therapeutic approaches to PMS/PMDD (see Table 11-13) (197) may be improved by increased understanding of its pathophysiology and the interaction of biologic and psychological factors. Biologic factors that cause PMS may be influenced by personal psychological and social factors (200). Alteration of the ovulatory menstrual cycle can alleviate symptoms, and thus drug therapy may be considered in adolescents with significant symptoms that have not responded to nonpharmacologic management. The health care provider should realize that most drug trials are hampered by the definition of PMS/PMDD, the sample size, and the strong placebo effect. In addition, adolescents are often at risk of unprotected intercourse and pregnancy, and many of the medications should not be prescribed to potentially pregnant adolescents. In most adolescents, premenstrual symptoms are mild, and the recognition that they are a real entity can be reassuring. For those troubled by their symptoms, the cyclic occurrence should be established by prospective recording symptoms on a special calendar for two to three cycles; many such calendars are in use by PMS clinics (220). Without documentation on a calendar, mood alterations and depression occurring throughout the cycle may be attributed to PMS, and adequate psychological intervention will not be undertaken. A calendar is also useful in deciding which symptoms are most troubling to the patient. Treatment options vary and are listed below according to the literature's support of efficacy.

TABLE 11-13. *Recommended treatment strategies for premenstrual dysphoric disorder[a].*

Medication	Starting dose (mg)	Therapeutic dose (mg)	Common side effects
First line: selective serotonin reuptake inhibitors			
Fluoxetine	10 to 20	20	Sexual dysfunction (anorgasmia and decreased libido), sleep alterations (insomnia, sedation, or hypersomnia), and gastrointestinal distress (nausea and diarrhea)
Sertraline	25 to 50	50 to 150	Same as fluoxetine
Paroxetine	10 to 20	20 to 30	Same as fluoxetine, not recommended in adolescents
Citalopram	10 to 20	20 to 30	Same as fluoxetine
Second-line			
Clomipramine	25	50 to 75	Dry mouth, fatigue, vertigo, sweating, headache, nausea
Alprazolam	0.50 to 0.75	1.25 to 2.25	Drowsiness, sedation
Third-line			
Leuprolide	3.75	3.75	Hot flashes, night sweats, headache, nausea

[a]For selective serotonin-reuptake inhibitors and clomipramine, the starting and therapeutic doses are administered once daily and are the same with luteal-phase and continuous administration. For luteal-phase administration, the medication should be initiated at time of ovulation (usually approximately 2 weeks before the expected onset of menses) and discontinued on the first day of menses. The therapeutic doses given for selective serotonin-reuptake inhibitors are those that were reported in the randomized clinical trials. However, clinical experience has shown that a subgroup of patients with premenstrual dysphoric disorder may require slightly higher doses (up to 60 mg of fluoxetine; up to 150 mg of sertraline; up to 40 mg of paroxetine; and up to 40 mg of citalopram). If a patient is taking another selective serotonin-reuptake inhibitor and tolerating it well but has a partial response at the doses listed, it would be appropriate to increase the dose of the specific selective serotonin-reuptake inhibitor before switching to another agent. Alprazolam is administered three times a day; treatment should begin at 0.25 mg three times a day. Clinical trials of leuprolide used the depot form; leuprolide should be administered intramuscularly each month. (From Grady-Weliky, TA. Premenstrual dysphoric disorder. *N Engl J Med* 2003;348:433; with permission.)

Treatments with Possible Benefit in PMS/PMDD

Exercise and Stress Reduction

Although no controlled studies have demonstrated the benefit of diet or exercise, most centers start with this approach because the lifestyle changes are healthy and undoubtedly give the adolescent a sense of control over her life. A program of aerobic exercise should be strongly encouraged as a first line of therapy. Patients are also instructed to avoid salty foods, alcohol, caffeine, chocolate, and concentrated sweets and to eat four to six smaller meals per day during the premenstrual period. A written sheet with foods to avoid (e.g., cola, coffee, hot dogs, canned foods, chips) and to add to the diet (e.g., unsalted popcorn, raw vegetables and fruits, skim milk, complex carbohydrates, high-fiber foods, low-fat meats) is helpful to the young woman. Additional dietary alternative therapies have been reported (27). Areas of stress should be identified. Stress-reduction programs such as biofeedback, self-hypnosis, or yoga may be helpful. Many patients experience an increased sense of well-being and control with a program of improved nutrition, exercise, and stress management. For adolescents who do not respond to lifestyle changes and have persistent and significant symptoms, pharmacologic therapies include NSAIDs, CHT, diuretics, SSRIs, and other options discussed below.

NSAIDs, Diuretics, CHT, and Agnus Castus Fruit Extract

Mefenamic acid (250 mg every 8 hours starting on day 16 of the cycle, increased to 500 mg on day 19 of the cycle) has been shown in one small study of 15 women with PMS to improve fatigue, headache, and general aches and pains; this medication may be especially useful in patients with severe dysmenorrhea as well (221). Other NSAIDs used in treating dysmenorrhea may be similarly useful, but none of them should be prescribed to the adolescent who is likely to become pregnant. A listing of NSAIDS, with dosages, can be found in Appendix 9 (17,18).

Although many patients complain of weight gain, actual daily measurements may reveal no change. Rather, fluid shifts and bowel wall edema may result in the symptoms. For true edema and weight gain from fluid retention, a diuretic such as spironolactone can be given (222,223).

Although CHT have given variable results in adult women with PMS, many adolescents, especially those with premenstrual exacerbation of seizures or headaches, show striking improvement on OCs with 30 to 35 µg of estrogen and a medium dose of progestin (see Chapter 20). Oral contraceptives may thus be effective in adolescents; the hormonal therapy can be utilized in either a cyclic or a continuous fashion. The continuous hormonal therapy can be effective in suppressing menses and it also creates a constant hormonal state without cyclic changes. A patient handout with instructions for taking combination hormonal therapy can be found in Appendix 3.

In a placebo-controlled trial of 170 women with PMS, the extract of the fruit of the *Vitex agnus castus* plant (one dry extract tablet daily) has been shown to significantly decrease irritability, anger, headache, and breast symptoms compared with placebo (224).

Treatments with Proven Benefit in PMS/PMDD

SSRIs have been beneficial in the treatment of PMS and PMDD (216,217, 225,226). In a randomized trial of women with PMS, fluoxetine in dosages from 20 to 60 mg per day continuously was superior to placebo (217,218). In addition, the researchers determined that the 20-mg dosage reduced the potential for side effects while maximizing therapeutic efficacy. Many dosing regimens for fluoxetine have been reported, including a single dose in the early luteal phase (216), a continuous daily dosage throughout the cycle (217), and daily dose only during the late luteal phase (216). Fluoxetine has been shown superior to placebo for relieving the most common physical symptoms of PMDD in addition to improving mood disturbances (227). Other SSRIs, including sertraline (50 to 150 mg to day) (228,229), paroxetine (20 to 30 mg per day) (should not be prescribed in adolescents) (230), and citalopram (20 to 30 mg per day) (231) have also been shown to be effective in treating PMS and PMDD. Venlafaxine (50 to 200 mg per day), which selectively inhibits the reuptake of both serotonin and norepinephrine, had been shown to be more effective than placebo (232). In addition to daily therapy, some SSRIs have been shown to be effective if taken only during the luteal phase of the cycle (231,233). Luteal therapy only can be challenging for some adolescents due to irregular cycles and issues relating to cyclic compliance.

Alprazolam (0.25 mg three times daily from day 20 until the second day of menstruation and then tapered by one tablet per day) relieved premenstrual symptoms in a double-blind study of women with PMS (234), but concern about patients' becoming dependent on this drug and having withdrawal symptoms has made us reluctant to use alprazolam in adolescents.

The GnRH-a can prevent the cyclic progesterone and estrogen production; however, this approach may be more useful as a probe in defining the cause of the problem than as a long-term treatment because of the potential for osteoporosis in estrogen-deficient patients. According to a hypothesis similar to Barbieri's estrogen threshold hypothesis (170), preventing ovulation and cyclic hormones but allowing some estrogen secretion might protect the bones from osteoporosis, treat PMS symptoms, and avoid the negative long-term effects of the GnRH-as. More recently, many studies have shown a beneficial effect of the long-term use of a GnRH-a with add-back therapy for the treatment of PMS (235–237). These therapies may be beneficial in the treatment of severe symptoms, but their unknown effects on adolescent bone density require caution for their use in the adolescent population.

Low-dose danazol (200 to 400 mg per day) has appeared beneficial in a small study (238) of adult women; however, reliable contraception is needed at doses of <400 mg per day. Danazol may inhibit ovulation and thus decrease cyclic hormonal responses, but it is likely to have undesirable side effects in adolescents and should be avoided.

Unproven Treatments of PMS/PMDD

Progesterone

Despite the widespread popularity of progesterone and many anecdotal reports of its success, only two of the nearly dozen prospective randomized, placebo-controlled studies have shown a benefit significantly greater than that of a placebo (239,240), and one recent large double-blind, placebo-controlled study of progesterone failed to demonstrate any effect that was greater than that of placebo (241). A recent review of the use of progesterone for PMS does not support its utilization (242).

Vitamins, Dietary Supplements, and Other Drugs

A large variety of vitamins and dietary supplements have been utilized for the treatment of PMS/PMDD but have generally been found to be no better than placebo. Vitamin B_6 has been popular with some self-help groups. Studies of its efficacy have been conflicting. One placebo-controlled study of 150 mg of vitamin B_6 found that while some premenstrual symptoms such as dizziness and behavioral symptoms were improved, most patients still experienced significant symptoms (243). Other studies have not found a beneficial effect. A recent review suggested some benefit of vitamin B_6 if taken in dosages of up to 100 mg per day, but the review is based on poor quality studies (244). In view of the concern about the toxic potential of this vitamin to cause sensory neuropathy, even in low doses, patients need to be cautioned about this risk.

Other studies have evaluated the use of evening primrose oil (245), essential free fatty acids (246), Ginkgo biloba (247), calcium (248), and magnesium (249,250), but these studies are not large randomized clinical trials and thus do not support the utilization of these products.

Bromocriptine has been used in some adult women to alleviate breast soreness, but this symptom is rarely a major complaint of adolescents, and this medication can have significant adverse side effects. In adolescents with breast soreness, we prefer to suggest reducing caffeine consumption and to prescribe a small dose of NSAIDs.

The plethora of drugs shown to be effective in small studies shows that more data are clearly needed to document their efficacy before adolescents are exposed to their potential risks. In addition, adolescents need to be asked whether they are taking over-the-counter medications.

Much more needs to be learned about PMS/PMDD and its causes; recent advances have improved the possibilities for drug therapy in the treatment of PMS/PMDD in adolescents.

REFERENCES

1. Klein JR, Litt IF. Epidemiology of adolescent dysmenorrhea. *Pediatrics* 1981;68:661.
2. Wilson C, Emans SJ, Mansfield J, et al. The relationship of calculated percent body fat, sports participation, age, and place of residence on menstrual patterns in healthy adolescent girls at an independent New England high school. *J Adolesc Health Care* 1984;5:248.
3. Pickles VR. A plain muscle stimulant in the menstruum. *Nature* 1957;180:1198.
4. Pickles VR, Cletheroe HJ. Further studies of the menstrual stimulant. *Lancet* 1960;2:959.
5. Pickles VR, Hall WJ, Best FA, et al. Prostaglandins in endometrium and menstrual fluid from normal and dysmenorrheic subjects. *Br J Obstet Gynaecol* 1965;72:185.
6. Halbert IR, Demers L, Fontana J, et al. Prostaglandin levels and endometrial jet wash specimens in patients with dysmenorrhea before and after indomethacin therapy. *Prostaglandins* 1975;10:1047.

7. Smith RE. Primary dysmenorrhea and the adolescent patient. *Adolesc Pediatr Gynecol* 1988;1:23.

8. Kaplan-Machlis B, Klostermeyer BS. The cyclooxygenase-2 inhibitors: safety and effectiveness. *Ann Pharmacother* 1999;33:979.

9. Buttar NS, Wang KK. The "aspirin" of the new millennium: cyclooxygenase-2 inhibitors. *Mayo Clin Proc* 2000;75:1027.

10. Fitzgerald GA, Patrono C. Drug therapy: the coxibs, selective inhibitors of cyclooxygenase-2. *N Engl J Med* 2001;345:433.

11. Fiorucci S, Meli R, Bucci M, Cirino G. Dual inhibitors of cyclooxygenase and 5-lipoxygenase. A new avenue in anti-inflammatory therapy. *Biochem Pharmacol* 2001;62:1433.

12. Alvin PE, Litt IF. Current status of the etiology and management of dysmenorrhea in adolescence. *Pediatrics* 1982;70:516.

13. Chan WY, Dawood MY, Fuchs F. Prostaglandins in primary dysmenorrhea. Comparison of prophylactic and nonprophylactic treatment with ibuprofen and use of oral contraceptives. *Am J Med* 1981;70:535.

14. Henzl MR, Buttram V, Segre EJ, et al. The treatment of dysmenorrhea with naproxen sodium. *Obstet Gynecol* 1977;127:818.

15. Larkin RM, Van Arden DE, Poulson AM. Dysmenorrhea: Treatment with an antiprostaglandin. *Obstet Gynecol* 1979;54:456.

16. Budoff PW. Use of mefenamic acid in the treatment of primary dysmenorrhea. *JAMA* 1979;241:2713.

17. Smith RP. Cyclic pelvic pain and dysmenorrhea. *Obstet Gynecol Clin North Am* 1993;20:753.

18. Ansani NT, Starz TW. Effective use of nonsteroidal anti-inflammatory drugs. *The Female Patient* 2002;27:25.

19. Klein JR, Litt IF, Rosenberg A, et al. The effect of aspirin on dysmenorrhea in adolescents. *J Pediatr* 1981;98:987.

20. DeLia JE, Emery MD, Taylor RH, et al. Flurbiprofen in dysmenorrhea. *Clin Pharmacol Ther* 1982;32:76.

21. Smith RP, Powell JR. Simultaneous objective and subjective evaluation of meclofenamate sodium in the treatment of primary dysmenorrhea. *Am J Obstet Gynecol* 1987;157:611.

22. Smith RP. The dynamics of nonsteroidal anti-inflammatory therapy for primary dysmenorrhea. *Obstet Gynecol* 1987;70:785.

23. Davis AR, Westhoff CL. Primary dysmenorrhea in adolescent girls and treatment with oral contraceptives. *J Pediatr Adolesc Gynecol* 2001;14:3.

24. DuRant RH, Jay MS, Shoffitt T, et al. Factors influencing adolescents'responses to regimens of naproxen for dysmenorrhea. *Am J Dis Child* 1985;139:489.

25. Pollison R. Nonsteroidal anti-inflammatory drugs: practical and theoretical considerations in their selection. *Am J Med* 1996;100:A31S.

26. Emery P. Cyclooxygenase-2: a major therapeutic advance? *Am J Med* 2001;110:42S.

27. Gladstar R. *Herbal healing for women.* New York: Simon & Schuster, 1993.

28. Muneyvirci-Delale O, Nacharaju VL, Altura BM, et al. Sex steroid hormones modulate serum ionized magnesium and calcium levels throughout the menstrual cycle in women. *Fertil Steril* 1998;69:958.

29. Benassi L, Barletta FP, Baroncini L, et al. Effectiveness of magnesium pidolate in the prophylactic treatment of primary dysmenorrhea. *Clin Exp Obstet Gynecol* 1992;19:176.

30. Laufer MR, Goitein L, Bush M, et al. Prevalence of endometriosis in adolescent women with chronic pelvic pain not responding to conventional therapy. *J Pediatr Adolesc Gynecol* 1997;10:199.

31. Laufer MR, Sanfilippo J, Rose G. Adolescent endometriosis: diagnosis and treatment approaches. *J Pediatr Adolesc Gynecol* 2003;16:S3.

32. Rapkin AJ, Reading AE. Chronic pelvic pain. *Curr Probl Obstet Gynecol Fertil* 1991;14:101.

33. Laufer MR. Endometriosis in adolescents. *Curr Opin Pediatr* 1992;4:582.

34. Velebil P, Wingo PA, Xia Z, et al. Rate of hospitalization for gynecologic disorders among reproductive-age women in the United States. *Obstet Gynecol* 1995;86:764.

35. Davis LG, Gerscovich EO, Anderson MW, et al. Ultrasound and Doppler in the diagnosis of ovarian torsion. *Eur J Radiol* 1995;20:133.

36. Davis AJ, Feins NR. Subsequent asynchronous torsion of normal adnexa in children. *J Pediatr Surg* 1990;25:687.

37. Eckler K, Laufer MR, Perlman SE. Conservative management of bilateral asynchronous adnexal torsion with necrosis in a prepubescent female. *J Pediatr Surg* 2000; 35:1248.

38. Vermesh M, Graczykowski JW, Sauer MV. Reevaluation of the role of culdocentesis in the management of ectopic pregnancy. *Am J Obstet Gynecol* 1990;162:411.
39. Quillin SP, Siegil MJ. Transabdominal color Doppler ultrasonography of the painful adolescent ovary. *J Ultrasound Med* 1994;13:549.
40. Tepper R, Lerner-Geva L, Zalel Y, et al. Adnexal torsion: the contribution of color Doppler sonography to diagnosis and post-operative follow-up. *Eur J Obstet Gynecol Reprod Biol* 1995;62:121.
41. Fleischer AC, Stein SM, Cullman JA, et al. Color Doppler sonography of adnexal torsion. *J Ultrasound Med* 1995;14:523.
42. Willms AB, Schlund JF, Meyer WR. Endovaginal Doppler ultrasound in ovarian torsion: a case series. *Ultrasound Obstet Gynecol* 1995;5:129.
43. American College of Obstetricians and Gynecologists (ACOG) Technical Bulletin. *Gynecologic ultrasonography.* 1995;215.
44. Shalev E, Mann S, Romano S, et al. Laparoscopic detorsion of adnexa in childhood: a case report. *J Pediatr Surg* 1991;26:1193.
45. Shalev E, Peleg D. Laparoscopic treatment of adnexal torsion. *Surg Gynecol Obstet* 1993;176:448.
46. Iwabe T, Harada T, Miura H, et al. Laparoscopic unwinding of adnexal torsion caused by ovarian hyperstimulation. *Hum Reprod* 1994;9:2350.
47. Styer AK, Laufer MR. Ovarian bivalving after detorsion. *Fertil Steril* 2002;7:1053.
48. Laufer MR, Billett A, Diller L, et al. A new technique for laparoscopic prophylactic oophoropexy prior to craniospinal irradiation in children with medulloblastoma. *Adolesc Pediatr Gynecol* 1995;8:77.
49. Goldstein DP. Acute and chronic pelvic pain. *Pediatr Clin North Am* 1989;365:573.
50. Wolner-Hanssen P, Svensson L, Mardh P-A, et al. Laparoscopic findings and contraceptive use in women with signs and symptoms suggestive of acute salpingitis. *Obstet Gynecol* 1985;66:233.
51. Heinonen PK, Miettinen A. Laparoscopic study on the microbiology and severity of acute pelvic inflammatory disease. *Eur J Obstet Gynecol Reprod Biol* 1994;57:85.
52. Bevan CD, Johal BJ, Mumtaz G, et al. Clinical, laparoscopic and microbiological findings in acute salpingitis: report on a United Kingdom cohort. *Br J Obstet Gynaecol* 1995;102:407.
53. Eschenbach DA, Wolner-Hanssen P, Hawes SE, et al. Acute pelvic inflammatory disease: association of clinical and laboratory findings with laparoscopic findings *Obstet Gynecol* 1997;89:184.
54. Kahn JA, Chiang VW, Shrier LA, et al. Microlaparoscopy with conscious sedation in adolescents with suspected pelvic inflammatory disease. *J Pediatr Adolesc Gynecol* 1999;12:149.
55. Faber BM, Coddington CC. Microlaparoscopy: a comparative study of diagnostic accuracy. *Fertil Steril* 1997;67:952.
56. Feste JR. Outpatient diagnostic laparoscopy using the optical catheter. *Contemp Obstet Gynecol* 1995;8:54.
57. Palter SF, Olive DL. Office microlaparoscopy under local anesthesia for chronic pelvic pain. *J Am Assoc Gynecol Laparosc* 1996;3:359.
58. Hann LE, Hall DA, Black EB, et al. Mittelschmerz: sonograph demonstration. *JAMA* 1979;241:2731.
59. Zondervan KT, Yudkin PL, Vessey MP, et al. Prevalence and incidence in primary care of chronic pelvic pain in women: Evidence from a national general practice database. *Br J Obstet Gynaecol* 1999;106:1149.
60. Howard F. Chronic pelvic pain. *Obstet Gynecol* 2003;101:594.
61. Mathias SD, Kuppermann M, Liberman RF, et al. Chronic pelvic pain: prevalence, health-related quality of life, and economic correlates. *Obstet Gynecol* 1996;87:321.
62. Harrop-Griffiths J, Katon W, Walker E, et al. The association between chronic pelvic pain, psychiatric diagnoses, and childhood sexual abuse. *Obstet Gynecol* 1988;71:589.
63. Rapkin AJ, Kames LD, Darke LL, et al. History of physical and sexual abuse in women with chronic pelvic pain. *Obstet Gynecol* 1990;76:92.
64. Reiter RC, Shakerin LR, Gambone JC, et al. Correlation between sexual abuse and somatization in women with somatic and nonsomatic chronic pelvic pain. *Am J Obstet Gynecol* 1991;165:104.
65. Walling MK, Reiter RC, O'Hara MW, et al. Abuse history and chronic pain in women: prevalences of sexual abuse and physical abuse. *Obstet Gynecol* 1994;84:193.
66. The International Pelvic Pain Society, Research Committee. Pelvic pain assessment form. Birmingham, Alabama: The International Pelvic Pain Society. Available at http://www.pelvicpain.org/pdf/FRM_Pain_Questionnaire.pdf Accessed 2003 Aug 17.

67. Goldstein DP, deCholnoky C, Leventhal JM, et al. New insights into the old problem of chronic pelvic pain. *J Pediatr Surg* 1979;14:675.
68. Goldstein DP, deCholnoky C, Emans SJ, et al. Laparoscopy in the diagnosis and management of pelvic pain in adolescents. *J Reprod Med* 1980;24:251.
69. Özaksit G, Cağlar T, Zorlu CG, et al. Chronic pelvic pain in adolescent women: diagnostic laparoscopy and ultrasonography. *J Reprod Med* 1995;40:500.
70. Bhoyryl S, Mori T, Way LW. Radially expanding dilatation. *Surg Endosc* 1996;10:775.
71. Mirhashemi R, Harlow BL, Ginsburg ES, et al. Predicting risk of complications with gynecologic laparoscopic surgery. *Obstet Gynecol* 1998;92:327.
72. Reese KA, Reddy S, Rock JA. Endometriosis in an adolescent population: the Emory experience. *J Pediatr Adolesc Gynecol* 1996;9:125.
73. Keltz MD, Peck L, Liu S, et al. Large bowel-to-pelvic sidewall adhesions associated with chronic pelvic pain. *J Am Assoc Gynecol Laparosc* 1995;3:55.
74. Alexander-Willimas J. Do adhesions cause pain? *Br Med J* 1987;294:659.
75. Meigs J. Endometriosis. *Ann Surg* 1948;127:795.
76. Wolfman W, Kreutner K. Laparoscopy in children and adolescents. *J Adolesc Health Care* 1984;5:251.
77. Motashaw N. Endometriosis in young girls. *Contrib Gynecol Obstet* 1987;16:22.
78. Ranney B. Etiology, prevention and inhibition of endometriosis. *Clin Obstet Gynecol* 1980;23:875.
79. Vercellini P, Fedele L, Arcaini L, et al. Laparoscopy in the diagnosis of chronic pelvic pain in adolescent women. *J Reprod Med* 1989;34:827.
80. Kontoravdis A, Hassan E, Hassiakos D. Laparoscopic evaluation and management of chronic pelvic pain during adolescence. *Clin Exp Obstet Gynecol* 1999;26:76.
81. Goldstein DP, deCholnoky C, Emans SJ. Adolescent endometriosis. *J Adolesc Health Care* 1980;1:37.
82. Chatman D, Ward A. Endometriosis in adolescents. *J Reprod Med* 1982;27:156.
83. Laufer, MR. Premenarcheal endometriosis without an associated obstructive anomaly: Presentation, diagnosis, and treatment. *Fertil Steril* 2000;74:S15.
84. Yamamoto K, Mitsuhashi Y, Takaike T. Tubal endometriosis diagnosed within one month after menarche: a case report. *Tohoko J Exp Med* 1997;181:385.
85. Sampson JA. Peritoneal endometriosis due to the menstrual dissemination of endometrial tissue into the peritoneal cavity. *Am J Obstet Gynecol* 1927;14:422.
86. Sampson JA. The development of the implantation theory for the origin of peritoneal endometriosis. *Am J Obstet Gynecol* 1940;40:549.
87. Halme J, Hammond MG, Hulka JF, et al. Retrograde menstruation in healthy women and in patients with endometriosis. *Obstet Gynecol* 1984;64:151.
88. Liu DTY, Hitchcock A. Endometriosis: its association with retrograde menstruation, dysmenorrhoea and tubal pathology. *Br J Obstet Gynaecol* 1986;93:859.
89. Blumenkrantz MJ, Gallagher N, Bashore RA, et al. Retrograde menstruation in women undergoing chronic peritoneal dialysis. *Obstet Gynecol* 1981;57:667.
90. Cramer DW, Wilson L, Stillman RJ, et al. The relationship of endometriosis to menstrual characteristics, smoking, and exercise. *JAMA* 1985;255:1904.
91. Schifrin BS, Erez S, Moore JG. Teen-age endometriosis. *Am J Obstet Gynecol* 1973;116:973.
92. Sanfilippo JS, Wakim NG, Schikler KN, et al. Endometriosis in association with uterine anomaly. *Am J Obstet Gynecol* 1986;154:39.
93. Meyer R. Über entzundliche neterope Epithelwucherungen im weiblichen Genetalgebiet und über eine his in die Wurzel des Mesocolon ausgedehnte benigne Wucherung des Darmepithel. *Virchows Arch Pathol Anat* 1909;195:487.
94. Halban J. Hysteroadenosis metastica. *Wien Klin Wochenschr* 1924;37:1205.
95. Foster DC, Stern JL, Buscema J, et al. Pleural and parenchyma pulmonary endometriosis. *Obstet Gynecol* 1981;58:552.
96. Thibodeau LL, Prioleau GR, Manuelidis EE, et al. Cerebral endometriosis: case report. *J Neurosurg* 1987;66:609.
97. Halme J, Becker S, Haskill S. Altered maturation and function of peritoneal macrophages: possible role in pathogenesis of endometriosis. *Am J Obstet Gynecol* 1987;156:783.
98. Dmowski W, Braun D, Gebel H. Endometriosis: genetic and immunologic aspects. *Prog Clin Biol Res* 1990;323:99.

99. Gleicher N, el-Roeiy A, Confino E, et al. Is endometriosis an autoimmune disease? *Obstet Gynecol* 1987;70:115.
100. Nothnick WB. Treating endometriosis as an autoimmune disease. *Fertil Steril* 2001;76:223.
101. Sinaii N, Cleary SD, Ballweg ML, et al. High rates of autoimmune and endocrine disorders, fibromyalgia, chronic fatigue syndrome and atopic diseases among women with endometriosis: a survey analysis. *Hum Reprod* 2002;17:2715.
102. Rier S, Foster WG. Environmental dioxins and endometriosis. *Toxicol Sci* 2002;70:161.
103. Ranney B. Endometriosis. IV. Hereditary tendency. *Obstet Gynecol* 1971;37:734.
104. Simpson JL, Elias S, Malinak LR, et al. Heritable aspects of endometriosis: I. Genetic studies. *Am J Obstet Gynecol* 1980;137:327.
105. Propst AM, Laufer MR. Endometriosis in adolescents: incidence, diagnosis, and treatment. *J Reprod Med* 1999;44:751.
106. Demco L. Mapping the source and character of pain due to endometriosis by patient-assisted laparoscopy. *J Am Assoc Gynecol Laparosc* 1998;5:241.
107. Cornillie FJ, Oosterlynck D, Lauweryns JM, et al. Deeply infiltrating pelvic endometriosis: Histology and clinical significance. *Fertil Steril* 1990;53:978.
108. Fedele L, Parazzini F, Bianchi S, et al. Stage and localization of pelvic endometriosis and pain. *Fertil Steril* 1990;53:155.
109. Koninckx PR, Meuleman C, Demeyere S. Suggestive evidence that pelvic endometriosis is a progressive disease, whereas deeply infiltrating endometriosis is associated with pelvic pain. *Fertil Steril* 1991;55:759.
110. Fukaya T, Hoshiai H, Yajima A. Is pelvic endometriosis always associated with chronic pain? A retrospective study of 618 cases diagnosed by laparoscopy. *Am J Obstet Gynecol* 1993;169:719.
111. Pittaway DE, Fayez JA. Use of CA-125 in the diagnosis and management of endometriosis. *Fertil Steril* 1986;46:790.
112. Ling FW, for the Pelvic Pain Study Group. Randomized controlled trial of depot leuprolide in patients with chronic pelvic pain and clinically suspected endometriosis. *Obstet Gynecol* 1999;93:51.
113. Gambone JC, Mittman BS, Munro MG. Consensus statement for the management of chronic pelvic pain and endometriosis: proceeding of an expert-panel consensus process. *Fertil Steril* 2002;78:961.
114. Walter AJ, Hentz JG, Magtibay PM, et al. Endometriosis: correlation between histologic and visual findings at laparoscopy. *Am J Obstet Gynecol* 2001;184:1407.
115. American Society for Reproductive Medicine. Revised American Society for Reproductive Medicine classification of endometriosis. *Fertil Steril* 1997;67:817.
116. Redwine DB. Age-related evolution in color appearance of endometriosis. *Fertil Steril* 1987;48:1062.
117. Stripling MC, Martin DC, Chatman DL, et al. Subtle appearances of pelvic endometriosis. *Fertil Steril* 1988;49:427.
118. Wiegerinck MAHM, Van Dop PA, Browns IA. The staging of peritoneal endometriosis by the type of active lesion in addition to the revised American Fertility Society classification. *Fertil Steril* 1993;60:461.
119. Redwine DB, Yocom LB. A serial section study of visually normal pelvic peritoneum in patients with endometriosis. *Fertil Steril* 1990;54:648.
120. Laufer MR. Identification of clear vesicular lesions of atypical endometriosis: a new technique. *Fertil Steril* 1997;68:739.
121. Nisolle M, Berliere M, Paindaveine B, et al. Histologic study of peritoneal endometriosis in infertile women. *Fertil Steril* 1990;53:984.
122. Murphy AA, Green WR, Bobbie D, et al. Unsuspected endometriosis documented by scanning electron microscopy in visually normal peritoneum. *Fertil Steril* 1986;46:522.
123. Martin DC, Hubert GD, Vander Zwaag R, et al. Laparoscopic appearances of peritoneal endometriosis. *Fertil Steril* 1989;51:63.
124. Hornstein MD, Harlow BL, Thomas PP, et al. Use of a new CA 125 assay in the diagnosis of endometriosis. *Hum Reprod* 1995;10:932.
125. Olive DL, Henderson DY. Endometriosis and müllerian anomalies. *Obstet Gynecol* 1987;69:412.
126. D'Hooghe TM, Bambra CS, Raeymaekers BM, et al. Serial laparoscopies over 30 months show that endometriosis in captive baboons (*Papio anubis, Papio cynocephalus*) is a progressive disease. *Fertil Steril* 1996;65:645.

127. Marcoux S, Maheux R, Bérubé S, et al. Laparoscopic surgery in infertile women with minimal or mild endometriosis. *N Engl J Med* 1997;337:217.

128. Schenken RS, Asch RH, Williams RE Hodgen GD. Etiology of infertility in monkeys with endometriosis: luteinized unruptured follicles, luteal phase defects, pelvic adhesions, and spontaneous abortions. *Fertil Steril* 1984;41:122.

129. Schenken RS, Asch RH. Surgical induction of endometriosis in the rabbit: effects on fertility and concentrations of peritoneal fluid prostaglandins. *Fertil Steril* 1989;34:581.

130. Kaplan CR, Eddy CA, Olive DL, et al. Effects of ovarian endometriosis on ovulation in rabbits. *Am J Obstet Gynecol* 1989;160:40.

131. Hornstein MD, Thomas PP, Sober AJ, et al. Association between endometriosis, dysplastic nevi and history of melanoma in women of reproductive age. *Hum Repro* 1997;12:143.

132. Redwine DB. Conservative laparoscopic excision of endometriosis by sharp dissection: life table analysis of reoperation and persistent or recurrent disease. *Fertil Steril* 1991;56:628.

133. Olive DL, Schwartz LB. Endometriosis. *N Engl J Med* 1993;328:1759.

134. Sutton J, Ewen SP, Whitelaw N, et al. Prospective, randomized, double blind, controlled trial of laser laparoscopy in the treatment of pelvic pain associated with minimal, mild and moderate endometriosis. *Fertil Steril* 1994;64:696.

135. Olive DL. Conservative surgery. In: Schenken RS, ed. *Endometriosis: contemporary concepts in clinical management.* Philadelphia: JB Lippincott Co, 1989:213.

136. Vancaillie T, Schenken RS. Endoscopic surgery. In: Schenken RS, ed. *Endometriosis: contemporary concepts in clinical management.* Philadelphia: JB Lippincott Co, 1989:249.

137. Beretta P, Franchi M, Ghezzi F, et al. Randomized clinical trial of two laparoscopic treatments of endometriomas: cystectomy versus drainage and coagulation. *Fertil Steril* 1988;70:1176.

138. Saleh A, Tulandi T. Reoperation after laparoscopic treatment of ovarian endometriomas by excision and by fenestration. *Fertil Steril* 1999;72:322.

139. Donnez J, Wyns C, Nisolle M. Does ovarian surgery for endometriomas impair the ovarian response to gonadotropin? *Fertil Steril* 2001;76:662.

140. Muzii L, Bianchi A, Croce C, et al. Laparoscopic excision of ovarian cysts: is the stripping technique a tissue-sparing procedure? *Fertil Steril* 2002;77:609.

141. Tamaya T, Motoyama T, Ohono Y. Steroid receptor levels and histology of endometrium and adenomyosis. *Fertil Steril* 1979;31:396.

142. Janne O, Kauppila A, Kokko E. Estrogen and progestin receptors in endometriotic lesions: comparison with endometrial tissue. *Am J Obstet Gynecol* 1981;141:562.

143. Fujishita A, Nakane PK, Koji T, et al. Expression of estrogen and progesterone receptors in endometrium and peritoneal endometriosis: an immunohistochemical and in situ hybridization study. *Fertil Steril* 1997;67:856.

144. Kistner RW. The treatment of endometriosis by inducing pseudopregnancy with ovarian hormones: a report of 58 cases. *Fertil Steril* 1959;10:539.

145. Vercellini P, Frontino G, De Giorgi O, et al. Continuous use of an oral contraceptive for endometriosis-associated recurrent dysmenorrhea that does not respond to a cyclic pill regimen. *Fertil Steril* 2003;80:560.

146. Miller L, Notter KM. Menstrual reduction with extended use of combination oral contraceptive pills: a randomized controlled trial. *Obstet Gynecol* 2001;98:771.

147. Moghissi KS, Boyce CR. Management of endometriosis with oral medroxyprogesterone acetate. *Obstet Gynecol* 1976;47:265.

148. Luciano AA, Turksoy N, Carleo J. Evaluation of oral medroxyprogesterone acetate in the treatment of endometriosis. *Obstet Gynecol* 1988;72:323.

149. Vercellini P, De Giorgio, Oldani S, et al. Depot medroxyprogesterone acetate versus an oral contraceptive combined with very low-dose danazol for long-term treatment of pelvic pain associated with endometriosis. *Am J Obstet Gynecol* 1996;175:396.

150. Ballweg ML. Tips on treating teens with endometriosis. *J Pediatr Adolesc Gynecol.* 2003; 163:27.

151. Cromer BA, Blair JM, Mahan JD. A prospective comparison of bone density in adolescent girls receiving depo-medroxyprogesterone acetate (Depo-Provera), levonorgestrel (Norplant), or oral contraceptives. *J Pediatr* 1996;129:671.

152. Berenson AB, Radecki C, Grady JJ. A prospective, controlled study of the effects of hormonal contraception on bone mineral density. *Obstet Gynecol* 2001;98:576.

153. Hammond MG, Hammond CB, Parker RT. Conservative treatment of endometriosis externa: the effects of methyltestosterone therapy. *Fertil Steril* 1978;29:651.
154. Barbieri RL, Hornstein MD. Medical therapy for endometriosis. In: Wilson EA, ed. *Endometriosis.* New York: Liss, 1987:111.
155. Barbieri RL. New therapy for endometriosis. *N Engl J Med* 1988;318:512.
156. Dmowski WP, Cohen MR. Antigonadotropin (danazol) in the treatment of endometriosis: evaluation of post-treatment fertility and three-year follow-up data. *Am J Obstet Gynecol* 1978;130:41.
157. Bayer SR, Seibel MM, Saffan DS, et al. Efficacy of danazol treatment for minimal endometriosis in infertile women. *J Reprod Med* 1988;33:179.
158. Hull ME, Moghissi KS, Magyar DF, et al. Comparison of different treatment modalities of endometriosis in infertile women. *Fertil Steril* 1987;47:40.
159. Burry KA. Nafarelin in the management of endometriosis: quality of life assessment. *Am J Obstet Gynecol* 1992;166:735.
160. Miller JD. Quantification of endometriosis-associated pain and quality of life during the stimulatory phase of gonadotropin-releasing hormone agonist therapy: a double-blind, randomized, placebo-controlled trial. *Am J Obstet Gynecol* 2000;182:1483.
161. Henzl MR, Corson SL, Moghissi K, et al. Administration of nasal nafarelin as compared with oral danazol for endometriosis. *N Engl J Med* 1988;318:485.
162. Kennedy SH, Williams IA, Brodribb J, et al. A comparison of nafarelin acetate and danazol in the treatment of endometriosis. *Fertil Steril* 1991;53:998.
163. Dlugi AM, Miller JD, Knittle J. Lupron depot (leuprolide acetate for depot suspension) in the treatment of endometriosis: a randomized, placebo-controlled, double-blind study. *Fertil Steril* 1990;54:419.
164. Dawood MY, Lewis V, Ramos J. Cortical and trabecular bone mineral content in women with endometriosis: effect of gonadotropin releasing hormone agonist and danazol. *Fertil Steril* 1989; 52:21.
165. Fogelman I. Gonadotropin-releasing hormone agonists and the skeleton. *Fertil Steril* 1992;57:715.
166. Lubianca JN, Gordon CM, Laufer MR. Addback therapy for endometriosis in adolescents. *J Reprod Med* 1998;43:164.
167. Agarwal SK. Impact of six months of GnRH agonist therapy for endometriosis. Is there an age-related effect on bone mineral density? *J Reprod Med* 2002;47:530.
168. Surrey ES, Gambone JC, Lu JKH, et al. Effects of combining norethindrone with a gonadotropin-releasing hormone agonist in the treatment of symptomatic endometriosis. *Fertil Steril* 1990;53.620.
169. Cedars MI, Lu JKH, Meldrum DR, et al. Treatment of endometriosis with a long-acting gonadotropin-releasing hormone agonist plus medroxyprogesterone acetate. *Obstet Gynecol* 1990; 75:641.
170. Barbieri RL. Hormone treatment of endometriosis: the estrogen threshold hypothesis. *Am J Obstet Gynecol* 1992;166:740.
171. Surrey ES, Judd HL. Reduction of vasomotor symptoms and bone mineral density loss with combined norethindrone and long-acting gonadotropin releasing hormone agonist therapy of symptomatic endometriosis: a prospective randomized trial. *J Clin Endocrinol Metab* 1992;75:558.
172. Ravn P, Bergqvist A, Hansen MA, et al. Treatment of endometriosis with the luteinizing hormone-releasing hormone agonist nafarelin. Effects on bone turnover and bone mass. *Menopause* 1994;1:11.
173. Surrey ES, Hornstein MD. Prolonged GnRH-a and add-back therapy for symptomatic endometriosis: long-term follow-up. *Obstet Gynecol* 2002;99:709.
174. Lindsay PC, Shaw RW, Bennick HJ, et al. The effect of add-back treatment with tibolone in patients treated with GnRHa, triptorelin. *Fertil Steril* 1996;65:342.
175. Keisel L, Schweppe KW, Sillem M, et al. Should add-back therapy for endometriosis be deferred for optimal results? *Br J Obstet Gynecol* 1996;103:15.
176. Taskin D, Yalcinoglv AI, Kucuk S, et al. Effectiveness of tibolone on hypoestrogenic symptoms induced by goserelin treatment in patients with endometriosis. *Fertil Steril* 1997;67:40.
177. Surrey ES, Fournet N, Voigt B, et al. Effects of sodium etidronate in combination with low-dose norethindrone in patients administered a long-acting GnRH-a: a preliminary report. *Obstet Gynecol* 1993;81:581.
178. Finkelstein JS, Klibanski A, Schaefer EH, et al. Parathyroid hormone for the prevention of bone loss induced by estrogen deficiency. *N Engl J Med* 1994;331:1618.

179. Kauppila A, Ronnberg L. Naproxen sodium in dysmenorrhea secondary to endometriosis. *Obstet Gynecol* 1985;65:379.
180. Greco CD. Management of adolescent chronic pelvic pain from endometriosis: a pain center perspective. *J Pediatr Adolesc Gynecol* 2003;16:S17.
181. Lichten EM, Bombard J. Surgical treatment of primary dysmenorrhea with laparoscopic uterine nerve ablation. *J Reprod Med* 1987;32:37.
182. Gürgan T, Urman B, Aksu T, et al. Laparoscopic CO_2 laser uterine nerve ablation for treatment of drug resistant primary dysmenorrhea. *Fertil Steril* 1992;58:422.
183. Lee RB, Stone K, Magelssen D, et al. Presacral neurectomy for chronic pelvic pain. *Obstet Gynecol* 1986;68:517.
184. Tjaden B, Schlaff WD, Kimball A, et al. The efficacy of presacral neurectomy for the relief of midline dysmenorrhea. *Obstet Gynecol* 1990;76:89.
185. Perez JJ. Laparoscopic presacral neurectomy. *J Reprod Med* 1990;35:625.
186. Candiani GB, Fedele L, Vercellini P, et al. Presacral neurectomy for treatment of pelvic pain associated with endometriosis: a controlled study. *Am J Obstet Gynecol* 1992;167:100.
187. Nezhat CH, Seidman DS, Nezhat FR, et al. Long-term outcome of laparoscopic presacral neurectomy for the treatment of central pelvic pain attributed to endometriosis. *Obstet Gynecol* 1998;91:701.
188. Chen FP, Soong YK. The efficacy and complications of laparoscopic presacral neurectomy in pelvic pain. *Obstet Gynecol* 1997;90:974.
189. Walters MD. Definitive surgery. In: Schenken RS, ed. *Endometriosis: contemporary concepts in clinical management.* Philadelphia: JB Lippincott Co, 1989:267.
190. Kettel LM, Liu JH, Murphy AA, et al. Endocrine responses to long-term administration of the antiprogesterone RU486 in patients with pelvic endometriosis. *Fertil Steril* 1991;56:402.
191. Barbieri RL. CA-125 in patients with endometriosis. *Fertil Steril* 1986;45:767.
192. Thomas PP, Higgins PH, Wolfe DH, et al. Development of a support network for adolescents with endometriosis. *J Pediatr Adolesc Gynecol* 1996;9:155.
193. Keltz MD, Kliman HJ, Arici AM, et al. Endosalpingiosis found at laparoscopy for chronic pelvic pain. *Fertil Steril* 1995;64:482.
194. Laufer MR, Heerema AE, Parsons KE, et al. Endosalpingiosis: description/classification of presentation and follow-up. *Gynecol Obstet Invest* 1998;46:195.
195. Campbell EM, Peterkin D, O'Grady K, et al. Premenstrual symptoms in general practice patients: prevalence and treatment. *J Reprod Med* 1997; 42:637.
196. Premenstrual dysphoric disorder. In: *Diagnostic and statistical manual of mental disorders,* 4th ed., Text rev. DSM-IV-TR.Washington, DC, American Psychiatric Association, 2000; 771.
197. Grady-Weliky, TA. Premenstrual dysphoric disorder. *N Engl J Med* 2003;348:433.
198. Clinical management guidelines for obstetricians-gynecologist: premenstrual syndrome. ACOG practice bulletin. No. 15. Washington, D.C.: American College of Obstetricians and Gynecologists, April 2000.
199. Fisher M, Trieller K, Napolitano B. Premenstrual symptoms in adolescents. *J Adolesc Health Care* 1989;10:369.
200. Keye W Jr, ed. *The premenstrual syndrome.* Philadelphia: WB Saunders, 1988.
201. Bargetzi MJ, Meyer UA, Birkhaeuser MH. Premenstrual exacerbations in hepatic porphyria: prevention by intermittent administration of an LH-RH agonist in combination with a gestagen. *JAMA* 1989;261:864.
202. Slater JE. Recurrent anaphylaxis in menstruating women: treatment with a luteinizing hormone-releasing hormone agonist: a preliminary report. *Obstet Gynecol* 1987;70:542.
203. Meggs WJ, Pescovitz OH, Metcalfe D, et al. Progesterone sensitivity as a cause of recurrent anaphylaxis. *N Engl J Med* 1984;311:1236.
204. Johnson SR, McChesney C, Bean JA. Epidemiology of premenstrual symptoms in a nonclinical sample: 1. Prevalence, natural history and help-seeking behavior. *J Reprod Med* 1988;33:340.
205. Muse KN, Cetel NS, Futterman LA, et al. The premenstrual syndrome: effects of "medical ovariectomy." *N Engl J Med* 1984;311:1345.
206. Schmidt PJ, Nieman LK, Danaceau MA, et al. Differential behavioral effects of gonadal steroids in women with and in those without premenstrual syndrome. *N Engl J Med* 1998; 338:209.
207. Maddocks S, Hahn P, Moller F, et al. A double-blind placebo-controlled trial of progesterone vaginal suppositories in the treatment of premenstrual syndrome. *Am J Obstet Gynecol* 1986;154:573.

208. Hammerback S, Damber JE, Backstrom T. Relationship between symptom severity and hormone changes in women with premenstrual syndrome. *J Clin Endocrinol Metab* 1989;68:125.
209. Rubinow DR, Hoban MC, Grover GN, et al. Changes in plasma hormones across the menstrual cycle in patients with menstrually related mood disorder and in control subjects. *Am J Obstet Gynecol* 1988;158:5.
210. Schmidt PJ, Nieman LK, Grover GN, et al. Lack of effect of induced menses on symptoms in women with premenstrual syndrome. *N Engl J Med* 1991;324:1174.
211. Reid RL, Yen SSC. Premenstrual syndrome. *Am J Obstet Gynecol* 1981;139:85.
212. Reid RL. Endogenous opiate peptides and premenstrual syndrome. *Semin Reprod Endocrinol* 1987;5:191.
213. Chuong CJ, Coulam CB, Bergstralh, et al. Clinical trial of naltrexone in premenstrual syndrome. *Obstet Gynecol* 1988;72:332.
214. Yonkers KA, Halbreich U, Freeman E, *et al.* Sertraline in the treatment of premenstrual dysphoric disorder. *Psychopharmacol Bull* 1996;32:41.
215. Freeman EW, Rickels K, Sondheimer SJ. Fluvoxamine for premenstrual dysphoric disorder. a pilot study. *J Clin Psychiatry* 1996;57:56.
216. Daamen MJ, Brown WA. Single-dose fluoxetine in management of premenstrual syndrome. *J Clin Psychiatry* 1992;53:211.
217. Steiner M. Fluoxetine in the treatment of LLPDD: a multi-center, placebo-controlled, double-blind trial. *Int J Gynecol Obstet* 1994;46[Suppl 2]:122.
218. Steiner M, Steinberg S, Stewart D, et al. Fluoxetine in the treatment of premenstrual dysphoria. *N Engl J Med* 1995;332:1528.
219. Roca CA, Schmidt PJ, Smith MJ, et al. Effects of metergoline on symptoms in women with premenstrual dysphoric disorder. *Am J Psychiatry* 2002;159:1876.
220. Mortola JF, Girton L, Beck L, et al. Diagnosis of premenstrual syndrome by a single, prospective and reliable instrument: the calendar of premenstrual experiences. *Obstet Gynecol* 1990; 76:302.
221. Mira M, McNeil D, Fraser IS, et al. Mefenamic acid in the treatment of premenstrual syndrome. *Obstet Gynecol* 1986;68:395.
222. Vellacott ID, Shroff NE, Pearce MY, et al. A double-blind, placebo-controlled evaluation of spironolactone in the premenstrual syndrome. *Curr Med Res Opin* 1987;10:450.
223. O'Brien PMS, Craven O, Selby C, et al. Treatment of premenstrual syndrome by spironolactone. *Br J Obstet Gynaecol* 1979;86:142.
224. Schellenberg R. Treatment for the premenstrual syndrome with agnus castus fruit extract: prospective, randomized, placebo controlled study. *BMJ* 2001;322:134.
225. Dimmonck PW, Wyatt KM, Jones PW, et al. Efficacy of selective serotonin-reuptake inhibitors in premenstrual syndrome: a systematic review. *Lancet* 2000;356:1131.
226. Wyatt KM, Dimmock PW, O'Brien PM. Selective serotonin reuptake inhibitors for premenstrual syndrome. *Cochrane Database Syst Rev* 2002;CD001396
227. Steiner M, Romano SJ, Babcock S, et al. The efficacy of fluoxetine in improving physical symptoms associated with premenstrual dysphoric disorder. *BJOG* 2001;108:462.
228. Yonkers KA, Halbreich U, Freeman E, et al. Symptomatic improvement of premenstrual dysphoric disorder with sertraline treatment. A randomized controlled trial. *JAMA* 1997;278:983.
229. Freeman EW, Rickels K, Sondheimer SJ, et al. Differential response to antidepressants in women with premenstrual syndrome/premenstrual dysphoric disorder: a randomized controlled trial. *Arch Gen Psychiatry* 1999;56:932.
230. Eriksson E, Hedberg MA, Andersch B, et al. The serotonin reuptake inhibitor paroxetine is superior to the noradrenaline reuptake inhibitor maprotiline in the treatment of premenstrual syndrome. *Neuropsychopharmacology* 1995;12:167.
231. Wikander I, Sundblad C, Andersch B, et al. Citalopram in premenstrual dysphoria: is intermittent treatment during luteal phases more effective than continuous medication throughout the menstrual cycle? *J Clin Psychopharmacol* 1998;18:390.
232. Freeman EW, Rickels K, Yonkers KA, et al. Venlafaxine in the treatment of premenstrual dysphoric disorder. *Obstet Gynecol* 2001;98:737.
233. Halbreich U, Bergeron R, Yonkers KA, et al. Efficacy of intermittent, luteal phase sertraline treatment of premenstrual dysphoric disorder. *Obstet Gynecol* 2002;100:1219.

234. Smith S, Rinehart JS, Ruddock VE, et al. Treatment of premenstrual syndrome with alprazolam: results of a double-blind, placebo-controlled, randomized crossover clinical trial. *Obstet Gynecol* 1987;70:37.
235. Mortola JF, Girton L, Fischer U. Successful treatment of severe premenstrual syndrome by combined use of gonadotropin-releasing hormone agonist and estrogen/progestin. *J Clin Endocrinol Metab* 1991;72:252A.
236. Leather AT, Studd JW, Watson NR, et al. The prevention of bone loss in young women treated with GnRH analogues with "add-back" estrogen therapy. *Obstet Gynecol* 1993;81:104.
237. Mezrow G, Shoupe D, Spicer D, et al. Depot leuprolide acetate with estrogen and progestin add-back for long-term treatment of premenstrual syndrome. *Fertil Steril* 1994;62:932.
238. Sarno AP, Miller EJ Jr, Lundblad EG. Premenstrual syndrome: beneficial effects of periodic, low-dose danazol. *Obstet Gynecol* 1987;70:33.
239. Dennerstein L, Spencer-Gardner C, Gotts G, et al. Progesterone and the premenstrual syndrome: a double-blind crossover trial. *Br Med J* 1985;29:1617.
240. Baker ER, Best RG, Manfredi RL, et al. Efficacy of progesterone vaginal suppositories in alleviation of nervous symptoms in patients with premenstrual syndrome. *J Assist Reprod Genet* 1995;12:205.
241. Freeman EW, Richels K, Sondheimer SJ, et al. A double-blind trial of oral progesterone, alprazolam, and placebo in treatment of severe premenstrual syndrome. *JAMA* 1995;274:51.
242. Wyatt K, Dimmock P, Jones P, et al. Efficacy of progesterone and progestogens in management of premenstrual syndrome: systematic review. *BMJ* 2001;322:776.
243. Kendall KE, Schnurr PP. The effects of vitamin B6 supplementation on premenstrual symptoms. *Obstet Gynecol* 1987;70:145.
244. Wyatt KM, Dimmock PW, Jones PW, et al. Efficacy of vitamin B-6 in the treatment of premenstrual syndrome: systematic review. *BMJ* 1999;318:1375.
245. Khoo SK, Munro C, Battistutta D. Evening primrose oil and treatment of premenstrual syndrome. *Med J Aust* 1990; 153:189.
246. Collins A, Cerin A, Coleman L, et al. Essential fatty acids in the treatment of premenstrual syndrome. *Obstet Gynecol* 1993; 81:93.
247. Tamborini A, Taurelle R. Value of standardized Gingko biloba extract (EGb 761) in the management of congestive symptoms of premenstrual syndrome. *Rev Fr Gynecol Obstet* 1993; 88:447.
248. Thys-Jacobs S, Starkey P, Bernstein D, et al. Calcium carbonate and the premenstrual syndrome: effects on premenstrual and menstrual symptoms. Premenstrual Syndrome Study Group. *Am J Obstet Gynecol* 1998;179:444.
249. Facchinetti F, Borella P, Sances G, et al. Oral magnesium successfully relieves premenstrual mood changes. *Obstet Gynecol* 1991;78:177.
250. Walker AF, De Souza MC, Vickers MF, et al. Magnesium supplementation alleviates premenstrual symptoms of fluid retention. *J Womens Health* 1998;7:1157.

12

Education of the Child and Adolescent

Phaedra Thomas, Vicki Burke, and Anne Jenks Micheli

Age-appropriate education is important for all aspects of pediatric and adolescent gynecology. This chapter outlines the most effective approach to educating girls and adolescents at various ages, their families, and health care providers, with particular focus on peri- and postoperative issues. A general knowledge of psychosocial development is essential in caring for infants, children, and adolescents. Assessing the child's cognitive level helps in the selection of effective methods of teaching and age-appropriate learning materials.

OFFICE EDUCATION

In each of the chapters of this text, the authors have indicated special educational approaches for children, adolescents, and their families. For each problem or diagnosis, the educational effort begins with the first appointment as history, physical examination, and treatment options are discussed. Diagnoses may range from vaginitis to menstrual disorders to vaginal agenesis to life-threatening cancers. Sometimes the diagnosis is apparent at the first visit, but often further tests are needed to confirm a suspected diagnosis. When testing is done following the initial consultation, health care providers are encouraged to meet with girls and their families for a follow-up visit to explain the results of the tests rather than conveying results and treatment over the telephone. Visual aids such as a pelvic model or diagrams can be extremely helpful when explaining the reproductive system to teens. A learning opportunity often follows with a discussion of treatment options and allows time for questions and answers by the patient and family. The second visit or post-consultation appointment is a key opportunity for dialogue of treatment options. During this visit the health care provider can also assess the adolescent's understanding of her diagnosis as well as her ability and desire to adhere to specific treatment strategies. For example, if the health care provider is considering continuous oral contraceptives for the treatment of endometriosis, it is important to understand the adolescent's lifestyle, her concerns, and any preconceived ideas that she may have. Having this knowledge will ultimately help the health care provider to assess whether she will be able to take her medication consistently.

Pamphlets and Internet materials (www.youngwomenshealth.org) can complement a discussion in the office about specific treatment options and provide patients and families material to review at a later time under less stressful conditions. It is helpful to ask teens how they learn best. Knowing whether a teen is an auditory or visual learner will determine how information should be delivered. The health care provider can then recommend audiotapes or videotapes, written materials, computer generated slide presentation learning modules, hands-on models, or contact with another teen or adult. In our practice we have found that young women who are given choices about learning modalities are more likely to be active participants in their treatment plan. Compliance with treatment plans often improves when myths are dispelled and medical information is clarified.

With the advancement of resources through the Internet, teens and families have access to a plethora of medical information. Unfortunately, not all of the information available online is accurate. It is therefore highly recommended that health care providers become familiar with on-line resources so that they can recommend reliable and teen friendly Web sites to young women and their families (see Appendix 1). Utilizing Internet health guides and other resources can greatly enhance a teen's awareness about her disease and proposed treatment plan. These resources, however, should not replace ongoing discussions with her health care provider. Reinforcement of information and ongoing dialogue are essential since questions may be repeated at each visit.

OUTPATIENT CONSIDERATIONS AND TEACHING

Comprehensive preoperative preparation of patients undergoing surgical procedures is essential to ensure a positive experience for the patient and her family. Preoperative teaching prepares the child, thus decreasing anxiety and the fear of the unknown that surrounds impending surgical procedures. Decreasing anxiety has a positive effect on both the patient's emotional and physical state (Fig. 12-1) (1). For patients undergoing pediatric and adolescent gynecologic surgery, the developmental issues of childhood and adolescence and issues of sexuality increase the need for comprehensive and sensitive teaching.

The need for surgical preparation is predicated on the belief that hospitalization and surgery are stressful experiences that can lead to long-term psychological problems in some children (1). Children entering the hospital for surgery leave the familiar surroundings of their home and enter a strange environment. In a study in the

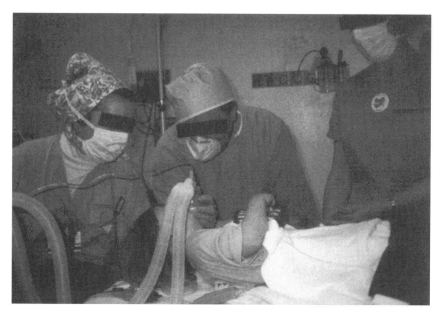

FIG. 12-1. A parent's presence and a favorite toy help children cope during the induction of anesthesia.

1970s, when there was less emphasis on teaching and involvement of families in the direct care of their children, Melamed and Siegal (2) noted that 10% to 35% of children exhibited immediate or sustained emotional and behavioral problems, night terrors, increased dependency, regression, eating disturbances, or increased fearfulness following hospitalization for surgery. Anxiety in both children and parents has been found to influence the child's response to medical care. The preparation of a child for surgery reduces psychological upset after hospitalization (1). In a study of different models of psychological preparation and supportive care designed to increase the adjustment of children hospitalized for elective surgery, systematic preparation, rehearsal, and supportive care prior to each stressful procedure resulted in significantly less upset and thus more cooperation from the children (3).

Effective preoperative and perioperative teaching in the pediatric setting must always include consideration of the parents' needs and fears. Children are very adept at sensing their parents' feelings and level of stress. The child's ability to remain calm is enhanced when the parents are calm, reassuring, and well prepared for upcoming events (Fig. 12-2). Because parents report that their own anxiety and stress may prevent them from understanding or remembering all of the information provided before surgery, health care providers should recognize the need to reintroduce concepts, repeat information, and provide Internet resources and printed material. Based on the parent's level of stress, it is best to obtain surgical informed consent prior to the day of the procedure (4).

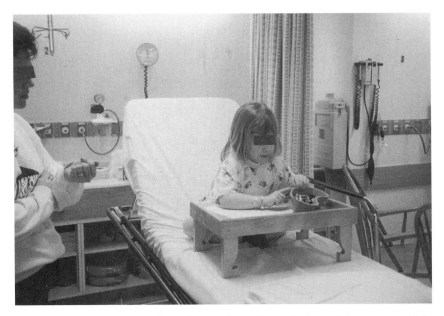

FIG. 12-2. Drawing during the immediate perioperative period can help younger children express feelings, fears, and experiences they may not be able to verbalize while providing a pleasant motor activity at an emotional time.

Procedures involving the reproductive organs, whether the patient is an infant, a child, or an adolescent, may create a higher level of anxiety than procedures involving other parts of the body. The social, cultural, and psychological effects of genital surgery can be significant and must be addressed preoperatively. Parents may have fears about a child's virginity during procedures such as a vaginal exam under anesthesia or repair of an imperforate hymen.

Generally the overall experience is much less stressful when books and props such as surgical masks are used to play out the upcoming hospital scenario. The details of the procedure, intraoperative care, and postoperative management should be clearly outlined and the risks and benefits of the surgery discussed with the child's parent(s). The patient or guardian should be given ample opportunity to express concerns and fears, and to ask questions, in a relaxed setting.

Education Modalities

Puppet shows, preoperative instructions, and tours of the operating room and hospital postoperative surgical recovery areas are some of the modalities that are effective for young children. Preparation is focused on familiarizing the child and parent with the hospital environment and providing clear instructions such as, arrival time, length of procedure, where to wait, when they can expect to talk with their surgeon, etc. In a study conducted by Ellerton and Merriam (5), children responded with decreased anxiety and were shown to cope positively with the perioperative course after watching a video depicting a child going through the preoperative and postoperative experience. Parents should be encouraged to participate in any preoperative program and/or tours offered by the hospital.

Patient education materials such as information guides, videos, audiotapes, and computer generated slide presentation learning modules can be very helpful when preparing the adolescent patient for surgery and provide an array of teaching modalities for different kinds of learners. Some pediatric hospitals may even offer a service whereby teens can talk with other teens who have undergone similar medical or surgical procedures. The older child and adolescent may struggle with how her medical condition, surgery, and recovery will impact her world, including school, sports, and social activities. Internet chats that are moderated by trained medical personnel are an alternative to traditional support groups and allow teens to chat about issues that are important to them.

Preoperative rehearsal play has been shown to reduce anxiety in children (6). Play is a way a child can control a situation and cope with stress. Parents can participate in play as a way to effectively teach the child about upcoming events. Parents should be made aware of the benefit of play, using toys, games, books, and hospital items such as surgical masks. Play gives children the opportunity to act out their fears. Parents can then offer reassurance in a nonthreatening way. Anatomically correct dolls help to teach older children about body parts and how they will be treated. Organized board games are available to provide information about health care or hospitalization and are appealing to children from preschoolers through teenagers (7).

DEVELOPMENTAL CONSIDERATIONS IN PREPARING FOR SURGERY

Stages of development are defined somewhat differently among textbooks. These descriptions and key concepts of general age group/developmental stages relating to gynecologic surgical procedures are summarized below (8–10).

Infancy: Birth until 1 Year

The provision of comfort and security should be the primary focus in meeting the developmental needs of infants. Long periods of preoperative fasting are not necessary for infants and young children (10), and the guidelines for fasting are often modified for the very young infant. For preoperative purposes, breast milk is considered a clear fluid, allowing mothers to breast-feed their children before surgery. Having the infant use a pacifier and/or bring a security object into the operating room is also very effective in decreasing the stress of separation during the perioperative period (11).

Early Childhood: Ages 1 to 5 Years

Early childhood spans the years from late infancy, through the toddler phase, until age 5, before entry into kindergarten. The toddler phase includes early language development and locomotion. Toddlers have a limited ability to communicate and reason and are threatened by changes in routine. The toddler may interpret separation from a parent as abandonment. She is often terrified by unfamiliar hospital staff dressed in unusual clothes or masks and benefits from having a parent present as much as possible. A parent's presence in the post-anesthesia care unit greatly reduces anxiety as the toddler emerges from the effects of anesthesia (Fig. 12-3).

The preschool period between toddler age and kindergarten is one of intellectual and emotional growth. The preschool child may be concerned with being in a new environment, disruption of routines, body mutilation, abandonment, and separation. Readiness for a new experience must be assessed, as well as the need for

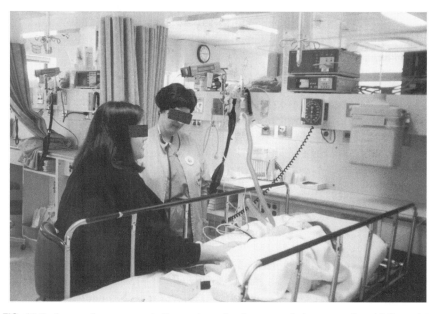

FIG. 12-3. A parent's presence in the postanesthesia care unit decreases the child's anxiety on emergence from the effects of anesthesia.

continued physical and emotional support in the new environment. Children in this age group become anxious with new sights and sounds and cannot distinguish between real and imagined dangers. Procedures such as injections or blood drawing can be very frightening. Children can become confused and stressed when large words are used and if the explanations are directed only to the parent. It is important for health care providers to ask the preschool child if she has any questions. Pretend play, in which the patient is "the doctor," addresses the child's fears and brings the child's concerns to the forefront. In a study of preoperative preparation of children, Ellerton and Merriam (5) found that many children are quite anxious about removing all of their clothing before a surgical procedure. The simple practice of allowing a child to wear her underwear into the operating room and replacing it before she leaves the operating room can help allay some of her fears. Preschoolers can often predict upcoming events by clues in the environment. Attempting to keep secrets from them only leads to misinterpretation and lack of trust in caregivers. Honesty is an important aspect of preoperative preparation.

Childhood: 5 to 11 Years

Children between five and 11 develop relationships with adults outside the family and with peers through school activities and learn to adapt to new environments and experiences. They generally have a good understanding of the external body but vague ideas about the structure and function of their internal body parts.

School-age children are eager to learn about the world and to find new ways to solve problems. They can adjust better to a variety of new experiences, and they are now capable of true cooperation. Fears are more reality based than during the preschool stage. Separation fears are less predominant, but other fears related to injury, mutilation, or death are important (12). School-age children often want to be brave and courageous and display bravado in threatening situations, but in fact they may require support. Consistency, clear limits, and avoidance of a power struggle are important in designing strategies.

Reading becomes easier for school-age children, and age-appropriate books that acknowledge feelings around hospital procedures can reduce anxiety. Booklets or pamphlets with specific hospital information about what to expect with the upcoming surgical procedure can be a fun way for parents to prepare their child for exams and surgical procedures. Encouraging the child to verbalize her concerns is important, since she may be shy or too embarrassed to ask certain questions (13). A few simple statements from a nurse or doctor such as "a lot of girls your age are concerned about whether this will hurt or not" can be helpful in getting the child to express her feelings. An appropriate response would be to explain if she will experience any discomfort and, if so, how the staff will comfort her. This method can be very effective with school-age children who are timid or socially inept at articulating their concerns or fears.

Older children seem to benefit from preparation several days before the surgery so they have time to think about how they will respond and what actions or behaviors they can use to cope with and/or participate in the experience (1). Research by Wolfer and Visintainer (14) in the 1970s indicated that older children who used home preparatory materials one week before hospital admission showed better adjustment than those receiving routine care. Meng and Zastowny (15) demonstrated that older children experienced a reduction in anxiety following a preadmission program a week prior to surgery, while younger children experienced increased anxiety until admission.

Adolescence

The onset of puberty is a major transition, as the adolescent begins to formulate attitudes and becomes an active participant in her health care. Motivation to learn is high when the adolescent is interested in the topic. Younger adolescents are concrete thinkers and need visual aids to understand the details of surgery. Older adolescents have the ability to think abstractly, which enhances learning and helps them to have realistic expectations of the consequences of their surgery.

Adolescents are developing values, ideals, and sexual identity. Peer relations, body image, sexuality, and fertility become increasingly important. Gynecologic surgical procedures directly affect these issues. Sometimes adolescent girls may articulate their concerns easily to parents or health care providers, but at other times they may be secretive, shutting down and not choosing to express their fears and anxieties. Defensive behavior may mask fears and anxiety. Thus, the health care provider faces the challenge and responsibility to initiate discussion.

Peer relations are paramount to most adolescents, but many may choose not to talk about their illness, chronic disease, congenital reproductive anomaly, or surgery with their friends. Adolescents may not want to share information with their siblings either. They may feel different and possibly ashamed of their diagnosis, or they may be deeply concerned about whether their friends and family will accept them and their new body image. The health care provider is encouraged to refer the adolescent for counseling when coping is compromised.

The possibility of a visible surgical scar can be very upsetting to a young woman. Although an increasing number of surgical procedures of the abdomen can be done through minimally invasive surgery (operative laparoscopy), decreasing the size of the visible scar, adolescents should still be given the opportunity to voice concerns around how the surgical procedure will impact their body image.

Perioperative Education and Management

In the eyes of a young child, a hospital is an unfamiliar environment filled with strangers. Historically, parents and children were separated during the immediate preoperative, intraoperative, and postoperative phases of care. Today, in many hospitals, there are opportunities in the preoperative and postoperative areas where a parent can stay with their child for support and to participate in their care. Efforts to minimize parent and child separation will promote a positive surgical experience.

Allowing a parent to participate in the induction process helps alleviate much of the fear and anxiety that is associated with anesthesia (16). Parent-present induction, whereby a parent dons a surgical gown, escorts the child into the operating room, and stays with her until induction of anesthesia has taken place, can aid in keeping a small child calm just before surgery. Conversely, very anxious parents may only heighten the child's anxiety (16). Careful assessment of the child and parent is imperative to ensure a positive outcome of this technique. Selection of the appropriate person to accompany the child to the operating room is individually based on the parent's comfort with their prospective role and their ability to be supportive to the child (4).

If the parent is present during induction of anesthesia and/or accompanies the child to the operating room, the parent is carefully prepared for the sights and sounds of the experience, including the child's response to the anesthetic agents. After the induction of anesthesia, the parent is escorted to a family waiting area, before the child undergoes positioning and surgical preparation.

Preoperative Counseling of the Adolescent

Maintaining confidentiality when dealing with adolescents and their parents is essential. To ensure accurate answers to sensitive questions about sexuality and peer relations, health care providers should speak to adolescents and their parents both separately and together before surgery. Careful preoperative teaching in the health care provider's office regarding the need for strict compliance with birth control methods must be stressed to the sexually active adolescent. Preoperative pregnancy testing on the day of surgery is important in the care of adolescents (17–19). In our institution, routine pregnancy tests are done on all girls who have reached menarche or are 12 years of age or over. Parents may initially react negatively to this testing in the belief that the health care provider or institution assumes that their daughter is sexually active. An explanation that this testing is hospital policy and not an assessment of sexual activity is necessary and usually quite effective. Policies and procedures surrounding confidentiality issues are further discussed in Chapters 1, 20, and 26 and must be clearly defined by individual health care facilities.

Parents of adolescents having gynecologic surgery most commonly voice concerns about their daughter's fertility. Additionally, some parents may feel guilty that they somehow are responsible for their daughter's condition. Health care providers can offer reassurance by providing an opportunity for parents to express their concerns and ask questions.

Postoperative Education and Management

The patient and her family should be prepared for expected postoperative events before they leave the hospital. Written postoperative instructions regarding wound care, diet, activity and pain management along with emergency contact numbers and a postoperative appointment are given to the parent/child or adolescent prior to hospital discharge. Ideally, prescriptions for postoperative analgesics or narcotics should be prescribed at the preoperative visit. In addition, parents of young children and adolescents should be informed of possible postoperative complications, indications for concern, and when to contact health care providers.

Internet Education

The Internet can be a safe and convenient way for teens to receive support if chat rooms are moderated by clinicians specializing in adolescent health. At Children's Hospital Boston, we have offered both traditional support groups and moderated Internet chats. Both forums allow teens to share common concerns; however, we have found participation to be higher in moderated Internet chats. Being able to remain anonymous and not worrying about transportation issues are among the factors that may contribute to the success of Internet chats. Since most teens have access to a computer either at home or at school, chatting on the Internet has quickly become a preferred way for teens to communicate. While teens are able to exchange in conversation with their peers from all over the world, it is critical that the chat be monitored by a health care professional, preferably by an adolescent gynecologist, adolescent medicine specialist, nurse educator, and/or mental health counselor. To protect privacy, teens should be required to register prior to the chat time. A designated "chat master" with expertise in moderating chat rooms is necessary to ensure a professional operation of the chats. While the Internet chat is a practical setting to dispel myths and clarify medical information, it is recommended that a disclaimer be posted on this type of Internet chat site informing the public that the Web site does not offer medical consultations nor does it replace the need for teens to discuss medical concerns with their health care provider.

SPECIFIC EDUCATIONAL CONSIDERATIONS

Colposcopy Education

In our practice, young women requiring colposcopy for treatment of an abnormal Pap test are referred to our resource center prior to their scheduled procedure date. They are offered learning modules about abnormal Pap tests, HPV, and specific information about what to expect with colposcopy. Written materials and computer generated slide presentations review the reproductive anatomy and explain facts at a reading level that most teens can easily comprehend. A teen can view a photograph of a colposcope and display text that explains that the colposcope is similar to a large microscope. When the teen reads on, she will learn that the colposcope is not inserted into the vagina but is placed outside the opening of the vagina. This and other informative statements reduce anxiety associated with the colposcope. Teens may also watch a video created by the Center for Young Women's Health at Children's Hospital Boston, of three young women discussing their own experience, from getting the news about their abnormal Pap test to how they personally coped with the colposcopy experience. All visitors to the resource center are taught how to access written materials on a variety of health topics that affect young women and are given health links to other reliable Web sites. Girls in other communities have access to materials on the www.youngwomenshealth.org Web site and other materials developed by ACOG and other professional groups to prepare for colposcopy.

When the patient arrives for colposcopy, she meets with a nurse and is asked if she has visited the resource center or Web site and reviewed the educational material. The nurse then asks the patient if she found the information to be helpful in preparing for today's visit and whether she has any questions or concerns. After quickly assessing the patients understanding of colposcopy, the nurse reviews basic information and gives an overview of the steps that will follow. A standard sexual history is used to elicit this information and care is taken to respect the sexual preferences. The patient is given the option of having her parent or partner present for the exam and procedure, explaining that the first part of the procedure consists of the visual exam, and the second part is the biopsy. The nurse remains present during the procedure and explains each step to the patient, such as "now the doctor is painting your cervix with a solution" and "you will feel a pinch as the doctor takes a biopsy of your cervix."

After the colposcopy, the patient is given the option of having her parent, partner, or friend return to her side. Discharge instructions are reviewed and written materials including a fact sheet about HPV are given to the patient to take home to reinforce the verbal discussion. Having the patient's partner in the exam room is an opportunity to reinforce that "nothing should be placed in the vagina for 2 weeks." When the patient is dressed and ready to exit, she is asked to schedule a return appointment to discuss her colposcopy results. At this visit, the results of the colposcopy are reviewed in detail and a follow-up plan for the patient is outlined. Abstinence or the consistent use of condoms should be advocated, especially with the immune-compromised patient.

Anomalies of the Reproductive Tract

Mayer-Rokitansky-Küster-Hauser Syndrome

Timing is very important when planning to teach a young woman about Mayer-Rokitansky-Küster-Hauser (MRKH) syndrome (see Chapter 10). This diagnosis can be devastating for an adolescent and her family. It is unlikely that she will be ready to learn about treatment options such as the use of dilators to create a vagina until she has had time to process, grieve, and finally accept her diagnosis. Education should therefore be individualized and offered when the adolescent is ready. Most often her gynecologist provides an explanation of MRKH to the adolescent and her family, once the findings have been confirmed. Since this visit can be quite emotional, it is recommended that a mental health counselor be present during the discussion if possible. If a counselor cannot be present, arrangements should be made to have a mental health counselor available as needed (20,21). Parents frequently ask many questions about their daughter's future fertility but newly diagnosed teens are initially overwhelmed with feeling "different." Some girls may ask a lot of questions and want to know what can be done to create a vagina. For young women who do not voice their concerns, it is helpful to acknowledge that many girls feel scared, confused, and sad when they are told about their diagnosis. Reassurance should be given along with an opportunity to talk at a later time. Written materials (www.youngwomenshealth.org/vaginalagenesis.html and www.MRKH.org) and information about Internet chats and, when possible, the chance to talk with other young women who share similar concerns are essential components of MRKH education.

When the adolescent is ready to learn more about her diagnosis and treatment options, models can be helpful when reviewing the reproductive system. Using the phrase "incomplete vagina" rather than saying "the absence of the vagina" is less threatening when explaining that MRKH is a congenital anomaly. It is recommended that a nurse, gynecologist, or practitioner with expertise in caring for adolescents with MRKH educate and counsel the teen. Education about creating a vagina can begin by explaining the advantages and disadvantages of nonsurgical and surgical methods for creation of a functional vagina. Teens typically are curious about how long it will take to create a vagina and if it will hurt. Teaching should be done in a private setting so that vaginal dilators can be viewed and handled without embarrassment. It is best to describe the dilators, showing the smallest dilator first. It is important to explain that the process begins by using a small dilator to create a "dimple" and as the vagina is created the next size dilator will be used. In our practice we place a rubber glove over the vaginal opening of a plastic model, then place the smallest dilator or pediatric blood drawing tube against it to demonstrate that gradual pressure causes the skin to stretch, similar to the rubber glove material. This concept has worked well to help teens understand how a vagina is created. Teens are told that a vagina can be created in 2 to 6 months if the dilators are used consistently but that it can take up to a year or more if the dilators are not used on a regular basis (www.youngwomenshealth.org/instructions.html).

Most teens have good results when they use the dilator at the same time every day, usually first thing in the morning or before they go to sleep. They are encouraged to take a warm bath for at least 10 minutes before they use the dilators, as the warm water helps to soften the skin, allowing it to stretch more easily. If a teen is using a glass blood drawing tube initially as the first dilator, she should be taught to inspect the glass tube for cracks or rough edges before proceeding. Samples of a water soluable jelly can be given to the teen with instructions on how to apply a small amount of lubricant on the tip of the dilator. A photo of a young women with her knees bent (similar to a pelvic exam) is useful to show the position for using the dilator. The insertion should be done in a comfortable location such as a bed or a reclining chair. The teen should be allowed to use a hand mirror to find where she will need to place the dilator. The clinician should stress that the dilator must be placed at an angle (toward the small of her back) when pressure is applied (see Fig. 10–79). Explain that she should feel pressure, but not pain. If she is not feeling anything, then she is not applying enough pressure. Support the teen by letting her know that it will feel like the right amount of pressure after using the dilators for a few times. Her progress will be checked at the next follow-up visit to make sure she is using the dilators correctly. The teen should be encouraged to call the office if she has any questions or concerns before her next appointment. Scheduling enough time for this teaching session is very important.

Follow-up visits are critical to ensure that the teen is using the dilator correctly, and that progress is being made. The follow-up visits help to establish a therapeutic relationship between teen and health care provider and offer ongoing teaching opportunities. Positive reinforcement must be given to teens who are making progress with dilation. Teens who have difficulty using dilators may not show for follow-up visits or feel ashamed at the next visit if they have not been compliant with the dilators. Care should be taken to reassure the teen that creating a vagina is her decision. She should not be forced by her parents or her health care provider to create a vagina until she is ready. Sometimes noncompliance with dilators can be due to constraints with school or sports or because of the lack of privacy at home. Offering ideas such as changing the time of day that the dilators are used or suggesting that a lock be installed on a teen's bedroom door to secure privacy may provide easy solutions. Encourage the teen to work out a plan with her family that will protect her privacy. Measures taken such as using a code word for the teen to say when she needs uninterrupted time or hanging something on her bedroom door to signal others she will not be available for a while are suggestions offered by teens who have had success with dilators.

Ongoing education and support from family members, the medical team, and other young women significantly help teens to cope with having MRKH. Issues surrounding this diagnosis are life long and will be revisited at various stages. For example, a teen at 16 may not desire information about surrogacy; however, she is likely to explore fertility options at another point in her life. The emotional impact of some gynecologic conditions can be devastating to a patient and her family. Poland and Evans (22) observed young women with vaginal agenesis through the course of diagnosis, surgical repair, and subsequent life events. A wide range of concerns were voiced by these young women, including anger, depression, and fear of rejection because of their altered fertility and sexuality. In this study, good relationships with parents and the ability to share feelings with family and friends seemed to be the best indicator of a good emotional outcome after diagnosis and vaginoplasty (22). Clearly young women also benefit from being counseled about the sensitive issues that surround the diagnosis of being a young woman with an incomplete vagina. Talking with other young women with the same diagnosis has proved beneficial in the immediate and long-term emotional and social health of these young women in our institution. Most patients create vaginas with the use of dilators, and a smaller number elect to have surgical vaginoplasty.

Vaginoplasty Education

Patients who will be using vaginal dilators after surgery for a pull-through vagino-plasty procedure for treatment of agenesis of the lower vagina or a transverse vagi-nal septum should be given the opportunity to view the dilators at the preoperative appointment (see Chapter 10). At this visit, we tell the patient/parents to purchase an elastic type panty girdle prior to the surgery. We explain that the panty girdle should be worn with a thick peripad following surgery and that the gentle pressure will keep the dilator in place. She is expected to wear the dilator 24 hours per day (removing only for urination, defecation, or bathing). Patients are also given Xylocaine Jelly to numb the irritation at the opening of the vagina that often occurs when using vaginal dilators for the first time. The patient should be told that she will have a vaginal dila-tor in place when she wakes up in the recovery room. On the first postoperative evening, the patient is taught by her nurse to insert and remove the dilator. Patient teaching is centered around promoting a comfort level with the insertion and removal of the dilators. When the patient is successful with inserting and removing the dila-tor, she has met the most important criteria for discharge.

The initial diagnosis and subsequent treatment of a gynecologic congenital anomaly can heighten adolescent concerns about sexuality and fertility. Facts and re-assurance given by the health care provider are necessary and helpful, but additional support in the form of peer group counseling and/or social services can be beneficial. Providing an opportunity for a newly diagnosed patient to talk confidentially with a teen who is at least one-year postdiagnosis has been particularly helpful in our prac-tice. Parents are also offered the opportunity to talk with parents of teen support vol-unteers. Internet resources and moderated chat rooms may provide other opportuni-ties for teens to receive support and learn more about their health condition.

EXAMINATIONS UNDER ANESTHESIA

An exam under anesthesia (EUA) may be indicated for the preschool age child who presents with vaginal discharge or bleeding of unknown etiology. If a visual exam and vaginal cultures cannot be obtained without trauma to the child in the office, an exam under anesthesia may be necessary to allow for an adequate examination of the vagina. The parent(s) should be told that the child is not having an "operation" but rather a "procedure" that is very brief and will allow the physician to examine the child without trauma. Parents should understand that while the child is sleeping, the doctor will use a fiberoptic scope and/or a small nasal speculum with a light source to visualize the vagina and cervix, in order to check for causes of the vaginal discharge such as a foreign body, and take necessary cultures to determine the cause of the discharge. Cultures and a Pap test or biopsy, when indicated, may be obtained. The child generally needs only 1 to 2 hours in the recovery room before going home and resuming normal activities.

Diagnostic Laparoscopy Education and Endometriosis

Teens who are scheduled for a laparoscopy for pelvic pain should be prepared for not only the procedure but also the possibility of receiving a diagnosis of endometriosis. Expectations of pain in the immediate postoperative period and a time frame for returning to normal school and social activities should be explained. In our practice, girls who have a diagnosis of pelvic pain and are scheduled for a diagnostic laparoscopy are also counseled about endometriosis using the resource center in our out-patient clinic staffed by a nurse educator. The materials are also available to the public at www.youngwomenshealth.org and are written in teen friendly format with a glossary of the medical terminology associated with endometriosis. Special considerations are made for various types of learners. For example, a teen is asked if she would prefer to view a short computer generated slide presentation on the computer, read a pamphlet, or listen to an audiotape that explains what endometriosis is and the possible causes and treatment (23).

If endometriosis is diagnosed at the time of surgery, basic facts about endometriosis are reviewed and an information packet including recommended reading and materials about the Endometriosis Association (www.endometriosisassn.org) is presented to patient and family prior to discharge. Patient teaching continues at the postoperative visit. At this visit, teens and parents generally ask specific questions about pain control, future fertility, and how the disease will impact their schoolwork and social life. Teens need to feel that they are not alone and that there is a pain management plan in place. In our practice, we have learned that teens who are 1 to 2 months postdiagnosis are becoming aware that they have a chronic disease and they usually want to know how other teens their age are coping at school, with sports, and with relationships. In response to this need, we created a video titled, "Teens Living with Endometriosis." In this video, four young women living with endometriosis are interviewed and share coping strategies such as working out at the gym to help increase energy to how to explain endometriosis to friends and significant others. Patients may view this video in the resource center or take a copy home to watch in the privacy of their home or dorm.

Teens who suffer from endometriosis and other chronic diseases benefit from talking with other girls approximately their own age. At Children's Hospital Boston, young women with certain chronic diseases such as endometriosis and vaginal agenesis who are at least 1 year post diagnosis may apply to become a support volunteer in a program called *Teen-to-Teen*. If accepted into the program, these young women receive a comprehensive training and are matched with newly diagnosed teens who desperately want to talk with someone their own age who knows first hand what it is like to live with the chronic disease. Typically, the support volunteer makes one to two phone calls to the younger teen. The support volunteer introduces herself by her first name but otherwise remains anonymous. Coping strategies are the primary focus of the discussion, and information about resources such as books and Internet chats are often shared. Parents of newly diagnosed teens are also given the opportunity to talk with other parents of teens who have successfully coped with their chronic illness. Parents who become support volunteers receive similar training and contact parents of newly diagnosed teens upon request. Issues around learning how to cope and support daughters with pain management issues are popular topics of discussion for parents.

In summary, the anxiety associated with visits to the doctor, hospitalization, and surgery can be challenging to the physical and emotional recovery of the child and adolescent. Children and adolescents, like adults, need information about impending procedures. The material must be age appropriate and thought should be taken whenever possible to provide a variety of resources for different types of learners. Pamphlets, audio and video tapes, and Internet materials complement learning but should not replace the need for a sensitive discussion among health care provider, patient, and parent(s). Special consideration must be given to the social, psychological, and developmental needs of patients and parents of patients undergoing gynecologic procedures in order to help reduce anxiety associated with the unknown and ensure a positive physical and emotional outcome.

REFERENCES

1. Keller F. Pre-operative teaching for children. *Neonatal Paediatr Child Health Nurs* 2001;4:4.
2. Melamed BG, Siegel LJ. Reduction of anxiety in children facing hospitalization and surgery by use of filmed modeling. *J Consult Clin Psychol* 1975;43:511.
3. Hatava P, Olsson GL, Lagerkranser M. Preoperative psychological preparation for children undergoing ENT operations: a comparison of two methods. *Paediatr Anaesth* 2000;10:477.
4. Larosa-Nash PA, Murphy JM, Wade LA, et al. Implementing a parent-present induction program. *AORN J* 1995;61:526.
5. Ellerton M, Merriam C. Preparing children and families psychologically for day surgery: an evaluation. *J Adv Nurs* 1994;19:1057.
6. Zahr LK. Therapeutic play for hospitalized preschoolers in Lebanon. *Pediatr Nurs* 1998;24:449.
7. Azarnoff P. Teaching materials for pediatric health professionals. *J Pediatr Health Care* 1990;4:282.
8. Mott SR, James SR, Sperhac AM. *Nursing care of children and families.* Redwood City, CA: Addison Wesley; 1990.

9. Wise BV, McKenna C, Garvin G, et al. Nursing care of the general pediatric surgical patient. Gaithersburg, MD: Aspen Publishers; 2000.
10. Dunn D. Preoperative assessment criteria and patient teaching for ambulatory surgery patients. *J Perianesth Nurs* 1998;13:274.
11. Frankville D. Preparing children for anesthesia and surgery. *West J Med* 1995;162:52.
12. Squires VL. Child-focused perioperative education: helping children understand and cope with surgery. *Semin Perioper Nurs* 1995;4:80.
13. Lynch M. Preparing children for day surgery. *Child Health Care* 1994;23:75.
14. Wolfer JA, Visintainer MA. Pediatric surgical patients' and parents' stress responses and adjustment as a function of psychologic preparation and stress-point nursing care. *Nurs Res* 1975;24:244.
15. Meng A, Zastowny T. Preparation for hospitalization: a stress inoculation training program for parents and children. *Matern Child Nurs* J 1982;11:87.
16. Kain ZN, Caldwell-Andrews A, Wang SM. Psychological preparation of the parent and pediatric surgical patient. *Anesthes Clin N Amer* 2002;20:29.
17. Azzam FJ, Padda GS, DeBoard JW, et al. Preoperative pregnancy testing in adolescents. [Comment]. *Anesth Analg* 1996;82:4.
18. Manley S, de Kelaita G, Joseph NJ, et al. Preoperative pregnancy testing in ambulatory surgery. Incidence and impact of positive results. [Comment]. *Anesthesiology* 1995;83:690.
19. Pierre N, Moy LK, Redd S, et al. Evaluation of a pregnancy-testing protocol in adolescents undergoing surgery. *J Pediatr Adol Gyn* 1998;11:139.
20. Laufer MR. Congenital absence of the vagina: in search of the perfect solution. When, and by what technique, should a vagina be created? *Curr Opin Obstet Gynecol* 2002;14:441.
21. Foley S, Morely GW. Care and counseling of the patient with vaginal agenesis. *The Female Patient* 1992;17:73.
22. Poland ML, Evans TN. Psychologic aspects of vaginal agenesis. *J Reprod Med* 1985;30:340.
23. Thomas P. Teaching teens about endometriosis. *J Pediatr Adolesc Gynecol* 2003;16:S29.

13

Pediatric Urology in the Pediatric and Adolescent Girl

Craig A. Peters

This chapter addresses urologic issues in girls and young women. Many urologic issues overlap with gynecologic issues, and thus some abnormalities are discussed in this chapter from a urologist's point of view, in addition to the discussion in other chapters.

In this chapter presenting symptoms, evaluation, and the differential diagnosis of the following entities will be discussed: incontinence, dysuria, urethral pain, pelvic pain, hematuria, flank pain and fever, renal colic, perineal mass, and congenital anomalies of the urinary tract. In addition we will focus on dysfunctional voiding, urinary obstruction, urinary tract infections, stones, reflux, ectopic ureter and ureterocele, renal masses, tumors, cloaca, exstrophy, epispadias, and urethral prolapse.

Commonly utilized diagnostic and imaging studies are also discussed. These include ultrasound, VCUG, IVP, DMSA renal scan, CT Scan, and urodynamics.

PRESENTING SYMPTOMS: EVALUATION AND DIFFERENTIAL DIAGNOSIS

Incontinence

Incontinence is a common complaint in girls, with a predominantly social rather than medical impact. The potential for underlying severe neurological and structural problems, however, cannot be ignored. Efficient screening for risk factors is the key to identifying the few patients with severe problems, and focusing therapy, as well as minimizing invasive evaluation, is the key for the remainder. Regular continence should develop in the third year of life in most children, with nighttime control developing more slowly. The range of normal is very wide and often culturally and socially influenced. Parents may be hesitant to bring children for evaluation, being unsure as to what is considered normal. Others are very aggressive and demand development of urinary control, often in response to childcare and school requirements.

Incontinence is the involuntary loss of urinary control and may have several forms. *Urge incontinence* is associated with the initial sense of the need to void, followed quickly by voiding. It may be of small amounts or dribbling or a complete emptying of the bladder. *Total incontinence* consists of constant leakage of urine, usually a substantial amount, yet may also be of limited amount in the case of an ectopic ureter. These children are truly "never dry." It is important to probe this symptom carefully, as the presence of total incontinence nearly always suggests a significant pathological process. Many parents will state that their child is never dry but will then admit if prompted, that they may be dry for an hour or so. Incontinence that occurs with the apparent lack of recognition by the child is frequent and might be best termed *wetting by neglect*. The child is rarely actually insensate to the void or the urine, but simply ignores the urge to void and the fact she is wet. Admitting the fact would necessitate a change in her behavior, and that is often the basis for the symptom in the first place. *Stress urinary incontinence* (SUI) is wetting associated with physical activity and is uncommon in young children, but becoming more recognized in teens, particularly those involved in high intensity athletics. It is usually of small amount and controlled by the use of pads, but very bothersome and embarrassing. *Urethral instability* is a more recently recognized form of wetting, which may be present in more children than previously recognized (1). It is best described in adults and may be amenable to surgical therapy. It is characterized by complete loss of bladder control associated with movement, but not so vigorous as with classic SUI. *Giggle incontinence* is an unusual form of wetting that is associated, as the name implies, with laughter (2,3). It is distinct from stress incontinence, which might occur with vigorous laughter or coughing, as well as physical activity. There is evidence of a familial tendency, but the etiology remains unknown.

Evaluation of the child with incontinence is founded on establishing the pattern of the wetting as described above, as well as the frequency of occurrence, the pattern over time, and any associated external factors. Patterns of fluid intake are important, as well as use of caffeinated drinks. The presence of any other urinary symptoms is important, particularly dysuria or known urinary infection. The child's neurodevelopmental status is relevant in terms of motor and cognitive function. Establishing the child's voiding patterns for both bowel and bladder is critical. Specific questions about bowel movement frequency and even size are important. Many children who are holders of urine are holders of bowel, and therapy will need to be directed toward both. Asking specific questions about how often the child voids will often reveal the cause or indicate that the family is actually unaware of the patterns. Specific questions must be asked of whether the wetting occurs associated with play and after witnessed episodes of squatting, crossing the legs, and other attempts to suppress a bladder contraction.

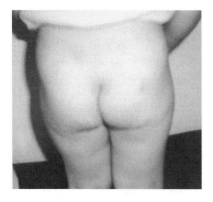

FIG. 13-1. Gluteal asymmetry in a 4-year-old girl with persistent wetting and recent UTI. She was found to have severe reflux, high-pressure bladder, and renal scarring due to a tethered spinal cord.

Physical examination is rarely revealing of any abnormality, but when it is, it usually suggests a major problem. The focus should be on any evidence of a neurological anomaly as evidenced by an abnormal sacral spine or lower extremities (Fig. 13-1). Since the sacral nerve roots control both the perineum and the feet, abnormalities of the latter may suggest neurological abnormalities of the bladder and bowel. An asymmetric gluteal cleft, a patch of hair, dermo-vascular malformation, or a sacral mass all point to a potential neurologic basis of incontinence (4,5). Examination of the perineum is important to exclude the rare condition of female epispadias, which is usually associated with total incontinence (Fig. 13-2). On occasion, one may be able to identify the ectopic ureteral orifice in the perineum leaking drops of urine. Palpating the abdomen can identify a distended bladder, often easily noted and with

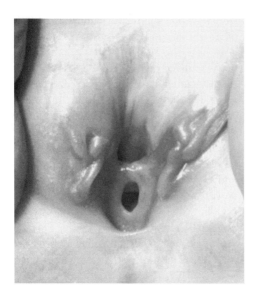

FIG. 13-2. External view of girl with epispadias. This is evident by the flattened mons pubis, the bifid clitoris, and patulous urethra. The vagina is normal but anteriorly displaced. This child is continually incontinent.

a child who claims they do not feel full. Similarly the full doughy sensation of an abdomen full of stool will suggest the association with constipation. It is also useful to observe the child's affect during the discussion about incontinence, as it will suggest their reaction to it. This can vary from total indifference to significant embarrassment. The interaction with the parent is also revealing for those in whom parental discipline may be overenthusiastic.

The presumed form of incontinence can usually be deduced from the history and physical examination. Further testing should be guided by recognition of what is likely to be demonstrated, as well as the therapeutic options available to those possible conditions. The child with voiding postponement with no signs of neurological abnormality can be treated with no further testing in most cases. A bladder ultrasound to show that she has a significant postvoid residual volume even when she is convinced she has emptied her bladder can confirm the diagnosis and also serves as an important teaching tool for both parent and child. It may also demonstrate bladder wall thickening, which is a frequent occurrence in these children (6). This is confirmatory and seldom suggests, in itself, a more complex underlying problem. In children with infection, a renal ultrasound is useful in ruling out any upper urinary tract pathology and is often very comforting to parents. Urodynamic studies, which are invariably invasive and may even aggravate symptoms, are seldom of value in these children. A simple urinary flow rate may help to identify an intermittent flow pattern. The child with infection and incontinence may need a cystogram to rule out reflux, and this may be used to assess bladder function. Urodynamic evaluation should be reserved for children with a clear suspicion of neurogenic dysfunction, any evidence of upper tract abnormality such as hydronephrosis, or in whom all measures have not produced any improvement in symptoms (7). Renal imaging with an intravenous pyelogram (IVP) or computed tomography (CT) scan is rarely indicated, and then in the unusual circumstance of a possible ectopic ureter. In those situations, an ultrasound may have demonstrated hydronephrosis of an upper pole but may also be normal. If there is strong suspicion based upon history of examination, an IVP will often reveal the ectopic ureter, usually from an upper pole moiety (Fig. 13-3). Rarely, a CT or DMSA scan will be needed to detect an occult duplex system or the small dysplastic renal unit in a child with constant wetting and an apparent solitary kidney (8) (Fig. 13-4). Cystoscopy is rarely indicated in the evaluation of the incontinent child.

Dysuria

Pain with urination or immediately afterward is usually due to infection of the bladder but may also be due to dysfunctional voiding patterns (Table 13-1). This is a widely variable complaint that occurs at all ages. Dysuria is not always due to infection, which carries several significant implications and therefore must be documented carefully. Patients are often given antibiotics without appropriate testing,

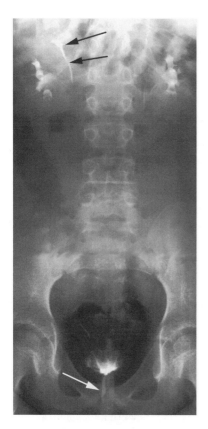

FIG. 13-3. Intravenous pyelogram of a child with continual wetting. The IVP reveals a duplicated right kidney and the upper pole ectopic ureter can be seen passing by the bladder toward the perineum.

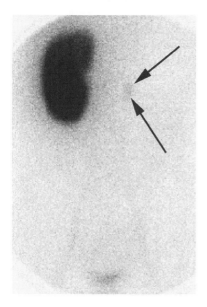

FIG. 13-4. DMSA scan in a child with continual wetting due to a small minimally functioning kidney drained by an ectopic ureter to the vagina. The small dysplastic renal unit is indicated by the *arrows*.

TABLE 13-1. *Differential diagnosis of dysuria in prepubertal girls.*

Common	Possible	Rare
Bacterial cystitis	Viral cystitis	Tuberculosis
Dysfunctional voiding	Endometriosis	Interstitial cystitis
—	Bladder stone	Eosinophilic cystitis
—	Foreign body	—
—	Bladder neoplasm	—

creating a confusing picture and clouding the decision-making process regarding further evaluation. In the patient with dysuria it should be determined if this occurs with every void or only after extreme delays in voiding. Is the pain relieved with voiding or actually aggravated? What was the appearance of the urine at the time of the episode? Was blood or red urine seen? Was the urine cloudy or foul smelling, all of which would point towards infection. Was there associated abdominal, flank or back pain, as well as fever? Voiding habits should be determined.

Evaluation should begin with a urinalysis and culture. Physical examination should assess any perineal lesions, bleeding, or discharge. The same assessment as for incontinence should be considered, as many patients with voiding dysfunction will have pain, with or without infection. Depending upon the degree of discomfort and the likelihood of infection, empiric therapy may be started, but the quality of the urine culture must be considered. If it is contaminated and antibiotics have been started, it is almost impossible to obtain an accurate culture. If infection is present, further evaluation will depend upon associated symptoms and age of the child. If the culture is negative, the urinalysis will guide therapy. If hematuria is present, imaging is essential to rule out neoplastic, structural, or calcific conditions, as discussed below. If pyuria alone is present, one should consider the rare possibility of an occult inflammatory condition such as tuberculosis, or infection with a fastidious organism such as *Ureaplasma*. Further cultures, imaging, or empiric therapy are used as suggested by the context. If the urinalysis is clear, dysuria is likely due to dysfunctional voiding. If recent in onset, reassurance and instruction are usually satisfactory. If chronic, more intensive behavioral therapy as described below is needed, often with anticholinergic medications.

Acutely symptomatic dysuria or pelvic pain may be debilitating, and an acute inflammatory or obstructive process should be ruled out by renal and bladder ultrasound. If normal, use of antispasmodic anticholinergics will usually relieve the symptoms. Pyridium (phenazopyridine) may occasionally help as well.

Endometriosis (see Chapter 11) can cause irritative bladder symptoms, although it is often difficult to detect direct vesical involvement. In a patient with known endometriosis and persistent dysuria, a search for intravesical involvement is appropriate, although rarely fruitful (9). In the absence of documented involvement, appropriate hormonal therapy (see Chapter 11) and symptomatic treatment of the dysuria is the best option.

Interstitial cystitis is a possible cause of dysuria in the adolescent, although the diagnosis is very problematic and controversial. There have been a few reports of IC in teens and younger children, although it remains a poorly defined entity, even in adults (10–13). Therapy is also limited. This is a diagnosis of exclusion.

Hematuria

Blood in the urine is one of the most disturbing symptoms, and while it may signal severe pathology, it is often due to infection and readily managed (Table 13-2). In girls the occurrence of gross, visible blood is usually noted in the toilet bowl, or the diaper; so there is little ability to recognize when in the voiding cycle it might have occurred, as can be done with males. It is important to make sure the blood is not menstrual or vaginal bleeding. Indeed, it may be assumed to be so, inappropriately. Associated symptoms are important, including dysuria or abdominal or flank pain. Presence of a recent viral illness may suggest immunological renal bleeding, as well might a recent streptococcal infection. Prior trauma, even relatively mild, may suggest upper tract structural bleeding. Urinalysis and culture are essential, with particular attention paid to the urinalysis. It is important to determine whether the bleeding is associated with pyuria, casts of red cells, or large numbers of crystals. Crystalluria, per se, is not pathological and occurs frequently in children, but it serves to focus attention on renal stone disease. An experienced observer with a phase contrast microscope can detect distorted RBCs associated with glomerular bleeding, in contrast to RBCs with normal morphology due to lower tract bleeding. Examination should seek any external lesions of the perineum that might be related to the bleeding, most of which would be obvious with inspection. Abdominal examination for masses and tenderness is needed, as well as a check for any spinal or lower extremity abnormalities in the setting of a UTI causing hematuria. Skin rashes may be present with immunological renal bleeding.

Ultrasound imaging of the entire urinary tract is the best first step in the evaluation of hematuria and may be done acutely. There are few lesions of immediate importance that will not be detected by ultrasound. The bladder wall may be

TABLE 13-2. *Differential diagnosis of hematuria in girls.*

Common	Possible	Rare
Urinary tract infection	Neoplasm: rhabdomyosarcoma, transitional cell carcinoma	Eosinophilic cystitis
Trauma	Viral cystitis	Endometriosis
Nephrolithiasis	Glomerulonephritis	Loin-pain hematuria syndrome

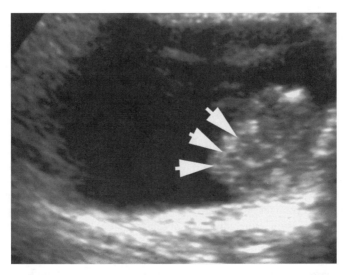

FIG. 13-5. Ultrasound (US) image of 15-year-old girl with gross painless hematuria and a bladder mass. The US shows an intravesical mass (*white arrows*). This is consistent with a transitional cell tumor and requires endoscopy to evaluate and resect the lesion.

abnormal in cases of inflammatory hematuria, ranging from mildly thickened and irregular, to having a pattern indistinguishable from a tumor. In the latter case it is occasionally necessary to perform cystoscopy and biopsy to determine the true nature of the lesion (Fig. 13-5). Most inflammatory bladder lesions are severely painful, while most tumors are not. In the setting of acute colicky flank pain consistent with a renal stone, spiral CT imaging is the best modality to identify the presence, location, and size of a stone, as well as determining the degree of hydronephrosis.

Renal Colic

Flank pain that is intermittent and in waves is termed *renal colic*, usually due to passage of a renal stone. It may also be due to intermittent obstruction of the ureter, usually at the uretero pelvic junction (UPJ). It may be associated with nausea and vomiting as well a fever, as discussed below. The description of the pain is fairly classic in the older child, being sharp and stabbing with radiation along the flank into the inguinal region and even felt in the perineum and coming in waves, often with complete resolution in between. The duration, intensity, and periodicity may be quite variable. Hematuria may be associated. A long-standing pattern of colic that might occur once or twice a month, often after meals or drinking, is suggestive of intermittent obstruction, often at the UPJ. Some of these children have already undergone extensive gastrointestinal evaluation. If stone is strongly suggested, a spiral CT may be the best modality (Fig. 13-6), but if uncertain, renal and bladder ultrasonography is the safest and simplest first step (Fig. 13-7). It can usually identify stones in the renal collecting system, the proximal or distal ureter, and if there is any hydronephrosis associated with them. It is a simple modality for serial follow-ups while waiting for stone passage.

Flank Pain and Fever

The association of flank pain and fever is almost always due to pyelonephritis, renal parenchymal infection, or a severe cystitis. It may occur with nausea and vomiting and sepsis in younger children. While it is likely due to infection, the possibility of an obstructive lesion, either structural or due to a stone, must be considered, since these children may become seriously ill if not treated promptly. The prior history of similar episodes, or a known diagnosis of vesicoureteral reflux or nephrolithiasis is important to extract. The duration and pattern of progression should be determined.

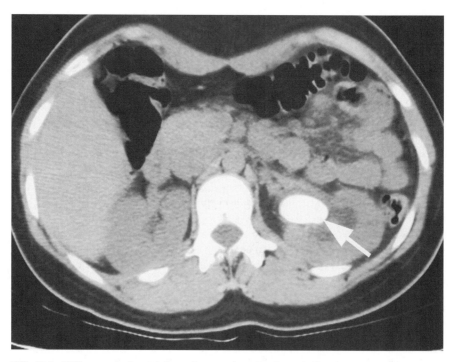

FIG. 13-6. CT image of a large left renal stone of cystine (*arrow*). There is some hydronephrosis of the kidney.

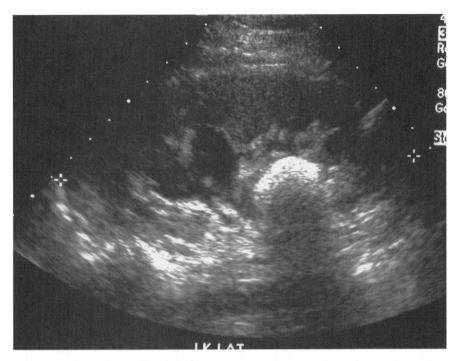

FIG. 13-7. Ultrasound image of a large cystine calculus in the renal pelvis of a teenage girl with periodic flank pain. The size of the stone is masked by the acoustic shadow it produces.

A urinalysis and culture are essential and should be done with great care or with a catheter to avoid a misdiagnosis or contaminated specimen. Since therapy will usually be started immediately, the one culture obtained is very important. Early imaging is usually not essential but should be considered if antibiotic therapy is not effective in reducing the pain and fever within 48 hours. Further imaging will depend upon the specific diagnosis and treatment response.

Perineal Mass

Diagnosis of an intralabial mass is based upon the age of the child and the physical appearance of the lesion. Table 13-3 lists the differential diagnosis of this condition. Each condition is characterized by its particular character and the clinical context. Urethral prolapse is typically in the African-American child who may have a predisposing factor to abdominal straining such as constipation, coughing, or an indwelling bladder catheter (Fig. 13-8). This condition is characterized as a circumferential edematous ring of tissue around the urethral meatus and distinct from the vagina. Occasionally the tissue is necrotic or dusky. A prolapsed ureterocele is

TABLE 13-3. *Intralabial mass in children.*

Diagnosis	Characteristics
Urethral prolapse	Circumferential, usually healthy tissue, some bleeding
Prolapsed ureterocele	Posterior urethral location, indurated and dusky
Periurethral cyst	Smooth white lateral
Imperforate hymen	Smooth, white or skin colored in midline posterior
Sarcoma botryoides	Posterior urethra or anterior vagina, irregular, may have tissue fragments
Gartner duct cyst	Smooth, fluid filled from vagina

typically in younger children and may be dusky with congestion. It will be emerging from the posterior aspect of the urethral meatus and will be smooth and rounded (Fig. 13-9). A tumor may emerge from the urethra but more commonly is from the vaginal opening and may be irregular, typical of sarcoma botryoides (see Color Plate 8). It may have been heralded by passage of tissue pieces. A periurethral cyst is seen almost exclusively in the neonate and is a smooth structure adjacent to the urethra but not involved with it and has a milky white appearance under the superficial epithelium (Fig. 13-10). An imperforate hymen (see Color Plate 21 and Chapter 10) is seen in the newborn as a midline smooth bulging posterior to the urethra, sometimes with a whitish appearance deep to the epithelium. The rare condition of a Gärtner duct cyst is most often noted in infancy and is a smooth cystic structure emanating from the vagina laterally with an appearance of being filled with clear fluid (Fig. 13-11).

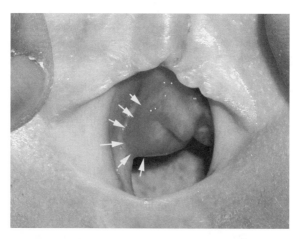

FIG. 13-8. Urethral prolapse in a 6-year-old girl. The edematous prolapsed tissue (*white arrows*) is seen surrounding the urethral meatus and anterior to the vaginal opening. The tissue is slightly erythematous but not necrotic.

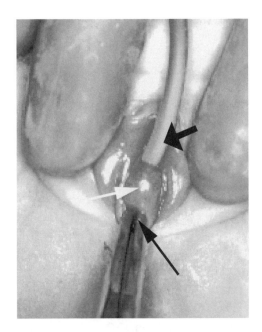

FIG. 13-9. Image of a prolapsed ureterocele in an infant. A Foley catheter (*thick
black arrow*) is in the urethra, anterior to
the bulging ureterocele (*white arrow*). A
clamp is pointing to the posterior aspect
of the ureterocele (*thin black arrow*).

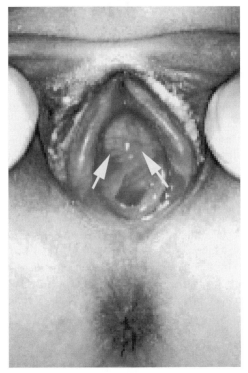

FIG. 13-10. Appearance of a paraurethral cyst in a newborn. The cystic
structure is posterior to the urethral meatus, anterior to the vaginal opening, and
covered by a thin membrane of skin. It
usually has a whitish coloration with deli-
cate blood vessels.

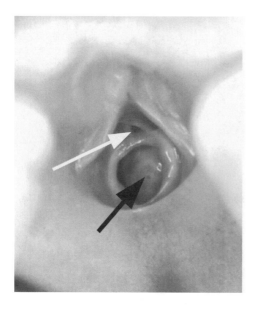

FIG. 13-11. External view of a neonate with a Gärtner duct cyst (black arrow) visible within the vaginal opening. She has a multicystic dysplastic kidney on the same side drained by the ectopic ureter associated with the cyst. The urethra is indicated by the white arrow.

Incidental: Congenital Anomalies of the Urinary Tract

A variety of congenital renal anomalies may be noted on routine or directed evaluation of the pediatric reproductive organs. These include renal duplications, solitary kidney, hydronephrosis, renal ectopia, and renal anomalies of shape and position. Many of these conditions are clinically insignificant, but it is important to recognize their presence and document the specific condition for future reference. The important parameters to be identified are obvious and include hydronephrosis and its degree, the possibility of vesicoureteral reflux, manifest by febrile UTI or hydronephrosis that arises during the examination. An ectopic kidney, if nonhydronephrotic, is seldom of any concern. It is important to recognize several important associations. One is that of a solitary normal kidney and a small, nondetected kidney that may be associated with an ectopic ureter and incontinence. These small dysplastic kidneys may be detected anywhere a normal kidney may be. Children with an ectopic ureter typically present with life-long constant wetting of small amount due to an ectopic ureter from the poorly functioning kidney draining into the perineum without any control from the bladder neck, which it misses entirely (Figs. 13-3 and 13-4). Any significant renal anomaly should raise the question of an associated cardiac or CNS abnormality. The value of screening for particular conditions is debatable, but the approach may be best viewed as having a high index of suspicion. In the setting of other known conditions, a more aggressive search for associated anomalies should be undertaken. Isolated renal abnormalities are usually not part of a syndrome. Horseshoe kidney is associated with Turner syndrome and the appropriate elements searched for. A two-vessel cord may be associated with renal and other anomalies of early development, yet the value of screening is debatable (14). A solitary kidney can be associated with müllerian anomalies such as unicornuate uterus, obstructed uterine segments, and vaginal malformations (see Chapter 10).

MAJOR CONDITIONS

Dysfunctional Voiding

Dysfunctional voiding (DV) represents a wide range of functional patterns and clinical symptoms. The term is usually reserved for conditions without an apparent structural or neurological basis, although that may be argued, as an inability to detect a neurological cause does not mean that one does not exist. Many of these patterns represent a behavioral abnormality but should not be viewed as merely behavioral, since the change in behavior can induce a functional and structural change in the bladder, which serves to perpetuate the clinical problem. Therapy should include consideration of both behavioral and functional or pathological elements. Voiding dysfunction is common. Depending upon definitions, it has been reported to be present in some form in as many as 29% of Danish 6- and 7-year-olds (15), in 8% of Belgian school-age children (16), and as many as 15% of teenage girls (17).

The clinical presentation of most dysfunctional voiding patterns includes aspects of incontinence, dysuria, UTI, pelvic pain, or urinary frequency. These patterns are often dynamic and may evolve or progress, yet they may also fade away. It is rare that they may cause permanent structural damage, but even mild symptoms are a significant bother to patients and family. There is no simple classification, but most patterns can be seen as being a manifestation of (a) small capacity bladder, (b) incomplete emptying of the bladder, (c) detrusor sphincter incoordination, and (d) large hypocontractile bladder. Identifying these patterns is key to targeting therapy. The goal of evaluation is to determine the pattern of dysfunctional voiding, which is usually apparent based upon history and physical, and to rule out underlying structural or functional abnormalities such as a neurogenic bladder.

Elements of history that should be covered include the voiding frequency and pattern, as well as any associated symptoms. Bowel history is important too, as many of these children have constipation. A voiding diary is helpful to make this more objective. A developmental history is important, as some children with mild learning disabilities will have an unstable bladder; handedness can give a clue to these subtle developmental issues as well. Nonfamilial left-handedness may suggest cross-dominance with mild upper CNS developmental abnormalities. If a child is left-handed without a family history and shows signs of cross-dominance, mild lower extremity hyperactivity and bladder instability may be seen. This association suggests that the child may have a small bladder capacity with instability as a cause of wetting, rather than the typical large bladder of the child who postpones voiding.

Age of onset is variable but is most often 1 to 3 years after toilet training, particularly in the child with voiding postponement. The child with bladder instability will have had trouble with toilet training and may never have been dry.

Social factors may play a role as well, although this may be difficult to discern (18). Major disruptions in the family can certainly trigger and aggravate dysfunctional voiding patterns. The dynamic of interaction between parent and child can be a major factor in these patterns and can present a major obstacle to correcting the dysfunctional patterns. On occasion, formal counseling may be appropriate.

The basic patterns of voiding dysfunction can be readily recognized as long as the practitioner is thinking about them. The most common is voiding postponement. The child simply waits too long to void and ends up wetting. This occurs most often in the 4- to 5-year-olds who do not want to interrupt play. They may have small wetting episodes or dampness with occasional flooding. They may be seen squatting or crossing their legs, all in an effort to avert wetting as they are responding to a bladder contraction. If asked, however, they will deny the need to void. Amazingly, many parents seem to believe them. All the while, they are developing a pattern where the bladder contraction has stimulated a responsive sphincteric contraction. This is detrusor-sphincter dyssynergy. When they ultimately choose to void, the same reflexive pattern occurs and voiding is inefficient, incomplete, and at high pressure. Many parents report an intermittent stream that is staccato or stop-and-start (Fig. 13-12).

Some of these children may have UTI, presumably due to incomplete emptying. The pain of the infection may prompt more vigorous holding behavior, aggravating the cycle. Pain may also occur with the bladder muscle contracting vigorously against the closed sphincter. It may be manifest as urethral or abdominal pain. It may be associated just with voiding and be sharp or may be more dull and steady or crampy. Constipation may of course be a contributing factor to this pain as well.

The urge syndrome is another variant of voiding dysfunction and is associated with a functionally small bladder capacity and instability on history. These children feel the urge to void with small volumes of urine in the bladder and may do so very frequently. The pattern may be life-long, but in some it develops after several infections or a period of voiding postponement. The specific etiology is unclear, but its association with subtle neurological abnormalities suggests an underlying neurodevelopmental basis. There is some suggestion of familial occurrence. It is likely that this pattern is aggravated by the child's response to the urge, in which case they will attempt to prevent voiding by contracting their pelvic floor muscles, creating a version of the voiding postponement pattern. This will tend to create an obstructed bladder, which will tend to be unstable, creating a vicious cycle of instability–holding–instability. If pain was a contributing trigger, as in prior UTIs, the pattern may be further aggravated by infection. The key to therapy is again to break a cycle of holding by preventing instability and infection, while retraining bladder patterns.

Therapy is aimed at breaking the holding cycle. Insight by the parents and child is important. It is critical to establish a realistic understanding that the basis of the problem exists and that a "quick fix" is not available. For most children, a program of reg-

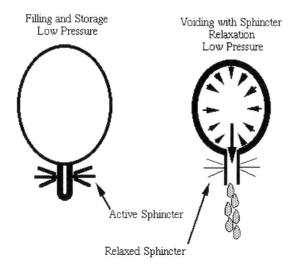

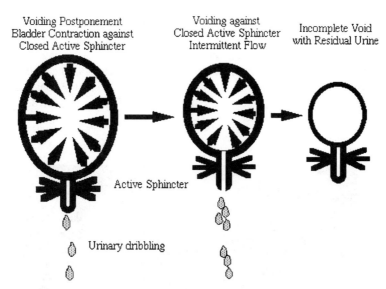

FIG. 13-12. Diagram illustrating the basic pattern of voiding dysfunction with voluntary holding by way of increased pelvic floor activity and subsequent poor bladder emptying at higher than normal pressures. This will lead to wetting, pain, infection, or a combination of all of these elements.

ular voiding is a cornerstone of successful therapy, coupled with relaxation measures to improve voiding efficiency (19). Initial approaches can be parent and child directed with a schedule of voiding every 2 to 3 hours with an attempt to relax by double voiding. In many cases, children may not initially be able to have a second void, but the time spent can help slow down and relax the overall process. Maintaining a record of performance and outcomes will help assess progress. In the child with urge syndrome, judicious use of anticholinergic medications will prevent the urge to which the child responds with holding. This must be used in the context of a voiding regimen as well. Prevention of UTI may be needed in the child with infection, which will only aggravate the urge pattern. Prophylactic antibiotics are appropriate until voiding patterns have normalized.

More formal behavioral modification and biofeedback measures have been described and are suitable for the refractory patient (20). They often entail multiple visits and complex equipment but have good reported success rates. Formal evaluation of reported trials of therapy, however, has not shown any true benefit (21). Focused voiding dysfunction clinics have been used to good effect in isolated circumstances and, if available, are a valuable resource (22).

Urinary Obstruction: UPJO and UVJO

Obstruction of the ureter is the most common cause of obstructive uropathy in girls. Proximal obstruction at the UPJ is far more common than that of the distal ureter or urethro vesical junction (UVJ). Most of these conditions are detected antenatally, with only a fraction presenting with symptoms in later life. That presentation is often quite impressive, however, and may be mistaken for gastrointestinal disorders manifest by severe intermittent abdominal pain and nausea. The association of these symptoms with hydronephrosis is strongly suggestive of UPJ obstruction. In the neonate with an ultrasound (US) picture of UPJO (Fig. 13-13), the decision re-

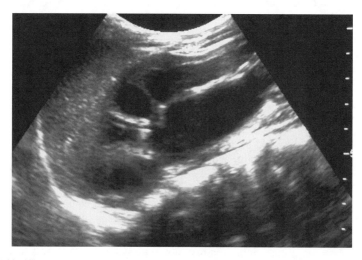

FIG. 13-13. Ultrasound image of hydronephrosis in the setting of a ureteropelvic junction obstruction. The renal pelvis and calyces are diffusely dilated. The renal parenchyma has normal echogenicity.

garding intervention is more difficult as these children appear asymptomatic and most probably are. The wide spectrum of severity, and the fact that some of these apparent obstructions will resolve without demonstrable sequelae in terms of renal injury, suggest that a uniform approach is inappropriate. Similarly, it should be cautioned that hydronephrosis is never "normal" and the functional impact should be assessed and monitored. There is great controversy regarding the appropriate identification of the child at risk for functional damage due to congenital UPJ or UVJO (23,24). There is no simple formula or gold-standard test to determine surgical candidates. Those most likely to benefit from surgery, and most at risk from the process, are those in whom the relative function of the affected kidney is depressed at diagnosis or in whom there is massive dilation of the kidney.

Moderate degrees of dilation seldom have functional depression and most will resolve with time. The interval may be several years, and UPJO seems to resolve more slowly than UVJO (25). The underlying etiologies are unknown. Protection against infection in the early months of life is reasonable, and it is important to rule out reflux as a contributing factor. Diuretic renography is usually used to assess the functional and obstructive effects of these conditions and can be used serially to monitor progress.

When function does deteriorate or is already low at diagnosis, surgical intervention is appropriate. For UPJ obstruction, surgical repair consists of a dismembered pyeloplasty performed through the flank or posteriorly, whereby the obstructing segment is removed and the renal pelvis and ureter reanastomosed. Overall outcomes are very good, approaching 97% success for all techniques. This has been performed laparoscopically with acceptable results. Endoscopic methods are less invasive but have lower success rates, about 75% (26). UVJ obstruction requires ureteral reimplantation with excision of the stenotic distal segment. The ureter may be so large as to require tapering by resecting part of the wall to permit successful tunneling in the bladder to prevent reflux and permit adequate urinary transport. This repair has a good success rate as well, even in the infant, but has been performed much less in recent years, due to the recognition of spontaneous resolution (25).

Urinary Tract Infection

Urinary tract infection (UTI) is one of the most common conditions affecting girls and may range from being a mild inconvenience to a major threat to health (27). UTIs are due to either abnormal anatomy or function of the urinary tract, with the latter being most common. The underlying principle in managing UTI is assessing the risk of damage to the kidneys with infection. This will not usually provide an explanation of the cause of UTI but of the effect, and it is important to guide the intensity of evaluation and therapy.

The question regarding evaluation of the child with a UTI is not simply answered, yet commonly raised. While the American Academy of Pediatrics has published guidelines as to the evaluation of UTI in the child under 2 years (28), even these have been questioned (29). In practice, a "better-safe-than-sorry" approach may be the most prudent, even if objective evidence supporting an approach may be difficult to find. The strongest indication would be the younger child with a well-documented infection and high fever. In these children, a renal ultrasound and voiding cysto ure-throgram (VCUG) are appropriate in nearly all cases. If the UTI is without fever, a simple ultrasound may be adequate, but obtaining the VCUG or radionuclide cystogram (RNC) is probably the best approach. In the older child in the toilet-training years, a well-documented febrile UTI warrants an ultrasound and cystogram in most cases. Repetitive UTIs, even if not febrile, also justify evaluation. A single UTI without fever can be evaluated with a renal ultrasound, looking for hydronephrosis, an anatomic abnormality of the kidney consistent with scarring, and to assess the bladder and its emptying. These children are then monitored for 6 months for subsequent UTI, and if this does not occur, it is unlikely that they are at risk of renal injury. In all cases of children after toilet training, assessment of their voiding function and education as to normal voiding are important.

For the child without reflux (reflux is discussed later) and no anatomic abnormality, the risk of renal injury is low and the role of management is to limit the symptomatic episodes and the exposure to antibiotics. The underlying cause is usually discernable from the history. If the UTIs are not associated with high fever, it is unlikely that they will be associated with reflux. Depending upon age and context, reflux may be ruled out with cystography. These children usually have infections due to dysfunctional voiding habits, described earlier.

Therapy is directed at correcting the dysfunctional voiding patterns. Often it will be necessary to use prophylactic antibiotics to allow the child to develop more normal voiding patterns without the parent telling them when and where to go. This is maintained for 4 to 6 months while the child is developing better voiding patterns. Assessing for bowel habits and treating constipation are important elements of managing these children. Vigorous hydration is encouraged, and probiotics such as yogurt and cranberry are used, albeit without hard evidence as to their efficacy (30–32).

There are children with a greater tendency toward UTI, and while this seems to extend into the adult years, the mechanisms remain unclear. Our ability to change this risk appears limited. It is rare that UTIs are due to an unrecognized anatomic abnormality that would not be detected by a well-performed renal bladder ultrasound and cystography. It is seldom, if ever, appropriate to perform cystoscopy for uncomplicated UTI, and even with recurrent pyelonephritis, this rarely yields any information to affect therapy. Urethral dilation for recurrent UTIs is still practiced but clearly misinterprets the pathophysiology of these infections. The result of the dilation is to temporarily injure the urethral sphincters to prevent the holding that the patient has learned. The dilation therefore will work for a period of time, but at risk of permanent injury and without addressing the underlying cause of the problem. It is therefore to be strongly discouraged. Retrograde pyelography in the child with recurrent UTI is also still performed, yet with no logical basis or a benefit.

Stone

Management of nephrolithiasis in children is a complex area that shares some elements with stone management in adults, yet differs in several unique ways. While uncommon, stones in children are not rare and have the potential for causing serious renal injury and morbidity.

Acute management is based upon the severity of symptoms, presence of fever, and renal obstruction. Most stones will pass, and as long as the child can be made comfortable and continue hydration, they may be cared for at home. If vomiting is present, intravenous hydration becomes necessary. A stone that is near the bladder may be observed for passage for a brief period of time in this context, perhaps 24 to 72 hours. At home this may be longer if pain control is adequate. In the presence of fever, the luxury of time is not usually afforded and antibiotics, with early decompression, is the safest approach. Decompression is usually with a double-J ureteral stent, as this provides for dilation of the ureter should ureteroscopic stone removal be required. It also permits extracorporeal shock wave lithotripsy (ESWL) to be performed. The child can be easily managed at home with a stent, in contrast to a percutaneous nephrostomy, which is not as readily cared for out of hospital. For a large proximal stone, however, percutaneous nephrostomy is the optimal decompression as it will likely be the route of stone removal. A very ill child with sepsis and obstruction is best served with a nephrostomy tube, due to the ease of placement and the efficacy of decompression. Subsequent stone management is discussed in detail elsewhere (33,34).

Long-term management of stone disease in children depends upon the metabolic basis of the stone disease. In the literature, it is often stated that a metabolic cause for stones can be found in most children, yet this does not seem to be the case in practice. It is also problematic in children to assume a metabolic cause, as this seems to suggest the need for medication in all children. There are no data regarding how long to maintain children on medication and what the long-term implications of this may be. With a regimen of vigorous hydration and moderating dietary changes, our experience has been that most children's stones do not recur. Those with clearly defined metabolic causes, such as cystinuria or primary hyperoxaluria, clearly require careful metabolic management, preferably by a physician experienced in stone disease.

Reflux

The presence of vesicoureteral reflux in a child with UTI places that child at risk for renal scarring and its long-term sequelae of hypertension, further UTIs, and renal insufficiency. There is much controversy regarding reflux management, and it continues to evolve. There are no simple rules that can be followed as to how long one should observe reflux and when surgery is "necessary." Recognition of this ambiguity is essential and parents of children with reflux must be counseled that there are no "rules" and that their preferences must be recognized in the care plan for their child (35).

The foundation of modern reflux management is the recognition that reflux does not cause UTIs, it only permits renal infection to develop from bladder infection. Most UTIs, as noted above, are due to bladder dysfunction, and reflux may well also be a product of dysfunctional voiding patterns. Reflux will resolve spontaneously, and it is therefore appropriate to observe patients with that expectation. During that time, however, they are at risk for further UTI and renal injury, so prophylactic antibiotics have become a standard part of management. There is controversy as to their need, but the risk of not using them seems unacceptably high for the small risk of using them. It is unpredictable when reflux will resolve, therefore periodic reassessment using cystography is needed, usually at intervals of 12 to 18 months. There is little value to stopping antibiotics to "see what will happen." The only recognizable outcome is another UTI with the potential for damage. The likelihood of resolution is inversely proportional to the grade of reflux, but all grades can resolve (35,36). It might take several years and for some families this is not reasonable. Surgical correction is therefore appropriate. Reflux rarely increases in grade unless there is significant bladder dysfunction. This may occur transiently at toilet training. The ultimate goal of reflux management is preservation of renal function and avoiding renal scarring. Assessing this damage is important and selective use of DMSA radionuclide renal scanning is necessary in those at risk, including recurrent infections, high grade of reflux, or those with nonresolution (Fig. 13-14).

Surgical therapy for reflux is appropriate if the goal of management is not being achieved with observational therapy. This includes the child with breakthrough UTIs or increasing scarring. It is also appropriate if reflux has not resolved after a reasonable period of time, or is very unlikely to do so. These are all value judgments and must reflect the statistical odds of resolution, as well as the family's perception of

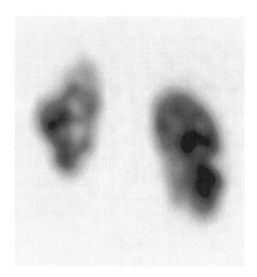

FIG. 13-14. Radionuclide image of the kidneys using DMSA to mark renal tubular mass. This image shows severe bilateral renal scarring due to pyelonephritis associated with reflux. This child is at high risk for developing hypertension as a young adult.

"reasonable." Standard surgical therapy remains open ureteral reimplantation using a transvesical procedure such as the transtrigonal or Leadbetter–Politano operation (35). An extravesical (Lich–Gregoir) technique is used frequently for unilateral reflux. Laparoscopic methods are emerging and will improve in the near term. Endoscopic methods of subureteric injection of bulking agents are available and are very simple. They are hindered by their lack of efficacy with one intervention, about 80%, their reduced efficacy with higher grades of reflux, and the uncertain durability of effect. The search for an acceptable injectable material is vigorously ongoing (37,38).

Ectopic Ureter and Ureterocele

The diagnosis of an ectopic ureter or ureterocele is well described and is usually in the context of prenatal detection or in the child with infection (39). Obstructed ectopic ureters and ureteroceles require surgical therapy. These are usually arising from the upper segment of a duplex kidney. If there is function in the affected segment, drainage into the lower moiety is the most effective approach, often with a proximal anastomosis. If there is little or no function, removal of the upper segment is preferred. In some ureteroceles, the system may be effectively drained with an endoscopic incision at the level of the bladder. If there is no subsequent reflux, this is definitive, even if there is little function of the affected upper pole. If reflux develops, a common sheath ureteral reimplantation of the upper and lower ureters side by side can be performed (Fig. 13-15).

The nonobstructed ectopic ureter is usually associated with incontinence, and this diagnosis may be difficult to make. As noted above, it should be suspected in the child with constant wetting of small amounts. A high index of suspicion will usually allow the diagnosis to be made, but this may require using CT scanning to detect a small, poorly functioning upper pole. Removal of the upper pole or upper to lower anastomosis is curative and very satisfying to the patient who is not dry. In the absence of reflux, the distal end of these ectopic ureters may be left in situ. An exception to this may be the vaginal-ectopic ureter. Several case reports of squamous cell carcinoma of the vagina and cervix have been published associated with an ectopic ureter (40). A recommendation that these children undergo life-long screening has been made, although the incidence of this association is unclear. It is also unclear if this is an age-dependent phenomenon, whereby the infant with this diagnosis may be at a lesser risk. The safe approach would be to recommend screening for all.

Renal Masses

A renal mass in a child represents a neoplasm until proven otherwise, but it is important to recognize the other causes of such masses. The likely diagnosis of a neoplastic mass is age dependent, with Wilms tumor being most likely from ages 1 to 5, but a renal cell carcinoma increasing in likelihood in the teen years. Its incidence is ac-

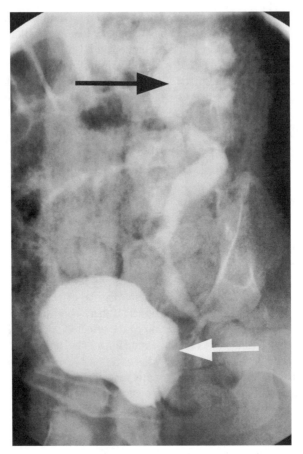

FIG. 13-15. Voiding cystogram in child with ureterocele showing the filling defect of the uretero-cele in the bladder (*white arrow*) and reflux into the lower pole (*black arrow*) of the duplicated left system.

tually equal to that of Wilms tumor in the adolescent, although both are rare. In the new-born, a congenital mesoblastic nephroma is most likely, while in the young infant neu-roblastoma must be considered. Its clinical appearance is usually distinct from Wilms, but this is not always obvious. Neuroblastoma typically presents in the younger child who appears ill. The mass is hard and irregular, may contain stippled calcifications and be so large as to cross the midline. Wilms tumor, in contrast appears in the well child with mild symptoms and a recently noted mass that is smooth, firm, and rarely so large.

In association with certain syndromes, particular tumors should be considered, in-cluding angiomyolipoma in a child with tuberous sclerosis. This is manifest by vari-able degrees of mental retardation, seizure activity, and facial adenoma sebaceum. These children may be at higher risk of Wilms tumor as well. The child with

Denys–Drasch syndrome (hermaphroditism, gonadal dysgenesis, and congenital nephropathy) is at high risk for Wilms tumor (40). The child with Beckwith–Wiedemann syndrome (hemihypertrophy, macroglossia, hypoglycemia) is at increased risk of Wilms tumor as well (41).

Cystic masses of the kidneys may present diagnostic confusion, as it is difficult to differentiate benign from malignant lesions. In general, these are masses with some element of solid tissue where there is consideration of them being part of the "Wilms tumor spectrum." The most common is congenital multilocular cystic nephroma, which is seen more often in girls with a bimodal distribution having peak incidences about 4 years and in late adolescence (42). Local resection is appropriate, but it remains unclear whether it really has malignant potential.

Inflammatory masses may mimic renal tumors, including the entity termed *focal lobar nephronia* (43). This is probably a misnomer, but the term is still used to indicate a focal area of acute pyelonephritis that appears as a mass in the kidney. It is often but not always associated with reflux and has been reported to prompt nephrectomy. The true identity can usually be discerned with careful imaging in the context of an acutely ill child.

Pelvic Tumors

The child with a solid pelvic mass should be considered to have rhabdomyosarcoma until tissue diagnosis can confirm this. The typical presentation of a prolapse of visible tumor protruding from the urethra or vagina, with the classic irregular botryoid (bunch of grapes) appearance supports this diagnosis (see also Chapter 3). Tissue biopsy is definitive and the histology is usually that of an embryonal pattern. Electro-resection should be avoided as it induces significant artifacts. Cold cup or scissor resection followed by cautery for hemostasis is appropriate. Most sarcomas are below the mucosa; so it is important to obtain a sufficiently deep tissue specimen. Staging is carried out with CT and conventional imaging of the chest, CT or MR imaging of the pelvis, bone scan, and bone marrow aspirate. Initial management is usually chemotherapy followed by surgical excision of residual disease, with or without radiotherapy (44). There is some controversy regarding the ability to preserve bladder function, as many patients in whom the bladder is preserved have bladder dysfunction due to chemo- and radiotherapy. In the Intergroup Rhabdomyosarcoma Study IV (1988–1996), only 13% of patients underwent surgical resection (45).

Cloacal Anomaly, Exstrophy, and Epispadias

Detailed discussion of the most severe congenital anomalies of the bladder and genitalia in girls, the cloacal anomaly, bladder and cloacal exstrophy, and epispadias is beyond the scope this chapter; a basic description will permit accurate identification and early management (see also Chapter 10). The cloacal anomaly entails genitourinary maldevelopment such that the urinary, genital, and gastrointestinal tracts do not separate (46). They create a common confluence, the cloaca that is a single opening for the urinary, intestinal, and genital structures. There are several variants possible and these are often associated with complex renal anomalies. The typical presentation is that of a child that appears to have imperforate anus only, but may have a pelvic mass. The mass is typically undrained urine in the vagina and bladder. On examination there is only one perineal orifice and often the clitoris is malformed, as with the external genitalia. Detailed diagnosis is by way of genitography and the child requires urinary drainage, usually by way of vaginal catheterization to prevent bladder outlet obstruction from pooled urine. The GI tract is decompressed with a colostomy to anticipate later functionalization. These children often require multiple reconstructive surgeries and may have associated congenital anomalies.

Sharing only a similar name, cloacal exstrophy is very different from the cloacal anomaly. It is the most extreme end of the exstrophy/epispadias spectrum (47,48). It is manifest by an abnormal communication between the GI tract and bladder with a lateral vesicoenteric fistula at the level of the cecum. The bladder is exstrophic and divided into two hemibladders by the fistula. It is on the lower abdominal surface, open and exposed. The ureteral orifices are exposed and may be seen dripping urine. The ileum often prolapses out the vesicoenteric fistula to create a protruding structure likened to an elephant truck (Fig. 13-16). Paired appendices may be seen

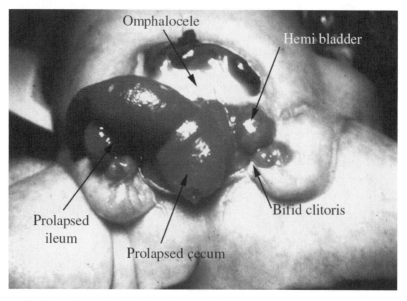

FIG. 13-16. View of neonate with cloacal exstrophy. The prominent tubular structure is the prolapsed ileum emerging from the prolapsed cecum, which is surrounded by two hemi-bladders. The clitoris is bifid. Many of these children will have neural tube defects as well.

prolapsing out as well. The distal end of the gut is the diminutive hind gut that is blind ending and small. The clitoris is bifid (see Fig 10-28) and widely splayed due to failure of pelvic closure. The vagina is anteriorly displaced and there is often an omphalocele. Spinal cord lesions such as myelomeningocele are common, occurring in about 50% of these children. The kidneys are usually normal but may be ectopic or malrotated. Other defects may be present as well. These children are very difficult to manage and one of the first challenges is determining the sex of rearing. Previous wisdom suggested that all should be raised as females, but this has recently shifted to where many are being raised according to their genetic sex (49). The basic principles of management are to separate the bowel and bladder and refunctionalize the bowel in continuity with an end colostomy. The bladder is closed to permit refunctionalization with posterior relocation of the bladder neck and vagina into the pelvis. This may be done with pelvic osteotomies to permit pelvic floor reconstruction.

Similar principles are involved in early management of classic bladder exstrophy, which includes an open bladder plate with no communication to the bowel, and a bifid clitoris, anteriorly located vagina and rectum. Bladder closure is performed with bladder neck reconstruction and posterior movement of the urogenital complex—the bladder neck and vagina—into the pelvic floor.

Neither cloacal exstrophy nor classic bladder exstrophy is difficult to recognize, yet epispadias in the female is not readily recognized (48). This is likely due to its rarity, yet it has significant implications on the child's continence. This is the mildest of the conditions in the exstrophy spectrum and appears as a bifid clitoris with an intact lower abdomen, but the urethral meatus is patulous and appears as large as the vaginal opening, which is also anteriorly displaced. These children may have a flattened mons pubis. Some have escaped recognition until examined for incontinence. Incontinence is due to the fact that these patients have very poorly developed bladder necks. Management is with bladder neck reconstruction in one stage or with a preliminary urethroplasty to permit bladder growth (50).

Urethral Prolapse

Urethral prolapse is readily recognized clinically and initial care is directed at relieving symptoms (51) (Fig. 13-8). Topical estrogen preparations are usually effective in settling the acute symptoms of bleeding and irritation, but do not often cause regression of the prolapse. If the tissues are not necrotic, elective resection can be planned if there is no regression. If the tissues are so congested as to be necrotic, acute resection is appropriate to avoid local infection. Resection is performed with circumferential resection of the internal and external mucosal tissues with reapproximation using interrupted or locked running suture. Tying the prolapse off over a catheter is not a reasonable approach as it requires an indwelling catheter for several days.

SUMMARY OF ESSENTIAL EVALUATION MODALITIES

Ultrasound

Ultrasound has become the mainstay of pediatric urological imaging and, when interpreted thoughtfully, can often provide the essential diagnostic information in most cases. It provides structural data regarding the kidneys including growth, character of the parenchyma, presence and degree of hydronephrosis and ureteral dilation. The bladder should not be ignored in this examination, as the degree of filling correlated with the child's sense of fullness, the thickness of the bladder wall, and the completeness of emptying are valuable in the assessment of many voiding disorders. US is excellent in evaluating for the presence of stone when it is not clearly present and for monitoring the progress of a passing stone. It also provides data on the state of the pelvic organs and ovaries. It is limited in its functional assessment, but this may often be inferred by the nature of the renal parenchyma, for example, or how well the bladder empties. It is excellent for identifying renal masses. It cannot, however, provide any definitive information on the presence or absence of reflux, only on the presence of severe renal scarring in the context of infection.

Voiding Cystourethrogram

Voiding cystourethrogram (VCUG) is indicated when determination of the presence and nature of vesicoureteral reflux is considered important. It should be used on the initial evaluation when the likelihood of reflux is high, as with a child with a febrile UTI. It will provide data as to the presence of reflux, the nature of the ureterovesical junction, which may indicate the likelihood of spontaneous resolution of the reflux, as well as providing information about bladder emptying, the character of the bladder wall, and any associated bladder or urethral abnormalities. The scout film may also suggest the extent of constipation, often associated with UTI. Radionuclide cystogram (RNC) may be used in place of the VCUG as a follow-up study or a screening test when the chance of reflux is low. It provides somewhat less radiation, depending upon how the VCUG is performed. There is no specific difference in the sensitivity of either study, and both may identify grade 1 reflux.

Intravenous Pyelogram

Intravenous pyelography (IVP) is becoming less used due to improved US imaging and functional renal scans. Its role is in clarification of complex anatomy, particularly in duplication anomalies. The IVP is both functional and anatomic as the rapidity of contrast appearance is dependent upon the ability of the kidney to extract and concentrate contrast, which is very similar to what is assessed in radionuclide renal scans. The IVP can show detailed anatomy in the setting of obstruction.

Radionuclide Renal Scans: DMSA and MAG-3

Radionuclide renal imaging provides functional and anatomic information dependent upon the tracer used. The two principle tracers in common use are DMSA and MAG-3. DMSA is used for detailed anatomic resolution of functional renal tissue. This is most often used to identify renal parenchymal scarring in the setting of possible reflux nephropathy. DMSA is probably the most accurate imaging test of relative function of the two kidneys, although in the setting of severe obstruction, it can overestimate relative function. In obstructive conditions, the MAG-3 scan is usually preferred to assess relative function based on early uptake, as well an indication of drainage. The latter is measured as a halftime for washout of tracer from the renal pelvis. This parameter has been heavily scrutinized and criticized, and it must be interpreted with caution (52). The appeal of a numerical indicator of a clinical process is strong, yet it must be recognized that making a clinical decision regarding surgical intervention for obstruction based upon a single number is fraught with risk.

Computed Tomography

The value of CT imaging cannot be overestimated, particularly in the urinary tract, but it should not be overused in children, particularly with US available. It is of great particular value in stone disease and is the study of choice for the new patient with a possible stone. CT does not provide any functional data unless contrast is used. Structural studies of the kidneys and pelvis are best done with contrast enhanced CT, especially in the setting of renal masses.

Urodynamics

The information gained for urodynamics (UDS) includes the compliance of the bladder during filling, the pressures generated with voiding, bladder capacity, coordination of the bladder detrusor muscle and sphincter muscle, the innervation pattern of the pelvic floor and sphincter, as well as the efficiency of voiding. Each of these may be important in some situations but may also be obtained by less invasive testing.

The use of UDS should probably be determined in close consultation with the specialist performing the study (53). Recognizing its moderate degree of invasiveness, a clear idea of how the findings of the study will influence therapy should be established. It is invaluable in the setting of complex neurologic disorders of bladder function, yet it is less important in simple dysfunctional voiding, which may be best assessed clinically (54). Therapy is often empiric and dependent upon response rather than by any set of quantitative parameters such as bladder pressure. It is often best reserved for those whose response to standard therapy is not adequate.

REFERENCES

1. Vereecken RL, Proesmans W. Urethral instability as an important element of dysfunctional voiding. *J Urol* 2000;163(2):585.
2. Williams DI. Giggle incontinence. *Acta Urol Belg* 1984;52(2):151.
3. Sher PK, Reinberg Y. Successful treatment of giggle incontinence with methylphenidate. *J Urol* 1996;156(2 Pt 2):656.
4. Satar N, Bauer SB, Shefner J, et al. The effects of delayed diagnosis and treatment in patients with an occult spinal dysraphism. *J Urol* 1995;154(2 Pt 2):754.
5. Keating MA, Rink RC, Bauer SB, et al. Neurourological implications of the changing approach in management of occult spinal lesions. *J Urol* 1988;140(5 Pt 2):1299.
6. Cvitkovi-Kuzmi A, Brkljaci B, Ivankovi D, Grga A. Ultrasound assessment of detrusor muscle thickness in children with nonneuropathic bladder/sphincter dysfunction. *Eur Urol* 2002;41(2):214; discussion 218.
7. Bauer SB. Special considerations of the overactive bladder in children. *Urology* 2002;60(5) [Suppl 1]:43; discussion 49.
8. Borer JG, Bauer SB, Peters CA, et al. A single-system ectopic ureter draining an ectopic dysplastic kidney: delayed diagnosis in the young female with continuous urinary incontinence. *Br J Urol* 1998;81(3):474.
9. Price DT, Maloney KE, Ibrahim GK, et al. Vesical endometriosis: report of two cases and review of the literature. *Urology* 1996;48(4):639.
10. Schuster GA. Interstitial cystitis in children: not a rare entity. *Urology* 2001;57(6) [Suppl 1]:107.
11. Park JM. Is interstitial cystitis an underdiagnosed problem in children? A diagnostic and therapeutic dilemma. *Urology* 2001;57(6 Suppl 1):30.
12. La Manna A, Polito C, Papale MR, et al. Chronic interstitial cystitis and systemic lupus erythematosus in an 8-year-old girl. *Pediatr Nephrol* 1998;12(2):139.
13. Close CE, Carr MC, Burns MW, et al. Interstitial cystitis in children. *J Urol* 1996;156(2 Pt 2):860.
14. Thummala MR, Raju TN, Langenberg P. Isolated single umbilical artery anomaly and the risk for congenital malformations: a meta-analysis. *J Pediatr Surg* 1998;33(4):580.
15. Hansen A, Hansen B, Dahm TL. Urinary tract infection, day wetting and other voiding symptoms in seven- to eight-year-old Danish children. *Acta Paediat* 1997;86(12):1345.
16. Bakker E, van Sprundel M, van der Auwera JC, et al. Voiding habits and wetting in a population of 4,332 Belgian schoolchildren aged between 10 and 14 years. *Scand J Urol Nephrol* 2002;36(5):354.
17. Alnaif B, Drutz HP. The prevalence of urinary and fecal incontinence in Canadian secondary school teenage girls: questionnaire study and review of the literature. *Int Urogynecol J Pelvic Floor Dysfunct* 2001;12(2):134.
18. Mazzola BL, von Vigier RO, Marchand S, et al. Behavioral and functional abnormalities linked with recurrent urinary tract infections in girls. *J Nephrol* 2003;16(1):133.
19. Wiener JS, Scales MT, Hampton J, et al. Long-term efficacy of simple behavioral therapy for daytime wetting in children. *J Urol* 2000;164(3 Pt 1):786.
20. Duel BP. Biofeedback therapy and dysfunctional voiding in children. *Curr Urol Rep* 2003;4(2):142.
21. Sureshkumar P, Bower W, Craig JC, et al. Treatment of daytime urinary incontinence in children: a systematic review of randomized controlled trials. *J Urol* 2003;170(1):196; discussion 200.
22. Schulman SL, Quinn CK, Plachter N, et al. Comprehensive management of dysfunctional voiding. *Pediatrics* 1999;103(3):E31.
23. Peters CA. Urinary obstruction in children. *J Urol* 1995;154:1874.

24. Koff SA. Postnatal management of antenatal hydronephrosis using an observational approach. *Urology* 2000;55(5):609.
25. McLellan DL, Retik AB, Bauer SB, et al. Rate and predictors of spontaneous resolution of prenatally diagnosed primary nonrefluxing megaureter. *J Urol* 2002;168(5):2177; discussion 2180.
26. Nicholls G, Hrouda D, Kellett MJ, et al. Endopyelotomy in the symptomatic older child. *BJU Int* 2001;87(6):525.
27. Riccabona M. Urinary tract infections in children. *Curr Opin Urol* 2003;13(1):59.
28. Anonymous. Practice parameter: the diagnosis, treatment, and evaluation of the initial urinary tract infection in febrile infants and young children. American Academy of Pediatrics. Committee on Quality Improvement. Subcommittee on Urinary Tract Infection. [Comment] [Erratum appears in 2000 Jan;105(1 Pt 1):141]. *Pediatrics* 1999;103(4 Pt 1):843.
29. Hoberman A, Charron M, Hickey RW, et al. Imaging studies after a first febrile urinary tract infection in young children [Comment]. *N Engl J Med* 2003;348(3):195.
30. Lowe FC, Fagelman E. Cranberry juice and urinary tract infections: What is the evidence? *Urology* 2001;57(3):407.
31. Stothers L. A randomized trial to evaluate effectiveness and cost effectiveness of naturopathic cranberry products as prophylaxis against urinary tract infection in women. *Can J Urol* 2002;9(3):1558.
32. Reid G. The role of cranberry and probiotics in intestinal and urogenital tract health. *Crit Rev Food Sci Nutr* 2002;42(3):293.
33. Cohen TD, Ehreth J, King LR, et al. Pediatric urolithiasis: medical and surgical management. *Urology* 1996;47(3):292.
34. Docimo SG, Peters CA. Pediatric endourology and laparoscopy. In: Walsh PC, Retik AB, Vaughan, ED, Jr, et al., eds. *Campbell's urology.* Philadelphia: WB Saunders, 2002:2564.
35. Elder JS, Peters CA, Arant BS, et al. Pediatric Vesicoureteral Reflux Guidelines Panel summary report on the management of primary vesicoureteral reflux in children. *J Urol* 1997;157(5):1846.
36. Connolly LP, Zurakowski D, Connolly SA, et al. Natural history of vesicoureteral reflux in girls after age 5 years. *J Urol* 2001;166(6):2359.
37. Lackgren G, Wahlin N, Skoldenberg E, et al. Endoscopic treatment of vesicoureteral reflux with dextranomer/hyaluronic acid copolymer is effective in either double ureters or a small kidney. *J Urol* 2003;170(4 Pt 2):1551; discussion 1555.
38. Puri P, Chertin B, Velayudham M, et al. Treatment of vesicoureteral reflux by endoscopic injection of dextranomer/hyaluronic acid copolymer: preliminary results. *J Urol* 2003;170(4 Pt 2):1541; discussion 1544.
39. Schlussel RN, Retik AB. Ectopic ureter, ureterocele, and other anomalies of the ureter. In: Walsh PC, Retik AB, Vaughan ED, Jr, et al., eds. *Campbell's urology.* Philadelphia: WB Saunders; 2002:2007.
40. Shimao Y, Nabeshima K, Inoue T, et al. Primary vaginal adenocarcinoma arising from the metanephric duct remnant. *Virchows Arch* 2000;436(6):622.
41. Borer JG, Kaefer M, Barnewolt CE, et al. Renal findings on radiological follow-up of patients with Beckwith-Wiedemann syndrome. *J Urol* 1999;161(1):235.
42. Canakli F, Tekdogan UY, Ergul G, et al. Cystic nephroma: a rare clinical entity. *Int Urol Nephrol* 2002;34(1):19.
43. Klar A, Hurvitz H, Berkun Y, et al. Focal bacterial nephritis (lobar nephronia) in children. *J Pediatr* 1996;128(6):850.
44. Andrassy RJ, Hays DM, Raney RB, et al. Conservative surgical management of vaginal and vulvar pediatric rhabdomyosarcoma: a report from the Intergroup Rhabdomyosarcoma Study III. *J Pediatr Surg* 1995;30(7):1034; discussion 1036.
45. Andrassy RJ, Wiener ES, Raney RB, et al. Progress in the surgical management of vaginal rhabdomyosarcoma: a 25-year review from the Intergroup Rhabdomyosarcoma Study Group. *J Pediatr Surg* 1999;34(5):731; discussion 734.
46. Hendren WH. Cloaca, the most severe degree of imperforate anus: experience with 195 cases. *Ann Surg* 1998;228(3):331.
47. Mitchell ME, Plaire C. Management of cloacal exstrophy. *Adv Exp Med Biol* 2002;511:267; discussion 270.
48. Gearhart JP. Exstrophy, epispadias, and other bladder anomalies. In: Walsh PC, Retik AB, Vaughan ED, Jr., et al. eds. *Campbell's urology.* Philadelphia: WB Saunders; 2002:2136.

49 Reiner WG, Gearhart JP. Discordant sexual identity in some genetic males with cloacal exstrophy assigned to female sex at birth. *N Engl J Med* 2004;350:333.
50. Peters CA, Gearhart JP, Jeffs RD. Epispadias and incontinence: the challenge of the small bladder. *J Urol* 1988;140(5 Pt 2):1199.
51. Valerie E, Gilchrist BF, Frischer J, et al. Diagnosis and treatment of urethral prolapse in children. *Urology* 1999;54(6):1082.
52. Connolly LP, Zurakowski D, Peters CA, et al. Variability of diuresis renography interpretation due to method of post-diuretic renal pelvic clearance half-time determination. *J Urol* 2000;164(2):467.
53. Bauer SB. The challenge of the expanding role of urodynamic studies in the treatment of children with neurological and functional disabilities. *J Urol* 1998;160(2):527.
54. Schewe J, Brands FH, Pannek J. Voiding dysfunction in children: role of urodynamic studies. *Urol Int* 2002;69(4):297.

14

Vulvovaginal Complaints in the Adolescent

Elizabeth R. Woods and S. Jean Emans

Vaginitis is a common gynecologic problem in the adolescent despite the fact that she has developed a more resistant, estrogenized vaginal epithelium, pubic hair, and labial fat pads. The striking difference between prepubertal and adolescent vaginitis is the shift in etiology. Vulvovaginitis in the prepubertal child is often nonspecific and results from poor perineal hygiene, whereas vaginitis in the adolescent usually has a specific cause, such as *Candida* or a sexually acquired infection. Vaginal discharge may also be the presenting symptom in the adolescent with cervicitis secondary to *Neisseria gonorrhoeae, Chlamydia trachomatis,* or herpes simplex (1). In addition to these true infections, physiologic discharge, a normal desquamation of epithelial cells secondary to estrogen effect, is a common complaint in the pubescent girl. This chapter includes a description of the various causes of vaginitis as well as of vulvar disease (2,3), toxic shock, and the urethral syndrome. Infections with *N. gonorrhoeae* and *C. trachomatis* are covered in Chapter 15 and human papillomavirus (HPV) in Chapter 17 (4).

VAGINAL DISCHARGE

The evaluation of vaginal discharge in the adolescent should include obtaining a history of symptoms (pruritus, odor, quantity), other illnesses such as diabetes or human immunodeficiency virus (HIV) infection (5), recent oral medications such as broad-spectrum antibiotics or oral contraceptive (OC) pills, previous similar episodes of vulvovaginal symptoms, and treatments. A history of broad-spectrum antibiotics or poorly controlled diabetes mellitus is frequently a clue to the diagnosis of *Candida* vaginitis. *Candida* vaginitis and bacterial vaginosis often recur despite compliance with a standard treatment course. The patient should be questioned about recent sexual relations, since treatment failure in an adolescent girl often occurs because of reexposure to an untreated contact. It should be remembered that several infections may coexist; a patient may be adequately treated for one infection and still have a second or third infection. For example, an adolescent may have *C. trachomatis* cervicitis, *Trichomonas* vaginitis, and vulvar condyloma. In addition, the use of oral broad-spectrum antibiotics for the treatment of one type of vaginitis may be followed by a second infection with *Candida*.

An adolescent may have symptoms for weeks or months before seeking medical help because of anxiety about a pelvic examination or because of guilt or trauma from a previous episode of rape, intercourse, or sexual abuse. Therefore, it is important to explain carefully to her both the details of obtaining vaginal swabs, and a speculum examination (if indicated), and the possible causes of vaginal discharge.

The microbiologic flora of the adolescent vagina and cervix are shown in Figure 14-1 (6). Assessment usually includes a visual inspection of the vulva, wet preparations of the vaginal discharge, pH, and testing for sexually transmitted diseases (STDs) as indicated. A speculum examination is usually omitted in the young virginal adolescent who has a whitish mucoid discharge. Samples for wet preparations can be obtained with a saline-moistened, cotton-tipped applicator or Calgiswab gently inserted through the hymenal opening to confirm the diagnosis of physiologic discharge and exclude *Candida* vaginitis. In sexually active patients, several different

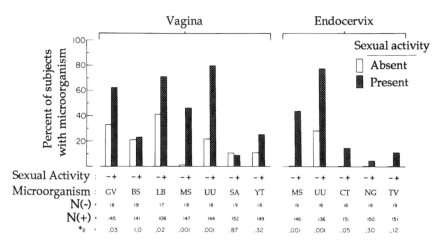

FIG. 14-1. Microbiologic isolations from vagina and endocervix in adolescent girls by presence or absence of sexual activity. BS, group B streptococcus; CT, *Chlamydia trachomatis;* GV, *Gardnerella vaginalis;* LB, lactobacillus; MS, *Mycoplasma* species; NG, *Neisseria gonorrhoeae;* SA, *Staphylococcus aureus;* TV, *Trichomonas vaginalis;* UU, *Ureaplasma urealyticum;* YT, yeast. *Chi-square statistic except for CT, NG, and TV Fischer exact test. (From Shafer MA, Sweet RL, Ohm-Smith MJ. Microbiology of the lower genital tract in postmenarcheal adolescent girls: Differences by sexual activity, contraception, and presence of nonspecific vaginitis. *J Pediatr* 1985;107:974; with permission.)

strategies for diagnosing vaginitis have been recommended. The most commonly used technique is to perform a speculum examination to obtain specimens of the vaginal discharge, pH, and endocervical tests for *N. gonorrhoeae* and *C. trachomatis* (see Chapters 1 and 15). Recent studies have focused on whether vaginal complaints can be diagnosed on the basis of urine testing for *N. gonorrhoeae* and *Chlamydia* (and *Trichomonas*) (7,8) and provider- or patient-obtained vaginal swabs for wet preps and pH (and, if available, *Trichomonas* culture) (9–13). Several studies have found that women can successfully obtain vaginal samples (a Dacron swab placed 1 inch into the distal vagina for 10 seconds) that have a high sensitivity and specificity for detection of gonorrhea, *Chlamydia,* and *Trichomonas* (14,15). Although this may have advantages, adolescents may provide less adequate vaginal pool self-sampling, and the vulva, vagina, and cervix are not visualized (missing dermatoses, condyloma acuminata, or genital herpes). Symptoms are not sufficient to distinguish between etiologies, although lack of itching makes candidiasis less likely, and lack of perceived odor makes bacterial vaginosis less likely (16). Endocervical sampling for *Chlamydia* and *N. gonorrhoeae* is preferred over urine testing if a speculum exam is being performed (4). Thus careful selection of patients with symptoms of vaginitis who might be appropriate for vaginal swabs, preferably done by a provider, without a speculum examination is important (17,18). Symptoms of abdominal pain and dyspareunia should lead to a full pelvic examination to assess the patient for pelvic inflammatory disease (PID) (18).

Inspection of the vulva is often helpful in the differential diagnosis of vulvovaginitis. A small magnifying glass can be of help. A red, edematous vulva with satellite red papules is characteristic of acute *Candida* vulvovaginitis. Fissures and excoriations are seen with subacute or chronic *Candida* infections. Vulvar dermatoses, such as psoriasis (Color Plate 20), may present with red, scaly, cutaneous plaques. Small vesicles or ulcers are typical of herpetic vulvitis (Color Plate 24). Symptomatic gonococcal cervicitis and pelvic inflammatory disease may be accompanied by a gray or greenish-yellow discharge from the vagina and urethra.

The appearance of the vaginal secretions often gives a clue to the diagnosis. A thick, curdy discharge is typical of *Candida;* a yellow or white, bubbly, frothy discharge can be typical of *Trichomonas vaginalis.* In patients with *Trichomonas* infections and those with cervicitis, the cervix may be friable and may bleed during collection of the samples. A cervical ectropion is present in many adolescents; large ectropions may be responsible for persistent vaginal discharge in adolescents, even in the absence of infection. Cervical ectopy has been associated with younger age, *C. trachomatis,* and OC use (19). Mucopurulent cervicitis (MPC) has been variably defined by the presence of mucopurulent discharge, quantitation of leukocytes in cervical exudate, easily induced cervical bleeding, and histologic examination of the cervix. The Centers for Disease Control and Prevention (CDC) definition of MPC is the presence of mucopurulent secretion visible in the endocervical canal or on an endocervical swab (1). Mucopus is evident if a yellow color is noted on a white cotton-tipped applicator inserted into the endocervical canal and twirled. The yellow color has been associated with *C. trachomatis* cervicitis in clinics that treat STDs but has a low positive predictive value (1). *N. gonorrhoeae* may also cause MPC, but often other infectious agents, not yet well-defined, cause persistent mucopus. Some women with MPC have an abnormal vaginal discharge or vaginal bleeding (such as after sexual intercourse) (1).

Microscopic examination of the wet preparations usually provides the diagnosis (see Chapter 1 and Fig. 14-2). On the saline preparation slide, trichomonads are seen as motile flagellated organisms. Sheets of normal epithelial cells are characteristic of physiologic discharge. So-called clue cells (epithelial cells coated with large numbers of refractile bacteria that obscure the cell borders) are seen in bacterial vaginosis. The potassium hydroxide (KOH) preparation is used to demonstrate the pseudohyphae of *Candida*. If the discharge is itchy or cheesy and yet no pseudohyphae are seen on the KOH preparation, a culture for *Candida* on Biggy agar is helpful.

Large numbers of leukocytes may be seen in the presence of *Trichomonas,* to a lesser extent with *Candida* vaginitis, and with cervicitis. The presence of leukocytes in the absence of a diagnosis suggests that further tests and a follow-up visit in 2 weeks may be necessary. For example, the wet preparation may miss the diagnosis of *Trichomonas* because of a sensitivity of only 50% to 75%.

An amine fishy odor when a drop of discharge is mixed with 10% KOH is a positive "whiff" test result; it occurs most commonly with bacterial vaginosis but may sometimes occur with *Trichomonas* as well. The pH of the vaginal secretions is helpful in the differential diagnosis. A normal pH of <4.5 is found in patients with normal discharge and *Candida* vaginitis, whereas the pH is elevated above 4.5 (4.7 in some studies) in patients with *Trichomonas* vaginitis and bacterial vaginosis. Gram stain of the vaginal discharge can be used to identify lactobacilli, typical of normal discharge, and to detect alterations in the flora seen in bacterial vaginosis in which gram-variable coccobacilli and curved gram-negative rods are observed. Gram stain of the endocervical mucopus can be examined for increased numbers of polymorphonuclear leukocytes and the presence of gram-negative intracellular diplococci (see Chapter 15). Tests should be done to detect *N. gonorrhoeae* and *C. trachomatis* in sexually active adolescents (4).

The Papanicolaou (Pap) test, if obtained, can sometimes be helpful in the diagnosis of discharge. Herpes simplex is associated with intranuclear inclusions and multinucleate giant cells. *Chlamydia* has been associated with inflammation, cytoplasmic inclusions, and transformed lymphocytes or increased histiocytes. *Trichomonas* may be seen on Pap test, but false-positives are not infrequent and should be confirmed with a wet preparation or culture in the asymptomatic patient. The Pap test has been noted to have a sensitivity of 17% to 58% for the detection of *C. trachomatis,* 3% to 49% for *Candida,* 25% for bacterial vaginosis, 33% to 79% for *Trichomonas,* and 25% to 66% for herpes simplex (20,21). Recent studies suggest that fluid from new liquid based Pap tests may be used to detect *C. trachomatis* (22–24). Multiple tests from the same specimen may be available in the future. In a study of STD patients, Paavonen and colleagues (25) found on colposcopic evaluation that endocervical mu-

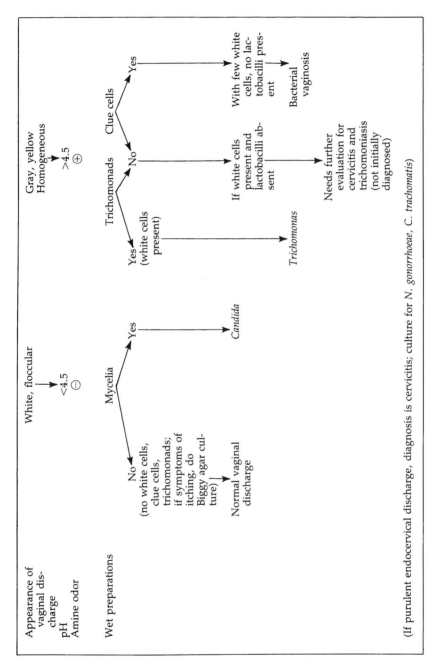

FIG. 14-2. Differential diagnosis of vaginitis.

copus was associated with *N. gonorrhoeae, C. trachomatis,* and herpes simplex; ulcers, necrotic areas, and increased surface vascularity with herpes simplex; strawberry cervix (uniformly arranged red spots or stippling of a few millimeters in size, located on the squamous epithelium covering the ectocervix) with *Trichomonas;* hypertrophic cervicitis with *C. trachomatis;* and immature metaplasia with *C. trachomatis* and cytomegalovirus.

Therapy is aimed at the specific cause. Patients should avoid douches because douching has been associated with an increased risk of PID (26) and reduced fertility (27). When one STD has been detected, the clinician should test the patient for others, including serology for syphilis. Counseling about prevention, abstinence, safer sex, and the use of condoms is essential.

In most situations, therapy should include the following:

1. Warm baths once or twice a day (baking soda may be added if the vulva is irritated). Only bland soaps should be used.
2. Careful drying after the bath and application of a small amount of baby powder (no talc) to the vulva.
3. Frequent changes of white cotton underpants or panty shields to absorb the discharge.
4. Good perineal hygiene (including wiping from front to back after bowel movements).
5. Avoidance of bubble bath or other chemical irritants.

Physiologic Discharge

Agent: A normal estrogen effect.

Symptoms: A whitish mucoid discharge that usually starts before menarche and may continue for several years. With the establishment of more regular cycles, the adolescent may notice a cyclic variation in vaginal secretions: copious mucoid or watery secretions at midcycle and then a stickier, scantier white discharge in the second half of the cycle associated with rising progesterone levels.

Diagnosis: The wet preparation reveals epithelial cells without evidence of inflammation.

Treatment: Most health classes that discuss puberty and menarche do not include an explanation of the change in vaginal secretions. The clinician can reassure the patient by explaining vaginal physiology and can suggest measures to help if she is bothered by the discharge—baths, cotton underpants, and, as needed, some form of panty shield that she can change frequently. If an older adolescent is troubled by excessive discharge, especially during jogging or athletics, evaluation of the cervix and vagina may be indicated. The use of a conventional tampon (not a superabsorbent tampon) during athletics for a few hours at midcycle can help the adolescent cope with the heavy discharge. It is extremely important that she not be overtreated with vaginal creams and given the impression that the physiologic discharge represents an infection. It is also important to discourage the daily use of tampons because of the possibility of vaginal ulcers and exacerbation of the discharge.

Trichomonal Vaginitis

Agent: Trichomonas vaginalis, a small, motile, flagellated parasite.

Symptoms: Frothy, malodorous, yellow or white discharge that may cause itching, dysuria, postcoital bleeding, dyspareunia, or any combination of these symptoms. May be asymptomatic and found on culture, Pap test, or wet preparation (21,28). *Trichomonas* infects the vagina, urethra, and Skene and Bartholin glands.

Source: Usually sexually acquired. Males are usually asymptomatic or have urethritis, but may reinfect the female after she is treated. Since *Trichomonas* may survive for several hours in urine and wet towels, the possibility of transmission by sharing wash cloths has been suggested but not proved; it is unlikely to occur frequently, given the association of this infection with other sexually transmitted diseases. The incubation time has been estimated to be between 4 and 20 days with an average of 7 days. The incidence of *Trichomonas* has decreased over the past two decades (1,29).

Diagnosis: The vulva may be erythematous or excoriated, with a visible discharge evident on inspection. The classic yellow-green discharge is seen in 20% to 35% of patients; more often the discharge is gray or white. A frothy discharge is seen in about 10% of women and may also occur with bacterial vaginosis. Grossly visible punctate hemorrhages and swollen papillae (strawberry cervix) are seen in only about 2% of patients (15% of a STD population evaluated by colposcopy). By colposcopy, this special finding had a 45% sensitivity and a 99% specificity for *Trichomonas* (25).

The wet preparation may show flagellated organisms moving under the coverslip along with an increase in the number of leukocytes, which can be visualized using both low and high power of the microscope (22,30,31). The vaginal wet mount is far from a perfect tool; it detects 64% of infections in asymptomatically infected women, 75% of those with clinical vaginitis, and 80% of those with characteristic symptoms. Philip and coworkers (32) found that the wet mount gave a positive result only in patients whose cultures had $>10^5$ colony-forming units/ml. The sensitivity of culture methods such as Diamond and Holander is higher (95% to 96%), as are newer tests such as DFA (85%), PCR (89% to 100%), and EIA (82%) (28,33,34). The office-based InPouch TV culture method also has higher sensitivity (84%) than the wet mount (35–37). The combination of wet mount and spun urine has a sensitivity of 85% compared to 73% for the vaginal wet mount alone (7). Recent studies show that

PCR has high detection rates and 97% to 98% specificity for vaginal samples (38,39). PCR for urine samples has a lower sensitivity of 64% to 83% with 99% to 100% specificity (38,39). Pap tests have a detection rate of only 50% to 86%, and false-positive results can occur with conventional Pap tests (21). If asymptomatic women are treated only on the basis of a positive Pap test, 20% to 30% may be treated unnecessarily (21,30). When the prevalence in the clinical population of *Trichomonas* is 10% or less, a positive Pap test should be confirmed with culture or other more sensitive test (21). If the prevalence is ≥20%, then treatment is suggested (21). Liquid-based Pap tests appear to provide higher sensitivity (61%) and specificity (99%) in an adult population with a prevalence of 21% (40). Monoclonal antibody staining has been reported to detect 86% of positive specimens, including 92% of those with positive wet mounts and 77% of those missed on wet mount (28). Bacterial vaginosis and *Trichomonas* vaginitis may occur simultaneously, and *Trichomonas* facilitates the growth of anaerobic bacteria.

Treatment: Metronidazole, 2.0 g orally all in one dose, is effective in 86% to 95% of patients (1). It is important that the sexual partner be treated with the same dose at the same time. The side effects of metronidazole include nausea, vomiting, headache, metallic aftertaste, and rarely blood dyscrasias. The patient should be instructed to avoid alcohol and intercourse until both partners have been treated. If the clinician does not wish to provide treatment for the partner, the partner can be referred to his own clinician (although trichomonads are difficult to document in the male).

If the organisms persist in the vagina after two courses of single-dose metronidazole, and if reinfection is not the cause, a longer course of metronidazole can be tried: 500 mg orally twice daily for 7 days (1). Recurrent infection necessitates retreating the partner(s) each time and making sure the relationship is monogamous; otherwise, the patient should understand the futility of repeated treatment. In an urban gynecology clinic in Atlanta, 2.4% of the isolates showed low level in vitro resistance; all treated women who returned for repeat examination had cleared the infection (41).

Rarely, a patient will have a *Trichomonas* infection that has relative resistance to metronidazole and is refractory to treatment (42,43). The patient can be treated with 2 g per day of metronidazole orally for 3 to 5 days. Patients not responding to the regimen should be managed in consultation with an expert (such as the CDC), and the susceptibility of the *Trichomonas* to metronidazole should be determined (1). Lossick and colleagues (42) reported the need for an average oral dose of 2.6 g per day of metronidazole for a mean period of 9 days to cure refractory *Trichomonas*. Neurologic side effects are common if >3 g is taken orally in a day. A complete blood count should be done before prolonged therapy is undertaken.

Pregnancy: No birth defects have been associated with the drug (1,44). Patients with symptoms may be treated with a single 2-g dose of metronidazole.

Candida Vaginitis

Agent: Candida albicans accounts for 60% to 80% of vaginal fungal infections; other *Candida* species, including *Candida glabrata* (20%) and *Candida tropicalis* (6% to 23%), also cause similar symptoms (45,46). Non-albicans species may be more difficult to eradicate with current therapies.

Symptoms: Thick, white, cheesy, pruritic discharge. The vulva may be red and edematous. Itching may occur before and after menses and, in some patients, seems to remit at midcycle. Patients may experience dyspareunia with an increase in symptoms after intercourse. Many patients have external irritation and dysuria.

Source: The predisposing factors to *Candida* vaginitis include diabetes mellitus, pregnancy, antibiotics, corticosteroids, obesity, and tight-fitting undergarments. The frequency of positive cultures rises from 2.2% to 16% by the end of pregnancy. The increase in clinical infections appears to be associated with the rise in pH that occurs in late pregnancy as well as premenstrually (47). Infections are more common in the summer. *Candida* may occur as part of the normal flora in 10% to 20% of women; eradication of *Candida* as determined by culture, however, appears to be important in patients with frequent recurrences. Recurrent *Candida* vaginitis may be the first presenting symptom of HIV disease in women. *Candida* is not seen more commonly in STD clinics than in other settings, and sexual transmission rarely plays a role (48,49). Males may have symptomatic balanitis or penile dermatitis.

Diagnosis: The vulva is usually red and may be edematous, with small satellite red papules or fissures at the posterior fourchette. The KOH preparation shows filamentous forms in 80% to 90% of symptomatic patients (Fig. 14-3A). In patients with suggestive signs or symptoms and especially in patients previously labeled as having recurrent *Candida* infections, it is important to obtain specimens for culture from the vagina before more aggressive therapy is undertaken. The easiest office culture medium is Biggy agar, which can be read for the presence of brown colonies after 3 to 7 days of incubation (Fig. 14-3B). Sabouraud agar can also be used. Most patients with symptomatic infections have a large number of colonies; however, even a few colonies may be significant in the woman with frequent infections who has recently finished a treatment course. In cases difficult to diagnose, the patient may be shown how to inoculate a culture at home with a cotton-tipped applicator when her symptoms increase.

Treatment: The options for therapy include intravaginal preparations and oral agents. The azoles are the mainstay of intravaginal treatment. Courses of therapy range from a single dose to 3 to 7 days of therapy with creams or suppositories for *uncomplicated infections* (mild to moderate, sporadic, normal host, susceptible *Candida albicans*). *Complicated infections* (severe local or recurrent infections in an ab-

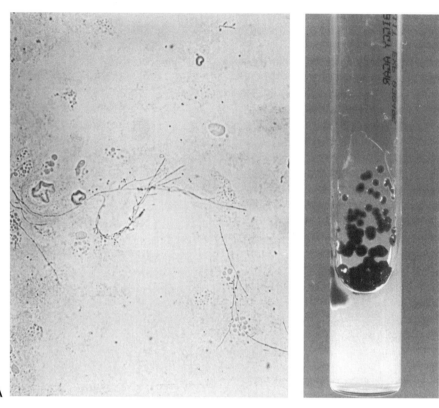

A

B

FIG. 14-3. *Candida* vaginitis. **A:** Potassium hydroxide preparation showing pseudohyphae. (From Syntex slide collection, Palo Alto, CA; with permission.) **B:** Biggy agar culture with multiple brown colonies.

normal host, such as diabetes, debilitation, immunosuppressed, or pregnant, or less susceptible pathogen such as *Candida glabrata*) require 10 to 14 days of topical or oral azoles. The suppositories are less messy than creams but may not treat vulvar infection as well. The symptomatic male partner can use the cream as well. Some packaging contains both suppositories and cream (e.g., Monistat Dual-Pak, Gyne-Lotrimin Combination Pack). The efficacy of treatment, as judged by symptomatic improvement and negative cultures after any of the available treatment courses with azoles, is approximately 85% to 90% at the end of therapy and 70% to 80% 3 weeks later. Allergic symptoms to the azoles are often manifested by increased burning and itching after several days of therapy. Nystatin is probably less effective because it requires the patient to comply with 2 weeks of therapy; however, it is useful in women who develop allergic symptoms to the azoles. A small study found topical boric acid (600 mg powder in a gelatin capsule administered intravaginally once daily for 14 days) to yield a moderate success rate in women with *T. glabrata,* which has been more difficult to treat with some antifungal creams (1,50). The intravaginal treatment doses are as follows (presented alphabetically) (1):

Butoconazole, 2% cream, one applicatorful (5 g) for 3 nights*
Butoconazole, 2% cream (5 g) (sustained release), for 1 night
Clotrimazole, 1% cream, one applicatorful (5 g) for 7 to 14 nights*
Clotrimazole, 100-mg vaginal tablet for 7 nights
Clotrimazole, 100-mg vaginal tablets, 2 tablets for 3 nights
Clotrimazole, 500-mg vaginal tablet for 1 night
Miconazole, 2% cream, one applicatorful (5 g) for 7 nights*
Miconazole, 200-mg vaginal suppository for 3 nights*
Miconazole, 100-mg vaginal suppository for 7 nights*
Nystatin, 100,000-unit vaginal tablet for 14 nights
Tioconazole, 6.5% ointment, one applicatorful (5 g) for 1 night*
Terconazole, 0.4% cream, 1 applicatorful (5 g) for 7 nights
Terconazole, 0.8% cream, 1 applicatorful (5 g) for 3 nights
Terconazole, 80-mg vaginal suppository for 3 nights

The base of some of these suppositories and creams may interact with latex products, including diaphragms and condoms, and thus the patient should be informed of this possibility.

Oral therapy with fluconazole 150 mg given as a single dose has the same efficacy as 3- and 7-day courses of the azole antifungal topical agents (1,51). The reported adverse effects of oral therapy have included headache (13%), nausea (7%), and abdominal pain (6%); rare cases of angioedema, anaphylaxis, and hepatotoxicity have been reported. The important drug interactions include those with terfenadine, rifampin, astemizole, phenytoin, cyclosporin A, tacrolimus, coumadin, protease inhibitors, oral hypoglycemic agents, calcium channel antagonists, theophylline, trimetrexate, and possibly OCs (1). In contrast, the primary side effects of topical agents are local burning and dysuria. Patients may prefer the ease of a single oral dose but should be counseled about the risks and benefits. For complicated infections, fluconazole can be given on days 1 and 4 or days 1, 4, and 7.

Only topical agents should be used during pregnancy (for significant symptoms); treatments that have been studied for use in the second and third trimesters include clotrimazole, miconazole, butoconazole, and terconazole. Absorption is negligible with tioconazole and clotrimazole and does not occur with nystatin (1). Pregnant patients should be treated for 7 days.

Recurrent vulvovaginal candidiasis, defined as four or more symptomatic episodes annually, can be very difficult to treat. The most important issue is to make sure that the diagnosis is in fact *Candida*. Patients may have inflammation of the minor vestibular glands, HPV infection, or allergies to soaps, spermicides, or rarely semen.

*Available over the counter.

Once the diagnosis of *Candida* has been confirmed, the clinician should check for predisposing factors such as diabetes. Looser-fitting clothing and nondeodorized panty shields can be recommended. Any douching equipment should be cultured or discarded. The potential for a gastrointestinal reservoir in the patient or partner should be considered. In addition, the patient may not have purchased the medication because of cost or may not have finished the previously prescribed dosage. In adolescents with recurrent *Candida* infections and risk factors, HIV infection should be considered.

Many patients who have experienced frequent recurrences of *Candida* vulvovaginitis in the past have symptomatic improvement with *one* of the following treatments: vaginal clotrimazole (500 mg) once a week *or* once a month *or* an antifungal vaginal cream for 2 to 3 days before and after each menses *or* a vaginal cream "always on Sunday" *or* a vaginal cream for 1 to 3 days at the first sign of itching or other symptoms. While prophylactic monthly clotrimazole treatment results in fewer episodes over a 6-month period, empiric self-treatment for symptoms is less expensive and is preferred by many (52).

Ketoconazole, itraconazole, and fluconazole have been studied as agents for chronic or recurrent candidiasis in women with a decrease in symptomatic recurrences (53,54). The doses given for 6 months have included fluconazole (100 to 150 mg once weekly or monthly), ketoconazole (100 mg daily) or itraconazole (400 mg once monthly or 100 mg daily) (1). Relapse after treatment is common even with long-term oral therapy, and the risks of using these and other oral agents needs to be carefully considered because of their potential for hepatotoxicity. Sexual partners are treated if they have symptomatic balanitis or penile dermatitis.

Bacterial Vaginosis

Agent. Bacterial vaginosis (BV) results from the complex alteration of microbial flora of the vagina. Although *Gardnerella vaginalis* is found in most patients with this diagnosis, it is also found in many asymptomatic patients, including nonsexually experienced young women. Bacterial vaginosis results from an increased concentration of *G. vaginalis,* anaerobic organisms (especially *Bacteroides* and *Mobiluncus* species) and *Mycoplasma hominis* with an absence of normal hydrogen peroxide-producing lactobacilli (31,55–59). The overgrowth results in an elevated vaginal pH and the production of amines, putrescine, and cadaverine, which cause the typical fishy malodor that patients experience. Gas–liquid chromatographic studies show an increase in acetate, propionate, isobutyrate, butyrate, and isovalerate, with an increase in the succinate/lactate ratio of 0.4. Bacterial vaginosis occurs in 4% to 15% of college students, 10% to 25% of pregnant women, and 30% to 37% of women attending an STD clinic. The presence of BV has been associated with postpartum endometritis, premature labor and premature rupture of membranes, preterm delivery of low-birthweight infants, irregular menstrual bleeding, and PID (especially following invasive procedures) (60–63). The treatment of bacterial vaginosis with antibiotics such as metronidazole appears to be effective in reducing preterm births in patients with a history of prematurity in the previous pregnancy (60–64).

Symptoms: Malodorous discharge; associated symptoms may be abdominal pain and irregular or prolonged menses.

Source: Occurs commonly in sexually active patients, but can occur in virginal patients and in lesbians. Risk factors have included absence of hydrogen peroxide–producing lactobacilli in the vagina, lack of condom use, douching, a new sexual partner, anal intercourse, uncleaned insertive sexual toys (65), an intrauterine device, prior STD, and smoking. Because semen binds hydrogen peroxide-producing lactobacilli, condom use is protective against getting BV. The anaerobes associated with bacterial vaginosis are commonly found in the rectum of women with this diagnosis (66).

Diagnosis: The pelvic examination reveals a homogeneous, malodorous, yellow, white, or gray discharge adherent to the vaginal walls, in contrast to the normal clumped or floccular discharge. Three of four criteria should be met to make the clinical diagnosis: (a) homogeneous white noninflammatory discharge adherent to the vaginal walls, (b) pH $\geq$ 4.5 (in one study, pH $\geq$ 4.7 [56]); (c) positive "whiff" test result (a fishy or amine odor noted before or after addition of 1 drop of 10% KOH to a sample of the vaginal discharge); and (d) the presence of clue cells, making up at least 20% of the cells (Fig. 14-4) (1).

Gram stain of the vaginal discharge can also be useful if available (58,67). A positive determination is made if four or fewer lactobacilli are seen per oil immersion field and if *Gardnerella* morphologic types plus one or more other bacterial morphologic types (gram-positive cocci, small gram-negative rods, curved gram-variable rod, or fusiforms) are detected. Making a diagnosis only on the basis of Gram stain findings or a Pap test may result in overdiagnosis of bacterial vaginosis. In a high-prevalence STD clinic population, the Gram stain had a 97% sensitivity, 79% specificity, and 69% positive predictive value for bacterial vaginosis (56). Homogeneous discharge was found in 69%, pH $\geq$ 4.7 in 97%, positive "whiff" test result in 43%, and clue cells ($\geq$20% of epithelial cells) in 78% of patients with bacterial vaginosis. The whiff test was the least sensitive test, and the pH was the least specific test, since 47% of patients without bacterial vaginosis had elevated pH. A pH of $\leq$4.4 and a predominance of lactobacilli on wet mount or Gram stain are useful in excluding the diagnosis of bacterial vaginosis. Cultures for *G. vaginalis* are not helpful and should not be obtained in diagnosing this condition. Simple point of care tests (such as Affirm, FemExam test card, and Pip Activity TestCard) may be useful in a setting with limited microscopic ability (1,11,37). A variety of tests including PCR, a rapid DNA hybridization test (85% to 94% and 96% to 98% specific), and immunofluorescent test are sensitive and are in development (68,69).

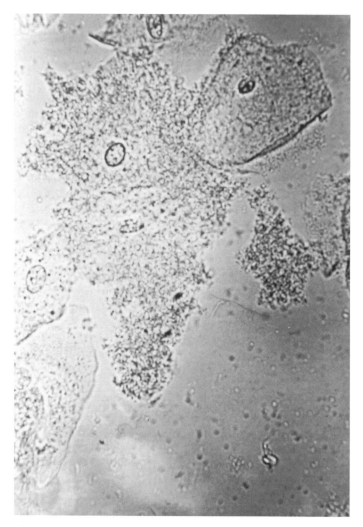

FIG. 14-4. Clue cells in bacterial vaginosis. (From Syntex slide collection, Palo Alto, CA; with permission.)

Treatment: Treatment is usually prescribed only to symptomatic women. However, because of the link between BV and PID and invasive procedures, as well as the evidence that metronidazole reduces postabortion PID, the treatment of symptomatic and asymptomatic BV may be considered before surgical abortion procedures are performed. The standard therapies for nonpregnant patients are oral metronidazole, 500 mg twice a day for 7 days, which results in cure rates of 95% (70); or metronidazole gel 0.75%, one applicatorful (5 g) intravaginally once a day for 5 days (71); clindamycin cream 2%, one applicatorful (5 g) intravaginally at bedtime for 7 days (1). Alternatives are clindamycin 300 mg, orally twice a day for 7 days (72), clindamycin ovules 100 mg once at bedtime for 3 days, or single-dose metronidazole (2 g), which is less effective (84%, with a range of 52% to 90% and even less effective in HIV positive women), especially if follow-up is done at 3 weeks instead of just 1 week after the completion of therapy (70,73). Treatment of the partner with metronidazole has not diminished recurrences in the woman and is not recommended, but the patient should not have intercourse during treatment. Condoms should be recommended for at least a month, with the hope of allowing the recolonization of the hydrogen peroxide-producing lactobacilli. Patients should be discouraged from douching. Recurrences are common in the year following treatment. For greater than three episodes, oral or vaginal metronidazole for 7 to 10 days and then twice a week (Sundays, Wednesdays) and use of condoms reduces recurrences. Although recolonizing the vagina with commercially available strains of lactobacilli has not proved effective, a trial of intravaginal colonization with hydrogen peroxide-producing *Lactobacillus crispatus* in addition to metronidazole has increased resolution of signs of BV at follow-up (74).

Low-risk pregnant women with symptomatic BV should be treated with metronidazole 250 mg 3 times a day for 7 days (alternatives: metronidazole gel; metronidazole 2 g single dose; or clindamycin 300 mg twice a day). Data has been conflicting on the use of clindamycin vaginal cream, but a recent study showed that a 3-day course decreased preterm birth (4%) compared to placebo (10%) (75). In general, antibiotics do not affect the likelihood of low-risk patients having a preterm birth but are helpful for high-risk women with a previous preterm delivery (59,76). Women in the later category who are asymptomatic may also be screened in the second trimester and treated with oral or topical medication (1).

Vaginitis Secondary to a Foreign Body

Agent: In adolescents, usually a retained tampon.

Symptoms: Foul-smelling, often bloody discharge.

Diagnosis: Examination.

Treatment: Removal of the foreign body, and if needed, gentle irrigation of the vagina with warm water.

Genital Herpes

Agent: Usually herpes simplex virus type 2 (HSV-2), but 5% to 15% of first episodes are caused by type 1 (HSV-1). Herpes infections can be divided into primary first episodes, in which the patient has no antibody to HSV-1 or HSV-2; nonprimary first episodes, in which the patient does have antibody to one type (usually a type 2 infection with antibodies to type 1); and recurrences. Primary first episodes are responsible for approximately 60% of first episodes and nonprimary infections for the other 40% of first episodes. Three percent of nonprimary first episodes and 2% of recurrences are caused by HSV-1 (77,78).

In patients with simultaneous oral and genital HSV infections, Lafferty and associates (79) showed that oral labial recurrences occurred in 5 of 12 patients with HSV-1 and 1 of 27 with HSV-2, whereas genital recurrences occurred in 2 of 27 with HSV-1 and 24 of 27 with HSV-2. Mean monthly recurrences were 0.33/month for genital HSV-2, 0.12/month for oral HSV-1, 0.02/month for genital HSV-1, and 0.001/month for oral HSV-2. Over the course of a year after the first episode, 14% of patients with HSV-1 and 60% of those with HSV-2 will have a recurrence. The recurrence rate may decrease after the first year (78–83).

Asymptomatic genital shedding of HSV has been reported in 1.6% to 8.0% of women in STD clinics and 0.25 to 1.5% of women in private gynecology practices. PCR has detected HSV DNA in genital specimens of HSV-2 seropositive women 28% of days (84). Although symptomatic patients are most infectious, asymptomatic patients may spread HSV to their partners (83–85). Seroepidemiologic studies in adults have suggested that the prevalence of HSV-2 is high (<1% in under-15-year-olds to 20% in 30- to 40 year olds) (86). Twenty-two percent of women attending a family planning clinic (87), 46% of women attending a STD clinic, and 8.8% of university students (88) had serologic evidence of HSV-2 infection. Among the HSV-2-seropositive women in the STD clinic, only 22% had symptoms, 4% had viral shedding without symptoms, 16% had formerly had symptomatic episodes, and 58% had neither shedding nor a history of clinical episodes (89). The characteristic external genital ulcers were present in only 66% of patients with positive HSV cultures. Atypical lesions included fissures, furuncles, excoriations, and nonspecific vulvar erythema. Also, HSV was noted to cause 29 of 33 cervical ulcers; anorectal infections were common. Herpes simplex may occur in 5% of women with dysuria and frequency.

Symptoms: In primary infections, vesicles appear on the labia, vestibule, vagina, and/or cervix; they rupture in 1 to 3 days and produce small painful ulcers (Color Plate 24). The patient experiences local burning and irritation, dysuria, and inguinal adenopathy. Systemic symptoms are often present, including headache, fever, myalgia, and malaise. Patients may also have neurologic symptoms such as aseptic meningitis, sacral anesthesia, urinary retention, and constipation that may last for 4 to 8 weeks. Anorectal symptoms in primary infections include discharge, pain, and tenesmus. Large numbers of virus are shed from the lesions and, usually, from the cervix. Positive cultures persist for 8 to 10 days and sometimes for as long as 2 weeks. Symptoms improve in 10 days to 3 weeks (Fig. 14-5).

The symptoms associated with recurrences are less marked and shorter in duration (3 to 5 days) than those of primary infections. The number of lesions is also less, and

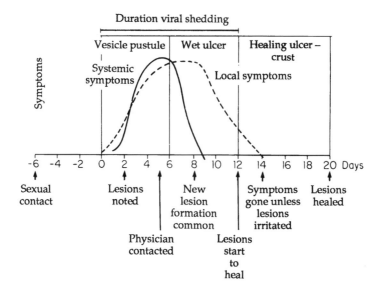

FIG. 14-5. The clinical course of primary genital herpes. (From Corey L, Adams HG, Brow ZA, et al. Genital herpes simplex virus infections: clinical manifestation, course, and complications. *Ann Intern Med* 1983;98:958; with permission.)

the lesions are generally external rather than vaginal or cervical and may be atypical (fissures as well as ulcers). The mean healing time was 8.0 ± 2.8 days in a study by Guinan and coworkers (90) of college students. Many patients experience a prodrome of neuralgia in the buttocks, groin, or legs and itching or burning 24 hours before the herpetic lesions recur. Virus is shed in lesser amounts for 4 to 5 days and is usually markedly diminished by the sixth to seventh day. Nonprimary first-episode infections with HSV have a time course for symptoms and viral shedding that is intermediate between those for primary herpes and recurrent herpes (Fig. 14–6). Extragenital sites may occur on the buttocks, groin, thighs, pharynx, fingers, and conjunctiva. HIV infected patients and other immunocompromised young women may have severe persistent herpes infection and often require prolonged therapy with antiviral agents.

Source: Sexually acquired. The incubation period is 2 to 10 days but may be 1 to 28 days or longer (91). The partner who transmits the genital herpes may be asymptomatic.

Diagnosis: Inspection and cultures. A tender, painful vesicle, pustule, or yellowish ulcer should make the clinician think of HSV. A scraping from the base of a lesion that is stained with Wright's stain (a Tzanck preparation), may reveal multinucleate giant cells and inclusions but the sensitivity is low (30% to 50%). The Pap test may show characteristic changes of intranuclear inclusions and multinucleated cells

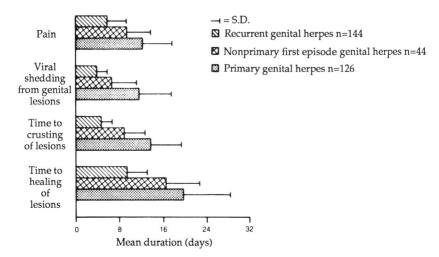

FIG. 14-6. Comparison of the mean duration of symptoms and signs in female patients with first episode, nonprimary first episode, and recurrent genital herpes. SD, standard deviation. (From Corey L, Adams HG, Brow ZA, et al. Genital herpes simplex virus infections: clinical manifestation, course, and complications. *Ann Intern Med* 1983;98:958; with permission.)

(40% to 50% sensitive). Colposcopy of the cervix may reveal ulcers and necrotic areas and increased surface vascularity (68% sensitive and 98.5% specific for the diagnosis of cervical HSV) (25).

The most common diagnostic technique is viral culture. The virus grows rapidly, and within several days a definitive diagnosis of HSV-1 or HSV-2 can usually be made (laboratories generally hold the culture for 2 weeks before reporting a negative). The rate of positivity of the culture depends on the timing and the type of infection. For example, HSV can be cultured from 94% of vesicles, 70% of ulcers (82% first episode, 42% recurrent), and 27% of crusted lesions (92). Culture of the cervix will yield HSV in 80% to 88% of primary first episodes, 65% of nonprimary first episodes, and 12% of recurrent episodes (81). In culturing a genital lesion, the vesicle should be unroofed and a sterile swab rubbed vigorously over the base. An ulcer can be similarly swabbed. The swab should then be placed immediately into viral transport media and processed as soon as possible. It is cost effective to swab several lesions and place the separate swabs into the same viral media (89).

Immunofluorescent techniques using fluorescein-labeled monoclonal antibodies are 50% to 80% sensitive, depending in part on the site of sampling; vulvar lesions are more likely to be positive than cervical swabs (83). The sensitivities of the commercial type-specific enzyme immunoassays are similar to that of the culture of early vesiculopustular lesions (91% to 100%), but better than that of the culture of later-stage, crusted lesions (58% vs. 26% culture positive) (83,93). PCR tests are likely to become the preferred method (1,92,94–96).

Documenting a conversion from negative titer (no antibodies detected) to a positive titer in a previously uninfected patient (no HSV-1 or HSV-2) can be useful in some clinical situations in which cultures are negative and primary infection is suspected. The absence of antibody on two occasions 2 to 3 weeks apart can help eliminate the diagnosis. A rise of IgM antibody followed by IgG antibody is most convincing of recent infection. A fourfold rise in titer is more difficult to interpret because it may indicate a new infection with a different type or a significant recurrence. In addition, the antibody tests done by many commercial laboratories have cross-reactivity between HSV-1 and HSV-2. Assays vary in sensitivity, and thus interpretation can be problematic. Titers with type-specific assays are useful in research settings and may soon be used as a more general screening test, especially for detection of possible discordant couples and for retrospective diagnosis (1). Viral shedding is variable (4% to 75% of days) and transmission is greatest when lesions are present (82). In discordant couples, when condoms were used more than 70% of the time, transmission was reduced by more that 60% (82). High titers of HIV are present in HSV genital lesions (84).

Treatment. Antiviral therapy with acyclovir and other similar drugs can shorten the duration of symptoms and viral shedding, prevent the formation of new lesions, reduce transmission and reduce systemic symptoms, but it is not curative, and initial therapy does not prevent later recurrences. Oral acyclovir 200 mg five times a day, or 400 mg three times a day (1), or oral valacyclovir 1 g twice daily and famciclovir 250 mg three times a day for 7 to 10 days (or until clinical resolution) are recommended for symptomatic primary genital herpes. Acyclovir 400 mg five times a day for 10 days (or until clinical resolution) is recommended for herpes proctitis (1). Higher doses of acyclovir for genital herpes do not decrease the symptoms or modify the time to first recurrence (97). Adjunctive measures include sitz baths in tepid water or Burow solution, dry heat (low or cool setting on a hair dryer), and/or lidocaine jelly 2% applied to the genital area. Patients may need to void in the shower or into a sitz bath if the lesions cause urinary retention. Analgesics may be necessary, but narcotics have the potential to worsen urinary retention. Occasionally, patients with severe genital lesions and systemic symptoms require hospitalization and treatment with oral or intravenous acyclovir, urinary catheterization, and bed rest. The side effects of intravenous acyclovir include phlebitis and transient reversible elevation of serum creatinine. Care must be taken to ensure adequate hydration. Nausea, vomiting, diarrhea, and headache may occur with intravenous or oral acyclovir. *Candida* vaginitis often accompanies or follows genital HSV infection.

Recurrences can usually be treated symptomatically with local measures in immunocompetent patients. However, if recurrences are severe and treatment can be started during the prodrome, acyclovir 400 mg three times a day for 5 days, or 800 mg twice a day for 5 days, or 200 mg five times a day for 5 days, valacyclovir 500 mg twice daily or 1.0 gram once a day for 3–5 days can be prescribed or famciclovir 125 mg twice a day for 5 days (1,98). Early treatment of recurrences for 3 to 5 days reduces the episode duration and development of lesions (99). Frequent recurrences (at least six times per year) can be suppressed with acyclovir, 400 mg twice a day for 1 year; however, recurrences may begin anew after the treatment has ended (1). Other options are famciclovir 250 mg twice a day and valacyclovir 500 mg or 1 g once a day. Toxicity of acyclovir does not appear to be a problem even when treatment lasts as long as 3 years, but treatment should be stopped once a year so that the clinical course can be reassessed. Suppressive therapy with valacyclovir 500 mg daily reduces transmission of genital herpes by 48% in HSV-2 discordant couples (100). Acyclovir-resistant strains can be recovered from healthy immunocompetent patients but have not been a treatment problem (101). Resistant strains among immunosuppressed and HIV-positive patients require alternative therapy. Acyclovir should not be used for recurrent herpes in pregnancy. New treatments with Interferon-α and $-\beta$, immune response modifiers (Resiquimod), and nucleoside analogues are being developed. Vaccines are also being studied.

Cultures from pregnant women with a previous history of HSV have not been found to be cost effective in preventing neonatal HSV. Women at high risk of transmitting infection to their newborns are those with a primary infection during the third trimester and those with active genital lesions at the time of vaginal delivery. Unfortunately, many mothers who give birth to babies with severe HSV are asymptomatic. In identifying HSV-2-seropositive patients, a detailed history of genital symptoms has not been found to be superior to a simple question asking the woman whether she has ever had genital herpes (102). The current guidelines of the American College of Obstetrics and Gynecology should be followed.

Patients with genital lesions from HSV should not have intercourse until the lesions heal. Although condoms can prevent the transmission of virus, the location of the lesions makes protection with barrier methods difficult. Patients should be educated about the risk of recurrence, the possibility of transmission, the availability of antiviral suppression (84), and the avoidance of self-inoculation to the mouth, eyes, and fingers.

Molluscum Contagiosum

Agent: Molluscum contagiosum virus (a pox virus).

Symptom: Firm, umbilicated lesions on the vulva, groin, thighs, and buttocks (Fig. 14-7).

Source: Close contact.

Diagnosis: Typical pearly surface with central umbilication.

Treatment: Curettage is definitive for individual lesions but can scar. Liquid nitrogen is effective but can be painful, and cantherone has been used topically.

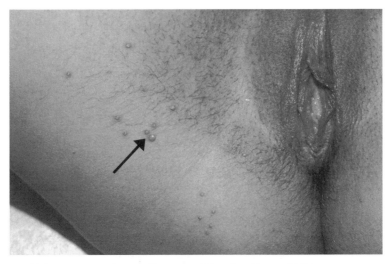

FIG. 14-7. Molluscum contagiosum. (Courtesy of Jonathan Trager, M.D.)

Imiquimod 5% cream (Aldara) has been used in similar dosing schedules (or 5 times per week) as for genital warts and in a small series appeared effective in 6 of 13 children and 14 of 19 adults (103). Lesions can spread with scratching and new lesions can appear after treatment.

Pediculosis Pubis (Crabs)

Agent: Phthirus pubis (crab lice).

Symptom: Pruritus.

Source: Close physical contact, infested blankets and clothing.

Diagnosis: On inspection, small, moving adult lice or minute, firmly attached flakes (1- to 2-mm nits, eggs) are visible on the pubic hair, often near the base of the hair follicle.

Treatment: One percent permethrin creme rinse (Nix) is applied and washed off after 10 minutes or 0.5% malathion lotion applied to dry hair and washed off in 8 to 12 hours. Alternatively, pyrethrins (RID, A-200 Pyrinate, Lice) may be applied and washed off after 10 minutes. After rinsing, the hair should be cleaned with a fine-tooth comb. If symptoms persist, the patient should be reevaluated in 1 week to check for lice or nits at the hair-skin junction; if lice or nits are found, the patient is retreated. Sex partners within the last month should be treated. Clothing and blankets should be laundered and machine-dried using the heat cycle or dry-cleaned or set aside for at least 72 hours (1,104). Some resistant strains are appearing worldwide and appear to be sensitive to malathion.

Scabies

Agent: Sarcoptes scabiei (scabies).

Symptom: Pruritus, especially at night. Lesions most commonly occur in the interdigital spaces and flexor surfaces of the waist, axillae, feet, wrist, and ankles; they can also occur in the lower abdomen and groin. Sensitization precedes pruritus and can take weeks to develop, but symptoms return with recurrences within 24 hours.

Source: Sexually acquired in adults, but not in children.

Diagnosis: Inspection of linear burrows. Unroofing of lesion to look for characteristic eggs and parasite.

Treatment: Five percent permethrin cream applied to body from neck down and washed off after 8 to 14 hours. The alternative treatment is ivermectin 200 μg/kg, orally, repeated in 2 weeks (1). Another option is 10% crotamiton once a day for two days with a cleansing bath 48 hours after last application, but there are frequent treatment failures (105). Bedding and clothing should be machine washed with hot water or dry-cleaned, or removed for at least 72 hours. Scabies epidemics in institutional settings have been controlled by oral treatment of the entire population. Crusted scabies (Norwegian scabies) occurs in immunodeficient, debilitated or malnourished persons. A combination of topical scabicide and oral ivermectin treatment is optimal for crusted scabies (1,104,106). Reinfection is common from partial treatment, family members, or fomites. Some recommend treatment 1 to 2 weeks later if symptoms persist, others suggest only if mites are observed. Some resistant organisms exist and may need an alternative or combination therapy (1). Persistent dermatitis and secondary infection are also possible (104).

Pinworms

Agent: Enterobius vermicularis (pinworm).

Symptom: Pruritus, mostly around the anus.

Source: Oral-anal spread; more common in young children.

Diagnosis: The parent or patient may have observed the actual pinworms, especially in the middle of the night. The diagnosis by observation of the characteristic ova can be made using a piece of Scotch tape or a commercial pinworm tape blotted around the anus as soon as the patient awakens in the morning. The tape is affixed to a glass slide and examined for the ova. Rarely, an adult pinworm may be seen in the vagina during an examination and can cause vaginitis.

Treatment: Mebendazole, 100 mg orally once, repeated in 2 weeks. Alternatives are pyrantel pamoate and albendazole as single dose and repeated in two weeks (105).

VULVAR DISORDERS

The differential diagnosis of vulvar dermatosis is shown in Table 14-1. Psoriasis, allergic and irritant reactions, lichen sclerosus (Color Plate 22) (94), seborrheic dermatitis, and vesiculobullous disease can cause symptoms in the adolescent. Lichen

TABLE 14-1. *Differential diagnosis of the common vulvar dermatoses.[a]*

Condition	Clinical appearance	Diagnostic test	Therapy
Psoriasis	Well-demarcated erythematous plaques with or without silvery scale; scaly plaques on knees, elbows, scalp; nail pitting	Clinical appearance; cutaneous biopsy	Topical steroids (low-to-mid potency) Tacrolimus (Protopic) ointment—avoids steroid side-effects (not FDA-approved for psoriasis)
Seborrheic dermatitis	Scaly, erythematous plaques; also on eyebrows, nasolabial folds, hairline, occasionally axillae	Clinical appearance; KOH preparation of scale negative	Low-potency topical steroid cream Antiseborrheic (dandruff) shampoos
Tinea cruris (dermatophyte)	Annular plaques with central clearing and peripheral scale; moist erythematous plaques in inguinal folds	KOH preparation of scale positive	Topical imidazole creams b.i.d. until clear for 1 week; avoid combination steroid-antifungal creams (steroid may worsen dermatophyte infection)

(continues)

TABLE 14-1. *Continued*

Condition	Clinical appearance	Diagnostic test	Therapy
Chronic dermatitis (contact or irritant)	Often eczematous and oozing; may involve congruent areas; eyelids; may generalize	Clinical appearance; careful history; patch test to common allergens if indicated	Cool compresses. Mild cleanser (Cetaphil) Topical steroid (low- to mid-potency) Avoid allergens
Lichen simplex chronicus	Thick, furrowed vulva; other common sites are ankles, wrists, nape of neck.	Clinical appearance; cutaneous biopsy	Topical steroid (mid- to-high potency) until clinical improvement, then wean to low-potency topical steroid p.r.n.; monitor for topical steroid side-effects; rule out vaginal *Candida*
Lichen planus	"Pruritic, purple, polygonal papules and plaques;" lacy white pattern or erosions on oral and vulvar mucosa; wrist and shins also common sites	Cutaneous biopsy	Topical steroid (mid- to-high potency) until clinical improvement, then wean to low-potency topical steroid p.r.n.; monitor for topical steroid side-effects; suppositories for vaginal involvement
Lichen sclerosus	White, wrinkly (atrophic); involves vulva, anus ("keyhole" or "hourglass" pattern); pruritus causes scratching, which results in erosions, petechiae, fissures, small purpura	Clinical appearance; cutaneous biopsy	Topical steroid (high potency: clobetasol propionate 0.05% ointment) b.i.d. for 6 weeks; then taper; monitor for topical steroid side effects. Proper hygiene; emollients Consider tacrolimus (Protopic) ointment—avoids steroid side-effects.

(aCourtesy of Jonathan Trager, MD, adapted and updated from McKay M. Vulvitis and vulvo-vaginitis: cutaneous considerations. *Am J Obstet Gynecol* 1991:165:1176.)

simplex chronicus and lichen planus can also occur; lichen planus may present with ulcers and can be associated with pain (106). Vesiculobullous conditions include erythema multiforme, pemphigus, benign familial pemphigus, bullous and cicatricial pemphigoid, linear IgA disease, and dermatitis herpetiformis (2,3,107). The definitive diagnosis of most vulvar disorders is made by biopsy.

Recent trends in adolescent grooming have increased vulvar symptoms. The use of shaving, depilatories, laser hair removal, and waxing in the vulvar area has led to more complaints: irritation; folliculitis; bacterial, HIV, and molluscum infections; and skin abscesses. Laser hair removal may be less traumatic but can cause pain, erythema, and pigment change. Those not willing to stop shaving and waxing can be encouraged to use a mild shaving gel and sharp triple-blade razor, to shave with the grain, and if needed to use 3 to 7 days of twice a day topical steroid (eg. Desonide 0.05% lotion) and clindamycin lotion 1%. For more severe infections, systemic antibiotics or incision and drainage may be required.

Multiple recurrent abscesses may indicate hidradenitis. *Hidradenitis suppurativa* is a disorder involving apocrine glands. This condition develops after puberty, and usually involves the breasts, axillae, and the anogenital region. The etiology is unclear. The earliest lesions present as subepithelial swellings that may be firm or appear fluctuant, but if incised, they are usually fleshy and do not drain purulent material. Initial therapy should include local care with warm baths and loose fitting clothing. Patients should be instructed to wear nonelasticized underwear. Oral antibiotics such as ciprofloxacin, levofloxacin, or amoxicillin-clavulanate and topical antiseptics may be helpful; intralesional steroids can be helpful. Maintenance therapy usually includes a daily cleaning with an antibacterial agent, such as chlorhexidine, and application of a topical antibacterial such as clindamycin. Oral contraceptives, antiandrogens and isotretinoin may also improve the condition. For severe cases, surgery is the best treatment with incision and healing secondarily. Local excision of affected areas can also be performed with primary closure of the surrounding nonaffected tissue. The current styles of piercing and tattooing may have local adverse effects as well including infection, bleeding, edema, swelling, foreign body reaction, as well as exposure to hepatitis and HIV (108).

The most common causes of vulvitis among adolescents are specific vaginal infections (e.g., *Candida*), genital herpes, and irritative vulvitis. Nonspecific vulvar irritation may be caused by hot weather, nylon underpants, tight blue jeans, obesity, or poor hygiene. The patient may also experience pruritus, pain, and dysuria. The vulva appears erythematous. The diagnosis is made by exclusion of a specific vaginitis, allergy, or HPV of the vulva (see Chapter 17). The application of hydrocortisone cream 2.5% applied twice daily to the vulva for several days to 1 week, white cotton underpants, and the avoidance of precipitating factors are usually effective in treating nonspecific irritation. Contact dermatitis from spermicides, depilatories, and hygiene products is common and can be treated with a low- to mid-potency steroid unless severe, in which case a high-potency steroid should be used for short course. Patients should be monitored for steroid side effects. Tinea corporis may occur in the vulvovaginal area, groin, and perianal area. *Vestibular papillomatosis* is a descriptive term for the presence of multiple papillae that may cover the entire mucosal surface of the labia minora (Fig. 14-8). It is a benign nonspecific finding but may be confused with multiple lesions from HPV. Normal sebaceous glands are shown in Fig. 14-9. *Lichen sclerosus* occurs in adolescents as well as young children (see Chapter 3 for treatment modalities) and can lead to significant loss of labia, narrowing of the introitus, and scarring of the clitoral hood, unlike *vitiligo*, which is associated with white color of the skin without the atrophic changes.

An entity that can be troubling to the adolescent is *vulvodynia*, characterized by vulvar discomfort and burning, stinging, and irritation. No one causative factor can be identified. The International Society for the Study of Vulvar Disease (ISSVD) has defined certain subsets. *Vulvar vestibulitis* is a chronic and persistent condition characterized by severe pain when the vestibule is touched or vaginal entry is attempted, tenderness to pressure localized within the vulvar vestibule, and physical findings confined to vestibular erythema of various degrees (108–110). Vulvar vestibulitis can be reliably diagnosed by a cotton-swab test showing severe pain limited to the vestibule (110). Some cases have been attributed to local inflammation, irritation, and/or infection with bacteria, *Candida,* or HPV, and possible increased association with OC use (111). The therapeutic options reviewed by the ISSVD found favorable results with vestibular resection and interferon therapy and less favorable results with laser therapy or local excision of sensitive lesions. There are no series dealing only with adolescent patients, but first-line therapy is twice daily plain-water rinsing; the avoidance of soaps, pads, and irritants; sparing use of topical 5% lidocaine ointment (108) or low-potency corticosteroids; the use of emollients, and the application of

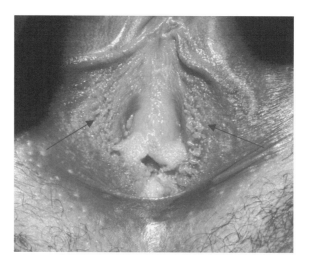

FIG. 14-8. Vestibular papillomatosis. (Courtesy of Jonathan Trager, M.D.)

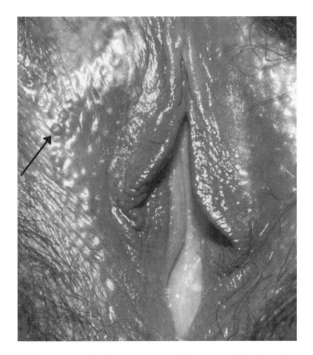

FIG. 14-9. Sebaceous glands on the vulva. (Courtesy of Jonathan Trager, M.D.)

vaginal lubricants for intercourse. Spontaneous remissions can be as high as 50%. While little data are available, medical and behavioral therapies for chronic pain including tricyclic medications, anticonvulsants such as gabapentin, physical therapy, biofeedback, acupuncture, and TENS, have had some benefit (112,113). Essential vulvodynia refers to a condition in which patients lack physical findings and complain of constant burning. These patients are more likely to be postmenopausal, and tricyclic antidepressants have been helpful for some patients. Idiopathic vulvodynia is characterized by dull, continuous pain; therapies have not been established (109,111).

VULVAR TRAUMA

Injuries to the vulva can result in large *vulvar hematomas* (Color Plate 25). Ice packs should be applied immediately, and if the injury is significant, a Foley catheter for urinary drainage should be inserted before genital anatomy is distorted by the swelling. Patients can be managed as "outpatients" with ice, narcotics, a leg bag for the Foley catheter, and bed rest. Surgical drainage should be avoided, if possible, in order to prevent the introduction of infection. The swelling and discoloration may take several weeks to resolve. Healing is usually complete without residual defect or long-term adverse effects. (See Chapter 3 for repair of lacerations.) Many vulvar in-juries heal after repair with little or no residual scarring or other sequelae.

VULVAR ULCERS

The diagnosis of vulvar ulcers is sometimes difficult; some helpful features are outlined in Table 14-2. The most common cause of ulcers in sexually active adoles-cents is genital herpes (oral–genital or genital–genital contact); other much less com-mon causes are chancroid, found in fewer than 1 in 1000 patients in the University of Washington STD clinic (89), and syphilis. All three have been associated with an in-creased risk of HIV infection. Syphilis is characterized by a nonpainful hard ulcer (see Chapter 15). Genital herpes is characterized by painful, usually multiple, and shallow ulcers (discussed earlier).

Vulvar ulcers may also occur in non-sexually active girls. The ulcers may be large and deep with a mixed aerobic and anaerobic flora and may be recurrent. They may be severe enough to require hospitalization and treatment with intravenous broad spectrum antibiotics. The etiology is often unclear. In addition, we frequently see painful ulcers in young adolescents caused by Epstein-Barr virus infection (mononu-cleosis) (114). The ulcer may be the presenting symptom of the girl with mononu-cleosis or she may have exudative pharyngitis, lymphadenopathy, and fever more suggestive of mononucleosis. Patients with myelocytic leukemia receiving chemotherapy may develop genital ulcers (115). Varicella zoster rarely causes ulcers. Ulcers can also occur with chronic fistulas or Crohn disease (Color Plate 23); the lo-cal application of zinc oxide paste may help alleviate symptoms. Some girls with Crohn disease have persistent shallow vulvar ulcers which may often have persistent purulent oozing; they often respond to an extended course of metronidazole. The mouth should always be examined in patients with vulvar ulcers. *Behcet disease* is a multisystem disorder characterized by recurrent oral and genital ulcers, often associ-ated with uveitis (70% to 80%) and, less commonly, arthritis, thrombophlebitis, and rashes. Although the disease usually does not appear until the third decade of life, cases in young children and adolescents do occur uncommonly (116,117). Therapy is often unsatisfactory and has included oral contraceptives, corticosteroids, colchicine, and immunosuppressive agents.

Chancroid typically appears as multiple purulent ulcers, often with ragged edges, and tender unilateral or bilateral inguinal adenopathy (118). Suppurative inguinal adenopathy is almost pathognomonic. The diagnosis is made by excluding the diag-nosis of genital herpes or syphilis, although these diseases may occur simultaneously. If the diagnosis is unclear, or if the patient resides in a community with a high preva-lence or outbreak of chancroid (119), treatment for both syphilis and chancroid may be indicated, as well as follow-up serology tests for syphilis. Culture of *Haemophilus ducreyi* is the only sure means of diagnosis, but special media and conditions are nec-essary. Detection from the direct smears of the base of the genital lesion is a method

TABLE 14-2. Clinical features of genital ulcers

	Syphilis	Herpes	Chancroid	Lymphogranuloma venereum	Donovanosis
Incubation period	9–90 days	2–7 days	1–14 days	3 days–6 weeks	1–4 weeks (up to 6 months)
Primary lesion	Papule	Vesicle	Pustule	Papule, pustule, or vesicle	Papule
Number of lesions	Usually one	Multiple, may coalesce	Usually multiple, may coalesce	Usually one	Variable
Diameter (mm)	5–15 mm	1–2 mm	Variable	2–10 mm	Variable
Edges	Sharply demarcated, elevated, round, or oval	Erythematous	Undermined, ragged, irregular	Elevated, round, or oval	Elevated, irregular
Depth	Superficial or deep	Superficial	Excavated	Superficial or deep	Elevated
Base	Smooth, nonpurulent, relatively nonvascular	Serous, erythematous, nonvascular	Purulent, bleeds easily	Variable, nonvascular	Red and velvety, bleeds readily
Induration	Firm	None	Soft	Occasionally firm	Firm
Pain	Uncommon	Frequently tender	Usually very tender	Variable	Uncommon
Lymphadenopathy	Firm, nontender, bilateral	Firm, tender, often bilateral with initial episode	Tender, may suppurate, loculated usually unilateral	Tender, may suppurate, loculated, usually unilateral	None; pseudobuboes

(From Ballard RC. Genital ulcer adenopathy syndrome. In: KK Holmes, P Mardh, Sparling PF, et al eds. *Sexually Transmitted Diseases*, 3rd ed. New York: McGraw-Hill, 1999:888; with permission.)

used by clinicians, although the sensitivity and specificity are lower than those of cultures. The specimen is obtained from the ulcer base, which may involve peeling off the crust or wiping away excess pus (but not extensive cleaning). The cotton swab is used to touch first the base and then the edges of the ulcer. The swab is then rolled onto a slide in a circle about the size of a dime, and the slide is allowed to air dry and is Gram stained. Enzyme immunoassays, DNA probes, and new PCR tests are promising techniques (118,120). Thus, patients with ulcers without a history of blisters who do not have herpes or syphilis (no evidence of *Treponema pallidum* on darkfield examination or by serologic test at least 7 days after the onset of ulcers, and no evidence of herpes by clinical presentation or HSV tests) and who have significant painful inguinal adenopathy should be treated for chancroid with azithromycin 1 g orally in one dose, or ceftriaxone 250 mg IM in a single dose, erythromycin base 500 mg orally three times a day for 7 days, or ciprofloxacin 500 mg twice a day for 3 days (only in nonpregnant and nonlactating patients) (1). A clinical response should be evident within several days; patients should be seen in 7 days to make sure that ulcer healing is occurring and that adenopathy is less painful. Nodes may become fluctuant in spite of adequate medical therapy and require needle aspiration or incision and drainage (1). If a response to therapy has not occurred by day 7, the diagnosis may be different (e.g., herpes), the patient may be noncompliant with medication, the organisms may be resistant to the antibiotic chosen, or the patient may be infected with HIV. Sexual contacts within the 10 days preceding the onset of symptoms should be examined and treated. Serologic testing for syphilis and HIV should be performed at the time of diagnosis and 3 months after therapy. Syphilis is less common than previously, but it is still important to keep in mind in the differential diagnosis of painless ulcers, adenopathy, and rashes. Screening is advisable in patients at high risk for STDs and those with STDs or HIV (1). Syphilis is discussed further in Chapter 15.

Lymphogranuloma venereum is caused by three serotypes (L-1, L-2, and L-3) of *C. trachomatis.* The ulcer is usually transient, and the patient is usually seen by the clinician for the late sequelae: enlarged inguinal nodes and rectal strictures. Diagnosis is made by isolation of the organism, immunofluorescence of inclusion bodies in leukocytes of a node aspirate, or most commonly serologic test. Treatment is doxycycline 100 mg twice a day for 21 days. An alternative treatment choice is erythromycin base 500 mg four times a day for 21 days (1). The diagnosis of carcinoma, pemphigus, or granuloma inguinale generally requires a biopsy specimen. *Granuloma inguinale*, a rare disease, causes painful ulcerations with red granulation tissue or keloid-like depigmented scars, elephantoid enlargement of the external genitalia, and fistulas.

NEVI

Although most darkly pigmented lesions on the vulva of adolescent girls represent lentigo (a benign freckle-like increase in the concentration of melanocytes in the basal layer of the epithelium) or a compound, functional, or intradermal nevus, the rare occurrence of melanoma or other forms of carcinoma makes it important to perform an excisional biopsy to establish a diagnosis with any suspicious lesion. Large or atypical vulvar nevi and nevi on the vulvar mucosa should be considered for removal (121).

TOXIC SHOCK SYNDROME

Toxic shock syndrome (TSS) received much publicity in the early 1980s as a disease that was occurring in young women primarily in association with one brand of tampon (Rely). Since that time, there has been recognition of milder cases than the original CDC definition as well as newer information on toxin production and risk factors (122).

Although the original description of TSS by Todd and associates (123) suggested that it was a disease of boys and girls, the increased awareness of TSS in the early 1980s stemmed from the recognition that it occurred in young menstruating women who used tampons (124). Subsequently, both menstrual and nonmenstrual cases were recognized. Almost all cases in men and nonmenstruating women have been associated with a focal infection such as an infected wound, abscess, augmentation mammoplasty, or pneumonia (especially associated with influenza); similar presentations have also been linked to toxin-producing strains of *Streptococcus pyogenes*. The disease in menstruating young women is associated with the elaboration of toxic-shock syndrome-1 toxin (TSST-1) in 84% to 100% of cases, and nonmenstrual cases with TSST-1, staphylococcal enterotoxin serotype A (SEA) or B (SEB), or streptococcal pyrogenic exotoxin C (SPE C) (122,124). *S. aureus* has been cultured from the vagina of 98% of women with TSS versus 7% of controls. TSS has a peak occurrence on the fourth day of the menses and has been associated with continuous tampon use.

In a study of time intervals based on the change in tampon types, Pettiti and Reingold (125) reported the incidence of TSS per 100,000 women to be 0.4 from 1972 to 1977 (tampon absorbency low), 1.5 from 1977 to 1979 (superabsorbent tampons, not Rely), 2.4 from 1979 to 1980 (Rely and other superabsorbent tampons), and 2.2 from 1980 to 1985 (Rely off the market). The incidence from April 1985 to December 1987 was 1.5 in 100,000 women (95% CI: 0.8, 2.6) in the interval after the removal of polyacrylate rayon products from the market and reductions in absorbency (126); further decreases occurred with the present incidence of about 1.0 in 100,000 (122,127,128). Factors that appear to promote TSS are the neutral pH of the vagina during menstruation and the introduction of oxygen into the vagina when tampons are inserted. Cases of TSS do, however, occur during menses in women not using tampons. Contraceptive sponges and, to a lesser extent, diaphragms have been associated with rare cases of TSS. Most individuals develop antibody to TSST-1 by the age of 20 years. Toxic shock syndrome occurs predominantly in the population that lacks antibody, because of either a genetic factor or lack of exposure. Although colonization rates and antibody titers maybe similar in adolescents and adults, young patients are at increased risk for TSS. Almost half of the 30 patients studied by Bergdoll and associates (129) had no antibody to this toxin during convalescence. This toxin appears to block B-lymphocytes from making antibody. Women who have not made antibody to TSST-1 by the time of follow-up are at a high risk of recurrence with future menses and tampon use.

Milder cases of TSS have also been described; physicians and patients need to be aware of the more minor symptoms occurring with tampon (or rare diaphragm) use in order to intervene effectively. The criteria set up by the CDC to study the epidemiology of TSS is for the more severe manifestation of the syndrome. Toxic shock syndrome requires three major criteria and at least three organ systems involved (130):

Major criteria:

1. Fever of $\geq 38.9°C$
2. Rash (diffuse macular erythroderma that looks like a sunburn) with desquamation (1 to 2 weeks after the onset of the illness, particularly of palms and soles)
3. Hypotension (systolic blood pressure ≤ 90 mm Hg for adults, or below the fifth percentile by age for children under 16 years, or orthostatic decrease ≥ 15 mm Hg in diastolic blood pressure, or orthostatic syncope or orthostatic dizziness)

Involvement of three or more of the following organ systems:

1. Gastrointestinal (vomiting or diarrhea)
2. Hepatic (total bilirubin, AST, ALT at least two times the upper limit of normal)
3. Muscular (severe myalgia or creatine phosphokinase level at least two times the upper limits of normal)
4. Mucous membranes (vaginal, oropharyngeal, or conjunctival hyperemia)
5. Renal (blood urea nitrogen or creatinine at least two times the upper limit of normal or >5 leukocytes/high-power field in the absence of urinary tract infection).
6. Cardiovascular
7. Central nervous system (disorientation or alterations in consciousness when fever and hypotension are absent)

In addition, if cultures from blood and cerebrospinal fluid are obtained, they must be negative (except for *S. aureus*). Serologic tests for Rocky Mountain spotted fever, leptospirosis, or measles also must be negative. Adolescents with any of these symptoms or with vomiting, diarrhea, and a rash during menstruation should be instructed to remove the tampon and go to the emergency room. Toxic shock syndrome should be managed in the same way as other forms of shock; the administration of fluid is most important. Laboratory tests include hematology and chemistry profiles, along with coagulation parameters. Hypocalcemia and hypomagnesemia and elevated creatine phosphokinase are common findings. A vaginal examination should be done, and the tampon should be removed if it is still in place and sent for culture. Gram stain of the vaginal pool should be performed. Cultures from the blood, rectum, vagina, oropharynx, anterior nares, and urine should be obtained. Penicillinase-resistant antistaphylococcal antibiotics should be administered for 2 weeks (IV, p.o.). Although evidence is lacking, many clinicians favor irrigating the vagina with saline, povidone-iodine solution, or vancomycin or gentamicin solution. In patients with deep abscesses in which the toxin-producing staphylococci are unlikely to be eradicated rapidly, or in particularly severe cases of TSS, therapy with immunoglobulin (which has high levels of antibody to TSST-1) and possibly steroids may improve the outcome. Inhibiting the binding of M protein to fibrinogen in streptococcal toxic shock is a new area of research (131).

Because there is an approximately 30% risk of recurrence, patients should be warned to avoid tampons for at least 6 months. The presence of high levels of antibody to TSST-1 at followup in a patient with no antibody at presentation is reassuring. Serial cultures of the vagina may be difficult to interpret, since other strains of S. *aureus* may be present. Testing for TSST-1 producing strains requires a specialized laboratory. Sources of antibody testing to TSST-1 at baseline and follow-up can be arranged through some academic centers or the CDC. Tampon use can be resumed when seroconversion occurs. There is insufficient knowledge on which to base absolute guidelines to patients, but we suggest that patients (a) avoid superabsorbent tampons, (b) use tampons intermittently and use pads at night, (c) change tampons every 4 to 6 hours, and, especially, (d) remove tampons and call a physician if vomiting, diarrhea, rash, or fever occur. The recommendation about the frequency of changing tampons has not been subjected to critical study.

DYSURIA

Dysuria is common in adolescent girls and is discussed in this section because vaginitis and vulvar lesions may produce symptoms usually associated with a urinary tract infection (UTI) (Table 14-3). The clinician needs to do a careful gynecologic assessment of adolescents with dysuria (7,8,132,133). In one study, only one-half of

TABLE 14-3. *Differential diagnosis of dysuria in adolescent girls*

Bacterial urinary tract infection
Vulvovaginitis/cervicitis/urethritis
   Candida
   Trichomonas
   Bacterial vaginosis
   N. gonorrhoeae
   C. trachomatis
   Herpes simplex
Vulvar dermatoses
Skene's gland abscess
Traumatic urethritis
Urethral syndrome of unclear etiology

adult women with dysuria had bacteriuria with more than 10^5 organisms/ml (133). Vaginitis, vulvitis, genital herpes, *N. gonorrhoeae, C. trachomatis*, and bacteriuria with fewer than 10^5 organisms per milliliter are responsible for most of the remaining group. Pyuria on urinalysis can occur with a UTI, *Trichomonas* vaginitis, and gonococcal or chlamydial infections. In early classic studies, Stamm and associates (133,134) suggested that women with dysuria and pyuria who do not have bacteriuria of $>10^4$ organisms per milliliter, gonorrhea, or vaginitis have either low counts of bacteriuria (coliforms or *Staphylococcus saprophyticus*) or infection with *C. trachomatis*. In contrast, of the undiagnosed group of women with dysuria but no pyuria, few had demonstrable infection. In women with dysuria and frequency (in whom the usual causes were excluded), doxycycline 100 mg orally twice a day for 10 days led to improvement only in those with pyuria (8 or more leukocytes/mm^3 of urine on hemocytometer chamber) (135).

In assessing dysuria in an adolescent, the clinician should take a history about the onset of symptoms, sexual activity (recent and past), symptoms of urethritis in the male partner(s), previous UTIs, and internal dysuria (pain felt inside the body such as symptoms of bladder spasm and end voiding pain) versus external dysuria (pain felt as urine passes over the inflamed labia) (Fig. 14-10). If the patient reports a clear-cut history of external dysuria and discharge, her symptoms are likely due to vaginitis or a vulvar cause. Although adult women who have internal dysuria and frequency usually have a UTI (136), many adolescent girls have vaginitis, gonorrhea, or *Chlamydia* infection alone or in combination with a UTI. In contrast to

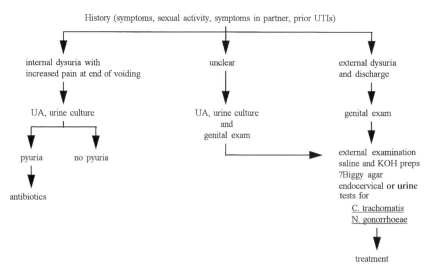

FIG. 14-10. Evaluation of dysuria in the adolescent girl. UTI, urinary tract infection; UA, urinalysis; KOH, potassium hydroxide.

older women, adolescents may be less able to differentiate internal versus external dysuria (132). Pain occurring only at the end of urination and/or hematuria suggests a UTI.

The laboratory evaluation of dysuria in an adolescent should include urinalysis, urine culture (if UTI is suspected), wet preparations of the vaginal secretions, and, in sexually active patients, endocervical or urine tests for gonorrhea and *C. trachomatis* (137). A 1+ or 2+ leukocyte esterase, red blood cells, and a positive nitrite result on the urine dipstick favor a diagnosis of UTI, as does a positive Gram stain (1 organism per high-power field) of unspun urine. However, many adolescents with a UTI do not have a positive urine nitrite test. Inspection of the genitalia should be done to exclude urethral or vulvar pathology such as genital herpes. Samples for wet preparations should be obtained as noted earlier. A culture for *Candida* should be done in patients with itching, vulvar erythema, or external dysuria in whom the KOH preparation does not reveal *Candida*.

The adolescent with dysuria usually has a UTI and/or a specific gynecologic infection (132). In patients with undiagnosed dysuria and persistent pyuria on urinalysis, a course of antibiotics effective against both low-count UTIs and *C. trachomatis* is recommended. Patients without pyuria or a diagnosis fall into the small category of urethral syndrome of unclear etiology, and antibiotics are not beneficial. Treatment, evaluation, and follow-up of urinary tract infections are discussed in Chapter 13. Patients often have recurrent UTIs in relation to coitus. Use of diaphragms, condoms, and spermicides are associated risk factors; spermicides change vaginal flora (see Chapter 20) (138). Coitus-related UTI can be treated with increased fluid intake, voiding every 2 hours during the day; voiding after intercourse (although no effect was noted in one study [138]); and suppressive antibiotics (139).

REFERENCES

1. Center for Disease Control and Prevention, 2002 Sexually Transmitted Disease Treatment Guidelines. *MMWR* 2002;52(RR-6);1.
2. Quint EH, Smith YR. Vulvar disorders in adolescent patients. *Pediatr Clin North Am* 1999;46:593.
3. Piippo S, Lenko H, Vuento R. Vulvar symptoms in pediatric and adolescent patients. *Acta Paediatr* 2000;89:431.
4. Centers for Disease Control and Prevention, Screening tests to detect *Chlamydia trachomatis* and *Neisseria gonorrhoeae* Infections—2002. *MMWR* 2002;51(RR-15):1.
5. Duerr A, Heilig CM, Meidle SF, et al. Incident and persistent vulvovaginal candidiasis among Human Immunodeficiency Virus-infected women: risk factors and severity. *Obstet Gynecol* 2003;101:548.
6. Shafer MA, Sweet RL, Ohm-Smith MS, et al. Microbiology of the lower genital tract in postmenarchal adolescent girls: differences by sexual activity, contraception, and presence of nonspecific vaginitis. *J Pediatr* 1985;107:974.
7. Blake, D, Duggan A, Joffe A. Use of spun urine to enhance detection of *Trichomonas vaginalis* in adolescent women. *Arch Pediatr Adolesc Med* 1999;153:1222.
8. Blake D, Woods ER. The future is here: Noninvasive diagnosis of STDs. *Contemporary Pediatrics* 2001;18:71.
9. Garrow SC, Smith DW, Harnett GB. The diagnosis of *chlamydia*, *gonorrhoea*, and *trichomonas* infections by self obtained low vaginal swabs, in remote northern Australian clinical practice. *Sex Transm Infect* 2002;78:278.

10. Tanaka M, Nakayama H, Sagiyama K, et al. Evaluation of a new amplified enzyme immunoassay (EIA) for the detection of *Chlamydia trachomatis* in male urine, female endocervical swab, and patient obtained vaginal swab specimens. *J Clin Pathol* 2000;53:350.

11. Chernesky M, Morse S, Schachter J. Newly available and future laboratory tests for sexually transmitted diseases (STDs) other than HIV. *Sex Transm Dis* 1999;26:S8.

12. Blake DR, Duggan A, Quinn T, et al. Evaluation of vaginal infections in adolescent women: can it be done without a speculum? *Pediatrics* 1998;102:939.

13. Rompalo AM, Gaydos CA, Shah N, et al. Evaluation of use of a single intravaginal swab to detect multiple sexually transmitted infections in active-duty military women. *Clin Infect Dis* 2001;33:1455.

14. Serlin M, Shafer MA, Tebb K, et al. What sexually transmitted disease screening method does the adolescent prefer? Adolescents' attitudes toward first-void urine, self-collected vaginal swab, and pelvic examination. *Arch Pediatr Adolesc Med* 2002;156(6):588.

15. Smith K, Harrington K, Wingood G, et al. Self-obtained vaginal swabs for diagnosis of treatable sexually transmitted diseases in adolescent girls. *Arch Pediatr Adolesc Med* 2001;155:676.

16. Anderson MR, Klink K, Cohrssen A. Evaluation of vaginal complaints. *JAMA* 2004;291:1368.

17. Shafer MB, Pantell RH, Schachter J. Is the routine pelvic examination needed with the advent of urine-based screening for sexually transmitted diseases? *Arch Pediatr Adolesc Med* 1999;153:119.

18. Blake DR, Fletcher K, Joshi N, et al. Identification of symptoms that indicate a pelvic examination is necessary to exclude PID in adolescent women. *J Pediatr Adolesc Gynecol* 2003;16:25.

19. Critchlow CW, Wolner-Hanssen PW, Eschenbach DA, et al. Determinants of cervical ectopia and of cervicitis: age, oral contraception, specific cervical infection, smoking, and douching. *Am J Obstet Gynecol* 1995;173:534.

20. Roongpisuthipong A, Grimes DA, Hadgu A. Is the Papanicolaou smear useful for diagnosing sexually transmitted diseases? *Obstet Gynecol* 1987;69:820.

21. Wiese W, Patel SR, Patel SC, et al. A meta-analysis of the Papanicolaou smear and wet mount for the diagnosis of vaginal trichomoniasis. *Am J Med* 2000;108:301.

22. Bianchi A, Moret F, Desrues JM, et al. PreservCyt transport media used for the ThinPrep Pap test is a suitable medium for detection of *Chlamydia trachomatis* by the COBAS Amplicor CT/NG test: results of a preliminary study and future implications. *J Clin Microbiol* 2002;40:1749.

23. Inhorn SL, Wand PJ, Wright TC, et al. *Chlamydia trachomatis* and Pap testing from a single, fluid-based sample. A multicenter study. *J Reprod Med* 2001;46:237.

24. Anguenot JL, de Marval F, Vassilakos P, et al. Combining screening for *Chlamydia trachomatis* and squamous intra-epithelial lesions using a single liquid-based cervical sample. *Hum Reprod* 2001;16:2206.

25. Paavonen J, Stevens CD, Wohler-Hanssen P, et al. Colposcopic manifestations of cervical and vaginal infections. *Obstet Gynecol Survey* 1988;43:373.

26. Wolner-Hanssen P, Eschenbach DA, Paavonen J, et al. Association between vaginal douching and acute pelvic inflammatory disease. *JAMA* 1990;263:1939.

27. Baird DD, Weinberg CR, Voight LF, et al. Vaginal douching and reduced fertility. Am J Public Health 1996;86:844.

28. Patel SR, Wiese W, Patel SC, et al. Systematic review of diagnostic tests for vaginal trichomoniasis. *Inf Dis Obstet Gynecol* 2000;8:248.

29. Krieger JN, Alderete JF. *Trichomonas vaginalis* and trichomoniasis. In: Holmes KK, Sparling PF, Mardh P, et al, eds. *Sexually transmitted diseases*, 3rd ed. New York: McGraw-Hill, 1999;587.

30. Weinberger MW, Harger JH. Accuracy of the Papanicolaou smear in the diagnosis of asymptomatic infection with *Trichomonas vaginalis*. *Obstet Gynecol* 1993;82:425.

31. Wathne B, Holst E, Hovelius B, et al. Vaginal discharge-comparison of clinical, laboratory and microbiological findings. *Acta Obstet Gynecol Scand* 1994;73:802.

32. Philip A, Carter-Scott P, Rogers C. An agar culture technique to quantitate *Trichomonas vaginalis* in women. *J Infect Dis* 1987;155:304.

33. Wendel KA, Erbelding EJ, Gaydos CA, et al. *Trichomonas vaginalis* polymerase chain reaction compared with standard diagnostic and therapeutic protocols for detection and treatment of vaginal trichomoniasis. *Clin Infect Dis* 2002;35:576.

34. Kaydos SC, Swygard H, Wise SL, et al. Development and validation of a PCR-based enzyme-linked immunosorbent assay with urine for use in clinical research settings to detect *Trichomonas vaginalis* in women. *J Clin Microbiol* 2002;40:89.

35. Barenfanger J, Drake C, Hanson C. Timing of inoculation of the Pouch makes no difference in increased detection of *Trichomonas vaginalis* by the InPouch TV method. *J Clin Microbiol* 2002; 40:1387.

36. Ohlemeyer CL, Hornberger LL, Lynch DA, et al. Diagnosis of *Trichomonas vaginalis* in adolescent females: InPouch TV culture versus wet-mount microscopy. *J Adolesc Health* 1998;22:205.

37. Burstein GR, Workowski KA. Sexually transmitted diseases treatment guidelines. *Curr Opin Pediatr* 2003;15:391.

38. Mayta H, Gilman RH, Calderon MM, et al. 18S ribosomal DNA-based PCR for diagnosis of *Trichomonas vaginalis*. *J Clin Microbiol* 2000;38:2683.

39. Lawing LR, Hedges SR, Schwebke JR. Detection of Trichomonas in vaginal and urine specimens from women by culture and PCR. *J Clin Microbiol* 2000;38:3585.

40. Lara Torre E, Pinkerton JS. Accuracy of detection of *Trichomonas vaginalis* organisms on a liquid-based Papanicolaou smear. *Am J Obstet Gynecol* 2003;188:354

41. Schmid G, Narcisi E, Mosure D, et al. Prevalence of metronidazole-resistant *Trichomonas vaginalis* in a gynecology clinic. *J Reprod Med* 2001;46:545.

42. Lossick JG, Muller M, Garrell TE. In vitro drug susceptibility and doses of metronidazole required for cure in cases of refractory vaginal trichomoniasis. *J Infect Dis* 1986;153:948.

43. Grossman JH, Galask RP. Persistent vaginitis caused by metronidazole-resistant *Trichomonas*. *Obstet Gynecol* 1990;76:521.

44. Piper JM, Mitchel EE, Ray WA. Prenatal use of metronidazole and birth defects: no association. *Obstet Gynecol* 1993;82:348.

45. Horowitz BJ, Edelstein SW, Lippman L. Candida tropicalis vulvovaginitis. *Obstet Gynecol* 1985;66:229.

46. Robertson WH. Mycology of vulvovaginitis. *Am J Obstet Gynecol* 1988;158:989.

47. Galask RP Vaginal colonization by bacteria and yeast. *Am J Obstet Gynecol* 1988;158:993.

48. Horowitz BJ, Edelstein SW, Lippman L. Sexual transmission of Candida. *Obstet Gynecol* 1987; 69:883.

49. Bisschop MP, Merkus JM, Scheygrand H, et al. Cotreatment of the male partner in vaginal candidiasis: a double blind randomized control study. *Br J Obstet Gynaecol* 1986;93:79.

50. Sobel JD, Chaim W. Treatment of Torulopsis glabrata vaginitis: retrospective review of boric acid therapy. *Clin Infect Dis* 1997;24:649.

51. Sobel JD, Brooker D, Stein GE, et al. Single oral dose fluconazole compared with conventional clotrimazole topical therapy of *Candida* vaginitis. *Am J Obstet Gynecol* 1995;172:1263.

52. Fong IW. The value of prophylactic (monthly) clotrimazole versus empiric self-treatment in recurrent vaginal candidiasis. *Genitourin Med* 1994;70:124.

53. Sobel JD. Recurrent vulvovaginal candidiasis: a prospective study of the efficacy of maintenance ketoconazole therapy. *N Engl J Med* 1986;315:1455.

54. Creatsas GC, Charalambidis VM, Zagotzidou EH, et al. Chronic or recurrent vaginal candidiasis: short-term treatment and prophylaxis with itraconazole. *Clin Ther* 1993;15:662.

55. Speigel CA, Amsel R, Eschenbach D, et al. Anaerobic bacteria in nonspecific vaginitis. *N Engl J Med* 1980;303:601.

56. Eschenbach DA, Hillier S, Critchlow C, et al. Diagnosis and clinical manifestations of bacterial vaginosis. *Am J Obstet Gynecol* 1988;158:819.

57. Larsson PB, Bergman BB. Is there a causal connection between motile curved rods, *Mobiluncus* species, and bleeding complications? *Am J Obstet Gynecol* 1986;154:107.

58. Speigel CA, Amsel R, Holmes KK. Diagnosis of bacterial vaginosis by direct gram stain of vaginal fluid. *J Clin Microbiol* 1983;18:170.

59. Briselden AM, Moncla BJ, Stevens CE, et al. Sialidases (neuraminidases) in bacterial vaginosis and bacterial vaginosis-associated microflora. *J Clin Microbiol* 1992;30:663.

60. Leitich H, Brunbauer M, Bodner-Adler BA. Antibiotic treatment of bacterial vaginosis in pregnancy: a meta-analysis. *Am J Obstet Gynecol* 2003;188:752

61. Hillier SL, Nugent RP, Eschenbach DA, et al. Association between bacterial vaginosis and preterm delivery of a low birth weight infant. *N Engl J Med* 1995;333:1737.

62. Koumans, EH, Markowitz LE, Hogan V, for the CDC Working Group. Indications for therapy and treatment recommendations for bacterial vaginosis in nonpregnant and pregnant women: a synthesis of data. *Clin Infect Dis* 2002;35 (Suppl 2):S152.

63. Morales WJ, Schorr S, Albritton J. Effect of metronidazole in patients with preterm birth in preceding pregnancy and bacterial vaginosis: a placebo-controlled, double-blind study. *Am J Obstet Gynecol* 1994;171:345.
64. Hauth JC, Goldenberg RL, Andrews WW, et al. Reduced incidence of preterm delivery with metronidazole and erythromycin in women with bacterial vaginosis. *N Engl J Med* 1995;333:1732.
65. Marrazzo JM, Loutsky LA, Eschenbach DA, et al. Characterization of vaginal flora and bacterial vaginosis in women who have sex with women. *J Infect Dis* 2002;185;1305.
66. Holst E. Reservoir of four organisms associated with bacterial vaginosis suggests lack of sexual transmission. *J Clin Microbiol* 1990;28:2035.
67. Nugent RP, Krohn MA, Hillier SL. Reliability of diagnosing bacterial vaginosis is improved by a standardized method of Gram stain interpretation. *J Clin Microbiol* 1991;29:297.
68. Makarova LN, Kratsov EG, Vasil'eva EA, et at. Modern methods for diagnosis of gardnerella infection. *Bulletin Exp Biol Med* 2000;130:196.
69. Witt A, Petricevic L, Kaufman U, et al. DNA hybridization test: rapid diagnostic tool for excluding bacterial vaginosis in pregnant women with symptoms suggestive of infection. *J Clin Microbiol* 2002;40:3057.
70. Swedberg J, Steiner JF, Deiss F, et al. Comparison of single-dose vs. one week course of metronidazole for symptomatic bacterial vaginosis. *JAMA* 1985;254:1046.
71. Hillier SL, Lipinski C, Briselden AM, et al. Efficacy of intravaginal 0.75% metronidazole gel for the treatment of bacterial vaginosis. *Obstet Gynecol* 1993;81:963.
72. Greaves WL, Chungafung J, Morris B, et al. Clindamycin versus metronidazole in the treatment of bacterial vaginosis. *Obstet Gynecol* 1988;72:799.
73. Lugo-Miro VI, Green M, Mazur L. Comparison of different metronidazole therapeutic regimens for bacterial vaginosis. *JAMA* 1992;268:92.
74. Hillier SL, Wiesenfeld C, Murray P, et al. A trial of intravaginal *Lactobacillus crispatus* as an adjunct to metronidazole therapy for the treatment of bacterial vaginosis. *Inf Dis Obstet Gynecol* 2002;10:S20.
75. Lamont RF, Duncan SLB, Mandal D, et al. Intravaginal clindamycin to reduce preterm birth in women with abnormal genital tract flora. *Obstet Gynecol* 2003;101:516.
76. Lamont RF. Infection in the prediction and antibiotics in the prevention of spontaneous preterm labour and preterm birth. *Int J Obstet Gynaecol* 2003;110:71.
77. Reeves WC, Corey L, Adams HG, et al. Risk of recurrence after first episodes of genital herpes. *N Engl J Med* 1981;305:315.
78. Corey L. First episode, recurrent, and asymptomatic herpes simplex infections. *J Am Acad Dermatol* 1988;18:169.
79. Lafferty WE, Coombs RW, Benedetti J, et al. Recurrences after oral and genital herpes simplex virus infection: influence of site of infection and viral type. *N Engl J Med* 1987;316:1444.
80. Ballard RC. Genital ulcer adenopathy syndrome. In: Holmes KK, Sparling PF, Mardh P, et al., eds. *Sexually transmitted diseases,* 3rd ed. New York: McGraw-Hill, 1999:887.
81. Corey L, Holmes KK. Genital herpes simplex virus infections: current concepts in diagnosis, therapy, and prevention. *Ann Intern Med* 1983;98:973.
82. Corey, L. Challenges in genital herpes simplex virus management. *J Infect Dis* 2002;186 (Suppl 1):S29.
83. Wald A. Testing for genital herpes: how, who, and why. *Curr Clin Top Infect Dis* 2002;22:166.
84. Kimberlin DW, Rouse DJ. Genital Herpes. *N Engl J Med* 2004;350:1970.
85. Wald A, Zeh J, Selke S, et al. Virologic characteristics of subclinical and symptomatic genital herpes infections. *N Engl J Med* 1995;333:770.
86. Johnson RE, Nahmias AJ, Magdar LS, et al. A seroepidemiologic survey of the prevalence of herpes simplex virus type 2 infection in the United States. *N Engl J Med* 1989;321:7.
87. Breinig MK, Kingsley LA, Armstrong JA, et al. Epidemiology of genital herpes in Pittsburgh: serologic, sexual, and racial correlates of apparent and inapparent herpes simplex infections. *J Infect Dis* 1990;152:299.
88. Koutsky LA, Ashley RL, Holmes KK, et al. The frequency of unrecognized type 2 herpes simplex virus infection among women, implications for the control of genital herpes. *Sex Trans Dis* 1990;17:90.
89. Koutsky LA, Stevens CE, Holmes KK, et al. Underdiagnosis of genital herpes by current clinical and viral-isolation procedures. *N Engl J Med* 1992;326:1533.

90. Guinan ME, MacCalman J, Kern ER. The course of untreated recurrent genital herpes simplex infection in 27 women. *N Engl J Med* 1981;304:759.
91. Thin RN. Does first episode genital herpes have an incubation period? A clinical study. *Int J STD AIDS* 1991:2:285.
92. Scoular A. Using the evidence base on genital herpes: optimizing the use of diagnostic tests and information provision. *Sex Trans Infect* 2002;78:160.
93. Cone RW, Swenson PD, Hobson AC, et al. Herpes simplex virus detection from genital lesions: a comparative study using antigen detection (HerpChek) and culture. *J Clin Microbiol* 1993;31:1774.
94. Powell J, Wojnarowska F. Childhood vulvar lichen sclerosis: the course after puberty. *J Reprod Med* 2002;47:706.
95. Scoular A, Gillespie G, Carman WF. Polymerase chain reaction for diagnosis of genital herpes in a genitourinary medicine clinic. *Sex Transm Infect* 2002;78:21.
96. Marshall DS, Linfert BS, Draghi BS, et al. Identification of herpes simplex virus genital infection: comparison of a multiplex PCR assay and traditional viral isolation techniques. *Mod Pathol* 2001;14:152.
97. Wald A, Benedetti J, Davis G, et al. A randomized, double-blind, comparative trial comparing high- and standard-dose oral acyclovir for first-episode genital herpes infections. *Antimicrob Agents Chemother* 1994;38:174.
98. Sacks SL, Aoki FY, Diaz-Mitoma F, et al. Patient-initiated twice-daily oral famcyclovir for early recurrent genital herpes. *JAMA* 1996;276:44.
99. Strand A, Patel R, Wulf HC, Coates KM, and the International Valaciclovir HSV Study Group. Aborted genital herpes simplex virus lesions: findings from a randomized controlled trial with valaciclovir. *Sex Transm Infect* 2002;78:435.
100. Corey L, Wald A, Patel R, et al. Once-daily valacyclovir to reduce the risk of transmission of genital herpes. *N Eng J Med* 2004;350:11.
101. Lehrman SN, Douglas JM, Corey L, et al. Recurrent genital herpes and suppressive oral acyclovir therapy: relation between clinical outcome and in-vitro drug sensitivity. *Ann Intern Med* 1986;104:786.
102. Brown ZA, Benedetti JK, Watts DH, et al. A comparison between detailed and simple histories in the diagnosis of genital herpes complicating pregnancy. *Am J Obstet Gynecol* 1995:172:1299.
103. Liota E, Smith K, Buckley R, et al. Imiquimod therapy for molluscum contagiosum. *J Cutaneous Med Surg* 2000;4:76.
104. Wendel K, Rompalo A. Scabies and pediculosis pubis: an update of treatment regimens and general review. *Clin Infect Dis* 2002;35(Suppl 2):S146.
105. American Academy of Pediatrics, Pickering LK, ed. *Red Book: 2003 Report of the Committee on Infectious Diseases.* 26th ed. Elk Grove Village, IL: American Academy of Pediatrics, 2003.
106. Rosen T. Update on genital lesions. *JAMA* 2003;290:1001.
107. Marren P, Wojnarowska F, Venning V, et al. Vulvar involvement in autoimmune bullous diseases. *J Reprod Med* 1993;38:101.
108. Zolnoun DA, Hartman KE, Steege JF. Overnight 5% lidocaine ointment for treatment of vulvar vestibulitis. *Obstet Gynecol* 2003;102:84.
109. McKay M, Frankman O, Horowitz BJ, et al. Vulvar vestibulitis and vestibular papillomatosis report of the ISSVD committee on vulvodynia. *J Reprod Med* 1991;36:413.
110. Bergeron S, Binik YM, Khalife S, et al. Vulvar vestibulitis syndrome: reliability of diagnosis and evaluation of current diagnostic criteria. *Obstet Gynecol* 2001;98:45.
111. Bouchard C, Brisson J, Fortier M, et al. Use of oral contraceptive pills and vulvar vestibulitis: a case-control study. *Am J Epidemiol* 2002;156:254.
112. Stewart EG, Spencer P. *The V book: A doctor's guide to complete vulvovaginal health.* New York: Bantam Books, 2002:301.
113. Ryan KJ, Berkowitz RS, Barbieri RL, et al. *Kistner's gynecology and women's health.* 7th ed. St. Louis: Mosby, 1999:71.
114. Portnoy J, Ahronheim GA, Ghibu F, et al. Recovery of Epstein-Barr virus from genital ulcers. *N Engl J Med* 1984;311:966.
115. Muram D, Gold SS. Vulvar ulcerations in girls with myelocytic leukemia. *South Med J* 1993;86:293.
116. Silber TJ, Olsen J. Recurrent genital ulcer in an adolescent as a manifestation of Behçet's disease. *J Adolesc Health Care* 1988;9:231.

117. Ammann AJ, Johnson A, Fyfe G, et al. Behçet syndrome. *J Pediatr* 1985;107:41.

118. Sehgal VN, Srivastaca G. Chancroid: contemporary appraisal. *Int J Dermatol* 2003;42:182.

119. Flood JM, Sarafian SK, Bolan GA, et al. Multistrain outbreak of chancroid in San Francisco, 1989–1991. *J Infect Dis* 1993;176:1106.

120. Lewis DA. Diagnostic tests for chancroid. *Sex Trans Infect* 2000;76(2):137.

121. Egan CA, Bradly RR, Logsdon VK, et al. Vulvar melanoma in childhood. *Arch Dermatol* 1997;133:345.

122. McCormick JK, Yarwood JM, Schlievert PM. Toxic shock syndrome and bacterial superantigens: an update. *Ann Rev Microbiol* 2001;55:77.

123. Todd J, Fishaut M, Kapral F, et al. Toxic shock syndrome associated with phage group-1 staphylococci. *Lancet* 1978;2:1116.

124. Berkley SF, Hightower AW, Broome CV, et al. The relationship of tampon characteristics to menstrual toxic shock syndrome. *JAMA* 1987;258:917.

125. Petitti DB, Reingold A. Tampon characteristics and menstrual toxic shock syndrome. *JAMA* 1988;259:686.

126. Petitti DB, Reingold AL. Recent trends in the incidence of toxic shock syndrome in Northern California. *Am J Public Health* 1991;81:1209.

127. Centers for Disease Control. Reduced incidence of menstrual toxic-shock syndrome United States, 1980–1990. *MMWR* 1990;39:421.

128. Hajjeh RA, Reingold A, Weil A, et al. Toxic shock syndrome in the United States: surveillance update, 1979–1996. Emerg Infect Dis J 1999;5(6). Available from: www.cdc.government/nicdod/EID/vol5no6/hajjehG.htm

129. Bergdoll MS, Reiser RF, Crass BA, et al. A new staphylococcal enterotoxin F, associated with toxic-shock-syndrome *Staphylococcus aureus* isolates. *Lancet* 1981;1:1017.

130. Matsuda Y, Kato H, Yamada R, et al. Early and definitive diagnosis of toxic shock syndrome by detection of marked expansion of T-cell-receptor vβ2-positive T cells. *Emerg Infect Dis* (serial online) 2003 Mar;9(3). Available from www.cdc.government/ncidod/EID/vol9no3/02-0360.htm

131. Herwald H, Cramer H, Matthias M, et al. M Protein, a classical bacterial virulence determinate, forms complexes with fibrinogen that induce vascular leakage. *Cell* 2004;116:367.

132. Demetriou E, Emans SJ, Masland RP. Dysuria in adolescent girls. *Pediatrics* 1982;80:299.

133. Stamm WE, Wagner KF, Amsel R, et al. Causes of the acute urethral syndrome in women. *N Engl J Med* 1980;303:409.

134. Stamm WE, Counts GW, Running KR, et al. Diagnosis of coliform infection in acutely dysuric women. *N Engl J Med* 1982;307:463.

135. Stamm WE, Running K, McKevitt M, et al. Treatment of acute urethral syndrome. *N Engl J Med* 1981;304:956.

136. Bent S, Nallamothu BK, Simel DL, et al. Does this woman have an acute uncomplicated urinary tract infection? *JAMA* 2002;287:2701.

137. Gaydos CA, Quinn TC, Willis D, et al. Performance of the Aptima Combo2 assay for detection of Chlamydia trachomatis and Neisseria gonorrhoeae in female urine and endocervical swab specimens. *J Clin Microbiol* 2003;41:304.

138. Fihn SD. Acute uncomplicated urinary tract infections in women. *N Engl J Med* 2003;349:259.

139. Hooten TM, Scholes D, Hughes JP, et al. A prospective study of risk factors for symptomatic urinary tract infection in young women. *N Engl J Med* 1996;335:468.

Further Reading

Kaufman RH, Friedrich EG, Gardner HL. *Benign diseases of the vulva and vagina.* 4th ed. St. Louis: Mosby—Year Book, 1994.

Stewart EG, Spencer P. *The V book: A doctor's guide to complete vulvovaginal health.* New York: Bantam Books, 2002.

Wilkinson EJ, Stone IK. *Atlas of vulvar disease.* Baltimore: Williams & Wilkins, 1995.

15

Bacterial Sexually Transmitted Infections: Gonorrhea, *Chlamydia*, Pelvic Inflammatory Disease, and Syphilis

Lydia A. Shrier

Sexually transmitted diseases (STDs) are epidemic among adolescents in the United States. Of the 15 million new cases of STDs identified each year, approximately one-fourth occur in adolescents (1). The high prevalence of STDs in teens is the result of many behavioral, biological, social, and epidemiological factors. Adolescents are more likely than adults to engage in a variety of sexual risk behaviors, including sexual intercourse with multiple and high-risk sexual partners; inconsistent, incorrect, or lack of condom use; and risky sexual practices such as rectal intercourse (often to preserve virginity). Early onset of sexual activity predisposes adolescents to STDs due to lack of immunity from prior exposure and, in girls, cervical ectopy (extension of endocervical columnar epithelium onto the exocervix). Sexual violence, secrecy, poor sexuality education, lack of ability to pay for services and treatment, lack of access, discomfort with facilities and services designed for adults, and concerns about confidentiality may increase the rates of STD acquisition and augment the dearth of preventive services and prompt treatment for adolescents (2).

Many pediatricians are not aware of confidentiality laws existing in every state that permit adolescents to consent to their own health care related to STDs; in a survey by the American Academy of Pediatrics, 28% of pediatricians identified "issues with confidentiality" as a barrier to care for adolescent patients (3). Increased health facilities for teenagers and the advent of noninvasive STD testing (4) have permitted better diagnosis and reporting, and the recognition of asymptomatic infections in males and females has resulted in increased screening, factors that have also contributed to higher reported rates in adolescents. Adolescent girls infected with *Neisseria gonorrhoeae* and *Chlamydia trachomatis* are at particular risk of upper genital

tract infections including pelvic inflammatory disease (PID) and the possible sequelae of infertility, ectopic pregnancy, and chronic pain. Although the highest number
of gonococcal and chlamydial infections occur in young women between 15 and 24
years of age (1), very young teenagers who are sexually active have an especially
high risk of acquiring these pathogens. The health consequences and costs associated
with the high prevalence of STDs are substantial, yet they remain largely hidden (2).

More widespread screening to detect asymptomatic infections of *N. gonorrhoeae*
and *C. trachomatis* and improved recognition of the symptoms of upper genital tract
infections are needed to enhance the health care of teenage women. The finding of
one STD should lead to the diagnostic suspicion of other potential STDs, including
syphilis and human immunodeficiency virus (HIV). Given the risk of transmitting
and acquiring hepatitis B infection during the adolescent years, all adolescents deserve appropriate immunization to prevent this infection. Family planning clinics
should provide adequate screening and treatment for STDs, and STD clinics should
counsel their clients about appropriate methods of contraception if pregnancy is not
desired. Potential effects of contraceptives on STDs are considered in Chapter 20.

GONOCOCCAL INFECTIONS

Following implementation of a national program in the mid-1970s to reduce gonococcal disease, the annual estimated rate of new infections with *N. gonorrhoeae* declined from 1 million in 1977 to 650,000 in 1996 (5). However, reported rates of
gonococcal infections increased by more than 8% from 1997 to 1999, then declined
slightly in 2000 to 2001 (6–8). Approximately 24% to 30% of the reported morbidity from gonorrhea is in adolescent age groups, and adolescent women ages 15 to 19
years have higher rates of gonorrhea than any other sex-age group (703.2 per 100,000
in 2001) (6).

The incubation period for *N. gonorrhoeae* is approximately 1 week, with symptoms
generally appearing within 10 days after exposure (9,10). Although it has been estimated that 75% to 90% of all gonococcal infections in women and 10% to 40% of infections in men are asymptomatic (9), many of these patients on careful questioning
do, in fact, have symptoms. Screening endocervical tests indicate that the asymptomatic rate of gonorrhea ranges from 0% to 13% in adolescent women, depending on
the clinical setting (11). Adolescents seen in private practices in the suburbs (11) and
in high schools (12,13) tend to have lower rates than adolescents seen in emergency
departments (14), large outpatient hospital clinics serving an inner city population
(15,16), or in juvenile detention centers (17,18) (Table 15-1). Risk markers for infection with gonorrhea include a history of sexual abuse, sexual behaviors such as early
onset of sexual intercourse, high numbers of casual partners, selection of partners at
high risk of gonorrhea, and "survival sex" (sex for food, money, drugs, or shelter), and
health behaviors such as failure to recognize symptoms, delay in seeking treatment,
delay in notifying partners, nonuse of barrier contraception, and noncompliance with

TABLE 15-1. *Prevalence of Urogenital Infection with* Neisseria gonorrhoeae *and* Chlamydia trachomatis *in Different Female Adolescent Samples*

Source	Sample Size (number of females)	Sample Characteristics	Prevalence	
			N. gonorrhoeae	C. trachomatis
Biro FM et al. (1995)	477	Patients 12–21 years-old attending an urban, hospital-based, adolescent clinic	6.3%	15.7%
Oh MK et al. (1996)	216	Urban adolescents	11.6%	23.2%
Oh MK et al. (1998)	46	Adolescents admitted to a short-term juvenile detention center	13.1%	28.3%
Gaydos C et al. (1998)	13,204	New female U.S. Army recruits	—	9.2%
Bunnell RE et al. (1999)	650	Sexually active patients of 4 teen clinics ages 14–19 years	6%	27%
Cohen DA et al. (1999)	1883	Urban high school students	2.5%	11.5%
Embling ML et al. (2000)	37	Adolescents 14 years and older seeking care in an urban emergency department	8%	8%
Kelly PJ et al. (2000)	200	Adolescents in 2 juvenile detention centers	—	22.2%
Mertz KJ et al. (2001)	141,336	Women 16–24 years of age enrolled in national job training program from 1990 to 1997	—	12.5%
Best D et al. (2001)	505	Adolescent patients of 2 pediatric private practices	<0.1%	0.9%
		Sexually active patients	<0.1%	2.7%
Mertz KJ et al. (2002)	621–8,658	Adolescents entering juvenile detention centers	3.4–10.0%	8.0–19.5%
Niccolai L et al. (2003)	200	Pregnant adolescents ages 14–19 years	3.4%	18.2%
Nsuami M et al. (2003)	200	Urban high school students	2.0%	6.5%
Moens V et al. (2003)	492	Adolescents 12–21 years of age attending a contraceptive and psychotherapy service	—	10.6%

therapy (19–21). Although clear recommendations do not exist (8), screening sexually active adolescents at low risk once a year or less often may be considered, depending on local population prevalence of gonorrhea. Adolescents at high risk should be screened once or twice a year. A young woman who has recently changed sexual partners, has symptoms, or has another STD should be tested for gonorrhea.

Diagnosis

N. gonorrhoeae, a fastidious gram-negative intracellular diplococcus, may be cultured using a selective (e.g., Thayer–Martin or Martin–Lewis) or nonselective (e.g., chocolate agar) medium. Specimens for culture must be transported under anaerobic conditions to maintain the viability of organisms. Culture is highly sensitive and specific, inexpensive, and yields an isolate that may be retained for additional testing for legal purposes, antimicrobial susceptibility determination, and subtyping (7). It is critical that *N. gonorrhoeae* be confirmed and properly identified in prepubertal girls, since cultures of vaginal discharge may yield other *Neisseria* species such as *N. cinerea*.

Two nucleic acid hybridization assays for the detection of *N. gonorrhoeae* are available, Gen-Probe PACE 2 and Digene Hybrid Capture II. With the PACE 2 assay, a DNA probe that is complementary to a specific sequence of *N. gonorrhoeae* rRNA hybridizes with any complementary rRNA found in the specimen. The Hybrid Capture II assay involves RNA hybridization probes that are specific for DNA sequences of *N. gonorrhoeae*. Specimens collected for testing using a hybridization assay may be stored and transported for up to 7 days without refrigeration before testing. Compared to culture, the sensitivity of the PACE 2 probe ranges from 90% to 100% (22–27); sensitivity for Hybrid Capture II is 87% to 93% (28–30). Both nucleic acid hybridization assays can test for *C. trachomatis* as well as *N. gonorrhoeae* using a single swab.

Nucleic acid amplification tests (NAATs) for gonorrhea in urine, endocervical, and urethral specimens have become increasingly sensitive, specific, and available. Although initial studies appear promising, currently no tests have been approved by FDA for use with vaginal specimens (7). Specimens, especially of urine, can contain amplification inhibitors that result in false-negative results on NAAT testing (31,32). However, in general, sensitivities among NAATs, nonamplified nucleic acid hybridization tests, and culture are not substantially different when using endocervical swabs. False-positive results may occur because of contamination or because the primers used with some NAATs for *N. gonorrhoeae* may cross-react with nongonococcal *Neisseria* species (31,33). Currently, polymerase chain reaction (PCR; Amplicor, Roche), transcription-mediated amplification (TMA; Aptima, Gen-Probe, Inc.), and strand displacement amplification (SDA; BDProbeTec ET, Beckton Dickinson) are available for testing of endocervical swabs, and the TMA and SDA assays may be performed with female urine specimens. As a result of the limitations of

NAAT testing for gonorrhea, PCR for gonorrhea on female urine specimens is not FDA approved and the ligase chain reaction (LCR) test (LCx, Abbott) for gonorrhea is no longer available for use with any specimen type (34).

There is currently no adequate point-of-care test for gonorrhea. Gram stains of endocervical specimens are not recommended for testing for *N. gonorrhoeae* infection among women because the sensitivity is low (9,35,36) and skilled microscopy must be performed to ensure adequate specificity (7). Gram stains of pharyngeal specimens are not recommended because the pharynx is colonized with *N. meningitidis* and commensal *Neisseria* species (37).

Culturing the endocervix remains the best screening test for detecting gonococcal infection because of optimal specificity compared with other test types, ease of additional testing, and ability to provide antimicrobial-resistance monitoring (Table 15-2) (7). If culture cannot be obtained from the endocervix or culture sensitivity might be compromised because of problems in maintaining appropriate transport and storage conditions, then NAAT or nucleic acid hybridization testing of an endocervical swab specimen is recommended. NAAT testing of a urine specimen may be conducted if a pelvic examination otherwise is not being performed, with the recognition that sensitivity may be slightly compromised (31,32). Additional testing after a positive nonculture result on screening for *N. gonorrhoeae* is generally recommended when screening in a population with a low prevalence of gonococcal infection (7). NAAT testing of urine or endocervical specimens is appropriate for diagnostic testing of symptomatic patients, who are more likely to have infection (7). NAATs are not recommended for use with rectal and pharyngeal specimens, and routinely culturing the rectum and pharynx is not cost-effective in asymptomatic adolescent populations (38,39). Pharyngeal gonorrhea was reported in 2.2% of an adolescent clinic population in 1982, but a follow-up of the same clinic 8 years later showed that 0 of 319 had pharyngeal gonorrhea (the earlier study may have included some *Neisseria* species that were misidentified) (38). Treatment regimens currently used generally will eradicate *N. gonorrhoeae* at all sites.

TABLE 15-2. *Recommended tests for screening for* Neisseria gonorrhoeae *and* Chlamydia trachomatis *in women (7)*

Order of Test Preference	N. gonorrhoeae	C. trachomatis
First choice	Culture of endocervical swab specimen	NAAT of endocervical swab
Second choice	NAAT or nucleic acid hybridization testing of endocervical swab specimen	NAAT of urine specimen
Third choice	NAAT of urine specimen	Non-culture, non-NAAT of endocervical swab specimen

NAAT = Nucleic acid amplification test

Urogenital Gonococcal Infection

The endocervix is the primary site of urogenital gonococcal infection. In 70% to 90% of cases, the urethra is also infected. Patients with urogenital gonococcal infection may be asymptomatic or they may present with vaginal discharge, dysuria, urinary frequency, dyspareunia, irregular or heavy vaginal bleeding, and/or suprapubic pain. On examination, the cervix may be friable and tender to palpation with a purulent discharge. Purulent exudate may be expressed from the urethra, periurethral (Skene) glands, or Bartholin gland ducts. Labial pain and swelling may be present with a *Bartholin gland abscess* (see Fig. 15-1), which is usually treated with incision and drainage using a Ward catheter. Marsupialization is necessary for recurrent infections. Treatment for gonorrhea can be instituted on the basis of symptoms and risk for infection, although the diagnosis should be confirmed by culture, nucleic acid hybridization probe, or NAAT testing from the endocervix. Although the urethra, Skene glands, and Bartholin gland ducts are frequently also infected, they are rarely the only site of infection and therefore do not need to be tested (9).

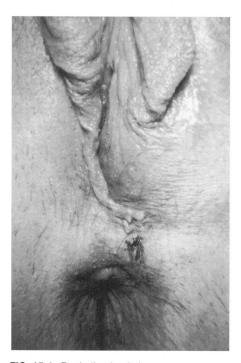

FIG. 15-1. Bartholin gland abscess.

Treatment of Asymptomatic Infections, Contacts, Urethritis, and Cervicitis

Treatment of *N. gonorrhoeae* must take into account the sites infected, the prevalence of antibiotic resistance, the high rate of coexisting *C. trachomatis* infections in adolescents, allergies, pregnancy, and the likelihood of compliance. Important variations currently identified in the United States are plasmid-mediated penicillin resistance (β-lactamase-producing *N. gonorrhoeae*), plasmid-mediated tetracycline resistance, and chromosomally mediated resistance to penicillin or tetracycline (40). In addition, quinolone resistance, established in Asia and the Pacific, has recently emerged in California and Hawaii and then Massachusetts, New York, Seattle, and Michigan, particularly among men who have sex with men (40–43). Resistance to broad-spectrum cephalosporins and to spectinomycin is rare (40).

The Centers for Disease Control and Prevention (CDC) 2002 Sexually Transmitted Diseases Treatment Guidelines recommends that one of the following regimens be used for treatment of uncomplicated urogenital gonococcal infection (42): ceftriaxone 125 mg IM single dose or cefixime 400 mg orally in a single dose (if available) or ciprofloxacin 500 mg orally single dose or ofloxacin 400 mg orally single dose or levofloxacin 250 mg orally single dose, *plus* treatment for *C. trachomatis*, such as azithromycin 1 g orally single dose or doxycycline 100 mg orally twice a day for seven days. A single intramuscular injection of ceftriaxone 125 mg is effective against gonorrheal infection of the cervix, urethra, rectum, and pharynx and is the regimen of choice when quinolone resistance (e.g. women whose partners have sex with men or who have acquired the infection in an area with quinolone resistance) or intolerance is a concern and in pregnant or nursing women. A 250-mg dose of ceftriaxone should be administered IM if treatment for incubating syphilis is indicated. Ceftriaxone can be mixed with 1% lidocaine (without epinephrine) to reduce patient discomfort with the injection (44). History and nature of allergy to penicillin and cephalosporins should be obtained before initiating treatment. Fortunately, the cross-reactivity between third-generation cephalosporins and penicillin is rare. An oral suspension of cefixime 100mg/5ml became available in 2004, and it is hoped tablets will also be made. Although irreversible articular cartilage damage has been seen in young animals treated with very high doses of fluoroquinolones, no permanent joint damage has ever been attributed to fluoroquinolone therapy in children (45). The CDC has stated that children weighing more than 45 kg can be treated with any regimen recommended for adults (42).

Spectinomycin, 2.0 g IM, is useful in patients who cannot tolerate cephalosporins or quinolones and is an alternative to ceftriaxone in pregnant patients; it is not effective against *Treponema pallidum* or for pharyngeal gonococcal infections. Other alternatives for the treatment of gonorrhea for which there are fewer data include single-dose ceftizoxime 500 mg IM, cefoxitin 2 g IM (with probenecid 1 g orally), or cefotaxime 500 mg IM. Although data are limited, alternative single-dose quinolone regimens presumed to be effective include gatifloxacin 400 mg orally, norfloxacin 800 mg orally, and lomefloxacin 400 mg orally. Although a single oral dose of azithromycin 2 g has an efficacy of 99.2% for urogenital infections and 100% for pharyngeal infection, it is not recommended because the dose is costly and poorly tolerated.

Because of the prevalence of coexisting *C. trachomatis* infections in heterosexual patients with gonorrhea of up to 42% (46,47), the single-dose therapy for gonorrhea is generally followed by medication effective against chlamydial infection. However, if the prevalence of coinfection with *C. trachomatis* is known to occur in less than 10% of cases of gonorrhea or if the results of a highly sensitive NAAT for *C. trachomatis* are known and are negative, then dual therapy may not be warranted (42).

A serologic test for syphilis should be sent at the time of therapy. If the initial test result is negative, a follow-up blood test 1 month later may be considered if the patient was treated with spectinomycin or a quinolone. HIV counseling and availability of testing as well as individual counseling about risk reduction and "safer sex" are important parts of care. Patients are instructed to abstain from sexual relations for 7 days. Since treatment failure is rare with the recommended regimens, test-of-cure is not necessary. However, a rescreening test for gonorrhea done 3 to 4 months after treatment allows the opportunity to test for reinfection. Among teens with an *N. gonorrhoeae* infection in our clinics, 23% developed one or more additional infections with *N. gonorrhoeae* and 19% developed a chlamydial infection in the ensuing 8 to 14 months of follow-up (48). Persistent symptoms also call for retesting and any *N. gonorrhoeae* isolates identified should undergo susceptibility testing.

Every patient should be interviewed to find contacts within 60 days before symptoms or diagnosis. If a patient's last sexual intercourse was more than 60 days before onset of symptoms or diagnosis, her most recent sexual partner should be sought. Regardless of their symptoms, all sexual contacts of infected patients should be tested and treated presumptively for both *N. gonorrhoeae* and *C. trachomatis*.

Gonococcal Pharyngitis

Pharyngeal infection, acquired via orogenital contact, may be detected in 10% to 20% of women with gonorrhea (9). Because pharyngeal gonorrhea is asymptomatic in more than 90% of cases, self-limited (spontaneously resolves by 12 weeks) and poorly transmitted through heterosexual contact, routine testing of the pharynx is generally not recommended (9,10). The exception is in prepubertal and peripubertal children, for whom the isolation of an organism is critical for documentation of sexual abuse. Only ceftriaxone 125 mg IM or ciprofloxacin 500 mg orally is recommended for the treatment of gonococcal pharyngeal infection.

Gonococcal Proctitis

Rectal infection may be seen in 35% to 50% of women with gonococcal cervicitis, generally from perineal contamination with infected cervical secretions; isolated rectal infection occurs in only 5% of women with gonorrhea (9). Women with rectal gonorrhea may present with anal pruritus, rectal pain, bleeding, or mucopurulent discharge, tenesmus, and/or constipation (9). In symptomatic patients and in cases of suspected childhood sexual abuse, a cotton-tipped applicator should be inserted into the rectum to obtain a sample of the pus for culture; the specimen should be obtained by direct visualization if possible (49). Proctitis can be more difficult to treat than urethritis, but the treatment courses for women are the same as noted for cervicitis.

Disseminated Gonococcal Infection

Disseminated gonococcal infection (DGI) results from gonococcal bacteremia. Affected patients may present with skin lesions, migratory arthralgias, tenosynovitis, arthritis, and rarely hepatitis, meningitis, or endocarditis. The diagnosis of gonococcal arthritis depends largely on clinical suspicion because the source of the gonococcus in adolescent girls is usually an asymptomatic or low-grade cervicitis or pharyngeal infection (50).

Unlike nongonococcal bacterial arthritis, which usually involves a single inflamed joint, gonococcal arthritis typically manifests with tenosynovitis and polyarthritis (51). The wrists, ankles, and small joints are commonly involved. Monoarthritis or oligoarthritis occurs in less than 50% of patients with DGI (52). In young women, DGI begins at the onset or just following a menstrual period in 50% and is characterized by migratory polyarthralgias, tenosynovitis, fever, chills, and, in two-thirds of patients, skin lesions (most commonly pinpoint erythematous papules that may progress to purpuric vesiculopustular lesions, although all forms of skin lesions have been seen) (see Fig. 15-2). There are usually <20 skin lesions, chiefly in a peripheral distribution. Gram stain and culture from these lesions are rarely positive. Blood cultures may be positive if taken within 2 days of the onset of symptoms. Joint fluid, usually scanty, is negative by culture for gonorrhea in about 75% of cases. PCR is a sensitive detection technique that may be useful in detecting *N. gonorrhoeae* in synovial fluid (53,54). In a study of 41 cases of gonococcal arthritis from 1985 to 1991, Wise and colleagues (55) reported positive cultures from 86% of urogenital samples, 14 (44%) synovial fluid samples, 7 rectal samples (39%), 4 blood samples (12%), and 2 throat samples (7%). Clinical features included migratory arthralgias in 27, urogenital symptoms or signs in 26, fever in 21, and skin lesions in 16.

Hospitalization is recommended for initial therapy and is essential in those who may not adhere to treatment or follow-up recommendations, have purulent joint effusions, an uncertain diagnosis, or evidence of meningitis, endocarditis, or other complications. The recommended treatment of DGI is ceftriaxone 1 g IV or IM daily (42). Alternative regimens include cefotaxime 1 g IV every 8 hours, ceftizoxime 1 g IV every 8 hours, ciprofloxacin 400 mg IV every 12 hours, ofloxacin 400 mg IV every 12 hours, levofloxacin 250 mg IV daily, or spectinomycin 2 g IM every 12 hours. All

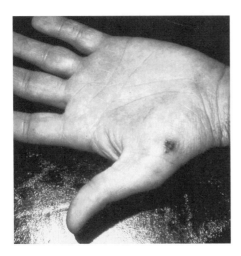

FIG. 15-2. Skin lesion of gonococcemia.

regimens should be continued for 24 to 48 hours after clinical improvement, and then therapy may be changed to one of the following regimens to complete 7 days of antimicrobial therapy (42): cefixime 400 mg orally twice a day (if available), ciprofloxacin 500 mg orally twice a day, ofloxacin 400 mg orally twice a day, or levofloxacin 500 mg orally once a day. Patients who are pregnant, unable to tolerate quinolones, or children <45 kg will need to remain on an IV or IM medication if cefixime is not available; in these cases, ceftriaxone 1 g IM once a day as an outpatient is a reasonable choice. Immobilization of the joint is helpful. Although open drainage of joints other than the hip is not indicated, repeated aspiration may be necessary (50). All patients receiving treatment for DGI should be treated presumptively for concurrent chlamydial infection unless NAAT testing excludes this infection (42).

Gonococcal endocarditis and meningitis should be treated with ceftriaxone 1 to 2 g intravenously every 12 hours; therapy should continue for 10 to 14 days in meningitis and 4 weeks in endocarditis. Complement deficiency may predispose individuals to disseminated gonococcal infection. However, because only a small proportion of patients with DGI have complement deficiency syndromes, routine screening for complement deficiencies is not indicated (9).

Reiter Syndrome

Reiter syndrome is characterized by the triad of arthritis, urethritis, and ocular abnormalities, frequently following a disease such as *N. gonorrhoeae* or *C. trachomatis* urethritis, or enteric infections such as *Shigella*, *Salmonella*, or *Yersinia*. Evidence of chlamydial infections has been found in 42% to 69% of patients with Reiter syndrome (40). Reiter syndrome is associated with HLA-B27 and -B7 determinants. The joints affected are primarily knees, ankles, feet, and wrists in an oligo- or monoarticular pattern; sacroiliitis and spondyloarthropathies can also occur. Ocular problems include iritis and conjunctivitis. Dermatologic findings include keratoblennorrhagia, mucocutaneous lesions, erosive vulvitis, nail changes, and oral ulcers. Treatment should aim at the detection and antimicrobial therapy of the genital infection and the use of nonsteroidal antiinflammatory agents for the reactive arthritis. The eyes should be carefully monitored by an ophthalmologist and treated with topical and systemic agents as indicated (56).

Gonococcal Eye Infections

Although gonococcal ophthalmia in the newborn is well known to pediatricians, adolescents can develop purulent discharge from gonococcal conjunctivitis. Periorbital edema and pain, gaze restriction, keratitis, and preauricular adenopathy can occur. A single dose of ceftriaxone 25 to 50 mg/kg (maximum 125 mg in neonates and 1 g in adults) IM should be administered, and the patient should be referred for evaluation and follow-up with an ophthalmologist. The possibility of concurrent chlamydial eye infection or genital infections with *N. gonorrhoeae* or other STDs should be evaluated.

Gonococcal Infections in the Prepubertal Child

After the newborn period, gonococcal infection in children is almost always transmitted via sexual contact. Vaginal instead of cervical infection is seen in pre- and peripubertal girls because *N. gonorrhoeae* infects columnar and transitional epithelia lining the vagina. As many as 44% of children with a positive gonorrhea culture may be asymptomatic (10). However, in a study of children less than 12 years of age presenting for evaluation of suspected sexual abuse who were cultured for gonorrhea ($n = 316$), none of the children who did not have vaginal or urethral discharge had a positive vaginal/urethral, oral, or rectal culture (57). Symptomatic children infected with gonorrhea may present with vulvar erythema, purulent vaginal discharge, pruritus, and/or dysuria. If untreated, the vaginal discharge may become serous and can persist for several months. In one recent study of girls younger than 12 years of age, 4 of 37 (11%) with a chief complaint of vaginal discharge were diagnosed with gonorrhea by vaginal culture (58). Rectal infections occur in about half of girls with gonococcal vaginitis and may be asymptomatic or cause perianal itching, burning, purulent discharge, and tenesmus. Oropharyngeal infections have been rarely reported alone (59,60). Conjunctivitis may occur alone or in association with vulvovaginitis.

Once a diagnosis is made, an experienced social worker, psychologist, nurse practitioner, or pediatrician should try to elicit a history of sexual abuse from the child (see Chapter 24). Culturing all family members and caretakers of the child can be helpful in determining the source of the infection, frequently an older male relative or caregiver. Although it is potentially possible that *N. gonorrhoeae* can be transmitted by sexual play with siblings and peers, the clinician should assume that sexual abuse is involved in all cases of prepubertal gonorrhea. Since sexual abuse often involves vulvar coitus or oral sex rather than vaginal penetration, a physical examination in many abused girls shows a normal hymen. Cases of gonorrhea in children must be reported to the mandated state agency.

Because of the frequency of infection at multiple anatomic sites and the importance of identifying pediatric cases for medicolegal purposes, cultures for gonorrhea should be obtained from the pharynx, vagina, and rectum prior to treatment of children who are symptomatic or in whom penetration or contact with a high-risk perpetrator has occurred. Cultures should be confirmed with two tests using different principles (biochemical, enzyme substrate, or serologic). Isolates should be preserved to permit additional testing if needed. Although the Gram stain is helpful in diagnosing gonorrhea, it must be noted that *Neisseria meningitidis* and other *Neisseria* species also can be associated with vaginal discharge. Other nonculture tests such as nucleic acid hybridization probes should not be used for diagnosis in children. A vaginal culture for *C. trachomatis* and a serology for syphilis should also be obtained. HIV counseling and testing should be considered initially and at follow-up.

Treatment is recommended for confirmed cases and in symptomatic children suspected of having gonococcal infection (once cultures have been obtained); prophylactic treatment of asymptomatic children being evaluated for sexual abuse is not recommended. For children who weigh ≥45 kg (99 lb), adult regimens for treating cervicitis and urethritis are used. For children under 45 kg, the recommended regimen is ceftriaxone, 125 mg IM in a single dose. Children allergic to cephalosporins are treated with spectinomycin, 40 mg/kg (maximum dose, 2 g) IM once, although this therapy is unreliable for treatment of pharyngeal infections. Patients with bacteremia or arthritis are treated with ceftriaxone, 50 mg/kg (if <45 kg, maximum dose, 1 g) once daily for 7 days. Treatment of coinfection with Chlamydia is discussed in the Chlamydia Treatment section.

Repeat cultures of the throat, rectum, and vagina should be taken 7 to 14 days after treatment. Reinfection is likely if the source is not identified and treated. Persistent vaginal discharge in a girl who has been adequately treated and had negative cultures for gonorrhea may result from a coinfection with *C. trachomatis* that was not adequately treated.

Only a few cases of salpingitis secondary to *N. gonorrhoeae* have been reported in prepubertal girls (61,62) and thus no data exist on the best form of treatment (59,62). Antibiotics with similar spectrum to those used in adolescent and adult PID are appropriate. Disseminated gonococcal disease has also been rarely reported in children.

CHLAMYDIA TRACHOMATIS INFECTIONS

With 783,242 cases reported to the CDC in 2001, *C. trachomatis* infections are the most frequently reported notifiable disease in the United States (6). In 2001, highest rates were reported from the southern United States and among women, especially those 15 to 19 years old (2,536.1 per 100,000 females) and 20 to 24 years old (2,447.0 per 100,000 females). Chlamydial infections in women may result in pelvic inflammatory disease and subsequent chronic pelvic pain, ectopic pregnancy, and tubal infertility. The rates of reported chlamydial infection increased in the 1990s, likely due to increased screening, use of more sensitive tests, and increased reporting. Where large-scale screening programs have been instituted, such as the West and Midwest, prevalence rates have declined. However, chlamydial infections are usually asymptomatic and screening is not universal, so the rate of new chlamydial infections each year in the United States is closer to an estimated 3 million (5).

It is estimated that sexually active women less than 20 years old have chlamydial infection rates two- to threefold higher than adult women. Prevalence figures vary depending on the population studied, with rates from 2.7% in sexually active adolescent patients of two suburban pediatric private practices to 28.3% in adolescents admitted to a short-term juvenile detention center (6,11–13,15,16,63–68) (Table 15-1).

Several factors contribute to increased risk of chlamydial infection among adolescent girls, including increased number of sexual partners, inconsistent condom use, nonwhite race, having a partner ≥2 years older, and marijuana use (69). Many adolescent girls have a significant cervical ectropion, the columnar cells of which are exposed to the vaginal environment and are thus more easily colonized with *C. trachomatis*. If the patient has an ectropion, the presence of infecting *C. trachomatis* is also more easily detected. Oral contraceptives have been reported to be associated with chlamydial infections in some studies, but not others. Oral contraceptives may affect the prevalence by contributing to the persistence of the ectropion. Adolescents also may be at increased risk of developing a chlamydial infection because of their "immunologic immaturity" and lower levels of antichlamydial antibodies. Younger age (69) is also an independent predictor of STDs, including *C. trachomatis*.

Although in STD clinics patients may present with signs and symptoms of chlamydial infection, in lower risk settings such as college health centers, most patients are asymptomatic and detected only by screening tests. Results of a randomized controlled trial of chlamydial screening indicated that routine screening can reduce the incidence of PID by as much as 60% (70). Because more adolescents with endocervical infection with *C. trachomatis* go on to develop salpingitis than do adult women, screening in this age group is particularly important. The CDC recommends at least annual screening for sexually active women <25 years of age (42) and in young populations with a high prevalence of *C. trachomatis*, twice-yearly screening may be warranted (71,72). It is also prudent to consider screening young women after a change in sexual partners and with any suggestive symptoms (73).

Recurrent chlamydial infections are problematic because of the increased incidence of resulting tubal damage and subsequent infertility. Adolescents are at particularly high risk for recurrent chlamydial infection (15,74,75). In one study, adolescents less than 15 years of age had an eightfold increased risk, those 15 to 19 years of age had a fivefold increased risk, and young adults 20 to 29 years had a twofold increased risk of recurrent *C. trachomatis* infection, compared to older women (74). Recurrence occurred in 54% of adolescents under 15 years and 30% of those 15 to 19 years old.

C. trachomatis is an obligate intracellular parasite of primarily squamocolumnar epithelial cells. Serotypes D through K have been associated with inclusion conjunctivitis, pneumonia, and vaginitis, most commonly in infants, nongonococcal urethritis and epididymitis in men, and mucopurulent cervicitis, salpingitis, urethritis, postabortal and postpartum endometritis, and perihepatitis in women. Both men and women may have conjunctivitis, Reiter syndrome, and rectal infections. Cervical infection with *C. trachomatis* has been associated with spontaneous abortion, intrauterine infection of the fetus, premature rupture of membranes, preterm labor, low birth weight, stillbirth, and postpartum endometritis (76,77). Chlamydial DNA or antigen is found in the fallopian tubes of a high percentage of women with tubal infertility (78). Current or past chlamydial infection may cause uterine inflammation that impairs embryo implantation or facilitates immune rejection after uterine transfer of in vitro–fertilized embryos (79).

Serotypes L1, L2, and L3 are associated with lymphogranuloma venereum (LGV), a systemic infection involving lymphoid tissue. Types A, B, Ba, and C are responsible for ocular trachoma, the most common cause of blindness in developing countries.

Transmission of *C. trachomatis* occurs via direct contact with infective material. Men who become infected with non-LGV strains will generally develop nongonococcal urethritis 1 to 3 weeks after infection. Perinatal chlamydial infection involves mucous membranes of the eye, oropharynx, urogenital tract, and rectum, and may present with or without symptoms. *C. trachomatis* is the most frequently identified infectious cause of ophthalmia neonatorum, which typically develops 5 to 12 days after birth. *C. trachomatis* may also cause a subacute, afebrile pneumonia in infants age 1 to 3 months.

Diagnosis

Female patients may be tested for *C. trachomatis* with culture; nonculture, nonamplification tests, including direct immunofluorescent smears (DFA, MicroTrak), enzyme immunoassays (Chlamydiazyme, Abbott; IDEIA, Dako), and DNA probes (PACE 2, Gen-Probe; Hybrid Capture II, Digene); and NAATs, including ligase chain reaction (LCR, Abbott), PCR (Amplicor, Roche), TMA (Aptima, Gen-Probe), and SDA (BDProbeTec ET, Becton Dickinson) (80).

Cell culture involves inoculation of McCoy cells and identification of characteristic intracytoplasmic inclusions with fluorescent antibody stain after 48 to 72 hours of growth. Culture has been the traditional "gold standard" for the diagnosis of *C. trachomatis* and is the test of choice for legal investigations because, barring laboratory error, the specificity is 100%. However, compared to newer NAAT technology, culture is suboptimal for most testing situations because of its relatively low sensitivity (80% to 90%), difficulties associated with transport and laboratory technique, and relatively high cost. Culture will not detect nonviable organisms of the lower genital tract while viable organisms may coexist in the upper genital tract. Care must be taken when cultures are obtained to use a Dacron swab and to scrape the endocervix to obtain cells, since *C. trachomatis* is an intracellular organism.

The Syva MicroTrak system includes urethral and cervical swabs and a cytobrush for making a direct smear. After applying a fluorescein-conjugated monoclonal antibody, the microscopist looks for the presence of yellow–green elementary bodies. The value of this test depends on the prevalence of *C. trachomatis* in the population studied, whether single- or double-pass cultures are used as the standard, and whether 1, 5, or 10 elementary bodies are considered a positive test result. Studies using a newer, expanded diagnostic standard that includes NAATs have found the sensitivity of this test to be as low as 38.7% (80).

Enzyme immunoassays include Chlamydiazyme and IDEIA. Chlamydiazyme is an enzyme-linked immunoabsorbent assay and requires a spectrophotometer. Its approximately 63% sensitivity is low relative to other nonculture tests (81). Sensitivity of the conventional IDEIA is 68.6% to 85% (82,83). The IDEIA PCE is a new, qualitative dual amplified EIA for the detection of chlamydial specific LPS antigens. The IDEIA PCE demonstrates improved test characteristics, with a sensitivity of 85.7% to 95% and a specificity, 98.2% to 99%, compared to conventional EIA and LCR or PCR (83,84). The new IDEIA PCE test can be performed on vaginal specimens, with a sensitivity of 88.8% and a specificity of 99.2% when a diagnostic standard that includes PCR is used and the population has a high prevalence of chlamydial infection (82). IDEIA PCE is less costly than NAATs.

The DNA probes can provide testing for both gonorrheal and chlamydial infection with a single swab. Sensitivities have been reported for chlamydial DNA tests to be 65% to 96.3% with specificities of 95% to 99.9%, when compared to culture and other nonculture, non-NAATs (85–87). Biro and colleagues (85) reported that the Gen-Probe PACE 2 system had a specificity of 96% and sensitivities of 72% and 65% in adolescent girls who were asymptomatic (prevalence 11%) and symptomatic (prevalence 20.7%), respectively. However, studies using a diagnostic standard that includes the highly sensitive NAATs have found sensitivities of the Gen-Probe PACE 2 test to be lower and specificities to be a little higher, 60.8% to 86.5% and greater than 99%, respectively (87–89).

NAATs are highly sensitive and specific for the detection of *C. trachomatis* in female urine and endocervical specimens (90–93). Although not FDA approved, the NAATs also perform well on both self-collected and clinician-collected vaginal specimens (69,94–96). PCR (Amplicor, Roche), TMA (Aptima GC/CT Combo 2 and AMP CT, Gen-Probe), and SDA (BDProbeTec, Becton Dickinson) are all available for detecting *C. trachomatis* in both endocervical swabs and female urine specimens. The LCR assay (LCx, Abbott) is no longer available. Compared with culture, the sensitivity of PCR is 82.6% for endocervical swab specimens and 84.4% for urine specimens (97). When *chlamydial infection* is defined as a positive culture or two positive NAATs, the sensitivity and specificity of PCR on urine have been high, 97.1% and 99.8%, respectively (98). TMA is similarly highly sensitive and specific on endocervical and urine specimens (sensitivities, 91.4% to 100%, specificities 99.5% to 100% (98,99). Compared to positive endocervical culture or two positive nonculture tests, the sensitivity and specificity of SDA was 92.8% and 98.8% in endocervical swabs and 80.5% and 98.4% in urine specimens, respectively (100). Depending on the prevalence of *C. trachomatis* infection in the population under study and the diagnostic standard being used for comparison, sensitivities of the NAATs may be lower than reported in the package inserts or in previous studies (69).

Rapid, point-of-care tests for *C. trachomatis* produce qualitative results while the patient is still present. However, these tests tend to be less sensitive, less specific, and more costly than laboratory-based *C. trachomatis* tests. Serology has limited utility in diagnosing *C. trachomatis* because previous chlamydial infection can produce long-lasting antibodies that cannot be readily distinguished from antibodies due to current infection (7). A conversion from lack of antibody to the presence of a titer three weeks after PID, the presence of IgM, and a fourfold rise in antibody titer have been used to confirm the role of *C. trachomatis* retrospectively in clinical cases of salpingitis and some sexual abuse cases. Antibodies to *C. trachomatis* are more common in women with PID, tubal infertility, and ectopic pregnancy than in women without these disorders.

While abnormalities may be seen on the Pap tests of women with chlamydial infection, the sensitivity, specificity, and predictive values are too low to merit recommendation of this test for the diagnosis of *C. trachomatis* (101). In a study of 257 sexually active adolescent women, 24 (9.3%) had a positive culture for *C. trachomatis* and 58 (22.6%) had significant cervical smear abnormalities (102). There were no significant differences in the prevalence of an abnormal Pap smear between adolescents with or without chlamydial infection.

In choosing a test for office practice, clinicians need to look at the comparison of the test with culture, the expense, the time to obtain results, and the sensitivity and predictive value in the population of patients for whom they will be providing care (7). In most instances, a NAAT is the preferred test for screening and diagnosis of *C. trachomatis*. NAATs may be performed on endocervical, urethral, and urine specimens (Table 15-2). No tests have been cleared yet for use with vaginal specimens, although several studies assessing vaginal specimens have shown promising sensitivity and specificity (94,95,103,104) and found the method to be highly acceptable among adolescents (96,105,106). NAAT testing should be performed on an endocervical swab specimen, if a pelvic examination is being performed; otherwise, an

NAAT performed on urine is recommended (7). The advent of routine urine testing has permitted screening to be conducted in nontraditional venues where pelvic examinations cannot be performed, such as schools, jails, street outreach programs, etc. If NAAT testing is not available, a nonculture, non-NAAT test such as a DNA hybridization probe or EIA may be performed on an endocervical specimen.

Culture is suitable for routine screening and diagnosis of *C. trachomatis*, but is generally used for chlamydial testing only in specific circumstances. In prepubertal children, in whom the diagnosis of sexual abuse must be considered and in adolescents, if specimens are being obtained for medico-legal purposes, culture is essential because of the possibility of false-positive results with nonculture tests. If culture is not readily available, some clinicians use NAAT tests, then culture the very few patients who have positive results before initiating antibiotic therapy. Culture is also indicated for rectal or pharyngeal swab specimens because there is limited data on the use of nonculture tests and the increased potential for cross-reactivity with other organisms (7).

Regardless of the test used, a positive result for *C. trachomatis* must be considered a true positive and the patient treated appropriately. However, all tests for *C. trachomatis*, even culture in rare instances, can yield false-positive results. In a low prevalence population, the proportion of total positive tests that are truly positive (i.e., the positive predictive value, or PPV) is reduced. For this reason, the CDC recommends that if the prevalence of chlamydial infection is less than 5%, a confirmatory test should be performed on patients with a positive screening test (107). Routine additional testing to further evaluate a positive *C. trachomatis* result is recommended in asymptomatic patients from such a population (7). Additional testing should also be considered if a false-positive screening test result would have substantial adverse medical, social, or psychological impact for a patient. After a potentially false-positive NAAT, only another NAAT has a sufficiently high sensitivity to be used for additional testing. Culture with a *C. trachomatis*–specific antimajor outer membrane protein (MOMP) stain or competitive probe and blocking antibody formats can be used after a positive non-NAAT (7).

In addition to genital tract infections, *C. trachomatis* is a major etiologic agent in perihepatitis or *Fitz–Hugh–Curtis syndrome,* with or without concurrent salpingitis (108,109). The patient typically presents with right upper quadrant pain, often pleuritic, and laboratory evaluation reveals an increased erythrocyte sedimentation rate (ESR) and may have a positive endocervical test for *C. trachomatis* (note that endocervical tests can be negative in patients with upper genital tract chlamydial infection). Ultrasonography may be necessary to exclude biliary tract disease in patients with this type of pain. Liver function tests are usually normal in chlamydial perihepatitis, in contrast to the elevated liver function tests that may accompany gonococcal perihepatitis.

Although asymptomatic pharyngeal colonization has been noted among men with urogenital *C. trachomatis* infection, the prevalence of chlamydial infection in the pharynx is low (110). On Amplicor PCR testing, *C. trachomatis* was detected in 11 ano-rectal specimens (5.6%) from 196 women attending an STD clinic and was not predicted by the presence of anorectal signs or symptoms (111). Proctitis may be seen in women as part of the anorectal syndrome of lymphogranuloma venereum, a chronic chlamydial infection that is seen primarily in Africa, Asia, and South America (112).

Treatment

The following regimens are recommended for the treatment of *C. trachomatis* cervical and urethral infections in women (42): azithromycin 1 g orally in a single dose or doxycycline 100 mg orally 2 times a day for 7 days. Alternate regimens include erythromycin base 500 mg 4 times a day for 7 days or erythromycin ethylsuccinate 800 mg 4 times a day for 7 days or ofloxacin 300 mg 2 times a day for 7 days or levofloxacin 500 mg orally once a day for 7 days.

Azithromycin and doxycycline are similar in efficacy and side effects, which are primarily gastrointestinal (113). In general, azithromycin is preferred in adolescents, because it can be administered by a health professional in a single oral dose. Azithromycin is more costly from the perspective of the public health clinic, but for the third-party payer and for the health care system as a whole, it is more cost-effective than doxycycline owing to improved compliance with the single dose and subsequent reduction in costly sequelae from infection (114). Erythromycin is less efficacious than either azithromycin or doxycycline and is often poorly tolerated due to gastrointestinal side effects. Ofloxacin has similar efficacy to azithromycin and doxycycline and can also be used to treat *N. gonorrhoeae* (115). Levofloxacin has similar pharmacology and *in vitro* microbiologic activity to ofloxacin and thus may be used for treatment of both chlamydial and gonococcal infections, although it has not been fully evaluated (116). Other quinolones either do not adequately treat *C. trachomatis* or have not been fully evaluated. Quinolones are more expensive than the other alternative regimens and they cannot be used in pregnancy or lactation. Children should be treated with erythromycin 50 mg/kg per day in four divided doses for 14 days (children <45 kg and <8 years), azithromycin 1 g orally single dose (children ≥45 kg of any age), or doxycycline 100 mg twice a day for 7 days (children >8 years). Clindamycin is effective against *C. trachomatis in vitro*, results in clinical and bacteriologic cure, and may be used in pregnant women, but is significantly more costly than alternative regimens (117).

Pregnant patients are treated with erythromycin 500 mg 4 times a day for 7 days or amoxicillin 500 mg 3 times daily for 7 days (42). Alternative regimens include erythromycin base 250 mg or erythromycin ethylsuccinate 400 mg 4 times daily for 14 days or erythromycin ethylsuccinate 800 mg 4 times a day for 7 days, or azithromycin 1 g orally in a single dose (117). Erythromycin estolate has been associated with hepatotoxicity and should not be used in pregnant women. Azithromycin is secreted in breast milk (118).

Patients being treated for chlamydial infection should be examined for other STDs and partners should receive adequate diagnosis and treatment at the same visit. It is important to remember that *C. trachomatis* can remain asymptomatic in the cervix for months and probably years (119,120), and pinpointing the source can be problematic in some adolescents. Thus, the recommendation is to evaluate and treat partners within 60 days of the onset of symptoms or identification in the asymptomatic patient. If the last intercourse was more than 60 days previously, the last sexual partner should be assessed and treated. Patients and their partners should abstain from intercourse until they have all completed the treatment course and are without symptoms. As with all STDs, patients should be thoroughly counseled about the need to have monogamous relationships and the use of barrier contraception or abstinence.

Because of the high risk of reexposure to an untreated partner, the possibility of noncompliance, the risk of persistent chlamydial infection despite treatment (120), and the substantial morbidity associated with chlamydial infection in young women, clinicians should rescreen adolescents 3 to 4 months after treatment and continue to advise ongoing screening on at least an annual basis thereafter (42). In general, patients treated with azithromycin or doxycycline do not need a test of cure. A test of cure may be considered 3 weeks after a course of erythromycin in nonpregnant patients. Repeat testing 3 weeks after treatment should be performed in all pregnant patients because of the reduced efficacy and frequent side effects (with associated decreased compliance) seen with regimens used in these patients. Nonculture tests performed less than 3 weeks after completing treatment may give false-positive results due to continued excretion of dead organisms.

PELVIC INFLAMMATORY DISEASE

Pelvic inflammatory disease involves infection of the female upper genital tract, including any combination of parametritis, acute salpingitis, oophoritis, tubo-ovarian abscess (TOA), and pelvic peritonitis. PID may occur as a sexually acquired acute salpingitis, a postpartum or postabortal infection, or the chronic sequela to a previous acute or silent salpingitis.

Over one million women are diagnosed with PID every year in the United States, with 16% to 20% of cases occurring in teenagers. The highest age-specific rates are for ages 15 to 19 years, with the risk of PID in sexually active 15 year olds 1:8 (versus 1:80 for age 24 years) (121). The highest rates of increase are also seen in adolescents (122).

The cost of acute PID was estimated to increase from over $4.2 billion (for medical services and lost work) in 1990 to $9 billion by 2000 (123). Declining rates of PID and a shift from inpatient to less costly outpatient management have reduced the estimates, although the costs are still substantial. The direct medical expenditures for PID and its three major sequelae, chronic pelvic pain, ectopic pregnancy, and infertility, were estimated to be $1.88 billion per year in 1998 dollars (124). This estimate does not include costs related to decreased quality of life the emotional consequences of sequelae, or lost productivity, which are several times the direct costs. Asymptomatic pelvic infection and minimally symptomatic PID can also lead to adhesions, infertility, and ectopic pregnancy and thus have additional costs.

Determinants of risk of PID include the size of inoculum, the number of infecting pathogens, the virulence of infecting organisms, host susceptibility, and environmental factors. There are several risk factors (possibly causative variables) unique to adolescents that predispose them to PID. First, adolescents are exposed to and become infected by nongonococcal agents at a disproportionate rate. *C. trachomatis* in particular is associated with asymptomatic infection, which can then develop into PID without warning. Second, adolescents have low levels of local protective antibody as they often had no previous exposure to the pathogens that can cause PID, and thus they are more likely than adults to develop a serious infection upon exposure. Third, many adolescent girls have a cervical ectropion, an erythematous area surrounding the os that is caused by columnar epithelium on the exocervix, to which many STD pathogens readily adhere. Fourth, adolescents are more likely than adults to engage in certain sexual behaviors that put them at risk for STDs and PID, including having unprotected intercourse, frequent intercourse, multiple sex partners, and intercourse during menses. Smoking and douching, common among adolescents, are also risk factors for PID. Risk markers (variables that are associated with PID but not in the causal pathway) include demographic and social indicators, such as black race, low socioeconomic status, substance abuse, and history of involvement with a child protective agency (122,125).

Oral contraceptive pills, a common choice for contraception among adolescents, are associated with scant cervical mucus, one of the natural barriers to ascension of bacteria into the upper tract, and increased rates of chlamydial infection (although not consistently across studies) (126–128). However, oral contraceptive pill use has been associated with a reduced risk of PID in women with chlamydial infection (129). The most recent data from the PID Evaluation and Clinical Health (PEACH) study of 563 women with pelvic pain showed a lack of an association between upper genital tract infection and the use of oral contraceptives or medroxyprogesterone (130). Inconsistent condom use was associated with a two to three times greater risk of upper tract infection. Invasive procedures, such as insertion of an intrauterine device (IUD) within the past 30 days or a therapeutic abortion, are associated with PID.

Cervicitis with *N. gonorrhoeae* or *C. trachomatis* is clearly associated with PID, particularly in adolescents. It has been estimated that adolescents with a gonococcal or chlamydial endocervical infection have a 30% chance of developing PID, compared to a 10% risk in older women. *N. gonorrhoeae* or *C. trachomatis* has been isolated from 77% of patients with laparoscopically confirmed acute salpingitis (131). In a study of 556 women at risk for PID, 1 in 4 of those with lower genital tract gonorrheal or chlamydial infection and 1 in 7 of those with bacterial vaginosis had subclinical PID (132). In approximately 30% of women with PID, only anaerobic and/or facultative bacteria have been isolated (133). The polymicrobial flora include coliforms, *Gardnerella vaginalis*, *Haemophilus influenzae*, group B streptococci, *Bacteroides* species (e.g., *Bacteroides fragilis*, *disiens*, and *bivius*), *Peptostreptococcus*,

Peptococcus, *Mycoplasma hominis*, and *Mycoplasma genitalium* (133–136). The presence of bacterial vaginosis, the most common infectious cause of vaginal discharge, may facilitate ascension of pathogenic organisms (137). The aerobic and anaerobic flora of PID are similar to those occurring in bacterial vaginosis (131), suggesting that bacterial vaginosis may be a risk factor for PID. Severe PID with abscess is invariably a polymicrobial infection that involves anaerobic bacteria (121,134). A previous episode of PID predisposes a woman to future episodes, due to scarring and impaired local barriers to infection.

PID has been reported to be temporally related to menses (138). Sweet and coworkers (139) found that 81% of women with PID occurring within 7 days of the onset of menses had gonorrheal or chlamydial infection. In contrast, of the occurrences of PID seen more than 14 days after the onset of menses, 66% were nongonococcal, nonchlamydial infections. Overall, 55% of gonococcal PID and 57% of chlamydial PID occurred in the first 7 days of the cycle. Among women with cervical *N. gonorrhoeae*, *C. trachomatis*, or bacterial vaginosis, the proliferative phase of the menstrual cycle was also associated with endometritis (140). In a case-control study of women with and without PID, women who reported sexual intercourse during the previous menses had more than five times the risk of PID (138). Slap and colleagues (141) found that adolescent patients with tubo-ovarian abscess tended to present later in their menstrual cycle (more than 18 days from the last menstrual period) than those without TOA. The increased risk of ascending infection during the menses may occur because of loss of the cervical mucus plug, shedding of the endometrium, which may have offered protection from infection, the presence of menstrual blood, which is an excellent culture medium, and the reflux of blood into the fallopian tubes.

STD-associated PID is caused by canalicular spread of microorganisms along mucosal surfaces from the vagina, through the cervix, to the endometrium, fallopian tubes, and abdominal cavity (121). In gonococcal PID, once the bacteria reach the tubal epithelium, they penetrate the nonciliated cells, where they are protected from immune defense factors, and eventually are released from the basal surfaces of the cells by exocytosis. Antibody binding to gonococcal lipoligosaccharides and peptidoglycan in the fallopian tubes activates complement and initiates the prostaglandin cascade, producing acute inflammation with purulent exudate, edema, vasodilatation, and tissue destruction. Antibody against *N. gonorrhoeae* likely offers some protection against recurrent gonococcal PID. The incidence of isolation of gonococcus is inversely proportional to the number of episodes of salpingitis, with no *N. gonorrhoeae* recovered from women with three or more previous episodes of salpingitis (142).

Chlamydial infection spreads in a similar fashion to gonococcal infection. *C. trachomatis* attaches to tubal epithelial cells and is transported into the cells, where it replicates protected from immune response (121) and cellular damage ensues. Local and systemic humoral immune responses, as well as cell-mediated immunity, are involved in chlamydial PID (143). In a prospective study of female sex workers, women with antibody to chlamydial heat shock protein-60 (CHsp60) had a two- to threefold increased risk for PID (144). It appears that *C. trachomatis* has an acute phase with influx of polymorphonuclear leukocytes and a chronic or persistent phase that involves the presence of mononuclear cells (delayed hypersensitivity) (145). Once chlamydial growth is inhibited by the acquired immune response, tissue damage may continue owing to autoimmune inflammation (143). Long-term damage may occur because of recurrent infection, which stimulates host responses. Protective immunity against reinfection appears to be serovar specific, so women may experience repeated episodes of chlamydial PID despite a normal immune response. Simultaneous infection with gonorrhea appears to facilitate replication of chlamydial organisms in cervical epithelium. Other postulated modes of spread for bacteria include transport via attachment to sperm or *Trichomonas vaginalis*, transfer with retrograde menstruation, or perhaps lymphatic spread (which may occur with *Mycoplasma*).

If the infection reaches the fimbriated ends of the tubes, it can cause pelvic peritonitis. If the tubes are blocked, a pyosalpinx may develop; if the ovaries are involved, a TOA may occur. About one-fourth of hospitalized PID patients have palpable adnexal swelling, and 3% to 17% develop an abscess. Anaerobic bacteria, which thrive in the environment created by facultative bacteria present early in PID, are the predominant pathogens in abscesses (121).

Diagnosis

The diagnosis of PID is generally made on the basis of clinical criteria, which have an accuracy of 65% to 90% when compared to laparoscopy. It is always important to weigh the consequences of a false-positive diagnosis ("overcalling" PID)—financial burden, risk of missing other diagnoses, exposure to unnecessary antibiotics, psychological stigma, bias towards making future diagnoses of PID—against the consequences of a false-negative diagnosis (missing the diagnosis of PID) and exposing the patient to undue risk of the complications and sequelae.

The classic picture of acute salpingitis which includes lower abdominal pain, vaginal/cervical discharge, and fever, with leukocytosis and increased ESR, following the onset of menses in a sexually active young woman, is seen in only about 20% of laparoscopically verified cases of PID. Symptoms may be much less specific and include menstrual irregularities, dyspareunia, nausea, vomiting, diarrhea, constipation, dysuria, and urinary frequency. Historical symptoms are usually not statistically significant indicators of PID and when they are, they have low sensitivity and specificity (146). However, compared to women with a visually normal pelvis, women with PID report longer duration of pain and irregular bleeding (147). A history of urethritis or an STD in the patient's sexual partner helps the clinician to make the appropriate diagnosis. Note that many women with laparoscopically confirmed PID may have only some or none of these signs and symptoms and women with mild pain, tenderness, and fever may have severe tubal disease (148). It is likely that subclinical infection accounts for most cases of PID; of women with infertility due to bilateral tubal occlusion, 71% have serum antibodies to *C. trachomatis* (149) and approximately 60% report no history of PID (121).

In 2002, the CDC recommended initiating empiric treatment of PID in sexually active young women and other women at risk for STDs who have uterine/adnexal tenderness or cervical motion tenderness and no other cause(s) for the illness can be identified (Table 15-3) (42). These criteria are less stringent, recognizing that many episodes of PID go undiagnosed. Requiring lower abdominal tenderness, cervical motion tenderness, *and* adnexal tenderness, as recommended in previous guidelines (150), likely resulted in low sensitivity in patients at high risk for infection. The PEACH study found that the finding of adnexal tenderness was 95.5% sensitive for the diagnosis of endometritis, which was significantly higher that the 83.3% sensitivity of the previously recommended CDC criteria (151).

Because of the low specificity of the new diagnostic criteria, it is important to consider the extensive differential diagnosis and excluded alternative explanations for

TABLE 15-3. *Criteria for the diagnosis of pelvic inflammatory disease (PID).*

Minimum criteria

Empiric treatment of PID should be initiated in sexually active young women if all of the following criteria are met *and no other cause(s) for the illness can be identified*:
- Uterine/adnexal tenderness or
- Cervical motion tenderness

Additional criteria

These criteria may be used to enhance the specificity of the minimum criteria but are not required to make the diagnosis of PID:
- Oral temperature >101°F (>38.3°C)
- Abnormal cervical or vaginal mucopurulent discharge[a]
- Presence of white blood cells (WBCs) on saline microscopy of vaginal secretions[a]
- Elevated erythrocyte sedimentation rate
- Elevated C-reactive protein
- Laboratory documentation of cervical infection with *N. gonorrhoeae* or *C. trachomatis*

Definitive criteria
- Endometrial biopsy with histopathologic evidence of endometritis
- Transvaginal sonography or magnetic resonance imaging techniques showing thickened, fluid-filled tubes with or without free pelvic fluid or tubo-ovarian complex
- Laparoscopic abnormalities consistent with PID

[a]Most women with PID have either mucopurulent cervical discharge or evidence of WBCs on a microscopic evaluation of a saline preparation of vaginal fluid. If the cervical discharge appears normal and no white blood cells are found on the wet prep, the diagnosis of PID is unlikely.

Sexually transmitted diseases treatment guidelines 2002. Centers for Disease Control and Prevention. *MMWR Recomm Rep* 2002;51(RR-6):1.

the patient's presentation before making the diagnosis of PID. Differential diagnoses for pelvic pain are numerous and include: other gynecologic causes (rupture or torsion of ovarian cyst, endometriosis, dysmenorrhea, ectopic pregnancy, normal pregnancy, mittelschmerz, ruptured follicle, septic or threatened abortion), gastrointestinal causes (appendicitis, constipation, diverticulitis, gastroenteritis, inflammatory bowel disease, irritable bowel syndrome), disease of the urinary tract (cystitis, pyelonephritis, urethritis, nephrolithiasis), as well as orthopedic, rheumatologic/ autoimmune, and psychiatric disorders.

Additional criteria may be used to enhance the specificity of the minimum criteria but are not required to make the diagnosis of PID (Table 15-3). Most women with PID have either mucopurulent cervical discharge or evidence of white blood cells (WBCs) on a microscopic evaluation of a saline preparation of vaginal fluid. If the cervical discharge appears normal and no WBCs are found on the wet prep, the diagnosis of PID is unlikely (42). The presence of neutrophils on saline wet mount of vaginal secretions is 90.9% sensitive, although only 26.3% specific, for the diagnosis of upper genital tract infection; the absence of any leukocytes in the cervical secretions and vaginal discharge suggests a different diagnosis from PID (negative predictive value 94.5%) (152). The most predictive additional criterion is a positive test result for *N. gonorrhoeae* or *C. trachomatis* (151). The combination of an elevated WBC count ($>$10,000 cells) and an elevated temperature ($>$100.4°F) also increases the risk of endometritis (151). The probability of endometritis is 82.8% when abnormal discharge, elevated WBC count, fever, and positive bacterial test result are all present (151).

The evaluation of a patient with possible PID includes vital sign measurement, abdominal examination, and pelvic examination with a bimanual examination. Abdominal tenderness and adnexal tenderness are typically bilateral, although Falk (153) reported an 8% incidence of unilateral salpingitis confirmed by laparoscopy. Although it is 95.5% sensitive, adnexal tenderness is only 3.8% specific for PID (151). Pain on cervical motion is usually present but is nonspecific and may also occur with other pathologic conditions such as appendicitis, gastroenteritis, urinary tract infection, pyelonephritis, and an ovarian cyst. Rebound tenderness may not be present early in the disease if peritonitis is not present. Liver tenderness caused by perihepatitis (Fitz–Hugh–Curtis) may occur in both gonococcal and chlamydial infections (108,109); the patient may complain of pleuritic right upper quadrant pain with radiation to the right shoulder and back. A palpable adnexal mass is 48% sensitive and 74% specific for PID (146). Fever is present in only 33% of patients with PID (temperature greater than 38°C has a sensitivity of 24% to 39% and a specificity as high as 94.7%) (146,151). Abnormal cervical or vaginal discharge has a 79.7% sensitivity and 29.8% specificity for PID (151).

The laboratory tests should include a complete blood count (CBC), ESR, serologic test for syphilis, Gram stain of the endocervical discharge, cultures or other tests for *N. gonorrhoeae* and *C. trachomatis*, urinalysis, urine culture (if any symptoms suggest pyelonephritis or cystitis), and a sensitive urine or serum pregnancy test. No one test is sensitive and specific enough for the diagnosis of PID. The CBC may show a normal or elevated leukocyte count; a WBC count $>10,000/mm^3$ has relatively high specificity (76.1% to 88%) but low sensitivity (41.1% to 57%) for PID (151,154). In a study of adolescents with PID, Oginski and colleagues (155) found that, depending on the cause of the PID, 33% to 71% of patients had normal leukocyte counts. The ESR is >15 mm per hour in 75% to 80% of patients. *C-reactive protein (CRP)* has a sensitivity of 71% to 93% and a specificity 50% to 90%; and ESR >15 mm per hour has a sensitivity of 70% to 81% and a specificity of 35% to 57% (146,154). Women with severe PID and PID complicated by anaerobic infection, TOA, or perihepatitis may have a higher ESR and CRP level than those with mild PID; ESR $\geqslant 40$ mm per hr and CRP > 60 mg/L is 97% sensitive and 61% specific for detecting severe PID (156). However, one study found that adolescents with PID complicated by TOA had a lower ESR and lower WBC than adolescents with uncomplicated PID (141).

Cervical discharge has not been found to be discriminating (146); the Gram stain of a purulent cervical discharge reveals gram-negative intracellular diplococci in only about half of patients with gonococcal PID. A pregnancy test should always be obtained and the possibility of an ectopic pregnancy considered in the adolescent with acute abdominal pain; it is important to remember that an adolescent may have more than one diagnosis, such as chlamydial PID and ectopic pregnancy. Although pregnancy and PID are rarely coincident, Acquavella and colleagues (157) reported a series of adolescents with both diagnoses in the first trimester.

Several groups have tried to examine whether clinical or historical indicators can help differentiate types of PID before the culture or other endocervical tests for gonorrhea and Chlamydia return. Patients with chlamydial PID have been observed to be less likely to be febrile and more likely to have long-standing milder symptoms and breakthrough bleeding on oral contraceptives than those with gonococcal or mixed aerobic–anaerobic PID (158). The markedly elevated ESR may contrast with the mild symptoms of chlamydial PID (158). Golden and colleagues (159) found that adolescent patients with *Chlamydia*-associated PID in contrast to girls with gonococcus-associated PID had a longer duration of symptoms (6.2 vs. 3.1 days), lower temperature (37.8°C vs. 38.5°C), and lower WBC count (11,055 vs. 14,648/mm³). Such associations have not been found in all studies (155).

Ultrasonography may be considered if the clinician cannot assess the adnexae (e.g., the patient is anxious or obese), an adnexal mass is palpated, or there is a question of an ectopic pregnancy or TOA. Ultrasonography (especially transvaginal) can be useful in ruling out other diagnoses and defining adnexal masses, but has relatively low sensitivity for the diagnosis of PID (160). Some experts recommend routine use of ultrasonography for all women hospitalized for treatment of PID (161). Clinicians may prefer to use the patient's history, physical examination, and laboratory findings, such as markedly elevated ESR or CRP, to guide the decision to obtain ultrasonography. TOAs should be monitored serially with ultrasound. Magnetic resonance imaging appears to be more accurate than transvaginal ultrasonography in diagnosing PID (162), but its use has not been fully evaluated and is not currently routinely recommended.

Laparoscopy has proved invaluable in clarifying the etiologic agents and the clinical accuracy of diagnosis in PID. Laparoscopy is 100% specific for PID (160), and thus it is indicated if the diagnosis is in doubt, especially in patients recurrently labeled with PID but never meeting satisfactory criteria and not responding to antibiotic therapy. Laparoscopy also may useful for management of complications of PID, such as lysis of adhesions and percutaneous drainage of TOAs (163). Laparoscopic studies of patients with a presumptive diagnosis of acute salpingitis have concluded that the clinical diagnosis is confirmed by visual inspection in only 60% to 70% of cases (164–168). An additional 5% of patients with negative examinations by laparoscopy do have gonococci present in the cervical culture. Jacobson (164,165) found that 12% of patients with "clinical PID" had in fact a different diagnosis on laparoscopy—acute appendicitis, ectopic pregnancy, ruptured corpus luteum, ovarian abscess, or endometriosis. In a significant number of patients, no pathologic condition of the pelvis was found. Laparoscopy, however, does not detect endometritis and may miss tubal inflammation (169). Endometrial biopsy also improves the accuracy of the diagnosis of PID but is not used in the routine clinical diagnosis. Histologic diagnosis of endometritis based on the presence of plasma cells had a sensitivity of 89% and specificity of 67% in detecting laparoscopically confirmed PID (170).

Previously, hospitalization for PID was frequently recommended for supervised parenteral treatment, especially in adolescents, for whom noncompliance with therapy and the risk of future reproductive problems were of special concern (150,171,172). However, there is no evidence that hospitalization with parenteral therapy is superior to outpatient treatment with oral and intramuscular medications. In the Pelvic Inflammatory Disease Evaluation and Clinical Health (PEACH) study, Ness and colleagues randomly assigned 831 women with uncomplicated PID ages 14 to 37 years to receive either inpatient or outpatient treatment (173). They found no differences between the groups in rates of long-term outcomes (mean 35 months), including pregnancy, infertility, self-reported recurrent PID, hysterectomy, ectopic pregnancy, tubal obstruction, or chronic pelvic pain.

The CDC recommends that the decision to hospitalize be at the discretion of the treating clinician (42). Hospitalization should be initiated for patients with suspected PID if any of the following are present: surgical emergency (cannot be excluded), pregnancy, clinical failure of oral therapy, inability to follow or tolerate outpatient oral regimen, severe illness, nausea/vomiting, high fever, or TOA (42). In addition, we recommend hospitalization be considered for young women who are <15 years of age (and possibly for those ages 15 to 17 years), had abortion or other gynecologic surgery procedure within previous 14 days, have a history of a previous episode of PID, or have other extenuating medical or social circumstances that may preclude receipt of appropriate treatment as an outpatient (see Fig. 15-3). Although outpatient treatment may be effective (174), we also recommend hospitalization and parenteral treatment of immunodeficient HIV-infected adolescent women with PID because of their increased risk of complications such as TOA. Other organizations continue to advocate for hospitalization of all adolescent

Children's Hospital Boston PID Clinical Practice Guidelines Committee August 30, 2002

Management of the Patient with Uncomplicated Pelvic Inflammatory Disease (PID)

2002 CDC Diagnostic Criteria

Minimum Criteria:

Institute empiric treatment for PID if at least one of the following is present and no other cause for the illness (refer to Differential Diagnosis below) can be identified *(Check all that apply)*:

❑ Uterine/Adnexal tenderness **OR** ❑ Cervical motion tenderness

Additional Criteria to enhance the specificity of the minimum criteria *(Check all that apply)*:

- ❑ Oral temperature >101 F
- ❑ Abnormal cervical or vaginal mucopurulent discharge
- ❑ Presence of white blood cells on saline microscopy of vaginal secretions
- ❑ Elevated erythrocyte sedimentation rate
- ❑ Elevated C-reactive protein
- ❑ Laboratory documentation of cervical infection with *N. gonorrhoeae* or *C. trachomatis*

Evaluation *(All of the following are recommended)*

- ❑ Pelvic examination
- ❑ Endocervical specimen for *N. gonorrhoeae* (culture)
- ❑ Endocervical specimen for *C. trachomatis* (culture or DNA probe)
- ❑ CBC with differential
- ❑ ESR or C-reactive protein
- ❑ RPR
- ❑ Urine dipstick or urinalysis
- ❑ Urine culture
- ❑ Urine BhCG (pregnancy test)

In Addition, Consider:

- ❑ *Pelvic ultrasonography* if any one of the following:
  - ❑ Pelvic mass
  - ❑ Adnexal tenderness and at least one of the following *(Check all that apply)*:
    - ❑ High fever ❑ Elevated WBC ❑ Elevated ESR
    - ❑ Other clinical indication________________________________
  - ❑ Unable to adequately assess gynecologic structures on bimanual examination
- ❑ *Serum BhCG and type & hold* if suspect ectopic pregnancy and urine BhCG negative
- ❑ *Gynecology consult* if patient is pregnant or ordering an ultrasound for pelvic mass, TOA, or other urgent gynecologic diagnosis
- ❑ *Surgery consult* if suspect appendicitis or other surgical diagnosis

*** Differential Diagnosis**

- GI: Appendicitis, constipation, diverticulitis, gastroenteritis, inflammatory bowel disease, irritable bowel syndrome
- Gyn: Ovarian cyst (intact, ruptured, or torsed), endometriosis, dysmenorrhea, ectopic pregnancy, mittelschmerz, ruptured follicle, septic or threatened abortion, TOA
- Urinary tract: Cystitis, pyelonephritis, urethritis, nephrolithiasis

FIG. 15-3. Forms used at Children's Hospital Boston in the management of the patient with uncomplicated pelvic inflammatory disease (PID). (Principal authors are L Shrier, Chair; M Laufer, SJ Emans, E Woods, D Goldmann, S Moszczenski, and M Harper.)

Criteria for Hospitalization *(Check all that apply)*
❑ Age less than 15 years (may consider for ages 15-17 years)
❑ Abortion or other gynecologic surgery procedure within previous 14 days
❑ Previous episode of PID
❑ Surgical emergencies cannot be excluded
❑ Patient is pregnant
❑ Patient does not respond clinically to oral antimicrobial therapy
❑ Patient is unable to follow or tolerate an outpatient oral regimen
❑ Patient has severe illness, nausea and vomiting, or high fever
❑ Patient has a tubo-ovarian abscess (TOA)
❑ Other extenuating medical or social circumstances_____

Considerations for Outpatient Management *(Complete all of the following prior to discharge)*
❑ Primary care provider (PCP) notified by phone
❑ This form faxed to PCP's office
❑ Follow-up appointment in 48-72 hours scheduled (if during daytime hours) or recommended (if after hours) – with PCP, if identified, or Adolescent Clinic
❑ Social situation assessed *(Social work consulted if assistance is needed to make this assessment)*
   • Ability to
     - fill prescriptions
     - abstain from sexual intercourse
     - notify partner of his need for treatment
     - make follow-up appointment in 48-72 hours
   · Substance use, other risk behaviors
   · Personal safety
   · Living situation
   · Financial situation, medical insurance
❑ Confidential patient contact information obtained
   • Home phone_____
   • Cell phone_____
   • School name_____
   • E-mail address_____
   • Alternative phone number_____
❑ Patient education sheet provided
❑ Prescriptions provided:
   Levofloxacin 500 mg PO QD x 14 days <u>and</u>
   Metronidazole 500 mg PO BID x 14 days
   OR
   Ceftriaxone 250 mg IM in a single dose (given at visit) <u>and</u>
   Doxycycline 100 mg PO BID x 14 days <u>and</u>
   Metronidazole 500 mg PO BID x 14 days
❑ Three days' worth of medications provided

Recommended Follow-up
• Telephone call at 24 hours
  - Filled prescription?
  - Knows when follow-up appointment is?
  - Notified partner(s) of need for evaluation and treatment?
  - Abstaining from sexual intercourse?
• Visit at 48-72 hours
  - Assess for clinical improvement (e.g., defervescence; reduction in abdominal tenderness; reduction in uterine, adnexal, and cervical motion tenderness)
  - Admit if no clinical improvement or if not able to tolerate/follow outpatient regimen

FIG. 15-3. *(Continued)*

women for both therapy and education of this high-risk group (175), despite the recent change in the CDC's treatment guidelines.

If an adolescent with PID is to be treated as an outpatient, the treating clinician should assess the psychosocial situation, including the patient's ability to fill prescriptions, abstain from sexual intercourse, notify her partner(s) of the need for treatment, and make a follow-up appointment in 48 to 72 hours; substance use and other risk behaviors; personal safety and living situation; and financial situation, including medical insurance. Confidential patient contact information should be obtained, including home, cell, and alternative telephone numbers, school name, and electronic mail and street addresses.

Inpatient (Parenteral) Therapy for Acute Pelvic Inflammatory Disease/ Tubo-ovarian Abscess (TOA)

Broad-spectrum antibiotics result in the resolution of symptoms in most patients; however, the long-term results of treatment are still far from satisfactory. Effectiveness of therapy for PID is improved with prompt institution of antibiotic therapy. Hillis and colleagues found that women who delayed seeking care for PID were three times more likely to have subsequent infertility or ectopic pregnancy than women who sought care promptly (within the first 3 days after the onset of symptoms) (176).

In selecting antibiotics for treatment of PID, the clinician needs to take into account the frequently polymicrobial nature of the disease (177), regardless of whether a test for *N. gonorrhoeae* or *C. trachomatis* is positive. It is especially important to make sure that the antibiotics are known to be effective against *C. trachomatis*, since clinical improvement may occur in spite of persistence of positive endometrial cultures for *C. trachomatis*. In a study of women treated with parenteral second- and third-generation cephalosporins, 94% showed prompt clinical improvement, yet *C. trachomatis* was recovered from 87% of the posttreatment endometrial aspirates (178). In contrast, patients treated with clindamycin plus tobramycin had negative posttreatment cultures for *C. trachomatis*. Additional anaerobic coverage is subject to some debate. The 2002 CDC treatment guidelines leave the addition of metronidazole optional (42), whereas the World Health Organization regimens include metronidazole (179). Addition of an antibiotic especially effective against anaerobes (e.g., metronidazole or clindamycin) is recommended if the patient has severe PID, a TOA, concomitant bacterial vaginosis (metronidazole only), or HIV.

The 2002 CDC treatment guidelines recommend one of the following two parenteral regimens (42):

Regimen A: Cefotetan, 2 g IV every 12 hours, or cefoxitin, 2 g IV every 6 hours, plus doxycycline, 100 mg orally or IV every 12 hours. The doxycycline should be given orally if gastrointestinal function is normal owing to pain associated with infusion. The above regimen is continued for at least 24 hours after the patient improves clinically. After discharge from the hospital, the patient is continued on doxycycline 100 mg orally twice daily for a total of 14 days. Limited data are available on the use of alternative cephalosporins, such as ceftizoxime, cefotaxime, and ceftriaxone, which give adequate coverage of gonococci and facultative gram-negative aerobes, but are less active against anaerobes (42).

Regimen B: Clindamycin, 900 mg IV every 8 hours, plus gentamicin, 2.0 mg/kg loading dose IM or IV followed by a maintenance dose of 1.5 mg/kg every 8 hours (in patients with normal renal function). Single daily dosing of gentamicin has been shown to be effective in the treatment of postpartum endometritis (180,181) and may be substituted for thrice-daily dosing (42). The regimen is continued for at least 24 hours after the patient improves clinically. After discharge from the hospital, the patient is continued on doxycycline, 100 mg orally twice daily or clindamycin, 450 mg orally 4 times a day, for a total of 14 days.

The recommended parenteral regimens for PID have demonstrated comparable efficacy and safety (182,183). At least two parenteral antibiotics are required to adequately cover both *N. gonorrhoeae* and *C. trachomatis*. Even though clindamycin provides better anaerobic coverage than doxycycline and both *in vitro* and *in vivo* data suggest efficacy against chlamydial infection, doxycycline is the preferred therapy when *C. trachomatis* is known or highly suspected to be present (184). There is synergism between gentamicin and clindamycin, but the magnitude does not appear to be sufficient to explain the beneficial clinical effect against gonococci.

The alternative regimens for parenteral treatment of PID include ofloxacin 400 mg IV every 12 hours or levofloxacin 500 mg IV once daily *with or without* metronidazole 500 mg IV every 8 hours, or ampicillin/sulbactam 3 g IV every 6 hours plus doxycycline 100 mg orally or IV every 12 hours.

Most patients with PID respond well clinically to broad-spectrum antibiotics. However, patients with TOA can be difficult to manage. Ultrasonography, and in some cases computed tomography (CT) and magnetic resonance imaging (in patients for whom ultrasonography does not provide adequate information), can be used along with clinical assessment to make the diagnosis and document improvement (Fig. 15-4). Anaerobic organisms, in particular *Bacteroides fragilis*, are strongly associated with abscess formation. In a study of 105 women with uncomplicated PID and 74 women with PID complicated by TOA, McKneeley and colleagues compared Regimen A (cefotetan and doxycycline), Regimen B (clindamycin and gentamicin), and triple therapy (clindamycin, gentamicin, and ampicillin) (161). The three antibiotic regimens had comparable efficacy to effect clinical improvement for uncomplicated PID. However, triple therapy was superior to the other two regimens for effective treatment of TOA. In contrast, a study of 232 women with TOA by Landers and Sweet (185) found that 68% of patients treated with a regimen that included clindamycin responded to medical management. The combination of tobramycin and clindamycin covers most organisms cultured from abscesses, and clindamycin has excellent penetration into abscess cavities. Other antibiotics with good activity against the anaerobes and good penetration of abscesses include cefoxitin and metronidazole. Although a trial of metronidazole plus tobramycin gave equivalent results in the treatment of a va-

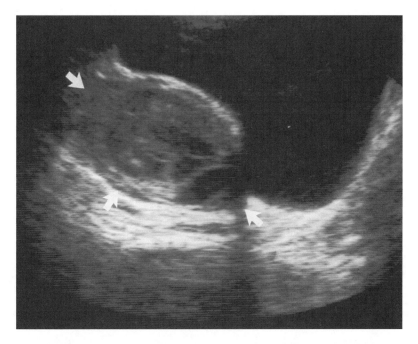

FIG. 15-4. Pelvic ultrasonograms of an adolescent referred to Children's Hospital Boston, after 1 month of pelvic pain, negative pregnancy test result, elevated sedimentation rate, a positive cervical culture for *C. trachomatis*, and noncompliance with outpatient antibiotics. **A:** Longitudinal sonogram of the right adnexa, showing a complex mass behind the bladder (*arrows*). A right ovary separate from this structure could not be identified. These findings can be seen with several disorders, including tubo-ovarian abscess, hemorrhagic ovarian cyst, ectopic pregnancy, or inflammation of nongynecologic origin, such as appendicitis. The patient was treated with cefoxitin and doxycycline for 10 days as an inpatient and then took an additional 14-day course of oral metronidazole and doxycycline as an outpatient.

riety of pelvic infections as did clindamycin and tobramycin, metronidazole in combination with an aminoglycoside does not provide adequate coverage against aerobic streptococci, *N. gonorrhoeae*, or microaerophilous streptococci (185). Reed and colleagues (186) found that both recommended PID regimens had equal efficacy for TOA with a 75% success rate. However, this study may have been biased because patients who were changed to a clindamycin-containing regimen due to physician preference were included among the responders.

Approximately 20% to 40% of women with TOA fail to respond to antibiotic therapy within 48 to 72 hours as defined by persistent fever, increasing size of the abscess, persistent leukocytosis, increasing sedimentation rate, or suspicion of rupture (161,186–188). It should be noted that the ESR may lag several days behind clinical improvement and may even rise initially. Bilateral abscesses and those >8 cm in diameter may be less likely to respond to medical management alone; more than 50% of patients with TOAs >10 cm require surgical therapy.

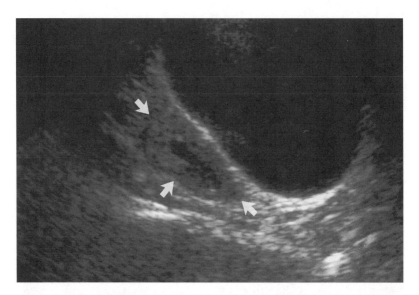

FIG. 15-4. *(Continued)* **B:** Resolution of the tubo-ovarian abscess 4 weeks after therapy. The right ovary is now well-visualized and is normal, except for a small amount of residual fluid within it *(arrows)*. (Readings of scans courtesy of Jane Share, M.D., Children's Hospital Boston.)

Surgical intervention for TOA may include percutaneous drainage (anterior abdomen, posterior transgluteal, transvaginal or transrectal) guided by CT or real-time ultrasound (188–191) (the majority that have been drained have been unilocular abscesses), transabdominal laparotomy with drainage or extirpation of the abscess, with or without unilateral adnexectomy, open laparoscopy (192), or total abdominal hysterectomy and bilateral salpingo-oophorectomy. Although long-term data are not available on fertility outcomes and are critically needed to evaluate new approaches, some centers have advocated a more aggressive early surgical approach to large TOAs with aspiration of the abscess, gentle washing of the abscess cavity, instillation of antibiotics, and closed drainage to gravity. Other centers (including ours) have taken a more conservative surgical approach and feel that preservation of fertility is more likely if the patient is treated medically with appropriate antibiotics with performance of surgery only if the patient does not improve with medical therapy. Fertility after treatment of TOAs may be 20% to 50% with conservative medical and surgical approaches. Patients with severe disease including TOAs are usually treated for a longer course with oral clindamycin or a two-drug regimen such as oral doxycycline plus metronidazole.

HIV-infected patients appear to be at increased risk for acquiring PID and may also have serious infections. However, HIV-positive women with PID, but no other acute illnesses, can be respond to standard therapeutic regimens (174,193). Jacobson and

Westrom (165) have questioned whether bias has confounded studies on the recognition of PID incidence, clinical presentation and course, and microbiology of PID in HIV-infected women. It is unclear whether the management of HIV-infected women with PID requires more aggressive intervention such as hospitalization or parenteral antimicrobial regimens (42).

Pregnant adolescents require aggressive inpatient management (parenteral therapy for 7 to 14 days is often recommended). Gonococcal infection during pregnancy is associated with septic abortion, preterm delivery, postpartum infection, and transmission to the newborn. Both chlamydial and gonococcal infections increase the risk for postabortal infection.

Following discharge from the hospital, the patient should be seen in 1 week to monitor for continued improvement and adherence to treatment. Male sexual contacts within 60 days of the onset of the patient's symptoms should be identified and treated with regimens effective against both *C. trachomatis* and *N. gonorrhoeae* to prevent reinfection, regardless of their symptoms, their STD test results, or results from the woman's STD tests. For women with documented infection with *C. trachomatis* and/or *N. gonorrhoeae*, rescreening at 4 to 6 weeks may be considered owing to the possibility of reinfection in these young women. STD counseling is important to minimize the chance of reinfection and to protect against acquisition of other infections.

Outpatient (Oral) Therapy for Acute Pelvic Inflammatory Disease

Patients with uncomplicated PID can be treated with oral therapy, ofloxacin 400 mg orally twice a day for 14 days or levofloxacin 500 mg orally once daily for 14 days *with or without* metronidazole 500 mg twice a day for 14 days. Oral ofloxacin (and, presumably, oral levofloxacin) treats both *N. gonorrhoeae* and *C. trachomatis* and is effective for PID (194,195). Because ofloxacin does not adequately cover anaerobes, clinicians may consider including metronidazole in the treatment regimen, especially if bacterial vaginosis is present. Ceftriaxone 250 mg IM (or cefoxitin 2 g IM plus probenecid, 1 g orally, or another parenteral third-generation cephalosporin) plus doxycycline 100 mg orally twice daily for 14 days *with or without* metronidazole 500 mg orally twice a day for 14 days, is an equivalently effective regimen, (195,196). Without metronidazole, this regimen provides less coverage for facultative and anaerobic bacteria.

It is essential that the clinician feel comfortable that the patient has the resources to purchase the antibiotics and will return in 48 to 72 hours to assess whether the treatment is effective. A lack of response, vomiting of the antibiotics, or noncompliance should prompt hospitalization since timely therapy is felt to be critical to fertility outcome. The patient is advised to abstain from intercourse for 3 to 4 weeks and her sexual partner(s) should be seen for appropriate testing and treatment as noted above. It cannot be overemphasized that the severity of the clinical presentation does not predict the degree of tubal damage; close follow-up and monitoring for adherence to therapy and clinical improvement is critical to minimize the likelihood of adverse sequelae from PID.

Consequences of Acute Pelvic Inflammatory Disease

Infertility, ectopic pregnancies, and chronic abdominal pain are the principal sequelae of acute PID. Thus, the aim of the clinician must be to treat the infection adequately and promptly to prevent recurrences. Women with a first episode of PID have a two- to threefold increased risk of a second episode of PID compared to women who have never had PID. During the treatment of the infection, it should be explained to the patient how the disease is sexually transmitted and how to prevent recurrences. The importance of monogamous relationships, consistent use of the condom, and treatment of all partners should be stressed. Patients can be reassured that a single episode of gonococcal salpingitis promptly and appropriately treated carries a low risk of later infertility.

Tubal occlusion may be more common in nongonococcal infections, although newer data have questioned this. Longer duration of abdominopelvic pain before admission, delayed care, and younger age at first intercourse have been associated with infertility and subsequent PID (176,197). The clinician needs to be skillful at counseling adolescents about the risks of infertility. If the issue of possible infertility is overemphasized, the teen may discontinue effective contraception and take risks to prove her own fertility. Westrom and colleagues have reported tubal occlusion in 8% to 12.8% after 1 episode, 19.5% to 35.5% after 2, and 40% to as high as 75% after 3 or more episodes of PID (198,199). In general, the more severe the PID is, the higher the risk of future infertility.

In addition to infertility, previous salpingitis is a major cause of ectopic pregnancy. Women who have had PID have a three- to tenfold increase in ectopic pregnancy (199–202). Adolescents who have had PID should be counseled about this risk, and ectopic pregnancy should always be considered in the differential diagnosis of the adolescent with acute abdominal pain (see Chapter 11). The clinician should maintain a high index of suspicion in monitoring the pregnancy of an adolescent with a history of PID. Women with nongonococcal PID, especially from *C. trachomatis*, and women with TOA are at increased risk of adverse reproductive outcomes (203).

PID may also result in chronic pain. Safrin and colleagues (197) found that 24% of patients with PID had pelvic pain for 6 months or more post hospitalization. Physical examination may reveal adnexal tenderness or masses. The sedimentation rate may be normal or elevated. Laparoscopy is necessary to establish the diagnosis and to evaluate the extent of the disease. Adolescents with endometriosis (see Chapter 11) can be incorrectly diagnosed as having PID, and they may receive multiple courses of antibiotics before the correct diagnosis is made by laparoscopy.

Therapy for chronic PID must be individualized. Treatment may include an extended course of oral antibiotics such as doxycycline, clindamycin, amoxicillin/clavulanate, or metronidazole, and nonsteroidal antiinflammatory drugs for pain. The patient should be cultured and treated with appropriate antimicrobial agents for subsequent episodes of PID and the sexual partner also examined and treated.

Prevention of PID is key and must include prevention of exposure to *C. trachomatis* and *N. gonorrhoeae* (e.g., delaying the age of intercourse), prevention of acquisition of chlamydial and gonorrheal infections (e.g., condoms, investigations of methods of transmission), prevention of PID (e.g., screening, antibiotic regimens), and prevention of PID sequelae (172). Adolescents at risk of PID need education to be able to assess symptoms, to access health care services for screening and evaluation of symptoms, to receive therapy that is effective and takes into account compliance issues, and to be able to refer sexual partners for treatment in a timely manner.

SYPHILIS

Syphilis is a genital ulcerative disease caused by *Treponema pallidum*, a spirochete bacterium. *T. pallidum* is an obligate human parasite; therefore, virtually all cases of syphilis are transmitted via direct genital contact or from mother to fetus across the placenta.

In the 1990s through 2000, the rates of primary and secondary syphilis declined to the lowest since recording began in 1941. From 2000 to 2001, rates continued to decline among women (1,967 reported cases, 1.4 cases per 100,000 women), although among men, an increase of 2.1% was noted (4,134 reported cases, 3.0 cases per 100,000 men) (204). Rates of congenital syphilis have followed rates of primary and secondary syphilis in women, declining to a low of 11.1 cases per 100,000 live births. Because of the declining rates and concentration of infection in specific geographic areas (e.g., the South) and populations (e.g., men who have sex with men), the Surgeon General launched a National Plan to Eliminate Syphilis from the United States in 1999 (205). Although most other STDs are most prevalent in adolescents and young adults, syphilis is primarily seen among women aged 20 to 24 years and men aged 35 to 39 years (204). However, as many as 1.6% of female adolescents in juvenile correction facilities have reactive tests for syphilis. African Americans are disproportionately affected by syphilis, with rates 16 times more than those seen among whites (204).

Guidelines have not been developed for the routine screening of adolescent patients for syphilis; however, clinical criteria have been used for both symptomatic and asymptomatic teens. Sexually active adolescents should be tested for syphilis when they present with any suspicious oral or genital lesions, unexplained skin rash or lymphadenopathy, other STDs, or pregnancy. Asymptomatic adolescents with multiple partners, nonuse of barrier methods, involvement in prostitution, drug abuse, or juvenile delinquency, and/or a history of STDs may be considered for annual syphilis screening since adolescents frequently do not present at the time of symptoms (206). However, because the rates of syphilis have declined dramatically in some communities, even among high-risk youth, local prevalence estimates should guide screening efforts. In 2001, 80.2% of 3,139 counties in the United States reported zero cases of infectious syphilis (204).

The presence of genital ulcers increases the risk of acquiring HIV infection, and adolescents at risk for HIV acquisition are also at risk for syphilis exposure. In a blinded study of sera from a comprehensive adolescent health center and two school-based clinics in an area of New York with a high seroprevalence of HIV, McCabe and associates (207) reported that of the 59 specimens positive for syphilis, 15% were HIV seropositive; 84% of the patients with positive syphilis serology (positive rapid plasma reagin [RPR] and fluorescent treponemal antibody absorbed [FTA-ABS] or just positive FTA-ABS) were female and 80% of these young women had had a prior STD, most commonly chlamydial infection (35%).

The nontreponemal tests, such as the Venereal Disease Research Laboratory (VDRL) and RPR, are very sensitive and can be accurately quantitated, making these tests useful for screening and to monitor response to therapy and progression of disease. The VDRL is used for cerebrospinal fluid (CSF) determinations. A rising titer on a nontreponemal test is indicative of recently acquired infection, reinfection, or relapse. However, patients with primary syphilis frequently have nonreactive tests. At the time of the appearance of the primary lesion of syphilis, the chancre, only about 25% of patients will have a reactive test; this proportion increases to 50% after 1 week and 75% after 2 weeks. Almost all untreated patients will have a reactive test 3 to 4 weeks after the appearance of the chancre and almost certainly by the time secondary syphilis develops. A decline in titer of at least fourfold is generally indicative of adequate treatment of early syphilis. Patients with primary syphilis will often have a nonreactive RPR within 1 year; patients with secondary syphilis can become nonreactive within 2 years; those in the macular and maculopapular stage of the rash at diagnosis and treatment return to seronegativity more rapidly than patients with papular and/or pustular rashes (208). Patients who are reinfected with syphilis also take longer to revert to a nonreactive RPR test. Patients who have early latent syphilis for <1 year generally revert to a negative test result within 4 years, whereas only 20% to 45% of late latent patients become nonreactive within 5 years. Many in the latter group remain serofast (209). Successful treatment of primary and secondary syphilis results in a fourfold decrease in serum RPR by 6 to 12 months. The same laboratory and the same nontreponemal test should be used to monitor a patient after therapy.

Both false-positive and false-negative results may occur with the nontreponemal tests. As noted, the nontreponemal tests may be negative early in the disease. In less than 2% of patients with secondary syphilis, the RPR or VDRL test may appear to give a false-negative result despite very strong reactivity because of a prozone reaction. HIV infection is also associated with false-negative results (210). Most laboratories do not do titers unless the undiluted specimen gives a positive result. Thus, if syphilis is suspected clinically and the nontreponemal test appears nonreactive or weakly reactive, a second serum specimen should be sent with instructions to dilute the serum. Biologic false positivity occurs in 1 out of 3000 to 5000 healthy patients; in some populations it may be 1% to 2% (211). Conditions such as autoimmune disease, injection drug use, tuberculosis, vaccinations, pregnancy, infectious mononucleosis, HIV, rickettsial infections, spirochetal infections other than syphilis, bacterial endocarditis, and hepatitis may result in false-positive RPR tests (212,213). If a false-positive result is suspected, a treponemal test, such as the FTA-ABS test or the microhemagglutination test (MHA-TP), should be performed to confirm the diagnosis.

Darkfield examination and direct fluorescent antibody test for *T. pallidum* (DFA-TP) of the lesion exudate or tissue are definitive methods for diagnosing early syphilis. The specific or treponemal tests are useful to make the diagnosis in situations in which false-positive reactions might occur and in the diagnosis of late syphilis. False-positive results for FTA-ABS and MHA-TP are infrequent but have been reported in patients with elevated globulins, Lyme disease, leprosy, malaria, infectious mononucleosis, relapsing fever, leptospirosis, and systemic lupus erythematosus (214). The FTA-ABS and MHA-TP tests are not recommended for screening, or for monitoring disease progression or therapeutic response because the test results remain positive for life in most individuals whether the syphilis has been treated or not. Because these tests are almost always positive in secondary syphilis, the principal use of these tests is to exclude the diagnosis of syphilis after the primary stage (215). However, negative results on treponemal tests may be seen in patients who have been treated for syphilis. Romanowski and colleagues found that the FTA-ABS result became negative in 24% of patients treated for primary syphilis and the microhemagglutination assay for antibody to *T. pallidum* (MHA-TP) negative in 13% of these patients (216). False-negative treponemal test results may also be seen with HIV infection (210,217). Special tests, which include DNA and Reiter absorptions for the FTA-ABS test, eliminate most of the false-positive results and can be performed by the STD Laboratory Program of the CDC upon request (which may sometimes be indicated in the diagnosis and treatment of the pregnant woman). If a patient has a reactive nontreponemal test and a nonreactive treponemal test and no clinical or epidemiologic evidence of syphilis, no treatment is necessary but both tests should be repeated in 4 weeks.

In caring for seropositive women, the clinician should always attempt to document previous titers and forms of treatment. A fourfold change in titer, equivalent to two dilutions (1:16 to 1:4 or 1:8 to 1:32) is necessary to demonstrate a change in status (reinfection, treatment failure, or response to treatment) (42). Patients should be retreated and reevaluated for HIV infection if they have persistent or recurrent signs or symptoms or a sustained fourfold increase in nontreponemal test titer (42). In general, high-risk seropositive women should be considered infected and treated unless the clinician is certain about recent therapy. The diagnosis and treatment of syphilis during pregnancy is particularly urgent to prevent congenital syphilis.

No single test can be used to determine if neurosyphilis is present. The diagnosis is made on the basis of reactive CSF-VDRL, CSF leukocyte count >5 leukocytes/mm^3, and elevated CSF protein. The sensitivity of the CSF-VDRL is 30% to 70%, but the test is very specific. Thus, a positive result is sufficient to diagnose neurosyphilis, but a negative result is not sufficient to exclude the diagnosis. FTA-ABS on CSF is more sensitive but less specific (more false positives); a negative test result appears to exclude the diagnosis (42). Lukehart and colleagues (218) reported that 41% of 39 patients with untreated primary and secondary syphilis had pleocytosis and 24% of 33 patients with secondary syphilis (compared to none of seven primary syphilis patients) had reactive CSF VDRL tests. It is essential that patients with syphilis have appropriate counseling and testing for HIV infection because of the difficulty with potential failed treatment and persistent neurosyphilis.

Stages of Syphilis

Patients with syphilis may present with primary infection (i.e., ulcer or chancre at the site of infection), secondary infection (i.e., skin rash, mucocutaneous lesions, and/or lymphadenopathy), tertiary infection (i.e., cardiac, ophthalmic, or auditory abnormalities, and/or gummatous lesions), or latent infection (i.e., no clinical manifestations) (42).

Primary Syphilis.   Ten to 90 days (average, 3 weeks) after oral or genital exposure to an infected partner, the young woman may develop a hard, painless chancre on her vulva, vagina, cervix, or anal area, or extragenital sites, such as the mouth, fingers, and breast. The lesion begins as a macule/papule that erodes into a clean-based ulcer with smooth, firm borders. Although there is usually a solitary chancre, multiple lesions may occur. The chancre is accompanied by nontender lymphadenopathy, but is often asymptomatic and may be missed. Since the serologic test for syphilis may not give a positive result until several weeks after exposure, a negative test result at the time a lesion is first noted does not rule out the diagnosis. If the result of the initial VDRL or RPR result is negative but the lesion arouses suspicion, repeat tests are indicated at 1 week, 1 month, and 3 months to exclude syphilis. If possible, a darkfield examination of clear fluid expressed from the chancre or a DFA-TP of the lesion should be done by an experienced clinician. The darkfield examination can be repeated for 3 consecutive days. Systemic antibiotics or local antiseptics may produce a negative result on darkfield examination. Even without therapy, the lesion(s) will heal spontaneously in one to five weeks, leaving a small scar.

Secondary Syphilis.   If the chancre is untreated, 6 weeks to several months later the patient may experience the symptoms of secondary syphilis, including a generalized rash (often present on the palms and soles), fever, malaise, alopecia, weight loss, lymphadenopathy, condyloma latum, or mucous membrane lesions. The rash generally progresses from macular to maculopapular to papular and lastly, to pustular lesions. The serum RPR test result at this time is positive.

Latent Syphilis.   By definition, this is the state of syphilis in which the patient has no symptoms and the spirochete is "hidden." However, the patient may be infectious and may later develop symptoms of tertiary syphilis. This stage is divided by history and serology into early latent (acquired within the previous year), late latent of >1 year duration, and latent syphilis of unknown duration. Patients can be documented to have acquired syphilis within the preceding year on the basis of documented seroconversion, unequivocal symptoms of primary or secondary syphilis, or a sex partner with primary, secondary, or early latent syphilis (42). All others are considered to have late latent syphilis or latent syphilis of unknown duration. Nontreponemal titers are usually higher in early latent versus late latent syphilis, but cannot be reliably used to distinguish between the two.

Late Syphilis.   Except for gummas, which are probably a hypersensitivity phenomenon, the late manifestations of syphilis (neurologic and cardiovascular problems) are the result of a vasculitis. Late syphilis usually occurs in patients beyond the adolescent age group, although very rarely neurosyphilis or cardiovascular lesions can develop in adolescents as a sequela of untreated congenital syphilis.

Treatment

Parenteral penicillin is the drug of choice for all stages of syphilis. Alternative therapy should be selected only for nonpregnant patients in whom there is documented penicillin allergy and for whom compliance is not a problem. Some patients will experience the Jarisch–Herxheimer reaction to the penicillin therapy—an acute febrile reaction with headache and myalgia that may occur within the first 24 hours of therapy for syphilis (antipyretics can be recommended) (42).

Primary or Secondary Syphilis or Contact History

Benzathine penicillin G, 2.4 million units IM as a single dose is the treatment of choice. Nonpregnant penicillin-allergic patients should be treated with doxycycline, 100 mg orally twice a day for 2 weeks or tetracycline, 500 mg orally 4 times a day for 2 weeks. Compliance with this regimen is extremely important, as is serologic follow-up. Patients who cannot tolerate doxycycline or tetracycline should have their penicillin allergy confirmed; choices are ceftriaxone 250 mg IM or IV for 8 to 10 days or azithromycin 2 g orally as a single dose with very close serologic follow-up because of reported failure with azithromycin, or penicillin desensitization so that benzathine penicillin can be used.

If signs or symptoms suggestive of neurologic or ophthalmic disease are present, CSF analysis and ophthalmic slit-lamp examination should be performed. Patients should be reexamined clinically and have serologic tests checked at 6 and 12 months. Patients who have persistent or recurrent signs or symptoms or who have a sustained fourfold increase in nontreponemal test titer compared with baseline or subsequent result can be considered to have failed therapy or be reinfected. They should be re-treated for syphilis and tested for HIV infection. Because treatment failure cannot be distinguished from reinfection and unrecognized CNS infection, CSF should be evaluated in these patients. If the CSF examination is negative, patients should be treated with benzathine penicillin G 2.4 million units IM for 3 weeks. Additional therapy is not necessary if serologic titers do not decline despite negative CSF and re-treatment.

Latent Syphilis

Early latent syphilis of <1 year duration can be treated with a single dose of penicillin, as above for primary syphilis.

Syphilis of >1 year duration or unknown duration, except neurosyphilis, should be treated with 2.4 million units of benzathine penicillin G, IM once a week for 3 consecutive weeks. Ideally, all patients with syphilis of >1 year duration should have a CSF examination. A CSF examination is also indicated in patients with neurologic or ophthalmic signs and symptoms, treatment failure, other evidence of active syphilis (aortitis, gumma, iritis), or a positive HIV antibody test result (with late latent syphilis or latent syphilis of unknown duration). If neurosyphilis is found, then patients should be treated with the regimen discussed next.

The efficacy of alternative drugs to penicillin in the treatment of syphilis of >1 year duration is less well established. Penicillin-allergic, nonpregnant patients who have had neurosyphilis excluded may be treated with doxycycline, 100 mg orally twice a day for 4 weeks or tetracycline, 500 mg orally 4 times a day for 4 weeks. The duration of therapy is 2 weeks for infections known to be <1 year (42). In patients who cannot tolerate doxycycline or tetracycline, penicillin allergy should be confirmed by history and testing, and penicillin desensitization should be considered.

Neurosyphilis

Neurosyphilis can occur at any stage, so any clinical evidence of central nervous system involvement in a patient being evaluated for syphilis should prompt examination of the CSF. Aqueous penicillin G, 18 to 24 million units per day is administered as 3 to 4 million units IV every 4 hours or continuous infusion for 10 to 14 days (42). If outpatient compliance can be ensured, an alternative treatment is procaine penicillin, 2.4 million units IM daily plus probenecid, 500 mg orally 4 times a day, both for 10 to 14 days. Because the duration of this regimen is shorter than the regimen recommended for the treatment of late syphilis without neurologic involvement, some experts follow the above neurosyphilis regimens with benzathine penicillin G, 2.4 million units IM weekly for one to three doses. If pleocytosis was initially present in the CSF, CSF examination should be repeated every 6 months until the cell count is normal. If the CSF cell count does not decrease after 6 months or is not normal after 2 years, re-treatment should be considered.

Syphilis and HIV Infection

Although unusual serologic responses may occur in HIV-infected patients, both treponemal and nontreponemal tests are usually accurate for most patients. HIV-infected patients have an increased risk of treatment failure and neurosyphilis (219). Current recommendations call for the usual treatment schedule for early syphilis, although some specialists treat with up to 3 injections, as for late syphilis (42). Following treatment, HIV-infected patients should be reevaluated clinically and serologically 3, 6, 9, 12, and 24 months. If the titer does not decrease fourfold in 6 to 12 months, the patient should undergo CSF examination and be re-treated. Some experts recommend CSF examination before initiating treatment of HIV-infected patients with early syphilis, with a follow-up CSF examination 6 months after treatment. HIV-infected individuals with latent syphilis and neurosyphilis should be managed as for HIV-negative patients, with the exception that HIV-infected patients with late latent syphilis or latent syphilis of unknown duration should have their CSF examined prior to treatment, regardless of signs, symptoms, or treatment history.

Syphilis in Pregnancy

Pregnant patients should be screened at their first prenatal visit and, in some states, at delivery. High-risk patients should also be screened at 28 weeks and at delivery. Women should be tested for syphilis if they deliver a stillborn infant after 20 weeks gestation. Pregnant patients with syphilis should be treated as soon as the diagnosis is made to prevent fetal death and congenital syphilis. Patients who are not allergic to penicillin should be treated with the same dosage schedules recommended for nonpregnant patients (42). Some experts recommend a second dose of benzathine penicillin 2.4 million units IM 1 week after the initial dose in women with primary, secondary, or early latent syphilis. There are no alternatives to penicillin, so pregnant women who have a history of penicillin allergy should have confirmation with skin testing, then be desensitized and treated with penicillin. Ziaya and colleagues (220) have described an intravenous method of penicillin desensitization that was used successfully in a pregnant woman. Desensitization should be used only in consultation with an expert and in a facility with emergency procedures available. Tetracycline and doxycycline are not recommended during pregnancy because of adverse effects on the fetus, and erythromycin is not optimal because of the possibility of inadequate treatment of the fetus. Following treatment, pregnant women should have serologic titers repeated in the third trimester and at delivery. Pregnant women at high risk for reinfection or those who reside in areas with a high prevalence of syphilis may be evaluated serologically each month for the remainder of the pregnancy.

Follow-up

Patients should have careful tracing of contacts performed by the state health department. Sexual partners exposed within the 90 days preceding the diagnosis of primary, secondary, or early latent syphilis in the index patient may have negative test results in spite of infection and should be presumptively treated. Partners exposed >90 days before the index patient's diagnosis can await the results of serologic tests if follow-up is certain; otherwise they should be presumptively treated. For the purposes of partner management, patients with syphilis of unknown duration with serologic titers >1:32 may be considered to have early syphilis. Long-standing partners of patients with latent syphilis should be evaluated clinically and serologically and treated for syphilis in accordance with this evaluation. The time periods for determining at-risk sex partners are 3 months plus duration of symptoms for primary syphilis, 6 months plus duration of symptoms for secondary syphilis, and 1 year for early latent syphilis (42). Contacts should be evaluated clinically and with serologic tests.

REFERENCES

1. Tracking the Hidden Epidemics. Trends in STDs in the United States 2000. Atlanta: Centers for Disease Control and Prevention. 2001.
2. Eng T, Butler W, eds. *The hidden epidemic: confronting sexually transmitted diseases.* Washington, DC: National Academy Press. 1997.
3. Fleming GV, O'Connor KG, Sanders JM, Jr. Pediatricians' views of access to health services for adolescents. *J Adolesc Health* 1994.15:473.
4. Orr DP. Urine-based diagnosis of sexually transmitted infections using amplified DNA techniques: a shift in paradigms? *J Adolesc Health* 1997;20:3.
5. Sexually transmitted diseases in America: how many cases and at what cost? Research Triangle Park: American Social Health Association, 1998:27.
6. Centers for Disease Control and Prevention. *Sexually transmitted disease surveillance, 2001.* Atlanta: US Department of Health and Human Services, 2002.
7. CDC. Screening tests to detect *Chlamydia trachomatis* and *Neisseria gonorrhoeae* infections—2002. *MMWR* 2002;51(RR-15):1.
8. Control of *Neisseria gonorrhoeae* Infection in the United States. Centers for Disease Control and Prevention, Division of STD Prevention. 2003.
9. Hook E, Handsfield H, Sparling PF, Mardh PA, et al. Gonococcal infections in the adult. In: Holmes K, et al. eds. *Sexually transmitted diseases.* New York: McGraw-Hill, 1999;451.
10. Muram D. Sexually transmitted diseases in adolescents. In: Muram, D, Sanfilippo JS, Dewhurst J, et al. eds. *Pediatric and adolescent gynecology*, 2nd ed. New York: WB Saunders, 2001;357.
11. Best D, Ford CA, Miller WC. Prevalence of *Chlamydia trachomatis* and *Neisseria gonorrhoeae* infection in pediatric private practice. *Pediatrics* 2001;108:E103.
12. Cohen DA, Nsuami M, Martin DH, et al. Repeated school-based screening for sexually transmitted diseases: a feasible strategy for reaching adolescents. *Pediatrics* 1999;104:1281.
13. Nsuami M, Elie M, Brooks BN, et al. Screening for sexually transmitted diseases during preparticipation sports examination of high school adolescents. *J Adolesc Health* 2003;32:336.
14. Embling ML, Monroe KW, Oh MK, et al. Opportunistic urine ligase chain reaction screening for sexually transmitted diseases in adolescents seeking care in an urban emergency department. *Ann Emerg Med* 2000;36:28.

15. Oh MK, Cloud GA, Fleenor M, et al. Risk for gonococcal and chlamydial cervicitis in adolescent females: incidence and recurrence in a prospective cohort study. *J Adolesc Health* 1996;18:270.

16. Bunnell RE, Dahlberg L, Rolfs R, et al. High prevalence and incidence of sexually transmitted diseases in urban adolescent females despite moderate risk behaviors. *J Infect Dis* 1999;180:1624.

17. Oh MK, Smith KR, O'Cain M, et al. Urine-based screening of adolescents in detention to guide treatment for gonococcal and chlamydial infections. Translating research into intervention. *Arch Pediatr Adolesc Med* 1998; 152(1):52.

18. Mertz KJ, Finelli L, Levine WC, et al. Gonorrhea in male adolescents and young adults in Newark, New Jersey: implications of risk factors and patient preferences for prevention strategies. *Sex Transm Dis* 2000;27(4):201.

19. Vermund SH, Alexander-Rodriguez T, Macleod S, et al. History of sexual abuse in incarcerated adolescents with gonorrhea or syphilis.[Erratum appears in *J Adolesc Health Care* 1991;12:214.] *J Adolesc Health Care* 1990;11:449.

20. Rice RJ, Roberts PL, Handsfield HH, et al. Sociodemographic distribution of gonorrhea incidence: implications for prevention and behavioral research. *Am J Public Health* 1991;81:1252.

21. Diclemente RJ, Wingood GM, Sionean C, et al. Association of adolescents' history of sexually transmitted disease (STD) and their current high-risk behavior and STD status: a case for intensifying clinic-based prevention efforts. *Sex Transm Dis* 2002;29:503.

22. Nohara M, Sugase M, Kawana T. Evaluation of DNA probe test for clinical diagnosis of chlamydial and gonococcal infections of the uterine cervix. *Nippon Sanka Fujinka Gakkai Zasshi—Acta Obstetrica et Gynaecologica Japonica* 1991;43:459.

23. Vlaspolder F, Mutsears JA, Blog F, et al. Value of a DNA probe assay (Gen-Probe) compared with that of culture for diagnosis of gonococcal infection. *J Clin Microbiol* 1993;31:107.

24. Stary A, Kopp W, Zahel B, et al. Comparison of DNA-probe test and culture for the detection of *Neisseria gonorrhoeae* in genital samples. *Sex Transm Dis* 1993;20:243.

25. Schwebke JR, Zajackowski ME. Comparison of DNA probe (Gen-Probe) with culture for the detection of *Neisseria gonorrhoeae* in an urban STD program. *Genitourinary Medicine* 1996;72:108.

26. Ciemins EL, Borenstein LA, Dyer IE, et al. Comparisons of cost and accuracy of DNA probe test and culture for the detection of *Neisseria gonorrhoeae* in patients attending public sexually transmitted disease clinics in Los Angeles County. *Sex Transm Dis*, 1997;24:422.

27. Hale YM, Melton ME, Lewis JS, et al. Evaluation of the PACE 2 *Neisseria gonorrhoeae* assay by three public health laboratories. *J Clin Microbiol* 1993;31:451.

28. Modarress KJ, Cullen AP, Jaffurs WJ Sr, et al. Detection of *Chlamydia trachomatis* and *Neisseria gonorrhoeae* in swab specimens by the Hybrid Capture II and PACE 2 nucleic acid probe tests. *Sex Transm Dis* 1999;26:303.

29. Schachter J, Hook EW 3rd, McCormack WM, et al. Ability of the digene hybrid capture II test to identify *Chlamydia trachomatis* and *Neisseria gonorrhoeae* in cervical specimens. *J Clin Microbiol* 1999;37:3668.

30. Van Der Pol B, Williams JA, Smith NJ, et al. Evaluation of the Digene Hybrid Capture II Assay with the Rapid Capture System for detection of *Chlamydia trachomatis* and *Neisseria gonorrhoeae*. *J Clin Microbiol* 2002; 40(10):3558.

31. Martin DH, Cammarata C, Van Der Pol B, et al. Multicenter evaluation of AMPLICOR and automated COBAS AMPLICOR CT/NG tests for *Neisseria gonorrhoeae*. *J Clin Microbiol* 2000;38:3544.

32. Crotchfelt KA, Welsh LE, DeBonville D, et al. Detection of *Neisseria gonorrhoeae* and *Chlamydia trachomatis* in genitourinary specimens from men and women by a coamplification PCR assay. *J Clin Microbiol* 1997;35:1536.

33. Van Der Pol B, Martin DH, Schachter J, et al. Enhancing the specificity of the COBAS AMPLICOR CT/NG test for *Neisseria gonorrhoeae* by retesting specimens with equivocal results. *J Clin Microbiol* 2001;39:3092.

34. CDC. Recall of LCx *Neisseria gonorrhoeae* assay and implications for laboratory testing for *N. gonorrhoeae* and *Chlamydia trachomatis*. *MMWR* 2002;51:709.

35. Jephcott AE. Microbiological diagnosis of gonorrhoea. *Genitourinary Medicine* 1997;73:245.

36. Ison CA. Laboratory methods in genitourinary medicine. Methods of diagnosing gonorrhoea. *Genitourinary Medicine* 1990;66:453.

37. Knapp J, Koumans E, Jorgensen JH, et al. *Neisseria* and *Branhamella*. In: Murray PR, Baron EJ, Pfaller MA, et al., eds. *Manual of clinical microbiology*, 7th ed. Washington, DC: American Society of Microbiology, 1999;586.

38. Roochvarg LB, Lovchik JC. Screening for pharyngeal gonorrhea in adolescents. A reexamination. *J Adolesc Health* 1991;12:269.

39. Brown RT, Lossick JG, Mosure DJ, et al. Pharyngeal gonorrhea screening in adolescents: is it necessary? *Pediatrics* 1989; 84:623.

40. Fox KK, Knapp JS, Holmes KK, et al. Antimicrobial resistance in *Neisseria gonorrhoeae* in the United States, 1988–1994: the emergence of decreased susceptibility to the fluoroquinolones. *J Infect Dis* 1997;175:1396.

41. CDC. Increases in fluoroquinolone-resistant *Neisseria gonorrhoeae*—Hawaii and California, 2001. *MMWR* 2002;51:1041.

42. Sexually transmitted diseases treatment guidelines 2002. Centers for Disease Control and Prevention. *MMWR* 2002;51(RR-6):1.

43. CDC. Increases in fluoroquinolone-resistant Neisseria gonorrhoeae among men who have sex with men—United States, 2003, and revised recommendations for gonorrhea treatment, 2004. MMWR 2004;53:335.

44. Schichor A, Bernstein B, Weinerman H, et al. Lidocaine as a diluent for ceftriaxone in the treatment of gonorrhea. Does it reduce the pain of the injection? *Arch Pediatr Adolesc Med* 1994;148:72.

45. Burstein GR, Berman SM, Blumer JL, et al. Ciprofloxacin for the treatment of uncomplicated gonorrhea infection in adolescents: Does the benefit outweigh the risk? *Clin Infect Dis* 2002;35(Suppl 2):S191.

46. Lyss SB, Kamb ML, Peterman TA, et al. *Chlamydia trachomatis* among patients infected with and treated for *Neisseria gonorrhoeae* in sexually transmitted disease clinics in the United States. *Ann Int Med* 2003;139:178.

47. Creighton S, Tanant-Flowers M, Taylor CB, et al. Co-infection with gonorrhoea and chlamydia: how much is there and what does it mean? *Int J STD AIDS* 2003;14:109.

48. Laras L, Craighill M, Woods E, et al. Epidemiologic observations of adolescents with *Neisseria gonorrhoeae* genital infections treated at a children's hospital. *Adolesc Pediatr Gynecol* 1994;7:9.

49. Felman Y, Nikitas J. Anorectal gonococcal infection. *NY State J Med* 1980;80:1631.

50. Guinto-Ocampo H, Friedland LR, Disseminated gonococcal infection in three adolescents. *Pediatr Emerg Care* 2001;17(6):441.

51. Rice P, Handsfield H, Mardh PA, Sparling PF, et al. Arthritis associated with sexually transmitted diseases. In: Holmes KK, et al., eds. *Sexually transmitted diseases.* New York: McGraw-Hill, 1999;921.

52. O'Brien JP, Goldenberg DL, Rice PA. Disseminated gonococcal infection: a prospective analysis of 49 patients and a review of pathophysiology and immune mechanisms. *Medicine* 1983;62(6):395.

53. Muralidhar B, Rumore PM, Steinman CR. Use of the polymerase chain reaction to study arthritis due to *Neisseria gonorrhoeae. Arthritis Rheum* 1994;37(5):710.

54. Liebling MR, Arkfield DG, Michelini GA, et al. Identification of *Neisseria gonorrhoeae* in synovial fluid using the polymerase chain reaction. *Arthritis Rheum* 1994;37:702.

55. Wise CM, Morris CR, Wasilauskas BL, et al. Gonococcal arthritis in an era of increasing penicillin resistance. Presentations and outcomes in 41 recent cases (1985–1991). *Arch Int Medicine* 1994;154:2690.

56. Banares A, Hernandez-Garcia C, Fernandez-Gutierrez B, et al. Eye involvement in the spondyloarthropathies. *Rheumatic Dis Clin North America* 1998;24:771,ix.

57. Sicoli RA, Losek JD, Hudlett JM, et al. Indications for *Neisseria gonorrhoeae* cultures in children with suspected sexual abuse. *Arch Pediatr Adolesc Med* 1995;149:86.

58. Shapiro RA, Schubert CJ, Siegel RM. *Neisseria gonorrhoeae* infections in girls younger than 12 years of age evaluated for vaginitis. *Pediatrics* 1999;104:e72.

59. Ingram DL. *Neisseria gonorrhoeae* in children. *Pediatr Ann* 1994;23:341.

60. Christian CW, Pinto-Martin JA, McGowan KL. The management of prepubertal children with gonorrhea. *Clin Pediatr* 1995;34:415.

61. Auman GL, Waldenberg LM. Gonococcal periappendicitis and salpingitis in a prepubertal girl. *Pediatrics* 1976;58:287.

62. Kulhanjian JA, Hilton NS. Gonococcal salpingitis in a premenarchal female following sexual assault. *Clin Pediatr* 1991;30:53.

63. Biro FM, Rosenthal SL, Kiniyalocts M. Gonococcal and chlamydial genitourinary infections in symptomatic and asymptomatic adolescent women. *Clin Pediatr* 1995;34:419.

64. Oh MK, Smith KR, O'Cain M, et al. Urine-based screening of adolescents in detention to guide treatment for gonococcal and chlamydial infections. Translating research into intervention. *Arch Pediatr Adolesc Med* 1998; 152:52.

65. Gaydos CA, Howell MR, Pare B, et al. *Chlamydia trachomatis* infections in female military recruits. *N Engl J Med* 1998; 339:739.

66. Kelly PJ, Bair RM, Baillargeon J, et al. Risk behaviors and the prevalence of Chlamydia in a juvenile detention facility. *Clin Pediatr* 2000;39:521.
67. Mertz KJ, Ransom RL, St Louis ME, et al. Prevalence of genital chlamydial infection in young women entering a national job training program, 1990–1997. *Am J Public Health* 2001;91:1287.
68. Niccolai LM, Ethier KA, Kershaw TS, et al. Pregnant adolescents at risk: sexual behaviors and sexually transmitted disease prevalence. *Am J Obstet Gynecol* 2003;188:63.
69. Shrier L, Dean D, Klein E, et al. Limitations of screening tests for the detection of *Chlamydia trachomatis* in asymptomatic adolescent and young adult women. *Am J Obstet Gynecol* 2004;190:654.
70. Scholes D, Stergachis A, Heidrich FE, et al. Prevention of pelvic inflammatory disease by screening for cervical chlamydial infection. *N Engl J Med* 1996;334:1362.
71. Burstein GR, Gaydos CA, Diener-West M, et al. Incident *Chlamydia trachomatis* infections among inner-city adolescent females. *JAMA* 1998;280:521.
72. Orr DP, Johnston K, Brizendine E, et al. Subsequent sexually transmitted infection in urban adolescents and young adults. *Arch Pediatr Adolesc Med* 2001;155:947.
73. Mosure DJ, Berman S, Fine D, et al. Genital Chlamydia infections in sexually active female adolescents: Do we really need to screen everyone? *J Adolesc Health* 1997;20:6.
74. Hillis SD, Nakashima A, Marchbanks PA, et al. Risk factors for recurrent *Chlamydia trachomatis* infections in women. *Am J Obstet Gynecol* 1994;170:801.
75. Fortenberry JD, Brizendine EJ, Katz BP, et al. Subsequent sexually transmitted infections among adolescent women with genital infection due to *Chlamydia trachomatis, Neisseria gonorrhoeae,* or *Trichomonas vaginalis. Sex Transm Dis* 1999;26:26.
76. Mardh PA. Influence of infection with *Chlamydia trachomatis* on pregnancy outcome, infant health and life-long sequelae in infected offspring. *Best Pract Res Clin Obstet Gynaecol* 2002;16:847.
77. Rastogi S, Das B, Salhan S, et al. Effect of treatment for *Chlamydia trachomatis* during pregnancy. *Int J Gynaecol Obstet,* 2003;80:129.
78. Patton DL, Askienazy-Elbhar M, Henry-Suchet J, et al. Detection of *Chlamydia trachomatis* in fallopian tube tissue in women with postinfectious tubal infertility. *Am J Obstet Gynecol* 1994;171:95.
79. Witkin SS, Sultan KM, Neal GS, et al. Unsuspected *Chlamydia trachomatis* infection and *in vitro* fertilization outcome. *Am J Obstet Gynecol* 1994;171:1208.
80. Van Dyck E, Ieven M, Pattyn S, et al. Detection of *Chlamydia trachomatis* and *Neisseria gonorrhoeae* by enzyme immunoassay, culture, and three nucleic acid amplification tests. *J Clin Microbiol* 2001;39:1751.
81. Wylie JL, Moses S, Babcock R, et al. Comparative evaluation of Chlamydiazyme, PACE 2, and AMP-CT assays for detection of *Chlamydia trachomatis* in endocervical specimens. *J Clin Microbiol* 1998;36:3488.
82. Tanaka M, Nakayama H, Yoshida H, et al. Detection of *Chlamydia trachomatis* in vaginal specimens from female commercial sex workers using a new improved enzyme immunoassay. *Sex Transm Infect* 1998;74:435.
83. Tanaka M, Nakayama H, Sagiyama K, et al. Evaluation of a new amplified enzyme immunoassay (EIA) for the detection of *Chlamydia trachomatis* in male urine, female endocervical swab, and patient obtained vaginal swab specimens. *J Clin Pathol* 2000;53:350.
84. Chernesky M, Jang D, Corpes D, et al. Comparison of a polymer conjugate-enhanced enzyme immunoassay to ligase chain reaction for diagnosis of *Chlamydia trachomatis* in endocervical swabs. *J Clin Microbiol* 2001; 39:2306.
85. Biro FM, Reising SF, Doughman JA, et al. A comparison of diagnostic methods in adolescent girls with and without symptoms of *Chlamydia* urogenital infection. *Pediatrics* 1994;93:476.
86. Iwen PC, Walker RA, Warren KL, et al. Evaluation of nucleic acid-based test (PACE 2C) for simultaneous detection of *Chlamydia trachomatis* and *Neisseria gonorrhoeae* in endocervical specimens. *J Clin Microbiol* 1995;33:2587.
87. Modarress KJ, Cullen AP, Jaffurs WJ Sr, et al. Detection of *Chlamydia trachomatis* and *Neisseria gonorrhoeae* in swab specimens by the Hybrid Capture II and PACE 2 nucleic acid probe tests. *Sex Transm Dis* 1999;26:303.
88. Carroll KC, Aldeen WE, Morrison M, et al. Evaluation of the Abbott LCx ligase chain reaction assay for detection of *Chlamydia trachomatis* and *Neisseria gonorrhoeae* in urine and genital swab specimens from a sexually transmitted disease clinic population. *J Clin Microbiol* 1998;36:1630.
89. Black CM, Marrazzo J, Johnson RE, et al. Head-to-head multicenter comparison of DNA probe and nucleic acid amplification tests for *Chlamydia trachomatis* infection in women performed with an improved reference standard. *J Clin Microbiol* 2002;40:3757.
90. Lee HH, Burczak JD, Muldoon S, et al. Diagnosis of *Chlamydia trachomatis* genitourinary infection in women by ligase chain reaction assay of urine. *Lancet* 1995;345:213.
91. Goessens WH, Mouton JW, van der Meijden WI, et al. Comparison of three commercially available

amplification assays, AMP CT, LCx, and COBAS AMPLICOR, for detection of *Chlamydia trachomatis* in first-void urine. *J Clin Microbiol* 1997;35:2628.

92. Pasternack R, Vuorinen P, Pitkajarvi T, et al. Comparison of manual Amplicor PCR, Cobas Amplicor PCR, and LCx assays for detection of *Chlamydia trachomatis* infection in women by using urine specimens. *J Clin Microbiol* 1997;35:402.

93. Oh MK, Richey CM, Pate MS, et al. High prevalence of *Chlamydia trachomatis* infections in adolescent females not having pelvic examinations: utility of PCR-based urine screening in urban adolescent clinic setting. *J Adolesc Health* 1997;21:80.

94. Domeika M, Bassiri M, Butrimiene I, et al. Evaluation of vaginal introital sampling as an alternative approach for the detection of genital *Chlamydia trachomatis* infection in women. *Acta Obstet Gynecol Scand* 1999;78:131.

95. Polaneczky M, Quigley C, Pollock L, et al. Use of self-collected vaginal specimens for detection of *Chlamydia trachomatis* infection. *Obstet Gynecol* 1998;91:375.

96. Wiesenfeld HC, Lowry DL, Heine RP, et al. Self-collection of vaginal swabs for the detection of Chlamydia, gonorrhea, and trichomoniasis: opportunity to encourage sexually transmitted disease testing among adolescents. *Sex Transm Dis* 2001;28:321.

97. Vincelette J, Schirm J, Bogard M, et al. Multicenter evaluation of the fully automated COBAS AMPLICOR PCR test for detection of *Chlamydia trachomatis* in urogenital specimens. *J Clin Microbiol* 1999;37:74.

98. Pasternack R, Vuorinen P, Miettinen A. Evaluation of the Gen-Probe *Chlamydia trachomatis* transcription-mediated amplification assay with urine specimens from women. *J Clin Microbiol* 1997;35:676.

99. Crotchfelt KA, Pare B, Gaydos C, et al. Detection of *Chlamydia trachomatis* by the Gen-Probe AMPLIFIED Chlamydia Trachomatis Assay (AMP CT) in urine specimens from men and women and endocervical specimens from women. *J Clin Microbiol* 1998;36:391.

100. Van Der Pol B, Ferrero DV, Buck-Barrington L, et al. Multicenter evaluation of the BDProbeTec ET System for detection of *Chlamydia trachomatis* and *Neisseria gonorrhoeae* in urine specimens, female endocervical swabs, and male urethral swabs. *J Clin Microbiol* 2001;39:1008.

101. Roongpisuthipong A, Grimes DA, Hadgu A. Is the Papanicolaou smear useful for diagnosing sexually transmitted diseases? *Obstet Gynecol* 1987;69:820.

102. Edelman M, Fox A, Alderman E, et al, Cervical papanicolaou smear abnormalities and *Chlamydia trachomatis* in sexually active adolescent females. *J Pediatr Adolesc Gynecol* 2000;13:65.

103. Wiesenfeld HC, Heine RP, Rideout A, et al. The vaginal introitus: a novel site for *Chlamydia trachomatis* testing in women. *Am J Obstet Gynecol* 1996;174:1542.

104. Tabrizi SN, Paterson B, Fairley CK, et al. A self-administered technique for the detection of sexually transmitted diseases in remote communities. *J Infect Dis* 1997;176:289.

105. Holland-Hall CM, Wiesenfeld HC, Murray PJ, Self-collected vaginal swabs for the detection of multiple sexually transmitted infections in adolescent girls. *J Pediatr Adolesc Gynecol* 2002;15:307.

106. Serlin M, Shafer M, Tebb K, et al. What sexually transmitted disease screening method does the adolescent prefer? Adolescents' attitudes toward first-void urine, self-collected vaginal swab, and pelvic examination. *Arch Pediatr Adolesc Med* 2002;156:588.

107. Recommendations for the prevention and management of Chlamydia trachomatis infections, 1993. CDC. *MMWR* 1993;42(RR-12):1.

108. Wang SP, Eschenbach DA, Holmes KK, et al. *Chlamydia trachomatis* infection in Fitz-Hugh-Curtis syndrome. *Am J Obstet Gynecol* 1980;138:1034.

109. Katzman DK, Friedman IM, McDonald CA, et al. *Chlamydia trachomatis* Fitz-Hugh-Curtis syndrome without salpingitis in female adolescents. *Am J Dis Child* 1988;142:996.

110. Jebakumar SP, Storey C, Lusher M, et al. Value of screening for oro-pharyngeal *Chlamydia trachomatis* infection. *J Clin Pathol* 1995;48:658.

111. Ostergaard L, Agner T, Krarup E, et al. PCR for detection of *Chlamydia trachomatis* in endocervical, urethral, rectal, and pharyngeal swab samples obtained from patients attending an STD clinic. *Genitourinary Medicine* 1997;73:493.

112. Perine P, Stamm W. Lymphogranuloma venereum. In: Holmes K, et al. eds. *Sexually transmitted diseases.* McGraw-Hill: New York, 1999;423.

113. Lau CY, Qureshi AK. Azithromycin versus doxycycline for genital chlamydial infections: a meta-analysis of randomized clinical trials. *Sex Transm Dis* 2002;29:497.

114. Lea AP, Lamb HM. Azithromycin. A pharmacoeconomic review of its use as a single-dose regimen

in the treatment of uncomplicated urogenital *Chlamydia trachomatis* infections in women. *Pharmacoeconomics* 1997;12:596.

115. Onrust SV, Lamb HM, Balfour JA. Ofloxacin. A reappraisal of its use in the management of genitourinary tract infections. *Drugs* 1998;56:895.

116. Mikamo H, Sato Y, Hayasaki Y, et al. Adequate levofloxacin treatment schedules for uterine cervicitis caused by *Chlamydia trachomatis*. *Chemotherapy* 2000;46:150.

117. Miller JM, Martin DH. Treatment of *Chlamydia trachomatis* infections in pregnant women. *Drugs* 2000;60:597.

118. Kelsey JJ, Moser LR, Jennings JC, et al. Presence of azithromycin breast milk concentrations: a case report. *Am J Obstet Gynecol* 1994;170:1375.

119. Joyner JL, Douglas JM Jr, Foster M, et al. Persistence of *Chlamydia trachomatis* infection detected by polymerase chain reaction in untreated patients. *Sex Transm Dis* 2002;29:196.

120. Dean D, Suchland RJ, Stamm WE. Evidence for long-term cervical persistence of *Chlamydia trachomatis* by omp1 genotyping. *J Infect Dis* 2000;182:909.

121. Westrom L, Eschenbach D. Pelvic inflammatory disease. In: Holmes K, et al. eds. *Sexually transmitted diseases*. McGraw-Hill: New York, 1999;783.

122. Simms I, Stephenson JM. Pelvic inflammatory disease epidemiology: What do we know and what do we need to know? *Sex Transm Infect* 2000;76:80.

123. Washington AE, Katz P. Cost of and payment source for pelvic inflammatory disease. Trends and projections, 1983 through 2000. *JAMA*, 1991;266:2565.

124. Rein DB, Kassler WJ, Irwin KL, et al. Direct medical cost of pelvic inflammatory disease and its sequelae: decreasing, but still substantial. *Obstet Gynecol* 2000;95:397.

125. Ellen JM, Kohn RP, Bolan GA, et al. Socioeconomic differences in sexually transmitted disease rates among black and white adolescents, San Francisco, 1990 to 1992. *Am J Public Health* 1995;85:1546.

126. Park BJ, Stergachis A, Scholes D, et al. Contraceptive methods and the risk of *Chlamydia trachomatis* infection in young women. *Am J Epidemiol* 1995;142:771.

127. Jacobson DL, Peralta L, Farmer M, et al. Relationship of hormonal contraception and cervical ectopy as measured by computerized planimetry to chlamydial infection in adolescents. *Sex Transm Dis* 2000;27:313.

128. Baeten JM, Nyange PM, Richardson BA, et al. Hormonal contraception and risk of sexually transmitted disease acquisition: results from a prospective study. *Am J Obstet Gynecol* 2001;185:380.

129. Wolner-Hanssen P, Eschenbach DA, Paavonen J, et al. Decreased risk of symptomatic chlamydial pelvic inflammatory disease associated with oral contraceptive use. *JAMA* 1990;263:54.

130. Ness RB, Soper DE, Holley RL, et al. Hormonal and barrier contraception and risk of upper genital tract disease in the PID Evaluation and Clinical Health (PEACH) study. *Am J Obstet Gynecol* 2001;185:121.

131. Soper DE, Brockwell NJ, Dalton HP, et al. Observations concerning the microbial etiology of acute salpingitis. *Am J Obstet Gynecol* 1994;170:1008.

132. Wiesenfeld HC, Hillier SL, Krohn MA, et al. Lower genital tract infection and endometritis: insight into subclinical pelvic inflammatory disease. *Obstet Gynecol* 2002;100:456.

133. Jossens MO, Schachter J, Sweet RL. Risk factors associated with pelvic inflammatory disease of differing microbial etiologies. *Obstet Gynecol* 1994;83:989.

134. Heinonen PK, Miettinen A. Laparoscopic study on the microbiology and severity of acute pelvic inflammatory disease. *Eur J Obstet Gynecol Reprod Biol* 1994;57:85.

135. McCormack WM. Pelvic inflammatory disease. *N Engl J Med* 1994;330:115.

136. Simms I, Eastick K, Mallinson H, et al. Associations between Mycoplasma genitalium, Chlamydia trachomatis, and pelvic inflammatory disease. *Sex Transm Infect* 2003;79:154.

137. Peipert JF, Montagno AB, Cooper AS, et al. Bacterial vaginosis as a risk factor for upper genital tract infection. *Am J Obstet Gynecol* 1997;177:1184.

138. Jossens MO, Eskenazi B, Schachter J, et al. Risk factors for pelvic inflammatory disease. A case control study. *Sex Transm Dis* 1996;23:239.

139. Sweet RL, Blankfort-Doyle M, Robbie MO, et al. The occurrence of chlamydial and gonococcal salpingitis during the menstrual cycle. *JAMA* 1986;255:2062.

140. Korn AP, Hessol MA, Padian NS, et al. Risk factors for plasma cell endometritis among women with cervical *Neisseria gonorrhoeae*, cervical *Chlamydia trachomatis*, or bacterial vaginosis. *Am J Obstet Gynecol* 1998;178:987.

141. Slap GB, Forke CM, Cnaan A, et al. Recognition of tubo-ovarian abscess in adolescents with pelvic inflammatory disease. *J Adolesc Health* 1996;18:397.

142. Sweet RL, Draper DL, Hadley WK. Etiology of acute salpingitis: influence of episode number and duration of symptoms. *Obstet Gynecol* 1981;58:62.

143. Cohen CR, Brunham RC. Pathogenesis of Chlamydia induced pelvic inflammatory disease. *Sex Transm Infect*, 1999;75:21.

144. Peeling RW, Kimani J, Plummer F, et al. Antibody to chlamydial hsp60 predicts an increased risk for chlamydial pelvic inflammatory disease. *J Infect Dis* 1997;175:1153.

145. Rice PA, Schachter J. Pathogenesis of pelvic inflammatory disease. What are the questions? *JAMA* 1991;266:2587.

146. Kahn JG, Walker CK, Washington AE, et al. Diagnosing pelvic inflammatory disease. A comprehensive analysis and considerations for developing a new model. *JAMA* 1991;266:2594.

147. Wolner-Hanssen P, Mardh PA, Svensson L, et al. Laparoscopy in women with chlamydial infection and pelvic pain: a comparison of patients with and without salpingitis. *Obstet Gynecol* 1983;61:299

148. Eschenbach DA, Wölner-Hanssen P, Hawes SE, et al. Acute pelvic inflammatory disease: associations of clinical and laboratory findings with laparoscopic findings. *Obstet Gynecol* 1997;89:184.

149. Anonymous. Tubal infertility: serologic relationship to past chlamydial and gonococcal infection. World Health Organization Task Force on the Prevention and Management of Infertility. *Sex Transm Dis* 1995;22:71.

150. CDC. 1998 guidelines for treatment of sexually transmitted diseases. *MMWR* 1998;47(RR-1):1.

151. Peipert JF, Ness RB, Blume J, et al. Clinical predictors of endometritis in women with symptoms and signs of pelvic inflammatory disease. *Am J Obstet Gynecol* 2001;184:856.

152. Yudin MH, Hillier SL, Wiesenfeld HC, et al. Vaginal polymorphonuclear leukocytes and bacterial vaginosis as markers for histologic endometritis among women without symptoms of pelvic inflammatory disease. *Am J Obstet Gynecol* 2003;188:318.

153. Falk V. Treatment of acute non-tuberculous salpingitis with antibiotics alone and in combination with glucocorticoids. *Acta Obstet Gynecol Scand* 1965;44:65.

154. Peipert JF, Boardman L, Hogan JW, et al. Laboratory evaluation of acute upper genital tract infection. *Obstet Gynecol* 1996;87:730.

155. Oginski W, Rosenfeld W, Bijar P. Acute pelvic inflammatory disease in adolescents. *Adolesc Pediatr Gynecol* 1992;5:243.

156. Miettinen AK, Heinonen PK, Laipalla P, et al. Test performance of erythrocyte sedimentation rate and C-reactive protein in assessing the severity of acute pelvic inflammatory disease. *Am J Obstet Gynecol* 1993;169:1143.

157. Acquavella AP, Rubin A, D'Angelo LJ. The coincident diagnosis of pelvic inflammatory disease and pregnancy: are they compatible? *J Pediatr Adolesc Gynecol* 1996;9:129.

158. Svensson L, Westrom L, Ripa KT, et al. Differences in some clinical and laboratory parameters in acute salpingitis related to culture and serologic findings. *Am J Obstet Gynecol* 1980;138:1017.

159. Golden N, Neuhoff S, Cohen H. Pelvic inflammatory disease in adolescents. *J Pediatr* 1989; 114:138.

160. Gaitan H, Angel E, Diaz R, et al. Accuracy of five different diagnostic techniques in mild-to-moderate pelvic inflammatory disease. *Infect Dis Obstet Gynecol*, 2002;10:171.

161. McNeeley SG, Hendrix SL, Mazzoni MM, et al. Medically sound, cost-effective treatment for pelvic inflammatory disease and tuboovarian abscess. *Am J Obstet Gynecol* 1998;178:1272.

162. Tukeva TA, Aronen HJ, Karjalainen PT, et al. MR imaging in pelvic inflammatory disease: comparison with laparoscopy and US. *Radiology* 1999;210:209.

163. Molander P, Cacciatore B, Sjoberg J, et al. Laparoscopic management of suspected acute pelvic inflammatory disease. *J Am Assoc Gynecol Laparosc* 2000;7:107.

164. Jacobson L. Laparoscopy in the diagnosis of acutes salpingitis. *Acta Obstet Gynecol Scand* 1964; 43:160.

165. Jacobson L, Westrom L. Objectivized diagnosis of acute pelvic inflammatory disease. Diagnostic and prognostic value of routine laparoscopy. *Am J Obstet Gynecol* 1969;105:1088.

166. Jacobson L. Differential diagnosis of acute pelvic inflammatory disease. *Am J Obstet Gynecol* 1980;138:1006.

167. Westrom L. Incidence, prevalence, and trends of acute pelvic inflammatory disease and its consequences in industrialized countries. *Am J Obstet Gynecol* 1980;138:880.

168. Hager WD, Eschenbach DA, Spence MR, et al. Criteria for diagnosis and grading of salpingitis. *Obstet Gynecol* 1983;61:113.

169. Sellors J, Mahony J, Goldsmith C, et al. The accuracy of clinical findings and laparoscopy in pelvic inflammatory disease. *Am J Obstet Gynecol* 1991;164:113.

170. Paavonen J, Aine R, Teisala K, et al. Comparison of endometrial biopsy and peritoneal fluid cytologic testing with laparoscopy in the diagnosis of acute pelvic inflammatory disease. *Am J Obstet Gynecol* 1985;151:645.

171. Rome ES, Moszczenski SA, Craighill M, et al. A clinical pathway for pelvic inflammatory disease for use on an inpatient service. *Clin Perform Qual Health Care*, 1995;3:185.

172. Shrier LA, Moszczenski SA, Emans SJ, et al. Three years of a clinical practice guideline for uncomplicated pelvic inflammatory disease in adolescents. *J Adolesc Health* 2000;29:57.

173. Ness RB, Soper DE, Holley RL, et al. Effectiveness of inpatient and outpatient treatment strategies for women with pelvic inflammatory disease: results from the Pelvic Inflammatory Disease Evaluation and Clinical Health (PEACH) Randomized Trial. *Am J Obstet Gynecol* 2002;186:929.

174. Bukusi EA, Cohen CR, Stevens CE, et al. Effects of human immunodeficiency virus 1 infection on microbial origins of pelvic inflammatory disease and on efficacy of ambulatory oral therapy. *Am J Obstet Gynecol* 1999;181:1374.

175. Hemsel DL, Ledger WJ, Marten M, et al. Concerns regarding the Centers for Disease Control's published guidelines for pelvic inflammatory disease. *Clin Infect Dis* 2001;32(1):103.

176. Hillis SD, Joesoef R, Marchbanks PA, et al. Delayed care of pelvic inflammatory disease as a risk factor for impaired fertility. *Am J Obstet Gynecol* 1993;168:1503.

177. Baveja G, Saini S, Sangwan K, et al. A study of bacterial pathogens in acute pelvic inflammatory disease. *J Comm Dis* 2001;33:121.

178. Sweet RL, Schachter J, Robbie MO. Failure of beta-lactam antibiotics to eradicate *Chlamydia trachomatis* in the endometrium despite apparent clinical cure of acute salpingitis. *JAMA* 1983;250:2641.

179. Anonymous. Guidelines for the management of sexually transmitted infections. 2001, World Health Organization.

180. Sunyecz JA, Wiesenfeld HC, Heine RP., The pharmacokinetics of once-daily dosing with gentamicin in women with postpartum endometritis. *Infect Dis Obstet Gynecol* 1998;6:160.

181. Del Priore G, Jackson-Stone M, Shim EK, et al. A comparison of once-daily and 8-hour gentamicin dosing in the treatment of postpartum endometritis. *Obstet Gynecol* 1996;87:994.

182. Walters MD, Gibbs RS. A randomized comparison of gentamicin-clindamycin and cefoxitin-doxycycline in the treatment of acute pelvic inflammatory disease. *Obstet Gynecol* 1990;75:867.

183. Hemsell DL, Little BB, Faro S, et al. Comparison of three regimens recommended by the Centers for Disease Control and Prevention for the treatment of women hospitalized with acute pelvic inflammatory disease. *Clin Infect Dis* 1994;19:720.

184. Peterson HB, Walker CK, Kahn JG, et al. Pelvic inflammatory disease. Key treatment issues and options. *JAMA* 1991;266:2605.

185. Landers DV, Sweet RL. Current trends in the diagnosis and treatment of tuboovarian abscess. *Am J Obstet Gynecol* 1985;151:1098.

186. Reed SD, Landers DV, Sweet RL. Antibiotic treatment of tuboovarian abscess: comparison of broad-spectrum beta-lactam agents versus clindamycin-containing regimens. *Am J Obstet Gynecol* 1991;164:1556.

187. Landers DV, Wolner-Hanssen P, Paavonen J, et al. Combination antimicrobial therapy in the treatment of acute pelvic inflammatory disease. *Am J Obstet Gynecol* 1991;164:849.

188. Perez-Medina T, Huertas MA, Bajo JM. Early ultrasound-guided transvaginal drainage of tuboovarian abscesses: a randomized study. *Ultrasound Obstet Gynecol* 1996;7:435.

189. Caspi B, Zalel T, Or Y, et al. Sonographically guided aspiration: an alternative therapy for tubo-ovarian abscess. *Ultrasound Obstet Gynecol* 1996;7:439.

190. Harisinghani MG, Gervais DA, Maher MM, et al. Transgluteal approach for percutaneous drainage of deep pelvic abscesses: 154 cases. *Radiology*, 2003;228:701.

191. Casola G, vanSonnenberg E, D'Agostino HB, et al. Percutaneous drainage of tubo-ovarian abscesses. *Radiology* 1992;182:399.

192. Yang CC, Chen P, Tseng JY, et al. Advantages of open laparoscopic surgery over exploratory laparotomy in patients with tubo-ovarian abscess. *J Am Assoc Gynecol Laparosc* 2002;9:327.

193. Barbosa C, Macasaet M, Brockmann S, et al. Pelvic inflammatory disease and human immunodeficiency virus infection. *Obstet Gynecol* 1997;89:65.

194. Peipert JF, Sweet RL, Walker CK, et al. Evaluation of ofloxacin in the treatment of laparoscopically documented acute pelvic inflammatory disease (salpingitis). *Infect Dis Obstet Gynecol* 1999;7:138.

195. Martens MG, Gordon S, Yarborough DR, et al. Multicenter randomized trial of ofloxacin versus cefoxitin and doxycycline in outpatient treatment of pelvic inflammatory disease. *Ambulatory PID Research Group. Southern Med J* 1993;86:604.

196. Arredondo JL, Diaz V, Gaitan H, et al. Oral clindamycin and ciprofloxacin versus intramuscular ceftriaxone and oral doxycycline in the treatment of mild-to-moderate pelvic inflammatory disease in outpatients. *Clin Infect Dis* 1997;24:170.

197. Safrin S, Schachter J, Dahrouge D, et al. Long-term sequelae of acute pelvic inflammatory disease. A retrospective cohort study. *Am J Obstet Gynecol* 1992;166:1300.

198. Westrom L, Effect of acute pelvic inflammatory disease on fertility. *Am J Obstet Gynecol* 1975; 121:707.

199. Westrom L, Joesoef R, Reynolds G, et al. Pelvic inflammatory disease and fertility. A cohort study of 1,844 women with laparoscopically verified disease and 657 control women with normal laparoscopic results. *Sex Transm Dis* 1992;19:185.

200. Westrom L. Pelvic inflammatory disease: bacteriology and sequelae. *Contraception* 1987;36:111.

201. Marchbanks PA, Annegers JF, Coulam CB, et al. Risk factors for ectopic pregnancy. A population-based study. *JAMA* 1988; 259:1823.

202. Coste J, Job-Spira N, Fernandez H, et al. Risk factors for ectopic pregnancy: a case-control study in France, with special focus on infectious factors. *Am J Epidemiol*, 1991;133:839.

203. Brunham RC, Binns B, Guijon F, et al. Etiology and outcome of acute pelvic inflammatory disease. *J Infect Dis* 1988; 158:510.

204. Primary and secondary syphilis—United States, 2000–2001. *MMWR* 2002;51:971.

205. Centers for Disease Control and Prevention. The national plan to eliminate syphilis from the United States. Atlanta: US Department of Health and Human Services, 1999;1.

206. Silber TJ, Niland NF. The clinical spectrum of syphilis in adolescence. *J Adolesc Health Care* 1984; 5:112.

207. McCabe E, Jaffe LR, Diaz A. Human immunodeficiency virus seropositivity in adolescents with syphilis. *Pediatrics* 1993;92:695.

208. Fiumara NJ. Treatment of primary and secondary syphilis. Serological response. *JAMA* 1980; 243:2500.

209. Fiumara NJ. Serologic responses to treatment of 128 patients with late latent syphilis. *Sex Transm Dis* 1979;6:243.

210. Hicks CB, Benson PM, Lupton GP, et al. Seronegative secondary syphilis in a patient infected with the human immunodeficiency virus (HIV) with Kaposi sarcoma. A diagnostic dilemma. *Ann Intern Med,* 1987;107:492.

211. Judson FN, Ehret J. Laboratory diagnosis of sexually transmitted infections. *Pediat Ann* 1994;23:361.

212. Golden MR, Marra CM, Holmes KK. Update on syphilis: resurgence of an old problem. *JAMA* 2003; 290:1510.

213. Thomas DL, Rompalo AM, Zenilman J, et al. Association of hepatitis C virus infection with false-positive tests for syphilis. *J Infect Dis* 1994;170:1579.

214. Hook EW, 3rd, Marra CM. Acquired syphilis in adults. *N Engl J Med* 1992;326:1060.

215. Musher D. Early syphilis. In: Holmes KK, Mardh PA, Sparling PF, eds. *Sexually transmitted diseases*. New York:McGraw-Hill, 1999:479.

216. Romanowski B, Sutherland R, Fick GH, et al. Serologic response to treatment of infectious syphilis. *Ann Intern Med* 1991;114:1005.

217. Erbelding EJ, Vlahov D, Nelson KE, et al. Syphilis serology in human immunodeficiency virus infection: evidence for false-negative fluorescent treponemal testing. *J Infect Dis* 1997;176:1397.

218. Lukehart SA, Hook EW 3rd, Baker-Zander SA, et al. Invasion of the central nervous system by Treponema pallidum: implications for diagnosis and treatment. *Ann Intern Med* 1988;109:855.

219. Schofer H, Imhof M, Thoma-Greber E, et al. Active syphilis in HIV infection: a multicentre retrospective survey. The German AIDS Study Group (GASG). *Genitourinary Medicine* 1996;72:176.

220. Ziaya PR, Hankins GD, Gistrap LC 3rd, et al. Intravenous penicillin desensitization and treatment during pregnancy. *JAMA* 1986; 256:2561.

Further Reading

Holmes KK, Mardh P, Sparling PF, et al, eds. *Sexually transmitted diseases*, 3rd ed. New York: McGraw-Hill, 1999.

16

Human Immunodeficiency Virus in Young Women

Cathryn L. Samples

INTRODUCTION

Young people worldwide are continuing to be impacted by the human immuno-deficiency virus (HIV)/acquired immune deficiency syndrome (AIDS) pandemic, with most of the 4.8 million persons newly infected in 2002 under the age of 25, or about 6000 new infections among youth daily. There are now more than 10 million teens and young adults age 15 to 24 living with HIV/AIDS worldwide, 62% of them female (1,2). The global impact of HIV has continued to increase, with at least 95% of the world's cases occurring in resource poor countries where treatment is rarely available (1). Worldwide, HIV is spread primarily as a sexually transmitted disease, with women and men equally at risk. As of December 31, 2002, 859,000 cases of AIDS had been reported in the United States, and there were an estimated 384,906 people living with AIDS in the United States (3). In the past decade, there have been major advances in our understanding of the pathogenesis and natural history of HIV in children and adolescents, and breakthroughs in antiretroviral treatment leading to improved morbidity and mortality and decreased perinatal transmission, though many of these benefits are not yet attainable in resource poor countries. With adoles-cents and young adults continuing to develop HIV, and youth born with HIV increasingly surviving to and beyond adolescence, the clinician caring for young women will need to be aware of risk factors for acquisition, to be able to offer HIV counseling and testing and risk reduction advice to young women, and to consider HIV as part of the differential diagnosis for many signs and symptoms. Those pro-viding health and reproductive health care services to young women should be pre-pared to inform and provide care for young women who test positive for HIV infec-tion, to provide appropriate reproductive health care and counseling to girls and young women born with HIV, and to manage the routine and episodic health care of adolescents and young adults with HIV infection acquired during or after puberty.

This chapter updates current epidemiologic information, describes the characteristics of AIDS and HIV infection in young women, and reviews recent developments in treatment and care and our understanding of the natural history of HIV among adolescents. It also reviews recent guidelines impacting the treatment of women with or at risk of HIV. We discuss the clinician's role in case finding, prevention, diagnosis, and management, and review the impact of HIV and its treatment on reproductive health, contraception, and pregnancy options.

EPIDEMIOLOGY

Description of the HIV epidemic in adolescents in the United States relies on information from several sources: AIDS case reports, seroprevalence studies, surveys of risk behavior and of indicator diseases, mortality data, and voluntary testing data. AIDS case reporting was introduced in the early 1980s, but HIV case reporting was introduced more recently. After a Centers for Disease Control and Prevention (CDC) recommendation for universal HIV reporting in 1994, 33 states were conducting confidential name-based surveillance by the end of 2001 (3–5). CDC currently reports HIV cases and estimates of incidence and prevalence only for 30 states or areas with established name based reporting, so national HIV reporting gives a substantial underestimate of incidence and prevalence of HIV nationally. Back calculation, serosurveillance, use of specialized assays to identify recent infection, and household surveys have been used to estimate both new cases and the number of people living with HIV infection in the United States (6).

AIDS Case Reports

A 1995 review of the first 500,000 cases of AIDS in the United States revealed an increase in the proportions of persons with AIDS who are female, persons of color, injection drug users, and alive at the time of the report (7). In 1995, there were 189,929 persons estimated to be living with an AIDS diagnosis. Since 1996, dramatic declines in both AIDS incidence and deaths have been reported. New cases have leveled at about 40,000 per year since 1999, with lesser decreases in incidence among non-whites, and persons with heterosexual contact risk. The estimated AIDS incidence in 13- to 24-year-old females dropped from 911 to 705 cases per year between 1994 and 2000 (a 23% decline), while the incidence in males 13 to 24 years old fell by 46%; for all adults and adolescents, the cases fell by 44% (8). By the end of 2002, an estimated 384,906 people in the United States were living with AIDS, nearly double the 1995 number. Of the 42,167 people less than 25 years of age reported through 2001 with AIDS in the United States, 35% have been female, and 84% of those were young women of color (4,9) (Table 16-1), while 83.1% of 13- to 24-year-old young women reported with AIDS have been Black or Hispanic. Because the time from

TABLE 16-1. *AIDS[a] cases in girls and young women, United States, reported through December 2001.[d]*

Categories	Age (years)		
	<13	*13 to 19*	*20 to 24*
Proportion of cases female			
Females (*n*)	4,463	1873	26,865
Females (%)	48.6	42.3	29
Female race/ethnicity category (%)			
White/non-Hispanic	15.8	15.8	21.3
Black/non-Hispanic	60.6	66.7	58.2
Hispanic	22.5	16.9	19.5
Other/unknown	0.9	0.6	1.0
HIV[b] exposure category (%)			
Injection drug use	—	13	25
Hemophilia	—	1	0
Heterosexual	—	51	55
Blood products	—	5	1
Other/unknown[c]	—	30	18

[a]AIDS, acquired immunodeficiency syndrome.
[b]HIV, human immunodeficiency virus.
[c]Risk not reported or identified. Includes women not yet interviewed and those with heterosexual contacts not known to be at risk or infected.
[d]Adapted from CDC. HIV/AIDS Surveillance Report, 2002.

infection with HIV to the development of AIDS-defining conditions or criteria averages five to 10 years, even without treatment, almost all 20- to 24-year-olds with AIDS acquired their infection during childhood or adolescence. Using CDC exposure categories, most girls less than 13 years of age were infected through their mothers, and most young women aged 13 to 24 years were infected through heterosexual transmission. A small number of 13- to 24-year-old women reported with AIDS are girls with perinatal HIV who have survived into adolescence before having an AIDS diagnosis. In the past 8 years, the advent of new antiretroviral treatments and improved understanding of their use have produced marked decreases in mortality and improved survival and quality of life. Thus, AIDS case reports give little insight to current spread of the virus among young women.

HIV Case Reports

A helpful picture of girls and young women known to have HIV can be obtained from examining data from recent reporting of HIV infection without AIDS. The addition of New York State to name reporting data in 2000 produced a dramatic but artificial increase in pediatric cases reported. Young women comprised 56.7% of HIV cases reported in the year 2001 among 13- to 19-year-olds, and 40.5% of cases among 20- to 24-year-olds. For 13- to 19-year-old females with reported HIV infection through 2001, 1% were infected by blood products, 7% had injection drug use (IDU) as their primary mode of transmission, 49% were heterosexual contacts of a known infected or high-risk partner, and 43% were other (most presumably heterosexual contacts of partners whose risk or HIV status was unknown) (4).

HIV and AIDS in Selected Areas with Established HIV Name Reporting

CDC combined HIV and AIDS reporting data in the 25 states with name based HIV reporting between 1994 and 2000 to develop a profile of HIV of people living with HIV (PLWH) with or without AIDS in those locales. Those states then accounted for 24% of all reported AIDS cases. The proportion of the 128,813 HIV-infected persons with AIDS at time of diagnosis went from 27% in 1994 to 24% in 2000 (9). People who already had AIDS at diagnosis were more likely to be male, older age, of an ethnicity other than black. Fifteen percent of all people reported with HIV and 5% of persons with AIDS were under 25. Among children under 13, 17% of children with HIV had AIDS at diagnosis, while among 13- to 24-year-olds, 8% had AIDS at time of their diagnosis. This data have been used to infer that 25% of all adults living with HIV in the United States do not know their diagnosis, and that among youth, HIV infection without AIDS is much more prevalent than AIDS (10).

HIV Seroprevalence

Although unlinked seroprevalence studies of cord blood (revealing serostatus of their mothers giving birth) were suspended, other studies of HIV antibody prevalence in selected populations continue to provide useful information. These use unlinked, blinded samples of blood obtained for other reasons or results of routine linked testing in special populations such as the military and Job Corps. Among Job Corps entrants aged 16 to 21 years, rates were highest in urban northeast and rural southern women and nonwhite women (11–13). Job Corps data for a seven-year period ending in 1996 showed a higher prevalence of HIV among young women than young men (3/1000 vs. 2/1000), and a rate of 4.9/1000 in African-American females age 16 to 21, increasing with each year of age (14). In 1997, African American females entering the Job Corps continued to have the highest rates of seroprevalence, and young women of all ethnic groups were twice as likely to be HIV-infected (15). Studies of homeless youth have shown seroprevalence rates ranging from 0.41% to 7.4% (13,16). In Baltimore sexually transmitted disease (STD) clinics, the greatest age-specific increases in seroprevalence in STD clinic users were among teenagers (from 0.18% in 1979 to 1983 to 2.1% in 1987 to 1989) (17). More recent studies have shown no decline in HIV seroprevalence among STD clinic users in nine cities between 1991 and 1997 (18,19). Few studies have documented the rate of HIV in healthy adolescents, but a study in Washington, DC, showed the highest seroprevalence rate (0.47%) in females attending an adolescent clinic (20). Overall, CDC sero-prevalence studies showed higher seroprevalence rates and ranges among girls than among boys under 20 years old in adolescent clinics, correctional facilities, and STD clinics, with heterosexual sex with a partner of unknown risk as the only risk factor for most young women. HIV seroprevalence increases proportionately with age during adolescence, but few have looked at seroincidence or seroconversion (21–23). A 1995–1997 vaccine preparedness study among 4,892 adults at high risk for HIV infection in nine U.S. cities found 90 incident HIV-1 infections (1.31/100 person-years [PY]), 1.24/100 PY among female intravenous drug users, and 1.13/100 PY among women at heterosexual risk (22). Recently serologic studies on stored HIV positive serum using a sensitive/less sensitive assay are being used to differentiate recent infection from established infection (24). A California STD clinic study using these assays demonstrated no decline in new HIV cases (23). A recent blinded serosurvey in an urban emergency department found that prevalence among adults was 8.9%, with 11.8% having recent infection (25). Ignorance of HIV status or never testing occurred in 18.6% of HIV positive participants, and was most common among those of younger age and female gender. Recent concern has been expressed about the high rates of new HIV among young men who have sex with men (YMSM). In a seven-city study of youth 15 to 21, the highest new infection rates were among YMSM who identified themselves as African American or mixed race/ethnicity, transgender or heterosexual, or who had sex with both men and women (26). A more recent study comparing HIV-infected YMSM who were or were not disclosing their sexual identity found nondisclosers more likely to be unaware of their HIV status (98% vs. 75%; $p < 0.01$); to have one or more female sex partners (35% vs. 10%; $p < 0.01$); and to have unprotected vaginal or anal intercourse with female sex partners (20% vs. 5%; $p = 0.01$) compared to disclosers (27). This suggests a risk for the young women, especially young women of color, who are their partners.

CLINICAL CHARACTERISTICS OF YOUNG WOMEN WITH ACQUIRED HIV

REACH Study

Much of our knowledge of the natural history of HIV and its progression, as well as treatment response, is based on studies in adult men (28). In addition to AIDS case reports, mortality rates, and seroprevalence data, recent observational and descriptive research has added greatly to our understanding of young women with HIV. The REACH Project (Reaching for Excellence in Adolescent Care and Health) of the Adolescent Medicine HIV/AIDS Research Network enrolled 367 HIV-infected and 211 HIV-negative adolescents (74% and 78% of each cohort, respectively, was female) in a prospective observational study between 1996 and 1999 (29–31). The study took place at 15 sites in 13 U.S. cities. Youth were between 12 and 19 years of age at enrollment and had behaviorally acquired infection or were HIV negative youth of similar age, gender and care site. Evaluations included face to face interviews, audio computer-assisted self interviews (ACASI), laboratory analyses, gynecologic examinations, STD screening, and record abstractions (30). Young women in the study were mostly Black or Hispanic, uninsured or had public insurance. Table 16-2 describes characteristics of the young women in this study at baseline.

TABLE 16-2. *Characteristics of REACH female study population by HIV status.[h]*

Characteristics	HIV infected N = 217 n (%)	HIV-negative N = 125 n (%)	Total N = 342 (%) n
Demographic characteristics			
Mean age in years (SD)	16.8 (1.1)	16.5 (1.2)	16.7 (1.2)
Race/Ethnicity			
African-American	171 (78.8)	85 (68.0)	256 (74.9)
Hispanic/Latina	20 (9.2)	18 (14.4)	38 (11.1)
White/Others	26 (12.0)	22 (17.6)	48 (14.0)
Dropped out of high school	61 (28.2)	19 (15.2)[e]	80 (23.4)
Living at home with parents	146 (67.6)	105 (84.0)[e]	251 (73.6)
Financial situation of household			
Always have more than necessities	68 (31.5)	34 (27.2)	102 (29.9)
Have necessities but not much more	74 (34.2)	59 (47.2)	133 (39.0)
Have necessities some of the time	33 (15.3)	20 (16.0)	53 (15.6)
Barely paying the bills	23 (10.7)	5 (4.0)	28 (8.2)
Struggling to survive	18 (8.3)	7 (5.6)	25 (7.3)
Behavioral and clinical characteristics			
Mean number of partners in past 3 mo (SD[a])	1.3 (1.7)	1.2 (1.4)	1.3 (1.6)
Mean age in years of first consenting vaginal sex (SD)	13.3 (1.4)	14.1 (1.6)[f]	13.6 (1.5)
Douching at least once in the past 3 mo	123 (56.7)	56 (44.8)[g]	179 (52.3)
Abstinent from sexual activities past 3 mo	40 (19.4)	17 (15.9)	57 (17.3)
Reproductive tract infections[b]			
BV (clinical definition)	25 (12.8)	18 (15.4)	43 (13.7)
BV (Gram stain definition)	93 (53.8)	51 (46.8)	144 (50.0)
Chlamydia, positive	33 (15.9)	17 (13.9)	50 (15.2)
Gonorrhea, positive	13 (6.3)	6 (4.9)	19 (5.8)
HPV infection, positive	144 (77.4)	59 (56.73)[f]	203 (70.0)
Syphilis	7 (3.2)	3 (2.4)	10 (2.9)
Trichomoniasis, positive	31 (14.3)	4 (3.2)[e]	35 (10.2)
Vulvovaginitis (Clinical definition)	57 (39.9)	20 (45.5)	77 (42.8)

[a] SD = standard deviation.
[b] Based on available data; missing values excluded from calculations of percentages.
[c] BV = bacterial vaginosis.
[d] HPV = human papillomavirus.
[e] $p < 0.01$.
[f] $p < 0.001$.
[g] $p < 0.05$.
[h] Adapted from Vermund SH, et al. Douching practices among HIV infected and uninfected adolescents in the United States. *J Adolesc Health* 2001;29[Suppl 3]:80; with permission. Copyright, Society for Adolescent Medicine.

Although the prevalence of sexual and substance-using risk behaviors and reproductive tract infections was high and similar in both groups, HIV-infected women were significantly more likely to be high school dropouts, to be living away from parents, to have had earlier sexual debut, and to have human papillomavirus (HPV) of high-risk types, anal HPV, cervical squamous intraepithelial lesions (70% vs. 30% of HPV-infected young women had cervical SIL, $p < 0.001$), or trichomonas infection (32,33). HIV-infected, sexually active females in REACH were also significantly more likely to have partners who were 4 to 6 years older, and a greater mean partner age difference. Although HIV-infected females used condoms more than uninfected young women, a lower rate of condom use was associated with greater age of partner, longer relationships, and perceived HIV-infected partner status (34). A higher proportion of infected females had been in detention at some time, had living children and/or current pregnancy, or had multiple sexual partners, while uninfected women were less likely to be using condoms (29). Most of the HIV-infected youth in the study were healthy at baseline (Table 16-3) and not on antiretroviral therapy. Few

TABLE 16-3. *HIV-1 disease data of REACH HIV-1-infected cohorts.[c]*

Variables	Female HIV infected N = 242		Male HIV infected N = 83	
	n	*(%)[b]*	*n*	*(%)[b]*
HIV-1 RNA viral load (copies/ml)				
Below detection	62	26	11	13
400 to 10,000	116	48	34	42
10,000 to 50,000	42	17	18	22
50,000	22	9	19	23
Not yet evaluated	0	—	1	—
CD4$^+$ T-cell counts (cells/mm^3)				
0 to 199	17	7	10	12
200 to 500	99	42	45	54
500	122	51	28	34
Missing	4	—	0	—
History of AIDS at entry				
Yes	39	16	15	18
CD4$^+$ T cell only	34	14	12	14
Other conditions	5	2	3	4
No	203	84	68	82
Antiretroviral therapy (ART) at entry				
No ART	134	55	49	59
Monotherapy	19	8	4	5
>1 ART excluding PI[a]	53	22	13	16
>1 ART including PI	36	15	17	20

[a]PI = protease inhibitor.
[b]Missing values are excluded in the calculation of percentages.
[c]From Wilson CM, et al. The REACH (Reaching for Excellence in Adolescent Care and Health) project: study design, methods, and population profile. *J Adolesc Health* 2001;29[Suppl 3]:8; with permission.

had an AIDS diagnosis, but, while young women had lower viral loads and higher CD4 T-cell counts than young men, they had a higher death rate during the study (1.1 vs. 0.49/100 PY) (29). Consistent with the very low rates of IDU in REACH, only 1.6% of HIV-infected young women were seropositive for hepatitis C (HCV), but 15% had evidence of active hepatitis B (HBV) (33).

In addition to baseline analyses, some longitudinal analyses have now been published from the REACH data. When 1212 visits were analyzed for 323 HIV-infected REACH subjects (240 female), 65% were sexually active across six visits, with 43% consistently reporting their last intercourse as unprotected (35). There was a significant decline in frequent alcohol and marijuana use over time, and some psychological correlates were observed (depression with frequent alcohol use and unprotected sex, and health anxiety with frequent marijuana use and a number of sexual partners). There were no significant differences in incident pregnancy rates between HIV-infected and uninfected young women over a 3-year period, but HIV-infected young women who were already mothers of a living child were significantly less likely than uninfected mothers to have additional pregnancies. Among HIV-infected young women, a previous pregnancy increased the risk of subsequent pregnancy, while those with higher spiritual hope had fewer pregnancies in a multivariate analysis (36). Univariate analysis showed hormonal contraceptive use, and problem solving skills to be protective, and being a high school dropout or older than 18 predictive of future pregnancy. Another study analyzed predictors of initiating highly active antiretroviral therapy for 219 HIV-infected REACH subjects (167 female) who were initially not on therapy. Fifty-five percent of the young women and 44% of young men initiated HAART during the period 1996–1999 with no significant gender difference (37). HAART initiation was more likely in youth with low CD4 T cells and higher viral loads, and associated with having a high school diploma or GED and with perceived health status. Another longitudinal analysis looked at response to HBV immunization among REACH participants, and found lower response rates among HIV-infected youth (38). REACH has offered both positive and concerning insight into the natural history of HIV infection in adolescents and more specifically young women.

Susceptibility and Transmissibility

Young women have increased susceptibility to sexually transmitted infections due in part to cervical ectopy. The same immaturity makes them more susceptible to acquisition of HIV. The REACH study found number of lifetime sex partners to be an inverse independent predictor of cervical ectopy (39). Although studies of HIV serotypes prevalent in Asia and sub-Saharan Africa report equivalent male/female and female/male transmission until recently, in Europe and the U.S. studies of couples discordant for HIV status have repeatedly shown that women are more susceptible to seroconversion due to vaginal sex than men, though consistent use of condoms dramatically lowers that risk (2,40–42). The likelihood of a woman sero-converting in a discordant couple or in an area of high seroprevalence is increased by factors such as sexual trauma, current or prior genital ulcer disease (syphilis, chancroid, herpes), atrophic vaginitis, *Chlamydia, trichomonas,* oral contraceptive use, vaginal sex during menses, and receptive anal sex (41,43–45). Host factors of the transmitting partner included recent infection, viral load, severity of HIV disease, presence of genital ulcer disease or untreated STI, and lack of circumcision (43,46). Recent studies have used techniques such as cervicovaginal lavage (CVL), Sno-strips, and Weck-Cel sponges (the latter ophthalmologic devices modified to collect cervical secretions without disruption) to quantify the presence of HIV ribonucleic or deoxyribonucleic acid (RNA or DNA) in the female genital tract. They have identified host factors (bacterial vaginosis, herpes simplex virus, HPV, gonorrhea, *Chlamydia, Candida,* nonspecific vaginal ulcers, and vaginitis) leading to shedding in the female genital tract and to likely increased transmission in discordant couples (46, 47). Although virologic control of HIV replication by antiretroviral treatment can decrease shedding in genital secretions, 20% of women with nondetectable viral loads in one study still had measurable HIV RNA in the genital tract. These data provide important background for counseling young women with vertically or recently acquired HIV about risks of transmission, and the continued need to use barrier methods.

Clinical Manifestations of HIV Infection and AIDS

Clinical manifestations discussed here include those that are AIDS defining, specific to girls and women, or likely to be seen as presenting conditions. Acute infection, likely to be seen by primary care and urgent care clinicians, is a nonspecific viral syndrome occurring 5 to 30 days after exposure. Symptoms may include fever, malaise, rash, headache, sore throat, lymphadenopathy, diarrhea, and occasionally night sweats, oral ulcers, thrush, and opportunistic infection (48). Diagnosis requires an index of suspicion and knowledge of appropriate tests including viral cultures and HIV antigen tests such as qualitative DNA polymerase chain reaction (PCR) or quantitative RNA PCR (viral load in copies per mm^3) to detect the viral antigen. Acute infection can be temporarily characterized by high viral loads, which then drop, as immune response takes place over several weeks or months, to a relatively stable level or set point. In general, young women with more severe symptoms and higher acute viral loads are more likely to have higher set points and more destruction of CD4 T-lymphocytes, with rapid progression to AIDS, so early treatment should be considered. During the subsequent period of minimal symptoms and clinical stability characterized by low or nondetectable viral loads and relatively normal immune function, acute illness can cause transient changes in viral burden. The list of AIDS-defining diagnoses (mostly opportunistic infections [OI]) for adults and adolescents has been expanded twice, in 1987 and 1993, adding cervical cancer and immunosuppression (CD4+ T-lymphocyte count [CD4 count] < 200 cells/mm^3, or <14%) as AIDS defining conditions (49). *Pneumocystis carinii* pneumonia (PCP), candidal esophagitis, chronic herpes simplex infection, and wasting syndrome have been more common among women than men, and Kaposi sarcoma much less common. Many young women have no unusual symptoms or illness during the first few years of their infection or have only mild constitutional signs and laboratory markers (e.g., a high erythrocyte sedimentation rate or immunoglobulins) suggesting chronic infection or inflammation. The complete blood cell count and differential usually reflect a viral process. Natural history studies (primarily of men) inform us that the probability of developing AIDS as well as survival is related to both immune function (measured by the CD4 count) and viral load (Fig. 16-1) (50). Other manifestations of early HIV infection seen months to years later, usually when CD4 counts fall to 250 to 500 cells/mm^3, may include lymphadenopathy, increased acne and other dermatitis or skin infection (seborrhea, zoster, molluscum, warts), parotid swelling, malaise,

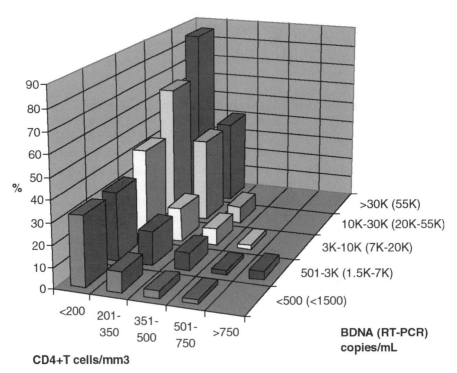

FIG. 16-1. Likelihood of developing acquired immunodeficiency syndrome within 3 years after becoming infected with human immunodeficiency virus type 1. (Adapted from Mellors JW, Muñoz A, Gigorgi JV, et al. Plasma viral load and CD+ lymphocytes as prognostic markers of HIV-1 infection. *Ann Intern Med* 1997;126(12):946. Source: March, 2004 Guidelines; http://www.aidsinfo.nih.gov/guidelines.)

persistent diarrhea, cholelithiasis, weight loss (or growth failure), and recurrent bacterial infections such as sinusitis, pneumonia, pelvic infection and pyelonephritis. OI are rare at CD4 counts >200 cells/mm^3.

Gynecologic Manifestations

Several common gynecologic conditions are more aggressive, severe, persistent, or likely to recur in women with HIV infection. Some young women present with these symptoms early in the disease, often with the initial drop in immune function that occurs during seroconversion but also years later, as cell-mediated immunity is gradually lost. Vulvovaginal candidiasis that is recurrent or resistant to brief treatment is extremely common, though increased use of antibiotics may be a cofactor. *Trichomonas* was more common among infected young women in REACH (Table 16-2) (32). Baseline human papillomavirus (HPV) prevalence was different, but HPV acquisition over time was similar in the infected and uninfected REACH cohorts. However cervical dysplasia was more common and persistent in young women with HIV infection, perhaps because of decreased ability to respond to the HPV infection (see Chapter 17). Young women with HIV need earlier initiation of cytology screening and more frequent follow-up (51). Women with cervical cancer and severe dysplasia have higher HIV seroprevalence, and several studies have concluded that there is an increased risk and rate of progression in women with HIV that is related to loss of immune function (CD4 count < 200) and viral interaction (52–55). Among 200 REACH subjects with at least two Pap smears, SIL was more common in infected youth than uninfected youth (50.7% vs. 19%), despite the fact that only 6.5% had low (<200) CD4 counts (56). Vulvovaginal and anal condylomata acuminata and neoplasia are also more common in HIV-infected girls and women and more difficult to treat. Pelvic inflammatory disease is reported more frequently in HIV-infected women, and is more likely to recur or cause chronic symptoms or complications such as tubo-ovarian abscess, but may also be atypical in presentation with lower white blood cell counts (57) (see Chapter 15). Genital ulcer diseases such as syphilis and herpes simplex (HSV) and zoster are more common and extensive in women with HIV infection and may have atypical presentations and require more prolonged or higher dose treatments according to CDC guidelines (58). Vulvar molluscum contagiosum and chancroid may also occur. The severity of these diseases may be exacerbated by declining immune function and lessened by immune reconstitution with successful antiretroviral therapy. Hospitalization and intravenous therapy and consultation with an infectious disease specialist should be considered in young women with significant immunosuppression who have PID, severe genital herpes, or zoster. Menstrual disorders are common in girls and young women with HIV. Girls infected since birth or infancy may be referred for short stature, delayed puberty or menarche, or growth failure, but many progress normally through puberty. Dysfunctional uterine bleeding may occur, especially in women with thrombocytopenia as a result of HIV disease or therapy, and severe bleeding may require hormonal therapy (Chapter 8). Young women with wasting syndrome or OI may present with oligomenorrhea or menorrhagia.

IDENTIFYING HIV BY COUNSELING AND TESTING

Testing for HIV only in people who are symptomatic or members of previously defined risk groups is inadequate for both prevention and access to care and support, especially for young women and for youth of color. Specific HIV prevention counseling and offering of testing are essential components of reproductive health care. HIV testing should include informed consent, assessment of sexual behavior, substance use and abuse, and psychosocial issues, as well as attention to the skills needed for risk reduction and personal protection. Guidelines and recommendations have been developed to address these issues in adolescents (59–61). Early detection of HIV is increasingly beneficial and justified, but many people presenting with a new diagnosis of symptomatic AIDS had recent medical or urgent care and missed opportunities for testing. When counseling and testing is encouraged and cost free in an urgent care setting, a significant number of people are diagnosed and enter care (62). Combination highly active antiretroviral therapy has produced dramatic declines in morbidity and mortality; perinatal transmission has been dramatically reduced by identification and treatment of pregnant women and their infants; transmission of HIV can be reduced by testing and risk reduction counseling, especially among youth with recent infection; and new technologies may improve the ease of testing and the proportion of youth receiving their results (63,64). The CDC announced in 2003 a new initiative focusing HIV prevention efforts on: the identification of people with HIV (by both routine offering of testing to all in clinical settings and outreach using new technologies to encourage testing among those at high risk); and increased efforts to promote reduced transmission risk by behavioral interventions for infected persons and prenatal screening (64,65). Special efforts are still needed to promote a sense of risk and vulnerability and to aid access to care and testing among youth. Primary prevention and the universal provision in schools and health promotion programs of concrete skill-based prevention education, risk reduction counseling, and access to effective contraceptive, sexual health and substance abuse services remain critical to prevention of new infections among youth.

Indications for Testing

In 1995 and 2001, the CDC issued and updated guidelines recommending routine HIV counseling and voluntary testing for all pregnant women, and the Institute of Medicine issued a strong 1999 report urging prenatal testing (60,66,67). Some states now mandate testing for pregnant women or children born to women without recent

HIV testing or lacking prenatal care (68). In addition, confidential or anonymous HIV testing with appropriate pre- and posttest counseling and referral services should be available (without parental permission or financial barriers) to any sexually active young woman who requests it. HIV testing should be recommended for all young women seeking pregnancy or seen with risk behaviors (including unprotected vaginal or anal sex), indicator conditions such as PID or STI, and life circumstances (partner characteristics, victimization by sexual assault or childhood sexual abuse) suggestive of increased risk for HIV. Young women are more likely to seek HIV testing if encouraged by their clinician (69,70). When new relationships, STI, pregnancy, or preconception counseling prompt testing, testing of sex partners should be encouraged and available. It is important to assess the timing of potential risk exposure and to recommend consistent condom use for both partners, as well as repeat testing in three to six months if an initial test is negative. The care provider must be aware of applicable state laws regarding HIV testing, consent, confidentiality, release of information, and reporting, as well as available sources of anonymous and/or free testing. Most states either have specific laws or policies allowing adolescents to access testing without parental or guardian consent, or the right to testing is assumed to be part of a youth's right to confidential STD diagnosis and treatment. Testing of younger children usually requires parental or guardian consent, but may need assent and education for the pubertal child.

Pretest and Posttest Counseling and Testing Methods

All sexually active adolescents should receive information about HIV testing from their health care providers. Pre- and posttest counseling usually take place in two visits (Table 16-4), but may be accomplished in a reasonable time with the use of screening tools and targeted counseling. Some offices train nursing or family planning or health educators to assist in this task, or offer rapid or noninvasive testing in nonmedical settings for at-risk youth. Results of standard HIV enzyme-linked immunosorbent assay (ELISA) antibody tests (blood or oral mucosal transudate [OMT] OraSure) should not be given until the result of the confirmatory test (usually a Western blot done on the same specimen) returns, as a positive ELISA with negative Western blot is a negative test. OMT testing is noninvasive, accurate, has sensitivity (99.9%) and specificity (>99.9%) comparable to serum testing, and has proved to be a useful technique for youths with needle phobia or in nonclinical settings (71). Recently, rapid screening for HIV antibody has become available, and the most recently licensed rapid test (Ora-Quick) now has a CLIA waiver, and may be done on venous or finger-stick samples in 15 to 30 minutes, and the FDA approved an OMT rapid test in March, 2004 (72). Rapid tests, which are preliminary and require prompt confirmation by a standard test if positive, should have great utility in labor and delivery, urgent care, and perhaps outreach settings in high prevalence areas, but require an altered counseling approach,

TABLE 16-4. *Components of HIV counseling and testing for adolescents.*

	Pretest	Posttest Negative	Posttest Positive or Ind.	Rapid test
Information about the HIV test, its benefits and consequences. (Include testing options on site and elsewhere.)	x			x
Ways HIV is transmitted—ways client is at risk.	x			x
Ways to prevent transmission— personalized based on risk assessment	x	x	x	x
Meaning of test results:	x			
Negative (Include window period and retesting need.)	x	x		x[a]
Indeterminate (retest)	x			
Positive—ELISA and Western blot	x			x
Positive—rapid test (Needs confirmation.)	x			x
Discuss confidentiality and reporting issues and availability of anonymous testing.	x			x
Obtain adolescent consent and test.	x			x
When and how test results will be available. Today for rapid test.	x			x[a]
Whether retest or confirmatory test is necessary.		x		x
Offer partner testing and or notification help.	x	x	x	x
Discuss resources for prevention.	x	x		x
Discuss treatment and care resources.	x		x	x
Discuss pregnancy implications (if applicable).	x		x	x
Schedule follow-up visit.	x	If need retesting	x	x

[a]For rapid test, preliminary results are available in less than an hour. A negative test is treated the same as a negative standard test: "You have no evidence of HIV infection today, but if you recently had unprotected sex or other risk, you will need to repeat the test in 2 to 3 months." A positive rapid test is preliminary and needs to be confirmed promptly with a standard antibody test.

guidance for which is available from CDC (http://www.cdc.gov/hiv/rapid_testing) and at the Project Respect-2 Web site (72,73) (Table 16-4). Positive predictive value of the rapid test is lower in low prevalence populations, so standard testing remains the recommended method today for screening most adolescents in the clinician office. An Assess, Counsel/Consent, Test, Support (ACTS) tool kit for simplifying office based testing for adolescents is currently being tested in New York (74). Giving positive or indeterminate HIV test results may have a serious impact and requires counseling time, in addition to clear instructions on future risk reduction and future testing. Information and support may need to be provided over several visits. Many HIV positive youths go through a period of denial in which they are unable or unwilling to seek care. Discussion of treatment and care options as part of the pretest counseling process and involvement in ongoing medical care may promote both the decision to test and the receipt of results as well as rapid baseline evaluations to assess prognosis and assist entry to ongoing care.

Prenatal Screening for HIV

CDC guidelines recommending testing of all pregnant women for HIV infection were developed in response to the 1994 results of Protocol 076 of the AIDS Clinical Trials Group (60,66,75). In this trial, treatment of asymptomatic pregnant women with zidovudine beginning in the second trimester, as well as intrapartum intravenous administration and 6-week treatment of the newborn child with oral drug, resulted in a highly significant drop in transmission rates to the infants (from 25.5% to 8.3%) of the treated mothers. Breast-feeding is contraindicated in HIV positive women in developed countries, and should also be discouraged if the young woman and her partner(s) have not been HIV tested. The use of antenatal zidovudine and the advent of HAART and combination therapy to improve effective viral suppression has led to rapid reduction in the incidence of perinatal transmission to 2% or less in the United States, lower if the viral load can be effectively controlled (60). Current minimal recommendations for treatment of newly diagnosed pregnant women and their offspring are discussed in Table 16-5. However, most treatment naive women require combination antiretroviral therapy during pregnancy (78). HIV education and pre- and posttest counseling of young women who are pregnant or seeking pregnancy (or not using effective contraception) and their partners should incorporate this information. A negative HIV test early in pregnancy does not eliminate the possibility of recent or

TABLE 16-5. *Zidovudine perinatal transmission prophylaxis regimen.[a,b]*

Antepartum	Initiation at 14 to 34 wk gestation and continued throughout pregnancy A. PACTG 076 regimen: ZDV 100 mg five times daily B. Acceptable alternative regimen: + ZDV 200 mg three times daily or ZDV 300 mg two times daily
Intrapartum	During labor, ZDV 2 mg/kg intravenously over 1 h, followed by a continuous infusion of 1 mg/kg intravenously until delivery.
Postpartum	Oral administration of ZDV to the newborn (ZDV syrup, 2 mg/kg every 6 h) for the first 6 wk of life, beginning at 8 to 12 h after birth.

[a]This regimen is directed only to prevention of perinatal transmission in women with very low (<1000 copies) or nondetectable viral load, who are not on or do not need antiretroviral therapy for their own health or to lower HIV-1 viral load. Women who require antiretroviral treatment or become pregnant while on antiretroviral therapy should receive a combination regimen including zidovudine and be treated in consultation with a perinatal expert. See scenarios at http://www.aidsinfo.nih.gov/guidelines.
[b]From Perinatal HIV Guidelines Working Group. Public Health Service Task Force Recommendations for use of antiretroviral drugs in pregnant HIV-1 infected women for maternal health and interventions to reduce perinatal HIV-1 transmission in the United States. 2004 June 23. (Accessed at http://aidsinfo.nih.gov/guidelines/)

future antenatal infection, so partner testing is important, and repeat testing of the pregnant woman and/or continued condom use is recommended if the partner's serostatus is positive or unknown, or his risk high. Young women presenting in labor with no prenatal care or no prenatal HIV test may be consented to receive HIV testing by a rapid point of care testing method, and then receive intrapartum intravenous zidovudine or oral zidovudine/lamivudine or nevirapine, with postpartum infant prophylaxis to prevent transmission (76–78).

HIV CARE AND SUPPORT

Caregivers providing routine, urgent or reproductive health care to young women and girls with HIV infection should be familiar with current developments in HIV care or have the consultative support of providers with HIV primary care and infectious disease experience. Providers of gynecologic, family planning, and prenatal care services may be seeing patients whose primary HIV care provider is elsewhere, necessitating close communication and care coordination, and an understanding of the implications of immune status, viral load, and treatment regimens for care and counseling. Many young women with HIV do not learn their status until they or their child become seriously ill with AIDS. For patients testing positive or entering care in the absence of life-threatening illness, a methodical baseline evaluation assists in establishing the current state of the patient's general health and immune function, identifying the timing of seroconversion, determining symptoms attributable to HIV, identifying coexisting infections and/or neoplastic disorders, assessing protection against vaccine-preventable diseases, ascertaining the need for antiretroviral treatment, and identifying and preventing opportunistic infections. Identification of barriers to care and treatment adherence, education and support, and discussion of sex, sexuality, and reproductive health issues and plans are also critical to both the initial evaluation and ongoing care of young women with HIV. Better understanding of the pathogenesis of HIV has demonstrated persistent viral replication during all stages of HIV infection and a correlation between viral load (quantitative HIV RNA or bDNA PCR as numbers of copies per mm^3 of plasma) and prognosis. Viral load should be assessed as part of the initial baseline evaluation and routine care, and the results incorporated into patient education and treatment recommendations (49,50). Viral load may be increased and CD4 count decreased during acute illnesses or shortly after immunizations; so two baseline values are often obtained. Many adolescents with recently diagnosed HIV infection will be asymptomatic or have mild nonspecific symptoms when initially diagnosed, though they may have high viral load or detectable alterations of immune function indicating need for antiretroviral treatment. The initial evaluation and subsequent monitoring should focus on a thorough history and physical detecting and treating illnesses that may hasten the progression of HIV, screening for latent infections that may reactivate as immune function fails, and assessing immune function, viral load, and immunization and nutrition status. Details of the baseline evaluation are described in Table 16-6 (79–81). This staging, along with careful assessment of immune function and viral load, is essential to advising the patient and family about likely disease progression over time, to recommending appropriate treatment and prophylaxis, and to aiding quality of life.

Baseline Evaluation and Routine Care for Newly Diagnosed Young Women

Care providers should pay particular attention to past medical history (hospitalizations, transfusions, surgery, lymphadenopathy) that may determine the timing of acquisition of infection, history of STDs and other infectious and parasitic diseases,

TABLE 16-6. *Baseline evaluation of young women with HIV.[a]*

History and physical examination
- Medical, family, social, psychiatric, reproductive history
- Review of systems
- Risk behavior assessment (sexual, substance use)
- Prevention counseling and risk reduction
- Immunization review

Laboratory evaluations and procedures
- Confirm HIV diagnosis (usually with ELISA and Western blot)
- CD4 count
- Viral load
- Chemistry panel: including liver and renal function
- Hematology panel: including white blood cell count, differential, platelets
- Lipid profile: total cholesterol, HDL, LDL, triglycerides
- Serologies: syphilis, toxoplasmosis, CMV, varicella-zoster virus (if no history of chickenpox or shingles), hepatitis A, hepatitis B, hepatitis C
- Urinalysis
- PPD
- G6PD (in selected patients)
- STD screening (all applicable sites)
- Pap smear; HPV typing
- Pregnancy test (if applicable)
- Resistance testing (sometimes recommended to guide treatment in pregnancy)
- Chest x-ray (if high risk of tuberculosis or symptomatic)

Referrals to HIV-experienced specialists or support staff
- Case management and support
- Dental examination and care
- Ophthalmology (urgent if AIDS or CD4 < 100 or visual problems)
- HIV specialist or infectious disease specialist with HIV experience

(Urgent if symptomatic, seroconversion syndrome, AIDS diagnosis, CD4 count < 350, interested in or needs antiretroviral treatment, pregnant or considering pregnancy, co-infections or interest in clinical trials)

[a]Modified from Feinberg J, Maenza J. Primary medical care. In: Anderson J, ed. *A guide to the clinical care of women with HIV.* Rockville, MD: HIV/AIDS Bureau, HRSA; 2001:77.; Samples CL, et al. Epidemiology and medical management of adolescents. In: Pizzo PA, Wilfert CM, eds. *Pediatric AIDS: the challenge of HIV infection in infants, children and adolescents.* 3rd ed. Baltimore, MD: Lippincott, Williams & Wilkins; 1998:615.

immunizations, drug allergies, growth and development, menstrual history, and sexual and reproductive history. The elements of the physical examination and baseline and periodic laboratory evaluations for HIV primary care are described in Table 16-6 and elsewhere (80). A more detailed review can be downloaded without charge from A Guide to the Clinical Care of Women with HIV, which is posted on the federal HIV/AIDS Bureau Web site, or available as a paperback text (79). The asymptomatic nonpregnant young woman who has no history of opportunistic infections or thrush, and no significant comorbidities, is managed according to her viral burden and immune function. As Fig. 16-1 demonstrates, a young woman with a CD4 count >500 cells/mm^3 (or 25%) and a low viral load (<1500 copies/mL) has little likelihood of rapid progression of disease to AIDS in the next 3 years, offering opportunities for stabilizing her health and supports, discussing reproductive issues and options, promoting a healthy lifestyle, and engaging her in ongoing supportive care (80–82). She should be offered standard immunization against childhood diseases (avoiding oral poliovirus vaccine), if not already immunized. Other recommended immunizations include *Haemophilus influenzae* type B conjugate vaccine and pneumococcal vaccine. Hepatitis B vaccine should be offered if there is no evidence of immunity and subsequent serologic testing may be necessary to document seroconversion (38). Hepatitis A vaccine is recommended for gay and bisexual men and their contacts and for young women who travel to endemic areas, and annual influenza virus vaccine is recommended for the patient and for household contacts. Varicella vaccine is currently being tested in HIV-infected children, youth, and adults.

Psychosocial Care and Support

Other components of care include assessment of cognitive function, mental status, and language and literacy, as well as reviews of biologic and practical family relationships and social supports (including disclosure—who does and does not know about the HIV diagnosis), continuing risk reduction, partner notification needs and plans, substance use and abuse and treatment history, criminal justice involvement, legal guardianship, practical needs (housing, food, income, health insurance), and education and school status (including disclosure preferences). Patient (and sometimes family or support person) education to promote self-care should cover HIV natural history, signs and symptoms of progression, currently available treatment alternatives and standards of care, frequency of visits, nutrition, exercise, importance of regular dental care and ophthalmologic examinations, sources of information about HIV and treatment, assistance with disclosure, reproductive options, hygiene and blood precautions, support services available, assistance with disclosure, dating, and safe sex and harm reduction, as well as education and counseling specific to the patient's problems. Peer support groups, when available, may be important local resources for young women and their families. Introduction to another adult or peer living with HIV infection may be more acceptable than a group approach, and involvement with other positive youth in recreational or community advisory or health promotion activities may be more affirming and attractive than a traditional support group approach. Several Internet Web sites such as Advocates for Youth's http://www.youthhiv.org offer access to the stories of youth in similar situations. Programs funded through the Ryan White Care Act or other local and state programs may offer opportunity for involvement in national and state consumer conferences and advocacy activities. Given the rapid changes in HIV treatments, clinicians should regularly update clients on changing standards of care and new developments in research. When youth are diagnosed in outreach or urgent care settings, the initial focus is supportive, with the goal of transitioning the young woman into care.

Follow-up and Primary Care

Follow-up examination frequency for recently infected youth, as well as vertically infected adolescents, is dependent on the patient's psychological and health status, CD4 count, illnesses present, and treatment being monitored, but is at least three to four visits annually for monitoring immune function and viral load, targeted review of symptoms and physical examination, and preventive care and counseling in asymptomatic immunocompetent youth. These factors, as well as practice location and available resources, may determine which services take place in a primary or reproductive health care setting, and which are provided by an HIV care specialist. Each time the adolescent is seen, sexual and substance using behavior and life circumstances should be assessed and risk reduction and importance of healthy practices reinforced. Clinicians also play a vital role in preventing transmission by regular screening and treatment for STI and recurrent discussions of childbearing plans and by partner notification and testing (64). Most studies have shown a survival benefit to care by an HIV-experienced clinician, but clinicians providing primary care and urgent care to young women with HIV can feel comfortable providing care to immunocompetent youth (CD4 count >500, or 25%) who are not on medications, and to others with adequate information to inform consultation and care (Table 16-7). Whether the HIV was acquired perinatally or recently, information available to the primary care or urgent care clinician should include questions designed to inform decision making about symptomatic illness, drug interactions and adverse reactions, and the likelihood of opportunistic infection. In general, young women who have never had an opportunistic infection or an AIDS diagnosis and have recent low viral loads and stable immune function (CD4 count >350) are not at risk of OI (unless they have recently discontinued antiretroviral medication). They may be at risk of diarrhea, dermatologic complaints, or recurrent bacterial infections (such as sinusitis, community-acquired pneumonia, pyelonephritis, PID). Nomograms for management of acute illnesses in young women with significant immunocompromise or AIDS (anemia, cough with dyspnea and fever, fever of unknown origin, acute and chronic

TABLE 16-7. *Questions to aid care of HIV-infected young women.*

- When were you diagnosed? How long have you known your diagnosis?
- Who is aware of your diagnosis? [family, household, sex partner(s), school, job, friends, health care providers, no one]
- Any hospitalizations related to HIV?
- What medications are you on?
  ○ Antiretroviral
  ○ Prophylaxis against PCP, other OI
  ○ Other prescribed medications
  ○ Over the counter medications
  ○ Illicit drugs and alcohol
- Do you know your CD4 T-cell count?
  ○ Lowest ever? When?
  ○ Most recent? When?
- Do you know your viral load?
  ○ Highest ever? When?
  ○ Most recent? When?
  ○ Were you taking antiretroviral medications last time you were checked?
  ○ Are you taking them now?
- Where do you get your HIV care? When last seen?
- What are your symptoms?
- Are you having sex or using drugs or alcohol?
  ○ Risk assessment and prevention counseling
- Are you pregnant or considering pregnancy?

diarrhea, headache, altered mental status, odynophagia) are available to guide consultation, referral, and management (79).

Reproductive Health Issues

As better treatment has improved the survival and quality of life of young women living with HIV, and as children infected with HIV perinatally reach adolescence, proactive HIV prevention education and pre-conceptual counseling of infected youth and their partners has become important. Most young women infected with HIV have given birth to healthy children, and CDC is collecting information on pregnancies to vertically infected young women as the first cohort of young women born with HIV become adults (83). Clinicians may also be caring for young women who are considering childbearing with HIV-infected male partners. Techniques such as artificial insemination, combined with careful antiretroviral management for HIV-infected young men and women to decrease viral burden, sperm washing, in vitro fertilization, intracytoplasmic insemination, and HIV PCR testing of semen samples are being practiced or studied in adult populations (84). Pregnancy, child bearing and parenthood are an expected future option for most young women, including those who have survived HIV since infancy, many of whom are now reaching adolescence and are healthy. However, currently most pregnancies to these long-term survivors of pediatric HIV are unintended, according to a recent report on 10 such pregnancies in Puerto

Rico (83). Any seropositive patient who is or might become sexually active should be counseled about the risks posed by intercourse and intimacy, including pregnancy and childbearing and exposure to STDs and new HIV strains, and they should be offered both barrier and hormonal methods of contraception. Seropositive women considering pregnancy should be offered alternatives (e.g., artificial insemination) to unprotected intercourse for conception and counseled about current transmission risks and aided in achieving optimum health and virologic control prior to attempting a pregnancy. Young women who are pregnant should be managed according to the latest guidelines (available at http://aidsinfo.nih.gov/guidelines/) (78,81). Although some antiretroviral medications or combinations are contraindicated in pregnancy, most are Category B or C. Young women on antiretrovirals usually need the care of an HIV-experienced obstetrical team and to receive combination therapy including zidovudine. Scenarios for treatment are shown in the latest perinatal treatment guidelines for women of varying treatment histories and clinical status, and the zidovudine treatment regimen is shown in Table 16-5. Obstetric care to minimize transmission can also include avoidance of invasive monitoring techniques and prolonged labor or rupture of membranes, and elective cesarean section. Infants born to HIV-infected mothers with advanced disease or higher viral loads are at increased risk, but all should receive postpartum prophylaxis with zidovudine, receive PCP prophylaxis beginning at 1 month of age until proved HIV negative, and receive care or consultation from a team with expertise in pediatric HIV and infectious diseases. Only long-term studies will determine the potential long-term impact of intrauterine exposure to HIV and the antiretroviral medications used to treat it, though they are minimal to date. The Pediatric AIDS Clinical Trials Group is now following such infants to age 24 years. Finally, seropositive pregnant and parenting adolescents should be given support for planning for the future care of their children in the event of their incapacitation or death.

Contraception

Intrauterine devices have not usually been recommended for HIV-positive teens because of the possible increased risk of pelvic infection and bleeding. Oral contraceptives and other estrogen containing regimens such as the contraceptive patch or ring metabolized in the cytochrome P-450 system may have interactions with some of the medications used for treating HIV (especially nelfinavir, ritonavir, amprenavir, lopinavir/ritonavir, and efavirenz) or opportunistic infections. These may decrease contraceptive efficacy, alter antiretroviral efficacy, or cause increased side effects, making use of a second barrier method essential. Other methods such as depot medroxyprogesterone injections and levonorgestrel subdermal implants have efficacy, but the accompanying spotting experienced by some young women may pose an increased risk of transmission and again stress the need for additional barrier methods. All HIV-infected youth (and young women who are partners of HIV-infected men) who use barrier methods or are considering sexual activity should be counseled about the availability of urgent care for both emergency contraception

(Chapter 20) and nonoccupational postexposure prophylaxis (N-PEP; discussed further in the case of sexual assault in Chapter 24), using the same principles and treatment plan as for occupational PEP (Fig. 16-2) (85–87). CDC has established a national registry (http:www.hivpepregistry.org) in an attempt to define the cost and efficacy of N-PEP.

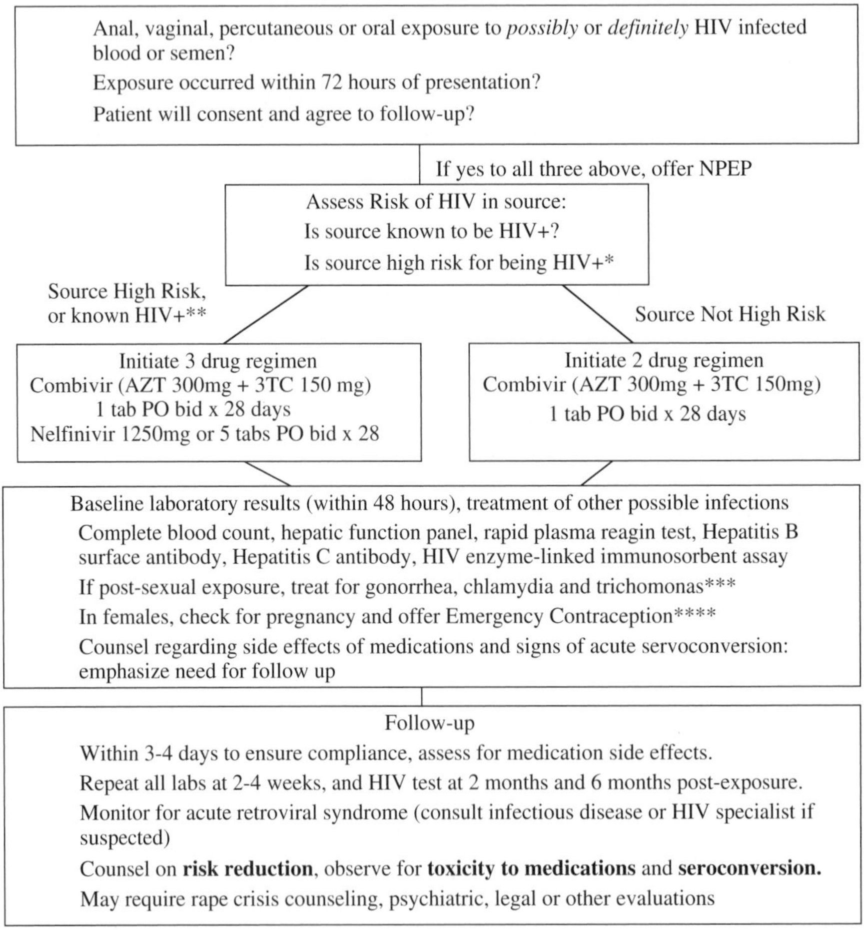

Anal, vaginal, percutaneous or oral exposure to *possibly* or *definitely* HIV infected blood or semen?

Exposure occurred within 72 hours of presentation?

Patient will consent and agree to follow-up?

If yes to all three above, offer NPEP

Assess Risk of HIV in source:
Is source known to be HIV+?
Is source high risk for being HIV+*

Source High Risk, or known HIV+**

Source Not High Risk

Initiate 3 drug regimen
Combivir (AZT 300mg + 3TC 150 mg)
1 tab PO bid x 28 days
Nelfinivir 1250mg or 5 tabs PO bid x 28

Initiate 2 drug regimen
Combivir (AZT 300mg + 3TC 150mg)
1 tab PO bid x 28 days

Baseline laboratory results (within 48 hours), treatment of other possible infections

Complete blood count, hepatic function panel, rapid plasma reagin test, Hepatitis B surface antibody, Hepatitis C antibody, HIV enzyme-linked immunosorbent assay

If post-sexual exposure, treat for gonorrhea, chlamydia and trichomonas***

In females, check for pregnancy and offer Emergency Contraception****

Counsel regarding side effects of medications and signs of acute servoconversion: emphasize need for follow up

Follow-up

Within 3-4 days to ensure compliance, assess for medication side effects.

Repeat all labs at 2-4 weeks, and HIV test at 2 months and 6 months post-exposure.

Monitor for acute retroviral syndrome (consult infectious disease or HIV specialist if suspected)

Counsel on **risk reduction**, observe for **toxicity to medications** and **seroconversion.**

May require rape crisis counseling, psychiatric, legal or other evaluations

*High risk for being HIV+ includes persons who: use intravenous drugs, engage in male-male sex, have multiple sexual partners, exchange sex for money or drugs or who have sex with persons presumed to be HIV+

**If source known HIV+ should initiate a three drug regimen as soon as possible and consult with infectious disease/HIV specialist

***We recommend: Ceftriaxone 125mg IMx1, Azithromycin 1g PO x1, and Metronidazole 2g PO x1

****We recommend Plan B 1 pill immediately, 1 pill 12 hours later

FIG. 16-2. Recommendations for initiating NPEP in adolescents. (From Olshen E, Samples CL. Postexposure prophylaxis: an intervention to prevent human immunodeficiency virus infection in adolescents. *Curr Opin Pediatr* 2003;15:379; with permission.)

Gynecologic Management

Frequent monitoring for cervical dysplasia, sexually transmitted diseases, and reproductive tract infections is needed. In general, HIV-infected patients require more prolonged and aggressive therapy for cervical dysplasia and genitourinary infections, with hospitalization usually indicated for pelvic inflammatory disease and primary herpes infection. Recurrent vulvovaginal candidiasis (Chapter 14) may be treated by monthly short courses of topical medication or oral fluconazole treatment or prophylaxis. In addition to cervical cancer and neoplasia (Chapter 17), young women with HIV may be more susceptible to other reproductive malignancies (e.g., ovarian cancer) and lymphoma. Immune reconstitution through effective antiretroviral therapy can help to prevent or aid in the management of these conditions.

TREATMENT AND PROPHYLAXIS

Highly Active Antiretroviral Therapy

The striking changes in understanding of HIV pathogenesis and care and treatment effectiveness in the past decade has brought the ability to prevent immunologic deterioration by suppressing viral replication, along with the ability to partly or fully restore the immune system (and thus the prognosis for longevity and health) through successful antiretroviral therapy (88). While highly active antiretroviral therapy has changed HIV from a fatal to a chronic disease for many young women, side effects, toxicity, drug interactions, metabolic complications, rapid development of drug resistance without near perfect adherence, and the failure of current treatments to eliminate viral reservoirs have led to increased complexity of HIV care and to some discouragement among consumers and care providers. Adding to this disillusionment is the fact that 97% of the world's HIV-infected population resides in areas where effective treatments are not available. The standard of care for management of HIV infection is constantly changing, with 22 antiretroviral drugs and fixed-dose combinations currently approved for combination antiretroviral therapy. For the past several years, a federally constituted panel has developed and posted annual updated guidelines for HIV treatment, which are an essential starting point to care provision for those involved in caring for or counseling HIV positive young women. The most recent guidelines, March 2004 (available at http://aidsinfo.nih.gov/guidelines/), provide an overview of the principles of treatment initiation, available agents and their toxicities and drug interactions, with drug interaction and side effect tables available for personal digital assistant download (89). Pediatric guidelines are also available for children under thirteen, and were updated January, 2004 (90). The goals of antiretroviral therapy are maximal and durable reduction in viral replication and viral load, and restoration or preservation of immune function with resultant improvements in survival and quality of life. These goals are tempered by the need to maximize adherence, sequence therapy in a way that preserves future options, and to utilize resistance testing to guide some therapeutic choices (89). Combinations of at least three potent antiretrovirals, taken consistently before significant loss of immune function or morbidity occur, are key to these goals, but young women with chronic HIV infection who have AIDS or are symptomatic may achieve clinical and survival benefit from treatment even if optimal virologic control is not achieved. Management of sick or significantly immunocompromised adolescents and adolescents on or meeting guidelines for initiation of antiretroviral treatment should be done in conjunction with infectious disease or other specialists knowledgeable about HIV management and new developments. Initiation of antiretroviral therapy is strongly recommended for youths with AIDS-defining conditions or CD4 count of <200 or symptomatic HIV disease (89) (Table 16-8). Therapy is also recommended for the asymptomatic patient with decreased or rapidly declining cellular immunity and a high viral load if the youth is ready, willing, and able to adhere to treatment. Some experts have previously recommended aggressive treatment for any detectable viral loads and higher T cells (the hit early, hit hard approach) but recent recommendations for treatment initiation are more conservative, with drug-related toxicities and reduction in quality of life, drug resistance, and the unknown factor of long-term treatment morbidities and impact seen as risks of early therapy. The clinician, patient, and family need to weigh the risks and benefits of delayed versus early therapy carefully and repeatedly. Treatment of symptomatic seroconversion may improve prognosis but requires careful follow-up and expert input, as clinical trials are in progress to determine the optimal agents and duration. For young women, additional expertise in the care of youth and reproductive health issues are also important to an effective

TABLE 16-8. *Indications for initiation of antiretroviral therapy in the HIV-infected young woman.[a]*

Clinical category	CD4+ cell count	Plasma HIV RNA	Recommendation
Symptomatic (AIDS or severe symptoms)	Any value	Any value	Treat
Asymptomatic, AIDS by CD4	CD4+ T cells <200/mm^3	Any value	Treat
Asymptomatic or mild symptoms	CD4+ T cells >200/mm^3 but ≤350/mm^3	Any value	Treatment should be offered, although controversial.
Asymptomatic	CD4+ T cells >350/mm^3	>55,000	Consider treatment: Some recommend. (3 year risk AIDS >30%)
Asymptomatic	CD4+ T cells >350/mm^3	<55,000	Defer and monitor. (3 year risk AIDS <15%).

[a]Adapted from Panel on Clinical Practices for Treatment of HIV Infection. Guidelines for the use of antiretroviral agents in HIV-1-infected adults and adolescents. Rockville, MD: Department of Health and Human Services, 2004 March 23.

treatment team. The Adolescent Medicine HIV/AIDS Research Network developed a treatment readiness intervention, Project TREAT, based on the stages of change model of behavioral intervention (91). Beginning antiretroviral therapy in a young person who is not ready to consider therapy (precontemplation) may in the long run be without much benefit. Once treatment is begun, viral load is a better indicator of treatment efficacy than CD4 count, and both should be monitored before and after antiretroviral therapy is initiated or changed. A drop of at least 1 log in viral load (e.g., from 100,000 to 10,000 copies/mm^3) is the criterion for measuring efficacy of a new treatment. Currently available antiretroviral agents have different sites of action, and include seven nucleoside analog reverse transcriptase inhibitors (RTIs): zidovudine, zalcitabine (ddC), didanosine (ddI), stavudine, lamivudine, abacavir and emtricitabine (FTC, licensed July 2003), as well as two RTI combinations, Combivir (zidovudine/lamivudine) and Trizivir (zidovudine, lamivudine, abacavir) were the first combination products licensed. Tenofovir, a once a day agent licensed in 2002, is the first nucleotide RTI. Eight available protease inhibitors (PI) now include saquinavir, indinavir, ritonavir, nelfinavir, amprenavir, lopinavir/ritonavir (Kaletra), with atazanavir (the first once a day PI) and fosamprenavir just approved in 2003. Nonnucleoside RTIs (NNRTI) include nevirapine, delavirdine and efavirenz, and have proven to be as potent as PIs when combined with two RTIs, and are simpler to take, but poor adherence can invoke classwide resistance. The first fusion inhibitor, enfuvirtide, was also recently licensed for twice daily subcutaneous administration. Regimens combining two PIs or using a PI "boosted" by a small dose of ritonavir to take advantage of drug interactions may also be beneficial, especially for treatment experienced patients. In most cases, adolescent treatment doses are empirically the same as those for adults for youths who are Tanner stage 4 or greater, and pediatric doses are used for youth who are Tanner stages 1 to 2. Young women less than 60 kg or on regimens with additive toxicity may warrant reduced doses of some medications. The currently recommended first line therapies for treatment naïve patients generally use two RTIs and either a potent NNRTI or a PI or boosted PIs shown in Table 16-9 (89). Several once a day medications and concentrated formulations have recently become available, allowing simplification of treatment, reduction of pill burden, and the possibility of once a day treatment regimens more consistent with the lifestyle of the young. In addition, about 60 new drugs and combinations are in development.

Adherence and Treatment Failure

HAART demands excellent adherence and may impose a heavy pill and side effect burden. In our experience, simpler regimens, lower pill burden, and once or twice a day frequency are best tolerated in adolescents. Since inconsistency in adherence and even dose timing variation can result in resistance, treatment failure, and diminution of future options, matching the regimen to the lifestyle and routine schedules (both weekday and weekend) is critical. A regimen that does not effect a decreased

TABLE 16-9. *Recommended antiretroviral regimens for treatment naive young women.[e]*

NNRTI-Based Regimens		No. pills/day
Preferred Regimens	**Efavirenz + lamivudine + (zidovudine or tenofovir DF or stavudine[a])—except for pregnant women or women with pregnancy potential**	**3–5 pills/d**
Alternative Regimens	Efavirenz + emtricitabine + (zidovudine or tenofovir DF or stavudine[a])—except for pregnant women or women with pregnancy potential	3–4 pills/d
	Efavirenz + (lamivudine or emtricitabine) + (didanosine or abacavir)—except for pregnant women or women with pregnancy potential	3–5 pills/d
	Nevirapine + (lamivudine or emtricitabine) + (zidovudine or stavudine[a] or didanosine)	4–5 pills/d

PI-Based Regimens		No. pills/day
Preferred Regimens	**Kaletra (lopinavir+ ritonavir) + lamivudine + (zidovudine or stavudine[a])**	**8–10 pills/d**
Alternative Regimens	Atazanavir + (lamivudine or emtricitabine) + (zidovudine or stavudine[a] or abacavir)	4–5 pills/d
	Fosamprenavir + (lamivudine or emtricitabine) + (zidovudine ostavudine[a] or abacavir)	6–8 pills/d
	Fosamprenavir + ritonavif[b] + (lamivudine or emtricitabine) + (zidovudine or stavudine[a] or abacavir)	6–8 pills/d
	Indinavir + ritonavir[b] + (lamivudine or emtricitabine) + (zidovudine or stavudine[a] or abacavir)	8–11 pills/d
	Kaletra (lopinavir + ritonavir), + emtricitabine + (zidovudine or stavudine[a] or abacavir)	8–9 pills/d
	Kaletra (lopinavir + ritonavir) + emtricitabine + abacavir	8–9 pills/d
	Nelfinavif[c] + (lamivudine or emtricitabine) + (zidovudine or stavudine[a] or abacavir)	12–14 pills/d
	Saquinavir (sgc or hgc)[d] + ritonavir + (lamivudine or emtricitabine) + (zidovudine or stavudine[a] or abacavir)	14–16 pills/d

Triple NRTI Regimen—Only when preferred or alternative above regimens can or should not be used as initial therapy		No. pills/day
	Abacavir + lamivudine + zidovudine (or stavudine[a])	2–6 pills/d

[a]Higher incidence of lipoatrophy, hyperlipidemia and mitochondrial toxicity reported with stavudine than with other NRTIs.

[b]Low-dose (100–400 mg) ritonavir.

[c]Less if nelfinavir 625 mg tablet—soon to be available

[d]sgc = soft gel capsule; hgc = hard gel capsule.

[e]Adapted from Panel on Clinical Practices for Treatment of HIV Infection. Guidelines for the use of antiretroviral agents in HIV-1-infected adults and adolescents. Rockville, MD: DHHS, 2004 March 23.

viral load (by at least 1 log) or improved immunologic and clinical status after 4 to 6 weeks should probably be changed to another combination regimen with at least two new drugs once nonadherence is ruled out. If adherence is an issue, a simpler regimen may produce a dramatic response. Early combination therapy with the goal of obtaining a nondetectable viral load is now the standard of care, and prolongs both survival and time before progression to AIDS if successful (89). Protease inhibitors can induce rapid development of resistance when used intermittently, and some have a high incidence of side effects and serious interactions with medications and street drugs, so their use in young women requires a level of motivation and compliance rare in our experience. In addition, the impact of a complex medication regimen on a patient's mental health and quality of life must also be considered. Management of HIV treatment requires constant patient education and input; shared knowledge of the doses, side effects, drug interactions, and monitoring needed for each regimen; and constant efforts to monitor changes in treatment guidelines and standards of care. Successful treatment of youths with HIV infection should include the young women as partners, with the clinicians explaining strategies and offering hope, as well as options and choices and empowering links to consumer resources, with attention to lifestyle issues that impact compliance and tolerance. As the generation of youth infected vertically with HIV transitions into and through adolescence, the development of a provider patient and family relationship fostering increasing autonomy and transitions to adult roles is sometimes complicated by the exhaustion of therapeutic options, treatment morbidity, and the development of advanced disease, as well as by reproductive health issues, including pregnancy and parenting. Many young women who are long-term survivors of HIV are extremely treatment experienced and may have multidrug resistance. Recently, genotypic and phenotypic resistance testing have become critical tools in the HIV care provider's management of treatment experienced patients and treatment failure.

Opportunistic Infection Prevention and Treatment

As immune function declines with CD4 counts $<14\%$, or <200 cells/mm^3, patients become vulnerable to a cascade of life-threatening opportunistic infections. Guidelines for primary (prevent first occurrence) and secondary (prevent recurrence) prevention of opportunistic infections in pregnant and nonpregnant persons living with HIV infection were last updated in 2001, adding criteria for discontinuation of prophylaxis following immune reconstitution and successful antiretroviral therapy (92,93). Prophylaxis designed to prevent PCP is recommended for all seropositive individuals who have a CD4 count <200 cells/mm^3, or 14%, an AIDS diagnosis, or a history of Pneumocystis disease. Prophylaxis with oral trimethoprim-sulfamethoxazole or alternatively with oral dapsone and pyrimethamine or aerosolized pentamidine is currently recommended. The first two regimens also prevent toxoplasmosis. Prophylaxis against *Mycobacterium avium-intracellulare* (MAI) infection is recommended for youths with a CD4 count of <50 cells/mm^3. The most commonly recommended MAI infection prophylaxis option is weekly azithromycin. Vigorous preventive treatment of tuberculin-positive individuals with HIV infection is also recommended, with 12 months of isoniazid as the standard treatment. Other primary and secondary prophylactic regimens as well as treatment recommendations for OI are listed in the USPHS/IDSA guidelines (92). For other OI such as cytomegalovirus (CMV) there are indicated secondary prophylactic regimens, but the evidence supporting primary prophylaxis is less strong. Until recently, secondary prophylaxis of people with AIDS experiencing OI such as PCP, MAI, or CMV was presumed to be lifelong. As new potent antiretroviral combinations produce dramatic CD4 cell count increases, studies have shown that primary and secondary prophylaxis can be safely discontinued after a period of several months of significant immune reconstitution and continued virologic control (92). With adolescents, poor adherence or treatment failure may lead to decline in CD4 counts and necessitate resumption of OI prophylaxis, however.

PREVENTION, CARE COORDINATION, RESEARCH, AND ADVOCACY

All health care professionals should be knowledgeable about HIV infection and comfortable doing individual risk assessments and providing counseling and testing and access to care. Every family planning, gynecology, prenatal, health maintenance, or urgent medical visit is an opportunity to engage in active prevention and case finding. Familiarity with community resources available for children, youths, and families affected by HIV is essential. Consultation with infectious disease or other experts experienced in HIV management improves awareness of current therapeutic and prophylactic guidelines, assists in the diagnosis and management of opportunistic infections, and helps to assess eligibility for clinical research. DiClemente has reviewed adolescent HIV risk, prevention research, and policy and legal issues, as well as the implications of parental monitoring for HIV prevention (94,95). Children and women have traditionally been considered more difficult research subjects, and trials of therapeutic modalities in adolescents, children, and women have generally lagged behind those for adults and men. In the early years of HIV research, adolescents were systematically excluded from treatment protocols, but in the past decade involvement of adolescents and women has been encouraged, with special protections against risk.

The REACH study was noninterventional, but intensive, and had retention rates of 91% among HIV-infected females. Many of the Institutional Review Boards for REACH sites allowed enrollment with parental permission waived. Although most legal and ethical experts feel adolescents are entitled to diagnosis and treatment of HIV as an STI, minors cannot generally consent alone to treatment research of greater than minimal risk, unless they meet the legal definition of emancipated minor or are consenting to treatment research of greater than minimal risk on their offspring or during pregnancy. The Society for Adolescent Medicine has issued guidelines for research participation among adolescents that are helping in designing research projects aimed at improving prevention and treatment for young women or assessing those already available (96,97). Building upon work of the REACH Project, in 2001 a new NIH funded domestic multicenter research network was formed specifically to develop and implement interventions for HIV treatment, care, and prevention among youth aged 12 to 24 (31). The Adolescent Trials Network (ATN) for HIV/AIDS Interventions is developing and conducting clinical trials and behavioral interventions for primary prevention and to promote adherence and behavioral change. Unlike other HIV multicenter research networks, ATN has as its agenda both improving treatment and care and improving prevention among HIV-infected and at-risk youth. It is also mapping HIV risk and forming community partnerships mobilized for broader implementation of effective prevention interventions, and preparation for adolescent vaccine trials in a hopeful future. ATN research efforts, in 15 adolescent HIV programs in 14 cities (each with at least 75 HIV-infected youth aged 12 to 24 in care), have included both vertically and recently infected young women. Studies include trials of structured treatment interruption or short cycle treatment, vaccine readiness trials in communities at risk, and novel approaches to adherence, behavior change to prevent transmission, and venue-based sero-incidence. The PACTG, successful in reducing both pediatric AIDS and maternal transmission and the birth of newly infected infants in the United States but faced with an increasing number and proportion of perinatally infected adolescents and young adults, has also focused recent and future clinical trials efforts on adolescent issues. These include the impact of puberty on HIV-infected youth and on treatment morbidity, novel treatment options for advanced disease and heavily treatment experienced youth, and assessment of pharmacokinetics of HIV drugs. Both research networks and treatment centers serving HIV-infected young women are integrating gynecologic and reproductive health issues into their services capabilities and areas of exploration. Research is also needed to define the impact of HIV infection on the social, cognitive, and behavioral functioning of youths, and to optimize mental and physical health and quality of life as well as long-term health. The Health Resources and Services Administration's Special Projects of National Significance (SPNS) program has funded several innovative programs assisting these efforts. There have been two generations of SPNS projects focusing on developing effective models of adolescent HIV prevention, case finding, and care. The first, from 1993 to 1997, featured 10 sites with four major models of care: two focused on youth involvement; two focused on outreach; three focused on case management and linkage to care; and three with a model featuring a comprehensive continuum of care for youth (98). The second SPNS cycle, which funded five programs from 1996 to 2000, built on that prior experience to address barriers to HIV testing, treatment seeking, and effective treatment among youth (99–102). Both of these efforts stressed the importance of a client-centered approach, which offers ease of access (one-stop shopping if possible), staff readily available for questions and consultation, feasible schedules, and case management and support.

Health care providers have an essential role as advocates and spokespersons on behalf of youth, who are often undervalued and disenfranchised. We often have unique opportunities to impact not only the young women in our care, but their families, partners, and peers. We can promote youth-friendly community policies, advocate for adolescent access to services, and become involved in prevention, education, and intervention at the community level through schools and community-based programs. Care providers can use their experience with the health care needs of at-risk and HIV-infected youths to advocate with local, state, and national policy makers for increased funding of research and early intervention efforts targeting adolescents and joint efforts to unify adolescent data collection efforts, clarify definitions, and include adolescents as a target group in federally funded programs. Epidemiologic studies have shown high rates of HIV risk among young women of color, and the neighborhoods most impacted are often those with high rates of STD, teen pregnancy, and health disparities, making coalition building among adolescent and reproductive health providers beneficial. Especially in resource poor settings, access to contraceptive and fertility options and to diagnosis and treatment of other sexually transmitted infections are essential to curbing transmission and promoting case finding and care. Young women living with HIV infection need the support and assistance of health professionals sensitive to their needs, knowledgeable about their disease, and willing to engage as active partners in sustaining health and optimizing quality of life with responsive, individualized and age-appropriate care and guidance.

REFERENCES

1. UNAIDS. 2004 Report on the Global AIDS Epidemic, 2004 July.
2. The Global Impact of HIV/AIDS on Youth: HIV/AIDS Policy Fact Sheet. Henry J. Kaiser Family Foundation, 2004. (Accessed July 18, 2004, at http:www.kff.org.)
3. Centers for Disease Control and Prevention. Cases of HIV Infection and AIDS in the United States, 2002. HIV/AIDS Surveillance Report 2003;14:1
4. Centers for Disease Control and Prevention. U.S. HIV and AIDS cases reported through December 2001 Year End Edition. HIV/AIDS Surveillance Report 2002;13(2):1.
5. Centers for Disease Control and Prevention. HIV Infection in Areas Conducting HIV Reporting Using Coded Patient Identifiers, 2000. HIV/AIDS Surveillance Technical Report 2002;1:3.
6. Karon JM, Rosenberg PS, McQuillan G, et al. Prevalence of HIV infection in the United States, 1984 to 1992. *JAMA* 1996;276:126.
7. Centers for Disease Control and Prevention. First 500,000 AIDS cases—United States, 1995. *MMWR Morb Mortal Wkly Rep* 1996;44:849.
8. Centers for Disease Control and Prevention. AIDS Cases in Adolescents and Adults, by Age—United States, 1994–2000. HIV/AIDS Surveillance Supplemental Report 2002;9:8.
9. Center for Disease Control and Prevention. Diagnosis and Reporting of HIV and AIDS in States with HIV/AIDS Surveillance—United States, 1994–2000. *MMWR Morb Mortal Wkly Rep* 2002; 51:595.
10. Fleming P, Byers R, Sweeney PA, et al. HIV Prevalence in the United States, 2000. In: Ninth Conference on Retroviruses and Opportunistic Infections; 2002; Seattle, WA; 2002.
11. Conway GA, Epstein MR, Hayman CR, et al. Trends in HIV prevalence among disadvantaged youth. Survey results from a national job training program, 1988 through 1992. *JAMA* 1993;269: 2887.
12. St Louis ME, Conway GA, Hayman CR, Miller C, Petersen LR, Dondero TJ. Human immunodeficiency virus infection in disadvantaged adolescents. Findings from the U.S. Job Corps. *JAMA* 1991;266:2387.
13. Sweeney P, Lindegren ML, Buehler JW, et al. Teenagers at risk of human immunodeficiency virus type 1 infection. Results from seroprevalence surveys in the United States. *Arch Pediatr Adolesc Med* 1995;149:521.

14. Valleroy LA, MacKellar DA, Karon JM, et al. HIV infection in disadvantaged out-of-school youth: prevalence for US Job Corps entrants, 1990 through 1996. *J Acquir Immune Defic Syndr Hum Retrovirol* 1998;19:67.

15. Centers for Disease Control and Prevention. National HIV Prevalence Surveys, 1997 Summary. Atlanta, GA: Centers for Disease Control and Prevention; 1998.

16. Stricof RL, Kennedy JT, Nattell TC,et al. HIV seroprevalence in a facility for runaway and homeless adolescents. *Am J Public Health* 1991;81(Suppl 50).

17. Quinn TC, Groseclose SL, Spence M, et al. Evolution of the human immunodeficiency virus epidemic among patients attending sexually transmitted disease clinics: a decade of experience. *J Infect Dis* 1992;165:541.

18. Weinstock H, Dale M, Gwinn M, et al. HIV seroincidence among patients at clinics for sexually transmitted diseases in nine cities in the United States. *J Acquir Immune Defic Syndr* 2002;29:478.

19. Weinstock H, Dale M, Linley L, Gwinn M. Unrecognized HIV infection among patients attending sexually transmitted disease clinics. *Am J Public Health* 2002;92:280.

20. D'Angelo LJ, Getson PR, Luban NL, et al. Human immunodeficiency virus infection in urban adolescents: Can we predict who is at risk? *Pediatrics* 1991;88:982.

21. Weinstock H, Sweeney S, Satten GA, et al. HIV seroincidence and risk factors among patients repeatedly tested for HIV attending sexually transmitted disease clinics in the United States, 1991 to 1996. STD Clinic HIV Seroincidence Study Group. *J Acquir Immune Defic Syndr Hum Retrovirol* 1998;19:506.

22. Seage GR, 3rd, Holte SE, Metzger D, et al. Are U.S. populations appropriate for trials of human immunodeficiency virus vaccine? The HIVNET Vaccine Preparedness Study. *Am J Epidemiol* 2001;153:619.

23. Schwarcz S, Kellogg T, McFarland W, et al. Differences in the temporal trends of HIV seroincidence and seroprevalence among sexually transmitted disease clinic patients, 1989–1998: application of the serologic testing algorithm for recent HIV seroconversion. *Am J Epidemiol* 2001;153:925.

24. Constantine NT, Sill AM, Jack N, et al. Improved classification of recent HIV-1 infection by employing a two-stage sensitive/less-sensitive test strategy. *J Acquir Immune Defic Syndr* 2003; 32:94.

25. Henson C, Laeyendecker O, Horne B, et al. HIV incidence, prevalence, and behavior of inner city indivuals attending the Johns Hopkins Emergency Department. In: 10th Conference on Retroviruses and Opportunistic Infections; 2003 February 11; Boston, MA; 2003.

26. Centers for Disease Control and Prevention. HIV incidence among young men who have sex with men—seven U.S. cities, 1994–2000. *MMWR Morb Mortal Wkly Rep* 2001;50:440.

27. Centers for Disease Control and Prevention. HIV/STD risks in young men who have sex with men who do not disclose their sexual orientation—six U.S. cities, 1994–2000. *MMWR Morb Mortal Wkly Rep* 2003;52:81.

28. Hewitt RG, Parsa N, Gugino L. Women's health. The role of gender in HIV progression. *AIDS Read* 2001;11:29.

29. Wilson CM, Houser J, Partlow C, et al. The REACH (Reaching for Excellence in Adolescent Care and Health) project: study design, methods, and population profile. *J Adolesc Health* 2001;29[Suppl 3]:8.

30. Rogers AS, Futterman DK, Moscicki AB, et al. The REACH Project of the Adolescent Medicine HIV/AIDS Research Network: design, methods, and selected characteristics of participants. *J Adolesc Health* 1998;22:300.

31. Rogers AS. HIV research in American youth. *J Adolesc Health* 2001;29(Suppl 3):1.

32. Vermund SH, Sarr M, Murphy DA, et al. Douching practices among HIV infected and uninfected adolescents in the United States. *J Adolesc Health* 2001;29(Suppl 3):80.

33. Vermund SH, Wilson CM, Rogers AS, Partlow C, Moscicki AB. Sexually transmitted infections among HIV infected and HIV uninfected high-risk youth in the REACH study. Reaching for Excellence in Adolescent Care and Health. *J Adolesc Health* 2001;29(Suppl 3):49.

34. Sturdevant MS, Belzer M, Weissman G, et al. The relationship of unsafe sexual behavior and the characteristics of sexual partners of HIV infected and HIV uninfected adolescent females. *J Adolesc Health* 2001;29(Suppl 3):64.

35. Murphy DA, Durako SJ, Moscicki AB, et al. No change in health risk behaviors over time among HIV infected adolescents in care: role of psychological distress. *J Adolesc Health* 2001;29(Suppl 3):57.

36. Levin L, Henry-Reid L, Murphy DA, et al. Incident pregnancy rates in HIV infected and HIV unin-

fected at-risk adolescents. *J Adolesc Health* 2001;29(Suppl 3):101.

37. Schwarz DF, Henry-Reid L, Houser J, et al. The association of perceived health, clinical status, and initiation of HAART (highly active antiretroviral therapy) in adolescents. *J Adolesc Health* 2001;29(Suppl 3):115.

38. Wilson CM, Ellenberg JH, Sawyer MK, et al. Serologic response to hepatitis B vaccine in HIV infected and high-risk HIV uninfected adolescents in the REACH cohort. Reaching for Excellence in Adolescent Care and Health. *J Adolesc Health* 2001;29(Suppl 3):123.

39. Moscicki AB, Ma Y, Holland C, et al. Cervical ectopy in adolescent girls with and without human immunodeficiency virus infection. *J Infect Dis* 2001;183:865.

40. Nicolosi A, Correa Leite ML, Musicco M, et al. The efficiency of male-to-female and female-to-male sexual transmission of the human immunodeficiency virus: a study of 730 stable couples. Italian Study Group on HIV Heterosexual Transmission. *Epidemiology* 1994;5:570.

41. Plourde PJ, Pepin J, Agoki E, et al. Human immunodeficiency virus type 1 seroconversion in women with genital ulcers. *J Infect Dis* 1994;170:313.

42. Peterman TA, Stoneburner RL, Allen JR, et al. Risk of human immunodeficiency virus transmission from heterosexual adults with transfusion-associated infections. *JAMA* 1988;259:55.

43. Quinn TC, Wawer MJ, Sewankambo N, et al. Viral load and heterosexual transmission of human immunodeficiency virus type 1. Rakai Project Study Group. *N Engl J Med* 2000;342:921.

44. Plummer FA, Simonsen JN, Cameron DW, et al. Cofactors in male-female sexual transmission of human immunodeficiency virus type 1. *J Infect Dis* 1991;163:233.

45. Anderson J, ed. A Guide to the Clinical Care of Women with HIV. Rockville, MD: HIV/AIDS Bureau, Health Resources and Services Administration; 2001.

46. Coombs RW, Reichelderfer PS, Landay AL. Recent observations on HIV type-1 infection in the genital tract of men and women. *AIDS* 2003;17:455.

47. Cummins JE, Jr., Villanueva JM, Evans-Strickfaden T, et al. Detection of infectious human immunodeficiency virus type 1 in female genital secretions by a short-term culture method. *J Clin Microbiol* 2003;41:4081.

48. Schacker T, Collier AC, Hughes J, et al. Clinical and epidemiologic features of primary HIV infection. *Ann Intern Med* 1996;125:257.

49. Centers for Disease Control and Prevention. Guidelines for national human immunodeficiency virus case surveillance, including monitoring for human immunodeficiency virus infection and acquired immunodeficiency syndrome. *MMWR* 1999;48(RR-13):1.

50. Mellors J W, Muñoz A, Gigorgi J V, et al. Plasma viral load and CD+ lymphocytes as prognostic markers of HIV-1 infection. *Ann Intern Med* 1997;126:946.

51. Kahn J, Hillard P. Tips for Clinicians: Cervical cytology screening and management of abnormal cytology in adolescent girls. *J Pediatr Adolesc Gynecol* 2003;16:167.

52. Maiman M, Fruchter RG, Guy L, et al. Human immunodeficiency virus infection and invasive cervical carcinoma. *Cancer* 1993;71:402.

53. Maiman M. Management of cervical neoplasia in human immunodeficiency virus-infected women. *J Natl Cancer Inst Monogr* 1998:43.

54. Moscicki AB, Ellenberg JH, Farhat S, et al. Persistence of human papillomavirus infection in HIV-infected and -uninfected adolescent girls: risk factors and differences, by phylogenetic type. *J Infect Dis* 2004;190:37.

55. Mandelblatt JS, Fahs M, Garibaldi K, et al. Association between HIV infection and cervical neoplasia: implications for clinical care of women at risk for both conditions. *AIDS* 1992;6:173.

56. Moscicki AB, Durako SJ, Ma Y, et al. Utility of cervicography in HIV-infected and uninfected adolescents. *J Adolesc Health* 2003;32:204.

57. Barbosa C, Macasaet M, Brockmann S, et al. Pelvic inflammatory disease and human immunodeficiency virus infection. *Obstet Gynecol* 1997;89:65.

58. Centers for Disease Control and Prevention. Sexually Transmitted Disease Treatment Guidelines 2002. *MMWR* 2002;51(RR-6).

59. Recommendations of the Work Group: AIDS testing and epidemiology for youth. *J Adolesc Health Care* 1989.;10(3s).

60. Centers for Disease Control and Prevention. Revised Guidelines for HIV counseling, testing, and referral and revised recommendations for HIV screening of pregnant women. *MMWR Morb Mortal Wkly Rep* 2001;50(RR-19):1.

61. Futterman D, Hein K, Kunins H. Teens and AIDS: identifying and testing those at risk. *Contemp*

Pediatr 1993:68.

62. Centers for Disease Control and Prevention. Routinely recommended HIV testing at an urban urgent-care clinic—Atlanta, Georgia, 2000. *MMWR Morb Mortal Wkly Rep* 2001;50:538.

63. Rotheram-Borus MJ, Futterman D. Promoting early detection of human immunodeficiency virus infection among adolescents. *Arch Pediatr Adolesc Med* 2000;154:435.

64. Centers for Disease Control and Prevention. Incorporating HIV prevention into the medical care of persons living with HIV. *MMWR Morb Mortal Wkly Rep* 2003;52(RR-12):1.

65. Centers for Disease Control and Prevention. Advancing HIV prevention: New strategies for a changing epidemic. *MMWR Morb Mortal Wkly Rep* 2003;52:329.

66. Centers for Disease Control and Prevention. US Public Health Service recommendations for human immunodeficiency virus counseling and voluntary testing for pregnant women. *MMWR Morb Mortal Wkly Rep* 1995;44(RR-1).

67. Reducing the Odds: Preventing perinatal transmission of HIV in the United States. Washington, DC: Institute of Medicine: National Research Council; 1999.

68. Charbonneau TT, Wade NA, Weiner L, et al. Vertical transmission of HIV in New York State: A basis for statewide testing of newborns. Aids Patient Care STDS 1997;11:227.

69. Goodman E, Tipton AC, Hecht L, Chesney MA. Perseverance pays off: health care providers' impact on HIV testing decisions by adolescent females. *Pediatrics* 1994;94(6 Pt 1):878.

70. Murphy DA, Mitchell R, Vermund SH, et al. Factors associated with HIV testing among HIV-positive and HIV-negative high-risk adolescents: the REACH Study. Reaching for Excellence in Adolescent Care and Health. *Pediatrics* 2002;110:e36.

71. Gallo D, George JR, Fitchen JH, et al. Evaluation of a system using oral mucosal transudate for HIV-1 antibody screening and confirmatory testing. OraSure HIV Clinical Trials Group. *JAMA* 1997; 277:254.

72. Centers for Disease Control and Prevention. Notice to Readers: Approval of a new rapid test for HIV antibody. *MMWR Morb Mortal Wkly Rep* 2002;51:1051.

73. Counseling Protocols and Counseling Prompt Cards. 2002. (Accessed September 21, 2003, at http://www.cdc.gov/hiv/projects/respect-2/counseling.htm)

74. ACTS (Assess, Counsel/consent, Test, Support): A Reality-based rapid HIV counseling and testing system. 2003. (Accessed October 1, 2003, at www.adolescentaids.org)

75. Centers for Disease Control and Prevention. Zidovudine for the prevention of HIV transmission from mother to infant. *MMWR Morb Mortal Wkly Rep* 1994;43:285.

76. Cohen MH, Olszewski Y, Branson B, et al. Using point-of-care testing to make rapid HIV-1 tests in labor really rapid. *AIDS* 2003;17:2121.

77. Centers for Disease Control and Prevention. Rapid point-of-care testing for HIV-1 during labor and delivery—Chicago, Illinois, 2002. *MMWR Morb Mortal Wkly Rep* 2003;52:866.

78. Perinatal HIV Guidelines Working Group. Public Health Service Task Force Recommendations for use of antiretroviral drugs in pregnant HIV-1 infected women for maternal health and Interventions to reduce perinatal HIV-1 transmission in the United States. 2004 June 23.

79. Feinberg J, Maenza J. Primary medical care. In: Anderson J, ed. *A guide to the clinical care of women with HIV*. Rockville, MD: HIV/AIDS Bureau, HRSA; 2001:77.

80. Samples CL, Goodman E, Woods ER. Epidemiology and medical management of adolescents. In: Pizzo PA, Wilfert CM, eds. *Pediatric AIDS: The challenge of HIV infection in infants, children and adolescents.* 3rd ed. Baltimore, MD: Lipincott Williams & Wilkins; 1998:615.

81. Anderson JA. HIV and Reproduction. In: Anderson JA, ed. A guide to the clinical care of women with HIV. Rockville, MD: HIV/AIDS Bureau, HRSA, 2001:213.

82. Carpenter CCJ, Fischl MA, Hammer SM, et al. Antiretroviral therapy for HIV infection in 1996: Recommendations of an international panel. *JAMA* 1996;276:146.

83. Centers for Disease Control and Prevention. Pregnancy in Perinatally HIV-infected Adolescents and Young Adults—Puerto Rico, 2002. *MMWR Morb Mortal Wkly Rep* 2003;52:149.

84. Al-Khan A, Colon J, Palta V, Bardeguez A. Assisted reproductive technology for men and women infected with human immunodeficiency virus type 1. *Clin Infect Dis* 2003;36:195.

85. Centers for Disease Control and Prevention. Updated U.S. Public Health Service Guidelines for the Management of Occupational Exposures to HBV, HCV, and HIV and Recommendations for Post-exposure Prophylaxis. *MMWR Morb Mortal Wkly Rep* 2001;50(RR-11).

86. Centers for Disease Control and Prevention. Management of possible sexual, injecting-drug-use, or other nonoccupational exposure to HIV, including considerations related to antiretroviral therapy: Public Health Service Statement. *MMWR Morb Mortal Wkly Rep* 1998;47(RR-17).

87. Olshen E, Samples CL. Postexposure prophylaxis: an intervention to prevent human immunodeficiency virus infection in adolescents. *Curr Opin Pediatr* 2003;15:379.
88. Centers for Disease Control and Prevention. Report of the NIH panel to define principles of therapy in HIV infection. *MMWR Morb Mortal Wkly Rep* 1998;47(RR-5):1.
89. Panel on Clinical Practices for Treatment of HIV Infection. Guidelines for the use of antiretroviral agents in HIV-1-infected adults and adolescents. Rockville, MD: Department of Health and Human Services; 2004 March 23.
90. Working Group on Antiretroviral therapy and medical management of HIV-infected children. Guidelines for the use of antiretroviral agents in Pediatric HIV infection. Rockville, MD: Department of Health and Human Services; 2004 January 20.
91. Rogers AS, Miller S, Murphy DA, Tanney M, Fortune T. The TREAT (Therapeutic Regimens Enhancing Adherence in Teens) program: theory and preliminary results. *J Adolesc Health* 2001;29(Suppl 3):30.
92. 2001 Guidelines for the prevention of opportunistic infections for persons infected with human immunodeficiency virus. 2001. (Accessed October 4, 2003, at http://aidsinfo.nih.gov/guidelines/)
93. Centers for Disease Control and Prevention. 1997 USPHS/IDSA Guidelines for the prevention of opportunistic infections in persons infected with human immunodeficiency virus. *MMWR Recomm Rep* 1997;46(R-12):1.
94. DiClemente RJ, ed. *Adolescents and AIDS, a generation in jeopardy.* 1st ed: Thousand Oaks, CA: Sage Publications Inc, 1992.
95. DiClemente RJ, Crosby RA, Wingood GM. Enhancing STD/HIV prevention among adolescents: the importance of parental monitoring. *Minerva Pediatr* 2002;54:171.
96. Santelli JS, Rosenfeld WD, DuRant RH, et al. Guidelines for adolescent health research: a position paper of the society for adolescent medicine. *J Adolesc Health* 1995;17:270.
97. English A. Guidelines for adolescent health research: legal perspectives. *J Adolesc Health* 1995;17:277.
98. Woods ER. Overview of the Special Projects of National Significance Program's 10 models of adolescent HIV care. *J Adolesc Health* 1998;23(Suppl 2):5.
99. Bell DN, Martinez J, Botwinick G, et al. Case finding for HIV-positive youth: a special type of hidden population. *J Adolesc Health* 2003;33(Suppl 2):10.
100. Johnson RL, Martinez J, Botwinick G, et al. Introduction: what youth need—adapting HIV care models to meet the lifestyles and special needs of adolescents and young adults. *J Adolesc Health* 2003;33(Suppl 2):4.
101. Dodds S, Blakley T, Lizzotte JM, et al. Retention, adherence, and compliance: special needs of HIV-infected adolescent girls and young women. *J Adolesc Health* 2003;33(Suppl 2):39.
102. Johnson RL, Botwinick G, Sell RL, et al. The utilization of treatment and case management services by HIV-infected youth. *J Adolesc Health* 2003;33(Suppl 2):31.

17

Human Papillomavirus Infection in Children and Adolescents

Jessica A. Kahn and Paula A. Hillard

BACKGROUND AND TERMINOLOGY

Human papillomavirus (HPV) infection is highly prevalent in sexually active adolescent and young adult women (1) and may be transmitted vertically from mother to infant. Although infection frequently is asymptomatic, it may be associated with serious sequelae. Infants exposed to HPV in utero or during delivery may develop recurrent respiratory papillomatosis, or warts in the upper respiratory tract (2). Children may develop condylomata acuminata (genital warts) through vertical transmission, sexual abuse, or close contact with a caregiver (3,4). In adolescent and adult women, HPV infection may cause condylomata acuminata, cervical dysplasia, and cervical carcinoma. The Papanicolaou test and other cytologic testing methods are used to screen cervical epithelial cells for evidence of cervical dysplasia, which is diagnosed histologically. Epithelial cell abnormalities found on cervical cytology that may indicate cervical dysplasia include atypical squamous cells of undetermined significance (ASC-US), atypical squamous cells cannot exclude high-grade squamous intraepithelial lesion (ASC-H), low-grade squamous intraepithelial lesion (LSIL), and high-grade squamous intraepithelial lesion (HSIL) (5). Cervical dysplasia may be a precursor of carcinoma in situ and invasive cervical carcinoma. Cervical dysplasia is classified as mild cervical intraepithelial neoplasia (or CIN 1), moderate (CIN 2), or severe (CIN 3, which includes carcinoma in situ).

Recent research has provided us with a tremendous amount of new information on the epidemiology and natural history of HPV infection and abnormal cytology (1,6,7), new techniques for cytologic screening and HPV testing (8–10) and strategies for cytologic screening and management of abnormal cytology (11,12) and treatment for genital warts (13). Strategies to prevent HPV infection and its sequelae, such as HPV vaccines, are also under active investigation (14).

BIOLOGY OF HPV INFECTION

Virology and Genetics

Human papillomaviruses are small, circular, double-stranded DNA viruses belonging to the papovavirus family. The virus infects and replicates in basal epithelial cells. The HPV genome is divided into two regions. The long control region (LCR) is noncoding, and contains transcription enhancer genes and promoter elements (15,16). The coding region consists of an early and a late coding region. The early region contains 6 open reading frames that encode for the proteins E1, E2, E4, E5, E6, and E7; these control viral replication, transcription, and cellular transformation. In cancer-associated (high-risk) HPV types, the E6 and E7 proteins interfere with cell cycle control and result in uncontrolled cell proliferation by binding to and inactivating the tumor suppressor gene products p53 and retinoblastoma protein (17). The late region encodes for L1 and L2, which are structural proteins. They self-assemble into the viral capsid, which interacts with a receptor on the target cell, facilitating entry of viral DNA.

HPV Typing

Human papillomaviruses are epitheliotropic, and each type preferentially infects a specific anatomic site. They are divided into cutaneous and mucosal types; the mucosal types are found in the anogenital tract and aerodigestive tract. HPVs are genotyped on the basis of their genetic similarities; different types share less than 90% homology (18). Over 100 different genotypes have been sequenced and classified, at least 30 of which infect the genital tract (18). These genital types have been classified into low risk and high risk based on their association with condylomata and cervical cancer, respectively (Fig. 17-1) (19). Although both types can regress spontaneously, persistent infection with low-risk types is associated with the development of genital warts (condylomata), and persistent HPV infection with high-risk types is associated with the development of cervical dysplasia and cervical cancer. When HPV infection occurs, the low-risk types remain extrachromosomal (episomal); in contrast, the genomes of high-risk types integrate into cellular host DNA in most human cervical carcinomas. High-risk HPV DNA, mRNA, and proteins are found in the vast majority of cervical dysplastic lesions and carcinomas and HPV is found in 99.7% of cervical cancer tissues (20,21); thus, high-risk HPV types are generally accepted as the etiologic agents of cervical cancer. Other anogenital cancers, oropharyngeal and tongue cancers, and a proportion of esophageal cancers have also been shown to be associated with HPV infection (22,23).

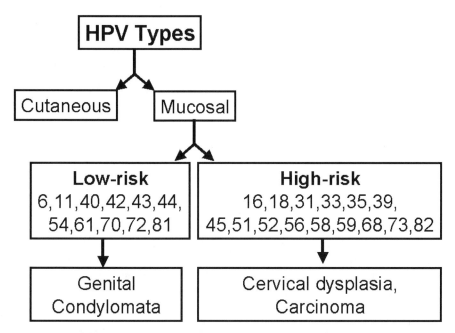

FIG. 17-1. Human papillomavirus (HPV) types.

EPIDEMIOLOGY AND NATURAL HISTORY OF HPV INFECTION

HPV in Children

HPV in children may be acquired perinatally or through sexual abuse (24–26). Other modes of transmission, including autoinoculation, heteroinoculation, and indirect transmission via fomites remain possible but controversial (27). Studies have demonstrated the presence of asymptomatic HPV on the skin of 50% to 70% of normal healthy infants from 1 to 4 months of age (28), and HPV has been found within the oral cavities of infants without disease (29,30). Sequelae of vertically transmitted HPV infection in infants are uncommon, but include respiratory papillomas and vulvar and anal condylomata. Development of vulvar condylomata due to vertical HPV transmission is rare after age three and should raise concern for sexual abuse (24). The risk of developing subsequent cervical, vulvar, or vaginal intraepithelial neoplasia after perinatal acquisition or sexual abuse is not known, although high-risk types have been shown to persist in some children (31). (See Fig. 3-1).

Recurrent respiratory papillomatosis (RRP) is a rare outcome of vertical transmission of HPV from mother to newborn, and is usually caused by HPV types 6 and 11 (32,33). Armstrong and colleagues estimated that there were 80 to 1,500 incident cases and 700–3,000 prevalent cases of RRP in the United States in 1999 (34). RRP is characterized by recurring papillomas in the upper respiratory tract, usually the larynx, and is most commonly diagnosed in children 2 to 3 years of age (Fig. 17-2) (2). Although RRP is rare, it may be associated with high morbidity in some children (35). For example, papillomas often recur, requiring repeated resections (2,34), which may cause chronic inflammation and vocal cord damage (2). RRP may be life-threatening if papillomas obstruct the airway.

HPV in Adolescents

HPV Infection

HPV infection is highly prevalent in the United States. Koutsky has estimated that 10% to 20% of 15- to 49-year-old men and women have molecular evidence of genital HPV infection (36). The data in Fig. 17-3, adapted from her reported results, demonstrate that 60% of men and women in this age group (approximately 81 million) have been infected by HPV previously, as evidenced by antibody positivity, and 15% are currently infected. Of the 15% who are currently infected, 10% (14 million)

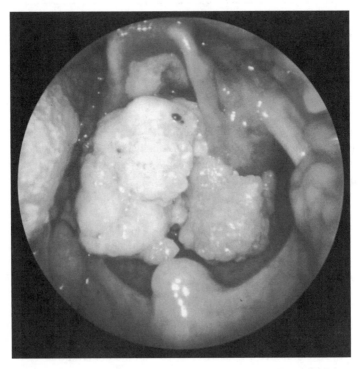

FIG. 17-2. Respiratory papillomas. (Photograph courtesy of Michael Rutter, M.D.)

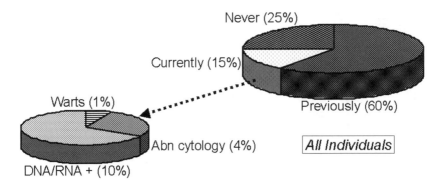

FIG. 17-3. Prevalence of genital human papillomavirus infection in the US population aged 15 to 49 years. (Adapted from Koutsky LA, Galloway DA, Holmes KK. Epidemiology of genital human papillomavirus infection. *Epidemiol Rev* 1988;10:122; with permission)

have subclinical infection and are positive for HPV DNA or RNA only, 4% (5 million) have abnormal cytology or colposcopy, and 1% (1.4 million) have genital warts (6,36). Figure 17-4 shows HPV prevalence by age as detected by polymerase chain reaction (PCR). The data are from a study of over 4000 women attending Planned Parenthood clinics in Washington State, and demonstrate that the prevalence rate is highest in women 18 to 24 years of age and then declines with age (37). There are few data on the prevalence of genital HPV infection in U.S. adolescents. Those studies which used sensitive tests for detection of multiple HPV DNA types demonstrate that the prevalence of HPV DNA in sexually active adolescent and young adult women appears to be in the range of 30% to 50% (1,38–40). Approximately 40% to 80% of the women in those studies who are HPV DNA positive had high-risk HPV types. Although the rates, types, and proportion of high-risk types are likely to vary depending on the population tested, these data demonstrate that HPV may be the most common sexually transmitted infection among U.S. adolescents.

Little was known about the natural history of HPV infection in adolescents until Moscicki and colleagues reported the results of a longitudinal cohort study of 618 HPV-positive young women 13 to 21 years of age (7). Participants were followed every 4 months with cytology, colposcopy, and HPV DNA testing. The investigators found that regression rates of HPV in these young women, defined as having at least three negative tests for HPV DNA by 30 months of follow-up, were high, particularly for those with low-risk HPV types. The regression rate for participants with low-risk HPV types was 90%, and for participants with high-risk HPV types was 75%. Of the young women who were HPV-positive at baseline or during a follow-up visit, only 22% developed LSIL over a median follow-up period of approximately 60 months (41). Those who had high-risk HPV types were at increased risk for developing high-

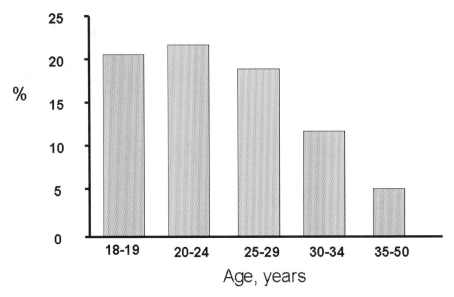

FIG. 17-4. Human papillomavirus DNA positivity by age. (Adapted from Kulasingam SL, Hughes JP, Kiviat NB, et al. Evaluation of human papillomavirus testing in primary screening for cervical abnormalities: comparison of sensitivity, specificity, and frequency of referral. *JAMA* 2002; 288:1749; with permission.)

grade squamous intraepithelial lesion (HSIL): the odds of developing HSIL for young women testing positive for high-risk HPV at more than or equal to three of four preceding visits were 14.1 compared to those who were negative for high-risk HPV (7). However, 88% of those subjects persistently positive for high-risk HPV for at least 1 year did not develop HSIL during the study period. The authors suggest that cofactors or more prolonged infection may be important in the development of HSIL.

A number of other studies similarly have demonstrated that persistence of high-risk HPV infection is associated with development of cervical dysplasia. Burk and colleagues conducted a longitudinal cohort study of HPV infection in college women and examined the risk of developing SIL in those with HPV infection at a previous and current visit (1). The investigators reported that the relative risk for developing SIL was 20.9% for participants who were HPV positive at both a previous and a current visit, regardless of whether these were the same types, compared to those who were HPV negative at either visit. The relative risk was higher if they had a high-risk type at the current visit (22.2%) than a low-risk type at the current visit (9.6%). Participants who were positive for high-risk HPV at both visits and had the *same* HPV type at both visits were at the highest risk for SIL (relative risk 37.2%). Results of studies in adult women similarly demonstrate that the highest risk for development of SIL is found in women with persistent high-risk HPV types, particularly with the same high-risk type (42,43).

Condylomata Acuminata

Condylomata acuminata, or genital warts, are a common clinical manifestation of genital HPV infection. The prevalence rate of symptomatic external genital warts in the general population is approximately 1% (36), though rates are likely to be higher in young women because HPV prevalence declines with age (37). Genital warts may resolve spontaneously without treatment, likely due to acquired cellular immune responses (13,44); some investigators report up to a 40% spontaneous resolution rate in those participating in treatment trials for genital warts who were treated with placebo agents (13,44). A higher wart burden at presentation is associated with longer time to clearance (45).

Abnormal Cytology

In adult women, the prevalence rates of ASC-US and LSIL mirror rates of HPV infection: rates are highest in 20 to 24 year-old women and decline with age (Fig. 17-5) (37). This is consistent with the hypothesis that LSIL in particular is thought to

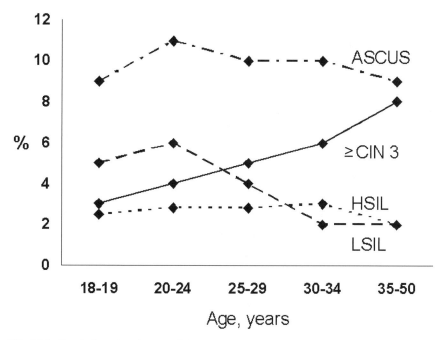

FIG. 17-5. Cervical cytology by age. (Adapted from Kulasingam SL, Hughes JP, Kiviat NB, et al. Evaluation of human papillomavirus testing in primary screening for cervical abnormalities: comparison of sensitivity, specificity, and frequency of referral. *JAMA* 2002;288:1749; with permission.)

represent active replication of HPV. The prevalence of HSIL rises slightly in 20- to 24-year-olds compared with 18 to 19 year-olds, but then remains fairly steady until age 35, when rates decline again. In contrast, the prevalence of CIN 3 or more severe abnormalities rises with age: this is consistent with the natural history of CIN.

There are few studies available that examine the prevalence of abnormal cytology in adolescents. In general, these studies demonstrate that although the prevalence of abnormal cytology is high in many adolescents, likely because of the high prevalence of HPV infection in this age group, relatively few have HSIL. Sadeghi and colleagues reviewed almost 200,000 Papanicolaou tests in the United States in the early 1980s. The investigators reported that 2% of smears were positive for CIN 1 or 2 and 0.1% were positive for CIN 3 (46). More recent studies involve fewer participants, but demonstrate higher rates of abnormal cytology (Table 17-1). Rates of ASC-US range from 4% to 13%, LSIL from 3% to 9%, and HSIL from 1% to 3% (47–50).

Data on the natural history of LSIL in adolescents have recently become available. Moscicki and colleagues reported that of all participants with LSIL in a longitudinal study, the regression rate after 3 years was very high—95% (51). This finding is in contrast to adult women, in whom only 50% to 80% of LSIL will regress. In the same study sample, the regression rate of LSIL in those with high-risk HPV was 80%, while only 6% progressed. The future risk of developing HSIL in adolescents with normal cytology at baseline was also low, even in those with high-risk HPV. The risk of developing HSIL within three years was 54% and in those with a low-risk type, was zero. Even in those with a high-risk type, the risk of developing HSIL was still only 3.2% (Barbara Moscicki, personal communication).

Finally, the progression of SIL generally takes several years and cervical carcinoma is exceedingly rare in adolescents. Nasiell reported that time from CIN 2 to CIS or carcinoma for women 25 years of age or younger was 54 to 60 months (52). Surveillance, Epidemiology and End Results (SEER) data from 1995 to 1999 demonstrated that the

TABLE 17-1. *Prevalence of abnormal cervical cytology in adolescents*

Author	Number of participants	Study population	% CIN 1-2		CIN 3
Sadeghi (46)	194,069	National sample in United States	2		0.1
			ASCUS	LSIL	HSIL
Mangan (47)	871	Outpatient department of urban public hospital	4	8	
Mount (48)	10,296	Vermont	10	3	1
Edelman (49)	271	Urban, hospital-based clinics in New York	12	9	1
Kahn (50)	490	Hospital-based clinic in Boston	13	9	3

incidence of cervical cancer was 0 per 100,000 women in the 10- to 19-year-old age group, and only 1.7 per 100,000 women in the 20- to 24-year-old age group (53).

EVALUATION AND MANAGEMENT OF HPV INFECTION

Evaluation and Management of HPV Infection in Children

Children who develop vulvar and genital condylomata that first appear after age three should be evaluated carefully for sexual abuse; sexual transmission of HPV should be considered even in younger children although perinatal and postnatal acquisition or autoinoculation are possible (3,26,54–56). Clinicians may wish to refer children who need treatment for condylomata to a specialist in pediatric and adolescent gynecology or pediatric dermatology. Treatment options depend on the child's symptoms, the extent of disease, and the clinician's experience in the use of topical and ablative therapies such as laser. Options include laser ablation therapy, surgical excision, imiquimod, trichloroacetic acid (TCA) 80% to 90% or bichloroacetic acid (BCA) 80% to 90%. The latter two are not always well tolerated in children. Some gynecologists obtain a biopsy for HPV typing at the time of laser ablation.

Children with RRP should be referred to an otorhinolaryngologist experienced in the surgical treatment of respiratory papillomas. Given the relatively high prevalence of vulvar condylomata and the rare occurrence of respiratory papillomatosis, cesarean delivery is thought to play only a very limited role and is not routinely indicated to prevent respiratory papillomatosis (57,58).

Risk factors for HPV in Adolescents

A number of recent studies have identified risk factors for HPV infection.

Behavioral risk factors include early age of first sexual intercourse, number of lifetime male sexual partners, partner's number of sexual partners, older age of male sexual partner, and cigarette use (39,59,60). Risk factors for incident LSIL include HPV infection and cigarette smoking (41). The efficacy of condoms in preventing HPV infection and its sequelae is more controversial. A recent meta-analysis demonstrated that condom use does not appear to reduce the risk of becoming HPV DNA-positive, but decreases the risk of genital warts, CIN 2/3, and invasive cervical carcinoma (61).

The primary *biological* risk factor for HPV infection is immunosuppression; for example, as a result of organ transplantation or HIV infection (62–64). Young women who have impaired host immune responses due to T-cell deficiency or T-cell dysfunction are at highest risk. Other biological risk factors specific to adolescence have been proposed. For example, compared to adults, adolescents have a relatively large area of cervical ectopy; those columnar and metaplastic cells may be particularly vulnerable to infection with sexually transmitted infections such as HPV (65–70). In addition, the adolescent cervix may be especially susceptible to minor trauma during sexual intercourse. Finally, preliminary data suggest that genital mucosal immunity may differ between adolescents and adults (71). *Sociodemographic* risk markers for HPV infection that have been identified to date are black and Hispanic race and having a black or Hispanic partner (1,59).

Evaluation of HPV in Adolescents

Condylomata

Anogenital condylomata, also referred to as condylomata acuminata or genital warts, are most commonly found on the vulva, perineum, perianal area, vagina or cervix in women (Fig. 17-6). Most are caused by types 6 and 11, and represent a be-

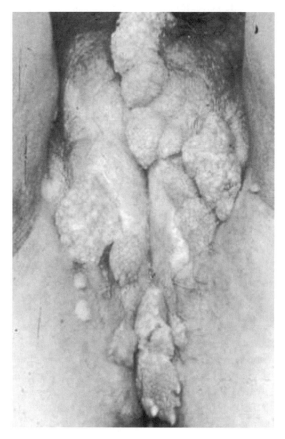

FIG. 17-6. Vulvar condylomata.

nign proliferation of cells. However, they may be a marker for possible exposure to high-risk HPV types or preneoplastic lesions of the cervix. HPV types 16, 18, 21, 33, and 35 occasionally are found in condylomata and have been associated with squamous vulvar intraepithelial neoplasia (VIN). Genital warts may present as single or multiple lesions; if multiple they may be clustered or plaquelike. They may be flat, cauliflower-shaped, dome-shaped, keratotic, or pedunculated. Diagnosis typically is based on clinical appearance using direct visual inspection with bright light and magnification if needed (13). The differential diagnosis in adolescents includes condyloma latum (syphilis), nevi, molluscum contagiosum, seborrheic keratoses, and high-grade intraepithelial lesions. Biopsy of vulvar and vaginal lesions should be considered if they are atypical or do not respond to treatment (13). Although condylomata often are asymptomatic, they may be uncomfortable or pruritic.

Cervical, Vaginal, and Vulvar Disease

HPV infection with either high-risk or low-risk types can cause abnormal cervical cytology. The traditional Papanicolaou smear and newer methods of examining cervical cytology assess exfoliated cervical cells. Cervical cytology results are classified using the Bethesda system, which was updated in 2001 to incorporate recent data about the natural history of HPV infection and CIN and make results more highly reproducible (5) (Table 17-2). The Bethesda system classifies epithelial cell abnormalities as ASC-US, ASC-H, LSIL, and HSIL. LSIL corresponds to the histologic diagnosis of CIN 1, and HSIL to the diagnoses of CIN 2, CIN 3, or carcinoma in situ. Figure 17-7 demonstrates cytology consistent with HSIL.

HPV infection of the vulva and vagina may lead to condylomata or dysplasia. Dysplastic lesions include VIN and vaginal intraepithelial neoplasia (VAIN), which occur uncommonly in adolescents (72–74). Vulvar dysplastic lesions (VIN) tend to be multifocal and have a variable appearance. Lesions may not be visible without application of acetic acid; if they are visible, lesions may appear as small papules, sessile lesions, or plaques and often have a keratinized, rough surface that may be pigmented or discolored (72). Lesions are usually asymptomatic, but may cause vulvar itching or irritation. Although VAIN is uncommon even in adults, the frequency of diagnosis is increasing, particularly in young women. Lesions are most commonly located in the upper third of the vagina and are often multifocal (75,76).

Limitations to Screening

Although cervical cytologic screening has been highly successful in reducing rates of cervical cancer worldwide, there are limitations to its use. General limitations to the traditional Papanicolaou (Pap) test include errors in sampling, slide preparation, and interpretation of results (77). A systematic review of the accuracy of cytology demonstrated that sensitivity for detecting abnormalities at least as severe as LSIL was relatively low, ranging from 30% to 87% (mean 47%), while the specificity was higher, ranging from 86% to 100% (mean 95%) (78). Some limitations are specific to adolescents; for example, the requirement for a speculum examination may discourage adolescents from seeking gynecologic services, because many find the examination to be painful or embarrassing (79,80). Another drawback to cytologic screening is the relatively low rate of adherence to screening and follow-up appointments in adolescents (81,82). Adherence is a critical factor in decreasing the incidence and mortality of cervical cancer among screened women (83); however, only 12 to 45% of sexually active adolescent girls have obtained Pap test screening (84–86). Although intentions to return for screening and follow-up are high in adolescents (50), many do not return for follow-up procedures (82). Poor compliance may be due to inadequate knowledge about HPV infection, lack of awareness of recommendations for cervical cancer screening, and attitudes about Pap screening and follow-up (82,87). An additional limitation of screening cytology in adolescents is the high rate of regression of LSIL. Adolescents with mildly abnormal cytology may

TABLE 17-2. *2001 Bethesda System Classification (adapted).*[a]

Specimen adequacy
  Satisfactory for evaluation
  Unsatisfactory for evaluation (specify reason)
General categorization (optional)
  Negative for intraepithelial lesion or malignancy
  Epithelial cell abnormality
  Other
Interpretation/result
Negative for intraepithelial lesion or malignancy
  Organisms (including *Trichomonas vaginalis*, fungal organisms consistent with *Candida* species, shift in flora suggestive of bacterial vaginosis, cellular changes consistent with herpes simplex virus)
  Other nonneoplastic findings (including reactive cellular changes associated with inflammation)
Epithelial cell abnormalities
Squamous cell
  Atypical squamous cells (ASC) of undetermined significance (ASC-US), cannot exclude high-grade SIL (ASC-H)
  Low-grade squamous intraepithelial lesion (LSIL) encompassing HPV, mild dysplasia, and cervical intraepithelial neoplasia (CIN 1)
  High-grade squamous intraepithelial lesion (HSIL) encompassing moderate and severe dysplasia, carcinoma *in situ*, CIN 2 and CIN 3
  Squamous cell carcinoma
Glandular cell
  Atypical glandular cells (AGC)
  Atypical glandular cells, favor neoplastic
  Endocervical adenocarcinoma *in situ* (AIS)
Other
Automated review and ancillary testing
Educational notes and suggestions (optional)

[a]From Kahn JA, Hillard PJ. Cervical cytology screening and management of abnormal cytology in adolescent girls. *J Pediatr Adolesc Gynecol* 2003;16:167, with permission. Copyright, North American Society Pediatric and Adolescent Gynecology.

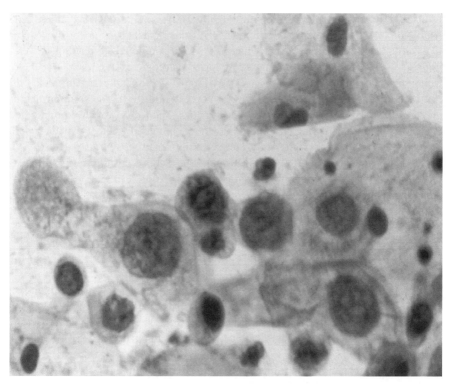

FIG. 17-7. Exfoliated cervical cells. Normal cervical cells are located at the top right, and cells with nuclear abnormalities typical of HPV infection and severe dysplasia, such as koilocytotic atypia, dyskeratosis, and multinucleation, are located in the center.

undergo procedures such as colposcopy for lesions that would likely have regressed spontaneously. New guidelines for cervical cancer screening, which will be described below, address many of these limitations (12).

New Technologies: Cervical Cytologic Screening and Cervicography

In response to the limitations of the traditional Papanicolaou test, new technologies for cytologic screening have been introduced. The Food and Drug Administration (FDA) has approved several new methods for liquid-based cytologic screening that are being used with increasing frequency in clinical practice. The ThinPrep 2000 (Cytyc-Sands, Boxborough, MA) and the Sure Path test (TriPath Imaging, Burlington, NC) are liquid-based slide preparation systems that filter out noncellular debris and blood and then deposit cells in a thin layer on a slide, thus preventing mucus or blood from obscuring visualization of cells. They have been shown to increase the sensitivity of screening in many, but not all, studies (8, 88). The supernatant can also be used to test for sexually transmitted infections, including HPV DNA. The AutoPap 300 QC (NeoPath Inc, Redmond, WA) and Papnet (Neuromedical Systems Inc, Suffern, NY) utilize automated microscopy and computerized reading of slides in order to detect abnormalities missed on initial cytologic examination. These two techniques may increase the sensitivity of cytologic screening, but at additional cost (89). Another technique, cervicography, involves taking a high-resolution photograph of the cervix after application of acetic acid. The film is reviewed by trained evaluators (National Testing Laboratories), who recommend whether women should be evaluated further. Cervicography increases the sensitivity of CIN detection in some studies, but the increased cost and high rate of false-positive results limit its utility (90,91). National organizations, including the American Cancer Society and American College of Obstetrics and Gynecology, have concluded that traditional Pap tests remain an acceptable screening technique. Guidelines for screening intervals differ depending on screening technique (11,12).

HPV Testing

Testing for HPV DNA has been developed in response to the importance of high-risk HPV infection in the development of cervical dysplasia. HPV infection is measured most sensitively by DNA-based testing, and results are highly reproducible. Currently, the only commercially available test is the Hybrid Capture II (Digene Corporation, Beltsville, MD), which can be performed on a liquid-based cytology specimen or co-collected at the screening visit using a swab. The Hybrid Capture II test identifies samples positive for high-risk HPV types but does not identify individual genotypes.

Recent evidence suggests that HPV DNA testing has the potential to be used as a test to augment cervical cytologic screening because of its high sensitivity and reasonable specificity in detecting high-grade lesions in women with ASC-US cytology (92–98). Data from six recent studies examining the utility of HPV testing to augment ASC-US cytology demonstrated that the sensitivity of HPV DNA testing for detection of high-grade lesions (83% to 100%) is higher than that of repeat cytology (67% to 85%) (93,99–103). In addition, HPV testing may spare women with abnormal results an additional clinical examination for repeat cytology and the anxiety of waiting for a repeat result. Results of a recent large, randomized trial demonstrated that HPV testing to augment ASC-US cytology was as sensitive as a strategy of immediate colposcopy in detecting HSIL while decreasing substantially the number of women referred for colposcopy (98). HPV testing may also decrease risk of loss to follow-up, because repeat cytology is not needed, and may be more cost-effective than repeat cytology, because it decreases the expense of repeated testing and office visits (104,105).

HPV testing also may be useful as a primary screen for dysplasia in adult women (37,106–109). A recent study examined the utility of HPV testing as a primary screen for CIN 3 or higher, comparing HPV testing to strategies involving cytology alone and cytology plus HPV testing (37). If a thin-layer Pap test was used alone, and the result was LSIL or more severe or was ASC-US with a repeat result of at least as severe as ASC-US, sensitivity for identifying women with CIN 3 or higher was 57% and specificity was 90%. If a thin-layer Papanicolaou test was combined with HPV DNA testing using the Hybrid Capture II method, and the result of the test was LSIL or more severe or was ASC-US with high-risk HPV, the sensitivity was similar (60%), and specificity was also similar (89%). In contrast, the sensitivity of HPV testing alone for identifying women with CIN 3 was higher (91%) while specificity dropped to 73%. In terms of referral for colposcopy, a higher percentage of women screened only with HPV would have been referred for colposcopy (29%) compared to women screened with cytology or a combination of cytology and HPV testing (12% to 13%). The negative predictive value was high for all strategies. Thus, in this study testing for HPV only has significantly higher sensitivity but significantly lower specificity than thin-layer Pap screening, and the authors suggest that it may be a reasonable alternative to cytology-based screening in some settings; for example, in developing countries where screening intervals are long or nonexistent (37).

According to data from several studies including the ASC-US–LSIL Triage Study (ALTS), a randomized multicenter trial designed to compare different management strategies for women with ASC-US or LSIL (107), HPV testing does not appear to be useful in making decisions about triage to colposcopy in those with LSIL cytology because approximately 80% of women with LSIL are positive for high-risk HPV (98).

Although HPV DNA testing may be useful in adult populations, either as an adjunct to ASC-US cytology or as a primary screening tool, the role of HPV testing in adolescents is still undefined. The relatively high rates of HPV infection and regression make it difficult to determine whether adolescents will benefit from HPV testing. Research is needed to examine strategies involving HPV testing in adolescents.

Recommendations for Cytologic Screening and Management of Abnormal Cytology

New information regarding the natural history of HPV infection and cytology in women and the availability of liquid-based cytology and HPV DNA testing have motivated a reassessment of strategies for cervical cancer screening and follow-up of abnormal cytology in women. The American Cancer Society (ACS) recently sponsored a committee to make recommendations regarding cytologic screening. Members of the committee were concerned that practitioners may be initiating cytologic screening too early in adolescents, resulting in the detection of too many lesions that were not clinically significant and would resolve spontaneously. They were also concerned that many of these adolescents were undergoing unnecessary colposcopy and/or destructive procedures. They stated that the goal of cervical screening in the United States is to identify and remove significant precancerous lesions such as HSIL, and to prevent mortality from invasive cancer (12). Because most HPV infections are transient in adolescents, the vast majority of low-grade lesions regress, the risk of HSIL is low even in those adolescents with high-risk HPV types, and low-grade lesions take several years to progress to high-grade dysplasia, the committee concluded that there is little risk of missing a high-grade cervical lesion until 3 to 5 years after initial exposure to HPV. Therefore, the committee recommended initiating screening approximately 3 years after initiation of sexual intercourse or by age 21, and continuing screening every year thereafter with regular Pap tests or every 2 years with liquid-based Pap tests. The authors noted that adolescents who may not need cervical cytology should still obtain preventive health care, including assessment of health risks, contraception, and prevention counseling, screening, and treatment of sexually transmitted infections. New American College of Obstetricians and Gynecologists (ACOG) recommendations state that while cervical screening should begin approximately 3 years after first vaginal intercourse, clinicians should take into account risk of noncompliance with follow-up, sexual behaviors, and history of sexual abuse in deciding when to initiate screening. In addition, ACOG recommends annual Pap testing in women less than 30 years old. Annual gynecologic visits beginning at approximately age 13 to 15 are suggested in order to address preventive health concerns and to assess gynecologic and sexual history in a confidential setting (110). (See also Chapter 1.)

Revised guidelines for management of abnormal cytology in women recently have been published by the American Society for Colposcopy and Cervical Pathology (ASCCP) (11) and are summarized in Table 17-3. Reflex HPV DNA testing is recommended for women with ASC-US when liquid-based cytology is used, with all women who test positive for high-risk HPV DNA referred for colposcopic evaluation. Colposcopy is recommended for all women with ASC-H, LSIL, and HSIL. An alternative option for adolescents with LSIL is repeat cytologic testing at 6 and 12 months with a threshold of ASC-US for referral for colposcopy, or HPV DNA testing at 12 months with a referral for colposcopy if testing is positive for high-risk HPV DNA.

Based on a review of all available data as well as the ASCCP and ACS guidelines, the following is a proposed strategy for screening cytology and management of abnormal cytology in adolescents (Fig. 17-8). We recommend annual cytologic screening in all sexually active adolescents beginning 3 years after sexual initiation. Screening may begin sooner at the discretion of the provider, after taking into account potential nonadherence to follow-up recommendations, sexual history (for example, number of sexual partners) and medical history. In young women with HIV infection or other immunocompromise, such as those who have had organ transplantation, we recommend earlier initiation of screening and follow-up cytology every 6 months. In those with a history of sexual abuse with penetration, we recommend initial screening when possible by a provider with experience in managing young women with a history of sexual assault, and then yearly follow-up if results are normal. Finally, in those with developmental delay and no history of sexual abuse, we recommend initiation of screening at approximately age 21, then every 2 years if results are normal.

TABLE 17-3. *Summary of 2001 Consensus Guidelines on Management of Abnormal Cytology.[g]*

Result	Recommendation for management

ASC-US[a]	**Preferred approach[b]**
	HPV DNA reflex testing
	 If high-risk HPV positive, then refer to colposcopy.
	  If high-risk HPV positive and colposcopy negative for CIN[c], then either cytology at 6 and 12 months (colposcopy if ASC-US or more severe) or HPV testing at 12 months (colposcopy if high-risk HPV positive).
	  If low-risk HPV positive or negative for HPV, then follow-up cytology in 12 months (refer to colposcopy if ASC-US or more severe).
	Acceptable approaches
	Repeat cytology.
	 Repeat at 4- to 6-month intervals until two consecutive results negative.
	  Refer to colposcopy if ASC-US or more severe
	  Return to annual screening if two consecutive results negative.
	Immediate colposcopy (recommended strategy if immunosuppressed)
	 If colposcopy negative for CIN, cytology in 12 months.

ASC-H[d]	**Preferred approach** Colposcopy If no lesion is identified, then review cytology, colposcopy, and histology results. If ASC-H diagnosis upheld, then cytology at 6 and 12 months (colposcopy if ASC-US or more severe) or HPV testing at 12 months (colposcopy if high-risk HPV positive) acceptable.
LSIL[e]	**Preferred approach** Colposcopy If biopsy does not confirm CIN and is satisfactory, acceptable options include repeat cytological testing at 6 and 12 months (refer to colposcopy if ASC-US or more severe) or HPV testing at 12 months (colposcopy if high-risk HPV positive). **Acceptable approach (adolescents)** Repeat cytologic testing at 6 and 12 months (colposcopy if ASC-US or more severe) or HPV testing at 12 months (colposcopy if high-risk HPV positive).
HSIL[f]	**Recommended strategy** Colposcopy with endocervical assessment. If no lesion is identified, review cytology, colposcopy, and biopsy results. If cytologic interpretation of HSIL upheld, review is not possible, or biopsy-confirmed CIN 1 identified, a diagnostic excisional procedure recommended (if not pregnant). In young women of reproductive age in whom biopsy-confirmed CIN 2,3 is not identified, may observe with colposcopy and cytology at 4–6 month intervals for 1 year if colposcopy satisfactory, endocervical sampling is negative, and patient accepts risk of occult disease.

[a] Atypical squamous cells of undetermined significance.
[b] When liquid-based cytology is used or when co-collection for HPV DNA testing can be done.
[c] Cervical intraepithelial neoplasia.
[d] Atypical squamous cells; cannot exclude high-grade squamous intraepithelial lesion.
[e] Low-grade squamous intraepithelial lesion.
[f] High-grade squamous intraepithelial lesion.
[g] From: Kahn JA, Hillard PJ. Cervical cytology screening and management of abnormal cytology in adolescent girls. *J Pediatr Adolesc Gynecol* 2003;16:167, with permission. Copyright, North American Society for Pediatric and Adolescent Gynecology.

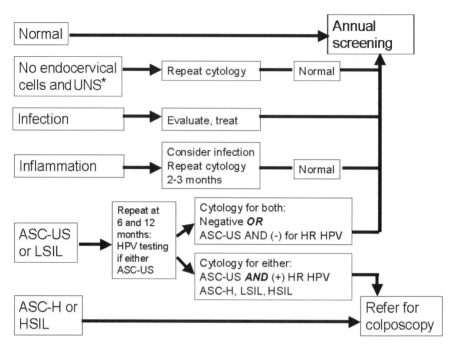

FIG. 17-8. A proposed management strategy for abnormal cytology in adolescents. (From Kahn JA, Hillard PJ. Cervical cytology screening and management of abnormal cytology in adolescent girls. *J Pediatr Adolesc Gynecol* 2003;16:167; reprinted with permission.) Other strategies for ASC-US and LSIL are in Table 17-3. *UNS-unsatisfactory for evaluation.

In healthy adolescents with initial results of ASC-US or LSIL, at Cincinnati Children's Hospital we repeat cytology at 6 and 12 months and perform reflex HPV testing if either result is ASC-US. This approach differs from the ASCCP guidelines, which recommend reflex HPV testing if the initial result is ASC-US and referral to colposcopy if results are positive for high-risk HPV. We modified our approach because of the high rate of regression of mildly abnormal cytology in adolescents. If the repeat tests at 6 and 12 months are negative or results are ASC-US but negative for high-risk HPV, we revert to annual screening. If either repeat cytology result is positive for ASC-US and HPV testing is positive for high-risk HPV, or if either repeat cytology result is ASC-H, LSIL or HSIL, we refer to colposcopy. If the initial cytology results are ASC-H or HSIL, we refer to colposcopy. Other clinicians obtain HPV testing with the first ASC-US results.

Colposcopy

The criteria for referral for colposcopic evaluation are described earlier. Given recent changes in recommendations for adolescent cytologic screening, decisions about whether or not to perform colposcopy in patients who have abnormal cytology, but who would not have even been screened using the new guidelines, are being made on a case-by-case basis.

The evaluation of abnormal cervical cytology in adolescents requires a special approach. Adolescent dysplasia clinics in which young women receive adolescent-specific education, an informed consent process that encourages patient-parent communication, an adolescent-specific approach to the colposcopic evaluation, and careful attention to follow-up care have been described (111). The procedure at our dysplasia clinic involves an educational visit one to two weeks prior to the scheduled colposcopy appointment. At that visit, a gynecologic nurse practitioner provides information about cytology, dysplasia, and colposcopy. Cervical testing for sexually transmitted infections is performed and colposcopy deferred if testing is positive for gonorrhea or Chlamydia. A wet preparation identifies bacterial vaginosis, which is treated prior to colposcopy to minimize risk for subsequent infection after cervical biopsy. A consent for biopsy is obtained with consent from both the adolescent and her parent or guardian if she is younger than 18 years of age at our hospital.

Colposcopy should be explained prior to every step of the procedure, proceeding slowing with the statements: "next you're going to feel me touch the outside of your vagina;" "next I'll be using vinegar to look at the outside area; it will feel cold and may sting a little; if it stings a lot we'll wash it off," etc. The colposcopic evaluation involves examination of the vulva/perineum/perianal area, vagina, and cervix to assess the entire genital area for HPV effects. A 3% to 5% solution of acetic acid (equivalent to common household vinegar) is used to soak the vulvar area. If areas of active inflammation, fissures, or broken epithelium are noted, the exam is typically deferred to allow healing of these areas, as the vinegar solution may cause severe burning.

The colposcope provides 3 to 20 × magnification of the area, which is examined for acetowhite staining and vascular patterns associated with HPV infection and intraepithelial neoplasia (Fig. 17-9). The vulva, vagina and cervix are examined in turn. Abnormal areas of the vulva are noted and biopsied, often after performance of the rest of the exam. A speculum examination (typically using a Graves speculum as opposed to the narrower Pederson speculum) is performed next. Again, acetic acid is sprayed or swabbed into the vagina; the speculum is rotated to allow visualization of the anterior and posterior vaginal walls that are typically obscured by the speculum (Fig. 17-10). Frequently, vaginal acetowhite micropapular projections described as asperities indicate subclinical HPV infection. More abnormal vascular changes suggesting vaginal intraepithelial neoplasia should be noted and biopsied. Attention is then turned to the cervix which is visualized using plain light as well as a green filter, highlighting vascular changes of condyloma and cervical intraepithelial neoplasia. A description of abnormal colposcopic features and features that guide biopsy of the most abnormal appearing area and helps to distinguish low-grade from high-grade lesions are summarized in Table 17-4. Biopsies are taken (typically from two or more sites) from the most abnormal appearing areas, preferably those areas that are closest to the squamo-columnar junction

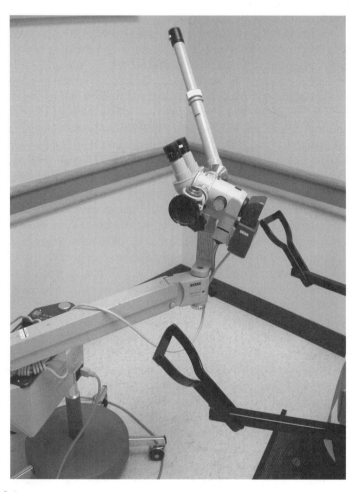

FIG. 17-9. Colposcope.

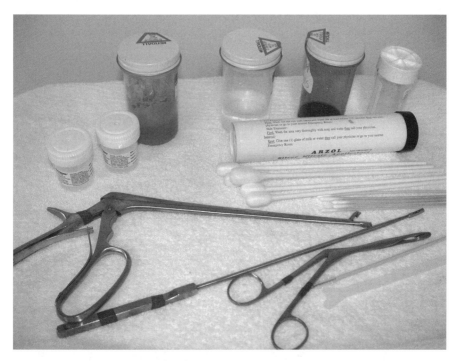

FIG. 17-10. Equipment tray for colposcopy.

TABLE 17-4. *Distinguishing characteristics between low-grade and high-grade squamous intraepithelial lesions.[e]*

	LSIL[a]	HSIL[b]
Color (degree of acetowhiteness)	More translucent (gray white), not shiny	More densely white/ opaque (oyster white)
Location	Peripheral (often with satellite lesions)	Central, close to SCJ[c]; larger
Vascular changes (mosaic, punctuations, atypical vessels)	Fine	Coarse and irregular; umbilicated; mosaic; atypical vessels
Margin of lesion	Geographic (irregular and uneven); may have satellite lesions	Distinct (straight and sharp); internal margins; rolling or peeling
Surface contour	Irregular (i.e., cerebriform condyloma)	Flat surface; rimmed glands/ cupping;
Speed of lesion fading	AW[d] changes transient	AW[d] changes persist

[a]Low-grade squamous intraepithelial lesion.
[b]High-grade squamous intraepithelial lesion.
[c]Squamo-columnar junction.
[d]Acetowhite.
[e]Adapted from Reid R. Biology and colposcopic features of human papillomavirus-associated cervical disease. *Obstet Gynecol Clin North Am* 1993;20;123.

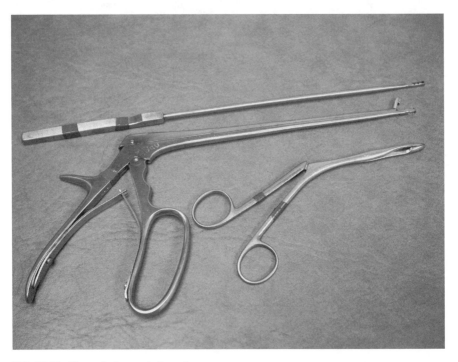

FIG. 17-11. Biopsy instruments for colposcopy.

(Fig. 17-11). The adequacy of the colposcopy is described; the colposcopic exam is considered adequate if the entire lesion is visualized and the entire squamo-columnar junction can be seen. An inadequate colposcopy requires further evaluation with a conization or a loop electrical excision procedure (LEEP) (Figs. 17-12 and 17-13). Many colposcopists routinely perform an endocervical curettage in all patients, although selective performance is also acceptable. A colposcopic impression is reached (mild, moderate, or severe dysplasia) based on the visual colposcopic appearance of the lesion, although biopsies are indicated to confirm this impression. The colposcopic findings are recorded.

Management of HPV in Adolescents

Condylomata

As there is no treatment currently available that eliminates HPV, therapy for condylomata is directed at destruction of affected tissue. It is unclear whether treatment decreases infectivity; therefore, the goal of treatment is to remove symptomatic warts (112). Without treatment, genital warts may resolve spontaneously, remain unchanged, or worsen; thus, some patients may prefer not to be treated. Patients who are immunosuppressed—those who have HIV infection or who are status post organ transplantation, for example—often do not respond well to treatment for condylomata and tend to have frequent recurrences. In addition, they are more likely to have squamous cell carcinomas that develop in or resemble genital warts.

Recommended provider-administered treatments include cryotherapy; podophyllin resin 10% to 25%; TCA or BCA 80% to 90%; surgical removal by excision, curettage, or electrosurgery; intralesional interferon; or laser surgery (113,114). Podophyllin resin is an antimitotic agent that causes tissue necrosis. Although it is as efficacious as other treatment modalities, the potential for adverse effects such as hematologic toxicity, central nervous system toxicity, and gastrointestinal symptoms have led some to recommend that its use be limited (115). Podophyllin resin should be washed off by 4 hours, and severe burns have been re-

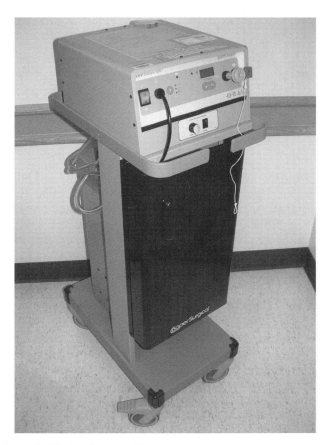

FIG. 17-12. Loop electrical excision machine.

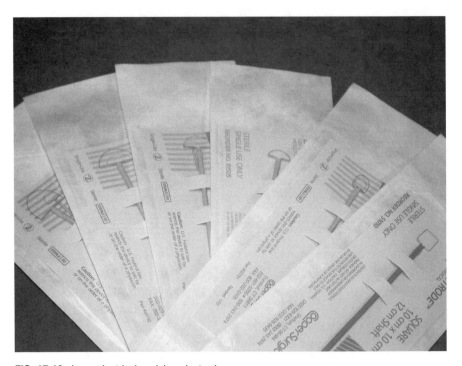

FIG. 17-13. Loop electrical excision electrodes.

ported. BCA and TCA also cause local destruction of warts, and effectiveness in clearing warts ranges from 63% to 70% (114). Podophyllin resin, TCA, and BCA may cause local irritation and pain if the agent spreads to adjacent skin; thus, they should be applied sparingly to the warts and then allowed to air dry. Treatment is repeated weekly with each of these modalities until clearance; up to six treatments may be needed.

Patient-administered treatments include podofilox 0.5% solution or gel and imiquimod 5% cream. Podofilox is applied to warts twice daily for three days, followed by four days of no therapy. The cycle is repeated as needed for up to four cycles. Local pain, usually mild or moderate, is common. Placebo-controlled trials demonstrate clearance in approximately 50% to 75% of treated patients within 4 to 6 weeks (116–118). Imiquimod is an imidazoquinolin heterocyclic amine that acts as a local immune enhancer by stimulating local production of interferon and other cytokines (119,120). Interferon inhibits human papillomavirus replication directly and enhances cell-mediated immune response against HPV (121). Imiquimod is applied at bedtime, three times a week for up to 16 weeks. The treatment area is washed with soap and water 6 to 10 hours after application. Randomized placebo-controlled trials have shown that approximately 30% to 55% of treated patients demonstrate clearance within 16 weeks (122,123). Advantages of imiquimod in comparison with other HPV treatments may include lower recurrence rates and self-application (13,122). Disadvantages include the need to visualize warts for proper application, the relatively long duration of treatment (124), the high cost relative to podofilox (125), and common local inflammatory reactions that may cause burning sensations, itching, or pain (126). In adolescents, follow-up may be helpful to assess response to treatment. If improvement does not occur after several treatments, the therapy should be changed.

Adolescents with vaginal or anal warts may be treated using cryotherapy with liquid nitrogen, TCA or BCA 80% to 90%. Urethral meatal warts may be treated with cryotherapy or topical podophyllin. Patient-applied podofilox and imiquimod, and provider-applied TCA and BCA, have also been used by some clinicians for distal meatal warts. Because of the increased risk of cervical dysplasia in women with a history of anogenital condylomata, it is recommended that all women who have genital warts undergo cervical cancer screening at regular intervals (13). Recurrences of warts are common, especially during the first 3 months after treatment. Imiquimod, podophyllin, and podofilox are not recommended in pregnancy.

Surgical therapy using laser ablation or sharp excision is indicated for large and extensive lesions, or for lesions that do not respond to topical treatments. Anesthesia (local for small lesions and regional or general for extensive lesions) is required and adds to the expense. Cryotherapy with liquid nitrogen, loop electrical excision procedure, or intralesional interferon have also been used but have varying drawbacks that limit widespread use.

Clinicians should recognize that a diagnosis of genital warts may be emotionally traumatic and should address specific patient concerns (127–129). Education of adolescents with genital warts should include a discussion of HPV transmission, the possibility of wart recurrence, treatment options, and the importance of regular cytologic screening. Providers should make sure that adolescents are able to visualize external warts so that they can monitor the progress of treatment, detect recurrences, recognize signs of infection, and use patient-applied therapies appropriately. Other measures that may promote healing and decrease discomfort are sitz baths and heat sources (such as a hair dryer on a low setting). Excellent educational resources on the internet include the Centers for Disease Control and Prevention and the American Social Health Association, and the Center for Young Women's Health at Children's Hospital Boston.

Cervical Dysplasia

Options for treatment of cervical dysplasia are listed in Table 17-5 and include cold knife conization, cryotherapy using a cervical probe (Fig. 17-14), laser, or LEEP. Factors that may play a part in the decisions about treatment of CIN in adolescents include issues of consent; cost; ability to understand the examinations, biopsies, and therapies given little previous experience; differences in cervical size and

TABLE 17-5. Treatment options for moderate or severe dysplasia

Treatment modality	Efficacy	Complications	Learning/skill	Expense	Pain	Specimen	Advantages/ disadvantages specific to method	Patient's perspective
Cold knife conization (CKC)	Equal to hysterectomy "gold standard"	Bleeding: immediate or delayed Uterine perforation Pelvic inflammatory disease Cervix scarring or distortion Cervical incompetence	Included in OB/Gyn residency training (fewer procedures performed than in the past)	Operating room/ anesthesia	Anesthesia (general or regional) required	+ + + +	Disadvantages Volume of tissue removed Risk to future reproduction Cervical distortion making subsequent evaluation difficult	Same day surgery Risk of bleeding Expense
Cryotherapy	Equal to laser in randomized studies; depends on skill of colposcopist to recognize carcinoma in situ or invasive disease	Cervical os narrowing and stenosis Pelvic inflammatory disease	Simple, but often not a part of residency training	Inexpensive Initial investment in equipment	Mild No anesthesia	None	Advantage: tissue conserving Disadvantage: "retreat" of squamo-columnar junction making subsequent colposcopic evaluation difficult Risk of missing invasive or microinvasive disease because no specimen	Mild-moderate cramps Watery discharge × 3 to 4 wk
Laser	Equal to cryotherapy in randomized studies; depends on skill of colposcopist to recognize carcinoma-in- situ or invasive disease	Bleeding risk > cryo Pelvic inflammatory disease	Significant experience is required for competency (training in OB/ Gyn residency)	Considerable for equipment	Greater than cryotherapy	± Vaporization vs. laser cone Margins with thermal injury for laser conization	Disadvantages: Cost of equipment and need for anesthesia Risks to future reproduction?	Pain greater than cryotherapy Risk of bleeding
Loop electrical excision procedure (LEEP)	Equal to laser and cryotherapy (similar to CKC)	Bleeding and operative times less than CKC Risk of cervical incompetence?	Less than laser; greater than cryotherapy OB/Gyn residency training now includes this experience	Less than laser; greater than cryotherapy and supplies billing codes	Intracervical or paracervical block	+ + + Margins may have thermal injury	Advantage: healing with accessible squamo-columnar junction Disadvantage: risk to future reproduction?	Pain greater than cryotherapy

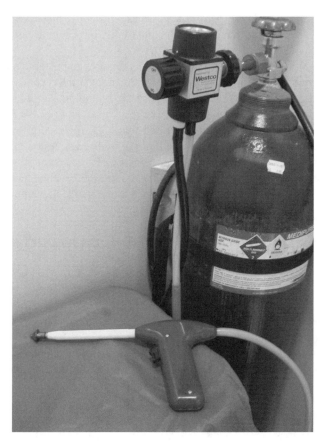

FIG. 17-14. Cryotherapy probe.

configuration (parous vs. nulliparous); threats or risks to future fertility and cervical competence posed by cold knife cone or LEEP; and the need to evaluate the cervix for recurrent disease for many years in the future.

In both adults and adolescents, generally there should be agreement in the following results: cervical cytology, colposcopic assessment, cervical biopsies, and endocervical curettage (if performed). If the results all suggest mild dysplasia, the recommended course of action is observation with periodic cervical cytology. This is based on the high likelihood of regression of low-grade lesions. If moderate/severe dysplasia or CIS are found, treatment generally is warranted. Evidence-based consensus guidelines for the management of women with CIN have been developed and adopted by a panel of experts (130). These guidelines note that some experts at the consensus conference expressed the opinion that "observation is appropriate for appropriately counseled adolescents with biopsy-confirmed CIN 2, considered to be reliable for follow-up." This assumes adequate colposcopy, negative endocervical sampling, and patient understanding of the possibility of occult disease. Ablation or excision is required for adolescents with CIN 3.

Multiple treatment modalities have been found to have comparable rates of "cure" or success in outcomes. A randomized clinical trial comparing cryotherapy, laser ablation, and LEEP as treatment for CIN of all grades found no significant difference in clearance rates or complications (131). The relative advantages and disadvantages of several treatment options are outlined in Table 17-5. If the colposcopy is inadequate and a high-grade lesion is suspected, or if a high-grade lesion is found on endocervical curettage, a cold knife conization or LEEP procedure is indicated. The management of vaginal and vulvar dysplasia and intra-epithelial neoplasia is beyond the scope of this chapter but may include excision or ablative procedures.

PREVENTION OF HPV INFECTION AND SEQUELAE

Strategies for primary prevention of HPV infection and its sequelae are based on established risk factors. Adolescents should be encouraged to delay sexual initiation, limit sexual partners, use condoms consistently, and avoid tobacco use.

Recent research concerning the genetics of HPV and immune response to infection has facilitated the development of HPV vaccines that may be useful in preventing HPV infection, genital warts, and cervical cancer. There is a clear biological rationale for HPV vaccine development. First, human papillomaviruses are the etiologic agents in almost all squamous intraepithelial lesions, cervical carcinomas, and condylomata (97). In addition, recent data suggest that HPV infection induces both humoral and cellular immunity, which correlates with lack of progression as well as regression of HPV infection (132). However, generation of HPV-specific immunity following natural infection is limited, perhaps because HPV infection is superficial and most virus genes are expressed at low levels. Over the last decade, however, investigators have succeeded in developing HPV vaccines that are highly immunogenic and induce HPV genotype-specific neutralizing antibodies. Vaccines may be prophylactic or therapeutic. Prophylactic vaccines are designed to prevent primary HPV infection. Therapeutic vaccines are designed to prevent progression of HPV infection or low-grade squamous intraepithelial lesions to high-grade lesions, achieve regression of CIN or condylomata, or eliminate residual cervical cancer after treatment.

Current vaccines primarily target types 6, 11, 16, and 18; these are the types that cause the majority of human condylomata and cervical carcinomas. Vaccines may be univalent (target one HPV type) or multivalent (target more than one type). There are two major types of vaccines under investigation. The first type is the viruslike particle, or VLP, vaccine. In the early 1990s, investigators found that by inducing expression of the major HPV capsid protein L1 (with or without L2) it was possible to produce HPV viruslike particles (133). These are identical to HPV virions morphologically but do not contain a viral DNA core, so they can be injected into a host to induce an antibody response without incurring any infectious or onco-genic risk. Phase I and II trials of HPV viruslike particle vaccines have demonstrated that they are highly immunogenic, well-tolerated, and safe (134). Several have entered clinical efficacy trials, and recently the first vaccine trial for preventing HPV infection was reported using a viruslike particle 16 vaccine (135). This randomized controlled trial involved >2,000 young women who received vaccine or placebo at 0, 2, and 6 months. The incidence of persistent HPV-16 infection was 0 in the HPV 16 vaccine group compared with 3.8% per 100 woman-years at risk in the placebo group, for an efficacy rate of 100%. The incidence of transient or persistent HPV 16 infection sim-ilarly was lower in the vaccine group (0.6% vs. 6.3%), for an efficacy rate of 91.2%. All nine cases of HPV-16 related CIN occurred among the placebo recipients. Of women who received HPV-16 vaccine, 99.7% seroconverted. Chimeric viruslike par-ticle vaccines (CVLP) are similar to viruslike particle vaccines, but also contain vari-ous combinations of early viral proteins attached in different ways to the major L1 or the minor L2 capsid proteins of the virus. Thus, chimeric viruslike particle vaccines have the potential to be used both as prophylactic as well as therapeutic vaccines, be-cause they target the early proteins such as E6 and E7 that are expressed in virtually all squamous intraepithelial lesions and cervical cancer cells.

Within the next 5 to 10 years, the results of additional phase III trials of HPV vac-cines will be available and it will be more apparent to what extent these vaccines will be instrumental in decreasing the disease burden of condylomata and cervical carci-noma worldwide. However, there are several important issues related to HPV vaccines that will require further attention in order to ensure successful vaccine implementation and prevention of HPV-related disease (136). First, HPV is spread as a sexually trans-mitted infection; therefore, vaccine coverage must reach high levels in the at-risk pop-ulation in order to eliminate infection. Second, there are multiple high-risk genotypes that may be involved in cervical carcinogenesis. Providers and patients will need to be informed that no vaccine will be 100% protective against cervical cancer. Third, there is concern about behavioral effects. If vaccine recipients believe that they are protected from HPV and cervical cancer, they may increase risky sexual behaviors and decrease routine gynecologic care visits. These effects are concerning because vaccine recipients may not be protected against HPV types not contained in the vaccine, the duration of protection may not be lifelong, and gynecologic exams are important for reasons other than cervical cancer screening. Fourth, vaccines in development may be prohibitively expensive for developing countries where the need for a preventive vaccine is most ur-gent. Finally, acceptability of the vaccine is a particularly important issue with HPV and other STD vaccines (137–139). The primary target population for HPV vaccine is likely to be school-aged children and early adolescents, but there may be barriers at sev-eral levels to vaccination of this population. At the individual level, concerns about con-fidentiality or lack of a sense of vulnerability may hinder vaccination. Parents may be reluctant to agree to immunization of their children against a sexually transmitted in-fection because they do not believe that their child is at risk for infection, may not be willing or ready to initiate the discussion about sexually transmitted infections that may arise as a result of giving permission for their child to be immunized, or may be concerned that immunization could increase rates of risky behaviors in their adolescent children. At the provider level, clinicians may have concerns about safety and efficacy of the vaccine. They may be reluctant to discuss issues of sexual activity and sexually transmitted infections with children and early adolescents.

CONCLUSIONS

HPV infection is highly prevalent in adolescent and adult women and may be associated with substantial morbidity and mortality. Recent research has increased greatly our understanding of the natural history and sequelae of HPV infection. This information has led to evidence-based revisions of the system for classifying cervical cytology and guidelines for screening and management of abnormal cytology. It has also facilitated the development of HPV vaccines, which hold promise for prevention of HPV infection, genital warts, and cervical cancer.

ACKNOWLEDGMENTS

Dr. Kahn was supported by a grant (K23 AI50923-01) from the National Institutes of Health, National Institute of Allergy and Infectious Diseases and would like to thank Diane Penny for assistance in preparation of the chapter.

REFERENCES

1. Ho GY, Bierman R, Beardsley L, et al. Natural history of cervicovaginal papillomavirus infection in young women. *N Engl J Med* 1998;338:423.
2. Armstrong LR, Derkay CS, Reeves WC. Initial results from the national registry for juvenile-onset recurrent respiratory papillomatosis. RRP Task Force. *Arch Otolaryngol Head Neck Surg* 1999;125: 743.
3. Armstrong DK, Handley JM. Anogenital warts in prepubertal children: pathogenesis, HPV typing and management. *Int J STD AIDS* 1997;8:78.
4. Armstrong DK, Bingham EA, Dinsmore WW, et al. Anogenital warts in prepubertal children: a follow-up study. *Br J Dermatol* 1998;138:544.
5. Solomon D, Davey D, Kurman R, et al. The 2001 Bethesda System: Terminology for reporting results of cervical cytology. *JAMA* 2002;287:2114.
6. Koutsky L. Epidemiology of genital human papillomavirus infection. *Am J Med* 1997;102:3.
7. Moscicki AB, Shiboski S, Broering J, et al. The natural history of human papillomavirus infection as measured by repeated DNA testing in adolescent and young women. *J Pediatr* 1998;132:277.
8. Hutchinson ML, Zahniser DJ, Sherman ME, et al. Utility of liquid-based cytology for cervical carcinoma screening: results of a population-based study conducted in a region of Costa Rica with a high incidence of cervical carcinoma. *Cancer* 1999;87:48.
9. Richart RM, Masood S, Syrjanen KJ, et al. Human papillomavirus. International Academy of Cytology Task Force summary. Diagnostic Cytology Towards the 21st Century: An International Expert

Conference and Tutorial. *Acta Cytol* 1998;42:50.

10. Cox JT. Clinical role of HPV testing. *Obstet Gynecol Clin North Am* 1996;23:811.

11. Wright TC, Cox JT, Massad LS, et al. 2001 consensus guidelines for the management of women with cervical cytological abnormalities. *JAMA* 2002;287:2120.

12. Saslow D, Runowicz C, Solomon D, et al. American Cancer Society guideline for the early detection of cervical neoplasia and cancer. *CA: Cancer J Clin* 2002;52:342.

13. Beutner KR, Reitano MV, Richwald GA, et al. External genital warts: report of the American Medical Association Consensus Conference. AMA Expert Panel on External Genital Warts. *Clin Infect Dis* 1998;27:796.

14. Lehtinen M, Dillner J. Preventive human papillomavirus vaccination. *Sex Transm Infect* 2002;78:4.

15. Severson JL, Beutner KR, Tyring SK. Genital papillomavirus infection. In: Stanberry LR, Bernstein DI, eds. *Sexually transmitted diseases: vaccines, prevention and control.* London: Academic Press, 2000:259.

16. Turek LP, Smith EM. The genetic program of genital human papillomaviruses in infection and cancer. *Obstet Gynecol Clin North Am* 1996;23:735.

17. Turek LP. The structure, function, and regulation of papillomaviral genes in infection and cervical cancer. *Adv Virus Res* 1994;44:305.

18. deVilliers EM. Human papillomavirus: introduction. *Semin Cancer Biol* 1999;9:377.

19. Munoz N, Bosch FX, de Sanjose S, et al. Epidemiologic classification of human papillomavirus types associated with cervical cancer. *N Engl J Med* 2003;348:518.

20. Bosch FX, Manos MM, Munoz N, et al. Prevalence of human papillomavirus in cervical cancer: a worldwide perspective. *J Natl Cancer Inst* 1995;87:796.

21. Walboomers JM, Jacobs MV, Manos MM, et al. Human papillomavirus is a necessary cause of invasive cervical cancer worldwide. *J Pathol* 1999;189:12.

22. Smith EM, Summersgill KF, Allen J, et al. Human papillomavirus and risk of laryngeal cancer. *Ann Otol Rhinol Laryngol* 2000;109:1069.

23. Bjorge T, Engeland A, Luostarinen T, et al. Human papillomavirus infection as a risk factor for anal and perianal skin cancer in a prospective study. *Br J Cancer* 2002;87:61.

24. Hammerschlag MR. Sexually transmitted diseases in sexually abused children: medical and legal implications. *Sex Transm Infect* 1998;74:167.

25. Rice PS, Cason J, Best JM, et al. High risk genital papillomavirus infections are spread vertically. *Rev Med Virol* 1999;9:15.

26. Stevens-Simon C, Nelligan D, Breese P, et al. The prevalence of genital human papillomavirus infections in abused and nonabused preadolescent girls. *Pediatrics* 2000;106:645.

27. Fairley CK, Gay NJ, Forbes A, et al. Hand-genital transmission of genital warts? An analysis of prevalence data. *Epidemiol Infect* 1995;115:169.

28. Antonsson A, Karanfilovska S, Lindqvist PG, et al. General acquisition of human papillomavirus infections of skin occurs in early infancy. *J Clin Microbiol* 2003;41:2509.

29. Chatterjee R, Mukhopadhyay D, Murmu N, et al. Correlation between human papillomavirus DNA detection in maternal cervical smears and buccal swabs of infants. *Indian J Exp Biol* 1998;36:199.

30. Summersgill KF, Smith EM, Levy BT, et al. Human papillomavirus in the oral cavities of children and adolescents. *Oral Surg Oral Med Oral Pathol Oral Radiol Endod* 2001;91:62.

31. Cason J, Kaye JN, Jewers RJ, et al. Perinatal infection and persistence of human papillomavirus types 16 and 18 in infants. *J Med Virol* 1995;47:209.

32. Rimell FL, Shoemaker DL, Pou AM, et al. Pediatric respiratory papillomatosis: prognostic role of viral typing and cofactors. *Laryngoscope* 1997;107:915.

33. Gabbott M, Cossart YE, Kan A, et al. Human papillomavirus and host variables as predictors of clinical course in patients with juvenile-onset recurrent respiratory papillomatosis. *J Clin Microbiol* 1997;35:3098.

34. Armstrong LR, Preston EJ, Reichert M, et al. Incidence and prevalence of recurrent respiratory papillomatosis among children in Atlanta and Seattle. *Clin Infect Dis* 2000;31:107.

35. Derkay CS, Darrow DH. Recurrent respiratory papillomatosis of the larynx: current diagnosis and treatment. *Otolaryngol Clin North Am* 2000;33:1127.

36. Koutsky LA, Galloway DA, Holmes KK. Epidemiology of genital human papillomavirus infection.

Epidemiol Rev 1988;10:122.
37. Kulasingam SL, Hughes JP, Kiviat NB, et al. Evaluation of human papillomavirus testing in primary screening for cervical abnormalities: Comparison of sensitivity, specificity, and frequency of referral. *JAMA* 2002;288:1749.
38. Fisher M, Rosenfeld W, Burk R. Cervicovaginal human Papillomavirus infection in surburban adolescents and young adults. *J Pediatr* 1991;119:821.
39. Winer RL, Lee SK, Hughes JP, et al. Genital human papillomavirus infection: incidence and risk factors in a cohort of female university students. *Am J Epidemiol* 2003;157:218.
40. Kahn JA, Slap GB, Huang B, et al. Comparison of adolescent and young adult self-collected and clinician-collected samples for human papillomavirus. *Obstet Gynecol* 2004;103:952.
41. Moscicki AB, Hills NK, Shiboski S, et al. Risks for incident human papillomavirus infection and low-grade squamous intraepithelial lesion development in young females. *JAMA* 2001;285:2995.
42. Wallin K, Wiklund F, Angstrom T, et al. Type-specific persistence of human papillomavirus DNA before the development of invasive cervical cancer. *N Engl J Med* 1999;341:1633.
43. Kjaer SK, van den Brule AJ, Gerson P, et al. Type specific persistence of high risk human papillomavirus (HPV) as indicator of high grade cervical squamous intraepithelial lesions in young women: population based prospective follow up study. *BMJ* 2002;325:572.
44. Beutner K, Wiley D, Douglas J, et al. Genital warts and their treatment. *Clin Infec Dis* 1998;28:S37.
45. Wilson JD, Brown CB, Walker PP. Factors involved in clearance of genital warts. *Int J STD AIDS* 2001;12:789.
46. Sadeghi S, Hsieh E, Gunn S. Prevalence of cervical intraepithelial neoplasia in sexually active teenagers and young adults. Results of data anaylsis of mass Papanicolaou screening of 796,337 women in the United States in 1981. *Am J Obstet Gynecol* 1984;148:726.
47. Mangan SA, Legano LA, Rosen CM, et al. Increased prevalence of abnormal Papanicolaou smears in urban adolescents. *Arch Pediatr Adolesc Med* 1997;151:481.
48. Mount SL, Papillo JL. A study of 10,296 pediatric and adolescent Papanicolaou smear diagnoses in northern New England. *Pediatrics* 1999;103:539.
49. Edelman M, Fox AS, Alderman EM, et al. Cervical Papanicolaou smear abnormalities in inner city Bronx adolescents: prevalence, progression, and immune modifiers. *Cancer* 1999;87:184.
50. Kahn JA, Goodman E, Slap GB, et al. Intention to return for Pap smears in adolescent and young adult women. *Pediatrics* 2001;108:333.
51. Moscicki AB, Hills NK, Shiboski S. High rate of regression of low-grade squamous intra-epithelial lesions in adolescents. Abstract presented at Pediatric Academic Societies Annual Meeting; Baltimore, MD; May 14, 2002.
52. Nasiell K, Roger V, Nasiell M. Behavior of mild cervical dysplasia during long-term follow-up. *Obstet Gynecol* 1986;67:665.
53. Ries LA, Eisner MP, Kosary CL, et al., eds. SEER Cancer Statistics Review, 1973–1999. Bethesda, MD: Natl Cancer Inst; 2002.
54. Handley J, Dinsmore W, Maw R, et al. Anogenital warts in prepubertal children; sexual abuse or not? *Int J STD AIDS* 1993;4:271.
55. Frasier LD. Human papillomavirus infections in children. *Pediatr Ann* 1994;23:354.
56. Moscicki AB. Genital HPV infections in children and adolescents. *Obstet Gynecol Clin North Am* 1996;23:675.
57. Kosko JR, Derkay CS. Role of cesarean section in prevention of recurrent respiratory papillomatosis—is there one? *Int J Pediatr Otorhinolaryngol* 1996;35:31.
58. Silverberg MJ, Thorsen P, Lindeberg H, et al. Condyloma in pregnancy is strongly predictive of juvenile-onset recurrent respiratory papillomatosis. *Obstet Gynecol* 2003;101:645.
59. Burk RD, Ho GY, Beardsley L, et al. Sexual behavior and partner characteristics are the predominant risk factors for genital human papillomavirus infection in young women. *J Infect Dis* 1996;174:679.
60. Kjaer SK, van den Brule AJ, Bock JE, et al. Determinants for genital human papillomavirus (HPV) infection in 1,000 randomly chosen young Danish women with normal Pap smear: are there different risk profiles for oncogenic and nononcogenic HPV types? *Cancer Epidemiol Biomarkers Prev* 1997;6:799.
61. Manhart LE, Koutsky LA. Do condoms prevent genital HPV infection, external genital warts, or cervical neoplasia? A meta-analysis. *Sex Transm Dis* 2002;29:725.
62. Ozsaran AA, Ates T, Dikmen Y, et al. Evaluation of the risk of cervical intraepithelial neoplasia and

human papillomavirus infection in renal transplant patients receiving immunosuppressive therapy. *Eur J Gynaecol Oncol* 1999;20:127.

63. Palefsky JM, Minkoff H, Kalish LA, et al. Cervicovaginal human papillomavirus infection in human immunodeficiency virus-1 (HIV)-positive and high-risk HIV-negative women. *J Natl Cancer Inst* 1999;91:226.

64. Massad LS, Riester KA, Anastos KM, et al. Prevalence and predictors of squamous cell abnormalities in Papanicolaou smears from women infected with HIV-1. Women's Interagency HIV Study Group. *J Acquir Immune Defic Syndr* 1999;21:33.

65. Harrison HR, Phil D, Costin M, et al. Cervical chlamydia trachomatis infection in university women: relationship to history, contraception, ectopy, and cervicitis. *Am J Obstet Gynecol* 1985;153:244.

66. Guijon FB, Paraskevas M, Brunham R. The association of sexually transmitted diseases with cervical intraepithelial neoplasia: a case-control study. *Am J Obstet Gynecol* 1985;151:185.

67. Moscicki AB, Winkler B, Irwin C, et al. Differences in biologic maturation, sexual behavior, and sexually transmitted disease between adolescents with and without cervical intraepithelial neoplasia. *J Pediatr* 1989;115:487.

68. Johnson BA, Poses RM, Fortner CA, et al. Derivation and validation of a clinical diagnostic model for chlamydial cervical infection in university women. *JAMA* 1990;264:3161.

69. Moss GB, Clemetson D, D'Costa L, et al. Association of cervical ectopy with heterosexual transmission of human immunodeficiency virus: results of a study of couples in Nairobi, Kenya. *J Infec Dis* 1991;164:588.

70. Moscicki AB, Burt VG, Kanowitz S, et al. The significance of squamous metaplasia in the development of low grade squamous intraepithelial lesions in young women. *Cancer* 1999;85:1139.

71. Shrier LA, Bowman FP, Lin M, et al. Mucosal immunity of the adolescent female genital tract. *J Adolesc Health* 2003;32:183.

72. Campion MJ, Greenberg MD, Kazamel TIG. Clinical manifestations and natural history of genital human papillomavirus infections. *Obstet Gynecol Clin North Am* 1996;23:783.

73. Stafford EM, Greenberg H, Miles PA. Cervical intraepithelial neoplasia III in an adolescent with Bowenoid papulosis. *J Adolesc Health Care* 1990;11:523.

74. De Silva AH, Sivapalan S, Harindra V, et al. Emerging incidence of vulval intraepithelial neoplasia in young women with genital warts. *Genitourin Med* 1992;68:346.

75. Cardosi RJ, Bomalaski JJ, Hoffman MS. Diagnosis and management of vulvar and vaginal intraepithelial neoplasia. *Obstet Gynecol Clin North Am* 2001;28:685.

76. Dodge JA, Eltabbakh GH, Mount SL, et al. Clinical features and risk of recurrence among patients with vaginal intraepithelial neoplasia. *Gynecol Oncol* 2001;83:363.

77. Koss LG. The Papanicolaou test for cervical cancer detection. A triumph and a tragedy. *JAMA* 1989; 261:737.

78. Nanda K, McCrory DC, Myers ER, et al. Accuracy of the Papanicolaou test in screening for and follow-up of cervical cytologic abnormalities: a systematic review. *Ann Int Med* 2000;132:810.

79. Kahn JA, Chiou V, Allen JD, et al. Beliefs about Papanicolaou smears and compliance with Papanicolaou smear follow-up in adolescents. *Arch Pediatr Adolesc Med* 1999;153:1046.

80. Serlin M, Shafer MA, Tebb K, et al. What sexually transmitted disease screening method does the adolescent prefer? Adolescents' attitudes toward first-void urine, self-collected vaginal swab, and pelvic examination. *Arch Pediatr Adolesc Med* 2002;156:588.

81. Lavin C, Goodman E, Perlman S, et al. Follow-up of abnormal Papanicolaou smears in a hospital-based adolescent clinic. *J Pediatr Adolesc Gynecol* 1997;10:141.

82. Kahn JA, Goodman E, Huang B, et al. Predictors of Papanicolaou smear return in a hospital-based adolescent and young adult clinic. *Obstet Gynecol* 2003;101:490.

83. IARC Working Group on the Evaluation of the Cervical Cancer Screening Program. Screening for squamous cervical cancer: duration of low risk after negative results on cervical cytology and its implications for screening policies. *BMJ* 1986;293:659.

84. Igra V, Millstein SG. Current status and approaches to improving preventive services for adolescents. *JAMA* 1993;269:1408.

85. Wilcox LS, Mosher WD. Factors associated with obtaining health screening among women of re-

productive age. *Public Health Rep* 1993;108:76.

86. Kahn JA, Colditz GA, Aweh GN, et al. Prevalence and correlates of pelvic examinations in sexually active female adolescents. *Ambul Pediatr* 2002;2:212.

87. Dell DL, Chen H, Ahmad F, et al. Knowledge about human papillomavirus among adolescents. *Obstet Gynecol* 2000;96:653.

88. Coste J, Cochand-Priollet B, De Cremoux P, et al. Cross sectional study of conventional cervical smear, monolayer cytology, and human papillomavirus DNA testing for cervical cancer screening. *BMJ* 2003;326:733.

89. Brown AD, Garber AM. Cost-effectiveness of 3 methods to enhance the sensitivity of Papanicolaou testing. *JAMA* 1999;281:347.

90. De Sutter P, Coibion M, Vosse M, et al. A multicentre study comparing cervicography and cytology in the detection of cervical intraepithelial neoplasia. *Br J Obstet Gynaecol* 1998;105:613.

91. Schneider DL, Herrero R, Bratti C, et al. Cervicography screening for cervical cancer among 8460 women in a high-risk population. *Am J Obstet Gynecol* 1999;180:290.

92. Fait G, Daniel Y, Kupferminc MJ, et al. Does typing of human papillomavirus assist in the triage of women with repeated low-grade, cervical cytologic abnormalities? *Gynecol Oncol* 1998;70:319.

93. Manos MM, Kinney WK, Hurley LB, et al. Identifying women with cervical neoplasia: Using human papillomavirus DNA testing for equivocal Papanicolaou results. *JAMA* 1999;281:1605.

94. Schneider A, Zahm DM, Kirchmayr R, et al. Screening for cervical intraepithelial neoplasia grade 2/3: Validity of cytologic study, cervicography, and human papillomavirus detection. *Am J Obstet Gynecol* 1996;174:1534.

95. Hatch KD, Schneider A, Abdel-Nour MW. An evaluation of human papillomavirus testing for intermediate- and high-risk types as a triage before colposcopy. *Am J Obstet Gynecol* 1995;172:1150.

96. Cox JT. Evaluating the role of HPV testing for women with equivocal Papanicolaou test findings. *JAMA* 1999;281:1645.

97. Nobbenhuis MA, Walboomers JM, Helmerhorst TJ, et al. Relation of human papillomavirus status to cervical lesions and consequences for cervical-cancer screening: a prospective study. *Lancet* 1999; 354:20.

98. The ASC-US–LSIL Triage Study (ALTS) Group. Results of a randomized trial on the management of cytology interpretations of atypical squamous cells of undetermined significance. *Am J Obstet Gynecol* 2003;188:1383.

99. Ferris DG, Wright TC, Litaker MS, et al. Triage of women with ASC-US and LSIL on Pap smear reports: management by repeat Pap smear, HPV DNA testing, or colposcopy? *J Fam Pract* 1998;46:125.

100. Bergeron C, Jeannel D, Poveda JD, et al. Human papillomavirus testing in women with mild cytologic atypia. *Obstet Gynecol* 2000;95:821.

101. Lin CT, Tseng CJ, Lai CH, et al. High-risk HPV DNA detection by Hybrid Capture II. An adjunctive test for mildly abnormal cytologic smears in women ≥50 years of age. *J Reprod Med* 2000;45:345.

102. Shlay JC, Dunn T, Byers T, et al. Prediction of cervical intraepithelial neoplasia grade 2–3 using risk assessment and human papillomavirus testing in women with atypia on Papanicolaou smears. *Obstet Gynecol* 2000;96:410.

103. Solomon D, Schiffman M, Tarone R. Comparison of three management strategies for patients with atypical squamous cells of undetermined significance: baseline results from a randomized trial. *J Natl Cancer Inst* 2001;93:293.

104. Association of Reproductive Health Care Professionals. Human Papillomavirus (HPV) and Cervical Cancer. AHRP Clinical Proceedings 2001:22.

105. Kim JJ, Wright TC, Goldie SJ. Cost-effectiveness of alternative triage strategies for atypical squamous cells of undetermined significance. *JAMA* 2002;287:2382.

106. Wright TC, Denny L, Kuhn L, et al. HPV DNA testing of self-collected vaginal samples compared with cytologic screening to detect cervical cancer. *JAMA* 2000;283:81.

107. Schiffman M, Herrero R, Hildesheim A, et al. HPV DNA testing in cervical cancer screening: Results from women in a high-risk province of Costa Rica. *JAMA* 2000;283:87.

108. Petry KU, Bohmer G, Iftner T, et al. Human papillomavirus testing in primary screening for cervical cancer of human immunodeficiency virus-infected women, 1990–1998. *Gynecol Oncol* 1999;75:427.

109. Cuzick J, Beverley E, Ho L, et al. HPV testing in primary screening of older women. *Br J Cancer* 1999;81:554.
110. ACOG Practice Bulletin No. 45. Cervical Cytology Screening. Obstet Gynecol 2003;102:417.
111. Hillard PJA, Biro FM, Wildey LS, et al. The value of an adolescent dysplasia clinic. *Adol Pediatr Gynecol* 1989;2:43.
112. Wilson J. Treatment of genital warts—what's the evidence? *Int J STD AIDS* 2002;13:216.
113. Centers for Disease Control and Prevention. Sexually transmitted diseases treatment guidelines 2002. *MMWR Morb Mortal Wkly Rep* 2002;51:No.RR-6.
114. Wiley DJ, Douglas J, Beutner K, et al. External genital warts: diagnosis, treatment, and prevention. *Clin Infect Dis* 2002;35:S210.
115. von Krogh G, Lacey CJ, Gross G, et al. European course on HPV associated pathology: guidelines for primary care physicians for the diagnosis and management of anogenital warts. *Sex Transm Infect* 2000;76:162.
116. Beutner KR, Conant MA, Friedman-Kien AE, et al. Patient-applied podofilox for treatment of genital warts. *Lancet* 1989;1:831.
117. Greenberg MD, Rutledge LH, Reid R, et al. A double-blind, randomized trial of 0.5% podofilox and placebo for the treatment of genital warts in women. *Obstet Gynecol* 1991;77:735.
118. Beutner KR, Wiley DJ. Recurrent external genital warts: a literature review. *Papillomavirus Rep* 1997;8:69.
119. Tyring SK, Arany I, Stanley MA, et al. A randomized, controlled, molecular study of condylomata acuminata clearance during treatment with imiquimod. *J Infect Dis* 1998;178:551.
120. Tyring S, Conant M, Marini M, et al. Imiquimod; an international update on therapeutic uses in dermatology. *Int J Dermatol* 2002;41:810.
121. Dahl MV. Imiquimod: An immune response modifier. *J Am Acad Dermatol* 2000;43:S1.
122. Edwards L, Ferenczy A, Eron L, et al. Self-administered topical 5% imiquimod cream for external anogenital warts. HPV Study Group. *Arch Dermatol* 1998;134:25.
123. Beutner KR, Spruance SL, Hougham AJ, et al. Treatment of genital warts with an immune-response modifier (imiquimod). *J Am Acad Dermatol* 1998;38:230.
124. Edwards L. Imiquimod in clinical practice. J Am Acad Dermatol 2000;43:S12.
125. Alam M, Stiller M. Direct medical costs for surgical and medical treatment of condylomata acuminata. *Arch Dermatol* 2001;137:337.
126. Owens ML, Bridson WE, Smith SL, et al. Percutaneous penetration of Aldara cream, 5% during the topical treatment of genital and perianal warts. *Prim Care Update Ob Gyns* 1998;5:151.
127. Filiberti A, Tamburini M, Stefanon B, et al. Psychological aspects of genital human papillomavirus infection: a preliminary report. *J Psychosom Obstet Gynaecol* 1993;14:145.
128. Persson G, Dahlof LG, Krantz I. Physical and psychological effects of anogenital warts on female patients. *Sex Transm Dis* 1993;20:10.
129. Chandler MG. Genital warts: a study of patient anxiety and information needs. *Br J Nurs* 1996;5:174.
130. Wright TC, Jr., Cox JT, Massad LS, et al. 2001 consensus guidelines for the management of women with cervical intraepithelial neoplasia. *Am J Obstet Gynecol* 2003;189:295.
131. Mitchell MF, Tortolero-Luna G, Cook E, et al. A randomized clinical trial of cryotherapy, laser vaporization, and loop electrosurgical excision for treatments of squamous intraepithelial lesions of the cervix. *Obstet Gynecol* 1998;92:737.
132. Tjiong MY, Out TA, Ter Schegget J, et al. Epidemiologic and mucosal immunologic aspects of HPV infection and HPV-related cervical carcinoma in the lower female genital tract: a review. *Int J Gynecol Cancer* 2001;11:9.
133. Kirnbauer R, Taub J, Greenstone H, et al. Efficient self-assembly of human papillomavirus type 16 L1 and L1–L2 into virus-like particles. *J Virol* 1993;67:6929.
134. Harro CD, Pang YY, Roden RB, et al. Safety and immunogenicity trial in adult volunteers of a human papillomavirus 16 L1 virus-like particle vaccine. *J Natl Cancer Inst* 2001;93:284.
135. Koutsky LA, Ault KA, Wheeler CM, et al. A controlled trial of a human papillomavirus type 16 vaccine. *N Engl J Med* 2002;347:1645.
136. Garnett GP, Waddell HC. Public health paradoxes and the epidemiological impact of an HPV vaccine. *J Clin Virol* 2000;19:101.
137. Zimet GD, Mays RM, Fortenberry JD. Vaccines against sexually transmitted infections: promise and problems of the magic bullets for prevention and control. *Sex Transm Dis* 2000;27:49.

138. Zimet GD, Mays RM, Winston Y, et al. Acceptability of human papillomavirus immunization. *J Women's Health Gender-Based Med* 2000;9:47.
139. Kahn JA, Rosenthal SL, Hamann T, et al. Attitudes about human papillomavirus vaccine in young women. *Int J STD AIDS* 2003;14:300.

18

Benign and Malignant
Ovarian Masses

Marc R. Laufer and Donald P. Goldstein

Ovarian masses in infants, children, and adolescents may result from functional cysts, or benign or malignant neoplasms. Ovarian tumors are the most common genital neoplasms that occur during childhood, accounting for about 1% of all malignant neoplasms found in the age range of 0 to 17 years (1,2). Historically, it was widely believed that all ovaries containing masses discovered in infants, children, and adolescents should be removed surgically, but with the identification of serum tumor markers and advances in radiologic imaging, a more rational and conservative fertility sparing approach to the management of these ovarian masses has been developed. The purpose of this chapter is to review the incidence, presentation, physical findings, evaluation, and management of various types of ovarian masses that are encountered in fetuses, neonates, children, and adolescents.

CLASSIFICATION OF OVARIAN MASSES

Ovarian masses may result from functional (nonneoplastic) cysts or benign or malignant neoplasms. The World Health Organization has classified ovarian neoplasms into nine major categories and 26 subtypes, based on histologic cell type and benign versus malignant state (3). An abbreviated and modified version is shown in Table 18-1 (3,4). In contrast to the adult experience, in which epithelial tumors account for the significant proportion of neoplasms, the majority of tumors in the younger population are of germ cell origin (Table 18-2) (5). Although the majority of lesions in childhood are benign, expedient diagnosis and management is important to lessen the possibility of ovarian torsion and loss of an adnexa and to improve the prognosis for malignant masses.

TABLE 18-1. *Modified World Health Organization's international histologic classification of ovarian tumors*

Common "epithelial" tumors	Sex cord tumor with annular tubules
Serous	Leydig (hilus) cell tumors
Mucinous	Lipid (lipoid) cell tumors
Endometrioid	Gynandroblastoma
Clear cell	**Germ cell tumors**
Brenner	Dysgerminoma
Transitional	Endodermal sinus tumor
Small cell	Embryonal carcinoma
Malignant mixed mesodermal	Polyembryoma
Unclassified	Choriocarcinoma
Sex cord-stromal tumors	Teratomas
Granulosa stromal cell	Immature
Granulosa cell	Mature (dermoid cyst)
Thecoma-fibroma	Monodermal (struma ovarii, carcinoid)
Sertoli stromal cell	Mixed forms
Sertoli cell tumors	Gonadoblastoma
Sertoli-Leydig cell tumors	**Metastatic**
Well differentiated	
Intermediately differentiated	**Other**
Poorly differentiated	
With heterologous element	

(Adapted from: Serov SF, Scully RE, Sobin LH. *International histological classification of tumours. No. 9. Histologic typing of ovarian tumours.* Geneva, World Health Organization, 1973; and Rice LW, Barbleri RL. The ovary. In: Ryan RJ, Berkowitz RS, Barbieri RL, eds. *Kistner's Gynecology,* 6th ed. Boston: Mosby-Year Book, 1995;187; with permission.)

TABLE 18-2. *Primary ovarian tumors treated at the Children's Hospital Boston (1928–1982)*

Tumor type	Number	%
Mature (benign) teratomas	78	47
Cystic (76)		
Solid (2)		
Common "epithelial" tumors	27	16
Mucinous (12)		
Serous (14)		
Mixed (1)		
Sex cord-stromal tumors	21	13
Granulosa cell (10)		
Thecoma (2)		
Fibroma (1)		
Sertoli-Leydig (7)		
Unclassified (1)		
Immature teratomas	17	10
Endodermal sinus tumor	14	8
Dysgerminoma	8	5
Choriocarcinoma[a]	1	<1

[a]Mixed malignant germ cell tumor with predominant element being choriocarcinoma.

(From: Lack EE, Goldstein DP. Primary ovarian tumors in childhood and adolescence. *Curr Probl Obstet Gynecol* 1984;8:1; with permission.)

Fetal Ovarian Cysts

Ovarian cysts have been detected prenatally on routine obstetric ultrasound in 30% to 70% of fetuses depending on the gestational age (6–9); the true incidence is unknown. The etiology of fetal ovarian cysts is unclear, but most likely they result from a combination of ovarian stimulation by maternal and fetal gonadotropins (see Fig. 4-4) (10,11). The differential diagnosis of fetal cystic intraabdominal masses is shown in Table 18-3 (12). An increased incidence of fetal and neonatal follicular cysts has been reported in association with preeclampsia, diabetes mellitus, polyhydramnios, and isoimmunization disease (9,10,13,14).

Management of Fetal Ovarian Cysts

The majority of antenatal ovarian cysts are unilateral, although both ovaries may be involved (13). Spontaneous regression occurs in both simple and complex fetal cysts both antenatally and postpartum, and thus the management of the patient with antenatally diagnosed ovarian cysts is observation (6–9,15–17). The risks to the fetus of an ovarian cyst may include intracystic hemorrhage, rupture of the cyst with

TABLE 18-3. *Differential diagnosis of fetal/neonatal intraabdominal cystic masses*

Genitourinary tract disorders
Ovarian cyst
Hydrometrocolpos
Cloacal anomaly
Urinary tract obstruction
Renal cyst
Megaloureter or megalocystis
Urachal cyst
Adrenal cyst

Gastrointestinal tract disorders
Mesenteric cyst
Enteric duplication cyst
Meconium cyst
Duodenal atresia
Volvulus

Miscellaneous disorders
Choledochal cyst
Pancreatic cyst
Splenic cyst
Presacral cystic teratoma
Anterior meningocele
Neuroblastoma
Lymphangioma

(From: Lack EE, Goldstein DP. Primary ovarian tumors in childhood and adolescence. *Curr Probl Obstet Gynecol* 1984;8:1; with permission.)

possible hemorrhage, gastrointestinal and urinary tract obstruction, ovarian torsion and necrosis, incarceration into a congenital inguinal hernia, difficulty with delivery due to abdominal dystocia, and respiratory distress at birth due to the mass effect (18,19). Antenatal aspiration of large (4 to 6 cm) ovarian cysts has been advocated to reduce the potential complications (20–22); however, the role of antenatal cyst aspiration is controversial due to potential misdiagnosis and complications of the aspiration procedure. In some fetuses with large cysts (>6 cm) or masses that are not cystic, elective cesarean section may be the preferred route to prevent rupture and/or dystocia. The rate of malignancy is so low that it need not be considered in making therapeutic decisions.

Neonatal Ovarian Cysts

The most common genitourinary cystic mass not related to the kidney is an ovarian cyst (23). The differential diagnosis of a neonate with a cystic intraperitoneal mass is extensive and includes a number of congenital cystic masses of other intraperitoneal organs, as well as congenital anomalies (see Table 18-3) (12,24). As noted above, the etiology of fetal and neonatal ovarian cysts is unknown, but is most likely the result of maternal hormonal stimulation in utero. If in utero ovarian torsion occurs, the ovary may undergo necrosis and develop into a calcified persistent mass or may be resorbed.

Clinical Presentation

Most neonatal cysts are asymptomatic and identified incidentally on antenatal neonatal ultrasound evaluation for another indication. As neonates have a shallow pelvis, the cysts are often displaced to the mid- or upper abdomen, at which time they are palpable abdominally. On abdominal examination, the ovary containing the cyst is generally freely mobile. Ultrasound reveals a cystic mass (Fig. 18-1) that may have a simple (clear, fluid-filled) or complex (fluid, debris, septa, solid components, echogenic wall) sonographic pattern. The complex appearance on ultrasound may make a precise diagnosis more difficult (12).

Management of Neonatal Ovarian Cysts

Spontaneous regression occurs in these cysts postpartum usually by 4 months of age. They should be followed with serial ultrasound examinations to ensure regression. The greatest concern in the neonate with an ovarian cyst is the possibility of torsion with subsequent ovarian loss. If the cyst does not resolve, then either neoplasia is present (unlikely) or torsion with hemorrhage and/or necrosis (see Fig. 11-1) has occurred (8,25).

The traditional management of neonatal cysts that persist for longer than 4 months and are greater than 5 cm, or increasing in size is surgery (9, 26–29). Although every

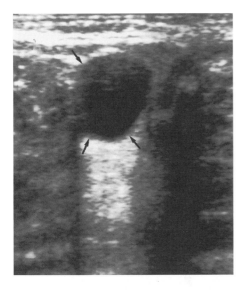

FIG. 18-1. Ultrasound shows a simple cyst (*arrows*) in a neonate. (Courtesy of Carol Barnewolt, M.D., Children's Hospital Boston)

attempt should be made to salvage the ovary in cases of persistent ovarian cysts, in some instances, especially in cases of torsion with ovarian necrosis, oophorectomy is necessary (10,22). Figures 18-2 to 18-4 demonstrate the preservation of some normal appearing ovarian tissue in a case of ovarian torsion. Whenever possible, every effort should be made to preserve any normal ovarian tissue with an ovarian cystectomy as opposed to an oophorectomy.

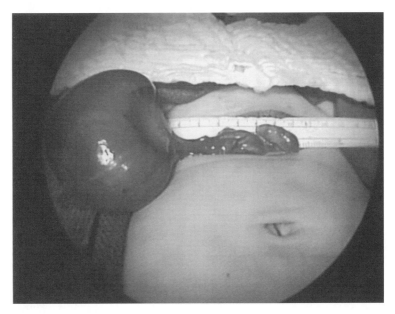

FIG. 18-2. Neonatal ovarian torsion.

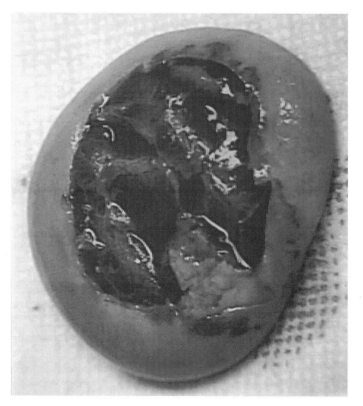

FIG. 18-3. Resection of torsed ovarian tissue seen in Fig. 18-2., An area of normal-appearing ovarian tissue was separated from the necrotic tissue and was preserved as seen in Fig. 18-4.

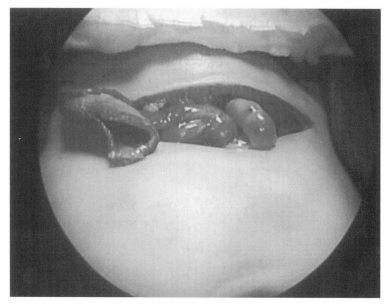

FIG. 18-4. Residual normal-appearing ovarian tissue conserved from the case in Fig. 18-2 and Fig. 18-3.

It should be noted that infants and children may also have torsion of normal ovaries (see Chapter 11) (30–32). It is possible to untwist the vascular pedicle in an attempt to salvage the ovary (33) (see Ovarian and Tubal Torsion below). Neonatal ovarian cysts can be managed preferentially by a laparoscopic approach, but may require a mini-laparotomy (34–38).

Postpartum cyst aspiration has been advocated to reduce the likelihood of torsion (39). In contrast to antenatal cyst aspiration, the use of neonatal cyst aspiration has been clearly established, because the diagnosis is more certain and the risk of complications is low (40). Aspiration of persistent large simple cysts (>5 to 6 cm) is recommended (9). If the cysts recur, surgical removal is indicated.

Ovarian Cysts in the Prepubertal Child

Childhood ovarian cysts develop as a result of gonadotropin stimulation of the ovary, and thus the incidence of ovarian cysts decreases in early childhood and then increases as puberty is approached (41,42). Most simple ovarian cysts in children result from failure of a follicle to involute.

Some functional cysts will be hormonally active and result in precocious pseudopuberty, with the patient presenting with an episode of vaginal bleeding or premature breast development (43–46). Hormone-secreting cysts may cause sexual precocity, as is seen in association with the McCune-Albright syndrome (47). These ovarian cysts may respond to medical therapy for McCune-Albright syndrome, but if they persist on therapy, needle aspiration under ultrasound guidance or laparoscopy may be indicated. Cysts may also occur in patients with idiopathic central precocious puberty and would be expected to resolve with the institution of gonadotropin-releasing hormone analog therapy (48) (see Chapter 5). When prepubertal ovaries are found to be enlarged and multicystic, an evaluation for thyroid disease is indicated (see Chapter 5). If a child has a cystic mass without precocity, the cyst may well be a para-ovarian (see Fig. 10-22) or mesothelial cyst and, if symptomatic, requires excision (see Figs. 10-23 to 10-25).

Clinical Presentation

In young children, an ovarian cyst is often discovered by a parent or clinician as an asymptomatic abdominal mass or as increasing abdominal girth. The embryologic ovary migrates from the level of 10th thoracic vertebrae (in early life it is characteristically abdominal in location) and during maturation descends to the true pelvis by puberty. Thus, ovarian tumors present as abdominal masses in the young child (1). Chronic abdominal aching pain, either periumbilical or located in one lower quadrant, may be present. Acute severe pain simulating appendicitis or peritonitis may develop secondary to torsion, perforation, infarction, or hemorrhage from or into a tumor or cyst (see Chapter 11). Patients may experience intermittent pain, presumably because of partial torsion, that subsequently resolves without therapy. This may also be the warning sign of impending torsion and the need for emergency surgery (see Ovarian and Tubal Torsion below). Nonspecific symptoms including nausea, vomiting, a sense of abdominal fullness or bloating, and urinary frequency or retention may signal the presence of a tumor.

Evaluation of Ovarian Cysts in Prepubertal Girls

Ultrasound is the best method for evaluation of ovarian cysts in prepubertal girls. The mass should be measured, and its characteristics determined (simple, complex, or solid). As discussed in Chapter 11, Doppler flow ultrasound may or may not be helpful in determining cases of ovarian torsion (see Fig. 11-3 and a discussion of torsion below).

Management of Ovarian Cysts in Prepubertal Girls

The management of an ovarian cyst in the prepubertal age group depends on the appearance of the cyst on ultrasound and the presence of significant symptomatology. Most likely these cysts will resolve spontaneously and require no intervention.

Rarely a simple ovarian cyst in a prepubertal child will rupture and may result in acute exacerbation of pain. This will most likely be self-limited and requires no surgical intervention.

If the prepubertal ovarian mass is purely cystic or has few internal echoes/debris suggestive of hemorrhage and no other complex features such as septation or calcification (Fig. 18-5), it is almost certainly benign and can be managed by observation (46,49). A follow-up ultrasound scan in 4 to 8 weeks should reveal a decrease in size. If the cyst has not resolved and the ultrasonic characteristics are still reassuring, then

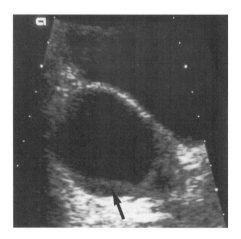

FIG. 18-5. Ultrasound shows an ovarian cyst containing debris (*arrow*). (Courtesy of Carol Barnewolt, M.D., Children's Hospital Boston.)

continued observation is still appropriate. Warner and associates (50) reported on the conservative management of 51 children with both simple and complex cysts, all >5 cm in diameter. Of these cysts, 90% spontaneously resolved, largely within 2 weeks. Of the 23 children treated surgically either because of initial ultrasonic appearance or for persistence, 10 were found to have neoplasms (six teratomas, two cystadenomas, one granulosa cell tumor, one Sertoli-Leydig cell tumor) (50). Thind and colleagues (51) found that in 64 children with simple cysts <5.5 cm in diameter, all of the cysts resolved. These girls, however, tended to have persistent symptoms for a few months followed by spontaneous resolution. The cysts sometimes recurred, although new ovarian cysts also occurred on the contralateral side (51).

If a prepubertal simple ovarian cyst persists and is symptomatic or is growing in size, then a surgical intervention is indicated. Laparoscopy can be safely performed in young girls and an ovarian cystectomy should be performed with preservation of normal ovarian cortex as opposed to an oophorectomy (see Figs. 18-6 to 18-9).

Ovarian masses in prepubertal girls associated with torsion are usually benign (52). In a series of 102 girls (aged 2 days to 20 years) who underwent 106 consecutive ovarian operations, the authors reported that 42% of those who presented with abdominal pain had ovarian torsion. In their series, the ovarian mass was malignant in only one patient. In comparison, 26% of those presenting with an asymptomatic mass were found to have an ovarian malignancy. The management of adnexal torsion is discussed below.

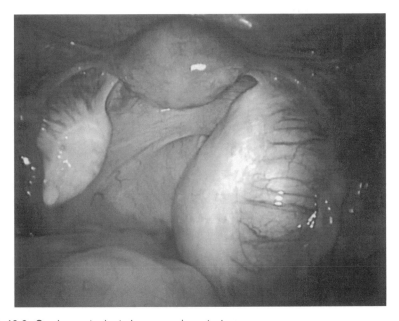

FIG. 18-6. Ovarian cyst prior to laparoscopic cystectomy.

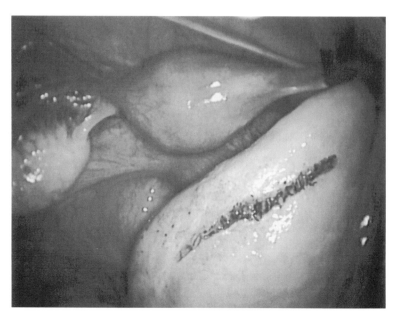

FIG. 18-7. Linear incision in normal ovarian cortex to initiate the ovarian cystectomy from Fig. 18-6.

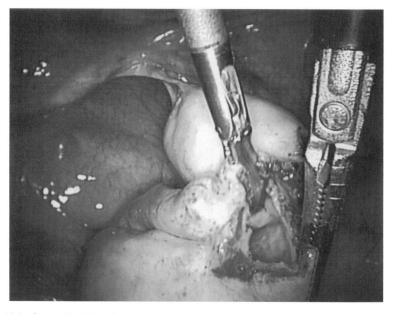

FIG. 18-8. Cyst wall visible after incision and drainage of ovarian cyst in Figs. 18-6 and 18-7.

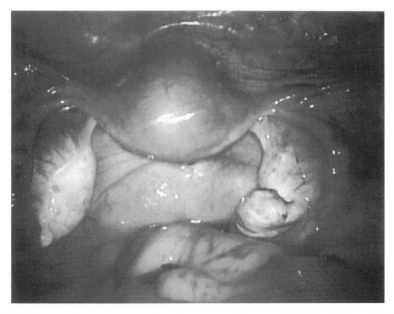

FIG. 18-9. Post-ovarian cystectomy view after removal of cyst wall in Figs. 18-6 to 18-8. Final pathology revealed a benign mucinous cystadenoma.

Postpubertal Ovarian Cysts

Functional Ovarian Cysts

Functional cysts (20% to 50% of ovarian tumors) are not true neoplasms but rather should be considered a variation of a normal physiologic process (see Chapter 4). Functional cysts include follicular, corpus luteum, and theca-lutein types, all of which are benign and usually self-limited. The incidence of cysts and nonmalignant tumors in the community is probably even higher than indicated in most series, as percentages are based on referred cases and it is not possible to determine the underlying incidence of nonidentified or asymptomatic cysts or masses (5,53).

The development of simple cysts is quite common in postpubertal girls and adolescents. Most simple cysts result from the failure of the maturing follicle to ovulate and involute. Adolescent ovaries may contain multiple follicles in different stages of development (see Fig. 11-4).

Clinical Presentation

Cysts in the postmenarchal adolescent may be asymptomatic or cause menstrual irregularities, pelvic pain, or, if large, urinary frequency, constipation, or pelvic heaviness. Cysts can rupture, causing intraabdominal hemorrhage (see Color Plate 38 and see Management of Cysts section, discussed next). Torsion of a cyst causes acute pain, nausea, vomiting, and pallor, often followed by less severe localized pain. The white blood cell count may be elevated with a shift to the left. Examination reveals pain, peritoneal signs, and a tender mass.

Management of Postpubertal Ovarian Cysts

Functional Simple Cysts   In most cases, follicular cysts found on routine examination resolve spontaneously in 1 to 2 months. Ovarian cysts less than 3 cm are usually normal follicles and require no further evaluation or intervention. If a cyst larger than 6 cm is palpated in an asymptomatic patient and ultrasound or pelvic examination confirms a simple, fluid-filled cyst, the patient may be observed with or without the addition of an oral contraceptive prescribed to suppress the hypothalamic-ovarian axis. The oral contraceptive pill does not "shrink" the existing cyst, but with suppression of the hypothalamic-ovarian axis another ovarian cyst is unlikely to develop and confuse the clinician as to whether the first cyst resolved and a new one formed or whether the original cyst has persisted. The patient should be examined monthly or follow-up ultrasound performed. Patients incidentally found to have small follicular cysts at the time of surgery (e.g., appendectomy) should not undergo cyst aspiration or cystectomy, as these cysts will resolve spontaneously and ovarian or paratubal adhesions may form from ovarian surgery and result in infertility and/or pelvic pain (see Chapter 11) (54,55).

If a fluid-filled cyst increases in size, is larger than 6 cm, or causes symptoms, then a laparoscopic cyst aspiration (with the cyst fluid sent for cytology) or cystectomy (with the cyst wall sent for pathologic evaluation) can be performed (see Color Plate 37 and Figs. 18-6 to 18-9) (56). If surgery is undertaken, ovarian cystectomy is preferred to cyst aspiration due to the high rate of recurrence after aspiration (57). If there is a contraindication to surgery, or if a nonsurgical approach is preferred, ultrasound-guided cyst aspiration can be performed; cyst aspiration does not require anesthesia or a laparoscopic approach.

It should be noted that asymptomatic simple cysts of 6 to 10 cm may also spontaneously resolve and can be safely observed in some patients. If the cyst recurs or operative intervention is needed, the procedure should be conservative with an ovarian cystectomy and not an oophorectomy so that as much ovarian tissue as possible is preserved.

Corpus Luteum   Corpus luteum cysts occur often and can reach 5 to 10 cm in diameter. These cysts are the result of the normal formation of a corpus luteum after ovulation (see Chapter 4). Ultrasound is useful to suggest the appearance of a corpus luteum cyst, which contains increased echoes (Fig. 18-10). There may be bleeding into the cyst or rupture with intraperitoneal hemorrhage. The hemorrhage needs to be assessed to determine whether the bleeding appears to be self-limited (in which case the patient can be observed with serial hematocrit readings and examinations) or

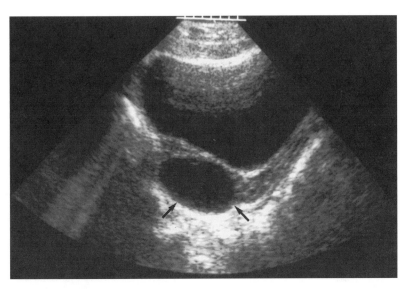

FIG. 18-10. Ultrasound shows a corpus luteum cyst (*arrows*) in a young woman reporting dull pain. (Courtesy of Carol Barnewolt, M.D., Children's Hospital Boston)

whether the bleeding is resulting in a significant decrease in hematocrit or changes in vital signs. If it is determined that the patient needs surgery, then she is stabilized and laparoscopy or laparotomy undertaken (49). Free blood and clots (see Color Plate 38) can be aspirated and hemostasis ensured by fulguration of areas of bleeding via laparoscopy. A hemoperitoneum is not a contraindication to laparoscopy. If the surgeon is not comfortable with laparoscopy for children or if the patient is hypotensive, then a laparotomy is undertaken. Most often the bleeding can be controlled with cauterization or ovarian cystectomy; oophorectomy is not indicated. Conservative management with conservation of normal ovarian tissue is the rule.

Corpus luteum cysts are often asymptomatic, they may cause pain. In the absence of pain or intraperitoneal bleeding, therapy with an oral contraceptive pill (to suppress a new cyst from forming) and observation for 3 months are indicated. If hemorrhage or severe pain occurs or the cyst is large (>6 cm) on initial examination, laparoscopy or laparotomy may be necessary. Due to increased ovarian size and weight, corpus luteum cysts may increase the risk of ovarian torsion (see Color Plates 40 and 41).

Ovarian and/or Tubal Torsion As mentioned above, the embryologic ovary migrates from the level of 10th thoracic vertebrae (in early life it is characteristically abdominal in location) and during maturation descends to the true pelvis by puberty (see Color Plate 31). Based on the abdominal location of the ovary, and the long utero-ovarian ligament, the normal adnexa of prepubertal girls are at increased risk of torsion. Torsion can occur with a cyst of any size, just as it does with normal adnexa, particularly when long pedicles are present (40,58). When known cysts are followed conservatively, parents or other caregivers should be made aware of the signs and symptoms of torsion (sudden onset of pain, nausea, vomiting, and possible low-grade fever) (see Chapter 11) and urged to contact the child's physician without delay.

As noted in Chapter 11, ultrasound may be helpful in determining the presence of ovarian torsion (59,60). The classic appearance of peripheral follicles with stromal edema may be helpful in making a diagnosis of torsion (see Fig. 11-3).

Adnexal torsion should be addressed as a surgical emergency (61–63). Patients usually experience sudden onset of pain, nausea, vomiting, and possible low-grade fevers and are found to have peritoneal signs with rebound and/or guarding and possibly a mild leukocytosis (64–66). Patients may also experience intermittent pain, presumably because of partial or incomplete torsion, that subsequently resolves without therapy or does not cause complete ischemia. This may also be the warning sign of impending complete torsion with ischemia and death of the ovary, and the need for emergency surgery. There should be no such condition as "chronic torsion" that is observed. If there is a concern for torsion, then a surgical procedure should be carried out for diagnosis and appropriate management.

In cases of ovarian torsion, surgery is indicated at the time of the diagnosis. Ovarian masses in girls and young women (age 2 days to 20 years) associated with torsion are usually benign (52). Torsed ovaries can thus be "detorsed" laparoscopically with conservation of the ovary (33,61,63,67–69). The historical concerns regarding blood clots and emboli from detorsion have been found to be untrue. The anatomy should be identified and the adnexa salvaged. Even in cases of a "black" tube and/or ovary, detorsion and preservation of the adnexa can be carried out (70). If the ovary appears "black," then a "bivalve" procedure may help facilitate increased blood flow to the ovary by decreasing the arterial blood pulse pressure and improving blood flow (71). Detorsion and oophoropexy (see below) may be all that is indicated, but if an ovarian cyst is present, then an ovarian cystectomy is performed and not an oophorectomy. Once again, preservation of normal ovarian tissue is the rule. It is our feeling that it is better to leave an ovary in place, even if it looks "dusky" after detorsion and bivalve procedures, as it will most likely maintain function. It is always possible to return to the operating room at a later date to remove an ovary that did not survive (patient has persistence of pain, fevers, increased WBC); it is not possible to replace a potentially viable ovary once an oophorectomy has been performed.

Ovarian torsion may occur without diagnosis and/or intervention (72). In this case, the ovary will most likely resorb and/or calcify. It is also possible for the ovary to "auto-amputate" and become a sessile complex mass within the abdominal cavity.

Several weeks to years after adnexal torsion, these same individuals may experience torsion of the other adnexa, and if the second torsed ovary is not salvageable, the individual is sterile (46–49,70). Based on this occurrence of bilateral asynchronous ovarian torsion, oophoropexy should be considered in all cases of ovarian torsion of a normal (ovary without a large cyst which caused the torsion) ovary.

Oophoropexy

Prophylactic oophoropexy (of the contralateral normal ovary) should be considered at the time of the surgery for detorsion of a torsed adnexa. Whether oophoropexy of the contralateral ovary can be helpful in preventing a second episode of ovarian torsion of a normal ovary needs additional evaluation, but there is no downside to performing the procedure. We offer an oophoropexy to all girls and young women who have or have had torsion of a normal ovary. If the torsion was associated and most likely due to an ovarian cyst, then an ovarian cystectomy can be performed after the detorsion and oophoropexy is not routinely offered.

If oophoropexy is elected, it can be safely accomplished by operative laparoscopy (73). There are varying techniques to accomplish the stabilization of the ovary. The utero-ovarian ligament can be sewn to itself to shorten the ligament, and/or the ovary can be sutured to the uterosacral ligament as shown in Fig. 18-11 (A–D).

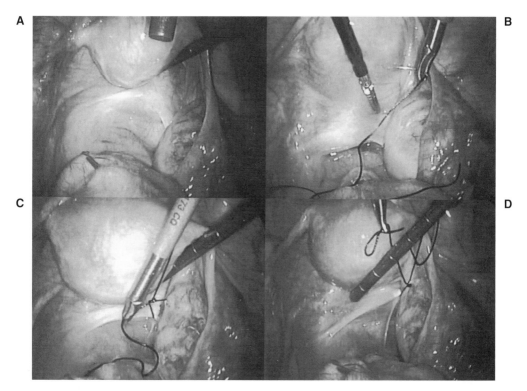

FIG. 18-11. A to **D**: Laparoscopic right oophoropexy with history of prior left salpingo-oophorectomy for torsion.

OVARIAN TUMORS/NEOPLASMS

Presentation and Examination

Patients with an ovarian tumor may present with abdominal pain or complaints of increasing abdominal girth, nausea, and vomiting, or they may be totally asymptomatic, with the mass being found on routine examination. The wide variety of symptoms caused by ovarian tumors suggests that abdominal palpation and rectal examination in the lithotomy position and a low threshold for obtaining an ultrasound evaluation are important in any girl with nonspecific abdominal or pelvic complaints (5,54). A large, thin-walled cyst may be confused with ascites. The size of the tumor is not indicative of its malignant potential. Exquisite tenderness suggests torsion or hemorrhage of the cyst but may also occur with appendicitis and rupture.

Imaging

Ultrasound is extremely helpful in the evaluation of an ovarian mass (23,49,51,74–78). Although ultrasound has revolutionized the management of patients with ovarian masses, not all tumors that are palpated will be visualized on ultrasound, and not all "masses" will turn out to be of significance. Ultrasound is routinely used to determine overall size and identify whether a mass is simple, complex, solid, bilateral, or associated with free fluid. This information is helpful in forming a differential diagnosis and correlating with age, presentation, and tumor markers to determine the appropriate therapy. Ultrasound and color flow Doppler imaging appearance of an ovarian mass help predict malignancy in older women (79–81). A solid ovarian mass in childhood is always viewed as malignant until proven otherwise by surgical removal (82). The differential diagnosis of solid tumors includes dysgerminoma, neuroblastoma, Wilms tumor, rhabdomyosarcoma, lymphoma, leukemia, or other nongenital tumors. For large tumors or those suspected of being malignant, additional information can be obtained with the use of computed tomography (CT) or magnetic resonance (MR) imaging to evaluate the tumor and identify liver or lung metastases (49,83–86).

Tumor Markers

Some ovarian neoplasms secrete protein tumor markers that can be assayed from peripheral blood samples (Table 18-4). These tumor markers are helpful in making a diagnosis of an ovarian tumor and in following clinical response and possible recurrences (87). Alpha-fetoprotein (AFP) is an oncofetal antigen that is a glycoprotein. It is produced by endodermal sinus tumors, mixed germ cell tumors, and immature teratomas (88,89). To assist with the interpretation of AFP levels in infants with

TABLE 18-4. *Serum tumor markers*

Serum Marker	Associated tumor
CA-125	Epithelial tumors (especially serous) Immature teratoma (rare)
Alpha-fetoprotein (AFP)	Endodermal sinus tumors Embryonal carcinomas Mixed germ cell tumors Immature teratoma (rare) Polyembryoma (rare)
Human chorionic gonadotropin (HCG)	Choriocarcinoma Embryonal carcinomas Mixed germ cell tumors Polyembryoma Dysgerminoma (rare)
Carcinoembryonic antigen (CEA)	Serous tumors Mucinous tumors
Lactate dehydrogenase (LDH)	Dysgerminoma Mixed germ cell tumors
Estradiol	Thecomas Adult granulosa cell tumors
Testosterone	Sertoli cell tumors Leydig (hilus) cell tumors
F9 embryoglycan	Embryonal carcinoma Yolk sac tumor Choriocarcinoma Immature teratoma
Inhibin	Granulosa-theca cell tumor
Müllerian inhibiting substance	Granulosa-theca cell tumor

ovarian masses, Table 18-5 shows serum AFP levels in normal infants (90). Lactate dehydrogenase (LDH) is found to be elevated in cases of dysgerminoma (91). CA-125, a marker for epithelial ovarian cancer (92), is highly sensitive but not very specific; it will be elevated with many intraperitoneal processes, such as endometriosis, pelvic inflammatory disease, pregnancy, Crohn disease, and other abdominal malignancies (93). Human chorionic gonadotropin (HCG) is produced by trophoblastic cells and thus will be elevated with pregnancy, hydatidiform moles, placental site tumors, choriocarcinoma, and embryonal ovarian carcinomas. Carcinoembryonic antigen (CEA) can be produced by epithelial and germ cell tumors. A human antibody against an embryoglycan present on the mouse teratocarcinoma cell line F9 (F9 embryoglycan) has been identified in the sera of patients with embryonal carcinoma, yolk sac tumor, choriocarcinoma, and immature teratoma, but it has not been identified in patients with dysgerminoma or mature teratoma (94). Levels of inhibin and müllerian inhibiting substance (MIS) have been shown to be elevated in children with granulosa-theca cell tumors (95,96).

TABLE 18-5. *Normal ranges of serum α-fetoprotein in infants.*

Age	No. points	Mean ± SD (ng/ml)
Premature	11	134,734 ±41,444
Newborn	55	48,406 ± 34,718
Newborn to 2 wk	16	33,113 ± 32,503
2 wk–1 mo	12	9,452 ± 12,610
2 mo	40	323 ± 278
3 mo	5	88 ± 87
4 mo	31	74 ± 56
5 mo	6	46.5 ± 19
6 mo	9	12.5 ± 9.8
7 mo	5	9.7 ± 7.1
8 mo	3	8.5 ± 5.5

(From Wu JT, Sudar K. Serum AFP levels in normal infants. *Pediatr Res* 1981;15:50; with permission.)

Thus we typically obtain AFP, HCG and LDH when evaluating for a germ cell tumor; CA-125 when evaluating for an epithelial tumor; and estradiol and testosterone are helpful in evaluating hormonally active tumors.

Surgery

Since most ovarian neoplasms of girls and young women are benign, minimally invasive surgery should be considered (97). Surgical planning is facilitated by appropriate preoperative evaluation including ultrasound imaging and tumor marker results (98). If surgical intervention is planned then a repeat imaging study should be performed close to the date for surgery to assure that the ovarian mass did not spontaneously resolve. Surgical intervention should aim, whenever possible, at preservation of reproductive potential. Surgery can be initiated laparoscopically; if the visual appearance of the mass yields concerns regarding malignancy, then a conversion to a laparotomy can be implemented. Unless a malignancy is diagnosed on frozen section at the time of the procedure, conservative surgery should be undertaken with excision of the lesion and ovarian reconstruction or unilateral salpingo-oophorectomy. It is preferable to subject the patient to a second procedure after the final pathology specimens are reviewed rather than perform unnecessary ablative procedures.

If, however, malignancy is found or suspected, adequate staging (see below), including abdominal and pelvic exploration, peritoneal washings, biopsies of suspicious areas, and periaortic and pelvic lymph node sampling, is crucial. Pathologic consultation may be invaluable in determining the exact diagnosis, so that appropriate therapy can be undertaken postoperatively, especially since advances in effective adjuvant chemotherapy for many ovarian tumors have improved the prognosis of many patients.

Staging

The staging of malignant ovarian tumors has been defined by the International Federation of Gynecology and Obstetrics (FIGO) and the American Joint Committee on Cancer (AJCC) (see Tables 18-6 and 18-7 and www.cancerstaging.org) (99–105).

TABLE 18-6. *The American Joint Committee on Cancer (AJCC) and the International Federation of Gynecology and Obstetrics (FIGO) staging of carcinoma of the ovary*

Staging of ovarian carcinoma is based on findings at clinical examination and by surgical exploration. The histologic findings are to be considered in the staging, as are the cytologic findings as far as effusions are concerned. It is desirable that a biopsy be taken from suspicious areas outside of the pelvis.

Stage I	Growth limited to the ovaries
Stage IA	Growth limited to one ovary; no ascites present containing malignant cells. No tumor on the external surface; capsule intact
Stage IB	Growth limited to both ovaries; no ascites present containing malignant cells. No tumor on the external surfaces; capsules intact
Stage IC[a]	Tumor classified as either stage IA or IB but with tumor on the surface of one or both ovaries; or with ruptured capsule(s); or with ascites containing malignant cells present; or with positive peritoneal washings
Stage II	Growth involving one or both ovaries, with pelvic extension
Stage IIA	Extension and/or metastases to the uterus and/or tubes
Stage IIB	Extension to other pelvic tissues
Stage IIC[a]	Tumor either stage IIA or IIB but with tumor on the surface of one or both ovaries; or with capsule(s) ruptured; or with ascites containing malignant cells present; or with positive peritoneal washings
Stage III	Tumor involving one or both ovaries with peritoneal implants outside the pelvis and/or positive retroperitoneal or inguinal nodes. Superficial liver metastasis equals stage III. Tumor is limited to the true pelvis but with histologically proven malignant extension to small bowel or omentum
Stage IIIA	Tumor grossly limited to the true pelvis with negative nodes but with histologically confirmed microscopic seeding of abdominal peritoneal surfaces
Stage IIIB	Tumor of one or both ovaries with histologically confirmed implants of abdominal peritoneal surfaces, none exceeding 2 cm in diameter; nodes are negative
Stage IIIC	Abdominal implants greater than 2 cm in diameter and/or positive retroperitoneal or inguinal nodes
Stage IV	Growth involving one or both ovaries, with distant metastases. If pleural effusion is present, there must be positive cytologic findings to allot a case to stage IV. Parenchymal liver metastasis equals stage IV

[a]To evaluate the impact on prognosis of the different criteria for allotting cases to stage IC or IIC, it would be of value to know whether the rupture of the capsule was spontaneous or caused by the surgeon and if the source of malignant cells detected was peritoneal washings or ascites.

(Adapted from: Greene FL, Page DL, Fleming ID, et al. AJCC Cancer Staging Manual, 6th Ed. New York: Springer-Verlag, 2002; International Federation of Gynecology and Obstetrics (FIGO) Cancer Committee. Staging announcement. *Gynecol Oncol* 1986;25:303; FIGO. Changes in definitions of clinical staging for carcinoma of the cervix and ovary. *Am J Obstet Gynecol* 1987;156:263–264; Creasman WT. Changes in FIGO staging. *Obstet Gynecol* 1987;70:138; FIGO. Annual report on the results of treatment in gynecological cancer. *Int J Gynaecol Obstet* 1989;28:189–190; Creasman WT. New gynecologic cancer staging. *Obstet Gynecol* 1990;75:287–288; and FIGO. Changes in gynecologic cancer staging by the International Federation of Gynecology and Obstetrics. *Am J Obstet Gynecol* 1990;162:610; with permission.)

TABLE 18-7. Modified FIGO staging classification for germ cell tumors

Stage	Extent of disease
I	Limited to ovary, peritoneal washings negative for malignant cells; no clinical, radiographic, or histologic evidence of disease beyond the ovaries. The presence of gliomatosis peritonei does not result in changing stage I disease to a higher stage. Tumor markers normal after appropriate half-life decline
II	Microscopic residual or positive lymph nodes <2 cm; peritoneal washings negative for malignant cells. The presence of gliomatosis peritonei does not result in changing stage II disease to a higher stage; tumor markers positive or negative
III	Lymph node involvement (metastatic nodule) >2 cm; gross residual or biopsy only; contiguous visceral involvement (omentum, intestine, bladder); peritoneal washings positive for malignant cells; tumor markers positive or negative
IV	Distant metastases, including liver

(Adapted from: International Federation of Gynecology and Obstetrics (FIGO) Cancer Committee. Staging announcement. *Gynecol Oncol* 1986;25:303; FIGO. Changes in definitions of clinical staging for carcinoma of the cervix and ovary. *Am J Obstet Gynecol* 1987;156:263–264; Creasman WT. Changes in FIGO staging. *Obstet Gynecol* 1987;70:138; FIGO. Annual report on the results of treatment in gynecological cancer. *Int J. Gynaecol Obstet* 1989;28:189–190; Creasman WT. New gynecologic cancer staging: *Obstet Gynecol* 1990;75:287–288; and FIGO. Changes in gynecologic cancer staging by the International Federation of Gynecology and Obstetrics. *Am J. Obstet Gynecol* 1990;162:610; with permission.)

This staging system standardizes nomenclature of ovarian malignancies for defining appropriate surgery and cytotoxic therapy and comparing outcome on the basis of clinical staging. The modified FIGO staging for germ cell tumors results in a significantly different grouping of patients, most notably that stage IC patients in the initial FIGO staging are now classified as stage III by the modified classification.

SPECIFIC BENIGN AND MALIGNANT OVARIAN TUMORS/NEOPLASMS

Endometriosis

Endometriosis is discussed in detail in Chapter 11, where it is noted that in the ovary large endometrial cysts may develop, so-called endometriomas or "chocolate cysts." Since endometrial tissue is dependent on hormones for growth, the ovary is an optimal site and has been reported to be the most common single site of endometriosis in adults (106). Endometriosis within the ovary (endometriomas), is much less common in adolescents and may represent disease progression (107). Ultrasound may be helpful in identifying an ovarian endometrioma (108). As noted in Chapter 11, endometriomas do not adequately respond to hormonal therapy and thus require surgical intervention. Laparoscopy is the surgical approach of choice, as endometriomas encountered in adolescent patients can safely be removed through the laparoscope (Fig. 18-12A). Adequate endometrioma surgery requires ovarian cystectomy with excision of the endometrioma's cyst wall (Fig. 18-12B and C). The normal ovarian cortex should be preserved as shown in Fig. 18-12B and C; there is no indication for an oophorectomy.

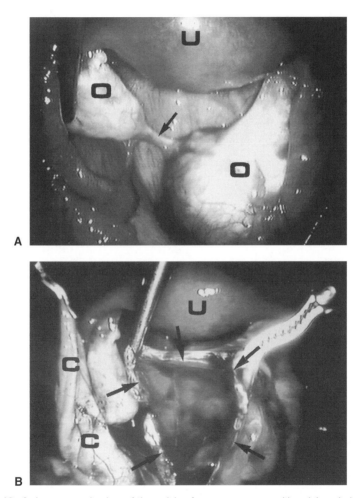

FIG. 18-12. A: Laparoscopic view of the pelvis of a young woman with pelvic pain in whom a nonresolving, 4-cm right ovarian endometrioma was identified on ultrasound. Note the abnormal dense adhesion between the right and left ovaries (*arrow*). This woman had previous surgery for a left ovarian dermoid cyst. **B:** After lysis of the adhesion, a right ovarian cystectomy of a 4-cm endometrioma has been performed. *Arrows* identify the edges of normal ovarian cortex remaining after the ovarian cystectomy. The endometrioma cyst wall has been removed from within the ovary and is now ready for removal from the intraperitoneal cavity. (U: uterus, O: ovary, C: cyst wall).

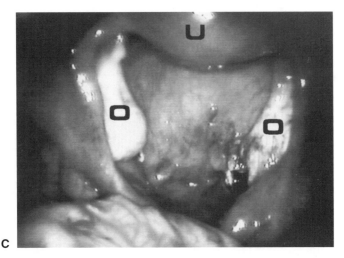

FIG. 18-12. (*Continued*) **C:** View of patient after lysis of adhesions and ovarian cystectomy. C, cyst wall; O, ovary; U, uterus.

Germ Cell Tumors

Germ cell tumors are the most common ovarian tumor in childhood and adolescence, accounting for two thirds of malignant tumors in children (82), and 55% of all ovarian cancers in adolescents (109). This diverse group of tumors is derived from germ cells (Fig. 18-13) (110) and includes both embryonic and extraembryonic tumors. The benign germ cell tumors include gonadoblastoma and teratoma; the malignant germ cell tumors include dysgerminoma, mixed germ cell tumor, endodermal sinus tumor, immature teratoma, embryonal tumor, choriocarcinoma, and polyembryoma.

Benign Germ Cell Tumors

Dermoids (Benign Teratomas)   The most common germ cell tumor is the *benign cystic teratoma,* more commonly known as a *dermoid cyst.* Dermoid cysts are mature cystic teratomas and are benign by definition; the malignant potential of teratomas (immature teratomas) is related to the histologic differentiation of the neural cells. Dermoids are the most common benign complex ovarian masses in children with an 18% incidence (111,112). Dermoid cysts are bilateral in 10% to 25% of cases in adults and 0% to 9% of those reported in children (7% of those in a series at Children's Hospital Boston) (5). Patients may present with abdominal pain or nausea or may be asymptomatic. Due to the weight of the dermoid contents, the ovary is at increased risk of torsion, and thus the patient may present with symptoms of torsion

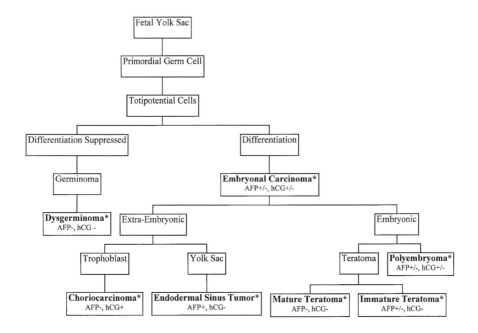

*Usual AFP and hCG tumor marker results.

FIG. 18-13. Germ cell tumor derivation. AFP, α-fetoprotein; HCG, human chorionic go-nadotropin. [Adapted from Teilum G. Classification of endodermal sinus tumour (mesoblastoma vitellinum) and so-called embryonal carcinoma of the ovary. *Acta Pathol Microbiol Scand* 1965;64:407; with permission.]

(see above and Chapter 11). An adnexal mass may be palpated on physical examination. Plain x-ray studies of the pelvis and abdomen may reveal a calcification in the pelvis. Ultrasonography can identify an ovarian mass as consistent with a dermoid cyst (Fig. 18-14A) due to the presence of thick sebaceous fluid, hair, and calcium (113,114). The contralateral ovary should also be examined carefully by ultrasound to exclude bilateral disease (115).

Management As dermoid cysts are germ cell tumors, they will not resolve spontaneously and thus require surgical intervention. Optimal treatment should preserve reproductive function, and thus there is much controversy of professional opinion as to the appropriate surgical approach (laparoscopy vs. laparotomy) (97,116–119). The endoscopic approach may be ideal with many of these tumors to shorten hospital

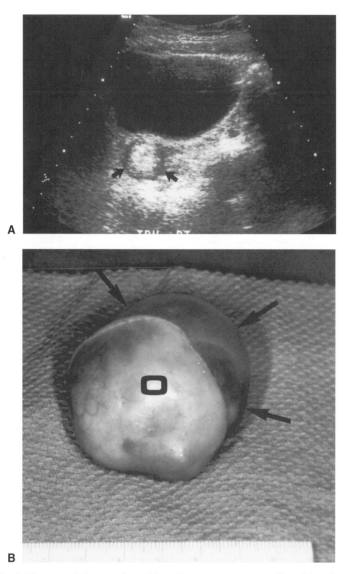

FIG. 18-14. A: Ultrasound shows a dermoid cyst in a young woman with pelvic pain and a palpable ovarian mass; *arrows* mark the edges of the cyst. (Courtesy of Carol Barnewolt, M.D., Children's Hospital Boston) **B:** The cyst is removed intact through a minilaparotomy incision. *Arrows* indicate the edges of the cyst; note the thin layer of ovarian cortex that remains on its surface.

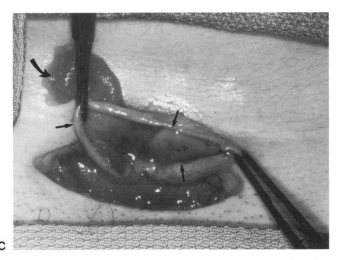

FIG. 18-14. *(Continued.)* **C:** After ovarian cystectomy, note the thin normal ovarian cortex that remains (*small arrows*) and the fimbriated end of the fallopian tube (*larger curved arrow*).

length of stay, improve cosmetic results (smaller incisions), and decrease overall cost; however, the risk of spillage of the cyst fluid may result in a chemical peritonitis with resulting adhesion formation and possible infertility (116). On the other hand, laparoscopic surgery itself may have a decreased risk of adhesion formation as compared to laparotomy (120,121). One study evaluating adhesion formation from release of dermoid contents in a rabbit model showed that spillage caused significant peritonitis, but with lavage inflammation and adhesion formation was reduced to control levels (122). No long-term human studies have been performed that evaluate long-term fertility. Due to the risk of spillage of cyst contents and the possible adverse effect on reproductive function, we recommend a minilaparotomy approach to these lesions. In addition, there is the possibility that what was thought to be a benign lesion is in fact a malignancy and that the tumor cells are spread intraperitoneally with spillage of the cyst contents (123–125). It is our practice to present the risks and benefits of each surgical approach to each patient and her parents in order to make an appropriate individual surgical plan. With either surgical approach, the dermoid cyst is excised and the remaining normal ovary salvaged (Fig. 18-14B and C). An ovarian cystectomy should thus be performed; there is no indication for an oophorectomy for benign teratomas.

Historically, it was recommended to bivalve the contralateral ovary in order to identify possible bilateral disease, but now with the use of preoperative ultrasound and careful inspection of the ovary intraoperatively, routine bivalving of the opposite ovary is no longer necessary.

Functional Teratomas (Struma Ovarii)   Functional teratomas are those that are hormonally active. When thyroid tissue is present, the term *struma ovarii* is applied (126,127). This condition is extremely rare (occurring in approximately 0.4% of teratomas), but when it does occur, thyrotoxicosis may develop. Carcinoma can also occur in functional teratomas (128). Management involves the removal of the affected ovarian tumor with an ovarian cystectomy and conservation of the remaining normal ovarian cortex.

Gonadoblastoma   Gonadoblastoma is a rare tumor composed of germ cells mixed with sex cord derivatives (129). Scully (130) regarded them as a type of *in situ* cancer from which a malignant germ cell tumor such as dysgerminoma can develop. Although this tumor is benign, it is associated with a malignant germ cell tumor (dysgerminoma) in approximately 25% to 50% of cases (131). Gonadoblastoma is almost always found in patients with gonadal dysgenesis associated with a Y chromosome or a Y-chromosomal fragment. Thus, if a Y chromosome or antigen is identified, the risk that patients who have this tumor will develop a malignancy is sufficiently high to require prophylactic bilateral gonadectomy. The exception to the need for immediate gonadectomy is the androgen insensitivity syndrome (AIS) (testicular feminization), in which the gonads should remain *in situ* until after puberty to allow normal secondary sexual development. The risk of a malignancy developing from a gonadoblastoma in AIS is low prior to the completion of the development of secondary sexual characteristics. Thus, in AIS, the gonads are removed once breast development is complete. In cases of 46,XY gonadal dysgenesis, the gonads appear as streaks as shown in Color Plate 47. Bilateral gonadectomy can be accomplished by either conventional laparotomy or laparoscopy (132–134); the best approach (laparoscopy vs. laparotomy) is controversial and not yet determined. It is known that germ cells can be present in the upper area of the infundibulopelvic ligament, and thus if a laparoscopic procedure is performed, there is a risk of persistence of gonadal tissue. In either approach, we recommend that frozen sections should be performed to determine whether residual gonadal tissue is present at the upper border of resection. At this time, we are currently recommending the laparoscopic approach, unless a large complex mass is present within the gonad.

Malignant Germ Cell Tumors

Immature Teratomas (Malignant)   The younger the patient is, the more likely it is that the teratoma will be of the immature germ cell type, so-called immature teratoma (5). Of complex masses in girls, 9.6% to 11.1% have been found to be malignant immature teratomas (112,135). Patients present with abdominal pain, a complaint of an abdominal mass, or nausea/vomiting. A mass may be palpable on abdominal (Fig. 18-15) or pelvic examination. Abdominal symptoms may occur acutely due to torsion or rupture of the tumor. MR imaging (Fig. 18-16) or CT may be helpful in further evaluation of the tumor and assessment for liver or lung metastases. Although levels of

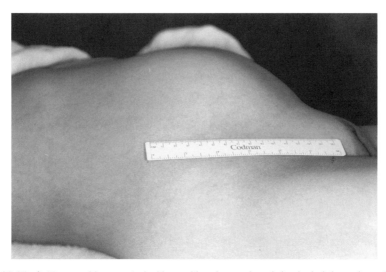

FIG. 18-15. A 12-year-old presented with vomiting, increasing abdominal girth, and a palpable abdominal mass. It was notable that the upper edge of the mass was not palpable as it extended under the rib cage.

tumor markers such as AFP and HCG are usually negative or slightly elevated, they should be measured preoperatively (see Table 18-4, and Fig. 18–13) (88,89).

Management in our institution involves preoperative imaging, testing for serum tumor markers, and a consultation with a pediatric oncologist. The surgical approach is a vertical midline skin incision, with standard staging procedure for ovarian cancer.

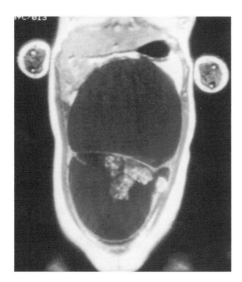

FIG. 18-16. MR image of the patient shown in Fig. 18-8. (Courtesy of Carol Barnewolt, M.D., Children's Hospital Boston)

After the pelvic washings, a unilateral salpingo-oophorectomy, distal omentectomy, and Papanicolaou test of the diaphragm, pelvic, and periaortic lymph node sampling are performed by a gynecologic oncologist or a pediatric surgeon (Fig. 18-17A and B). The malignancy is staged according to the modified FIGO staging classification for germ cell tumors (Table 18-7). Immature teratomas are graded based on a histol-

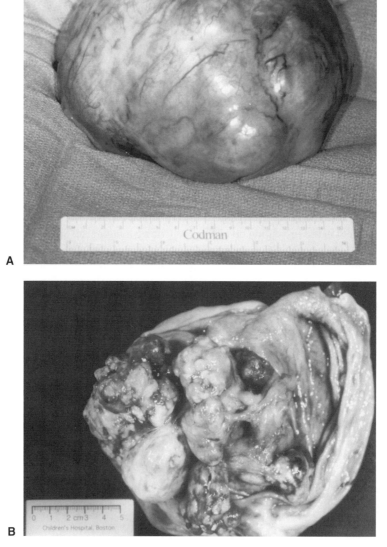

FIG. 18-17. A and **B:** Gross pathology of a large ovarian mass (immature teratoma) removed from a 9-year-old girl with increasing abdominal girth and a palpable abdominal mass.

TABLE 18-8. *Grading of immature ovarian teratomas*

Grade 0	All tissues mature; no mitotic activity
Grade 1	Some immaturity but with neuroepithelium absent or limited to one low-magnification field; no more than one focus in a slide
Grade 2	Immaturity present; neuroepithelium common but no more than three low-power microscopic fields in one slide
Grade 3	Immaturity and neuroectoderm prominent; no more than four low-power fields per section

[From: Norris HJ, Zirkin HJ, Benson WL. Immature (malignant) teratoma of the ovary: a clinical and pathologic study of 58 cases. *Cancer* 1976;37:2359–2372; with permission.]

ogy grading system (Table 18-8) (136), with grade 1 being the most differentiated (with the least risk of malignancy) and grade 3 being the least differentiated (with the greatest malignant potential). The immature component considered most important for grading is the neural component. Peritoneal implantation of mature glial tissue (gliomatosis peritonea) is thought to be a separate and distinct entity, does not represent malignant spread, and, if present, does not change the stage of the tumor (137,138). The grade and stage of the disease are determined by the final pathologic evaluation. Tumor size, stage, and histologic grade are factors in predicting survival (136,139–141). In the Air Force study of 1972 (142), all patients with tumors smaller than 10 cm at greatest dimension survived regardless of stage or grade. The survival rate fell to 67% for tumors 10 to 19.9 cm and to 54% for tumors larger than 20 cm. With pure immature teratomas, it has been observed that 5-year survival is based on stage (74% survival for all grades of stage I and 38% survival for stages II and III) and histologic grade (grade I, 81%; grade II, 60%; grade III, 30%) (136,140). Chromosomal analysis of the tumor suggests that immature ovarian teratomas of premeiotic origin show a greater malignant potential (143) and deviations in karyotype suggest a worse prognosis (144,145).

The current recommended therapy for immature teratomas from the Pediatric Oncology Group and the Children's Cancer Group has evolved (146). The report states that surgery alone is curative for most children and adolescents with resected ovarian immature teratoma of any grade, even when elevated levels of serum AFP or microscopic foci of yolk sac tumor are present. Their experience strongly supports avoiding chemotherapy in most children and reserving postoperative therapy for cases of relapse (146). If a serum tumor marker is positive, it can be followed pre- and postoperatively to detect early recurrence. Unilateral salpingo-oophorectomy and staging procedure is the treatment of choice. The prognosis for patients with higher stages has improved significantly in the last 20 years with the use of adjuvant chemotherapy (5,54,147,148). Most trials utilizing chemotherapy use a multiagent approach (Table 18-9) (138,139,149–154). In patients treated with surgery and who have a recurrence, the response to chemotherapy is excellent (138,146). In a report of 10 years' experience of 32 prospectively treated patients with pure immature teratoma, 30 patients had fertility-sparing surgery and were treated with chemotherapy only if they had stage I or II grade 3 or stage III disease; 10 patients who were initially

TABLE 18-9. *Examples of multiagent combination chemotherapy regimens (given in cycles intravenously every 3–4 weeks)[a]*

VAC	Vincristine
	Actinomycin
	Cyclophosphamide
PVB	Cisplatin
	Vinblastine
	Bleomycin
BEP	Cisplatin
	Etoposide
	Bleomycin
EP	Etoposide
	Cisplatin

[a]These regimens are provided as informational background; specific chemotherapy and dosages for individual patients should be determined by a medical or gynecologic oncologist.

treated with surgery alone relapsed and were treated with chemotherapy (138). Long-term follow-up studies of patients with malignant germ cell tumors report that the majority have normal menstrual function and a reasonable probability of having normal reproductive outcomes (155–157).

Dysgerminoma   Dysgerminoma is a malignant tumor derived from the primordial, sexually undifferentiated germ cells (see Fig. 18-13). Dysgerminoma accounts for 1% of all ovarian cancers and for 50% of all ovarian germ cell malignancies (158). In the Children's Hospital Boston series, the average age of patients was 14 years (range, 6.5 to 21 years) (5). Dysgerminoma has the same histology as seminoma in males. As mentioned above, it can occur in phenotypic females with abnormal karyotypes (pure gonadal dysgenesis—46,XY; mixed gonadal dysgenesis-45X/46XY; or complete androgen insensitivity—46XY) and abnormal gonads containing gonadoblastomas (131). Several cases of dysgerminoma have also been reported in girls with Turner syndrome, one of whom had male-specific sequences of the Y chromosome detected by DNA probes (159). The symptoms and signs associated with the tumor are similar to those discussed for other germ cell tumors. Rarely (2%), a pure dysgerminoma will contain syncytiotrophoblastic cells and produce low levels of HCG (160). In many instances, tumor cells are mixed with other cell types that may also produce HCG. LDH is elevated in some patients with dysgerminoma, and can also be helpful in postoperative follow-up (54,91,161). Other tumor markers such as AFP and CEA should be measured, although they are usually negative.

Management   At surgery, the tumor appears grossly as a lobulated, solid, yellow-white mass. Most patients (50%) with dysgerminoma have stage I disease, and thus surgery alone is adequate for cure (158,162). The mass should be removed intact, and an adequate staging procedure performed. A conservative surgical approach with unilateral salpingo-oophorectomy is usually undertaken in young women with stage IA tumors (<10 cm, removed unruptured, without evidence of metastatic spread) (54). Approximately 8% to 15% of dysgerminomas are bilateral, and thus the contralateral ovary is closely inspected, and any suspicious areas are biopsied (163). If there is bilateral ovarian involvement, then the uterus can be left *in situ* for reproduction options with donor oocytes and assisted reproductive technologies. Since the spread of this tumor is usually lymphatic with early involvement of pelvic and paraaortic lymph nodes followed by mediastinal and supraclavicular nodes, ipsilateral pelvic and paraaortic lymph nodes should be sampled to adequately stage the patient. Staging is critical for determining therapy and prognosis (162). In addition, some studies have shown a benefit with chromosomal analysis of the tumor in that deviations in karyotype suggest a worse prognosis (145).

All patients with greater than stage I disease should undergo cytoreductive surgery with removal of all operable tumor and require additional multiagent chemotherapy (158,162,164,165). The 10-year survival rates for patients with dysgerminoma confined to one ovary and treated with surgery alone was shown to be 92%; however, there was a 17% recurrence rate and a 6% mortality (163). The 5-year survival rate for patients with dysgerminoma confined to one or both ovaries is excellent (80% to 96%), and two-thirds of those with recurrences can be successfully treated later with radiation (5,54). Dysgerminoma is extremely radiosensitive; however, radiation therapy has adverse effects on reproductive endocrine function and fertility (see Chapter 23) and historically was reserved for cases of metastatic disease or recurrence (54,165). Because these tumors occur in young women and reproductive preservation is of great importance, multiagent chemotherapy (see Table 18-9) has replaced radiation therapy as the treatment of choice of advanced disease and appears helpful in preserving reproductive potential (82,152,153,155,158,162, 166–169). The 5-year survival of patients with dysgerminoma with extraovarian spread drops to 63%. Patients with advanced or bilateral disease should have abdominal hysterectomy, bilateral salpingo-oophorectomy, nodal biopsies, omental biopsy, and tumor debulking (54). A dysgerminoma with mixed elements of endodermal sinus tumor has an increased malignant potential and poorer prognosis.

Endodermal Sinus Tumor   Endodermal sinus tumor (EST), also termed *yolk sac tumor*, is of extraembryonic germ cell origin (see Fig. 18-13). It is rare, usually reported as 5% of malignant ovarian tumors, but in our series ranked second in frequency among germ cells tumors (5). The average age of our patients was 10 years (range, 18 months to 16 years), while other series have shown the average age at presentation to be 19 years (170,171). Endodermal sinus tumor is usually very aggressive, and patients usually seek medical attention rapidly due to abdominal pain (5). The serum tumor marker AFP can be useful during preoperative evaluation, as most of these tumors have a positive result, and can be used to follow the course of therapy. An unusual case of ataxia-telangiectasia and endodermal sinus tumor has been reported, emphasizing the association of both conditions with abnormal production of AFP (172). Yolk sac tumors are usually unilateral stage I (170,171), and thus appropriate surgery is a staging exploratory laparotomy with unilateral salpingo-oophorectomy. Intraperitoneal and hematogenous spread is common. The histology reveals Schiller-Duval bodies (a central capillary surrounded by simple papillary projections). Unlike dysgerminoma, these tumors are not radiosensitive (170,171), and prior to the use of multiagent chemotherapy they were usually uniformly fatal. Long-term outcomes have improved for patients with stage I tumor treated with unilateral salpingo-oophorectomy followed by aggressive chemotherapy (152–155,165,167,168,173–175). Unlike the highly treatable dysgerminoma, the EST can exhibit rapid lymphatic and peritoneal spread and has a propensity for metastases to the liver, lung and CNS; this aggressive nature accounts for the 15% survival rate (82).

Embryonal Carcinoma   Embryonal cell carcinoma (see Fig. 18-13) is a highly malignant and very rare germ cell tumor (176). In 60% of cases, the tumor is hormonally active and may produce precocious puberty in the child and menstrual irregularity or hirsutism in the adolescent (176). The markers AFP and HCG may be secreted by this tumor. It is rarely bilateral and tends to spread intraperitoneally. Standard staging laparotomy with unilateral salpingo-oophorectomy should be performed. Postoperative chemotherapy has been shown to be useful in reducing the likelihood of recurrence (162,165,173,175). This tumor is less aggressive than the EST, although it is still lethal, with a 50% survival rate for stage I disease (82).

Polyembryoma   This is a very rare tumor of germ cell origin (see Fig. 18-13) that usually presents in premenarchal patients. Elevated levels of both AFP and HCG have been documented (177). Prognosis is poor, as chemotherapy has only rarely induced remission.

Choriocarcinoma   Pure ovarian choriocarcinoma may develop without an association with a gestation. Although rare, this is a very aggressive tumor. As with gestational choriocarcinoma, HCG is an accurate tumor marker (178). Multiagent chemotherapy (see Table 18-9) is used in the treatment after surgical resection and staging (1,2,54,152,153,162). The nongestational form of choriocarcinoma, which appears in the brain or mediastinum as well as the gonads, is usually fatal (82).

Mixed Germ Cell Tumors   A mixed germ cell tumor consists of two or more germ cell tumors and usually has a prognosis based on the "worst" cell element. These tumors usually present as stage I disease, and the mean age at presentation is 16 years (179). Tumor markers should be measured, since HCG, AFP, and sometimes LDH are elevated. Appropriate surgical therapy includes a staging laparotomy with unilateral salpingo-oophorectomy. Postoperative multiagent chemotherapy (see

Table 18-9) is selected based on the pathologic elements identified (153,162,165, 179,180).

Non-Germ Cell Tumors

Sex Cord-Stromal Tumors

Thecoma-fibroma   Thecoma-fibroma is rare in the pediatric age group. Thecoma is uncommon before age 30. Fibromas account for less than 2% of all ovarian tumors of children and young women (181). Thecoma-fibroma is benign. Fibromas with ascites and pleural effusions (Meigs syndrome) have been seen in children. Gorlin syndrome is an autosomal-dominant disorder consisting of ovarian fibroma, basal cell nevi, dental cysts, and skeletal abnormalities. A thecoma can be hormonally active and produce estrogen, although there is a report of a testosterone-producing thecoma (182). It is highly unusual for this tumor to be malignant.

Sclerosing Stromal Tumor   Sclerosing stromal tumor (SST) of the ovary is a rare (approximately 100 cases reported in the literature), benign tumor that is distinct from the thecoma-fibroma group because of a predominant occurrence below age 30, lack of hormonal manifestations, and histologic heterogeneity (183,184). The youngest patient to date is 10 years of age (184). Imaging with ultrasound and CT is helpful. Conservative surgical resection is the treatment.

Granulosa Cell Tumors   Tumors of sex cord–stromal cell origin make up 10% to 20% of childhood ovarian tumors. Malignancy is related to the proportion of granulosa cells present; the pure granulosa cell tumors are highly malignant, mixed tumors are less so, and the pure thecoma is benign (82). Approximately one-half are hormonally active. Granulosa cell tumors are divided into adult and juvenile subtypes (Table 18-10) (185). Juvenile granulosa cell tumors secrete estrogen and in the young child may therefore produce pseudoprecocious puberty with breast enlargement and vaginal bleeding (186). In 2 of 10 patients in our series, pubic hair and clitoral enlargement were also noted (186). In the adolescent, these tumors may cause menstrual irregularities, including hypermenorrhea. Juvenile granulosa cell tumors have a more favorable prognosis than the typical adult tumor (5,54,185–190). Since less than 5% of tumors are bilateral, unilateral salpingo-oophorectomy with appropriate staging is usually adequate since almost all children have stage IA tumors (5,82,189,191,192). Call-Exner bodies are pathognomonic of the adult granulosa cell tumor but are rare in the juvenile type (185). Bilateral oophorectomy, chemotherapy, and/or radiation therapy have not been shown to improve outcome in patients with stage I disease (186). Postoperatively, estrogen levels and vaginal maturation index should return to normal prepubertal levels in young girls. Serum inhibin levels are helpful in follow-up for determining recurrent disease. Prognosis is excellent, with

TABLE 18-10. *Comparison of adult granulosa cell tumors (GCT) and juvenile GCT*

Adult GCT	Juvenile GCT
<1% prepubertal	50% prepubertal
Usual after age 30 years	Rare after age 30 years
Follicles usually regular, without mucin	Follicles often irregular, contain mucin
Call-Exner bodies common	Call-Exner bodies rare
Nuclei pale, commonly grooved	Nuclei dark, rarely grooved
Luteinization infrequent	Luteinization frequent
Recurrence rarely early, often very late	Recurrence typically early

(From Young RH, Dickersin GR, Scully RE. Juvenile granulosa cell tumor of the ovary: a clinicopathologic analysis of 125 cases. *Am J Surg Pathol* 1984;8:575–596; with permission.)

84% to 92% survival. More advanced disease may be treated with multiagent chemotherapy (189,193).

Sertoli-Leydig Cell Tumors   Sertoli–Leydig cell tumor was previously termed androblastoma or arrhenoblastoma, and is rare, accounting for less than 0.5% of all malignant ovarian neoplasms in children (82). The spectrum of Sertoli cell tumors in children covers a wide range of testis and ovarian tumors classified as sex cord-stromal tumors (194). In our pediatric series, the average age at diagnosis was 13 years (range, 5 to 17 years) (5). This tumor may secrete 17-hydroxyprogesterone, testosterone, and androstenedione producing heterosexual precocity in young children and hirsutism or virilization in adolescents (195). These girls or young women may present with oligomenorrhea, amenorrhea, breast asymmetry, hirsutism, deepening voice, male pattern baldness, acne, and clitoral enlargement. Two adolescents have been reported to have elevated levels of serum AFP, which initially suggested endodermal sinus tumor, but AFP returned to undetectable levels after surgery for Sertoli-Leydig cell tumor (196). Prognosis is dependent on the stage and degree of differentiation of the tumor; in most cases, it is a low-grade malignant tumor. Unilateral salpingo-oophorectomy and staging are important; prognosis is usually good. For advanced, metastatic, or recurrent disease, multiagent chemotherapy is utilized (197).

Gynandroblastoma   Gynandroblastoma is a rare ovarian tumor consisting of both male and female sex cord cells. It may cause premature breast development in girls and either hyperestrogenism or hyperandrogenism in adolescents (198–200).

Sex Cord Tumors with Annular Tubules   Sex cord tumors with annular tubules (SCTAT) have been associated with Peutz-Jeghers syndrome (gastrointestinal polyposis and oral cutaneous pigmentation), a condition also associated with adenocarcinoma of the cervix (198).

"Epithelial" (Coelomic) Tumors

Epithelial ovarian tumors account for approximately 15% of all pediatric ovarian masses. In a study of 240 ovarian masses in children, 16.2% were epithelial in origin (201). Of these tumors in Morowitz's study, 47% were serous cystadenomas, 16% were mucinous cystadenoma, 16% mucinous cystadenocarcinoma, and 21% serous tumors of borderline malignancy.

Benign Epithelial Tumors

Cystadenoma, an epithelial tumor filled with pseudomucinous (pseudomucinous cystadenoma) or cystic fluid (serous cystadenoma), accounts for 10% to 20% of ovarian tumors. In most cases, it is diagnosed after menarche, and the youngest patient in our series was 11.5 years old (5).

Borderline and Malignant Epithelial Tumors

Cystadenoma is usually benign, with about 7% being borderline and 4% malignant (202–205). Conservative surgery with unilateral salpingo-oophorectomy is appropriate for stage IA borderline tumors involving only one ovary in order to preserve future fertility (201–209). Biopsy of the contralateral ovary (with serous cystadenoma or if the ovary appears suspicious in cases of mucinous cystadenoma) and staging are important. Careful and prolonged follow-up is essential since recurrences may appear many years later. Tumors of borderline malignancy have a more favorable prognosis than higher-grade carcinomas (202–206,210). Long-term follow-up has shown that fertility interventions (ovulation induction and IVF) can be utilized if needed in survivors of borderline ovarian tumors (211).

In the rare invasive tumor, patients with other than stage IA should be managed, in similar fashion to adult women, with a staging laparotomy, cytoreductive surgery, and multiagent chemotherapy (212,213). With conservative management of stage II or III borderline ovarian tumors, fertility can be preserved (214).

Genetic Predisposition to Epithelial Ovarian Cancers

Families have been identified with increased rates of epithelial ovarian and breast cancers; affected individuals have been found to have a deletion of chromosome 17 in the q21–q23 region suggestive of a tumor suppressor gene (215–217) (see Chapter 19). This finding of genetic abnormalities initially related to an increased risk of breast cancer has been named breast cancer gene-1 (BRCA-1). It has been suggested that this gene may be mutated in 1 in 800 American women. An estimated 5% of ovarian cancer before age 70 years is associated with mutations in BRCA-1 (218). Of those carrying the BRCA-1 mutation, the ovarian cancer risk has been estimated to be 26% to

85% by age 70 years (219,220), although a more recent analysis found a lower risk of 16% (221). The BRCA-1 frameshift gene mutation (185delAG) in Ashkenazi Jewish women is believed to occur at a carrier frequency of 1% and to account for approximately 39% of ovarian cancer cases occurring prior to age 50 years (222). Ovarian cancer developed in 20% of women of Ashkenazi descent with the 185delAG mutation, as compared with none of the Jewish women without the mutation (223). Provisional recommendations for women with BRCA-1 mutations, published in 1997, included annual or semiannual screening using transvaginal ultrasonography (ideally with color flow Doppler and a morphologic index) and serum CA-125 levels beginning at age 25 to 35 years. These recommendations have been based on expert opinion and thus the efficacy has not been proved (220). However, since no surveillance regimen has been shown to be effective, prophylactic oophorectomy as soon as childbearing has been completed has been advocated (224). Salpingo-oophorectomy can reduce the risk of breast cancer and other gynecologic cancers; however, primary peritoneal cancers can occur (225). There are vast psychosocial issues and implications of testing for young women in families with this genetic gene defect (226–229).

Familial ovarian cancer centers currently exist in many locations throughout the world and provide families with genetic counseling and screening for both ovarian and breast cancer. Clinicians caring for adolescents will need to be involved in decision making with their patients to make the best use of the emerging genetic technology without increasing anxiety in these young women and their families. The optimal age for offering genetic testing has not been determined, but in general, genetic testing is best undertaken at earliest in young adulthood when the findings may alter screening strategies and follow-up.

Other Tumors

Lipid Cell Tumor

Lipid (lipoid) cell tumor is rare (230,231). Wentz and co-workers (232) reported a 17-year-old adolescent with hirsutism and oligomenorrhea in association with a lipid cell tumor.

Fibrosarcoma

Fibrosarcomas and undifferentiated sarcomas are rare and rapidly fatal.

Metastatic Disease to the Ovary

Tumors can be metastatic to the ovary. Lymphoma may occur as a primary ovarian tumor (233), or metastatic to the ovary. Rarely, leukemia will relapse with ovarian enlargement simulating an ovarian tumor (142,234). Gastric carcinoma has also been shown to be metastatic to the ovary (235).

REFERENCES

1. Breen JL, Maxson WS. Ovarian tumors in children and adolescents. *Clin Obstet Gynecol* 1977;20:607.
2. Breen JL, Bonamo JF, Maxson WS. Genital tract tumors in children. *Pediatr Clin North Am* 1981;28:355.
3. Serov SF, Scully RE, Sobin LH. *International histological classification of tumours. No. 9. Histologic typing of ovarian tumours.* Geneva: World Health Organization, 1973.
4. Rice LW, Barbieri RL. The ovary. In: Ryan RJ, Berkowitz RS, Barbieri RL, eds. *Kistner's gynecology,* 6th ed. Boston: Mosby-Year Book, 1995;187.
5. Lack EE, Goldstein DP. Primary ovarian tumors in childhood and adolescence. *Curr Probl Obstet Gynecol* 1984;8:1.
6. Nussbaum AR, Sanders RC, Hartman DS, et al. Neonatal ovarian cysts: sonographic-pathologic correlation. *Radiology* 1988;168:817.
7. Lindeque BG, du Toit J, Muller LM, et al. Ultrasonographic criteria for the conservative management of antenatally diagnosed fetal ovarian cysts. *J Reprod Med* 1988;33:196.
8. Brandt ML, Luks FI, Filiatrault D, et al. Surgical indications in antenatally diagnosed ovarian cysts. *J Pediatr Surg* 1991;26:276.
9. Bryant AE, Laufer MR. Fetal ovarian cysts: incidence, diagnosis and management. *J Reprod Med* 2004;49:329.
10. Kirkinen P, Jouppila P. Perinatal aspects of pregnancy complicated by fetal ovarian cyst. *J Perinat Med* 1985;13:245.
11. Speroff L, Glass RH, Kase NG. *Clinical gynecologic endocrinology and infertility,* 6th ed. Philadelphia: Williams & Wilkins, 1999.
12. Case records of the Massachusetts General Hospital. *N Engl J Med* 1995;332:522.
13. Bower R, Delmer LP, Ternberg JL. Bilateral ovarian cysts in the newborn: a triad of neonatal abdominal masses, polyhydramnios, and maternal diabetes mellitus. *Am J Dis Child* 1974;128:731.
14. Nguyen KT, Reid RL, Sauerbrei E. Antenatal sonographic detection of a fetal theca lutein cyst: a clue to maternal diabetes mellitus. *J Ultrasound Med* 1986;5:665.
15. Spence JEH, Domingo M, Pike C. The resolution of fetal and neonatal ovarian cysts. *Adolesc Pediatr Gynecol* 1992;5:27.
16. Murray S, London S. Management of ovarian cysts in neonates, children, and adolescents. *Adolesc Pediatr Gynecol* 1995;8:64.
17. Bagolan P, Giorlandino C, Nahom A, et al. The management of fetal ovarian cysts. *J Pediatr Surg* 2002;37:25.
18. Siegel M. Pediatric gynecologic sonography. *Radiology* 1991;179:593.
19. Armentano G, Dodero P, Natta A, et al. Fetal ovarian cysts: prenatal diagnosis and management. Report of two cases and review of literature. *Clin Exp Obstet Gynecol* 1998;25:88.
20. Giorlandino C, Bilancioni E, Bagolan P, et al. Antenatal ultrasonographic diagnosis and management of fetal ovarian cysts. *Int J Gynaecol Obstet* 1994;44:27.
21. Perrotin F, Potin J, Haddad G, et al. Fetal ovarian cysts: a report of three cases managed by intrauterine aspiration. *Ultrasound Obstet Gynecol* 2000;16:655.
22. Luzzatto C, Midrio P, Toffolutti T, et al. Neonatal ovarian cysts: management and follow-up. *Pediatr Surg Int* 2000;16:56.
23. Meizner I, Levy A, Katz M, et al. Fetal ovarian cysts: prenatal ultrasonographic detection and postnatal evaluation and treatment. *Am J Obstet Gynecol* 1991;164:874.
24. Teele RL, Share JC. The abdominal mass in the neonate. *Semin Roetgenol* 1988;23:175.
25. Croitoru DP, Aaton LE, Laberge JM, et al. Management of complex ovarian cysts presenting in the first year of life. *J Pediatr Surg* 1991;26:1366.
26. Crombleholme TM, Craigo SD, Garmel S, et al. Fetal ovarian cyst decompression to prevent torsion. *J Pediatr Surg* 1997;32:1447.
27. Mizuno M, Kato T, Hebiguchi T, et al. Surgical indications for neonatal ovarian cysts. *Tohoku J Exp Med* 1998;186:27.
28. Dolgin SE. Ovarian masses in the newborn. *Semin Pediatr Surg* 2000;9:121.
29. Chiaramonte C, Piscopo A, Cataliotti F. Ovarian cysts in newborns. *Pediatr Surg Int* 2001;17:171.
30. Schultz R, Newton WA, Clatworthy HW. Torsion of previously normal tube and ovary in children. *N Engl J Med* 1963;268:343.

31. Worthington-Kirsch R, Raptopoulos V, Cohen I. Sequential bilateral torsion of normal ovaries in a child. *J Ultrasound Med* 1986;5:663.
32. Davis AJ, Feins NR. Subsequent asynchronous torsion of normal adnexa in children. *J Pediatr Surg* 1990;25:687.
33. Shalev E, Mann S, Romano S, et al. Laparoscopic detorsion of adnexa in childhood: a case report. *J Pediatr Surg* 1991;26:1193.
34. van der Zee DC, van Seumeren IGC, Bax KMA, et al. Laparoscopic approach to surgical management of ovarian cysts in the newborn. *J Pediatr Surg* 1995;30:42.
35. Esposito C, Garipoli V, DiMatteo G, et al. Laparoscopic management of ovarian cysts in newborns. *Surg Endosc* 1998;12:1152.
36. Templeman CL, Reynolds AM, Hertweck SP, et al. Laparoscopic management of neonatal ovarian cysts. *J Am Assoc Gynecol Laparosc* 2000;7:401.
37. Colby C, Brindle M, Mass RL. Minimally invasive laparotomy for treatment of neonatal ovarian cysts. *J Pediatr Surg* 2001;36:693.
38. Ferro F, Iacobelli BD, Zaccara A, et al. Exteriorization-aspiration minilaparotomy for treatment of neonatal ovarian cysts. *J Pediatr Adolesc Gynecol* 2002;15:205.
39. Landrum B, Ogburn PL, Feinberg S, et al. Intrauterine aspiration of a large fetal ovarian cyst. *Obstet Gynecol* 1986;68(suppl):11S.
40. Salkala E, Leon Z, Rouse G. Management of antenatally diagnosed fetal ovarian cysts. *Obstet Gynecol Surv* 1991;46:407.
41. Cohen HL, Eisenberg P, Mandel F, et al. Ovarian cysts are common in premenarchal girls: a sonographic study of 101 children 2–12 years old. *AJR* 1992;159:89.
42. Cohen HL, Shapiro MA, Mandel FS, et al. Normal ovaries in neonates and infants: a sonographic study of 77 patients 1 day to 24 months. *AJR* 1993;160:583.
43. Kosloske AM, Goldthorn JF, Kaufman E, et al. Treatment of precocious pseudopuberty associated with follicular cysts of the ovary. *Am J Dis Child* 1984;138:147.
44. Chasalow Fl, Granoff AB, Tse TF, et al. Adrenal steroid secretion in girls with pseudoprecocious puberty due to autonomous ovarian cysts. *J Clin Endocrinol Metab* 1986;63:828.
45. Freedman SM, Kreitzer PM, Elkowitz SS, et al. Ovarian microcysts in girls with isolated premature thelarche. *J Pediatr* 1993;122:246.
46. Millar DM, Blake JM, Stringer DA, et al. Prepubertal ovarian cyst formation: 5 years' experience. *Obstet Gynecol* 1993;81:434.
47. Frisch LS, Copeland KC, Boepple PA. Recurrent ovarian cysts in childhood: diagnosis of McCune-Albright syndrome by bone scan. *Pediatrics* 1992;90:102.
48. Arisaka O, Shimura N, Nakayama Y, et al. Ovarian cysts in precocious puberty. *Clin Pediatr* 1989; 28:44.
49. Van Winter JT, Simmons PS, Podratz KC. Surgically treated adnexal masses in infancy, childhood, and adolescence. *Am J Obstet Gynecol* 1994;170:1780.
50. Warner B, Kuhn J, Barr L. Conservative management of large ovarian cysts in children: the value of serial pelvic ultrasonography. *Surgery* 1992;112:749.
51. Thind CR, Carty HM, Pilling D. The role of ultrasound in the management of ovarian masses in children. *Clin Radiol* 1989;40:180.
52. Cass DL, Hawkins E, Brandt ML, et al. Surgery for ovarian masses in infants, children, and adolescents: 102 consecutive patients treated in a 15-year period. *J Pediatr Surg* 2001;36:693.
53. Diamond M, Baxter J, Peerman C, et al. Occurrence of ovarian malignancy in childhood and adolescence: a community-wide evaluation. *Obstet Gynecol* 1988;17:858.
54. Kennedy AW. Ovarian neoplasms in childhood and adolescence. *Semin Reprod Endocrinol* 1988; 6: 79.
55. Goldstein DP, deCholnoky C, Emans SJ, et al. Laparoscopy in the diagnosis and management of pelvic pain in adolescents. *J Reprod Med* 1980;24:251.
56. Mettler L, Irani S, Semm K. Ovarian surgery via pelviscopy. *J Reprod Med* 1993;38:130.
57. Lipitz S, Seidman DS, Menczer J, et al. Recurrence rates after fluid aspiration from sonographically benign-appearing ovarian cysts. *J Reprod Med* 1992;37:845.
58. Mordehai A, Mares Y, Bakri R, et al. Torsion of uterine adnexa in neonates and children: a report of 20 cases. *J Pediatr Surg* 1991;26:1195.
59. Albayram F, Hamper UM. Ovarian and adnexal torsion: spectrum of sonographic findings with pathologic correlation. *J Ultrasound Med* 2001;20:1083.

60. Ben-Ami M, Perlitz Y, Haddad S, et al. The effectiveness of spectral and color Doppler in predicting ovarian torsion. A prospective study. *Eur J Obstet Gynecol Reprod Biol* 2002;104:64.
61. Cohen SB, Oelsner G, Seidman DS, et al. Laparoscopic detorsion allows sparing of the twisted ischemic adnexa. *J Am Assoc Gynecol Laparosc* 1999;6:139.
62. Panksy M, Abargil A, Dreazen E, et al. Laparoscopic detorsion allows sparing of the twisted ischemic adnexa. *J Am Assoc Gynecol Laparosc* 2000;7:121.
63. Cohen SB, Wattiez A, Seidman DS, et al. Laparoscopy versus laparotomy for detorsion and sparing of twisted ischemic adnexa. *JSLS* 2003;7:295.
64. Kokoska ER, Keller MS, Weber TR. Acute ovarian torsion in children. *Am J Surg* 2000;180:462.
65. Houry D, Abbott J. Ovarian torsion: A fifteen-year review. *Ann Emerg Med* 2001;38:1.
66. McGee DM, Connolly SA, Young RH. Case 24-2003: A 10 year old girl with recurrent bouts of abdominal pain. *N Engl J Med* 2003;349:486.
67. Gordon JD, Hopkins KL, Jeffrey RB, et al. Adnexal torsion: color Doppler diagnosis and laparoscopic treatment. *Fertil Steril* 1994;61:383.
68. Mage G, Canis M, Marshes H, et al. Laparoscopic management of adnexal torsion: a review of 35 cases. *J Reprod Med* 1989;34:520.
69. Shalev E, Peleg D. Laparoscopic treatment of adnexal torsion. *Surg Gynecol Obstet* 1993;176:448.
70. Eckler K, Laufer MR, Perlman SE. Conservative management of bilateral asynchronous adnexal torsion with necrosis in a prepubescent female. *J Pediatr Surgery* 2000;35:1248.
71. Styer AK, Laufer MR. Ovarian bivalving after detorsion. *Fertil Steril* 2002;7:1053.
72. Templeman C, Hertweck SP, Fallat ME. The clinical course of unresected ovarian torsion. *J Pediatr Surg* 2000;35:1385.
73. Laufer MR, Billett A, Diller L et al. A new technique for laparoscopic prophylactic oophoropexy prior to craniospinal irradiation in children with medulloblastoma. *Adolesc Pediatr Gynecol* 1995;8:77.
74. Wilson DA. Ultrasound screening for abdominal masses in the neonatal period. *Am J Dis Child* 1982; 136:147.
75. Wu A, Siegel MJ. Sonography of pelvic masses in children: diagnostic predictability. *AJR* 1987; 148: 1199.
76. Fleischer AC. Transabdominal and transvaginal sonography of ovarian masses. *Clin Obstet Gynecol* 1991;34:433.
77. Helmrath M, Shin C, Warner B. Ovarian cysts in pediatric population. *Semin Pediatr Surg* 1998;7:19.
78. Heling KS, Chaoui R, Kirchmair F, et al. Fetal ovarian cysts: prenatal diagnosis, management and postnatal outcome. *Ultrasound Obstet Gynecol* 2002;20:47.
79. Kawai M, Kano T, Kikkawa F, et al. Transvaginal Doppler ultrasound with color flow imaging in the diagnosis of ovarian cancer. *Obstet Gynecol* 1992;79:163.
80. Weiner Z, Thaler I, Beck D, et al. Differentiating malignant from benign ovarian tumors, with transvaginal color flow imaging. *Obstet Gynecol* 1992;79:159.
81. Timor-Tritsch IE, Lerner JP, MonteagudoA, et al. Transvaginal ultrasonographic characterization of ovarian masses by means of color flow-directed Doppler measurements and a morphologic scoring system. *Am J Obstet Gynecol* 1993;168:909.
82. Lazar E, Stolar C. Evaluation and management of pediatric solid ovarian tumors. *Semin Pediatr Surg* 1998;7:29.
83. Fedele L, Dorta M, Brioschi D, et al. Magnetic resonance evaluation of gynecologic masses in adolescents. *Adolesc Pediatr Gynecol* 1990;3:83.
84. Scoutt LM, McCarthy SM. Imaging of ovarian masses: magnetic resonance imaging. *Clin Obstet Gynecol* 1991;34:443.
85. Kim YH, Cho KS, Ha HK, et al. CT features of torsion of benign cystic teratoma of the ovary. *J Comput Assist Tomogr* 1999;23:923.
86. Pretorius ES, Outwater EK, Hunt JL, et al. Magnetic resonance imaging of the ovary. *Top Magn Reson Imaging* 2001;12:131.
87. Schwartz PE. Ovarian masses: serologic markers. *Clin Obstet Gynecol* 1991;34:423.
88. Perrone T, Steeper T, Delmer L. Alpha-fetoprotein localization in pure ovarian teratoma: an immunohistochemical study of 12 cases. *Am J Clin Pathol* 1987;88:713.
89. Kawai M, Furuhashi Y, Kano T, et al. Alpha-fetoprotein in malignant germ cell tumors of the ovary. *Gynecol Oncol* 1990;39:160.
90. Wu JT, Sudar K. Serum AFP levels in normal infants. *Pediatr Res* 1981;15:50.

91. Schwartz PE, Morris JMcL. Serum lactic dehydrogenase: a tumor marker for dysgerminoma. *Obstet Gynecol* 1989;32:191.

92. Bast RC, Klug TL, St. John E, et al. A radioimmunoassay using a monoclonal antibody to monitor the course of epithelial ovarian cancer. *N Engl J Med* 1983;309:883.

93. Rubal A, Encabo G, et al. CA-125 serum levels in non-malignant pathologies. *Bull Cancer (Paris)* 1988;71:751.

94. Kawata M, Sekiya S, Tamkamizawa H, et al. Molecular properties of F9 embryoglycan recognized by a unique antibody in sera from patients with germ cell tumors. *Cancer Res* 1987;47:2288.

95. Gustafson ML, Lee MM, Scully RE, et al. Müllerian inhibitory substance as a marker for ovarian sex cord tumor. *N Engl J Med* 1992;326:466.

96. Lappohn RE, Burger HG, Bouma J, et al. Inhibin as a marker for granulosa cell tumor. *Acta Obstet Gynecol Scand* (Suppl) 1992;155:61.

97. Elsheikh A, Milingos S, Kallipolitis G, et al. Ovarian tumors in young females. A laparoscopic approach. *Euro J Gynecol Oncol* 2001;22:243.

98. Piippo S, Mustaniemi L, Lenko H, et al. Surgery for ovarian masses during childhood and adolescence: a report of 79 cases. *J Pediatr Adolesc Gynecol* 1999;12:223.

99. Greene FL, Page DL, Fleming ID, et al. AJCC Cancer Staging Manuel, 6th Ed. New York: Springer-Verlag, 2002.

100. International Federation of Gynecology and Obstetrics (FIGO). Changes in definitions of clinical staging for carcinoma of the cervix and ovary. *Am J Obstet Gynecol* 1987;156:263.

101. Creasman WT. Changes in FIGO staging. *Obstet Gynecol* 1987;70:138.

102. International Federation of Gynecology and Obstetrics (FIGO). Annual report on the results of treatment in gynecological cancer. *Int J Gynaecol Obstet* 1989;28:189.

103. Creasman WT. New gynecologic cancer staging. *Obstet Gynecol* 1990;75:287.

104. International Federation of Gynecology and Obstetrics (FIGO). Changes in gynecologic cancer staging by the International Federation of Gynecology and Obstetrics. *Am J Obstet Gynecol* 1990; 162:610.

105. Heintz APM, Odicino F, Maisonneuve P, et al. Carcinoma of the ovary. *J Epidemiol Biostat* 2001;6:107.

106. Jerkins S, Olive DL, Haney AE. Endometriosis: pathogenetic implications of the anatomic distribution. *Obstet Gynecol* 1986;67:335.

107. Laufer MR, Sanfilippo J, Rose G. Adolescent endometriosis: diagnosis and treatment approaches. *J Pediatr Adolesc Gynecol* 2003;16:3.

108. Mais V, Guerriero S, Ajossa S, et al. The efficiency of transvaginal ultrasonography in the diagnosis of endometrioma. *Fertil Steril* 1993;60:776.

109. Wu XC, Chen VW, Steele B, et al. Cancer incidence in adolescents and young adults in the United States, 1992–1997. *J Adolesc Health* 2003;32:405.

110. Teilum G. Classification of endodermal sinus tumour (mesoblastoma vitellinum) and so-called embryonal carcinoma of the ovary. *Acta Pathol Microbiol Scand* 1965;64:407.

111. Templeman C, Fallat ME, Blinchevsky A, et al. Noninflammatory ovarian masses in girls and young women. *Obstet Gynecol* 2000;96:229.

112. Templeman CL, Hertweck SP, Scheetz JP, et al. The management of mature cystic teratomas in children and adolescents: a retrospective analysis. *Hum Reprod* 2000;15:2669.

113. Sisler CL, Siegel MJ. Ovarian teratomas: a comparison of the sonographic appearance in prepubertal arid postpubertal girls. *AJR* 1990;154:139.

114. Mais V, Guerriero S, Ajossa S, et al. Transvaginal ultrasonography in the diagnosis of cystic teratoma. *Obstet Gynecol* 1995;85:48.

115. Ayhan A, Aksu T, Develioglu O, et al. Complications and bilaterality of mature ovarian teratomas (clinicopathological evaluation of 286 cases). *Aust N Z J Obstet Gynaecol* 1991;31:83.

116. Howard FM. Surgical management of benign cystic teratoma: laparoscopy vs. laparotomy. *J Reprod Med* 1995;40:495.

117. Morgante G, Ditto A, La Marca A, et al. Surgical treatment of ovarian dermoid cysts. *Eur J Obstet Gynecol Reprod Biol* 1998;81:47.

118. Campo S, Garcea N. Laparoscopic conservative excision of ovarian dermoid cysts with and without an endobag. *J Am Assoc Gynecol Laparosc* 1998;5:165.

119. Zanetta G, Ferrari L, Mignini-Renzini M, et al. Laparoscopic excision of ovarian dermoid cysts with controlled intraoperative spillage. *J Reprod Med* 1999;44:815.

120. Nezhat CR, Nezhat FR, Metzger DA, et al. Adhesion reformation after reproductive surgery by videolaseroscopy. *Fertil Steril* 1990;53:1008.

121. Operative Laparoscopy Study Group. Postoperative adhesion development after operative laparoscopy: evaluation at early second-look procedures. *Fertil Steril* 1991;55:700.
122. Fiedler E, Guzick DS, Guido R, et al. Adhesion formation from release of dermoid contents in the peritoneal cavity and effect of copious lavage: a prospective, randomized, blinded, controlled study in a rabbit model. *Fertil Steril* 1996;65:852.
123. Maiman M, Seltzer V, Boyce J. Laparoscopic excision of ovarian neoplasms subsequently found to be malignant. *Obstet Gynecol* 1991;77:563.
124. Nezhat F, Nezhat C, Welander C, et al. Four ovarian cancers diagnosed during laparoscopic management of 1011 women with adnexal masses. *Am J Obstet Gynecol* 1992;167:790.
125. Canis M, Rabischong B, Botchorishvili R, et al. Risk of spread of ovarian cancer after laparoscopic surgery. *Curr Opin Obstet Gynecol* 2001;13:9.
126. Ayhan A, Yanki F, Tuncer R, et al. Struma ovarii. *Int J Gynecol Obstet* 1993;42:143.
127. Dunzendorfer T, de Las Morenas A, Kalir T, et al. Struma ovarii and hyperthyroidism. *Thyroid* 1999;9:499.
128. Young RH. New and unusual aspects of ovarian germ cell tumors. *Am J Surg Pathol* 1993; 17: 1210.
129. Scully RE. Gonadoblastoma: gonadal tumor related to dysgerminoma (seminoma) and capable of sex hormone production. *Cancer* 1953;6:455.
130. Scully RE. Gonadoblastoma: a review of 74 cases. *Cancer* 1970;25:1340.
131. Trochir V, Hernandez E. Neoplasia arising in dysgenetic gonads. *Obstet Gynecol Surv* 1988;41:74.
132. Droesch K, Droesch J, Chumas J, et al. Laparoscopic gonadectomy for gonadal dysgenesis. *Fertil Steril* 1990;53:360.
133. Shalev E, Zabari A, Romano S, et al. Laparoscopic gonadectomy in 46,XY female patient. *Fertil Steril* 1992;57:459.
134. Arici A, Kutteh WH, Chantilis SJ, et al. Laparoscopic removal of gonads in women with abnormal karyotypes. *J Reprod Med* 1993;38:521.
135. Quint EH, Smith YR. Ovarian surgery in premenarchal girls. *J Pediatr Adolesc Gynecol* 1999; 12:27.
136. Norris HJ, Zirkin HJ, Benson WL. Immature (malignant) teratoma of the ovary: a clinical and pathologic study of 58 cases. *Cancer* 1976;37:2359.
137. Nielsen SNJ, Scheithauer BW, Gaffey TA. Gliomatosis peritonea. *Cancer* 1985;56:2499.
138. Bonazzi C, Peccatori F, Colombo N, et al. Pure ovarian immature teratoma, a unique and curable disease: 10 years' experience of 32 prospectively treated patients. *Obstet Gynecol* 1994;84:598.
139. Ayhan A, Aksu T, Selcuk Tuncer Z, et al. Immature teratoma of the ovary. *Eur J Gynaecol Oncol* 1993;14:205.
140. O'Connor DM, Norris HJ. The influence of grade on the outcome of stage I ovarian immature (malignant) teratomas and the reproducibility of grading. *Int J Gynecol Pathol* 1994;13:283.
141. Ayhan A, Tuncer ZS, Yanik F, et al. Malignant germ cell tumors of the ovary: Hacettepe Hospital experience. *Acta Obstet Gynecol Scand* 1995;74:384.
142. Norris HJ, Jensen RD. Relative frequency of ovarian neoplasms in children and adolescents. *Cancer* 1972;30:713.
143. King ME, DiGiovanni LM, Yung JF, et al. Immature teratoma of the ovary grade 3, with karyotype analysis. *Int J Gynecol Pathol* 1990;9:178.
144. Ihara T, Ohama K, Satoh H, et al. Histologic grade and karyotype of immature teratoma of the ovary. *Cancer* 1984;54:2988.
145. Palmquist MB, Webb MJ, Lieber MM, et al. DNA ploidy of ovarian dysgerminomas: correlation with clinical outcome. *Gynecol Oncol* 1992;44:13.
146. Cushing B, Giller R, Ablin A, et al. Surgical resection alone is effective treatment for ovarian immature teratoma in children and adolescents: a report of the Pediatric Oncology Group and the Children's Cancer Group. *Am J Obstet Gynecol* 1999;181:353.
147. Pippin CH Jr, Cain JM, Hakes TB, et al. Primary chemotherapy and the role of second-look laparotomy in non-dysgerminomatous germ cell malignancies of the ovary. *Gynecol Oncol* 1988;31:268.
148. Ablin AR, Krailo MD, Ramsay NK, et al. Results of treatment of malignant germ cell tumors in 93 children: a report from the Children's Cancer Study Group. *J Clin Oncol* 1991;9:1782.
149. Nielsen SNJ, Gaffey TA, Malkasian GD. Immature ovarian teratoma: a review of 14 cases. *Mayo Clin Proc* 1986;61:110.
150. Gershenson DM, DelJunco G, Silva EG, et al. Immature teratoma of the ovary. *Obstet Gynecol* 1986;68:624.

151. Kouolos JP, Hoffman JS, Steinhoff MM. Immature teratoma of the ovary. *Gynecol Oncol* 1989;34:46.
152. Schwartz PE, Chambers SK, Chambers JT, et al. Ovarian germ cell malignancies: the Yale University experience. *Gynecol Oncol* 1992;45:26.
153. Schwartz PE. Combination chemotherapy in the management of ovarian germ cell malignancies. *Obstet Gynecol* 1984;64:564.
154. Wong LC, Ngan HYS, Ma HK. Primary treatment with vincristine, dactinomycin, and cyclophosphamide in nondysgerminomatous germ cell tumor of the ovary. *Gynecol Oncol* 1989;34:155.
155. Gershenson DM. Menstrual and reproductive function after treatment with combination chemotherapy for malignant ovarian germ cell tumors. *J Clin Oncol* 1988;6:270.
156. Wu PC Huang RL, Lang JH, et al. Treatment of malignant ovarian germ cell tumors with preservation of fertility: a report of 28 cases. *Gynecol Oncol* 1991;40:2.
157. Uzunlar AK, Yalinkaya A, Yaldiz M, et al. Survival and reproductive function after treatment of immature ovarian teratoma. *Euro J Gynecol Oncol* 2001;22:384.
158. Pawinski A, Favalli G, Ploch E, et al. PVB chemotherapy in patients with recurrent or advanced dysgerminoma: a Phase II study of the EORTC Gynaeological Cancer Cooperative Group. *Clin Oncol* 1998;10:301.
159. Shah KD, Kaffe S, Gilbert F, et al. Unilateral microscopic gonadoblastoma in a prepubertal Turner mosaic with Y chromosome material identified by restriction fragment analysis. *Am J Clin Pathol* 1988;90:622.
160. Kapp DS, Kohorn EL Merino MJ, et al. Pure dysgerminoma of the ovary with elevated serum human chorionic gonadotropin: diagnostic and therapeutic considerations. *Gynecol Oncol* 1985;20:234.
161. Pressley RI, Muntz HG, Falkenberry S, et al. Serum lactic dehydrogenase as a tumor marker in dysgerminoma. *Gynecol Oncol* 1992;44:281.
162. Suita S, Shono K, Tajiri T, et al. Malignant germ cell tumors: clinical characteristics, treatment, and outcome. A report from the study group for Pediatric Solid Malignant Tumors in the Kyushu Area, Japan. *J Pediatr Surg* 2002;37:1703.
163. Gordon A, Lipton D, Woodruff JD. Dysgerminoma: a review of 158 cases from the Emil Novak ovarian tumor registry. *Obstet Gynecol* 1981;58:497.
164. Thomas GM Dembo AJ, Hacker NF, et al. Current therapy for dysgerminoma of the ovary. *Obstet Gynecol* 1987;70:268.
165. Stern JW, Bunin N. Prospective study of carboplatin-based chemotherapy for pediatric germ cell tumors. *Med Pediatr Oncol* 2002;39:163.
166. Bjorkholm E, Lundell M, Gyftodimos A, et al. Dysgerminoma: the Radiumhemmet series 1927–1984. *Cancer* 1990;65:38.
167. Gershenson DM, Morris M, Cangir A, et al. Treatment of malignant germ cell tumors of the ovary with bleomycin, etoposide, and cisplatin. *J Clin Oncol* 1990;8:715.
168. Gershenson DM. Update on malignant ovarian germ cell tumors. *Cancer* 1993;71:1581.
169. Kanazawa K, Suzuki T, Sakumoto K. Treatment of malignant ovarian germ cell tumors with preservation of fertility: reproductive performance after persistent remission. *Am J Clin Oncol* 2000;23:244.
170. Kurman RJ, Norris HJ. Endodermal sinus tumor of the ovary: a clinical and pathologic analysis of 71 cases. *Cancer* 1976;38:2404.
171. Gershenson DM, DelJunco G, Herson J, et al. Endodermal sinus tumor of the ovary: the M. D. Anderson experience. *Obstet Gynecol* 1983;61:194.
172. Pecorelli S, Sartori E, Favalli G, et al. Ataxia-telangiectasia and endodermal sinus tumor of the ovary: report of a case. *Gynecol Oncol* 1988;29:240.
173. Williams SD, Birch R, Einhorn LH, et al. Treatment of disseminated germ-cell tumors with cisplatin, bleomycin, and either vinblastine or etoposide. *N Engl J Med* 1987;316:1435.
174. Athanikar N, Saikia TK, Ramkrishnan G, et al. Aggressive chemotherapy in endodermal sinus tumor. *J Surg Oncol* 1989;40:17.
175. Kawai M, Kano T, Furuhashi Y, et al. Prognostic factors in yolk sac tumors of the ovary: a clinicopathologic analysis of 29 cases. *Cancer* 1991;67:184.
176. Kurman RJ Norris HJ. Embryonal carcinoma of the ovary: a clinicopathologic entity distinct from endodermal sinus tumor resembling embryonal carcinoma of the adult testis. *Cancer* 1976;38:2420.
177. Takeda A, Ishizuka T, Goto S, et al. Polyembryoma of ovary producing alpha-fetoprotein and HCG: immunoperoxidase and electron microscopic study. *Cancer* 1982;49:1878.

178. Axe SR, Klein VR, Woodruff JD. Choriocarcinoma of the ovary. *Obstet Gynecol* 1985;66:111.
179. Gershenson DM DelJunco G, Copeland LJ, et al. Mixed germ cell tumors of the ovary. *Obstet Gynecol* 1984;64:200.
180. Carlson RW, Sikic BI, Turbow MM, et al. Cisplatin, vinblastine and bleomycin (PVB) therapy for ovarian germ cell tumors. *J Clin Oncol* 1983;1:645.
181. Bosch-Banyeras JM, Lucaya X, Bernet M, et al. Calcified ovarian fibroma in prepubertal girls. *Eur J Pediatr* 1989;148:749.
182. Givens JR, Andersen RN, Wiser WL, et al. A testosterone-screening gonadotropin-responsive pure thecoma and polycystic ovarian disease. *J Clin Endocrinol Metab* 1975;41:845.
183. Gupta S. Sclerosing stromal tumour of the ovary—a case report. *Ind J Pathol Microbiol* 1999;42:97.
184. Fefferman NR, Pinkney LP, Rivera R, et al. Sclerosing stromal tumor of the ovary in a premenarchal female. *Pediatr Radiol* 2003;33:56.
185. Young RH, Dickersin GR, Scully RE. Juvenile granulosa cell tumor of the ovary: a clinicopathologic analysis of 125 cases. *Am J Surg Pathol* 1984;8:575.
186. Lack EE, Perez-Atayde AR, Murthy ASK, et al. Granulosa theca cell tumors in premenarchal girls: a clinical and pathologic study of ten cases. *Cancer* 1981;48:1846.
187. Bjorkholm E, Silfversward C. Prognostic factors in granulosa-cell tumors. *Gynecol Oncol* 1981;11:261.
188. Biscotti CV, Kennedy AW. Ovarian juvenile granulosa cell tumors. *Adolesc Pediatr Gynecol* 1990;3:15.
189. Powell JL, Johnson NA, Bailey CL, et al. Management of advanced juvenile granulosa cell tumor of the ovary. *Gynecol Oncol* 1993;48:119.
190. Stuart GC, Dawson LM. Update on granulosa cell tumours of the ovary. *Curr Opin Obstet Gynecol* 2003;15:33.
191. Zaloudek C, Norris HJ. Granulosa tumors of the ovary in children: a clinical and pathologic study of 32 cases. *Am J Surg Pathol* 1982;6:503.
192. Fotious SK. Ovarian malignancies in adolescence. *Ann NY Acad Sci* 1997;816:338.
193. Erdreich-Epstein A, Monforte HL, Lavey RS, et al. Successful multimodality therapy of recurrent multifocal juvenile granulosa cell tumor of the ovary. *J Pediatr Hematol Oncol* 2002;24:229.
194. Borer JG. Tan PE, Diamond DA. The spectrum of Sertoli cell tumors in children. *Urol Clin North Am* 2000;27:529.
195. Young RH, Scully RE. Ovarian Sertoli-Leydig cell tumors: a clinicopathological analysis of 207 cases. *Am J Surg Pathol* 1985;9:543.
196. Mann WJ, Chumas J, Rosenwaks Z, et al. Elevated serum α-fetoprotein associated with Sertoli-Leydig cell tumors of the ovary. *Obstet Gynecol* 1986;67:141.
197. Gershenson DM, Copeland LJ, Kavanagh JJ, et al. Treatment of metastatic stromal tumors of the ovary with ciplastin, doxorubicin, and cyclophosphamide. *Obstet Gynecol* 1987;70:765.
198. Simmons PS, Backes RJ, Kaufman GIL, et al. Gynandroblastoma of the ovary in a young child. *Adolesc Pediatr Gynecol* 1988;1:57.
199. Scully RE. Sex cord tumor with annular tubules: a distinctive ovarian tumor of the Peutz-Jeghers syndrome. *Cancer* 1970;25:1107.
200. Young RI, Welch WR, Dickersin GR, et al. Ovarian sex cord tumor with annular tubules: review of 74 cases including 27 with Peutz-Jeghers syndrome and four with adenoma malignum of the cervix. *Cancer* 1982;50:1384.
201. Morowitz M, Huff D, von Allmen D. Epithelial ovarian tumors in children: a retrospective analysis. *J Pediatr Surg* 2003;38:331.
202. Deprest J, Moerman P, Corneillie P, et al. Ovarian borderline mucinous tumor in a premenarchal girl: review on ovarian epithelial cancer in young girls. *Gynecol Oncol* 1992;45:219.
203. Leake JF, Currie JL, Rosenshein NB, et al. Long-term follow-up of serous ovarian tumors of low malignant potential. *Gynecol Oncol* 1992;47:150.
204. Elchalal U, Dgani R, Piura B, et al. Current concepts in management of epithelial ovarian tumors of low malignant potential. *Obstet Gynecol Surv* 1995;50:62.
205. Barakat RR. Borderline tumors of the ovary. *Obstet Gynecol Clin North Am* 1994;21:93.
206. Casey AC, Bell DA, Lage JM, et al. Epithelial ovarian tumors of borderline malignancy: long-term follow-up. *Gynecol Oncol* 1993;50:316.
207. Morris RT, Gershenson DM, Silva EG, et al. Outcome and reproductive function after conservative surgery for borderline ovarian tumors. *Obstet Gynecol* 2000;95:541.

208. Morice P, Wicart-Poque F, Rey A, et al. Results of conservative treatment in epithelial ovarian carcinoma. *Cancer* 2001;92:2412.
209. Tsai JY, Saigo PE, Brown C, et al. Diagnosis, pathology, staging, treatment, and outcomes of epithelial ovarian neoplasia in patients age <21 years. *Cancer* 2001;91:2065.
210. Boruta D, Van Le L. Ovarian tumors of low malignant potential: current understanding and controversy. *Curr Probl Obstet Gynecol* 2002;25:45.
211. Beiner ME, Gotlieb WH, Davidson B, et al. Visual diagnosis: an adolescent female who has increasing hair growth. *Pediatr Rev* 2001;22:240.
212. Cannistra SA. Cancer of the ovary. *N Engl J Med* 1993;329:1550.
213. Parker LP, Ramirez PT, Broaddus R, et al. Low grade ovarian cancer in an adolescent patient. *Gynecol Oncol* 2001;80:104.
214. Camatte S, Morice P, Pautier P, et al. Fertility results after conservative treatment of advanced stage serous borderline tumour of the ovary. *BJOG* 2002;109:376.
215. Hall JM, Lee MK, Newman B, et al. Linkage of early-onset familial breast cancer to chromosome 17q21. *Science* 1990;250:1684.
216. Narod SA, Feunteun J, Lynch HT, et al. Familial breast-ovarian cancer locus on chromosome 17q21–q23. *Lancet* 1991;338:82.
217. Easton DF, Ford D, Bishop DT. Breast and ovarian cancer incidence in BRCA1-mutation carriers. *Am J Hum Genet* 1995;56:265.
218. Stratton JF, Gayther SA, Russell P, et al. Contribution of BRCA1 mutations to ovarian cancer. *N Engl J Med* 1997;336:1125.
219. Ford D, Easton DF, Bishop DT, et al. Risks of cancer in BRCA1-mutation carriers. *Lancet* 1994;343:692.
220. Burke W, Daly M, Garber J, et al. Recommendations for follow-up care of individuals with an inherited predisposition to cancer. *JAMA* 1997;277:997.
221. Struewing JP, Hartge P, Wacholder S, et al. The risk of cancer associated with specific mutations of BRCA1 and BRCA2 among Ashkenazi Jews. *N Engl J Med* 1997;336:1401.
222. Struewing JP, Abeliovich D, Peretz T, et al. The carrier frequency of the BRCA1 185delAG mutation is approximately one percent of Ashkenazi Jewish individuals. *Nat Genet* 1995;11:198.
223. Muto MG, Cramer DW, Tangir J, et al. Frequency of the BRCA1 185delAG mutation among Jewish women with ovarian cancer and matched population controls. *Cancer Res* 1996;56:1250.
224. Wooster R. Weber BL. Breast and ovarian cancer. *N Engl J Med* 2003;348:2339.
225. Kauff ND, Satagopan JM, Robson ME, et al. Risk-reducing salpingo-oophorectomy in women with a BRCA1 or BRCA2 mutation. *N Engl J Med* 2002;346:1609.
226. Biesecker BB, Ishibe N, Hadley DW, et al. Psychosocial factors predicting BRCA1/BRCA2 testing decisions in members of hereditary breast and ovarian cancer families. *Am J Med Genet* 2000; 93:257.
227. Elger BS, Harding TW. Testing adolescents for a hereditary breast cancer gene (BRCA1). *Arch Pediatr Adolesc Med* 2000;154:113.
228. Elger BS, Harding TW. Genetic testing of adolescents: is it in their best interest? [letter to the editor]. *Arch Pediatr Adolesc Med* 2000;154:851.
229. Ross LF. Genetic testing of adolescents: is it in their best interest? [letter to the editor]. *Arch Pediatr Adolesc Med* 2000;154:850.
230. Hayes MC, Scully RE. Ovarian steroid cell tumors (not otherwise specified): a clinicopathological analysis of 63 cases. *Am J Surg Pathol* 1987;11:835.
231. Padilla SL. Androgen-producing tumors in children and adolescents. *Adolesc Pediatr Gynecol* 1989;2:135.
232. Wentz AC, Gutai JP, Jones GS, et al. Ovarian hyperthecosis in the adolescent patient. *J Pediatr* 1976;88:488.
233. Fox H, Langley FA, Govan AD, et al. Malignant lymphoma presenting as an ovarian tumour: a clinicopathological analysis of 34 cases. *Br J Obstet Gynaecol* 1988;95:386.
234. Heaton DC, Duff GB. Ovarian relapse in a young woman with acute lymphoblastic leukemia. *Am J Hematol* 1989;30:42.
235. Cacciaguerra S, Miano AE, Di Benedetto A, et al. Gastric carcinoma with ovarian metastases in an adolescent. *Pediatr Surg Int* 1998;14:98.

19

The Breast: Examination and Lesions

Marc R. Laufer and Donald P. Goldstein

Breast development in the majority of girls begins between the ages of 8 and 13 years (see Chapter 4). As breast development is often regarded as a sign of feminine sexuality, young women and their families may worry about minor asymmetry or "inadequate" development. It is often difficult for the teenager to acknowledge smaller breasts as "normal." On the other hand, reassurance is in order only if the remainder of the examination and history excludes an endocrine or developmental disorder.

Increasing publicity about the frequency of breast cancer among women in the United States and the occurrence of breast cancer among relatives and mothers of adolescent patients has made many adolescents exceptionally nervous about breast masses, even though malignancy in this age group is rare (1,2). This concern may be used constructively to encourage young women to seek routine preventive health assessments and information about normal breast development and the techniques of breast self-examination.

BREAST EXAMINATION

All pediatric and adolescent patients should have a breast examination at the time of their annual physical examination regardless of whether specific complaints are mentioned. Examination of breasts is initiated during the newborn examination when breast tissue is usually evident secondary to stimulation from maternal hormones. In addition, neonates may have bilateral "white" nipple discharge ("witches' milk"), which is also due to maternal hormonal stimulation. Neonates and infants may have breast problems such as accessory nipples, infection, hemangioma, lipoma, and lymphangioma. For the prepubertal child, the assessment includes inspection and palpation of the chest wall for masses, pain, nipple discharge, or signs of premature thelarche or precocious development (see Chapter 5).

For the adolescent examination, the patient is asked to lie supine with one arm under her head. Breast development is recorded as Sexual Maturity Ratings (SMR), also

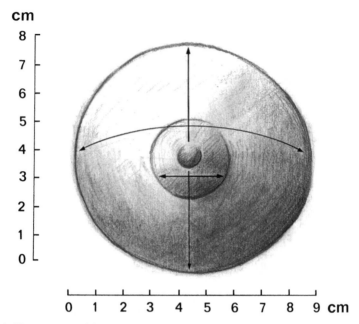

FIG. 19-1. Measurement of the developing breast (see text).

called *Tanner stages B1* to *B5* (see Fig. 4-7). If asymmetry or disorders of development are a concern, then exact measurements of the areola, glandular breast tissue, and overall breast size should be included at each examination (Fig. 19-1). For example, one might record the following:

	Areola (cm)	Breast gland (cm)	Overall (cm)
Right	2.5	5 × 6	9
Left	2.4	4 × 5	8.5

The first number in the breast gland figure is the upper-to-lower measurement; the second number is the right-to-left measurement. The overall size is the right-to-left measurement of the border of the fatty tissue of the breast mound.

Techniques for Breast Examination

There are several techniques for the orderly examination of the breast of the adolescent. In the first method, the examiner palpates the breast tissue in a pattern similar to spokes of a wheel, that is, in a straight line from the margin of the breast inward and clockwise around the breast starting with the tail of the breast in the axilla (Fig. 19-2). In a second method, the breast is palpated by the examiner using a circular clockwise pattern with either concentric circles or a spiral pattern inward. In a third method, the vertical or horizontal strip method, the breast is palpated in a linear systematic approach to cover all of the breast tissue. This last method appears to be particularly effective for self-examination (3). In all the methods, the flat finger pads should be moved in a slightly rotatory fashion (about the size of a dime) to feel for abnormalities. Each of these methods is acceptable and all have the goal of palpation of all breast tissue in a consistent uniform fashion. Normal glandular tissue has an irregular, granular surface (like tapioca pudding); a fibroadenoma feels firm, rubbery, or smooth. The areola should be compressed to assess for the existence of nipple discharge. As part of the overall health assessment, supraclavicular, infraclavicular, and axillary lymph nodes are palpated.

Breast Self-examination

Educating an older adolescent about the techniques of self-examination at the time of the breast examination may increase understanding of the ongoing examination and

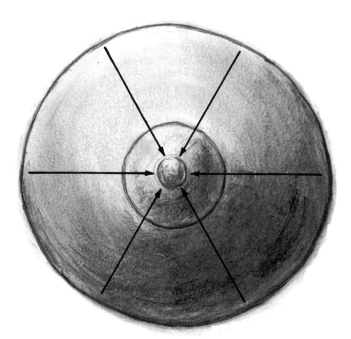

FIG. 19-2. Palpation of the breast. The fingers are moved in a straight line inward going clockwise around the breast.

make her feel more at ease (4). Breast self-examination is often taught in schools as part of health education classes and thus provides a link to examinations in the office. Although adolescents can become quite proficient in learning the necessary techniques, adolescents appear to practice self-examination only sporadically and often not at the end of menses (5). Studies on the value of self-examination during adolescence toward promoting lifelong health habits or early detection of breast cancer have been limited (6–10). The rationale for teaching breast self-examination is to contribute to an older adolescent's understanding and acceptance of her body, enhance her level of comfort with the clinical examination, and provide an opportunity for discussion about women's health issues (10,11). However, a number of authors have questioned whether early teaching of breast examination promotes anxiety, extra visits to health care facilities, and surgery in adolescents; these authors have also queried whether time in the office visit is better spent with other important risk-reduction strategies, given the extraordinary rarity of breast cancer in the adolescent age group (10–13). Thus teaching self-examination techniques is most appropriate for older adolescent and young adult women who are usually more interested in learning these techniques and want to participate in this aspect of their health care. There is some evidence that breast self-examination is the primary mode by which adolescent breast masses are detected; Hein and colleagues (4) found that 81% of a group of 95 teenagers with breast masses found them by self-detection. Nevertheless, adolescents should be reassured that cancer is extraordinarily unlikely in their age group but that a new breast mass that does not disappear after a menstrual period or is associated with pain, fever, or erythema should be evaluated in an expedient fashion.

With increasing knowledge about predisposing risk factors for breast cancer such as genetic markers, family history, and previous radiation and cancer, clinicians will be better able to target those with increased risks of developing breast cancer with appropriate in-office instruction and take-home educational materials. Adolescent women with previous radiation of the chest, who have an increased risk of second tumors including cancers of the breast (14–17), with a family history of BRCA1 or BRCA2 gene defects (18), and those with malignancies that may metastasize to the breast should have early teaching of breast self-examination during adolescence.

Breast self-examination should be performed at the end of each menstrual period. Instructions include having the young woman

1. Look in the mirror for asymmetry while undressing for a shower.
2. Examine the breasts while standing in the shower (soap on the hands facilitates the examination).
3. Reexamine the breasts that night supine (before going to sleep) with one hand behind the head and a small pillow under the shoulder.

She should be shown how to press gently with the middle three finger pads in one of the systematic approaches described previously. Patient information pamphlets, videos, or posters (such as those published by the American Cancer Society) should be available in the health care provider's office, additionally a guide to breast health and self-examination is available at *http://www.youngwomenshealth.org/ breast_health.html* It is particularly helpful for the patient to begin self-examination the night after a normal examination at the office visit so that she can be assured that she has a normal baseline for comparison. She can then continue to perform a breast self-examination after each annual checkup in addition to her monthly examinations to reinforce normal breast findings.

MASTALGIA (BREAST PAIN)

Mild breast tenderness often occurs premenstrually in association with fibrocystic changes or exercise or as a sign of early pregnancy. Girls initiating oral contraceptives (OCs) may also have mild breast symptoms in the first several months of use, with OCs containing 35 μg of ethinyl estradiol more likely to cause symptoms that 20 μg pills (see Chapter 20). Severe breast tenderness is not a major complaint of healthy adolescents. Breast pain has been shown to be a marker of emotional or physical abuse in some women (19).

The clinician providing office care to adolescents must be prepared to do a breast assessment and a pregnancy test in young women complaining of mastalgia. In spite of much anecdotal evidence that elimination of caffeine from the diet may benefit individual adolescents with fibrocystic changes and mastalgia, the majority of case-control studies have not demonstrated an association between benign breast disease and caffeine and methylxanthines (20,21) or benefit from elimination diets (20,22,23). We usually suggest that teenagers with cyclic or noncyclic breast discomfort wear a comfortable supporting bra, use NSAIDs as needed, and undertake a 3-month trial of elimination of substances such as coffee, tea, cola, and chocolate. Depending on the patient's self-assessment of how she is doing, she can continue to avoid caffeine as she wishes. Some adolescents also notice improvement of symptoms with switching to a lower dose 20 μg ethinyl estradiol oral contraceptive. Evening primrose oil (1,000 mg three times a day for 3 months) has been reported to have a response rate of 44% improvement in mastalgia (24,25); the mode of action is thought to be related to the high fatty acid content and its resulting action on the prostaglandin pathway, but more data are needed. Bromocriptine has been used in some adult women to alleviate breast soreness, but this symptom is rarely a major complaint of adolescents, and this medication can have significant adverse side effects. In adolescents with breast tenderness, we prefer not to suggest this therapy due to the side effect profile.

For young women active in sports, the utilization of a "sports bra" may be helpful to avoid pain and discomfort. This is particularly helpful to those with large breasts involved in activities such as jogging, basketball, and weightlifting (26).

PROBLEMS OF BREAST DEVELOPMENT

Asymmetry

Asymmetry of the breasts is a common complaint, especially from girls in the early stages of breast development. Since the breast bud may initially appear on one side as a tender, granular lump, parents are often concerned about the possibility of a malignancy. The etiologies of most breast asymmetries are unknown; however current theories of etiologies include endocrine, iatrogenic, and traumatic injury. Recently two cases of significant asymmetry were reported from sports injuries occurring at Tanner stage 1–2 (27).

In all individuals with breast asymmetry, a careful examination should be performed to rule out a breast mass, cyst, or abscess. Giant fibroadenomas or abscesses may blend into normal breast tissue and may be missed initially during palpation.

The clinician can play an important role in counseling the patient with true asymmetric breast development. The young adolescent needs to hear that many other adolescents and adult women have breast asymmetry; it should be pointed out that she may be unaware of the degree of asymmetry in other girls because her observations are based on seeing them fully clothed.

It is helpful to let the 13- or 14-year-old girl know that most 18- or 19-year-olds are coping well with the amount of breast asymmetry they have and that most elect not to have surgical intervention. The clinician should acknowledge that many younger adolescents (14 or 15 years old) are most anxious to have their body image equalized and "made normal" as quickly as possible without regard for the possible risks and long-term complications involved in augmentation or reduction mammoplasty. The young teenager can benefit from being told that the clinician understands that the asymmetry may cause worries for her and that an annual examination is important to determine the degree of asymmetry and to help her decide at the end of full growth (no further change in measurements) whether any consideration of intervention is warranted.

Since bathing suit fittings can be particularly difficult for girls with asymmetry, girls should be encouraged to try on a large number of styles that offer breast support, before coming to a final decision about the need for surgical intervention. For many youngsters, the use of slightly padded bras or simple bra pads also makes the asymmetry much less of a problem. A major difference in breast size can be treated with a prosthetic insert (available in department stores for mastectomy patients).

If asymmetry is still marked at age 15 to 18 years and serial measurements show no further increase in size of either breast, patients may wish to explore the option of augmentation or reduction mammoplasty. A plastic surgeon can delineate the risks and benefits. Potential long-term sequelae of implants have been an increasing concern, and newer materials are needed. Referral to a plastic surgeon willing to discuss the options without pushing the patient inordinately in the direction of surgery is essential. Success can be quite dramatic, as illustrated in Fig. 19-3.

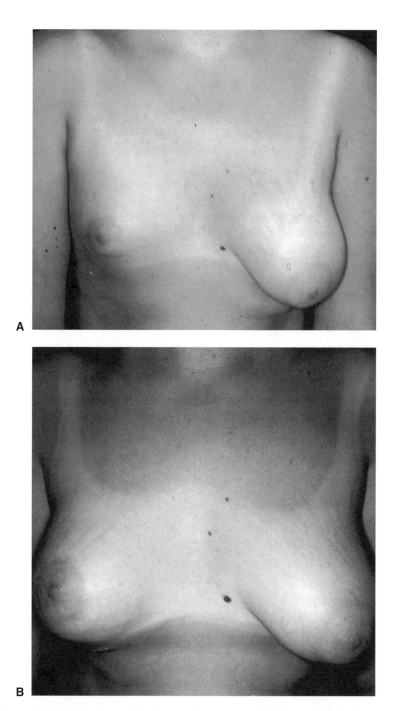

FIG. 19-3. A: Preoperative view of a 16-year-old girl with hypoplasia of the right breast. **B:** Appearance after augmentation mammoplasty with a prosthesis. (Courtesy of George E. Gifford, M.D., Children's Hospital Boston, MA.)

Hypertrophy

Some adolescents develop very large breasts that are associated with back pain, postural kyphosis, breast discomfort, shoulder soreness from bra straps, intertrigo, and psychological distress. Surgical reduction of large breasts at the end of breast growth can yield rewarding benefits to many young women. However, as is the case with augmentation mammoplasty, adolescents need to understand the results and risks of surgery, including infection, scars, and potential difficulty with breast-feeding.

True virginal hypertrophy occurs rarely in adolescents and causes the breasts to continue to enlarge in size beyond normal; unilateral or segmental enlargement may occur. The differential diagnosis includes juvenile fibroadenomas, nonbreast cancers, and phyllodes tumors (28–30). For cases of true virginal hypertrophy, surgical reduction should be delayed, if possible, until growth has ceased (Fig. 19-4).

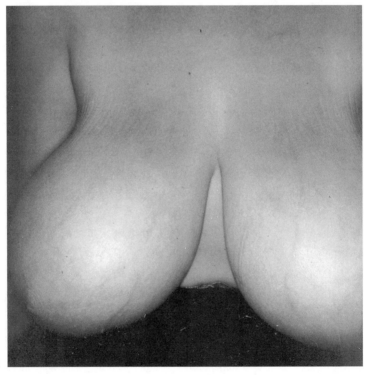

A

FIG. 19-4. A: Preoperative view of a 19-year-old woman with virginal hypertrophy of both breasts, resulting in back pain and kyphosis.

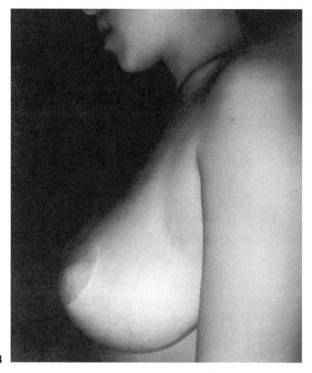

FIG. 19-4. Continued. B: Appearance after reduction mammoplasty. (Courtesy of George E. Gifford, M.D., Children's Hospital Boston, MA.)

Tuberous Breasts

Tuberous breasts are a variant of breast development in which the base of the breast is limited in size and the nipple–areola complex is overdeveloped, giving the appearance of a tuberous plant root (see Fig. 19-5). The etiology of this condition is unknown. The glandular tissue may be totally within the distended, enlarged areolae. This condition is sometimes associated with breasts that develop with the induction of secondary sexual characteristics from exogenous hormones prescribed for treatment of premature ovarian failure, abnormalities of gonadotropin-releasing hormone secretion, or gonadal dysgenesis. Plastic surgery may be undertaken for cosmetic reasons, and should be postponed until the completion of breast development in later adolescence.

Lack of Breast Development

Lack of breast development may be secondary to congenital absence of glandular tissue (amastia), a systemic disorder (e.g., malnutrition, Crohn disease), radiation

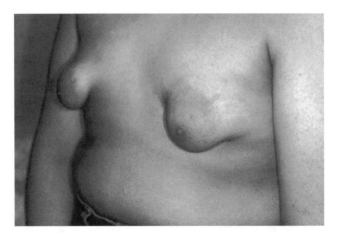

FIG. 19-5. Tuberous breasts.

therapy, congenital adrenal hyperplasia (CAH), gonadal dysgenesis, hypogo-nadotropic hypogonadism, or rarely an intersex disorder or 17α-hydroxylase defi-ciency. Amastia is extremely rare and usually unilateral; it also may be associated with Poland syndrome (aplasia of pectoralis muscles, rib deformities, webbed fin-gers, radial nerve aplasia). The congenital absence of one or both nipples (athelia) is very rare and may not be associated with absent breast tissue.

The evaluation of adolescents with amastia depends on the history and physical findings (see Chapter 6). Any evidence of androgen excess, such as mild enlargement of the clitoris, hirsutism, or severe acne, should suggest a disorder such as CAH, an intersex disorder, polycystic ovary syndrome, or possibly an adrenal or ovarian tu-mor (see Chapter 9). Figure 19-6 shows a 19-year-old patient who had irregular menses, lack of glandular breast development, normal pubic and axillary hair, mild clitoromegaly, and mild hirsutism. Adrenocorticotropic hormone testing was consis-tent with late-onset 21-hydroxylase deficiency (CAH) (see Chapter 9). Suppression of adrenal androgens with corticosteroids resulted in regular menses and normal breast development.

Despite the need to consider endocrinologic problems, the clinician should be aware that the great majority of adolescents with small breasts, normal sexual hair, and regular menses are healthy young women and deserve reassurance. Sports bras, which tend to compress the breast further, can be avoided. The oversized sweater and sweatshirt look can be reassuring to young teenagers who are often self-conscious in tank tops. Augmentation mammoplasty may be considered by some young women in their late teens and early 20s, and an understanding of the risks and benefits is essen-tial. Athletes with small breasts are generally counseled to avoid augmentation mam-moplasty until their careers are completed, since the change could potentially alter performance (26).

Premature Thelarche and Precocious Puberty

A discussion of premature thelarche and precocious puberty can be found in Chapter 5.

Accessory Nipples or Breasts

Accessory nipples (polythelia) or breasts (polymastia) occur in 1% to 2% of healthy patients. In some cases, all three components of the breast—glandular tissue, areola, and nipple—are present. More commonly, only a small areola and nipple are found, usually along the embryologic "milk line" between the axillae and groin. The most common sites are medial, just inferior to the normal breast tissue, and in the axilla. These abnormalities are usually asymptomatic, and no therapy is usually undertaken, unless at a later date the patient wishes to have the tissue removed for cosmetic reasons. If the patient is symptomatic with pain and/or nipple discharge, the supernumerary nipple or nipple (see Figs. 19-7 and 19-8) and breast (see Figs. 19-9 and 19-10) can be surgically removed. There have been reports of

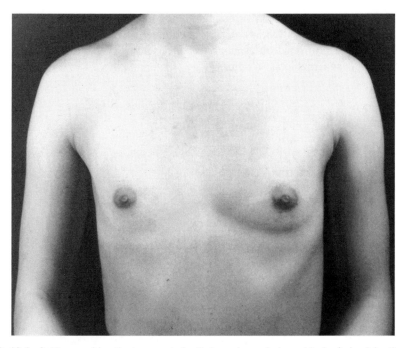

FIG. 19-6. A 19-year-old patient presented with irregular periods and lack of glandular tissue; late-onset 21-hydroxylase deficiency (CAH) was diagnosed.

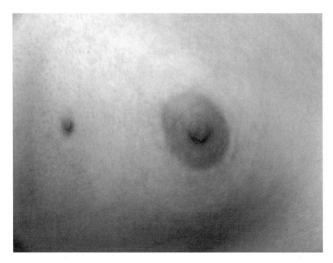

FIG. 19-7. Supernumerary nipple, (note that the supernumerary nipple occurs in the "milk line").

fibroadenomas and phyllodes tumors (discussed later) in supernumerary breast tissue (31,32).

Although studies have been conflicting on the association of supernumerary nipples and renal anomalies (33,34) and further studies are needed, a reasonable approach is to perform renal ultrasonography in an infant with multiple congenital anomalies and supernumerary nipples.

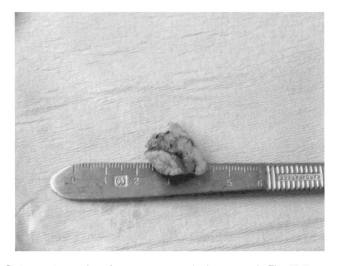

FIG. 19-8. Status post resection of supernumerary nipple as seen in Fig. 19-7.

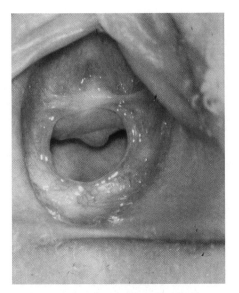

Plate 1. Normal hymen in prepubertal girl.

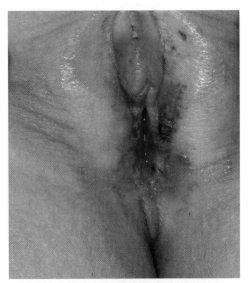

Plate 2. Lichen sclerosus in a prepubertal child (Courtesy of Drs. John Browning and Clifford Mishaw, Texas Children's Hospital, Houston TX).

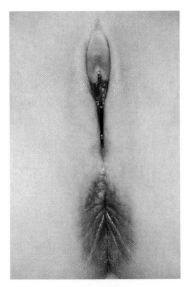

Plate 3. Lichen sclerosus in a prepubertal child.

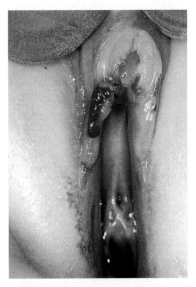

Plate 4. Close up of lichen sclerosus (Plate 3).

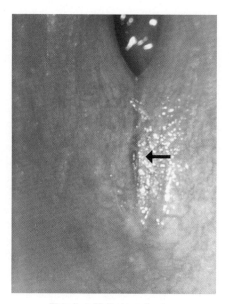

Plate 5. Labial/vulvar adhesion.

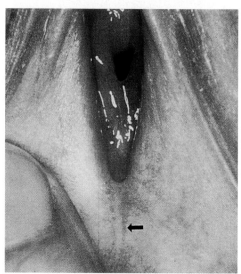

Plate 6. Linea vestibularis (midline sparing, midline avascular area) in a prepubertal girl. (From Heger A, Emans SJ, Muram D et al. Evaluation of the Sexually Abused Child. 2nd Ed. Oxford Press, New York, 2000. Reproduced by permission.).

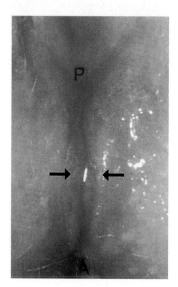

Plate 7. Failure of midline fusion (arrows) between the posterior fourchette (P) and the anus (A).

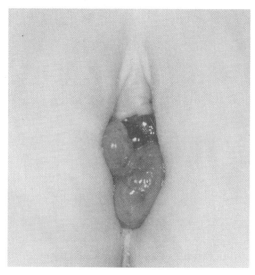

Plate 8. Rhabdomyosarcoma of the vagina (sarcoma botryoides).

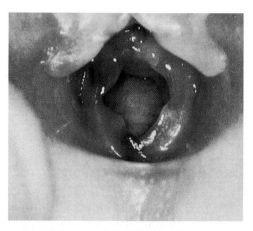

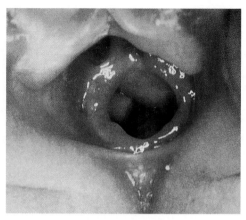

Plate 9. Three-year-old girl with submucosal hemorrhage at 6 o'clock and from 8 to 10 o'clock. Traumatic shallow transection at 9 o'clock from acute sexual abuse. (From Heger A, Emans SJ, Muram D et al. Evaluation of the Sexually Abused Child. 2nd Ed. Oxford Press, New York, 2000. Reproduced by permission.).

Plate 10. Same patient as Plate 9 with follow-up 10 days later showing a well healed hymen without any clear indication of previous trauma. (From Heger A, Emans SJ, Muram D et al. Evaluation of the Sexually Abused Child. 2nd Ed. Oxford Press, New York, 2000. Reproduced by permission.).

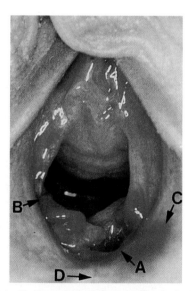

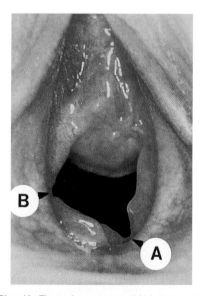

Plate 11. Three days post sexual assault of a 9-year-old girl. Supine traction with jagged edges at 5 o'clock (A). A second transection at 9 o'clock is obscured by edematous tissue (B). Contusion of the vestibular wall (C) and small midline posterior fourchette adhesion (D). (From McCann J, Voris J, Simon M. Genital injuries resulting from sexual abuse: A longitudinal study. *Pediatrics* 1992; 89:307-317. Reproduced by permission.).

Plate 12. Eleven days post assault in the patient described in Plate 11. Transections (complete clefts) of the hymen at 5 and 9 o'clock. (From McCann J, Voris J, Simon M. Genital injuries resulting from sexual abuse: A longitudinal study. *Pediatrics* 1992; 89:307-317. Reproduced by permission.).

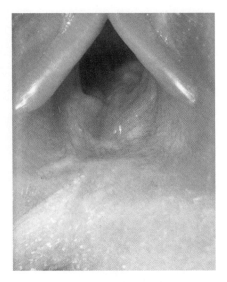

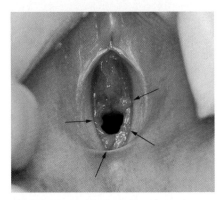

Plate 13. Dilated hymen orifice and transection of hymen at 6 o'clock in a 9-month-old sexually and physically abused infant.

Plate 14. Condyloma acuminata (at arrows) on the hymen of a prepubertal girl.

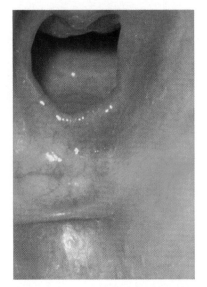

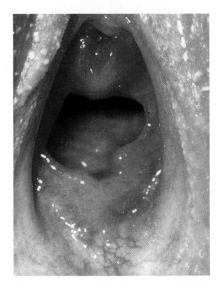

Plate 15. Scarring and rounding of the lower half of the hymen in a 9-year-old girl with a 2 year history of chronic sexual abuse. (From Emans SJ, et al. Genital findings in sexually abused, symptomatic and asymptomatic girls. *Pediatrics* 1987;79:778. Reproduced by permission.).

Plate 16. U-shaped indentation at 6 o'clock in an 11-year-old girl with a long history of sexual abuse.

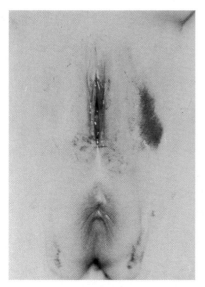

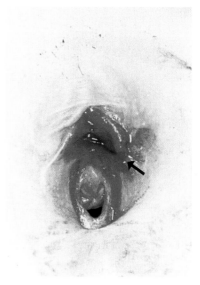

Plate 17. Ecchymoses and bleeding in a child following a straddle injury of the perineum.

Plate 18. Same child as Plate 17. Close-up of the vulva with laceration by the labia minora and periurethral tissues (arrow). (Note the normal hymen.).

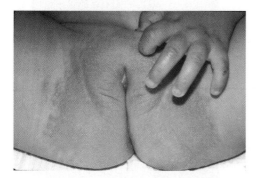

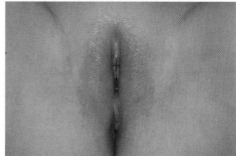

Plate 19. Candida vulvitis in a 10-month-old (Courtesy of Dr. Jonathan Trager, Mount Sinai Medical School, New York, NY.).

Plate 20. Psoriasis on the vulva of a 3-year-old (Courtesy of Dr. Jonathan Trager, Mount Sinai Medical School, New York, NY.).

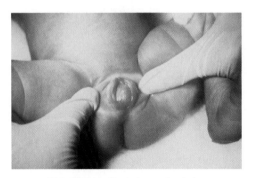

Plate 21. Imperforate hymen in a baby.

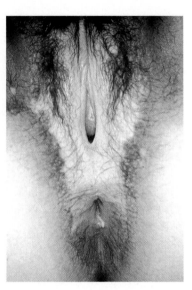

Plate 22. Postpubertal girl with lichen sclerosus.

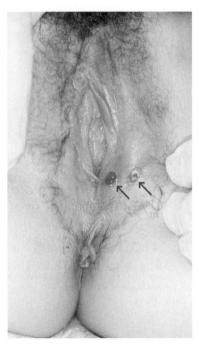

Plate 23. Vulvar Crohn disease (Note fistula track at arrows).

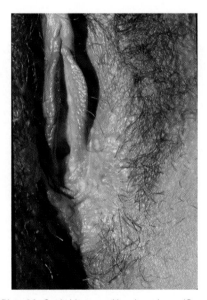

Plate 24. Genital herpes with vulvar ulcers. (Courtesy of Dr. Jonathan Trager, Mount Sinai Medical School, New York, NY.).

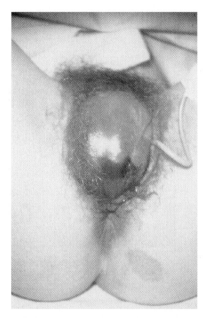

Plate 25. Vulvar hematoma from trauma.

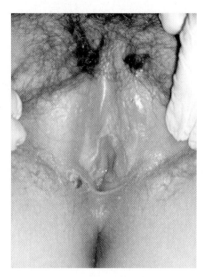

Plate 26. Non-herpetic non-specific vulvar ulcers (note eschar on right and active ulcer on left).

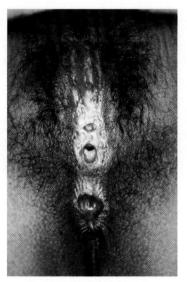

Plate 27. Status post ritual genital mutilation of a young woman from Somalia.

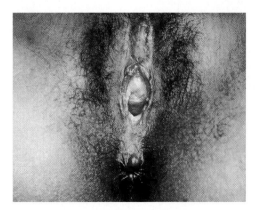

Plate 28. Re-creation of the introitus of the young woman's vulva from Plate 27, performed at the request and specifications of the young woman.

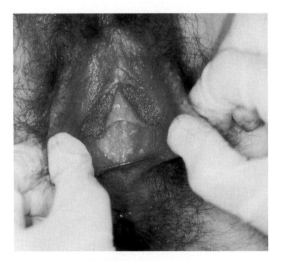

Plate 29. Vaginal agenesis.

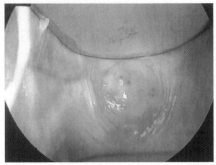

Plate 30. High transverse vaginal septum (note pin hole fenestration).

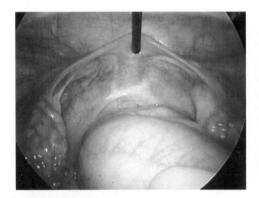

Plate 31. Laparoscopic view of normal anatomy in a prepubescent girl.

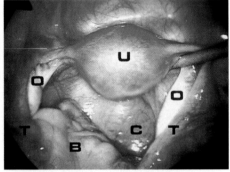

Plate 32. Laparoscopic view of normal pelvis. (U=uterus, C=cul-de-sac, O=ovary, T=fallopian tube, B=bowel).

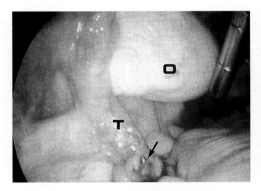

Plate 33. Laparoscopic view of normal ovary (O) and fallopian tube (T). Chromopertubation shows free spill of blue dye from fimbriae (arrow). Note that the distal end of the fallopian tube is not directly attached to the ovary.

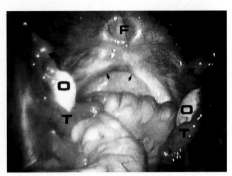

Plate 34. Seventeen year old with vaginal agenesis and bilateral rudimentary uterine horns. (F=Foley catheter balloon, O=ovary, T=fallopian tube, small arrows demonstrate uterosacral ligaments, large arrows demonstrate rudimentary uterine horns).

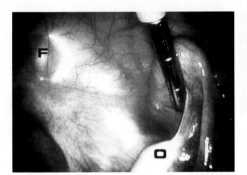

Plate 35. Close-up of rudimentary uterine horn (hemiuterus) shown in Plate 34 (O=ovary, F=Foley catheter balloon).

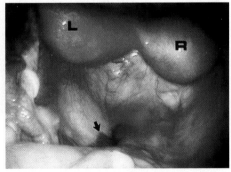

Plate 36. Laparoscopic view of left hemiuterus (L) communicating with single cervix as demonstrated by flow of blue dye injected through the cervix "freely spilling" from left fallopian tube (arrow). Right hemiuterus (R) does not communicate with the cervix and was removed laparoscopically as shown in Figures 10-93 to 10-95.

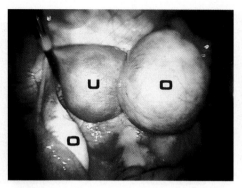

Plate 37. Right simple symptomatic ovarian cyst (U=uterus, O=ovary).

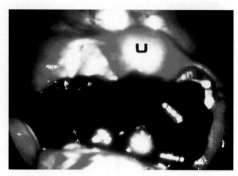

Plate 38. Laparoscopic view of blood and clot filling the pelvis from a ruptured corpus luteal cyst.

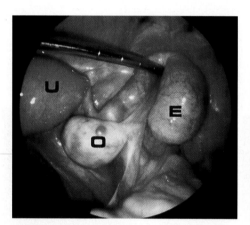

Plate 39. Laparoscopic view of right ectopic pregnancy. (U = uterus, O = ovary, E = ectopic pregnancy in right fallopian tube) [Courtesy of Dr. Robert B. Hunt, Department of Obstetrics, Gynecology, and Reproductive Biology, Harvard Medical School, Boston, Massachusetts].

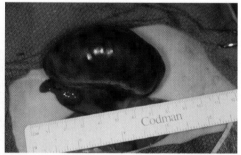

Plate 40. Ovarian torsion (ovary was detorsed, bilvalved and salvaged).

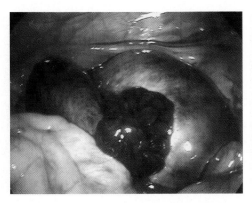

Plate 41. Ovarian and tubal torsion (both were salvaged).

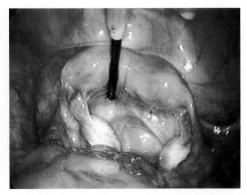

Plate 42. Uterus didelphys (bicollis as shown in Plate 43).

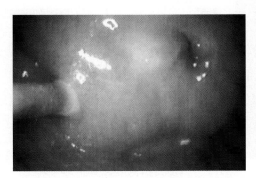

Plate 43. Bicollis (2 cervical os from uterus didelphys shown in Plate 42).

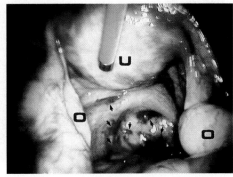

Plate 44. Endometriosis: flame lesions (arrows), (U = uterus, O = ovary).

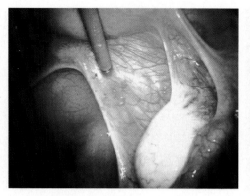

Plate 45. Clear lesions endometriosis.

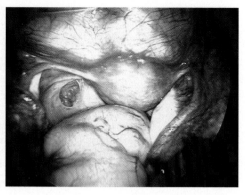

Plate 46. Peritoneal window.

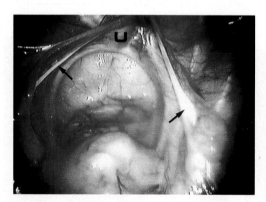

Plate 47. Streak gonads (small arrows) and "prepubertal" uterus (u) in a 15-year-old diagnosed with gonadal dysgenesis.

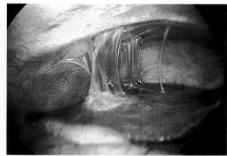

Plate 48. Fitz-Hugh-Curtis Syndrome.

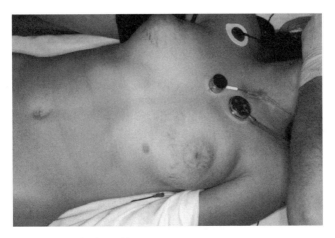

FIG. 19-9. Supernumerary nipple and breast.

Engorgement of accessory breasts is common during pregnancy and lactation. If no outlet is present, the breast tissue spontaneously involutes within several days to weeks after delivery.

NIPPLE DISCHARGE

Nipple discharge is uncommon during the teen years. The discharge may be milky, purulent, watery, serous, serosanguineous, or bloody. Most discharges, even bloody ones, do not signify cancer. A milky discharge is characteristic of galactorrhea, which

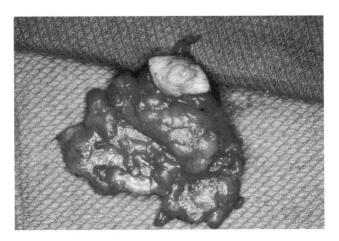

FIG. 19-10. Status post resection of supernumerary nipple and breast as seen in Fig. 19-9.

occurs in adolescents following a pregnancy (full term or after an abortion) or is associated with drug use (prescription and illicit), hypothyroidism, or prolactin-secreting tumors. The evaluation of galactorrhea and hyperprolactinemia is discussed in Chapter 7.

A purulent discharge is suggestive of infection. A sticky green or serosanguineous, brown, or a multicolored discharge may be associated with duct ectasia. A serosanguineous discharge may occur with intraductal papilloma, fibrocystic changes, or rarely cancer. A small amount of yellow, clear serous material can be expressed in early adolescence or in the later teen years, associated with fibrocystic changes.

A cytologic smear can be obtained on a frosted glass slide sprayed with cytologic fixative. Microscopic evaluation can be helpful in the evaluation of the discharge.

MontgomeryTubercles

Occasionally, a periareolar gland of Montgomery (Morgagni tubercles) will drain a small amount of clear to brownish fluid through an ectopic opening on the areola for several weeks. A small subareolar lump may be palpable. Usually no treatment is necessary, and the discharge and lump resolve spontaneously over several weeks to months (25,35). If the cyst persists, however, excision is advisable.

Intraductal Papillomas

Intraductal papillomas arise from abnormal proliferation of mammary duct epithelium projecting into a dilated lumen. Slight local trauma may rupture the vascular stalk and cause a bloody discharge. The mass may enlarge sufficiently to make it palpable. In adolescents, these masses may be subareolar or located in ducts in the periphery of the breast (36). In an extensive review of breast masses, Neinstein (25) found that intraductal papillomas accounted for only 1.2% of lesions biopsied in adolescents. In the review seen in Table 19-1, intraductal papillomas account for 0.82% of all breast disease in young women requiring breast surgery. Intraductal papillomas should be surgically excised.

Mammary Duct Ectasia

Ductal ectasia can be associated with a nipple discharge and/or breast mass usually occurring in the subareolar region. Ultrasound can be helpful in determining the diagnosis (37). These fluid collections will usually resolve spontaneously and do not require intervention. If the fluid with the subareolar cyst is dark, it sometimes appears as a blue mass under the nipple; this has been referred to as a *blue breast*. These blocked ducts are at risk of becoming infected and can lead to mastitis and breast

TABLE 19-1. Summary of studies involving breast disease in girls and young women

Reference	N	Age (yrs)	Normal	Cyst	Fibroadenoma	FC/Prolif	CP	Hypertrophy	IP	Other Benign Lesions/Tumors	Infection	Total Benign	Malignant
46	63	10 to 20	0	0	40	9	2	0	0	4	5	60	3
50	429	<21	0	0	338	76	0	0	2	2	10	428	1
51	118	10 to 20	0	0	0	118	0	0	0	0	0	118	0
52	53	8 to 20	2	2	41	4	0	0	1	3	0	53	0
53	225	10 to 20	0	8	169	25	0	0	13	5	2	222	3
54	111	<16	2	1	84	2	0	4	1	7	9	110	1
55	38	12 to 18	0	0	30	0	0	0	0	0	8	38	0
56	116	0 to 16	0	0	102	4	2	0	0	0	9	115	1
57	145	<21	0	0	104	26	0	0	4	4	4	144	1
48	117	11 to 20	0	0	103	9	0	0	0	0	4	116	1
58	59	10 to 20	0	0	42	9	1	5	0	0	5	56	3
59	40	12 to 22	0	0	19	11	0	0	0	2	0	38	2
60	209	11 to 30	0	0	167	37	0	0	0	5	0	204	5
61	151	<21	0	0	119	7	0	0	0	0	20	151	0
62	5	10 to 16	0	0	5	0	0	0	0	0	0	5	0
49	59	8 to 20	0	3	48	3	0	0	0	4	1	59	0
63	95	12 to 21	0	0	90	0	0	0	1	2	2	95	0
64	30	<21	0	0	18	9	0	1	0	1	1	30	0
20	33	12 to 18	0	1	29	1	0	0	0	0	1	32	1
65	95	12 to 21	0	9	71	0	2	0	0	2	11	95	0
13	185	<18	0	0	100	44	0	24	0	11	2	181	4
66	148	13 to 19	0	0	127	18	0	0	0	0	3	148	0
68	37	Prepub	0	0	31	0	1	3	1	0	1	37	0
67	242	14 to 20	0	0								236	6
Totals	**2803**		**4**	**24**	**1877**	**412**	**8**	**37**	**23**	**52**	**98**	**2771**	**32**
Percent	**100**		**0.14**	**0.86**	**66.96**	**14.70**	**0.29**	**1.32**	**0.82**	**1.86**	**3.50**	**98.86**	**1.14**

CP: cystosarcoma phyllodes.
FC/prolif: fibrocystic/proliferative.
IP: intraductal papillomas.

abscesses. Patients should be advised to watch for signs of erythema or pain, and if there is a concern of infection, oral antibiotic therapy should be initiated (see *Infection* below). If the abnormal duct leads to recurrent or persistent symptoms then it should be surgically excised. Identification of the blocked duct and surgical planning can be facilitated with the utilization of ductography (38).

Hyperprolactinemia has also been associated with mammary duct ectasia, a clinical syndrome of nipple discharge, nipple inversion, breast mass, and/or periareolar sepsis (nonpuerperal mastitis). In a study of 108 patients, Peters and Schuth (39) found that 27% of the patients had transiently elevated prolactin (42 ± 22 µg/L) during the period of inflammation with return to normal within 4 weeks and that 20% of the patients had more severe hyperprolactinemia (78 ± 56 µg/L), often associated with a previously undiagnosed prolactinoma. The authors suggested that the former group may have neurogenic hyperprolactinemia in response to the inflammation, whereas the latter group may be predisposed to the infection because nipple secretion might facilitate bacterial invasion. Of the patients in this study, 19 (18%) were between 12 and 20 years of age.

Apocrine Chromhidrosis

Apocrine chromhidrosis, the secretion of colored sweat by the apocrine glands of the areola, may sometimes be confused with bloody nipple discharge. Characteristically, the discharge occurs when the patient exercises or manually exerts pressure around the areola. Both cytologic examination and cultures are negative. No treatment is indicated for this condition (40).

PERIAREOLAR HAIR

Periareolar hair is not uncommon in the healthy adolescent. Cosmetic treatment (usually unnecessary) can be accomplished by cutting the hairs. Plucking or shaving may be uncomfortable and can lead to mastitis/cellulitis.

OTHER PROBLEMS

Joggers may experience sore or scaling nipples in response to friction. Lubrication of the nipple, a soft cotton bra without a seam in the cup, or Band-Aids over the nipples in the girl with small breasts not using a bra are often curative (26). Bicyclists may have difficulty with cold, painful nipples after several days of riding in the colder climates; a wind-breaking jacket and increased insulation over the chest should be advised.

Overweight girls with large pendulous breasts may have local infections on the undersurface of the breast with agents such as *Candida*, which results in a bright red rash. Topical antifungal drugs are usually sufficient, although florid cases with axillary involvement have responded better to oral antifungal agents.

BREAST CYSTS AND MASSES

Breast cysts/masses in adolescents, found either at the time of routine examination or during self-examination, provoke much anxiety for both the individuals and their families. The evaluation should include a history of previous breast disease, previous or intercurrent malignancy, chest radiation, menstrual history, pregnancy, constitutional symptoms, duration, size, symptoms associated with the breast mass, nipple discharge, and family history of breast disease and breast cancer. The workup includes a complete physical examination (checking for hepatosplenomegaly and lymphadenopathy) and assessment of the mass including evaluation of consistency, size, mobility, tenderness, warmth, overlying skin changes, and associated discharge. Importantly, the majority of adolescents who present to clinicians with the complaint of a "breast lump" have normal physiologic breast tissue or fibrocystic changes (2,10,41).

Breast Cysts

Breast cysts are fairly common in the developing adolescent breast. Usually the cysts result from ductal ectasia (discussed earlier), periareolar gland of Montgomery (Morgagni tubercles) (discussed earlier), or lymphangiomas (42). Physical exam is helpful in differentiating a cyst from a solid mass. Ultrasound is the imaging technique of choice for diagnosis (37). Usually these cysts will resolve spontaneously over a few weeks to months. If there is persistence of a symptomatic breast cyst, then needle aspiration can be utilized as a therapeutic intervention (discussed later).

Fibrocystic Breast Changes

Adolescents typically have very dense breast tissue. Fibrocystic changes are characterized by diffuse cordlike thickening and lumps that may become tender and enlarged prior to menses each month. Physical findings tend to change each month, so that suspected cysts can often be followed clinically. Love and colleagues (43) have questioned whether these findings should be characterized as a disease since the process occurs in 50% of women clinically and 90% histologically. The etiology of fibrocystic changes is unknown and, as noted earlier, does not appear to be related to methylxanthine consumption (44). One possible etiology is an imbalance of estrogen/progesterone (22,25).

In a survey of English-language articles published since 1960 on breast lesions evaluated by biopsy, Neinstein (25) determined that 18.5% showed fibrocystic changes. The long-term risk of cancer in women with fibrocystic changes relates to the histology of the lesions found. In a study of 10,366 consecutive breast biopsies followed up for a median duration of 17 years, DuPont and Page (45) reported that women having proliferative disease without atypical hyperplasia had a risk of cancer that was 1.9 (95% confidence interval [CI]: 1.2, 2.9) times the risk of women with nonproliferative lesions; the risk in women with atypical hyperplasia (atypia) was 5.5 (95% CI: 3.1, 8.8) times that in women with nonproliferative lesions. The risk in women with atypia and a family history of breast cancer was 11-fold that of women with no atypia and a negative family history. Seventy percent of the women undergoing breast biopsy for benign disease did not have risk factors detected and were not at increased risk of later breast cancer.

Fibroadenomas

Although most breast "lumps" seen in the office setting in adolescents are normal nodularity or fibrocystic changes, most breast masses that are surgically excised in this age group are fibroadenomas (13,46,47). Table 19-1 shows the data from 24 studies of the types of breast masses surgically removed in adolescents (13,20,25,46,48–68), and fibroadenomas were identified in 66.96% of cases. In a review of 51 patients, aged 8 to 20 years, who underwent excision of breast masses at Children's Hospital Boston, 81.4% of the masses were fibroadenomas (49). The pathology report on the remainder of the biopsy specimens showed fibrocystic disease, simple cysts, capillary hemangiomas, fat necrosis, adenomatous hyperplasia, and (in one patient) normal breast tissue. This is similar to the spectrum of breast disease reported by Daniel and Mathews (46), who found that fibroadenomas accounted for 94% of breast tumors in the 12- to 21-year age group. Neinstein's review (25) of 15 series in the literature demonstrated that fibroadenomas represented 68.3% of the lesions in 1,797 cases involving patients <22 years old. In clinical series of adolescents in office settings, the percentage of breast masses attributed to fibroadenomas is only 15% (41).

Fibroadenomas are typically firm or rubbery and mobile, and usually have a clearly defined edge. Pathologically, they have stromal proliferation surrounding aggregates of compressed or uncompressed, elongated and distorted ducts (56). They tend to be eccentric in position and occur more frequently in the lateral breast quadrants than the medial quadrants. The breast mass may remain unchanged or increase in size with subsequent menstrual cycles. The average duration of symptoms is 5 months (55), and the average size is 2 to 3 cm with a range of <1 cm to >10 cm. Recurrent or multiple fibroadenomas have been reported in 10% to 25% of cases (41). Giant fibroadenomas grow more rapidly to >5 cm and have a greater degree of stromal cellularity; they may replace and compress most of the normal breast tissue. Because of the soft consistency, these lesions may be mistaken initially for normal tissue. They accounted for 1.1% of lesions in Neinstein's review (25).

A question that has frequently been raised is whether patients with a history of fibroadenoma are at increased risk of breast cancer. In a retrospective cohort study of

1,835 patients with fibroadenoma diagnosed between 1950 and 1968, Dupont and colleagues (69) compared these patients with two control groups (Connecticut Tumor Registry) and women chosen from among patients' sisters-in-law. They reported that the risk of invasive breast cancer among patients with fibroadenoma was 2.15 (95% CI: 1.5, 3.2) times that of controls. The risk for complex fibroadenoma (cysts, sclerosing adenosis, epithelial calcifications, or papillary apocrine changes) was 3.1-fold (95% CI: 1.9, 5.1). Patients with benign proliferative disease in the parenchyma adjacent to the fibroadenoma had a risk of 3.88 (95% CI: 2.1, 7.3). In their series, two-thirds of the patients had noncomplex fibroadenomas, no family history of breast cancer, and no increased risk. However, among patients with a family history of breast cancer and either a complex fibroadenoma or proliferative disease, the incidence of breast cancer during the first 25 years after diagnosis of the fibroadenoma was 20%. In a follow-up to their initial study, these researchers showed that atypia confined to a fibroadenoma does not incur a clinically meaningful risk of future breast carcinoma development greater than that of fibroadenoma alone (70).

Phyllodes Tumors

Phyllodes tumor (previously known as *cystosarcoma phyllodes*) is a rare primary tumor that is usually benign but can be malignant (71). Phyllodes tumors have both stromal hypercellularity and benign glandular elements. This tumor accounted for 0.4% of cases in the Neinstein series (25), and 0.29% of all tumors shown in Table 19-1. The lesions are usually large and circumscribed; Briggs and coworkers (72) found an average size of 6 cm (range, 2 to 13 cm) in nine adolescents. Overlying skin may be taut and shiny with distended veins apparent; skin retraction, necrosis, nipple discharge, and retraction may occur. The tumor is usually large, painless, and rapidly growing. Classification of the lesion as benign or malignant is based on stromal findings (25).

Juvenile Papillomatosis

Juvenile papillomatosis is a rare breast tumor of young women, first described in 1980. The findings in 180 patients from the Juvenile Papillomatosis Registry were reported in 1985 (73). The tumor features atypical papillary duct hyperplasia and multiple cysts. The mean age at presentation was 23 years (range, 12 to 48 years). The localized tumor was often initially mistaken for a fibroadenoma. In 28% of cases, patients had a relative with breast cancer, and 7% had a first-degree relative with breast cancer. A small number of patients had breast cancer diagnosed concurrently with the juvenile papillomatosis, and several patients developed cancer at follow-up. Bilateral juvenile papillomatosis may especially increase the risk of later developing cancer, and thus careful surveillance is indicated in patients with this diagnosis based on excisional biopsy. Papillary hyperplasia without the cystic component of juvenile papillomatosis appears to be a more benign condition in young patients (74).

Primary Breast Cancer

Cancer of the breast is extremely rare in children and adolescents (46,50,75–78). In a series of 237 patients 10 to 20 years of age with breast lesions, Farrow and Ashikari (79) reported only one patient with primary breast carcinoma and two patients with sarcomas metastatic to breast tissue. In a retrospective review of surgically treated breast disease in 185 adolescents (11 to 17 years old) at the Mayo Clinic, four patients had malignant neoplasms (primary rhabdomyosarcoma, metastatic rhabdomyosarcoma, metastatic neuroblastoma, and non-Hodgkin lymphoma) (13). A report of breast cancer in women under age 20 from 1976 to 2000 identified four cases (one invasive ductal, two secretory carcinomas, and one invasive lobular) with three out of four disease free at follow-up (76 to 126 months post diagnosis) and one with metastatic disease (80). Only 0.2% of primary breast cancers occur before the age of 20 years, and the prevalence of breast cancer under age 18 years is 0 per 1,000,000 (10). Primary lymphoma may present as a breast mass in adolescents (29,81). In Neinstein's series (25), 0.9% of lesions were cancer (range, 0% to 2% in various series) with 5/16 adenocarcinoma. Up to 30% of teenagers with breast cancer have a family history. The size of tumors has varied from 1 cm to 2.5 cm. Patients with previous radiation therapy to the chest have an increased risk of developing cancer of the breast at a young age and therefore require careful ongoing surveillance including breast self-examination, clinical examination, and mammography (14–17).

Genetic Predisposition to Breast Cancers

It has been recognized that breast cancers cluster in families. There is an increased risk of breast cancer in women whose relatives have been found to have breast cancer. The risk is highest if there are multiple affected relatives and if the relatives are closer (mothers or sisters). It is thought that the risk of genetic transmission is greater from the maternal side than from the paternal side (82). Several genetic syndromes have been associated with an increased risk for breast cancer. The Li-Fraumeni syndrome includes brain, breast, and lung malignancies, lymphomas, and sarcomas that develop at an early age; this syndrome has been found to result from a germline mutation of the p53 tumor suppressor gene (83).

Families have been identified with increased rates of breast and/or ovarian cancers; these individuals have been found to have a deletion of chromosome 17 in the q21–q23 region suggestive of a tumor suppressor gene (84,85). This finding of genetic abnormalities related to an increased risk of breast cancer has been named breast cancer gene-1 (BRCA-1) (86). A second mutation, BRCA-2, has also been identified and other genetic patterns are likely to be delineated. An estimated 7% to 9% of breast cancers have been thought to be due to the BRCA-1 and BRCA-2 mutations, (87). Risks for carriers of these mutations were originally derived from high-risk families enrolled in protocols and required cautious interpretation. The cumulative risk for breast cancer for women with BRCA-1 mutations was originally estimated to be 3.2% by age 30, 19.1% by age 40 years, and 85% by age 70 years (88). Ovarian cancer risk with this mutation was estimated to be 26% to 85% by age 70. The risk of breast cancer for those with the BRCA-2 mutations appears to be less than the risk for women with the BRCA-1 mutation, and the ovarian cancer risk is <10% by age 70 years. A more recent analysis of Jewish women in the Washington area with a specific BRCA-1 or a BRCA-2 mutation found lower estimates of breast cancer (56%) and ovarian cancer (16%) by age 70 years (89). Recommendations for women with these mutations were published in 1997 and have included breast self-examination beginning at age 18 to 21 years, annual or semi-annual clinical breast examination beginning at age 25 to 35, and mammography screening beginning at age 25 to 35 years (88). Adult women may also choose to participate in MRI follow-up trials or elect prophylactic mastectomy (90). These recommendations have been based on expert opinion and thus the efficacy has not been proved (88). Clinicians caring for these adolescents will need to be involved in decision making with them to make the best use of emerging technology without increasing their anxiety (91–93).

Clinical Management of Breast Masses

History and Physical Exam

If the adolescent presents with the complaint of a breast mass, palpation may make the diagnosis evident with findings such as the thickening of fibrocystic disease or the tenderness and erythema consistent with a breast infection or abscess. Trauma may cause a breast mass, but examination immediately following a contusion may locate a preexisting lesion. If the differential diagnosis is a cyst or fibroadenoma, the lesion can be measured and the patient instructed to return after her next menstrual period. If the lesion has disappeared, then a cyst was probably present. If the lesion is still present and the patient is cooperative, needle aspiration of the mass can be performed as described later.

Breast Imaging (Ultrasound, Mammography, MRI)

Ultrasound is the imaging technique of choice for breast masses in children and adolescents (37). Ultrasound of the breast tissue can also be helpful in delineating a fibroadenoma (Fig. 19-11) from a phyllodes tumor, or a simple cyst (Fig. 19-12) or a galactocele (Fig. 19-13), as well as in localizing the extent of an abscess (37,94–96). Color Doppler ultrasound has also been shown to be helpful in the evaluation of fibroadenomas and breast abscesses (37). Three-dimensional (3-D) B-mode ultrasound techniques have not shown an advantage in differentiating breast masses (97). Mammography is rarely used to evaluate breast masses in the adolescent age group, since the breast tissue is very dense, the risk of the patient's having carcinoma is negligible,

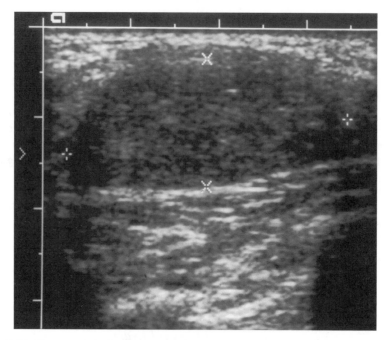

FIG. 19-11. Ultrasound of a fibroadenoma. (Courtesy of Carol Barnewolt, M.D., Children's Hospital Boston.)

and radiographic features have not influenced clinical management (98). MRI has been utilized for breast imaging, but additional studies in adolescents are needed (99).

Needle Aspiration of Breast Masses

Persistent breast masses can be aspirated although we find that this is a rarely utilized intervention in pediatric and adolescent breast disease. If elected, breast cyst/mass aspiration can be performed in the office using a 23-gauge needle on a 3-ml syringe (Fig. 19-14). A small amount of lidocaine can be used to infiltrate the skin with a 25-gauge needle (100). A cyst can be aspirated, whereas a fibroadenoma gives a characteristic gritty, solid sensation. Material obtained (even if just on the tip of the needle) may be smeared on a ground glass frosted slide, fixed, and sent for cytologic examination. Nonbloody fluid aspirates have not been found to be clinically helpful, as a study of aspirated fluid found that nonbloody fluid was acellular, inadequate for cytologic diagnosis, or had no malignant cells, and thus the authors suggest that only frankly bloody fluid should be submitted for cytologic analysis (101). If the mass collapses after aspiration, it is assumed to be a cyst and is reevaluated in 3 months. Fine needle aspiration has not been extensively studied in adolescents (102); however, it might allow prolonged observation in adolescents with fibroade-

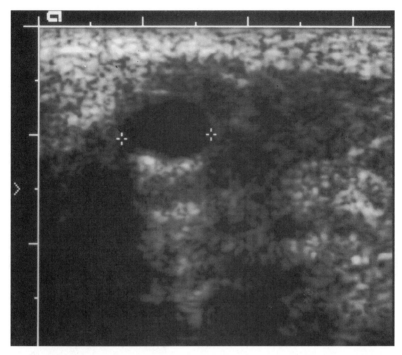

FIG. 19-12. Ultrasound of a simple cyst of the breast. (Courtesy of Carol Barnewolt, M.D., Children's Hospital Boston.)

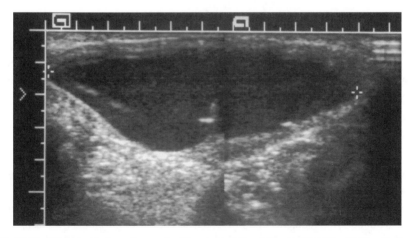

FIG. 19-13. Ultrasound of a galactocele. (Courtesy of Carol Barnewolt, M.D., Children's Hospital Boston.)

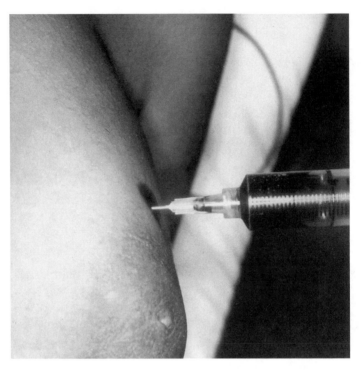

FIG. 19-14. Needle aspiration of simple cyst of the breast.

nomas or altered therapy in an adolescent diagnosed with a primary carcinoma and suspected of having metastatic disease to the breast.

Observation of Breast Masses

Asymptomatic breast masses that are small, and consistent with a fibroadenoma on imaging studies can be observed without surgical intervention. Interval ultrasounds should be obtained to determine if the mass is increasing in size. Recent studies have shown that a significant percentage of fibroadenomas will resolve spontaneously and do not require surgical resection if asymptomatic (103).

Surgical Resection of Breast Masses

When aspiration of a persistent, discrete mass is not feasible or is nonproductive or when masses are nonmobile and hard, enlarging, tender, or a source of considerable anxiety, the patient should have a surgical excision of the mass (Fig. 19-15). Unless there are underlying medical conditions, such as cardiac or pulmonary disease, an excisional biopsy can be done in an ambulatory surgical setting under local or general anesthesia, depending on technical considerations and the patient's preference and

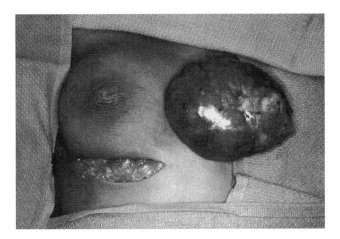

FIG. 19-15. Resection of a giant fibroadenoma.

ability to cooperate. Since breast scars can be cosmetically deforming, the optimal incision of the breast is circumareolar (Fig. 19-16). Tissue adjacent to the fibroadenoma should be obtained to examine for atypical proliferative changes (see previous discussion) (69). Curvilinear or semilunar incisions are superior to radial incisions in terms of wound healing and cosmetic results. Periareolar ectopic lobules, which often have clear or dark discharge from the areola (not the nipple), can be excised with a circumareolar incision. If the mass is too large to remove through a periareolar incision,

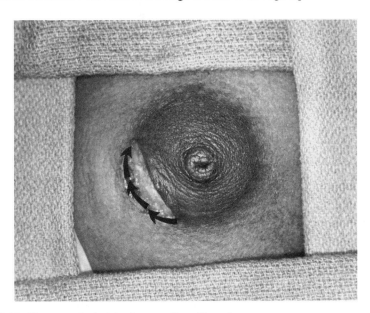

FIG. 19-16. Circumareolar incision for resection of breast mass.

then an incision can be made inferior to the breast, in the "bra line" in order to be more cosmetically pleasing (see Fig 19-15). It should be noted that even giant fibroadenomas can however be removed through small incisions (104). Follow-up is particularly important after excision because new cysts and fibroadenomas can occur.

Nonclassic Surgical Options

Recent reports of nonsurgical destruction of breast masses have been reported in the adult literature utilizing MRI guided focused ultrasound surgery (105). Office-based ultrasound guided cryoablation of biopsy proven breast fibroadenomas have been reported in adolescent and adult patients with excellent results (106).

Contusion

A contusion to the breast may result in a poorly defined, tender mass that resolves over several weeks. Trauma may result from sports or other accidental injuries or from physical or sexual abuse. As mentioned above, two cases of significant asymmetry were reported from sports injuries occurring at Tanner stage 1–2 (27). A hematoma resulting from trauma should be managed with pain medications, ice packs, and binding of the breast with a sports bra or elastic wrap. A mass from severe trauma may take several months to resolve, and occasionally scar tissue remains palpable indefinitely. Fat necrosis may also result from trauma, although the patient may not notice the growing lesion until several months later. Biopsy is frequently indicated in such circumstances. It should be remembered that the examination immediately following trauma to the breast may locate a preexisting lesion. A sharply delineated, nontender mass is probably unrelated to the recent injury.

Infection

Infection of the breast can occur in newborns, girls, and adolescents. These infections are most commonly seen in newborns and lactating adolescent women but can also occur in adolescents who are not pregnant or sexually active.

In a review of neonatal mastitis at Children's Hospital Boston, Walsh and McIntosh (107) found that infections occurred in full-term infants 1 to 5 weeks of age with a female/male sex ratio of 2:1. All but a few cases were caused by *Staphylococcus aureus*, and most infants (10 of 17) treated after 1971 responded to appropriate β-lactamase-resistant antibiotics without the need for incision and drainage. Recurrent infections or persistence of a mass after treatment for an infection may signal an underlying lesion such as a hemangioma, lymphangioma, or cystic hygroma.

Breast infections in adolescents are most common during lactation. Bacteria such as staphylococci and streptococci enter through cracks in the nipples; cellulitis is often associated with streptococci and abscesses with staphylococci. Nonlactating adolescents may also develop breast infections, usually beneath the areola or at the margin between the areola and the normal skin. The etiology of these infections is unclear, but they may occur because of duct ectasia or metaplasia of the duct epithelium. In addition, the adolescent may give a history of having recently shaved around the areola or having plucked a periareolar hair. Infections can also be the result of nipple piercing (108). Sexual play may also cause breast trauma. Subareolar inflammatory masses may occur secondary to rupture of an areolar gland. The patient may present with a tender mass or, in the early stages of infection, with erythema and warmth of the skin adjacent to the areola. In agreement with our experience, Beach (44) found that infections may be more extensive and deeper than initial superficial findings suggest. As in the neonate, staphylococci are the most common pathogens. Aspiration of the mass (with or without the aid of ultrasound) can help make the clinical and bacteriologic diagnosis. Mastitis associated with duct ectasia usually has a visible discharge, which can be Gram-stained and cultured. If diagnosed early when the predominant feature is cellulitis, most cases will respond to oral antibiotics such as dicloxacillin or a cephalosporin given for 7 to 10 days without need for surgical intervention. If the mass becomes fluctuant or if symptoms progress or fail to resolve, then aspiration of pus and a longer course of antibiotic therapy is indicated (109). In a study of 30 adolescent and adult women with breast abscesses, 60% required only a single aspiration, 30% required multiple aspirations, and the remainder required surgical incision and drainage (109). If the abscess continues to enlarge or fails to respond, then incision and drainage (Fig. 19-17) and packing are performed. Antibi-

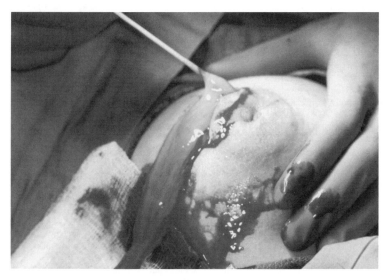

FIG. 19-17. Incision and drainage of a very large breast abscess.

otics should be continued postoperatively. Subareolar abscesses may become recurrent and require elective excision of the dilated milk ducts and associated inflammatory tissue (44,76,110,111).

REFERENCES

1. West KW Resoorla FJ, Schere LR III, et al. Diagnosis and treatment of symptomatic breast masses in the pediatric population. *J Pediatr Surg* 1995;30:182.
2. Johnson P. Breast lumps in the adolescent female. *J Pediatr Health Care* 2002;16:47.
3. Atkins JE, Solomon LJ, Worden JK, et al. Relative effectiveness of methods of breast self-examination. *J Behav Med* 1991;14:357.
4. Hein K, Dell R, Cohen MI. Self-detection of a breast mass in adolescent females. *J Adolesc Health Care* 1982;3:15.
5. Cromer BA, Frankel ME, Keder LM. Compliance with breast self-examination instruction in healthy adolescents. *J Adolesc Health Care* 1989;10:105.
6. O'Malley MS, Fletcher SW. Screening for breast cancer with breast self-examination: a critical review. *JAMA* 1987;257:2196.
7. Clark JK, Sauter M, Kotecki JE. Adolescent girls' knowledge of an attitudes toward breast self-examination: evaluating an outreach education program. *J Cancer Educ* 2000;15:228.
8. Wei G, Borum ML. Breast self-examination in women in two primary care settings: an evaluation of the impact of insurance status. *J Womens Health Gend Based Med* 2000;9:311.
9. Ludwick R, Gaczkowski T. Breast self-exams by teenagers: outcome of a teaching program. *Cancer Nurs* 2001;24:315.
10. Simmons PS. Breast disorders in adolescent females. *Curr Opin Obstet Gynecol* 2001;13:459.
11. Simmons PS. Diagnostic considerations in breast disorders of children and adolescents. *Obstet Gynecol Clin North Am* 1992;19:91.
12. Goldbloom R. Self-examination by adolescents. *Pediatrics* 1985;76:126.
13. Simmons PS, Weld LE. Surgically treated breast disease in adolescent females: a retrospective review of 185 cases. *Adolesc Pediatr Gynecol* 1989;2:95.
14. Bhatia S, Robinson LL, Oberlin O, et al. Breast cancer and other second neoplasms after childhood Hodgkin's disease. *N Engl J Med* 1996;334:745.
15. Ivins JC, Taylor WF, Wold LE. Elective whole-lung irradiation in osteosarcoma treatment: appearance of bilateral breast cancer in two long-term survivors. *Skeletal Radiol* 1987;16:133.
16. Tucker MA, Coleman CN, Cox RS, et al. Risk of second cancers after treatment for Hodgkin's disease. *N Engl J Med* 1988;318:76.
17. Diller L, Medeiros Nancarrow C, Shaffer K, et al. Breast cancer screening in women previously treated for Hodgkin's disease: a prospective cohort study. *J Clin Oncol* 2002;20:2085.
18. Templeman C, Hertweck SP. Breast disorders in the pediatric and adolescent patient. *Obstet Gynecol Clin North Am* 2000;27:19.
19. Colegrave S, Holcombe C, Salmon P. Psychological characteristics of women presenting with breast pain. *J Psychosom Res* 2001;50:303.
20. Lubin F, Ron E, Wax Y, et al. A case-control study of caffeine and methylxanthines in benign breast disease. *JAMA* 1985;253:2388.
21. Shairer C, Brinton LA, Hoover RN. Methylxanthines and benign breast disease. *Am J Epidemiol* 1986;124:603.
22. Vorherr H. Fibrocystic breast disease: pathophysiology, pathomorphology, clinical picture, and management. *Am J Obstet Gynecol* 1986;154:161.
23. Heyden S, Fopdor JG. Coffee consumption and fibrocystic breasts: an unlikely association. *Can J Surg* 1986;29:208.
24. Pye JK, Mansel RE, Hughes LE. Clinical experience of drug treatments for mastalgia. *Lancet* 1985;2:373.
25. Neinstein LS. Review of breast masses in adolescents. *Adolesc Pediatr Gynecol* 1994;7:119.
26. Haycock CE. How I manage breast problems in athletes. *Phys Sports Med* 1987;15:89.

27. Jansen DA, Spencer Stoetzel R, Leveque JE. Premenarchal athletic injury to breast bud as the cause for asymmetry: prevention and treatment. *Breast J* 2002;8:108.
28. Hays D, Donaldson S, Shimada H, et al. Primary and metastatic rhabdomyosarcoma in the breast: Neoplasms of adolescent females, a report from the intergroup rhabdomyosarcoma study. *Med Pediatr Oncol* 1997;29:181.
29. DiNoto A, Parcheco P, Vicala R, et al. Two cases of breast lymphoma mimicking juvenile hypertrophy. *J Pediatr Adolesc Gynecol* 1999;12:33.
30. O'Hare PM, Frieden IJ. Virginal breast hypertrophy. *Pediatr Dermatol* 2000;17:277.
31. Aughsteen AA, Almasad JK, Al-Muhtaseb MH. Fibroadenoma of the supernumerary breast of the axilla. *Saudi Med J* 2000;21:587.
32. Oshida K, Miyauchi M, Yamamoto N, et al. Phyllodes tumor arising in ectopic breast tissue of the axilla. *Breast Cancer* 2003;10:82.
33. Grossl NA. Supernumerary breast tissue: historical perspectives and clinical features. *South Med J* 2000;93:29.
34. Galli-Tsinopoulou A, Krohn C, Schmidt H. Familial polythelia over three generations with polymastia in the youngest girl. *Eur J Pediatr* 2001;160:375.
35. Watkins F, Giacomantonio M, Salisbury S. Nipple discharge and breast lump related to Montgomery's tubercles in adolescent females. *J Pediatr Surg* 1988;23:718.
36. Organ CH Jr, Organ BC. Fibroadenoma of the female breast: a critical clinical assessment. *J Natl Med Assoc* 1983;75:701.
37. Garcia CJ, Espinoza A, Dinamarca V, et al. Breast US in children and adolescents. *Radiographics* 2000;20:1605.
38. Dinkel HP, Trusen A, Gassel AM, et al. Predictive value of galactographic patterns for benign and malignant neoplasms of the breast in patients with nipple discharge. *Br J Radiol* 2000;73:706.
39. Peters F, Schuth W. Hyperprolactinemia and nonpuerperal mastitis (duct ectasia). *JAMA* 1989;261:1618.
40. Saff D. Apocrine chromhidrosis. *Pediatr Dermatol* 1995;12:48.
41. Diehl T, Kaplan DW. Breast masses in adolescent females. *J Adolesc Health Care* 1985;6:353.
42. Chung SY, Oh KK, Kim DJ. Mammographic and sonographic findings of breast cystic lymphangioma. *J Ultrasound Med* 2003;22:307.
43. Love SM, Gelman RS, Silen W. Fibrocystic "disease" of the breast—a nondisease? *N Engl J Med* 1982;307:1010.
44. Beach RK. Routine breast exams: a chance to reassure, guide, and protect. *Contemp Pediatr* 1987;70:100.
45. Dupont WD, Page DL. Risk factors for breast cancer in women with proliferative breast disease. *N Engl J Med* 1985;312:146.
46. Daniel W, Mathews M. Tumors of the breast in adolescent females. *Pediatrics* 1968;41:743.
47. Anyanwu SN. Fibro-adenoma of the breast in Nigerian Igbos. *S Afr Med J* 2000;90:1223.
48. Stone AM, Shenker IR, McCarthy K. Adolescent breast masses. *Am J Surg* 1977;134:275.
49. Goldstein DP, Miler V. Breast masses in adolescent females. *Clin Pediatr* 1982;21:17.
50. Simpson JS, Barson AJ. Breast tumors in infants and children: a 40-year review of cases at a children's hospital. *Can Med Assoc J* 1969;101:100.
51. Oberman HA Stephens PJ. Carcinoma of the breast in childhood. *Cancer* 1971;30:470.
52. Nichini FM, Goldman L. Inflammatory carcinoma of breast in a 12-year-old girl. *Arch Surg* 1972;105:505.
53. Kern WH, Clark RW. Retrogression of fibroadenomas of the breast. *Am J Surg* 1973;126:59.
54. Seashore JH. Breast enlargements in infants and children. *Pediatr Ann* 1975;4:542.
55. Turbey WJ, Buntain WL, Dudgeon DL. The surgical management of pediatric breast masses. *Pediatrics* 1975;56:736.
56. Bower R, Bell MJ, Ternberg JL. Management of breast lesions in children and adolescents. *J Pediatr Surg* 1976;11:337.
57. Ashikari R, Jun MY, Farrow JH. Breast carcinoma in children and adolescents. *Clin Bull* 1977;7:55.
58. Gogas J, Sechas M, Skalkeas GR. Surgical management of disease of the adolescent female breast. *Am J Surg* 1979;137:634.
59. Oberman HA. Breast lesions in the adolescent female. *Pathol Ann* 1979;1:175.
60. Ligon R, Stevenson D Diner W, et al. Breast masses in young women. *Am J Surg* 1980;140:799.

61. Seltzer MH, Skiles MS. Diseases of the breast in young women. *Surg Gynecol Obstet* 1980;150:360.
62. Hammar B. Childhood breast carcinoma: report of a case. *J Pediatr Surg* 1981;16:77.
63. Ernster VL, Goodson WH, Hunt T, et al. Vitamin E and benign breast "disease": a double-blind, randomized, clinical trial. *Surgery* 1985;4:490.
64. London RS, Sundaram GS, Murphy L, et al. The effect of vitamin E on mammary dysplasia: a double-blind study. *Obstet Gynecol* 1985;65:104.
65. Raju CG. Breast masses in adolescent patients in Trinidad. *Am J Surg* 1985;149:219.
66. El-Tamer MB, Song M, Wait RB. Breast masses in African-American teenage girls. *J Pediatr Surg* 1999;34:1401.
67. Elsheikh A, Keramopoulos A, Lazaris D, et al. Breast tumors during adolescence. *Eur J Gynaecol Oncol* 2000;21:408.
68. Inder M, Vaishnav K, Mathur DR. Benign breast lesions in prepubertal female children—a study of 20 years. *J Indian Med Assoc* 2001;99:619.
69. Dupont WD, Page DL, Parl FE, et al. Long-term risk of breast cancer in women with fibroadenoma. *N Engl J Med* 1994;331:10.
70. Carter BA, Page DL, Schuyler P, et al. No elevation in long-term breast carcinoma risk for women with fibroadenomas that contain atypical hyperplasia. *Cancer* 2001;92:30.
71. Hart J, Layfield LJ, Trumbull WE, et al. Practical aspects in the diagnosis and management of cystosarcoma phyllodes. *Arch Surg* 1988;123:1079.
72. Briggs RM, Waiters M, Rosenthal D. Cystosarcoma phyllodes in adolescent female patients. *Am J Surg* 1983;146:712.
73. Rosen PP, Holmes G, Lesser ML, et al. Juvenile papillomatosis and breast carcinoma. *Cancer* 1985;55:1345.
74. Rosen PE. Papillary duct hyperplasia of the breast in children and young adults. *Cancer* 1985;56:1611.
75. McNicholas NM, Mercer PM, Miller JC, et al. Color Doppler sonography in the evaluation of palpable breast masses. *AJR* 1993;161:765.
76. Ekland D, Zeigler M. Abscess in the nonlactating breast. *Arch Surg* 1971;107:398.
77. Oberman H, Stephens P. Carcinoma of the breast in childhood. *Cancer* 1972;30:470.
78. Karl SR, Ballantine TV, Zaino R. Juvenile secretory carcinoma of the breast. *Br J Surg* 1987;74:214.
79. Farrow JH, Ashikari H. Breast lesions in young girls. *Surg Clin North Am* 1969;49:261.
80. Rivera-Hueto F, Hevia-Vazquez A, Utrilla-Alcolea JC, et al. Long-term prognosis of teenagers with breast cancer. *Int J Surg Pathol* 2002;10:273.
81. Dixon JM, Lumsden AB, Krajewski A, et al. Primary lymphoma of the breast. *Br J Surg* 1987;74:214.
82. Smith BL. The breast. *Crr Probl Obstet Gynecol Fertil* 1996;19:1.
83. Levine AJ. The p53 tumor-suppressor gene. *N Engl J Med* 1992;326:1350.
84. Hall JM, Lee MK, Newman B, et al. Linkage of early-onset familial breast cancer to chromosome 17q21. *Science* 1990;250:1684.
85. Narod SA, Feunteun J, Lynch HT, et al. Familial breast-ovarian cancer locus on chromosome 17q21–q23. *Lancet* 1991;338:82.
86. Ford D, Easton DE Bishop DT, et al. Risks of cancer in BRCA1-mutation carriers. *Lancet* 1994;343:692.
87. Easton DF, Ford D, Bishop DT, et al. Breast and ovarian cancer incidence in BRCA1-mutation carriers. *Am J Hum Genet* 1995;56:265.
88. Burke W, Daly M, Garber J, et al. Recommendations for follow-up care of individuals with an inherited predisposition to cancer. *JAMA* 1997;277:997.
89. Struewing JP, Hartge P, Wacholder S, et al. The risk of cancer associated with specific mutations of BRCA1 and BRCA2 among Ashkenazi Jews. *N Engl J Med* 1997;336:1401.
90. Wooster R, Weber BL. Breast and ovarian cancer. *N Engl J Med* 2003;348:2239.
91. Elger BS, Harding TW. Testing adolescents for a hereditary breast cancer gene (BRCA1). *Arch Pediatr Adolesc Med* 2000;154:113.
92. Elger BS, Harding TW. Genetic testing of adolescents: is it in their best interest? [letter to the editor]. *Arch Pediatr Adolesc Med* 2000;154:851.
93. Ross LF. Genetic testing of adolescents: is it in their best interest? [letter to the editor]. *Arch Pediatr Adolesc Med* 2000;154:850.

94. Weinstein SP, Contant EF, Orel SG, et al. Spectrum of US findings in pediatric and adolescent patients with palpable breast masses. *Radiographics* 2000;20:1613.
95. Kronemer KA, Rhee K, Siegel MJ, et al. Gray scale sonography of breast masses in adolescent girls. *J Ultrasound Med* 2001;20:491.
96. Chao TC, Lo YF, Chen SC, et al. Sonographic features of phyllodes tumors of the breast. *Ultrasound Obstet Gynecol* 2002;20:64.
97. Hochmuth A, Boehm T, Bitzer C, et al. Differentiation of breast masses during 3-D sonographic and echo-enhancer-based evaluation of the vascular pattern: initial experiences. *Ultrasound Med Biol* 2002;28:845.
98. Williams SM, Kaplan PA, Peterson JC, *et al.* Mammography in women under age 30: is there clinical benefit? *Radiology* 1986;161:49.
99. Wedegartner U, Bick U, Wortler K, et al. Differentiation between benign and malignant findings on MR-mammography: usefulness of morphological criteria. *Eur Radiol* 2001;11:1645.
100. Hindle WH, Payne PA, Ran EY. The use of fine needle aspiration in the evaluation of persistent palpable dominant masses. *Am J Obstet Gynecol* 1993;168:1814.
101. Hindle WH, Arias RD, Florentine B, et al. Lack of utility in clinical practice of cytologic examination of non-bloody cyst fluid from palpable breast cysts. *Am J Obstet Gynecol* 2000;182:1300.
102. Markovic-Glamoçak M, Suçiç M, Hoban D. Fine-needle aspiration and nipple discharge cytology in the diagnosis of breast lesions in adolescent and young women: cytologic findings as compared with those obtained in older women. *Adolesc Pediatr Gynecol* 1994;7:205.
103. Greenberg R, Skornick Y, Kaplan O. Management of breast fibroadenomas. *J Gen Intern Med* 1998;13:640.
104. Maharaj D, Naraynsingh V, Ramdass M. Management of giant fibroadenomas: a case for small incisions for large tumors. *Breast J* 2003;9:141.
105. Jolesz FA, Hynynen F. Magnetic resonance image-guided focused ultrasound surgery. *Cancer J* 2002;8:S100.
106. Kaufman CS, Bachman B, Littrup PJ, et al. Office-based ultrasound-guided cryoablation of breast fibroadenomas. *Am J Surg* 2002;184:394.
107. Walsh M, McIntosh K. Neonatal mastitis. *Clin Pediatr* 1986;25:395.
108. Brook I. Recovery of anaerobic bacteria from 3 patients with infection at a pierced body site. *Clin Infect Dis* 2001;33:12.
109. Schwarz RJ, Shrestha R. Needle aspiration of breast abscesses. *Am J Surg* 2001;182:117.
110. Osuch JR. Benign lesions of the breast other than fibrocystic change. *Obstet Gynecol Clin North Am* 1987;14:703.
111. Greydanus DE, Parks DS, Farrell EG. Breast disorders in children and adolescents. *Pediatr Clin North Am* 1989;36:601.

20

Contraception

S. Jean Emans

Contraceptive counseling of adolescents requires knowledge of adolescent development and the available forms of contraception. The adolescent needs to be in partnership with the health care professional to make healthy choices, including postponement of sexual relationships and use of effective methods to lessen the risk of pregnancy and sexually transmitted diseases (STDs). Correct and effective use of contraception by adolescent girls and young women is dependent on a number of factors, including the personal characteristics of the user (age, educational level, socioeconomic status, parity, and social context), the characteristics of the method (dosage, side effects, ease of use, and cost), and the service system providing the method (access, counseling, provider characteristics, educational methods, and choices offered) (1). Too often, clinicians think only of the user without reflecting on the other two important areas that have a major impact on compliance.

Although clinicians providing health care to adolescents should promote postponement of sexual activity and secondary abstinence, many teenagers are engaging in sexual intercourse without the use of effective contraception. The number of teens initiating sexual intercourse before age 18 years increased in the 1980s compared to the early 1970s (2). However, data from the Youth Risk Behavior Survey (YRBS) (3) have shown a decline in sexual intercourse and an increase in condom use through the 1990s. Among ninth to 12th grade high school students, 50.8% of girls reported ever having had sexual intercourse in 1991 compared to 45.3% in 2003. Similarly, 57.4% of boys reported ever having had sexual intercourse in 1991 compared to 48.0% in 2003 (3). In 2003, 27.9% of ninth grade girls and 62.3% of 12th grade girls reported ever having had sexual intercourse. Among boys, 37.3% of ninth graders and 60.5% of 12th graders reported ever having had sexual intercourse. Condom use increased for girls from 38% in 1991 to 57.4% in 2003 and for boys from 54.5% to 68.8%. In 2003, 87% of high school students were characterized as having "responsible sexual behavior" (never had sexual intercourse, no sexual intercourse in past 3 months, or sexual intercourse in past 3 months and used a condom). Among currently sexually active students, 63% used condoms at last sexual intercourse, and 21% of girls used the oral contraceptive pill. Among high school students, 11.2% of girls report four or more sexual partners (3). These data capture youth in school, and it is important to remember that percentages are higher for out-of-school youths. The data from the YRBS are similar to the 1995 Survey of Family Growth, which found that 21.4% of 15-year-old, 38% of 16-year-old, 49.6% of 17-year-old, 62.7% of 18-year-old, and 72.4% of 19-year-old never-married girls/women reported ever being sexually active, with an overall rate for 15- to 19-year-old never-married girls/women of 48.1% (4). When adolescents are dissimilar from their partners—in age, grade, or school—they are less likely to use condoms and other contraceptive methods (5). Early onset of sexual behavior is associated with more lifetime partners and a higher number of recent partners (6). Adolescents who become sexually active in their early teens are often involved in other risk-taking activities such as substance abuse and smoking, and are especially likely to have an unplanned pregnancy or acquire a sexually transmitted disease (STD).

The U.S. teen birth rate has declined significantly throughout the 1990s, from 62.1 births/1000 women 15 to 19 years old in 1991 to 42.9/1000 in 2002 (7). This decline in pregnancy rates has been attributed to more teens choosing abstinence, the increased use of condoms, and the introduction of long-acting contraceptive options. However, many adolescents remain at risk of unplanned pregnancy because of method failure, inconsistent or incorrect use, or discontinuation of the method chosen without the selection of a new method (8). Comprehensive sexuality education in schools, faith based community programs, good parent–teen communication, and access to high quality adolescent health care including contraceptive services and STD screening are essential to assure that the declines in pregnancy rates and increases in responsible sexual behavior are sustained (see Chapter 22). Adolescents who have had sexuality education courses are less likely to become sexually active and more likely to use condoms. Enhanced parent–child communication fostered by specific joint homework assignments also appears to be helpful (9). Additionally, media literacy programs to help teens understand the sexual messages in their environment and peer education programs are promising interventions but need further evaluation. Males need to be involved early and included in abstinence and family planning educational programs and services. More holistic approaches to teenage pregnancy prevention are expensive but have long-term benefits to individuals and society (see Chapter 21). Office screening by history of each adolescent patient is equally important, as noted in Chapter 1. The adolescent patient should be asked about menses and sexual history at each visit to her health care provider. A 14- or 15-year-old teenager will rarely make a specific request for a contraceptive from her primary care clinician unless she knows that the topic can be discussed confidentially. A college student aged 18 or 19 years is much more likely to think abstractly, to plan ahead, and to seek gynecologic care on her own and deal with the issue of contraception. Too often, the first visit to a family planning clinic results from a pregnancy scare. It becomes particularly critical to combine the resources of family planning clinics and STD clinics so that teenagers accessing family planning services can be screened for STDs and those accessing STD clinics can discuss family planning needs.

The interval between first intercourse and clinic visit varies from 2 weeks to several years, with mean intervals of 9 to 23 months in different studies. In our 1987 study (10), the interval between first intercourse and a clinic visit to initiate oral contraceptive (OC) use was not different among patients seen in an urban adolescent clinic (10.7 months), a family planning clinic (8.5 months), and a suburban private practice of adolescent medicine (10.9 months). However, the suburban adolescents were much more likely to have used some type of contraceptive method (usually condoms) before making an appointment; 57% of urban adolescents compared to 14% of suburban adolescents had *never* used a method before coming to the clinic.

Rates of successful use of contraceptives can vary with the population of adolescents served (10–14). In a study of adolescents prescribed OCs, only 48% of those seen in the urban clinic returned for their 3-month follow-up visit and continued to take the pill, compared to 65% of patients seen in a family planning clinic and 84% of patients seen in a suburban private practice (10). At long-term follow-up (13.5 ± 3.7 months), 34% of urban and 55% of suburban teens continued to take the pill. Factors associated with OC compliance included health care in a private practice, suburban residence, white race, college-bound, higher level of father's education, satisfaction with the OC, and absence of side effects. Ten pregnancies occurred among noncompliant urban patients. Furstenberg and associates (12) made similar observations in a study of compliance among family planning patients, in which continuing use of contraception was associated with older age, white race, adolescents who had working parents with higher levels of education, being college bound, above-average grades, a steady sexual relationship, and satisfaction with the method chosen. A study of San Francisco teens found that intention to use contraception was related to actual use of contraception 1 year later (13,14).

In rethinking appropriate counseling, Oakley (15) has suggested that since demographic factors related to contraceptive compliance are difficult to change, counseling of women should focus on use behaviors and assessment of abilities and intentions to carry out those behaviors. The woman who is particularly in need of new counseling approaches is one without prior experience to draw on (no successful analogous behavior from which to generalize), no future plans, no support for avoiding unplanned pregnancy, previous unplanned pregnancies, short-term sexual relationships, cognitive impairment, having a visit not initiated by her, low self-evaluation, concerns about future fertility, and the acceptance of a pregnancy in the next 6 to 12 months. The emphasis of the counseling has to be on future orientation, reviewing the complex behaviors necessary for effective use, assessing intentions, interpreting problems with contraception correctly, and mobilizing self-planning so that effective actions can be taken to resolve problems. Before prescribing contraceptives, the health care provider should discuss the risks of being sexually active, including the emotional consequences, STDs, and pregnancy. Behavioral change is often slow. Some teenagers have not even thought that they could get pregnant with sexual intercourse and have not contemplated the use of contraception. Others have already thought about contraceptive options and made a choice. The adolescent may later forget about her commitment and no longer be using condoms or other protection because of sporadic relationships. Clinicians are challenged by assisting young people through the stages of change by education, personalizing the risk, and skills building (see Chapter 1).

The possibility of parental involvement should be assessed with the adolescent, because many adolescents can share the information with a parent, particularly the mother. Payment for the visit and laboratory tests and issues of confidentiality should be discussed early in the provision of contraceptive services. Involvement of the male partner is ideal but often not achieved in clinical practice. The teen using condoms alone should be knowledgeable about *emergency contraception* (EC) and have access to or a prescription for the progestin-only EC method. For the teen who has been successfully using condoms and now wishes to use hormonal contraception, discussion about the need for continuing protection against STDs is paramount. Although in one study two-thirds of patients stated that they planned to continue to use condoms after initiating hormonal contraception, Loeb and colleagues (16) found that only 28% were using condoms at last intercourse at the 3-month follow-up visit. An adolescent girl needs to discuss with the health care provider whether to tell her partner about her decision to initiate hormonal contraception. She may be concerned that his knowledge of her method will negatively affect his condom use.

Some states have passed laws that specifically allow minors to give their own informed consent for birth control. Adolescents who are emancipated minors or "mature minors" can consent to their own contraception (see Chapter 26). This important issue is best dealt with at the first visit. If the clinician is providing continuity of care from childhood to adolescence, a comprehensive clinical preventive services visit when the girl is 11 or 12 years old is an ideal time to explain the need for privacy and confidentiality in the adolescent years. The parents can understand that a new phase of health care is beginning and that the physician will share as much as possible, but that certain information about school, friends, drugs, and sexuality needs to remain confidential. The parents should be encouraged to call with any of their concerns. Most families welcome knowing that physicians and nurse practitioners are concerned about psychosocial and health issues. The clinician can explicitly state the confidentiality policy before contraceptive issues arise, letting families know that their input is valued and that issues will be shared as needed, and clearly if life threatening. In some situations, prescribing an OC for dysmenorrhea or irregular menses may be better accepted by parents and preserve confidentiality for the patient.

The teen who does not share the information about birth control with her parents needs to think through with the clinician what she would do if her parents found the contraceptive pills or device. In volatile situations, the clinician should offer to be the mediator to help both sides come to a solution around responsible sexuality. The clinician can facilitate communication by asking both the parents and the daughter to come in for counseling at the end of the office day. Each health care provider has his or her own style of communication, but it is helpful to empathize with and acknowledge the parents' genuine concerns for their daughter's health. Additionally, the clinician can discuss with parents the issues faced by teens such as media messages about sexuality and the challenges of establishing healthy relationships. Parents should be congratulated on raising a daughter who is being responsible about contraception instead of becoming pregnant, as with so many of her peers. Acknowledging to parents how difficult it is to raise adolescents and listening to their issues can facilitate solutions acceptable to parent and adolescent.

The pregnancy rates of 100 women using different contraceptive devices for 1 year (100 woman-years of use) are listed in Table 20-1 (17–20). Trussell and colleagues

TABLE 20-1. *Lowest expected and typical percentages of accidental pregnancy in the United States during the first year of use of a method.*

Method	% of women experiencing an unintended pregnancy within the first year of use	
	Typical use[a]	Lowest expected[b]
Chance[c]	85	85
Spermicides[d]	26 to 29	6 to 15
Periodic abstinence	25	—
Calendar	—	9
Ovulation method	—	3
Sympto-Thermal[e]	—	2
Postovulation	—	1
Cap[f]		
Parous women	32 to 40	26
Nulliparous women	16 to 20	9
Sponge		
Parous women	40	20
Nulliparous women	20	9
Diaphragm[f]	10 to 18	6

[a]Among *typical* couples who initiate use of a method (not necessarily for the first time), the percentage who experience an accidental pregnancy during the first year if they do not stop use for any other reason.

[b]Among couples who initiate the use of a method (not necessarily for the first time), and who use it perfectly (consistently and correctly), the percentage who experience an accidental pregnancy during the first year and who do not stop use for any other reason.

[c]The percents becoming pregnant in column titled "Typical use" is based on data from populations where contraception is not used and from women who cease using contraception in order to become pregnant. Among such populations, about 89% become pregnant within 1 year. This estimate was lowered slightly (to 85%) to represent the percent who would become pregnant within 1 year among women now relying on reversible methods of contraception if they abandoned contraception altogether.

[d]Foams, creams, gels, vaginal suppositories, and vaginal film.

[e]Cervical mucus (ovulation) method supplemented by calendar in the preovulatory and basal body temperature in the postovulatory phases.

[f]With spermicidal cream or jelly.

(continues)

TABLE 20-1. *Continued*

Method	% of women experiencing an unintended pregnancy within the first year of use	
	Typical use[a]	Lowest expected[b]
Withdrawal	19 to 27	4
Condom[g]		
Male	14	3
Female	21	5
Pill	5 to 8	
Combined estrogen/progestin pill	—	0.1
Progestin only pill	—	0.5
Vaginal ring (NuvaRing)[h]	—	0.65 to 1.0
Transdermal contraception patch (Ortho Evra)[h]	—	1.0
Intrauterine devices		
Copper T380A	0.8	0.6
Levonorgestrel IUS (Mirena)	0.1	0.1
Injectables		
Depot medroxyprogesterone acetate (DMPA, Depo-Provera)	3	0.3
Depot medroxyprogesterone acetate/estradiol cypionate (Lunelle)[i]	3	0.05
Subdermal implants		
Levonorgestrel implants (Norplant and Norplant-2)	0.2	0.05
Etonogestrel implant (Implanon)	—	0
Female sterilization	0.5	0.5
Male sterilization	0.15	0.10

Lactational amenorrhea method: LAM is highly effective, *temporary* method of contraception. [j]

[g]Without spermicides.
[h]Clinical trials. Typical use data not available.
[i]Not available in United States.
[j]However, to maintain effective protection against pregnancy, another method of contraception must be used as soon as menstruation resumes, the frequency or duration of breastfeeds is reduced, bottle feeds are introduced, or the baby reaches 6 months of age.
Sources: Trussell J, Contraceptive efficacy. In: Hatcher RA, Trussell J, Stewart F, et al. *Contraceptive technology,* 17th ed. New York, NY: Irvington, 1998. Trussell J, Hatcher R, Cates W, et al. Contraceptive failure in the United States: an update. *Stud Fam Plan* 1990;21. Trussell J, Vaughan B, Contraceptive failure, method-related discontinuation and resumption of use: Results from the 1995 National Survey of Family Growth. *Fam Plan Perspect* 1998;31:64. Hatcher RA, Nelson AL, Zieman M, et al. A Pocket Guide to Managing Contraception. Bridging the Gap Foundation, Tiger, Georgia, 2003. Speroff L, Darney PD. *A clinical guide for contraception.* Philadelphia: Lippincott Williams & Wilkins, 2001.

(18–20) and others (17,21) have written eloquently about the problems of developing these numbers, including the varying definitions and measurements of efficacy from study to study, the lack of randomized clinical trials of two methods at the same time, selection bias of compliant, nonobese women, concepts of use and exposure, sexual activity and fertility of women in the trial, assessment and self-reporting of failures (pregnancies by report versus monthly urine or blood pregnancy tests, frequency of reporting, lost-to-follow-up rates), acceptance of backup methods into the trial, recent

OC use, and conflict of interest of investigators. Estimates for use failure rates for a first year of contraception may be 30% higher because of underreporting of abortions. The two techniques commonly used to measure efficacy are the Pearl Index, required by the Food and Drug Administration (FDA), and the Life-Table Analysis (LTA). The Pearl Index provides the incidence of unintended pregnancies over total cycles, or months, of contraceptive usage (pregnancies per 100 woman-years of exposure). This Index does not take into account duration of exposure and thus may overestimate failure rates for methods in which the user is more likely to use the method correctly with longer duration of use. Because the studies are not randomized trials, the clinician cannot use the numbers to make comparisons. In contrast, the LTA accounts for duration of use and derives a cumulative failure rate. In addition, data from clinical trials do not mirror actual or typical use in different populations of patients. The design of the study itself with frequent visits and monitoring can encourage correct method use. For example, a study of a triphasic levonorgestrel (LNG) OC evaluating 13 cycles of use reported an overall Pearl Index of 2.18 and method failure Pearl Index of 1.25 per 100 woman-years (22), but a 5 year study of the same OC reported a failure rate of 0.22 and 0.06, respectively (23). Using the LTA for up to 13 cycles of use, the cumulative pregnancy rate for the LNG triphasic OC was 1.3% and the overall probability 1.8%, compared to the transdermal patch of 1.1% and 1.3%, respectively (22). In contrast, the 1-year typical use-failure rate for OCs in the 1995 NSFG study was 7% (18). For some teenagers, the pregnancy rate with the combined OC may climb to 9 to 12 pregnancies per 100 woman-years or even higher because of missed pills (frequently underreported [24]) and misunderstanding the directions. Continuation rates can also significantly impact pregnancy rates.

Thus it is critical for teens to know how to use backup methods and how to obtain EC. Regardless of what the patient initially states as her preferred form of contraception, it is important for the clinician to discuss all available forms of birth control, because method switching is common (25). She may well make other choices in the future depending on her need for contraception, the frequency with which she is having intercourse, her age, parity, and her partner's preferences. Writing the methods of contraception (including abstinence), the pregnancy rates, and the risks and benefits on a sheet of paper can help the patient make a good choice for a method that she will use. Unfortunately, many materials are written at a level that is above the reading level of adolescent patients, and thus care should be taken in selection of print and internet materials. Women with low reading skills are particularly likely to have inadequate knowledge about family planning (26). Almost half of teen girls use the Internet for reproductive health information, and authoritative websites should be recommended (Appendix 1). The mortality in sexually active women is shown in Table 20-2. The risk of combined OCs is substantially less than that of carrying a pregnancy to term. However, hormonal contraception offers no protection from acquiring a STD, and thus the use of condoms needs to be emphasized.

Health care providers also need to address the sexuality issues of adolescents with chronic diseases, disabilities, and developmental delay (see Chapter 23). Adolescents

TABLE 20-2. *Annual number of birth- or method-related deaths associated with control of fertility per 100,000 nonsterile women by fertility control method according to age (yr).*

Method of control and outcome	15 to 19	20 to 24	25 to 29	30 to 34	35 to 39	40 to 44
No fertility control methods[a]	7.0	7.4	9.1	14.8	25.7	28.2
Oral contraceptives, nonsmoker[b]	0.3	0.5	0.9	1.9	13.8	31.6
Oral contraceptives, smoker[b]	2.2	3.4	6.6	13.5	51.1	117.2
Intrauterine device[b]	0.8	0.8	1.0	1.0	1.4	1.4
Condom[a]	1.1	1.6	0.7	0.2	0.3	0.4
Diaphragm/spermicide[a]	1.9	1.2	1.2	1.3	2.2	2.8
Periodic abstinence[a]	2.5	1.6	1.6	1.7	2.9	3.6

[a]Deaths are birth-related.
[b]Deaths are method-related.
From: *Physicians' desk reference,* Montvale, NJ: Medical Economics Data, Inc., 2003. Adapted from: Ory HW. Mortality associated with fertility and fertility control: *Fam Plan Perspect* 1983;15:50.

with chronic diseases, especially those with delayed development and undernutrition, are frequently assumed to be too sick to be sexually active or may be infantilized by parents and health care providers. A discussion of sexuality and contraceptive methods is important for all adolescents. Many ill patients take chances because they falsely assume their disease has made them infertile. Patients who are immunosuppressed must be educated about their increased risks of persistent human papillomavirus (HPV) infection (see Chapter 17) and should be encouraged, as all adolescents, to use condoms with every sexual relationship. Permanent sterilization can be considered by young women with conditions such as severe heart disease or cystic fibrosis, depending on the wishes of the patient. Patients with disabilities need sensitive counseling to help them through a pelvic examination, reassurance about their normal anatomy, and provision of contraception that meets their needs. Insertion of female barrier methods, such as the diaphragm or female condom, may not be possible for some teens. Patients with myelodysplasia have an increased incidence of latex allergy, and thus use of polyurethane rather than latex condoms are important for these patients. Parents often bring in adolescent girls with developmental delay to discuss contraception or menstrual hygiene. These patients, especially those with mild retardation, appear to be at increased risk of sexual assault or abuse. Thus, depending on the social environment and available supervision, risk, and age of the adolescent, thoughtful discussion is needed about the choices: observation, prophylactic hormonal contraception (an OC, patch, injectable progestins, or implants), endometrial ablation, or sterilization (depending on the needs of the patient and the legal issues involved). Clinicians should identify local disability organizations and lawyers who have expertise in the area to assist young women and their families. These adolescents also benefit from education about hygiene, reproduction, contraception, and responsible sexuality.

EVIDENCE-BASED CONTRACEPTIVE PRACTICE: THE WHO GUIDELINES FOR MEDICAL ELIGIBILITY CRITERIA GUIDELINES FOR PRESCRIBING CONTRACEPTION

Over the past ten years, there has been a shift toward evidence-based contraceptive practice. In 1995, the World Health Organization (WHO) released medical eligibility criteria guidelines to assist family planning agencies and clinicians that prescribe contraception; these were updated in 2000 and 2004, and are available on the web and in print (27,28). The document was undertaken because of concern that women may be denied access to effective contraception if policies for prescribing are based on outdated medical information. Most medical conditions in and of themselves do not necessarily preclude use of combination OCs; the risks of a high-risk pregnancy to the mother and baby must be weighed against the risk of the contraceptive method. The WHO criteria for contraception were developed after a critical review of the existing medical literature. Although some domains lack rigorous trials and evidence, this comprehensive approach has been widely adopted (29). Levels 1 to 4 are noted in Table 20-3. With level 3, the method should not be used in parts of the world in which medical expertise and judgment are not readily available. However, in the United States, clinicians should weigh the risks and benefits with the individual woman and assess her ability to use other methods to prevent unintended pregnancies. For example, sickle cell disease (SS) is considered a Level 2 and epilepsy is a Level 1. Although smoking cessation is always important, smoking is designated Level 2 for women less than 35 years old. The summary of the full guideline is in Appendix 2. Table 20-4 includes selected level 3 and level 4 conditions for combined estrogen/progestin contraceptives. Other authors have also provided evidence based guidelines in articles, books, and on the Internet (including the Cochrane reviews) (30–32).

TABLE 20-3. *Four category classification for WHO guidelines. The framework can be used in situations in which clinical judgment is available and in those in which clinical judgment is not available in the field.*

Classification	Use with clinical judgment	Use with limited clinical judgment
1	Use method in any circumstances	Yes (Use the method)
2	Generally use the method	Yes (Use the method)
3	Use of method not usually recommended unless other more appropriate methods are not available or not acceptable	No (Do not use the method)
4	Method not to be used	No (Do not use the method)

From: World Health Organization. Medical eligibility criteria for contraceptive use. Geneva, 2004; with permission.

TABLE 20-4. *Selected WHO guidelines for combined hormonal contraceptives.*

<u>Category 3 WHO guidelines</u> (for combined hormonal contraceptives)
Use of method is usually not recommended unless other, more appropriate methods are not available or not acceptable.
- Smoking (<15 cigarettes/day) <u>and</u> age ≥35 years.
- Hypertension
  History of hypertension in which blood pressure cannot be monitored.
  Adequately controlled hypertension, where blood pressure can be evaluated.
  Systolic blood pressure 140 to 159 or diastolic 90 to 99[a] mmHg.
- Postpartum <21 days
- Primary breast-feeding, 6 weeks to 6 months
- Long-term use of enzyme inducing antibiotics or anticonvulsants (rifampin, phenytoin) because of drug interactions
- History of oral contraceptive-related cholecystitis
- Symptomatic biliary tract disease (not treated by cholecystectomy)
- Known genetic hyperlipidemia (category 2–3)
- Migraine <35 years, no aura (continuation)
- Diabetic nephropathy, retinopathy, neuropathy (category 3–4)

<u>Category 4 WHO guidelines</u> (for combined hormonal contraceptives)
Method is contraindicated.
- Smoking ≥15 cigarettes/day <u>and</u> age ≥35 years
- Hypertension
  Systolic blood pressure >160 or diastolic >100 mmHg
- History of or current deep vein thrombosis or pulmonary embolism
- Known thrombogenic mutations
- Complicated valvular heart disease (pulmonary hypertension, atrial fibrillation, history of subacute bacterial endocarditis)
- Migraine headaches with aura or other focal neurologic symptoms
- Major surgery with prolonged immobilization
- Active viral hepatitis
- Breast feeding <6 weeks postpartum

[a]The blood pressure ranges are for adults, and lower levels corresponding to 95% of age should be used in young teens.
Adapted from: the WHO recommendations. World Health Organization. Medical eligibility criteria for contraceptive use. Geneva, 2004.

PATIENT EVALUATION

The indications and contraindications of each method are discussed below. Adolescents deserve information on all methods, including emergency contraception (EC). A careful history, recent general physical examination, blood pressure, and, if indicated, urine pregnancy test, are first steps in providing hormonal contraception. Questions that are appropriate to ask the teen are shown in Table 20-5. The clinician should determine whether there are any specific indications or contraindications to the use of a particular form of contraception. If the patient has already practiced contraception, she may be more apt to comply with the method chosen. The degree to which one or both partners can take responsibility for avoiding an unplanned pregnancy should be assessed. In one study, adolescents with a previous pregnancy were more likely to choose hormonal methods than never-pregnant adolescents, but less likely to

TABLE 20-5. *Questions to pose to teens choosing a contraceptive method.*

What methods have you used before?
What are your worries about this method?
Do you have friends who have used this method?
What were their experiences? Did they have problems?
Do you think you can use this method effectively?
Have you ever had problems with your weight? Have you ever dieted?
Is your partner in favor or opposed to this method?
How will you be able to handle unexpected bleeding or extra bleeding?
Do you have any questions I haven't answered?

be consistent condom users (33). Clinicians should take a complete medical history including information on problems such as weight gain, headaches, acne, breast tenderness, dysmenorrhea, irregular menses, and nausea/vomiting, so that issues that arise at future visits can be better assessed. Additionally, a history of blood-clotting disorders within the family (Table 20-6) can further help with choice of contraceptive method. Screening for STDs and gynecologic assessment, including Pap smears, are part of general adolescent preventive care. Fear of the first pelvic examination has been shown to be a barrier to teens wishing to obtain contraceptives (34) and delaying the first pelvic examination in adolescents can be helpful in building trust (35). Decisions about the timing of the examination need to be individualized and should not be a prerequisite to the prescribing of OCs (See Chapter 1). Risk-taking behaviors (substance use, nonuse of seat belts, violence) should be assessed and addressed; providing effective counseling on tobacco avoidance and smoking cessation is particularly important. Whichever method is chosen should be demonstrated for the teen. Younger adolescents are concrete thinkers and need to have the OC package opened and the exact method of taking the pill demonstrated. Similarly, the use of condoms requires a hands-on demonstration. Any handouts that will be given should be read with the teen and open-ended questions asked. The various methods are outlined below. Extensive information on irregular bleeding, cancer, thrombosis, and other health issues are described in the section on oral contraceptives below but most of these data likely also apply to other combined estrogen/progestin methods such as patches and rings.

TABLE 20-6. *Questions to ask to ascertain a personal/family history of thromboembolism.*

Have you or a close family member (including uncles and aunts) ever had blood clots in the legs or lungs?
Have you or a close family member ever been hospitalized for blood clots in the legs or lungs?
Have you or a family member ever taken a blood thinner?
Under what circumstances did the clot form? How old was the relative? Was there cancer, airline travel, obesity, immobility, hormones, or some other illness that may have led to the clot?

COMBINED ORAL CONTRACEPTIVES

Many teenagers choose a hormonal method such as an oral contraceptive (OC) because of the low failure rate, the relief from dysmenorrhea, and the ease of use of a method that is not directly related to the episode of intercourse. Common pills and their hormone content are listed in Table 20-7. The majority of OCs are combination pills containing an estrogen and a progestin. The so-called minipill is a progestin-only pill.

The estrogen contained in the combination pills is either *mestranol* or *ethinyl estradiol* and varies in dose from 20 to 50 µg. Ethinyl estradiol (EE) is rapidly absorbed, with peak levels in 60 to 120 minutes (36). Mestranol is converted in the liver to ethinyl estradiol; therefore, peak serum levels of ethinyl estradiol are lower and occur later after ingestion of mestranol than after ingestion of the same dose of ethinyl estradiol. All of the low-dose OCs have ≤35 µg ethinyl estradiol. OCs with 50 µg estrogen have either mestranol or ethinyl estradiol. It is difficult to assess the exact potency of these two compounds in relation to each other because the progestin may potentiate or lessen the effects of a particular dose of the estrogen. However, many authors consider that 50 µg of mestranol is equivalent to 35 µg of ethinyl estradiol (37). The plasma levels of ethinyl estradiol seen with an OC containing 50 µg mestranol and 1 mg norethindrone were the same as those with a pill containing 35 µg ethinyl estradiol and 1 mg norethindrone (38). However, there is significant variability among individual women and even within the same woman at different sampling times.

Most of the progestins used in OCs are 19-nortestosterone derivatives and are related to 19-carbon androgens. These include norethindrone, norethindrone acetate, norethynodrel, ethynodiol diacetate, norgestrel, levonorgestrel, desogestrel, norgestimate, and gestodene. Norgestrel is a racemic mixture of dextro- and levonorgestrel with the levonorgestrel being the active isomer (thus 0.3 mg of norgestrel can be considered equivalent to 0.15 mg of levonorgestrel). These progestins have varying qualities of being estrogenic, antiestrogenic, progestational (anabolic), and androgenic. However, *none* of the progestins are truly androgenic in the quantities contained in OCs and when the estrogen content of the OC is taken into consideration. Potencies are extremely controversial because of the varying tests used, including animal models, delay of menses, and ability to induce glycogen vacuoles in human endometrium (38,39).

Generally, the estranes—norethindrone, norethindrone acetate, and ethynodiol diacetate—are considered fairly equipotent; norgestrel is estimated to be 5 to 10 times more potent, and levonorgestrel is 10 to 20 times more potent. Gestodene is considered less androgenic and more progestational than levonorgestrel. Norgestimate is estimated to have three times the potency of norethindrone on the test of percentage of rabbits ovulating (levonorgestrel is seven to eight times more potent than norethindrone on this test). Norgestimate has four to five times less binding affinity for rabbit uterine receptors than levonorgestrel and much less affinity for androgen receptors and sex hormone-binding globulin than levonorgestrel. Desogestrel is more progestational than levonorgestrel but less androgenic; this compound also binds to corticoid receptors (1,36). In general, the doses of progestins have been adjusted to be roughly equipotent across

TABLE 20-7. *Common Oral Contraceptives Available in the United States (other generics are available).*

Drug	Estrogen	Amount (mcg)	Progestin	Amount (mg)
Demulen 1/50 Zovia 1/50	Ethinyl estradiol	50	Ethynodiol diacetate	1
Ovral Ogestrel	Ethinyl estradiol	50	Norgestrel	0.5
Ovcon-50	Ethinyl estradiol	50	Norethindrone	1
Norinyl 1+50 OrthoNovum 1/50	Mestranol	50	Norethindrone	1
Norinyl 1+35 Necon 1/35 OrthoNovum 1/35 Norethin1/35 Nortrel 1/35	Ethinyl estradiol	35	Norethindrone	1
Demulen 1/35 Zovia 1/35	Ethinyl estradiol	35	Ethynodiol diacetate	1
Ortho-Novum 7/7/7	Ethinyl estradiol	35	Norethindrone	0.5 × 7d 0.75 × 7d 1.0 × 7d
Ortho-Cyclen Sprintec	Ethinyl estradiol	35	Norgestimate	0.25
Ortho-TriCyclen Tri-Sprintec	Ethinyl estradiol	35	Norgestimate	0.180 × 7d 0.215 × 7d 0.250 × 7d
Brevicon Necon 0.5/35 Modicon Norcept 0.5/35	Ethinyl estradiol	35	Norethindrone	0.5
Ovcon-35	Ethinyl estradiol	35	Norethindrone	0.4
Yasmin	Ethinyl estradiol	30	Drospirenone	3.0
Lo/Ovral Low-Ogestrel	Ethinyl estradiol	30	Norgestrel	0.3
Loestrin 1.5/30 Microgestin 1.5/30	Ethinyl estradiol	30	Norethindrone acetate	1.5
Nordette Portia Levlen Levora	Ethinyl estradiol	30	Levonorgestrel	0.15
Seasonale	Ethinyl estradiol	30	Levonorgestrel	0.15 × 84 d
Desogen Apri OrthoCept	Ethinyl estradiol	30	Desogestrel	0.15
Loestrin 1/20 Microgestin 1/20	Ethinyl estradiol	20	Norethindrone acetate	1
Estrostep	Ethinyl estradiol	20 × 5d 30 × 7d 35 × 9d	Norethindrone acetate	1
TriNorinyl	Ethinyl estradiol	35	Norethindrone	0.5 × 7d 1.0 × 9d 0.5 × 5d
Triphasil Trivora TriLevlen Enpresse	Ethinyl estradiol	30 40 30	Levonorgestrel	0.05 × 6d 0.075 × 5d 0.125 × 10d
Cyclessa	Ethinyl estradiol	25	Desogestrel	0.1 × 7d 0.125 × 7d 0.150 × 7d

(continues)

TABLE 20-7. *Continued*

Drug	Estrogen	Amount (mcg)	Progestin	Amount (mg)
Ortho Tri-Cyclen Lo	Ethinyl estradiol	25	Norgestimate	0.180 × 7d 0.215 × 7d 0.250 × 7d
Alesse Aviane Levlite Lessina	Ethinyl estradiol	20	Levonorgestrel	0.1
Mircette Kariva	Ethinyl estradiol	10 × 5d 20 × 21d	Desogestrel	0.15 × 21d
Ovrette			Norgestrel	0.075
Nor-Q.D. Camila Micronor Errin			Norethindrone	0.35

all OCs and androgenic activities of the progestins are insignificant. "Second generation" OCs are products containing norethindrone, levonorgestrel, and norgestimate and up to 35 μg EE; "third generation" OCs contain desogestrel and gestodene and 20 to 30 μg EE. Norgestimate has been classified as "second generation" because it is metabolized to levonorgestrel (LNG) and levonorgestrel metabolites. The half-lives of the progestins have been estimated to be about 7 to 8 hours (range, 4 to 11 hours) for norethindrone, 10 to 12 hours for gestodene, 16 hours (range, 8 to 30 hours) for levonorgestrel, 45 to 71 hours for norgestimate, and 20 hours (range, 11 to 24 hours) for desogestrel.

There are variations in elimination half-lives between subjects and within the same subject, as well as evidence of differences when the progestin is given alone, when it is given for multiple doses, and when it is administered with estrogen (38). Some progestins, such as norethindrone, have a loss of drug with the first pass through the liver after absorption, and others, such as levonorgestrel, do not. Long half-lives and other aspects of binding and metabolism of certain progestins likely contribute to the lowered incidence of breakthrough bleeding. Drospirenone is a new synthetic progestin chemically related to 21-carbon 17α-spironolactone with antimineralocorticoid (antialdosterone) and antiandrogenic activity (40,41). It blocks the stimulation of the renin-angiotensin-aldosterone system by estrogen (40). Serum half life is 31 to 33 hours (42). The 3 mg dose of drospirenone, equivalent to 25 mg spironolactone, may be helpful in the treatment of acne and mild water retention (43). Because of the possibility for potassium retention, drospirenone-containing OCs should be avoided in those with adrenal insufficiency, renal or hepatic disease, and used with monitoring of potassium in those taking potassium sparing diuretics, potassium supplements, ACE inhibitors, NSAIDs, heparin, or angiotensin-II receptor antagonists. Other progestins are under study.

The combination OCs prevent pregnancy by suppressing the ovarian-hypothalamic axis and thus inhibiting ovulation. In addition, they alter the endometrium, increase the viscosity of the endocervical mucus, and may have a direct effect on corpus luteum steroidogenesis. Fortunately, even with missed pills, ovulation usually remains suppressed (44). Women taking an OC with 35 μg EE with monophasic 1 mg norethindrone (NET) appear to have less follicular development than those taking the same dose of estrogen with 0.5 mg NET or a triphasic NET dose (Ortho-Novum 7/7/7) (45). Creinin and colleagues found that women taking a 20 μg EE/LNG who started their second cycle 2 days late had greater follicular activity than users of a triphasic norgestimate (NGM) 35-μg EE pill (46). A recent study has suggested that body weight may play a role in increasing the risk of OC failure (47). In a study of women in the Group Health Cooperative of Puget Sound, women of the highest body weight quartile (>70.5 kg) had increased risk of OC failure (OR 1.6, 95% CI 1.1 to 2.4) compared to women of the lower weight; higher risk was seen with the very low-dose OCs for the highest quartile (OR 4.5, 95% CI 1.4 to 4.4). However, the absolute risk of a pregnancy was very small. This observation needs further study.

Selection of a particular combined OC depends on the patient's needs and response, side effects with prior methods, the availability of samples and supplies to family planning clinics and physician offices, and cost (typically, $12 to $40 per cycle). Typical starter OCs contain 20 to 35 μg EE. OCs with 20 μg EE are generally associated with a higher rate of intermenstrual bleeding than 35 μg pills (depending on the progestin), but 20 μg EE formulations have been associated with lower rates of breast soreness and nausea (48). A progestin-dominant OC may be helpful in patients with dysmenorrhea, hypermenorrhea, previous breakthrough bleeding (BTB), or dysfunctional uterine bleeding. OCs with 50 μg EE should rarely be prescribed and are reserved for patients with persistent intermenstrual bleeding, concomitant use of anticonvulsants, which augments metabolism of the OC (see Epilepsy section), and those in whom ovarian cysts recur on a 35 μg EE OC. Although one study has suggested that OCs with 20 μg EE may have a less positive impact on bone density in adolescents than the 30- to 35-μg pills (see Bone density section), further studies are needed. A Cochrane review of biphasic versus triphasic OCs found that only two trials qualified for review. In one study, the biphasic NET pill had more problems with cycle control than the triphasic LNG OC, but was similar to the NET triphasic OC (49). Only one trial compared monophasic and biphasic OCs with NET, and no significant differences were found (50). In another trial, a triphasic norgestimate (NGM)/35 μg EE OC showed lower BTB and amenorrhea rates than a NET/20 μg EE OC. Despite this, there was no difference in satisfaction or compliance with the two pills (51). Similarly, although some adolescents may find the particular packaging or the presence of many different colored tablets in the triphasics confusing, most do well, and compliance rates for monophasics and triphasics are similar at 1-year follow-up (52). Patients also may desire to avoid the pill-free interval and take the pill continuously for 2, 3 or 4 cycles or continuously without interruption; in one study, taking 42 days of active pills resulted in fewer days of bleeding and fewer headaches and complaints of vaginal itch (53). An extended 84/7-day oral contraceptive (Seasonale), consisting of 0.15 mg LNG and 30 μg EE, has demonstrated similar efficacy and duration of withdrawal bleeding to a comparable, cyclic OC. Unscheduled bleeding was higher than the comparison group with the 84/7 initially, but improved so as to be comparable by the fourth cycle (54). A 12-month trial of a continuous 20 μg EE/0.1 mg LNG versus a cyclic pill showed fewer bleeding days for the continuous regimen (55). Other monophasics can be used similarly. Some patients may use a preset number of months of cycling and others use the pill continuously until menstrual bleeding occurs and then stop for 3 to 7 days and subsequently resume use.

Breakthrough bleeding (BTB) rates appear to be lower with some of the newer OCs, although studies are difficult to compare because of varying definition of bleeding and spotting. For example, the triphasic LNG pill has less BTB than NET triphasics. Desogestrel (DSG)– and NGM–containing pills have extremely low rates of BTB and amenorrhea. In a comparative study, Corson (56) reported that 11.3% of women taking a NGM/EE OC and 10.6% of women taking a norgestrel (NG)/EE pill experienced BTB in the first 6 months, and 1.1% and 1.8%, respectively, experienced amenorrhea in the same interval. Absence of side effects can be important for adolescents to enhance continued use of OCs.

Verbal counseling about risks and benefits should be documented in the medical record; some clinics use a standard informed consent form. Although physicians are usually concerned about the serious but highly unlikely side effects of OCs, patients often have very different worries related to pill use. Their intention to use and actual use of OC may be influenced by concerns about health and physical appearance (57). In our Boston study (10), urban teens were concerned about weight gain (32%), blood clots (22%), birth defects (11%), and future fertility (10%), whereas suburban teens were almost exclusively worried about the possibility of weight gain (86%). Although birth defects and future fertility are not related to OC use, failure to address a patient's worries may lead to noncompliance. The statements such as "Some adolescents I see are worried about gaining weight" or "Some adolescents are worried about not being able to have children" help initiate the dialogue between the adolescent and the health care provider. A number of studies have shown no significant increase in weight with OCs (For a discussion of weight, see weight change section). It is important to weigh the patient at each visit and provide appropriate assessment of diet and physical activity and counseling. Avoiding all fast foods and decreasing TV viewing time for the first 3 months of use of hormonal contraception can be an important preventive strategy. Encouraging the sedentary teen to increase her exercise level is also important.

A handout should be given to patients, and this can serve as an important point of discussion. To avoid confusion, the clinic handout should reflect the content of the Food and Drug Administration (FDA) patient package insert. Although written instructions and Internet sites can save phone calls, they are not a substitute for careful counseling in the office because many patients misplace their directions soon after the visit (10). The possible occurrence of intermenstrual bleeding for the first few cycles should be explained in detail, with patients being shown the actual pill package and where the bleeding might occur (usually the second week). Patients should be encouraged to call if any problems are worrying them and counseled not to stop taking the pill without calling. Patients are instructed in possible side effects using the acronym ACHES: Abdominal pain (severe); Chest pain (severe), cough, shortness of breath; Headache (severe), dizziness, weakness, numbness, speech problems; Eye problems (vision loss or blurring); Severe leg pain (calf or thigh). The benefits of the pill should be stressed. These include less iron-deficiency anemia, less dysmenorrhea, a lowered incidence of benign breast disease and uterine and ovarian cancers, less pelvic inflammatory disease (PID), and less acne. For example, among teens seen in an urban family planning clinic, those girls with severe dysmenorrhea who experienced a reduction of their symptoms on OCs were eight times more likely to be consistent users (58).

Patients should then be given a prescription or a 3-month supply of pills and asked to return to the clinic in 1 to 3 months to check weight, blood pressure, and side effects. The patient who is older and who sought medical care specifically to obtain a contraceptive may be seen in 3 months and encouraged to call if any special problems arise. It is helpful if each office has one professional designated to take patients' phone calls at the time they are initiated, as adolescents may be calling from school or another location where the call may be difficult to return. Younger teenagers, those who have been having intercourse for months to years without adequate contraception, and those with multiple partners, school failure, concerns about fertility, or other high-risk behaviors, or the sibling of a parenting teen should be encouraged to return in 6 weeks or even sooner to continue the dialogue on contraceptive choices and address other risky behaviors if present.

Most pills are available in 21- and 28-day packages; the latter have seven tablets that are placebos except for a few pills that have iron (e.g., Loestrin and Estrostep*) or 5 days of low-dose EE (e.g., Mircette). The majority of teenagers do best using a 28-day pill pack, since it is easier to remember to take a pill every day rather than for 21 days of hormones followed by a 7-day rest. In our experience, 21-day pills frequently result in confusion (unless being used as continuous pills). To start the first package of pills, patients may start on the Sunday following the first day of menses (unless menses starts on a Sunday, in which case the pills are started that day); on the first day of menses (some OCs are packaged only for Sunday starts; others have stickers or mechanisms that allow any day start); on day 5 of menses (to accommodate the timing of arrival of patients in the office); or any day ("Quick Start") (59). Teens using "Quick Start" with ingestion of the first pill at the time of the clinic visit (after excluding pregnancy) appear to be more adherent at 3 months than teens using Sunday start, but similar at 12 months (60). Immediate start of OCs does not appear to result in any more bleeding days than conventional start within the first 7 days of the cycle (61). Except for day 1 start, patient should be instructed to use backup contraception (condoms) for at least 7 days. Patients who are amenorrheic and desire to use OCs can refrain from intercourse for 2 weeks, a sensitive pregnancy test obtained, and then started. Alternatively, medroxyprogesterone (10 mg for 5 days) can be used (after a negative pregnancy test) to initiate withdrawal flow before starting an OC.

Patients are instructed to take one pill daily at about the same time each day, preferably after dinner or at bedtime. It is essential that adolescents cue pill taking to

---

* Names of pills do not imply endorsement of any particular brand.

a daily activity such as a meal or tooth brushing. A new chewable version of one OC (Ovcon-35) was approved by the FDA in November 2003. Adolescents frequently miss pills and thus should receive careful instructions on methods of dealing with this problem (Appendix 3). The importance of a backup method and emergency contraception (EC) should be stressed. Patients will likely experience breakthrough bleeding with missed pills. The follow-up visit includes a blood pressure measurement and weight check. Teens should be questioned about consistent use, concerns, and side effects of the method, and the benefits should be reviewed. Not infrequently, the nausea and intermenstrual bleeding that patients experience during the first cycle of pills have disappeared by the third cycle. Adjustments in pill dosage can be made as suggested in the section below on side effects. Adolescent patients' ability to obtain or pay for refills should be reviewed. Young adolescents are then seen at least every 6 months for renewal of the pill prescription, blood pressure and weight check, and counseling. Screening for *C. trachomatis* (and *Neisseria gonorrhoeae*) every 6 months in high-risk teens or with a change in sexual partner and every 12 months in lower-risk teens is appropriate. Older adolescents who are consistent contraceptive users can be seen annually for STD and Pap screening (as indicated). Teens at high risk for other problem behaviors need much more frequent visits to deal with not only contraceptive use but with the many other behavioral and social issues in their lives.

Side Effects, Contraindications, and Precautions

Weight Change

Weight gain or change in body composition has not been associated with low-dose OC use in a number of studies (1,10,62–65). Carpenter and Neinstein (63) reported no significant difference between an OC group and a control group in initial weight and weight after 1 year of use. A study by Lloyd and colleagues did not find any changes in body composition or weight among adolescent OC users versus comparison adolescents (65). Despite this, fear of weight gain is a source of major worry for teens, and weight should be checked at each visit. There do appear to be some teens, especially very young teens, who seem to be particularly prone to gain weight with the use of hormonal methods, perhaps because of increased appetite. Several studies have specifically looked at the new progestin drospirenone and have shown a mild decrease in weight or a smaller increase in weight compared to several other OCs but the magnitude is small (66–68). Teens may lose weight because of self-imposed dieting, nausea, or depression. Often an adolescent believes she has gained 5 to 10 lb, when in fact the gain is a perception and not an actual change. Thus, if teens call about significant weight gain, it is important to have them come to the office for a weight measurement. If weight gain occurs, a lower-calorie, lower-salt diet, an increase in exercise, a decrease in TV time, and, if needed, a change to a pill low in both estrogen and progestin usually solve the problem.

Nausea

Nausea is generally considered an estrogenic side effect. Many patients will experience mild nausea for the first few days of taking OCs and sometimes for the first day of the subsequent one or two cycles. Generally, this mild nausea disappears without treatment over the first three cycles, and most patients tolerate the low-dose OCs quite well. If patients take the pill a half-hour after dinner or with a snack at bedtime rather than in the morning, nausea is less likely to be a problem. However, if the nausea is persistent or bothersome, it is wise to reduce the amount of estrogen (from 30–35 μg to 20–25 μg), although the tradeoff may be more irregular cycles. Nausea and vomiting can obviously have many other etiologies, including pregnancy, viral syndromes, and gastrointestinal diseases, and thus may need further evaluation. Patients who have vomiting or gastroenteritis may risk pill failure and should use a backup method for 7 days. If vomiting occurs within 1 hour of taking the pill, taking an extra pill from a different pill pack is recommended.

Intermenstrual or Breakthrough Bleeding

Irregular vaginal bleeding while the patient is taking hormone tablets occurs most frequently in the first one or two cycles, often during the second week of the cycle; it usually diminishes with subsequent cycles on the same pill. In general, it is more common as the dose of EE is reduced from 35 to 20 μg. The patient should be told in advance about the possibility of breakthrough bleeding (BTB) so that she will not stop taking the pill because of excessive concern about this common side effect. In adolescents who develop bleeding after several months to years of use, missed pills are a common cause, but chlamydial infection should always be kept in mind, as this is another frequent etiology of the problem. Pregnancy should also be considered in the differential diagnosis. Thus, when patients call concerned about irregular bleeding, the clinician should assess the pill dose, duration of use, and possibility of missed pills ("Some patients find it hard to remember all their pills. Have you missed any?"), and whether there has been a recent change to a generic pill, as well as previous gynecologic problems, pelvic pain, new sexual partners, other medications, gastrointestinal problems, and symptoms of pregnancy. Usually, there is a benign explanation such as missed pills or the early months of pill use. In fact, among 15- to 17-year-old OC users, 28% had missed two or more pills in the previous 3 months. Among university women, self-report of missed pills was much lower than observed on the basis of electronic data (24). Rosenberg observed that, by the sixth cycle of OCs, those who smoked were almost threefold more likely to experience irregular bleeding than those who did not (69). If there are worrisome factors in the history, an evaluation should be undertaken to exclude pregnancy (including ectopic), chlamydial or gonococcal infection (70), pelvic inflammatory disease, neoplasia, and other gynecologic pathology.

For irregular bleeding in the early months of pill taking, patients can usually be reassured and observed. Patients who have skipped or missed pills should make them up, as indicated in Appendix 3, and consider using EC if appropriate timing. Condoms should be used for the rest of the cycle. If the BTB is a persistent problem after the first three cycles or lasts an entire cycle (despite good adherence), a change to a more progestin-dominant pill should be tried for those already on a 30- to 35 μg EE pill. For example, choices may include changing *from* a pill with 35 μg of EE/0.5 mg NET or a triphasic NET pill (Ortho-Novum 7/7/7) *to* a pill containing 1 mg NET/ 35 μg EE, or *from* a pill with 1 mg NET *to* a triphasic LNG pill (e.g., Triphasil or Tri-Levlen), a NG pill or LNG pill with 30 μg EE, or to a 35 μg NGM pill. If the patient is on a 20 μg EE pill, changing from a 20 μg EE pill to one with 30 to 35 μg EE may alleviate the problem. Occasionally, a 50 μg EE pill with NG is necessary for 1 to 2 cycles for several cycles to regain cycle control, after which patients can resume a 35 μg EE pill or a triphasic pill. Additional estrogen or estrogen/progestin is sometimes used for heavy bleeding or persistence. There are several approaches, none of which has been evaluated in clinical trials. Adding oral 20 μg ethinyl estradiol, conjugated estrogens (0.625 to 1.25 mg), or micronized estradiol (1.0 to 2.0 mg) 12 hours after the OC for 7 days at the first sign of breakthrough bleeding or daily with the active pills for one to three cycles may alleviate the problem (71,72). Another approach is to take one pill in the morning and another in the evening for several days until the breakthrough bleeding stops, with additional pills drawn from a separate package of pills; however, a number of authors feel that "doubling up" does not change the estrogen/progestin ratio and may not be as effective as estrogen. Using estrogen alone may be more likely to stabilize the endometrium, especially if it is atrophic. NSAIDs prescribed twice to three times daily for 7 days may also lighten flow. Irregular bleeding is not generally a sign of decreased efficacy or altered hormone levels, unless patients are taking medications that may interfere with metabolism, have gastroenteritis, or have missed pills. A backup method of contraception is advisable in these circumstances.

Headaches

Headaches occur in 10% to 30% of healthy adolescents on a weekly basis. Thus, it is important for the clinician to obtain a history of headache type, frequency, and severity before prescribing an OC. Headaches may be precipitated by caffeine and alcohol use, fatigue, stress at school, psychosocial issues, sinus infections, medications including hormones, or rarely an intracranial process. The majority of headaches can be divided into "tension" headaches, migraine without aura (common migraine), and migraine with aura (classic migraine). Recent studies have examined whether there is an increased risk of stroke with migraine headaches with or without the use of OCs (73–79). Of note, ascertainment and definition of migraine in studies are not uniform, and do not always use the International Headache Classification System (IHC) (80). In a study of 86 cases of ischemic stroke and 214 controls, Donaghy and colleagues (76) found that the adjusted risk of ischemic stroke was significantly associated with the following:

1. Migraine of more than 12 years duration, odds ratio (OR) 4.61 (95% CI 1.27 to 16.8)
2. Initial migraine with aura, OR 8.37 (95% CI 2.33 to 30.1)
3. Attacks more frequent than 12 times per year, OR 10.4 (95% CI 2.18 to 49.4).

Data from a WHO study found that the OR for ischemic stroke among women with migraine with aura to be 3.8 (95% CI 1.3 to 11.5) (74). A family history of migraine was associated with an OR of 5.0 (95% CI 2.0 to 12.3). In non-OC users reporting migraine, the risk of ischemic stroke was 2.3 (95% CI 0.7 to 7.5) (74). The absolute risk of stroke in women aged 20 years who have migraine and use OCs has been estimated to be 10/100,000 compared to 100/100,000 in women aged 40 years (75).

The WHO guidelines consider migraine headaches with aura or other focal neurologic symptoms to be Level 4; migraine headaches without focal neurologic symptoms in women <35 years old are considered to be Level 2 for initiation of OCs and Level 3 for continuation of OCs. Nonmigrainous headaches are considered Level 1 for initiation and Level 2 for continuation. Whenever patients call with an increase in or new onset of headaches, a history of associated factors, prior headaches, and the presence of neurologic symptoms should be obtained. A blood pressure reading should be obtained and a neurologic and physical examination performed, if indicated. Some patients, especially those with an increase in headaches in the premenstrual phase, may actually find that headaches are ameliorated with the use of monophasic pills (78). Other patients with migraine or other types of headaches experience an increase in headaches, especially during the pill-free interval (79). Some patients may have new onset of headaches associated with OC use. If headaches (without aura or neurologic symptoms) worsen during the menstrual period, providing estrogen during the placebo week (using a pill with EE during the fourth week, such as Mircette, or a transdermal estradiol patch) or using continuous OCs may alleviate symptoms (17). For some patients, lowering the dose of EE may alleviate headaches; if not, a progestin-only method is preferred. Further evaluation is needed if patients experience new sudden, severe, or persistent headaches, headaches with neurologic symptoms that persist after the headaches resolve, or headaches waking them from sleep.

Hypertension

A combination OC is not recommended for patients with untreated hypertension. At most 1% to 2% of normotensive individuals have been observed to develop hypertension (a blood pressure >140/90 mm Hg) within weeks to several months of starting an OC, with the risk of hypertension increasing with age, parity, and obesity (81). The WHO guidelines designate as Level 3 adequately controlled hypertension and systolic blood pressure 140 to 159 or diastolic 90 to 99 mmHg; Level 4 is systolic blood pressure over 160 or diastolic over 100 mmHg (these levels should be adjusted for adolescent blood pressure standards based on age) (82). The mechanism of development of the hypertension is still a matter of controversy and may be related to both the estrogen, progestin, and genetic susceptibility. In the rare adolescents in whom new-onset hypertension develops while taking OCs, the elevated blood pressure usually returns to normal within 2 to 12 weeks after the pill is discontinued. Preferably, nonhormonal contraception should be used until the blood pressure returns to normal, but in some patients effective contraception with a progestin-only method is indicated, given the evidence that this method does not alter blood pressure. For example, if mild hypertension develops in a patient taking a 35 μg ethinyl estradiol pill and subsequently resolves, a pill lower in estrogen (20 μg) and progestin or a progestin-only pill may be prescribed, with monitoring of the blood pressure. If hypertension recurs, the patient should use another form of contraception. Sustained hypertension requires an evaluation.

Vascular Thrombosis

The estimated risk of venous thromboembolism (VTE) associated with OC use has varied among studies (83–89). Studies of deep vein thrombosis (DVT) are particularly complicated by the difficulty of making a clinical diagnosis of thrombophlebitis, case ascertainment, and lack of controlling for confounding factors. The rate of false-positive clinical diagnosis varies from 25% to 83%. The large Puget Sound Study involving 37,807 woman-years of OC use found three cases of venous thrombosis with a relative risk (RR) of 2.8 (84). A number of factors have been identified as leading to elevated risks overall and in OC users, including family history, low antithrombin III, hypercoagulability states (e.g., polycythemia, protein C and protein S deficiency, factor V Leiden and prothrombin 20210 mutations (90), hyperhomocysteinemia (91), high factor VIII levels (92), smoking (OR 2.0 [95% CI 1.4 to 2.7]) (93), postpartum, lupus erythematosus, obesity (body mass index [BMI] >35; OR 3.8 [95% CI 1.8 to 8.0]) (93), chronic diseases such as diabetes, and immobility, especially leg fractures (94).

Slightly increased levels of coagulation factors II, VII, VIII, and X, unchanged or reduced antithrombin III activity and protein S levels, and mildly increased fibrinolytic activity are observed for some OCs. Even when changes do occur, the levels of factors are usually still within the normal range and the decrease in antithrombin III noted is not in the range noted in familial disorders associated with thrombophlebitis (88). Although studies on pills with the newer progestins have shown little or no impact on clotting factors, several epidemiologic studies in the mid 1990s suggested that DSG and gestodene ("third generation" pills) were associated with a higher risk (1.5 to 2.0) of VTE than norethindrone (NET) and levonorgestrel (LNG)-containing OCs ("second generation" pills) (95–98). These studies led to an estimated annual risk for nonfatal VTE to be approximately 4/100,000 for healthy women, 10 to 15/100,000 for women taking NE- and LNG-containing pills, 20 to 30/100,000 for women taking DSG- or gestodene-containing pills, and 60/100,000 for pregnant women. Using the UK General Practice Research Database, Vasilakis and colleagues (99) reported an incidence rate of 3/100,000 for new users, 5.3/100,000 person-years for OCs with less than 35 μg EE and LNG, 10.7/100,000 person-years for OCs with less than 35 μg EE and DSG or gestodene, and 15.5/100,000 person-years in pregnant or postpartum women. However, the issue of elevated risk for certain progestins continues to be debated along with the relevance of duration of use and estrogen dosage (100–103). Burnhill found the risks for OCs among young healthy women served by Planned Parenthood Federation of America to be considerably lower than a number of epidemiologic studies. The rates for DVTs, myocardial infarction (MI) and cerebrovascular accidents (CVAs) were 3/100,000 (1.9/100,000 for norgestimate [NGM] OC users to 3.97/100,000 for DSG users) with a death rate of 0.22/100,000 women-years of use (104). In a meta-analysis, Hennessey and colleagues indicated that confounding of all observational studies is problematic and estimated a summary RR of 1.7 (95% CI 1.3 to 2.1) for gestodene and DSG (105). In another meta-analysis, Kemmeren and colleagues reported an OR of VTE of 2.5 (95% CI 1.6 to 4.1) for short-term users and 2.0 (95% CI 1.4 to 2.7) for longer-term users (106). Bloemenkamp found similar results for increased risk in the early months of use (107). In a case control study in Denmark, Lidegaard and colleagues found that longer use of the OC is associated with decreased OR over time: <1 year 7.0 (95% CI 5.1 to 9.6), 1 to 5 years 3.6 (95% CI 2.7 to 4.8); and >5 years, 3.1 (95% CI 2.5 to 3.8), compared with OC nonusers (108). Thus, risk among current users decreased 50% during the first years of use. They found that there was a difference in ORs for VTE associated with second-generation progestins (LNG or NGM) of 2.9 (95% CI 2.2 to 3.8) and third-generation progestins (DSG or gestodene) 4.0 (95% CI 3.2 to 4.9) when compared with nonusers. The risk declined with lower estrogen dose. With 30 to 40 μg of ethinyl estradiol as a reference range, the ORs was 0.6 (95% CI 0.4 to 0.9) for 20 μg OCs and 1.6 (95% CI 0.9 to 2.8) for 50 μg OCs. After the authors corrected for duration of use and varying estrogen doses, they calculated the third/second-generation risk ratio was 1.3 (95% CI 1.0 to 1.8; $p < 0.05$). The risk of VTE for drospirenone containing OCs in relation to other OCs is not fully elucidated although additional studies are needed given a case report (109).

Among women who have a VTE, only half have an identified clotting disorder, with the majority related to the recently recognized and moderately prevalent factor V Leiden mutation. The carrier frequency of factor V Leiden, a mutation of factor V that renders activated factor V relatively resistant to degradation by activated protein C (APC), is 5.3% among Caucasian Americans, 2.2% among Hispanic Americans, 1.2% among African Americans, and 0.45% among Asian Americans (110). The risk of VTE is estimated to be 140/100,000 for OC users with factor V Leiden mutation (a 35-fold increase in risk) compared to 32/100,000 for OC nonusers and factor V Leiden (111). Since 1% of VTE events are fatal, OC users may experience 3 deaths/1 million, compared to those with factor V Leiden with 14 deaths/1 million (1/71,429), of which 10.8 deaths/1 million (1/92,593) can be attributed to OC use (111). Using data from a small case control study, Spannagl estimated a somewhat lower risk for the Factor V Leiden mutation and OCs (112). The OR for VTE for women using OCs *without* factor V Leiden was 4.1 (95% CI 2.1 to 7.8) and *with* Factor V mutation was 10.2 (95% CI 1.2 to 88.4). The OR for Factor V Leiden alone was 2.0 (95% CI 1.0 to 4.4). Thus the OR for OC users with Factor V mutation compared to those with no Factor V mutation and non OC users was 10.2 (95% CI 3.8 to 27.6). The WHO 2004 guidelines have given a Level 4 to known thrombogenic mutations; unfortunately, unintended pregnancy will also increase the risk of VTE. Screening the entire population before the use of OCs would not be cost effective (111). Young women who have a strong family history of thrombosis or who develop thrombosis on OCs should be evaluated for familial disorders. If at all possible, it is best to screen the relative who actually had the VTE so that appropriate testing can be carried out in the young woman requesting OCs.

Since prior thrombophlebitis is a contraindication to OC use, rigorous medical criteria should be used to determine whether a patient has VTE. Because studies have found an increased risk of postoperative thromboembolism in women using OCs prior to major (especially abdominal and lower extremity) surgery, discontinuing OC use 4 weeks before major elective surgery is recommended. Major surgery with prolonged immobilization is considered Level 4 (See WHO Guidelines, Appendix 2). The possibility of an unplanned pregnancy, however, is a significant risk for adolescents, and thus the risks and benefits need to be weighed for each procedure. It is not necessary to discontinue OCs for minor procedures such as laparoscopy (113). OCs are generally considered contraindicated in patients with cyanotic heart disease or pulmonary artery hypertension. The presence of varicose veins is not a contraindication to OC use. The WHO guideline has given a Level 2 designation for Sickle cell disease (27,28). Progestin-only methods such as depot medroxyprogesterone acetate may have a beneficial effect of decreasing sickle cell crises.

An association between OC use and stroke (including subarachnoid hemorrhage) has been reported by some studies, but not by others (77,114–123). Many studies have also focused on the contribution of other risk factors for strokes such as smoking, hypertension, migraine headaches, and illicit drug use (115) (See also Headache section). The Puget Sound Study (83) and the updated Oxford Study (117) found no increase in risk for cerebral vascular accident. The Nurses' Health Study (120) found no change in the risk of mortality from stroke in ever-users of OCs (OR: 1.05; 95% CI 0.75 to 1.45; multivariate RR: 1.03). A case-control study at Kaiser Health Plan (123) found that for current users of OCs, the odds ratio for ischemic stroke was 1.18 (95% CI 0.54 to 2.59) and for hemorrhagic stroke 1.14 (95% CI 0.60 to 2.16). For hemorrhagic stroke, there was an increased odds ratio for OCs and smoking of 3.64 (95% CI 0.95 to 3.87). Past users had a decreased risk of stroke. An increase in ischemic stroke in smokers and those with hypertension was also noted in the WHO international study but no increase was found in hemorrhagic stroke in women <35 years (121,122). A recent meta-analysis by Gillum and colleagues found a summary relative risk of ischemic stroke of 1.93 (95% CI 1.35 to 2.74) controlling for smoking and hypertension (118). Studies are conflicting as to whether there are no differences or less risk for "third generation" OCs (116,117,124). There may be a lower risk with lower doses of ethinyl estradiol (EE). The OR of cerebral thromboembolic attacks (strokes and transient ischemic attacks) among current OC users with nonusers as the reference group was: 4.5 (95% CI 2.6 to 7.7) for OCs with 50 μg EE; 1.6 (95% CI 1.3 to 2.0) for OCs 30 to 40 μg; 1.7 (95% CI 1.0 to 3.1) for OCs with 20 μg EE; and 1.0 (95% CI 0.3 to 3.0) for progestin-only pills. Factors that appear to contribute to the lowering of risk include a reduction of hormone doses, better screening of users, and better epidemiologic studies that control for confounding factors.

The data initially suggesting an association between myocardial infarction and OC use have been extensively reevaluated and new studies completed (83–85,120, 125–128). The Walnut Creek Study (84) found an increased incidence of acute myocardial infarction with OCs only in smokers over 40 years old. The Puget Sound Study (83) found no cases of myocardial infarction among 36,807 woman-years of use. A study of 119,061 women in the Nurses' Health Study found that past use of OCs did not increase the risk of subsequent cardiovascular disease (126). In a 12-year follow-up study of 166,755 nurses, Colditz (120) reported that ever use of OCs was associated with a RR of mortality from coronary heart disease of 0.82 (95% CI 0.66 to 1.02) and current use with a RR of 0.70 (95% CI 0.33 to 1.51). Smoking is a major contributing factor to elevated risk in older women. The increased risk of myocardial infarction is felt to be primarily related to thrombosis, not atherosclerosis, since the risk is not related to past use or duration of OC use. Most studies suggest that current or past use of OCs alone in young women has no effect on the incidence of myocardial infarction. Whether there is any difference between users of "second generation" progestins and "third generation" is debated, with perhaps a small advantage to third generation pills (129); however, smoking is the strongest risk factor (128,130). Rare case reports of mesenteric artery thrombosis, retinal artery thrombosis, and Budd Chiari syndrome have been reported (1,131–133).

Diabetes and Carbohydrate Metabolism

Early studies using older, higher-dose OC pills suggested that these compounds impaired glucose tolerance. More recent studies using the lower-dose formulations appear to show minimal, if any, impact (134–137). Studies of healthy, nonsmoking diabetic patients taking OCs have been reassuring (138). The WHO guidelines designate Level 1 for history of gestational diabetes, Level 2 for diabetes without vascular disease, and Level 3/4 for diabetics with nephropathy, retinopathy, neuropathy, or a duration of 20 years or more (27,28).

Lipid Metabolism

The interpretation of studies examining the role of OCs in altering plasma lipids has been difficult because of lack of knowledge as to whether changes observed have any relationship to long-term morbidity and mortality. Conclusions about the association of high-density lipoprotein (HDL) cholesterol on the lower incidence of myocardial infarction are drawn from epidemiologic studies in men in their midlife, not from young women taking OCs. In addition, the benefit of altering HDL cholesterol in a supposedly beneficial direction has not been demonstrated. Because factors other than triglycerides, total cholesterol, and HDL and low-density lipoprotein (LDL) cholesterol play roles in atherosclerosis, interest has emerged in studying subfractions of HDL cholesterol, apolipoproteins, and other factors. An elevated level of apolipoprotein (apo) B or depressed level of apo A-1 (or a high ratio of apo B to apo A-1) has been associated with coronary heart disease. Additionally, other factors such as inflammatory markers play a role in cardiovascular risk.

Oral estrogens in high doses can increase liver synthesis and release of very low-density lipoproteins (VLDLs), triglycerides, HDL cholesterol, and total cholesterol. Progestins are associated with a decline in HDL cholesterol. The balance of estrogen to progestin, the amount of contraceptive steroid, and the response of the individual patient determine the changes in lipid levels. Because of widely different protocols, including numbers and characteristics of subjects, duration of OCs, and nature of the lipoproteins studied, results must be interpreted with caution. Speroff and DeCherney (103) have pointed out that most studies are short term (a steady state may not be reached in 6 months), a number of factors are often not controlled (phase of menstrual cycle, postpartum state), and untreated controls are not included in the design. In general, the HDL/total cholesterol and HDL/LDL cholesterol ratios do not appear to change significantly with most OCs. For example, their review of 23 reports of desogestrel-containing pills found changes (some small or variable) in total cholesterol (+3%), HDL cholesterol (+13%), LDL cholesterol (+2%), triglycerides (+29%), apo B (+10%), and apo A-1 (+11%). Monophasic norgestimate pills showed changes in triglycerides (+4%), total cholesterol (+5%), LDL cholesterol (+3%), and HDL cholesterol (+7%). In a comparative 3-month trial, a 30-μg EE/levonorgestrel(LNG) triphasic pill appeared to increase LDL-C compared to desogestrel (139), but DSG OCs may have a less favorable effect on coagulation (140). LNG OC with 20 μg EE was noted to have a more "favorable" profile than one with 30 μg EE (137).

Of interest, women using the 20 μg EE/LNG OC over 24 cycles had only one change from baseline (HDL3) that remained at the end of the trial (141). However, the relevance of these small differences in measured lipid levels to clinical outcomes is questionable. In fact, contrary to assumptions that have been made on an epidemiologic basis in humans, studies in nonhuman primates have suggested that even a progestin-dominant combination pill that lowered HDL cholesterol reduced the amount of arteriosclerosis because the estrogen component appears to have a protective effect (142). Given the problems of epidemiology, controlled studies, and extrapolation of risks to women, the most prudent course for practitioners is to select a balanced contraceptive with a low dose of progestin and estrogen. Instruction in low-cholesterol, low-saturated fat, high-fiber diets, avoidance of smoking, and exercise are useful adjuncts in the care of young women. Combination OCs should not be used by patients with known hypertriglyceridemia (>350 mg/dL) because of the risk of pancreatitis (143). Progestin-only pills have a negligible effect on lipids and thus appear preferable in the presence of hypertriglyceridemia.

Changes in Laboratory Values

Several laboratory tests are potentially altered by the ingestion of OCs (17,144). Of particular importance to clinicians is the change observed in some thyroid function tests. Although there is no change in the free thyroxine (free T_4) level or the clinical status of patients, the increase in thyroid-binding globulin (TBG) leads to an increase in measured total T_4 and a decrease in resin triiodothyronine (resin T_3) levels and the TBG index. In some studies, but not others, the serum folate concentration has been reported to be decreased (145,146). This might be important in adolescents with inadequate diets and in women who become pregnant shortly after discontinuing OC use.

Gastrointestinal Diseases

Combined OCs may increase the risk of symptomatic gallbladder disease, and the WHO guidelines give a Level 3 for medically treated or current symptomatic gallbladder disease, and past OC related cholestasis, and a Level 2 for asymptomatic gallbladder disease and symptomatic disease treated by cholecystectomy. One review found a odds ratio of 1.36 for OC use and gallbladder disease (95% CI 1.15 to 1.62) (147); but the Oxford Family Planning Study found no association, with a RR of 1.1 (95% CI 0.9 to 1.3) (148). Grodstein and colleagues (149) found no increase for ever-users in symptomatic gallstones but did find a slight increase in long-term users (RR: 1.5, 95% CI 1.0 to 2.2 for 10 to 14 years of use). Increased body mass index was the strongest predictor of risk. Others have suggested that rather than increasing the lifetime risk, OCs might accelerate gallbladder disease in women with susceptibility to this problem (1).

Studies of the risk of OC use and inflammatory bowel disease have been conflicting (150,151). In one study, the RRs of Crohn disease and ulcerative colitis were higher in current users, but the results were not statistically significant (1). A Puget Sound Study found that women who had used OCs within 6 months of disease onset had a RR of 2.0 (95% CI 1.2 to 3.3) for ulcerative colitis and a RR of 2.6 (95% CI 1.2 to 5.5) for Crohn disease, compared to never-users. Use for over 6 years was associated with a RR of 5.1 for Crohn disease but no increased risk for ulcerative colitis (152). An estrogen dose over 35 μg also appears to increase the RRs (1). An Italian study (153) similarly found a higher risk for Crohn disease but not ulcerative colitis in OC users. Studies have been conflicting on whether the use of OCs is associated with a increased risk of relapse of Crohn disease with one study finding no association (RR 1.11, 95% CI 0.80 to 1.55) (154) and another finding an elevated risk (RR 3.0, 95% CI 1.5 to 5.9) (155). In both studies, smoking increased the risk of relapse.

Women who have reduced hepatic reserve because of an inherited or acquired defect may become jaundiced while taking OCs. WHO has given a Level 2 for women with a history of pregnancy-related cholestasis. A Level 4 has been assigned to the use of OCs in patients with active viral hepatitis and severe (decompensated) cirrhosis, and a Level 3 to mild compensated cirrhosis. However, it should be noted that patients with mononucleosis and hepatitis A are frequently completely recovered before the issue of OC use is raised or therapy altered. The potential risks and benefits need to be balanced in adolescents with chronic hepatitis, cystic fibrosis, or other conditions associated with changes in liver function tests. Patients with porphyria may have exacerbation of attacks in the premenstrual period and with the use of oral contraceptives (156); however, GnRH analogs and estrogen add-back have been helpful for some patients (157).

Collagen Vascular Disease

Women with systemic lupus erythematosus (SLE) have an increased risk of thrombosis that may be enhanced in those with antiphospholipid antibodies and in those taking OCs (158–160). Julkunen and colleagues (158,159) estimated a RR of 2.3 for thrombosis, but with a wide CI (0.5 to 10.3). Although progestin-only agents are often preferred, they reported that 25 (78%) of 32 women who used a progestin-only method discontinued use because of side effects (mostly gynecologic but one case of thrombosis was noted). There is conflicting evidence on whether OCs are associated with flares of SLE (160). Low-dose OCs have been prescribed for adolescents with SLE in the absence of active nephritis, thrombosis, or antiphospholipid antibodies. In a recent case control study of 240 women with SLE and 321 controls, no association was found between SLE and current use or duration of use of hormone replacement therapy or OCs (161). Most patients with rheumatoid arthritis tolerate OCs well. In addition, OC use does not influence the outcome of long term rheumatoid arthritis although there may a slight trend toward better functional outcome (162). Conflicting studies have shown either no effect or a protective effect of OCs on the development of rheumatoid arthritis (163,164).

Epilepsy

Several studies have demonstrated no increase in seizures with current formulations (73,165,166). In fact, patients with a history of an increase in seizures in the premenstrual and/or menstrual phase of the cycle may benefit from OC use. The major problem with the use of OCs in adolescents with seizure disorders is the potential for intermenstrual bleeding and possibly lowered efficacy of the OC and decreased anticonvulsant levels. Anticonvulsants such as phenobarbital, phenytoin, carbamazepine, primidone, and oxycarbazepine increase the metabolism of synthetic steroids by increasing conjugation in the gut and enzyme induction in the liver (167–170). In addition, these drugs increase the production of sex hormone-binding globulin to which the progestin is bound (165). Felbamate and topiramate also appear to have an effect on OC metabolism (171,172). Unlike Depo-Provera, use of progestin-only pills or levonorgestrel subdermal implants does not provide sufficient efficacy for patients on enzyme-inducing anticonvulsants. Sodium valproate has not been associated with OC failure (171,173). Most of the new antiepileptic agents such as gabapentin, lamotrigine, levetiracetam (174) and the benzodiazepines do not interfere with OCs. However, lowered plasma levels of lamotrigine have been associated with OC use in one small series (168), and pharmacokinetic studies of the new anticonvulsants have used low doses in clinical studies (113).

For patients on enzyme-inducing anticonvulsants, a pill with 35 to 50 μg ethinyl estradiol is generally prescribed. The patient should be counseled about the potential increased risk of pregnancy, and a backup method such as condoms strongly suggested. Although not proved, the persistence of intermenstrual bleeding in patients on anticonvulsant therapy may imply lowered efficacy and the need to change to a pill with more estrogen (50 μg) and a more potent progestin. A barrier method should be used in cycles with breakthrough bleeding. Some clinicians reduce the pill-free interval from 7 days to 4 to 5 days to further decrease the risk of ovulation; others advise prescribing only 50 μg EE OC pills; still others recommend four packs of 21-day hormone pills followed by a hormone-free interval of 5 to 6 days.

Drug Interactions

Drugs may interact with OCs by changing absorption, altering serum protein binding, and increasing hepatic metabolism with the induction of cytochrome P-450 enzymes (170,175,176). Some women are rapid metabolizers of steroids, and some women may have liver enzyme systems that are particularly likely to induction or experience changes in bowel flora (1,177). As noted, certain anticonvulsants reduce OC estrogen levels and can increase intermenstrual bleeding; the effect on efficacy is less certain. St John's wort has also been noted to increase clearance of OC steroids and decrease cycle control (178), and ongoing studies are assessing whether there is an impact on efficacy of OCs. Fluoxetine has not been shown to change the efficacy of OCs (179). Rifampin, which also induces cytochrome P-450 enzymes, was noted early to be associated with case reports of unintended pregnancies (180), and alternative or additional methods of contraception (such as condoms) should be used. Similarly, griseofulvin may accelerate metabolism of OC steroids (176,181). Antiretrovirals may have interactions with OCs. Itraconazole, fluconazole, and ketoconazole are inhibitors of the P-450 system and may cause increased EE levels and delayed withdrawal bleeding (182,183). Other antibiotics such as ampicillin or tetracycline are unlikely to diminish efficacy. Studies of clinical pharmacology have been unable to demonstrate altered kinetics in a small number of women (184–186), and a large study found no difference in pregnancy rates between OC users who had used antibiotics and those who had not (187). Because the OC package insert includes a statement about potential interactions, many clinicians still suggest patients use barrier method, especially if intermenstrual bleeding occurs. The clearance of benzodiazepines (such as chlordiazepoxide and diazepam), theophylline, prednisolone, caffeine, metoprolol, and cyclosporine is reduced in OC users (170). Levels of tricyclic antidepressants may be altered by OC use. Levels of these drugs should be monitored to avoid toxicity. Decreased concentrations of acetylsalicylic acid, clofibric acid, morphine, paracetamol, and temazepam have been observed in OC users (170). Although mineral oil and OC pills should not be taken at the same time, absorbents such as antacids and kaolin have not been shown to have any effect on OCs. Vitamin C does not appear to alter OC kinetics (188).

Oligomenorrhea or Amenorrhea

Scanty or absent withdrawal flow, most commonly associated with progestin-dominant and low-estrogen pills, may develop months or even several years after continuous use. If a patient becomes amenorrheic, she should continue taking her pills, and the possibility of pregnancy should be evaluated promptly. Menses may return spontaneously, or amenorrhea may persist. The patient should be reassured that the lack of menses is in no way harmful and is not associated with postpill amenorrhea. The options are to continue pregnancy tests every 1 to 2 months (it may be best to err of the side of more frequent tests in questionably compliant patients), to have the patient check basal body temperatures during the placebo week each month, or to change to an OC more likely to result in menstrual flow. For patients who can take their temperatures easily and understand the instructions (usually college students), the procedure involves checking basal body (oral) temperature for 3 days during the 7-day hormone-free interval (on placebos). If no pills have been missed and the temperature is less than 98°F, pill amenorrhea is likely and the pills can be continued. Temperatures greater than 98°F may imply a viral infection or incorrectly measured temperature, but a sensitive pregnancy test should be done.

If patients desire a change of pill, selecting one with less progestin is often helpful, for example, switching from a pill with 1.0 mg norethindrone (NET) to one containing 0.4 mg or 0.5 mg NET, or from a 30 μg EE/0.3 mg norgestrel OC to a triphasic levonorgestrel pill, or from any pill to a norgestimate pill. Some clinicians also add a small amount of supplemental estrogen (micronized estradiol 1 to 2 mg (72), ethinyl estradiol 20 μg, or conjugated estrogens 0.625 to 1.25 mg) for 21 days for one to three cycles, although it is clearly best to try to find a pill with 30 to 35 μg of estrogen for long-term use. Patients on OC therapy should be reassured that a 1- to 3-day light withdrawal flow is perfectly normal.

After discontinuation of the pill, 1% to 2% of patients have postpill amenorrhea, similar to the incidence of amenorrhea in control populations (189). Approximately 95% of these patients revert to regular periods within 12 to 18 months. Most patient with postpill amenorrhea have irregular cycles before initiating OC use, and thus the cause of oligomenorrhea should be investigated before an OC is prescribed. For example, a patient with polycystic ovary syndrome and hirsutism may appropriately be treated with an OC, but she will likely experience oligomenorrhea again after it is discontinued. Patients who lose weight or engage in endurance sports while taking OCs appear to be more susceptible to postpill amenorrhea just as they would be if they were not taking OCs. Patients with amenorrhea for more than 6 months after the cessation of OCs or with galactorrhea or headaches should have an appropriate evaluation (see Chapter 7). In adolescents, pregnancy must be an important consideration regardless of the number of weeks or months of amenorrhea.

Depression

Subjective symptoms such as depression, nervousness, sleep disturbance, or emotional lability have been associated with OC use in some studies, but not in others (1,190–192). In a review of research studies, Oinonen and Mazmanian concluded that OC users had less variability in mood across the cycle, but that some patients with a history of depression, psychiatric symptoms, and a family history of OC-related mood complaints were more likely to experience negative affect. They felt that monophasic pills were reported to have a greater "stabilizing effect" than triphasic pills (190). A study of a drospirenone OC suggested improvement in *premenstrual dysphoric disorder* (PMDD) for symptoms of appetite, acne, and food cravings but overall most endpoints did not reach statistical significance (193). Another study found lower scores on negative affect and water retention at cycle 6 in women treated with this OC (194). However, more data are needed to recommend a specific formulation for treatment of PMDD. Most adolescents do well on OCs without any impact on psychological well-being, but some—perhaps because of a predisposition (family history or personal history) or intervening life stresses—do feel symptoms of irritability or depression that appear to coincide with the initiation of OC use. Depressive symptoms are common during adolescence, and thus the clinician is often faced with trying to assess whether the OC is part of the problem and to determine the severity of the depression or other mood changes and the need for psychiatric intervention. It is crucial to have a baseline history of previous psychiatric symptoms as the adolescent begins OC use. Expectations about OC use may also play a role. After other causes for the depression or emotional lability are explored, the clinician can suggest a change to a different hormone preparation with less progestin or discontinuing the pill to see if the subjective effects are improved. Although some clinicians recommend supplementation with 20 mg vitamin B$_6$ daily, patients should be counseled about the potential for side effects with excessive doses.

Pregnancy Outcome

There is no increase in the incidence of congenital anomalies over the background rate of 2% to 3% in patients who have previously taken OCs or in those who have inadvertently taken OCs during early pregnancy (195). Dating of pregnancies is improved if patients wait a cycle or two after discontinuing OCs to attempt conception.

Ovarian Cysts

Benign ovarian cysts were less common in OC users who took the older, higher-dose pills (50 μg EE) than nonusers. Several studies have suggested that lower-dose OCs may not have the same effect (196,197). The Puget Sound study, a cross-sectional study, compared 100 women with history of functional ovarian cysts to 255 controls, using pharmacy records; the relative risk of an ovarian cyst for monophasic OC users was 0.8 (95% CI 0.4 to 1.8) compared to nonusers, and for those using triphasic OCs 1.3 (95% CI 0.5 to 3.3) (196). This study suggested that use of low-dose monophasic OCs did not substantially decrease risk of functional cyst formation, but also that use of triphasic OCs did not statistically increase the risk of cyst formation. One recent prospective study using transvaginal ultrasound, however, did find protection against the development of functional cysts >3 cm with low-dose monophasic pills (RR 0.22, 95% CI 0.13 to 0.39) compared to nonusers (198). OCs with higher doses of estrogen (199) and injectable and trans-dermal estrogen/progestin methods are more suppressive of ovarian cysts. Oral contraceptives do not hasten resolution of ovarian cysts. In one study in which patients were randomized to receive norethindrone 1 mg/mestranol 50 μg versus no treatment for 6 weeks, there were no differences in the rates of regression of functional ovarian cysts between the two groups (200). Therefore, OCs are probably best used to possibly prevent the formation of new cysts while allowing those already present to spontaneously regress (see Chapter 18).

Neoplasms

Most studies to date have found no increase in lifetime risk of breast cancer associated with the use of OCs, although this issue is a source of controversy and ongoing reassessments (201–205). Part of the difficulty with the epidemiologic studies is the issue of recall of use, the decreasing number of women who are never-users, the change in estrogen dose over the past 20 years, and the change in users to adolescents of younger age. The Cancer and Steroid Hormone (CASH) study (201) found a slightly increased RR for women 20 to 34 years old at diagnosis, no association for those aged 35 to 44 years, and a slightly decreased risk for women aged 45 to 54 years. In an analysis of 54 epidemiologic studies of over 53,000 women with breast cancer and over 100,000 women without breast cancer, the Collaborative Group on Hormonal Factors in Breast Cancer concluded that there was a small relative risk of having breast cancer diagnosed in current users of 1.24 (95% CI 1.15 to 1.33), which decreased to 1.16 (95% CI 1.08 to 1.23), 1 to 4 years after stopping OCs, and to 1.01 (95% CI 0.96 to 1.05) by 10 years after use (202,203). The cancers diagnosed in OC users were less advanced compared to never-users and more likely to be localized to the breast. It may be that women receiving OC prescriptions are more likely to have breast cancer diagnosed early. There was no effect on duration of use, age at first use, type of formulation, parity, reproductive or family history, or a number of other factors. In a large case control study of women 35 to 64 years old (4,575 with breast cancer and 4,682 controls), Marchbanks and colleagues found a relative risk of 1.0 (95% CI 0.8 to 1.3) for current users and 0.9 (95% CI 0.8 to 1.0) for previous users (204). Neither initiation of OCs at a young age nor a family history of breast cancer increased risk. Studies are conflicting on risk for women with known genetic markers (204,206). A case control study by Narod and colleagues found a small increased OR in BRCA1 mutation carriers for ever-use (OR 1.20, 95%CI 1.02 to 1.40), at least 5 years use (OR 1.33, 95% CI 1.11 to 1.60), use before age 30 (OR 1.29, 95% CI 1.09 to 1.52), and use of OCs before 1975 (OR 1.42, 95% CI 1.17 to 1.75) (206). In contrast, Heimdal found a RR of 2.0 but the 95% CI were wide at 0.36 to 10.9, precluding a conclusion (207). The numbers were too small to come to a conclusion about BRCA2 mutation carriers. A recent cohort study in Canada of women 40 to 59 years old suggests that OCs continue to provide a reduced risk of benign breast disease without atypia (208).

Although an increased incidence of cervical dysplasia and progression to carcinoma in situ have been reported in some studies of OC users, these women have higher rates of sexual activity, an increased number of partners, increased exposure to HPV, and an earlier age of beginning coitus, as well as more substance use (including cigarettes) (1). OC users are also under increased surveillance with Pap smears because of the need for a prescription, and thus detection bias in studies is also a problem. A WHO study (209) found that ever-users of OCs had a RR of 1.75 for carcinoma in situ with an even greater risk for long-term (>5 years) users. In an analysis of 28 studies, Smith and colleagues found that the relative risks of cervical cancer was increased in OC users with increasing duration of use; the risk for under 5 years was 1.1 (95% CI 1.1 to 1.2), 5 to 9 years, 1.6 (95% CI 1.4 to 1.7), and 10 or more years, 2.2 (95% CI 1.9 to 2.4) for all women. For HPV positive women the summary relative risks were 0.9 (95% CI 0.7 to 1.2), 1.3 (95% CI 1.0 to 1.9), and 2.5 (95% CI 1.6 to 3.9) for the same durations of use (210). Moreno and colleagues in an analysis of 8 case control non-U.S. studies reported that women who were OC users less than 5 years, compared to never-users, had an odds ratio of cervical cancer of 0.73 (95% CI 0.52 to 1.03). Risk was increased for longer use: 5 to 9 years, 2.82 (95% CI 1.46 to 5.42) and 10 years or more, 4.03 (95% CI 2.09 to 8.02) (211). However, a Scandinavian study found smoking was the most important contributor to increased risk for CIN 2 and 3 (OR 2.6, 95% CI 1.7 to 4.0); the smoking-related risk was not affected by adjusting for positivity for HPV (212).

Ever or current use of combination OCs reduces the incidence of endometrial cancer, with age-adjusted RRs of 0.2 to 0.7 (1,213–216). The CASH study (216) found a RR of 0.6 for ever-use, with the protective effect lasting over 15 years. The protective effect increases with duration of use. For a duration of use of at least 2 years, there appears to be a 38% reduction in risk, compared to estimated risk reduction of 51% with 4 years of use, 64% with 8 years, and 70% with 12 years. In a Scandinavian study, Weiderpass and colleagues found that combined OCs significantly reduced the risk of endometrial cancer at 3 years (OR 0.5, 95% CI 0.3 to 0.7), with even greater protection with 10 years of use (80% lower risk) (217). Reduction in risk lasted for at least 20 years after cessation. Progestin-only pills reduced the risk more than combined OCs at 3 years.

OCs have a strong protective effect against ovarian cancer (1,218–224), with the RR of 0.64 (95% CI 0.57 to 0.73) for ever-use of OCs in a meta-analysis (220). Using data from several sources, Gross and Schlesselman (220) have estimated that 5 years of OC use by nulliparous women can reduce their ovarian cancer risk to the level observed in parous women and that 10 years of use by women with a positive family history can reduce their risk below that of a never-user with a negative family history. OCs up to 50 µg EE have been shown to be protective with no difference between low estrogen, low progestin pills and high estrogen, high progestin pills (222). Another study suggested that OCs with high progestin potency might lead to a greater reduction (223). The protective effect occurred with as little as 3 to 6 months of use and continued for 15 years after use ended. Use of OCs also reduces the risk of ovarian cancer in those with a family history of ovarian cancer. In one small study, the risk reduction appeared to be greater in those with a family history than those without a history (224). By age 70, 4 to 8 years of OC use has been estimated to reduce the risk from 4/100 for not using OCs to 2/100 (225). Similarly, the risk is reduced approximately 50% in women with BRCA1 and BRCA2, with greater reduction with increased duration of use (225). In modeling the hypothetical incidence of all reproductive cancers ascribed to OC use, the net effect appears to be negligible (226). Coker and colleagues (227) suggested that for every 100,000 pill users there would be 44 fewer reproductive cancers. Schlesselman has estimated that 8 years of OC use would be associated with a reduction of five cancers per 1000 white women and less than 1 per 1000 black women (228).

Studies on the RR of liver cancer have yielded variable results in different populations (1,120,156,229). In the Nurses Health Study (120), ever-use of OCs was not related to an increased risk for liver cancer mortality (RR 0.43; 95% CI 0.08 to 2.42). Although the data have been interpreted in different ways, the development of benign liver adenomas has been found to be increased by OCs in some studies but not others (1,156,230). In British studies that included over a quarter million woman-years of use, no liver tumors were found (1). A study of 15 German liver centers did not find a statistically significant increased risk with longer duration of use (230). A study at the Armed Forces Institute of Pathology suggested that one type of hepatic tumor (fibrolamellar) occurs in the same age group that would be taking OCs, and thus an age-related bias may have occurred in establishing an association (231). Patients with hepatocellular adenoma may have an abdominal mass, vague upper abdominal pain, or acute pain with circulatory collapse following hemorrhage. A recent case report suggested that these tumors may regress with discontinuation of the OCs (232). There may be an increase in hepatic focal nodular hyperplasia associated with OC use (230). Most studies have demonstrated a reduced risk of colorectal cancer (233–238).

Skin

The majority of OC users note an improvement in acne and hirsutism. The principal metabolic effects of OCs that have implications for androgens and acne are:

1. A decrease in LH levels, therefore causing decreased androgen synthesis and a decrease in ovarian androgen production;
2. An increase in sex hormone binding globulin (SHBG) levels, which leads to increased binding of testosterone and a lower free testosterone, thus decreasing its bioavailability;
3. An inhibition of 5-α-reductase activity, which leads to decreased conversion of testosterone to dihydrotestosterone, which is the active androgen which causes acne and hirsutism.

There are differences in the magnitude of 5-α-reductase inhibition (239) (greater inhibition with norgestimate *in vitro*) and of the increase in SHBG (greater increase in SHBG with new progestins) (240), but a similar decrease in free testosterone for all OCs. OCs not only decrease free testosterone but also frequently decrease dehydroepiandrosterone sulfate (an adrenal androgen often elevated in polycystic ovary syndrome [PCOS]) (241). Although several pills have an FDA indication for acne, studies have found efficacy of a number of pills in decreasing total acne lesion count, including formulations that include the progestins norethindrone, norgestimate (242,243), levonorgestrel (244–246), desogestrel (245,247,248), and drospirenone (249). There are only a few trials comparing different pills (245,249) with minimal if any differences. Most clinicians select pills with lower doses of progestins, especially if acne does not respond over 2 to 3 months. Continuous OCs can be prescribed if there is an insufficient response. Of note, a recent study of lean and obese women with PCOS suggested that obese patients had less response of clinical androgenic symptoms to OCs than lean women (250). Familiarity with other acne therapies is important for clinicians providing care to teenagers since patients frequently benefit from topical agents and oral antibiotics, as needed.

Chloasma (the darkening of the upper lip and forehead and under the eyes) has been noted in a small number of OC users; it usually fades slowly after discontinuing OCs but may be permanent. It is more common in dark-skinned patients who are exposed to sunlight and taking higher-dose OCs. Occasionally patients have developed erythema nodosum in association with OC use. There is no association of OCs and melanoma (1), but all patients should be advised to use sunscreens. Hair loss may be due to many stresses; therefore, it is difficult to establish the OC as a definite cause in most cases. Most reports stem from the use of higher-dose pills, not current formulations.

Hot flashes are reported by some patients during the hormone-free week and can be ameliorated by continuous OCs or low-dose transdermal estradiol for the week (17).

Ocular Problems

Much of the literature on the occurrence of eye problems is related to case reports and experiences with higher-dose OCs (1), in which concern was raised about the possibility of dry eyes or corneal edema from combined OCs. In a review, Petursson and coworkers (251) found only seven cases of difficulty in wearing contact lenses; several studies have found no statistical differences in the rates of eye pathology or the ability to wear contact lenses (1). Optic nerve or retinal disease is a contraindication to OC therapy. The pill should be discontinued immediately if visual symptoms, especially transient loss of vision, occur, since retinal thrombosis, optic neuritis, and migraine with focal ophthalmic symptoms may occasionally be associated with OC use.

Bone Density

Although there are a number of studies on the relationship of OCs to bone density, the results are conflicting. Most show a beneficial effect, but some have found no effect (1,252–258). Additionally, there may be vitamin D receptor gene polymorphisms that determine response to OCs (259). In a prospective longitudinal study of up to 5 years in 156 college-aged women, Recker and associates (252) reported that OC use contributed a further, independent positive effect beyond physical activity and dietary calcium. If a beneficial effect is present, premenopausal OC users may enter menopause with 2% to 3% more bone density (252). A question has recently been raised as to whether 20 μg EE OCs have the same positive benefit on bone density as 30- to 40-μg EE pills and whether all progestins have similar effects (257,260, 261). In a prospective 12 month study, Berenson found an increase of 2.33% in lumbar spine bone mineral density in users of a 35 μg EE/1.0 mg NET OC, but not a similar gain with a 30-μg EE/desogestrel pill (257). In a study by Cromer et al, bone mineral apparent density decreased 1.0% for depot medroxyprogesterone acetate (DMPA) and increased 1.4% for a 20 μg EE OC, and 2.87% for nonusers (261). In a study of women 22 to 34 years old, there were no differences in bone mineral density after 1 year in controls compared to women taking a 15- and 20-μg EE pill (253). Another longitudinal study of women 18 to 39 years old found no differences in bone density of the spine, hip, and total body in OC users (80% 30 to 35μg EE) and nonusers over three years (255). If there is truly an effect in teens, it is possible that the low-dose pills decrease ovarian and adrenal androgens without raising estrogen levels to achieve peak bone mass. DeCherney suggests that progestins such as NET have a positive bone-sparing effect and that the response to estrogen is dose dependent (258).

Infections

Although OCs were earlier thought to be associated with an increased possibility of candidal vaginitis, more recent data on low-dose pills have not confirmed this association. Eschenbach and colleagues also found minimal effect of OC use on vaginal epithelium, vaginal and cervical discharge, and vaginal flora (262). Several studies have suggest that OC use lessens the risk of being hospitalized with PID (263), although a recent study of women suggests that upper tract genital infection is not associated with OC use (264). Adolescent OC users are at an increased risk of having *C. trachomatis* isolated from the cervix, thought to be secondary to factors such as the nonuse of barrier methods and the presence of a prominent and persistent cervical ectropion, which increases replication and detection of this organism. Studies are conflicting on the risk of acquiring HIV infection in OC users. Postulated causes have included persistence of the cervical ectropion, higher rates of chlamydial cervicitis, and immunologic changes.

PROGESTIN-ONLY PILL

Progestin-only oral contraceptive pills (POPs) are a good choice for teenagers who cannot tolerate the estrogen in the combined OC pill or have a medical contraindication to the use of the estrogen. The available options include a low-dose (0.35 mg) norethindrone pill (Micronor, Nor-QD) and a 0.075-mg norgestrel pill (Ovrette). There are other progestins such as desogestrel that are available in other countries (265). Because norethindrone is inactivated as it passes through the liver, it is roughly 60% bioavailable, whereas the norgestrel pill is 100% bioavailable. These two POPs are considered approximately equivalent in terms of progestin dose and effect on metabolism. POPs have several modes of action. Foremost, they alter the cervical mucus, inhibiting sperm penetration. They also alter the endometrium in most women, slow movement of the ovum in the fallopian tube, and prevent ovulation in about 50% of women.

POPs must be taken daily at approximately the same time to be effective in the prevention of pregnancy because serum progestin levels peak about 2 hours after oral administration and then rapidly decline because of rapid distribution and elimination (1) (Fig. 20-1). For increased effectiveness in the evening, it is thus preferable for a woman to take the pill in the late afternoon or what has been termed "tea time." If a woman is 3 hours late taking the pill, she should be instructed to use a backup method (e.g., condom) for 48 hours. The failure rate in typical use probably approaches 3% to 5%, but this rate is lower in older women (who are subfertile) and in women under 112 lb, who are more likely to have short cycles with ovulation inhibited (1). Since ovulation is not inhibited in many patients, pregnancy should be considered in patients with irregular bleeding or amenorrhea. If pregnancy does occur, ectopic pregnancy should be considered since the risk appears to be about 10% among POP failures. Ovarian cysts are also more likely to occur in POP users than combined OC pill users. Irregular menses are the usual reason that women decide to discontinue this method, and careful counseling in advance about menstrual changes is important for users. Often, the menses are most irregular in the first 3 to 4 months, after which the cyclicity improves.

A. Norethindrone

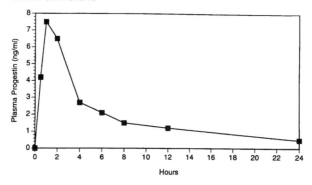

B. Levonorgestrel

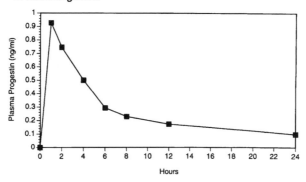

FIG. 20-1. Mean plasma levels during first 24 hours after oral intake: (**A**) Norethindrone 0.35 mg (*n* = 16). (**B**) Levonorgestrel 0.03 mg (*n* = 5). (From: McCann MF, Potter LS. Progestin-only oral contraception: comprehensive review. *Contraception* 1994; 50[Suppl 1]:S23; with permission.)

The risk of thrombophlebitis has not been established but appears to be minimal. A history of deep vein thrombosis (DVT) or pulmonary embolism (PE) is considered a Level 2, but current DVT/PE is a Level 3. The coagulation changes associated with combination pills are not evident with POPs in short-term studies. Hypertension is usually not a problem. Carbohydrate and lipid metabolism is probably not affected in most patients. Liver disease is not considered a contraindication to the use of POPs (1). POPs are acceptable choices for women with diabetes mellitus, SLE, sickle cell disease, hypertension, cyanotic and other cardiac disease, migraine headaches exacerbated by combined OCs, and lipid problems, as well as during lactation. Controversy exists on the best time to initiate POPs postpartum in the breast-feeding mother. The WHO guidelines assign a Level 3 to less than 6 weeks postpartum and a Level 1 to more than 6 weeks postpartum for breast-feeding women. However, a recent study found no adverse effect to initiation of progestin only methods within 3 days postpartum (266). POPs are not a good choice for patients taking anticonvulsants that enhance liver metabolism of contraceptive steroids, rifampin, or griseofulvin. In addition, POPs do not increase sex hormone-binding globulin production and lower free testosterone as effectively as combined OCs and thus are not as helpful in the treatment of patients with polycystic ovary syndrome. If teenagers are switching from a POP to a combined OC, they should be instructed to start on the first day of menses; if they are switching from an OC to a POP, the first POP should be taken at the end of the 21 active hormone tablets (discarding the placebos).

DEPOT MEDROXYPROGESTERONE ACETATE AND OTHER INJECTABLE HORMONES

Depot medroxyprogesterone acetate (DMPA or Depo-Provera) is a synthetic progestin derived from progesterone (267,268). A 150-mg dose of this aqueous micronized suspension is injected IM (deltoid or gluteus maximus) every 3 months (11 to 13 weeks); the site should not be massaged. DMPA suppresses the hypothalamic-ovarian axis and prevents the midcycle luteinizing hormone surge. In addition, it produces thinning and sometimes profound atrophy of the endometrium and increases the viscosity of the cervical mucus. The pregnancy rate of women given DMPA has been estimated at 0 to 0.4/100 woman-years (268). In a recent review of Planned Parenthood data, Borgatta and colleagues (269) reported a crude pregnancy rate of 0.42/1000 women using DMPA; there was no increase in ectopic pregnancies or fetal anomalies.

The first injection of DMPA is preferably given within the first 5 days of the menstrual cycle (after a pregnancy test) but can be given at other times if the patient is not pregnant and is counseled to use backup for 7 days (17). Postpartum women should be given the injection within 5 days of delivery if not breast-feeding or at the 6th week postpartum if breast-feeding (although one study has shown no effect on breast-feeding [266]). A reminder system that encourages patients to return at 12 weeks after the previous injection can be very helpful so that 1 week of "grace" period is provided. If the patient is late for injection but has her menses for up to 5 days *or* has not had sexual intercourse since her last menses, a pregnancy test is obtained and DMPA injected. If she does not fit these criteria, she should have a pregnancy test. If negative, she can be offered Emergency Contraception if she had intercourse within 5 days. She can then be counseled about several options: (1) waiting 14 days using barrier contraception or abstinence and having a repeat pregnancy test before injection; (2) switching to a different method; or (3) electing immediate injection (17).

The most important side effect of DMPA is menstrual irregularity; patients often experience irregular spotting and, occasionally, very heavy menses during the first few months of therapy. Weight gain can be another important side effect; it has been estimated that women gain about 5 lb each year for the first 3 years (although control groups have not been included in these studies). The package insert reports an average gain of 13.8 lb for 4 years of use and 16.5 lb for 6 years of use. However, several retrospective studies have shown that many adolescents lose or maintain weight on DMPA (270,271). Other side effects reported include depression, nervousness, breast tenderness, headaches, nausea, vomiting, decreased glucose tolerance, and lowered HDL cholesterol (1,272). Of note, a prospective study of adolescents using DMPA did not find significant changes in positive or negative mood affect using standardized questionnaires (273). The risk of thromboembolic disease is probably not increased (1); however, similar to POPs, past history of DVT/PE is a Level 2 and current DVT/PE is a Level 3 category. Liver cancer is not increased in humans, and DMPA has a protective effect on endometrial cancer (1). An analysis of a pooled data set of the WHO and New Zealand studies reported a RR of 1.1 (95% CI 0.97 to 1.4) for breast cancer in women who had ever used DMPA, with no increase in risk with increasing duration of use (274). However, recent or current use within the past 5 years was associated with a RR of 2.0 (95% CI 1.5 to 2.8), raising the possibility that enhanced detection of tumors or acceleration of the growth of preexisting tumors may be occurring. Another study of breast cancer by Shapiro and colleagues did not find an elevated risk for progestin only injectables (mostly DMPA): 0.9 (95% CI 0.7 to 1.2) (275).

A concern with special importance for teenagers is the potential impact of DMPA on bone density. Although estradiol levels are in the low follicular range, they are lower than those that occur during use of subdermal levonorgestrel implants. Since women acquire a major portion of their ultimate bone density during their adolescent years, especially between 11 and 16 years, it is critical to know whether the use of DMPA enhances, diminishes, or leaves unchanged the normal gains in bone density. A cross-sectional study in adult women suggested that bone density was lower in women given DMPA than in premenopausal control women, but no relationship to duration of use was observed (276). Based on small numbers, the researchers did find that bone density measurements increased after discontinuation. A cross-sectional study of adolescents 14 to 18 years old found no significant differences in adolescents using DMPA versus non-users, although mean bone density at the three sites was less; there was a trend of lower bone density with more injections (277). Merki-Feld and colleagues, using quantitative CT, did not observe accelerated bone loss at the distal radius in women 30 to 45 years old, but there was a wide range of responses in DMPA users and controls (278). They suggested that calcium intake and genetic susceptibility may play a role in the bone changes observed. Cundy and colleagues reported lower lumbar bone density in DMPA users than nonusers, especially in women who initiated use before age 20 years, those using it for more than 15 years, and those who were heavy smokers (279). In a longitudinal study of adolescents receiving DMPA, levonorgestrel implants (Norplant), OCs, or no hormonal therapy, Cromer and colleagues (280) reported that lumbar vertebral bone density decreased slightly in the DMPA users and increased in the other groups. Scholes and colleagues found recovery of bone density over 30 months in women, with less improvement in those 18 to 21 years old (281). Berenson found a mean decrease of lumbar spine bone mineral density of 2.74% over 12 months (257). While bone loss may occur, calcium supplementation may be protective and most importantly the degree of reversibility needs further study. These risks contrasted with the known benefits of pregnancy prevention with the use of DMPA need to be weighed by the clinician and the adolescent, particularly in the first few years after menarche and those at risk of low bone density.

DMPA is a good choice for teens who have difficulty remembering to take a daily pill or using a hormonal patch or ring and need long-term effectiveness. Injectable contraceptives may be particularly culturally acceptable to teens who have experience with the popularity of injectables in their native countries. Of importance, DMPA appears to lessen the risk of sickle cell crises in users (282), and there are no drug interactions with anticonvulsants in young women with epilepsy. The indications for DMPA include postpartum and lactating women and women with hypertension, hemoglobinopathies (SS disease), seizure disorders, and mental retardation (to help with menstrual hygiene problems). Women using teratogenic medications and those experiencing side effects with estrogen are also good candidates. Very little is known about continuation rates in adolescents; in a study of 50 teens, Smith and colleagues (283) reported that 72% continued to use DMPA at 1 year, 56% at 2 years, and 18% at 3 years.

Patients planning to use DMPA need to be counseled in advance about irregular menses. Most patients will have amenorrhea after three shots, but some have problems with frequent or heavy menses. By 12 months of use, 57% of women have amenorrhea, and by 24 months, 68% have amenorrhea. Most patients are happy about the amenorrhea. Adolescents are often concerned about irregular or heavy bleeding and may benefit from reassurance. If treatment is needed, a number of regimens have been advocated including 1 to 2 weeks of conjugated estrogens (1.25 mg) or micronized estradiol (2 mg) daily, 2 weeks of NSAIDs, 3 weeks of ethinyl estradiol (20 μg), or one or two packages of estrogenic OCs. For patients with mental retardation in whom the clinician wishes to ensure that the progestin is likely to be tolerated without significant mood change and the patient does not need immediate contraception, a 2- to 3-week course of oral medroxyprogesterone, 10 mg daily, can be helpful to assess side effects. After a 150-mg injection of DMPA, the mean interval before the return of ovulation is 4.5 months. In long-term users, the return of fertility is delayed, with a median time to conception of 10 months (range, 4 to 31 months). Of former DMPA users, 70% conceive within 12 months (compared to 94% for OCs) and more than 90% by 24 months.

A low-dose subcutaneous form of DMPA is in clinical trials and will allow self-administration. Another injectable contraceptive (not yet available in the United States) is norethindrone enanthate (Noristerat), with low pregnancy rates (two studies have found a rate of 0.4/100 and 0.6/100). Because a large WHO study showed a failure rate of 3.6 at 12 months, with pregnancies occurring 10 to 12 weeks following the last dose, the dosage was altered to 200 mg every 2 months for the first 6 months and then 200 mg every 2 to 3 months thereafter. Side effects are similar to those of DMPA, although bleeding tends to be more regular (284). Mean time to return of ovulation was 2.6 months.

Medroxyprogesterone Acetate/Estradiol Cypionate Injectable Contraceptive

A monthly injectable combined contraceptive, containing 25 mg of medroxyprogesterone acetate (MPA) with 5 mg of estradiol cypionate (E_2C) (Lunelle) has resulted in more regular menstrual cycles than DMPA (285–291), but is not currently available in the United States (voluntary withdrawal). The injections are given every 28 to 30 days (not to exceed 33 days). In a pharmacokinetic study of 77 women, the injection site (deltoid, gluteus maximus or anterior thigh muscles) did not have a significant impact on efficacy. In a multicenter, nonrandomized study comparing MPA/E_2C to norethindrone/EE triphasic (NET/EE) pill, there were no pregnancies in the MPA/E_2C group compared with one in the NET/EE group giving a pregnancy rate of 0.0 and 0.4 per 100 women-years, respectively (285). A large WHO study involving over 4,000 women and 40,000 woman-months of use reported a pregnancy rate of 0.1 per 100 woman-years (286). The manufacturer recommends that the first shot be given within 5 days of the start of a menstrual period, 5 days of an abortion, no earlier than 4 weeks if postpartum and not breastfeeding, or 6 weeks if breast-feeding. A patient who is over 33 days from her last injection should have pregnancy excluded before her late injection is given.

Withdrawal flow typically occurs 2 to 3 weeks after injection, with 4 menses in the first 3 cycles of use. After the initial 3 months, the majority of women have regular menstrual cycles lasting 6 days with the bleeding usually starting at day 22 (day 0 being the injection day). Women who received injections at evenly spaced intervals had more predictable bleeding patterns. Reasons given by women who discontinued MPA/E_2C have included weight gain (5.7%), metrorrhagia (2.5%), breast tenderness (1.8%), and acne (1.9%) (285). Kaunitz and colleagues found that among women weighing less than 150 lb at entry into the study the median weight gain was 2 to 4 lb; in contrast those weighing more than 150 lb had median of 3- to 8-lb weight gain (285). At 1 year, the intermenstrual/breakthrough bleeding/spotting rate was approximately 4% (289). Amenorrhea was noted by 1% to 4%. Women with a BMI over 27.3 were more likely to have missed periods or an irregular bleeding pattern than those at lower weight, possibly related to E_2 and/or MPA pharmacokinetics. Small differences in the mean area under the curve of serum MPA and serum MPA maximum were noted for BMI over 28 kg compared to those 28 kg or less with the levels higher for the group with lower BMI (289). However, the MPA minimum trough levels on day 28 were similar. Overall, body weight does not appear to have a clinically significant effect when comparing BMIs in the ranges of 18 to 28, 29 to 38, and over 38 (290). MPA/E_2C has been associated with decreased total cholesterol, HDL cholesterol, LDL cholesterol, triglycerides, apolipoprotein B, and apolipoproteins A-I and A-II, and maintenance of cholesterol/HDL-C ratio (291). In a randomized study of 30 women, MPA/E_2C resulted in a significantly lower incidence of follicular development up to 20-mm diameter compared to a low-dose oral contraceptive (20 µg EE and 0.1 mg levonorgestrel) (0% vs. 46.1%; $p < 0.05$) (292). MPA/E_2C appears to be particularly effective in the prevention of functional ovarian cysts (292). Ovulation returns 63 to

112 days following the last injection (293). Approximately 90% of MPA/E$_2$C users reported that they would recommend the injectable to a friend (294).

SUBDERMAL PROGESTIN IMPLANTS

Progestin implants are highly effective and have extremely low 5-year pregnancy rates. Levonorgestrel subdermal implants (Norplant System) were the first implants to be introduced in the United States, and were widely used through the 1990s (before voluntary discontinuation). The Norplant System has six nonbiodegradable Silastic rods that are implanted through a small incision in the upper or lower arm and slowly release levonorgestrel with efficacy for 5 years. Initially, 85 μg/day levonorgestrel is released with a decline to 50 μg/day by 9 months, 35 μg/day by 18 months, and 30 μg/day thereafter. The pregnancy rate is 0.03 to 0.4/100 woman-years of use. Insertion typically took 10 to 15 minutes and removal 15 to 30 minutes. Knowledge of different removal techniques is important (17). Potential complications with insertion have included infection, expulsion, hematoma/bleeding, increased pigmentation over the implant area, and scarring. Similar complications occur with removal and include breakage of the implants, scarring, and the need for a second incision or procedure.

The main reason for discontinuing the use of the Norplant System (as well as the Norplant II system, which has two rods) is menstrual irregularity. Other side effects include headache, mood change, acne, hirsutism, scalp hair loss, gallbladder disease, and weight gain (295). No unfavorable changes in carbohydrate metabolism, liver function, blood pressure, ectopic pregnancy rate, or total menstrual blood loss have been reported. It appears that the total cholesterol/HDL cholesterol ratio and other lipid parameters are unchanged or only minimally decreased (296,297). Norplant users have more functional ovarian cysts than do normally cycling women (1). Initial continuation rates in adults were reported at 85% to 90% at 1 year (298). After removal of the implants, women experience a prompt return of fertility; by 1 month, 25% are pregnant, by 3 months 49%, and by 12 months 86% (299).

Ease of use and high effectiveness were important benefits for teenagers and adult women (298,300–302), and teens were often influenced by their mothers to consider use (303). In a study of teenage mothers who selected OCs or Norplant, Polaneczky and colleagues (302) found that at 15 months 95% of 48 teens were using Norplant with only one pregnancy, compared to only 33% of 50 teens still using OCs, with 19 pregnancies having occurred. In some adolescents, the weight gain was minimal; in others, major weight gain occurred. Kozlowski and colleagues (304) found weight gain to be greater in heavy girls and African Americans (5.4 kg) than in white girls (2.6 kg) at ≥8 months of follow-up. Norplant also did not exacerbate postpartum depression in teen mothers with immediate insertion (305). Management of irregular menses has been accomplished through counseling and observation, with exclusion of diagnoses such as pregnancy or an STD. With persistent problems, a trial of a nonsteroidal antiinflammatory agent (e.g., ibuprofen) or several months of a combined

OC pill may improve the symptoms. Drug interactions are an important consideration with LNG implants, and lowered efficacy is noted with enzyme-inducing anticonvulsants and rifampin (1). Removal requests occurred because of side effects, desire for another pregnancy, a change in partners, and adverse publicity about implants.

Overall, there are four progestins in the subdermal implants that are in use or clinical trials: levonorgestrel in Norplant and Jadelle (also called Norplant II), etonogestrel in Implanon, nestorone in Elcometrine, and nomegestrol acetate in Uniplant and Surplant (306,307). The LNG two Silastic rod implant is currently available in Europe and China and is approved for 3 years in the United States. Sivin and colleagues found a 3 year cumulative pregnancy rate of 0.8 per 100 users and a mean annual continuation rate of 77/100; no pregnancies were noted in years 4 and 5. Mean removal time was 5.9 minutes (308,309). A single rod implant (40 mm long by 2 mm diameter) (Implanon) has 68 mg of etonogestrel embedded in a rod of ethylene vinyl acetate (EVA) copolymer membrane, which is covered by a thin EVA copolymer membrane. Implanon maintains contraceptive dose for 3 years with a Pearl Index of 0. It releases 60µg per day of etonogestrel after 3 months, which decreases to 30µg/day by the end of 2 years. Serum concentrations peak on day 4 at 813 pg/ml and decline to 196 pg/ml at the end of year one to 156 pg/ml by the end of year 3. Levels fall to undetectable by one week after removal (310). It has acceptable bleeding patterns with a incidence of amenorrhea of 30% to 40% in the first 3 months and prolonged bleeding in a similar percentage in the first 3 months, decreasing to 10% to 20% subsequently. Prolonged bleeding is similar with the LNG implants (Norplant) and Implanon, but amenorrhea is more common with Implanon (311). Implanon inhibits ovulation more than Norplant. Implanon is associated with few changes in lipid profile (312,313). A skin incision is needed for removal, but not insertion. Ovulation and fertility return within 3 months. Discontinuation rates vary greatly by country, with rates of 30% over 3 years in Europe and Canada and only 1% is Southeast Asia (313). Implanon may be available in the U.S. in 2005.

THE TRANSDERMAL CONTRACEPTIVE PATCH

The contraceptive patch (Ortho Evra) is 20 cm^2 and delivers transdermally norelgestromin 150 µg/d, the primary active metabolite of norgestimate, and ethinyl estradiol (EE) 20 µg/d (Fig. 20-2). The patch is applied once a week for three consecutive weeks; during the fourth week the patch is left off to allow for a withdrawal bleed. The mechanism of action is the same as combined oral contraceptives, and the options for starting the same (see p. 776). In pharmacokinetic studies, the serum concentrations of norelgestromin and EE are within the ranges seen with oral contraceptives containing norgestimate 250 µg and EE 35 µg for up to 10 days (Figs. 20-3 and 20-4) (314); however, the pattern is quite distinct. The transdermal release provides continuous serum concentrations of hormones, unlike the oral contraceptive pill in which there are daily peaks and troughs of hormones (315). The four application sites (upper arm, upper torso excluding the breast area, lower abdomen, and

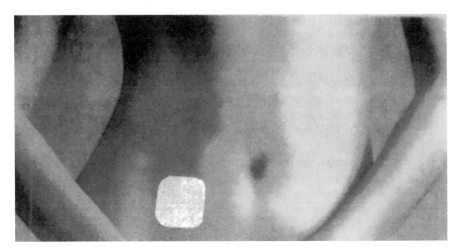

FIG. 20-2. Combined estrogen/progestin contraceptive patch (Ortho Evra). (Courtesy of Ortho Pharmaceutical Company, with permission.)

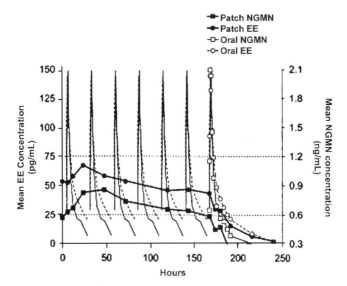

FIG. 20-3. Mean serum contraception versus time profile of norgestimate (NGM) and EE following patch application on the buttock during cycle 3, week 3, in the present study versus following administration of oral norgestimate 250 µg/ EE 35 µg (data on file RWJPRI). For oral dosing, actual steady-state serum concentrations of NGMN and EE are shown for cycle 3, day 21, and these results are replicated for the other days. Horizontal dashed lines indicate upper and lower limits of reference range for NGMN and EE. (From: Abrams LS, Skee DM, Natarajan J, et al. Multiple-dose pharmacokinetics of a contraceptive patch in healthy women participants. *Contraception* 2001;64:287–294; with permission).

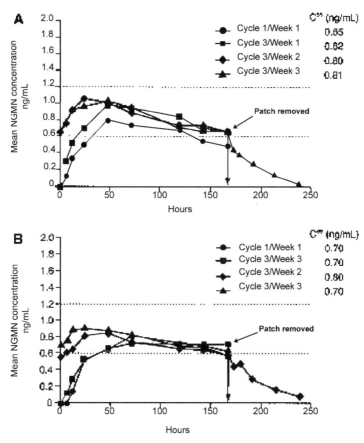

FIG. 20-4. A: Mean serum concentration versus time profile of NGMN following patch application on the abdomen for three consecutive cycles. **B:** Mean serum concentration versus time profile of NGMN following patch application on the buttock for three consecutive cycles. Horizontal dashed lines indicate upper and lower limits of reference range for NGMN. (From: Abrams LS, Skee DM, Natarajan J, et al. Multiple-dose pharmacokinetics of a contraceptive patch in healthy women participants. *Contraception* 2001;64:287; with permission).

buttocks) all deliver mean serum concentrations of norelgestromin and EE in the effective ranges during the entire 7-day period of use. However, the absorption from the abdominal site had resulted in serum levels 20% less than from other sites (316). The drug concentrations are not affected by gastrointestinal problems because the transdermal absorption avoids the first-pass metabolism (through the gastrointestinal tract and liver) that occurs with oral hormones (316). Of importance, drug levels remain in the reference range for the 7-day period even under conditions of exercise, heat, and humidity (315), and these conditions do not affect the adhesion of the patch (317). In a pooled analysis of 3 studies (≥3300 women 18 to 45 years old and

>22,000 treatment cycles), only 4.7% of patches were replaced because they fell off completely (1.8%) or partially (2.9%) (317). The percentage of detached patches was highest in the first cycle and decreased over treatment cycles, suggesting that application technique improves with continued use (317).

The overall Pearl Index (number of pregnancies per 100 woman-years) was 0.88 (95% CI 0.44 to 1.33) and method failure Pearl Index was 0.7 (95% CI 0.31 to 1.10) (318). No association was noted between pregnancy rate and either race or age. There was, however, an association between body weight of at least 90 kg ($\geq$198 lb) and pregnancy ($P < 0.001$), suggesting the patch may be less effective for overweight women. Despite this finding, pharmacokinetic studies revealed only 10% to 20% of the variability could be explained by body weight (318), and thus further research is needed. Rates of intermenstrual bleeding or spotting associated with patch use are low and decrease from cycle 1 to cycle 13, with no statistically significant difference between OCs and the patch (318). The incidence of adverse events including headache, nausea, and abdominal pain is similar between those using the patch compared to OCs. Patch users were noted to have a higher incidence of breast symptoms during the first 2 cycles and more dysmenorrhea (319). Breast symptoms decreased to 0% during cycle 13 of patch use. Twenty percent of patch users had application site skin reactions, but they were almost exclusively mild to moderate (94.5%) and did not increase over time. Only 2.6% of participants discontinued use because of skin reactions (319). The mean change in body weight was an increase of 0.3 kg and not different from users of a placebo patch or OC users (319). The patch can also be used continuously or as 9 weeks in a row followed by 7 days patch free.

Because nonadherence to a method is the greatest contributor to typical-use failure rates of contraceptives, particularly among adolescents, research has focused on rates of perfect use by age group. In a study examining use of OCs compared to the patch, perfect cycle use for oral contraceptives was significantly related to age ($p <$ 0.0001), with younger women under 20 years old having 67.7% perfect cycles; 20 to 24 year olds 74.4%; and women 25 years and older 79.8% to 85.2% (320). In comparison, rates of perfect use cycles for the patch were 88.1% to 91% across *all* age groups (320). It may be that the once-a-week dosing for the patch or the visibility of the patch on the body serves as a daily reminder has resulted in higher adherence rate for younger users compared with OCs in the clinical trials (320). Consumers have also voiced a desire, however, for smaller patches with clear options or variable colors. The contraceptive patch appears to have a number of advantages, including a convenient dosing schedule, improved compliance, user-controlled, and easily reversible (318). Patients are given the following instructions:

1. Choose a place on your body to put the patch—buttock, abdomen, upper outer arm, or upper torso—but never put the patch on your breasts. To avoid irritation, apply each new patch to a different place on your skin.
2. Open the foil pouch by tearing along the top edge and side edge. Peel the foil pouch apart and open it flat.

3. Using your fingernail, lift one corner of the patch, removing the patch *and* the plastic—it is important to keep them together, and sometimes patches can stick to the inside of the pouch.

4. Peel away half of the clear plastic from the patch and be careful not to touch the exposed sticky surface of the patch with your fingers.

5. Apply the sticky side of the patch to the skin you've cleaned and dried, then remove the other half of the clear plastic. Press firmly on the patch with the palm of your hand for 10 seconds, making sure the edges stick well.

6. Run your finger around the edge of the patch to make sure it is sticking properly. Check your patch daily to make sure all the edges are sticking. Avoid applying lotion directly over the patch to help adhesion. See instructions that come with the patch for what to do if it becomes loose or has fallen off.

7. Wear the patch for seven days, and on your "patch change day," day 8, remove the used patch. Even though the patch is used it still contains some medicine—fold it in half so that it sticks to itself before throwing it away.

8. Apply a new patch for week 2 and week 3 to a new area of skin. Do not wear a patch on week 4—your period should start during this week.

9. Begin your next 4-week cycle by applying a new patch on your normal "patch change day," the day after day 28—no matter when your period begins or ends.

10. If you are late applying your new cycle of patches, apply the patch and use backup for at least 7 days.

THE VAGINAL CONTRACEPTIVE RING

In October 2001, the FDA approved a contraceptive vaginal ring, NuvaRing (321), a soft, flexible, transparent polymer with an outer diameter that measures 2.1 inches (54 mm) and a cross section of 4 mm (322) (Fig. 20-5). The ring, self-inserted into the vagina, delivers an average of 120 µg of etonogestrel, the biologically active metabolite of desogestrel, and 15 µg of ethinyl estradiol (EE) per day over three weeks, after which the ring is removed for a week to allow menstruation. A new ring is then inserted. The levels are comparable to an OC pill containing 150µg desogestrel and 30 µg EE with lower overall exposure for EE from the ring (322,323) (Fig. 20-6), but as with the patch maintaining more constant levels on a day-to-day basis and avoiding the first pass through the gastrointestinal tract and liver. Maximum serum concentrations of etonogestrel are achieved by one week and decline from day 7 to day 21. EE levels reach a peak at 2 to 3 days and then decline (323,324). The advantages of the vaginal ring include ease of use, once a month insertion, lower hormone doses, and rapid onset of action (325). The contraceptive failure rate is similar to OCs and to the patch. The Pearl Index was 0.65 (95% CI 0.24 to 1.41) in a European study of 1145 woman 18 to 40 years old and 1.75 (95% CI 0.98 to 2.89) in a North American study that included user

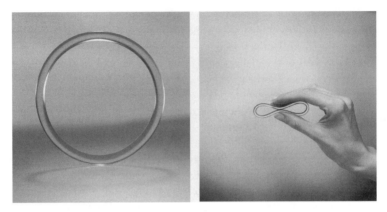

FIG. 20-5. Contraceptive vaginal ring (NuvaRing). (From: Organon website www.nuvaring.com; with permission.)

and method failure. If the failures due to noncompliance were excluded, the Pearl Index in the North American group was 0.77 (95% CI 0.37 to 1.40) (326,327).

In a study of 16 women between 18 and 35 years old, assessed by vaginal ultrasound and serum concentrations of FSH, LH, progesterone, and estradiol, complete inhibition of ovulation was noted throughout the normal 3-week period of use. Dur-

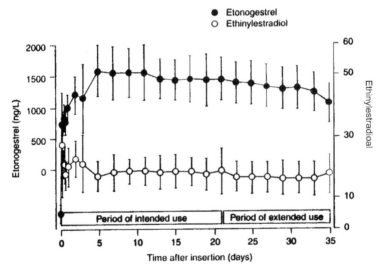

FIG. 20-6. Serum concentration–time curve (mean ± standard deviation; *n* = 16) of etonogestrel and ethinylestradiol during treatment with NuvaRing [day 1 to 21 (intended use) and days 22 to 25 (extended use)]. (From Timmer CJ, Mulders MT. Pharmacokinetics of etonogestrel and ethinyl estradiol released from a combined contraceptive vaginal ring. *Clin Pharmacokinet* 2000;39(3):233; with permission).

ing 2 weeks of extended use, inhibition of ovulation was also maintained (327). Follicular diameter and serum hormone concentrations on day 21 of an OC with desogestrel 150 μg and EE 30 μg indicated similar ovarian suppression to that observed after 3 weeks of the ring on day 20 (328). In a study of 45 woman ages 18 to 35, as few as 3 days of NuvaRing use suppressed the hypothalamic-pituitary-ovarian axis (322). Ovulation returned a median of 19 days after removal of the vaginal ring, with first ovulation occurring after 13 days. During patient use, if the ring is out of the vagina for more than 3 hours, a back up method is needed for 7 days.

In a study comparing NuvaRing to an OC with 150 μg levonorgestrel and 30 μg EE, the incidence of irregular bleeding was 5% or lower in all cycles, lower than the OC pill (5.4% to 38.8%) (325). Withdrawal flow occurred in 100% of women. The users of the vaginal ring were more likely to experience the "intended bleeding" pattern for the method (65.3% to 68.4%) than the OC users (28.4% to 46.8%). Withdrawal bleeding occurred in 97.9% to 99.4% of cycles, and women were compliant for 85.6% to 90.8% of cycles (326,327). The mean change in body weight was small at cycle 6: OC users experienced a slight mean increase ($+0.40$ kg) and ring users a slight mean decrease (-0.13 kg) (325). In a study of over 2000 women 18 to 40 years old, only 2.5% discontinued the ring because of the device, 85% were satisfied, and 90% would recommend it to others (327). Ninety-six percent of women said they never/rarely or occasionally felt the ring during intercourse and 90% of their partners never/rarely or only occasionally felt it (326). The most common side effects included vaginitis (5.8%), headache (5.8%), leukorrhea (4.8%), device–related events (4.4%), nausea (3.2%), breast tenderness (2.6%), and vaginal discomfort (2.4%) (327), which are comparable to OC users (326). In one small study, vaginal flora was not changed (329), and several studies have found no significant changes in the cervical or vaginal epithelium of users of various rings (330–332). Other progestin-only rings and rings with varying progestin/estrogen combinations are in clinical trials and have demonstrated good safety and efficacy (332–335). Patients are given the following instructions:

1. Wash and dry your hands before removing the NuvaRing from the reclosable foil pouch. Find a place to keep the pouch so that it can be used for proper disposal after use.
2. Choose the position for insertion that is most comfortable for you—lying down, squatting, or standing with one leg up. Hold the NuvaRing between your thumb and index finger and press the opposite sides of the ring together.
3. Gently push the folded ring into your vagina—the exact position is not important for NuvaRing to work. If you feel discomfort, NuvaRing is probably not inserted back far enough—use your finger to gently push it further into your vagina.
4. The NuvaRing cannot be pushed too far up in the vagina or get lost—it can only go as far as the end of the vagina where the cervix blocks it from going further.

5. Once inserted, keep NuvaRing in place for 3 weeks in a row.
6. Remove the ring 3 weeks after insertion on the same day of the week as it was inserted, at about the same time. For example, when NuvaRing is inserted on a Sunday at about 10:00 PM, the ring should be removed on the Sunday 3 weeks later at about 10:00 PM.
7. Remove the NuvaRing by hooking the index finger under the forward rim or by holding the rim between the index and middle finger and pulling it out.
8. Place the used ring in the foil pouch and dispose of it in a waste receptacle out of the reach of children and pets. Do not throw it in the toilet.
9. Your period should start this week. It may not have finished before the next ring is inserted—to continue to have pregnancy protection you *must* insert the new ring 1 week after the last one was removed, on the same day of the week around the same time.

INTRAUTERINE DEVICES AND SYSTEMS

The two intrauterine contraceptives available in the United States are the copper T-380A intrauterine device (ParaGard) and the levonorgestrel-releasing intrauterine system (LNG-IUS Mirena). Although the use of intrauterine devices (IUDs) is popular worldwide, it represents less than 2% of contraceptive use in the United States. The copper T-380A IUD is approved for 10 years of use with a pregnancy rate of 0.2 to 0.5/100 woman-years (2.6/100 women over 10 years of use) (336). The exact mechanism of action is unknown. IUDs lower the number of viable sperm, prevent fertilization of ova, increase leukocytes in the fallopian tubes, change tubal fluids, and cause a low-grade endometritis (17). Side effects of IUDs include increased vaginal discharge, heavy menses in nonhormonal devices, dysmenorrhea, uterine perforation, and pregnancy, as well as difficulty in removal because of loss of IUD strings. Bacterial vaginosis may be more common in IUD users (337). There is a reduction of ectopic pregnancies compared to women using no method (RR 0.2, 95% CI 0.1 to 0.4) (338). In a review of insertion timing, Stanwood and colleagues found that insertion of an IUD immediately following an induced or spontaneous abortion has a low risk of complications, and continuation rates were high (339); however, there were no randomized trials (340). Expulsion rates were higher for insertions after second trimester gestations.

The levonorgestrel-releasing intrauterine system (LNG-IUS), Mirena, releases a continuous sustained daily dose of 20 μg levonorgestrel into the lining of the uterus (Fig. 20-7). By 5 years, the dose of LNG release is still above 10 μg/24 hours (341). The device has several mechanisms of action including prevention of endometrial growth, thickening of cervical mucus, and inhibition of sperm mobility and function (342,343). It is considered one of the most effective long-term reversible contraceptive methods (344) with a Pearl Index (from 4 studies) of 0 to 0.6 (345,346). The cumulative pregnancy rate was 0.0 to 0.5 with up to 7 years of use (347). The estimated

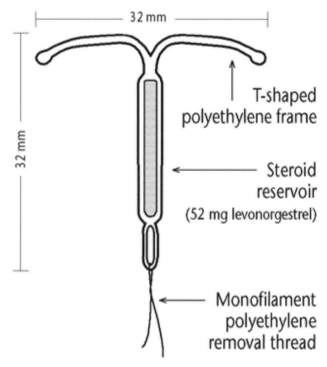

32 mm

32 mm

T-shaped
polyethylene frame

Steroid
reservoir
(52 mg levonorgestrel)

Monofilament
polyethylene
removal thread

FIG. 20-7. Levonorgestrel intrauterine system. (From: The Contraceptive Report, The LNG-IUS and menorrhagia treatment, *www.contraceptiononline.org/contrareport* June 2003, volume 14; source Berlex, with permission.)

risk of ectopic pregnancy is 1/5000, which is a 90% decrease in the risk of ectopic pregnancy compared to women not using contraception (340). Fertility rapidly returns after discontinuation of the IUS. Eighty-five percent of 203 women ages 29 to 45 years have reported that the LNG-IUS insertion was either not painful or resulted in only mild to moderate pain (348). The success of first insertion was 98.5% (348). Expulsion rate in one study was 5.6% (345). At 12 months, 71% to 88.7% of women continued use (345).

The striking difference between the LNG-IUS and prior IUDs is the reduction of blood loss associated with use. A number of studies have shown that the mean number of bleeding days decreases over the 12-month period and that 22.6% of women have amenorrhea of at least 90 days (348). By 8 months, approximately half have no menstrual bleeding. Ovulation frequently occurs in LNG-IUS users, and the bleeding pattern does not reflect ovarian function. Hemoglobin concentration, hematocrit, and serum ferritin levels rise with use (348). The reduction of menstrual flow that some women may view as a side effect resulting in discontinuation also makes it an effective medical treatment for woman with menorrhagia, reducing blood loss by 74% to 97% and helping to avoid surgical intervention (349,350). The LNG IUS has been found helpful in patients with chronic disease and menorrhagia (351). The occurrence of dysmenorrhea, breast pain, premenstrual syndrome, and headaches all decreased with IUS use (348). At 5 years, side effects were uncommon: lower abdominal pain (2.1%), headache (1.6%), acne (1.2%), and mastalgia (1.0%) (341). Those switching to the IUS from OCs had a decrease in serum triglycerides (348). The most common reasons for removing the device were (a) bleeding problems including spotting, frequent irregular bleeding, heavy menstrual flow, and amenorrhea and (b) pelvic, abdominal, and back pain and dysmenorrhea (348). The discontinuation rates due to pregnancy and expulsion of the device are higher among those with menorrhagia (349,352). Of note from a counseling perspective, women informed about the amenorrhea are more satisfied with the method than those who are less informed (353). Compared to nonhormonal IUDs, LNG IUS devices are associated with lower risk of ectopic pregnancy, higher risk of amenorrhea and expulsion, and more likely to be discontinued because of hormonal side effects (354). Compared to LNG implants, LNG IUS users are less likely to have prolonged bleeding and spotting.

A number of studies have reexamined the potential risk of infection related to IUDs. The increased risk of PID noted in early studies has been questioned because the results were based on the use of inappropriate controls (groups with lower risk, such as OC users), overdiagnosis of PID in IUD users, and lack of control for confounding factors such as number of sexual partners and exposure to STDs. Recent insertion within 20 days (or reinsertion) appears to be associated with a small increased risk of infection in those with STDs, which quickly declines to baseline levels; the risk is inversely associated with age (355,356). Shelton has estimated the risk of PID to be 0.15% (357). Although screening for STDs is important and in particular before insertion, prophylactic antibiotics (doxycycline or azithromycin) at the time of insertion do not appear to decrease the risk of PID or the likelihood of removal, but do decrease unscheduled visits (358,359). In a case control study of fertility and use of a copper IUD, the OR for tubal occlusion was 1.0 (95% CI 0.6 to 1.7) (360). Tubal infertility was associated with the presence of antibodies to Chlamydia but not with the reason for removal of the IUD, duration of use, or gynecologic problems associated with IUD use. Women under 25 years of age may be especially susceptible to complications, perhaps because they are more likely to have more than one sexual partner and have an increased risk of Chlamydia and gonorrhea. Although the risk of infection is low (352,361) and may actually be reduced with LNG-IUS (346), IUDs are not recommended for most adolescents due to their increased risk of STDs. However, monogamous young women who have a low risk of infection and desire long-term highly effective contraception are candidates for this new method. IUDs are often not recommended for HIV positive patients, although limited data show no increased risk (362). The Level 3 and 4 categories for the LNG-IUS are shown in Table 20-8.

TABLE 20-8. *Selected WHO guidelines for levonorgestrel-releasing IUD.*[a]

Category 3 WHO guidelines (for levonorgestrel-releasing IUD, 20 μg /24 h)
Use of method is usually not recommended unless other, more appropriate methods are not available or not acceptable.

- □ Postpartum <4 wk
- □ Current deep vein thrombosis or pulmonary embolism
- □ Current and history of ischemic heart disease (for continuation of use, category 2 for initiation)
- □ Headaches with focal neurologic symptoms at any age (for continuation of use, category 2 for initiation)
- □ Past breast cancer and no evidence of current disease for 5 years
- □ PID, current or within the last 3 months (for continuation of use)
- □ Increased risk of STIs
- □ AIDS (for initiation, category 2 for continuation)
- □ Active viral hepatitis
- □ Benign or malignant liver tumors.

Category 4 WHO guidelines (for levonorgestrel-releasing IUD, 20 μg /24h)
Method is contraindicated.

- □ Anatomical abnormalities: distorted uterine cavity incompatible with IUD insertion
- □ Unexplained vaginal bleeding before evaluation (category adjusted after evaluation)
- □ Cervical cancer awaiting treatment (for initiation of use, category 2 for continuation)
- □ Current breast cancer
- □ PID, current or within the last 3 months (for initiation of use)
- □ STIs, current or within 3 months

[a]Adapted from: the WHO recommendations. World Health Organization. Medical eligibility criteria for contraceptive use. Geneva, 2004.

A number of clinical trials of frameless IUDs are ongoing. These devices are anchored by one end of a nylon thread to the fundal myometrium to which the copper sleeves are attached. All three trials reviewed in the Cochrane database excluded nulliparous women (363). Expulsion rates were higher than the TCu380A for several devices. Pregnancy rates were extremely low and overall the devices performed similarly to the copper IUD. A frameless IUD with levonorgestrel delivery system has demonstrated reduction in blood loss, similar to the LNG IUS (364).

FEMALE BARRIER METHODS

Options for female-controlled barrier methods have increased in the past few years. Intravaginal nonhormonal methods include female condoms, diaphragms, cervical caps, sponges, and spermicides. Because of the increased concerns about STDs, including HIV infection, young women who might previously have selected a sponge, diaphragm, or cervical cap are now more likely to have their partner use condoms. Many of these methods are available over the Internet (365). All women using these methods should have easy access to emergency contraception.

Diaphragm

The diaphragm is fitted by the health care provider. There are three types of diaphragms available: arcing spring, coil spring, and wide-seal rim (Fig. 20-8). Diaphragms come in sizes 50 to 95, with sizes 60 to 75 most often used by adolescents. Actual diaphragms rather than fitting rings should be used so that the patient can practice in the clinic. The ring of the arcing spring diaphragm provides firm pressure on the lateral vaginal walls and is therefore especially good for patients with poor vaginal tone, mild uterine prolapse, or marked uterine anteflexion or retroversion. The coil spring rim, which folds flat for insertion, can be used for most women with average vaginal tone and a normal pubic notch. The wide-seal rim has a flexible flange on it to create a better seal and is available in arcing spring and coil spring.

The size of the diaphragm is estimated by the examiner's placing a gloved index finger and middle finger in the vagina until they reach the posterior vaginal wall behind the cervix. The thumb is then placed on top of the index finger to mark the point at which the index finger touches the pubic bone. The fingers are removed in this position, and the diaphragm size is determined by placing the tip of the middle finger against the rim and the opposite rim against the spot on the index finger previously marked with the thumb (Fig. 20-9). The diaphragm should fit snugly, since vaginal size increases with sexual stimulation and coitus. A too loose diaphragm will be displaced; a too large diaphragm can cause pressure, pain, and urinary tract infections.

The pregnancy rates reported with diaphragm use vary from 6 to 23/100 woman-years of use, with most studies reporting 10 to 18 pregnancies (17,366). Trussell and associates (366) reported a pregnancy rate of 8% for perfect use in nulliparous

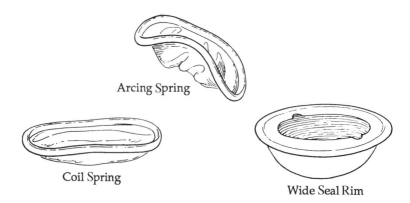

FIG. 20-8. Types of diaphragms. (From: Hatcher RA, Trussell J, Stewart F, et al. *Contraceptive technology,* 16th ed. Atlanta, GA: Irvington, 1994; with permission.)

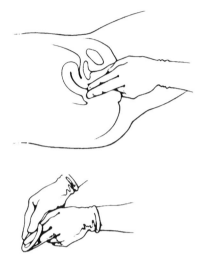

FIG. 20-9. Determining diaphragm size. (From: *Ortho diaphragms*. Raritan, NJ: Ortho Pharmaceutical Corp, 1981; with permission.)

women (15% for consistent use) versus 4% for perfect use in parous women (5% for consistent use). Causes of failure include nonuse, an incorrect fit, a flawed device, and failure to use a condom if there is a second episode of intercourse. Some women cannot use a diaphragm because of poor vaginal tone, congenital anomalies, uterine prolapse, rectovaginal or vesicovaginal fistulas, or allergy to latex or spermicide. A 2- to 2.5-fold increased risk of urinary tract infections has been noted (367,368). Vaginal colonization with *Escherichia coli* was significantly greater in diaphragm users. A change in diaphragm type or size, postcoital antibiotics, or a change to a different method of contraception may be necessary in adolescents with recurrent urinary tract infections associated with diaphragm use. Other problems with the diaphragm include foul-smelling vaginal discharge associated with prolonged wearing of the diaphragm, pelvic discomfort, vaginal ulceration from excessive rim pressure, and possible association with toxic shock syndrome (see Chapter 14). Before a prescription is given, young women should be shown how to feel for the cervix and should have an opportunity during the office visit to insert the diaphragm and remove it (Fig 20-10). Teaching aids such as the Ortho pelvic model are helpful. A return appointment 2 to 3 weeks later to check for proper fit of the prescribed size allows the clinician a chance to assess patients' understanding and acceptance of this form of contraception. Patients are given the following instructions:

1. Before inserting, urinate and wash hands with soap and water.
2. Place 2 tsp of contraceptive jelly or cream inside the cup of the diaphragm and spread a small amount around the entire rim. The diaphragm can be inserted up to 6 hours prior to intercourse. Check that the diaphragm is in a correct position

before each time you have sex. (Many women routinely insert the diaphragm every night.) Never use Vaseline or petroleum products on the diaphragm.

3. For insertion, hold the diaphragm with the dome facing down, and press together the opposite sides of the rim. After inserting the diaphragm, check the cervix to make sure that it is covered by the diaphragm and that the diaphragm is locked in place behind the pubic bone.

4. Leave the diaphragm in place for at least 6 hours but not more than 24 hours after intercourse, and do not douche during the 6 hours after intercourse.

5. To remove the diaphragm, place the index finger behind the front rim and pull the diaphragm down and out. If difficult to remove, insert a forefinger up and over the top side of the diaphragm to break the suction.

6. After removal, wash the diaphragm with mild soap, dry it thoroughly, and store it in a cool, dry place.

7. Before each use, hold the diaphragm up to the light and check for holes.

8. The diaphragm should be replaced at least every 2 years and at any time a small tear or puckered appearance near the rim is noted. If a woman has a weight change of 10 lb or has had a recent pregnancy, the clinician should be consulted to make sure that the diaphragm still fits.

9. If the diaphragm is displaced or not used correctly, use emergency contraception.

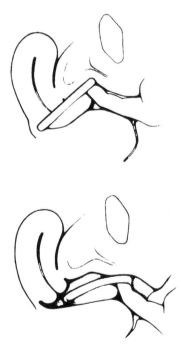

FIG. 20-10. A technique for removal of the diaphragm. (From *Ortho diaphragms.* Raritan, NJ: Ortho Pharmaceutical Corp, 1981; with permission.)

Cervical Cap

A cervical cap is similar to a diaphragm except that it is designed to cover only the cervix (369). The Prentif Cavity-Rim Cervical Cap is available in four sizes. One-tenth to one-third of women cannot be fitted, although the introduction of custom-molded caps may alleviate some of this problem. Patients need to feel comfortable with insertion of tampons or diaphragms into the vagina, before considering the cap. A small amount of spermicide is placed in the cap (about one-third full of 2% spermicidal jelly), and the cap is inserted onto the cervix; it is held in place by suction. The device can be left in place for at least 8 hours (maximum of 48 hours) and should not be worn during menses. It is not necessary to reapply spermicide with repeated intercourse, but the cap should be checked before and after intercourse (especially in the first month of use) to make sure it has not been dislodged. Use of additional spermicide in the vagina and/or use of a condom seems prudent in the first 2 months after fitting and with a new position or new partner. The pregnancy rates are similar to those with the diaphragm, with a range of 8 to 27/100 woman-years of use (366,370,371), with studies indicating a higher failure rate for parous women than nulliparous, unlike the diaphragm. In a study of over 3400 women, Richwald and colleagues (370) estimated first year pregnancy rate to be 11.3% (8.3% and 3.8% for user and method failure, respectively). "Near-perfect" users had half the pregnancy rate of others (6.1% vs. 11.9%). Trussell and co-workers (366) have estimated a pregnancy rate of 8% to 10% for perfect use in nulliparous women and 26% to 27% for perfect use in parous women. Because of questions in the initial trials related to Pap smear changes, the cap is contraindicated in patients with abnormal Pap tests. Other problems with the cap include odor, dislodgment, vaginal discharge, bacterial vaginosis, UTIs, partner discomfort, and difficulty with insertion or removal. Contraindications to use of a cap include known or suspected uterine or cervical malignancy and current cervicovaginal infections. Practitioners usually wait 6 to 8 weeks postpartum and 3 to 4 weeks postabortion to fit a cap.

Two other devices similar to the cervical cap are Lea's shield and Femcap. Lea's shield is a one-size-fits-all vaginal contraceptive that is made of silicone rubber and shaped like an elliptical bowl with a loop at the front end to aid removal; it has a valve to allow passage of cervical secretions and air to allow a better fit. It appears to be acceptable to some women (372). The adjusted 6-month failure rate was 5.6 per 100 woman-years when used with spermicide and 9.3 per 100 woman-years when used without spermicide (373). It should be left in place for 8 hours after intercourse and then washed with mild soap and air dried. The Femcap is another vaginal contraceptive made of silicone rubber that is shaped like a sailor's hat. The brim adheres and conforms to the vaginal walls. It can be used with a spermicide. Because it comes in two sizes, it requires fitting by a clinician. It appears to have a higher pregnancy rate than the diaphragm with typical use 6-month pregnancy rate of 13.5% in one trial (374).

Spermicides and Sponges

Spermicides are available over the counter and include vaginal creams, jellies, foams, suppositories, and films. The most well-known spermicide is nonoxynol-9. Recent data has concluded that nonoxynol-9 does not have efficacy against sexually transmitted infections and may increase the risk of HIV transmission in women who have multiple daily acts of intercourse (375). Frequent usage of spermicides in female sex workers did not decrease gonococcal or chlamydial infections and resulted in increased HIV transmission (376). Irritation of the vaginal mucosa may result in a reduced barrier protection. The use of spermicides in teens at low risk of HIV infection is preferable to no contraception at all, but condoms without spermicides are preferable for STD and pregnancy prevention. The pregnancy rates for spermicides alone are in the range of 3 to 30/100 woman-years of use; the lower rate can be achieved by educated, motivated women in their 30s who are given specific in-office demonstration of appropriate use and application (high in the vagina) of spermicides (377). Data from the 1995 National Survey of Family Growth suggest a failure rate of 10.5% at 6 months, 15.3% at 12 months, 22.1% at 18 months (18). Whenever possible, adolescents choosing a spermicide should also have their partners use a condom.

The jellies, creams, and foams should be inserted less than 60 minutes before intercourse and are effective within several minutes (foams are effective immediately, but gels and creams need a few minutes to reach body temperature to melt). Suppositories require 10 to 15 minutes to melt or effervesce and appear more unpredictable in their dispersion. A vaginal contraceptive film (VCF) consists of a 2-in. × 2-in. flat package with wax paperlike tissues, each containing 72 mg of nonoxynol-9. The film is inserted on a dry fingertip up into the vagina at least 5 minutes before intercourse and remains effective for 2 hours. Patients may have difficulty with odor and allergic reactions to the spermicides. Vaginal flora is altered with the use of spermicides and spermicide users have an increased risk of urinary tract infections. A prospective study of university women found that the prevalence of *E. coli* colonization and abnormal Gram stain scores (Nugent criteria) were more common among spermicide users than OC users (378). Studies have not found any link between spermicides and congenital anomalies (379,380). During counseling, specific names of foams (e.g., VCF Foam, Delfen), suppositories (e.g., Intercept), and film (e.g., VCF) should be mentioned. A demonstration of how to fill the applicator with foam is useful. Individual one-dose applicators (Conceptrol Jel, Advantage S) are convenient for adolescents but are also more expensive than the refillable applicators. For girls choosing to use spermicides, instructions include

1. Be sure to read the instructions for the product you use before insertion. For example, films and suppositories must be inserted 15 minutes before intercourse to allow time to dissolve.

2. Insert the contraceptive foam, suppository, or film high into the vagina so that it will cover the cervix. Use the foam 60 minutes or less prior to finishing intercourse—not after intercourse.
3. Do not douche for at least 6 hours after intercourse.
4. Wash the spermicide applicator with warm water and soap after each use.
5. Frequent daily use of spermicides may increase the risk of acquiring HIV infection.
6. Using a condom is the preferred method of pregnancy and STD prevention.

The Vaginal Contraceptive Sponge is a disposable polyurethane foam sponge impregnated with a high dose of nonoxynol-9 and may be available in 2004 or 2005. In a Cochrane review, Kuyoh and colleagues found that the sponge was less effective than the diaphragm and more likely to be discontinued; the pregnancy rate was 17.4 for the sponge versus 12.8 for the diaphragm in the US trial, and 24.5 and 10.9, respectively, for the UK trial (381). The Protectaid sponge is a barrier method that acts as a physical barrier absorbing semen and as a chemical barrier with three spermicides (sodium cholate, nonoxynol-9, and benzalkonium chloride); it is currently available in Canada and through the Internet. The reported efficacy in a trial of 129 women was 77% with high acceptability (382). The low concentrations of nonoxynol and the dispersing gel appear to markedly reduce vaginal irritation. It can be placed in the vagina up to 12 hours before intercourse.

Female Condom

The introduction of the female condom offers an additional alternative for patients for contraception and likely STD prevention (Fig. 20-11). The female condom is a prelubricated, loose-fitting, disposable polyurethane sheath with two diaphragm-like flexible rings at either end. The inner ring covers the cervix (similar to a diaphragm) and the outer ring fits against the vulva. In a 6-month trial involving 240 women, the pregnancy rate was estimated at 2.6% with perfect use and 12.4% with typical use (9.5% failure for women $\geq$25 years and 22.3% failure for women <25 years) (383,384). Trussell and colleagues (384) have estimated a 5.1% pregnancy/failure rate with perfect use; they also suggested that with perfect use the device would be 94% protective against HIV infection for women having intercourse twice a week with an infected partner. The female condom offers the advantage of female control over a barrier method that can aid in the prevention of STDs and does not change vaginal flora (385). Female condoms should be seen for the most part as an additional option, rather than a replacement for male condoms (386). A 6-month study of STD clinic patients showed that having the option of selecting to use male and female condoms at different times improved consistent condom use (387). Self-insertion practice in the clinic may build skills and aid in acceptance of the method (388). The cost ($2–3 each) and the unusual appearance may be barriers to the widespread usage by

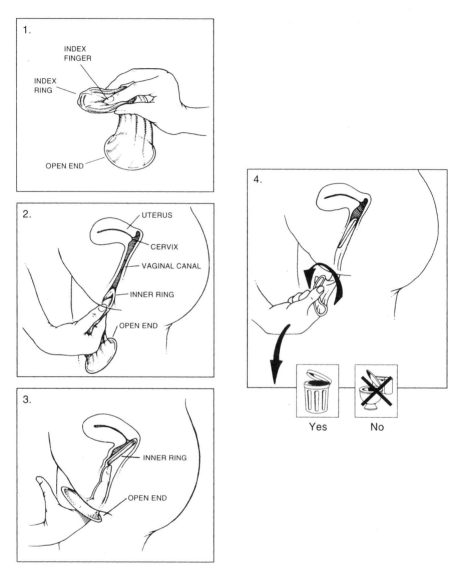

FIG. 20-11. The female condom. [From: *Contracept Rep* 1994;5(6):8; with permission].

teenagers. Reuse is *not* recommended, although one study showed no deterioration in up to eight uses of washing, drying, and relubricating (389). Some users may complain that there is a "squeaking" sound with intercourse or that the female condom seems to be sticking to the penis; both problems can be addressed by the use of additional vaginal lubricant (e.g., K-Y Jelly) on the inside of the device or on the penis.

A male condom should not be used at the same time. Our instructions to patients are the following:

1. Find a comfortable position. You may want to stand with one foot on a chair, squat with knees apart, or lie down with legs bent and knees apart.
2. Hold the female condom with the open end hanging down. Squeeze the inner ring with your thumb and middle finger.
3. Holding the inner ring squeezed together, insert the ring into the vagina and push the inner ring and pouch into the vagina past the pubic bone.
4. When properly inserted, the outer ring will hang down slightly outside the vagina. During intercourse, when the penis enters the vagina, the slack will lessen. One partner should assure proper adherence of the outer ring of the condom to the perineum during intercourse.
5. To remove the device, squeeze and twist the outer ring to keep the sperm inside the pouch. Pull the condom out gently. Throw away in the garbage; do not flush down the toilet. Do not reuse.
6. Male condoms should not be used at the same time as a female condom.

Other female condom designs under development include the Bikini condom (a panty with a covered perineal area), Women's Choice (which requires an applicator for insertion), and Reddy Female Condom, made of latex with the outer ring conforming more closely to female anatomy.

MALE CONDOMS

Recognition of the major threat posed by HIV infection and other STDs has markedly increased condom usage. Consistent condom use requires skills-based learning, practice, empowerment of women, overcoming cultural barriers, and peer support. Educational efforts to improve the image of condom users and increase the peer pressure to use condoms, as well as the availability of free condoms in drug stores, clinics, and schools, have increased usage in some settings. Adolescent girls frequently are not assertive about the use of condoms when the male rejects the notion. It is helpful for the health care provider to give patients some ideas to enhance their negotiating ability, as well as some catchy phrases, such as "You don't know how? Allow me," or "My doctor says I must protect my cervix." Cultural barriers need to be understood and efforts framed within the context of realistic change that can occur for a given adolescent. Some condoms are now marketed exclusively for women and are shelved in pharmacies with other feminine hygiene products. Adolescents may feel more comfortable purchasing contraceptive supplies from an unfamiliar pharmacy. Pregnant teenagers should also be encouraged to use condoms throughout pregnancy to prevent exposure to STDs.

The pregnancy rate of condoms has varied in studies from 2 to 20/100 woman-years of use, with good usage resulting in pregnancy rates of 3 to 4/100 woman-years of use (17,18). A survey of 20- to 39-year-old men who had used a condom in the preceding 6 months showed that the average condom breakage rate was 2.9% and that 1.9% of all condoms used broke during that time (390). Men with low incomes and infrequent use of condoms were more likely to experience condom breakage and slippage (391,392). Similar findings were noted in a study of 177 couples, with a breakage rate of 5% and a slippage rate of 3.5% (392). "Always" use of condoms provides significant protection against STDs, such as HIV, *N. gonorrhoeae,* and likely *C. trachomatis,* but is less protective for transmission of herpes and HPV (393,394). In a meta-analysis of 25 studies, Davis and colleagues found that the heterosexual transmission rates of HIV for discordant couples was 0.9/100 person-years for those who always used condoms and 6.9/100 person-years for male to female transmission (395). Spermicidal condoms are *not* recommended (See Spermicide section above). Condom use appears to increase the risk of UTI in women; an increased risk was observed for condoms coated with spermicide and for exclusive use of condoms (396). Polyurethane condoms (e.g., Durex Avanti, Trojan Supra) are an alternative for those who are latex allergic or prefer these condoms. Unlike latex condoms, which can be weakened by oil based lubricants and vaginal creams, polyurethane condoms can be lubricated with oil-based lubricants. They are thinner and potentially provide greater sensitivity and comfort. Polyurethane condoms are more expensive than latex condoms, have similar efficacy, and appear to be more likely to have slippage and breakage (8.5%) than latex condoms (1.6%) (397).

A latex-like styrene ethylene butylene styrene (SEBS) natural-rubber condom (Tactylon) is an option for latex-allergic patients in other countries. The breakage rates appear to be greater for the condoms made of Tactylon (3.5% to 4.2%) compared to latex condoms (0.86%), but the slippage rates were similar (0.7% to 1.3%) for Tactylon compared to 1.1% for latex condoms (398). A positive report of a phase I trial of a "baggy" condom suggests that alternative designs may increase acceptance with similar breakage and slippage rates (399). Because natural condoms have larger pores that can allow the smaller particles of hepatitis B virus or HIV to pass through, latex or polyurethane condoms should be used for the prevention of STDs. Condoms may be lubricated or unlubricated, with the former being preferred by most adolescents. It is unknown whether thick condoms offer any more protection than thin condoms with vaginal intercourse, although thin condoms may be more likely to tear. Instructions—with a demonstration if possible—are extremely important for adolescents to be able to use condoms correctly. Condoms should not be exposed to excessive heat (i.e., in a wallet for >2 months or in a glove compartment). Many clinicians suggest that couples relying on condoms should have a prescription or supply of emergency contraception levonorgestrel (1.5 mg) available for self-administration. Recommendations to teenagers using latex condoms include the following:

1. Latex condoms are preferred.
2. Condoms should be stored in a cool, dry place.
3. Condoms in damaged packages (brittle, sticky, discolored) should not be used.

4. Condoms should be put on before any genital contact. The tip of the condom should be held and the condom unrolled onto the erect penis, leaving 1/4 to 1/2 inch of space at the tip to collect semen yet ensuring that no air is trapped in the tip.

5. Adequate lubrication should be used. Only water-based lubricants (e.g., K-Y Jelly, Surgilube) should be used, not petroleum-based lubricants such as Vaseline.

6. If the condom breaks, it should be replaced. If ejaculation occurs after breakage, insert spermicidal foam if available (17), and use emergency contraception.

7. After ejaculation, the base of the condom should be held to prevent slippage. The penis should be withdrawn while still erect. Be careful not to let semen spill. Remove the condom, and dispose of it safely.

COITUS INTERRUPTUS

Withdrawal is a not an effective method of contraception for adolescents, although it is practiced widely by many who often believe that it offers significantly more protection than it does. Few adolescents have the ability to prevent ejaculation effectively, and thus even those who believe they can practice this method well often have difficulty. Couples are clearly not protected from STDs with the use of withdrawal, and pregnancy rates are high because the preejaculate may contain sperm from a previous ejaculation. The annual failure rate with typical use of this method has been estimated at 19% to 27% (17).

"NATURAL" FAMILY PLANNING OR FERTILITY AWARENESS

Calendars, basal body temperature charts, cervical mucus awareness, and hormonal testing have been used for both contraception and facilitation of conception in infertile couples. The advantages are the ease of the method and the fact that adolescents can be taught the method as a noncontroversial part of reproductive health. The major drawbacks of these methods are the high failure rate for pregnancies and the lack of protection against STDs. Although these methods do encourage communication between sexual partners, extensive records are required and sexual spontaneity is restricted. Calendar methods are less likely to help adolescents prevent pregnancy than adults because of the wider range of cycles in adolescents. The Standard Day Method has users avoid intercourse between cycle days 8 through 19. In one efficacy trial, the pregnancy rate was 12% over 13 cycles (400). The Billings method of cervical mucus awareness is based on determining ovulation by the change of mucus to abundant slippery mucus. Secretions can be affected by coitus, vaginitis, cervicitis, and vaginal medications and spermicides. Electronic handheld computers can boost the reliability of the rhythm method. Most of the high-technology methods of hormonal assays are more appropriate for the treatment of infertile couples. The pregnancy rates reported are variable, ranging from 6 to 38/100 woman-years of use (typical use 20), depending on the population studied and the method employed (401,402).

LACTATIONAL AMENORRHEA METHOD

Postpartum women who (a) breast-feed their infants exclusively (or nearly exclusively), (b) are amenorrheic and (c) under 6 months postpartum have less than a 2% chance of pregnancy in the first 6 months (403). A second method needs to be used if any of the three criteria change. Use of the lactational amenorrhea method (LAM) has a positive influence on women continuing to breastfeed. A multicenter trial of LAM ($n = 302$ acceptors) found no pregnancies at 7 months and the rate of continuation to another method of contraception at 7 months to be 67% (404).

EMERGENCY CONTRACEPTION (POSTCOITAL CONTRACEPTION)

Emergency contraception (previously known as postcoital contraception or the "morning after pill") is an important yet still underutilized method of contraception (405–421). The most common methods of emergency contraception (EC) are progestins alone or estrogen/progestin combinations, but mifepristone has been studied in trials and postcoital insertion of an IUD is a possible option. All adolescents should be educated about the availability of this method in situations of unexpected coitus, broken condoms, rape, missed OCs (any two consecutive pills), dislodged diaphragm or cervical cap, expulsion of IUD, late injection of DMPA, or exposure to a possible teratogen (406). Many clinicians provide a prescription or actual medication at the time of the visit to assure that the patient has access to the doses in a timely manner. Several states have the progestin only levonorgestrel (LNG) method (Plan B) available through the pharmacy, and over-the-counter status has been advocated by many.

In the past, the most commonly used hormonal dosing was the Yuzpe regimen (407,408), which utilizes 100 µg ethinyl estradiol (EE) *plus* either 1.0 mg norgestrel (NG) or 0.5 mg levonorgestrel (LNG) within 72 hours of unprotected intercourse, followed by the same dose 12 hours later. A specially marketed formulation (Preven) comes with a pregnancy test. Alternatively, a variety of oral contraceptives can be used to provide each dose, including 2 Ovral tablets, 4 tablets of Lo/Ovral, Levlen, or Nordette (slightly higher dose), or 5 tablets of Alesse, with each of these doses repeated 12 hours later. The pregnancy rate has varied from 1.1% to 2.9% versus an expected rate of 5% to 8% (406–410,412,413), depending in part on how the studies were done and whether the day of cycle was controlled. Trussell and colleagues (412) suggested that estimates of efficacy should consider the reduction in expected pregnancies. In reviewing 10 studies of the Yuzpe regimen that contained data on the cycle day of unprotected intercourse, they estimated that effectiveness was 74% (95% CI 68.2% to 79.3%). In a recent reanalysis, the effectiveness may be 51% to 62% (406). Side effects are primarily nausea (50%) and vomiting (20%), which can be lessened by preceding the dose with an antiemetic such as meclizine hydrochloride (Dramamine II or Bonine) 25 to 50 mg 1 hour before first dose. Meclizine may increase drowsiness. Extra doses of the estrogen/progestin should be available in case the patient vomits in one hour and needs to repeat the dosage. WHO and International Planned Parenthood list the contraindication of pregnancy to the use of the Yuzpe regimen. Others have suggested that migraine with neurologic symptoms at the time of the EC, clotting disorders, history of DVT/PE, and strokes are contraindications but there is no evidence in this regard. Plan B is preferable in these situations. A retrospective cohort study in the UK found no cases of thromboembolism among over 100,000 episodes of EC with the Yuzpe regimen (414). No adverse effects on fetuses have been found (415).

More recently, the introduction of progestin-only therapies has provided enhanced efficacy and fewer side effects such as nausea (14% to 23%) and vomiting (1% to 6%). The initial dosing was 0.75 mg levonorgestrel, followed 12 hours later by 0.75 mg. This dose is packaged as Plan B. Twenty tablets of Ovrette would be needed to simulate each dose. The use of LNG (Plan B) resulted in a 88% reduction in pregnancies, similar or better than the Yuzpe regimen (416). For both Yuzpe and LNG regimens, there was waning of efficacy with each day. For less than 24 hours, 25 to 48 hours, and 49 to 72 hours, LNG EC prevented 95%, 85%, and 58% of pregnancies, respectively, compared to the Yuzpe estrogen/progestin EC, which prevented 77%, 36% and 31%, respectively. Most recently, a multicenter WHO trial of over 4000 women, taking EC within 120 hours of unprotected intercourse, demonstrated equal efficacy for 0.75 mg LNG 12 hours (pregnancy rate 1.8%) apart versus 1.5 mg single dose (1.5%), with overall prevention of pregnancy 77% and 82%, respectively (417). There was efficacy in the prevention of pregnancy up to 5 days but large confidence intervals were noted at 4 to 5 days because of small numbers (Table 20-9). The only contraindication to the LNG method is pregnancy, but EC has no effect on a preexisting pregnancy.

There are multiple mechanisms of actions proposed for the Yuzpe regimen and Plan B; these include, among others, interrupting follicular maturation, delaying or preventing ovulation, and impairing sperm migration, fertilization, fallopian tube transport, endometrial receptivity, and corpus luteum sufficiency (310,418). A study of the Yuzpe regimen found a reduction in endometrial MUC-1 expression, an increase in endometrial estrogen receptor, lower luteal phase estrogen levels, reduced endometrial thickness, and more glandular supranuclear vacuoles (419). The mechanism varies with the stage of the menstrual cycle, with anovulation in 80% of participants who took the LNG on day 10 of the cycle compared to a change in progesterone levels in those who were in the late follicular phase but were pre-ovulatory. Endometrial histology was normal in all the women with ovulatory cycles (420).

Patients are counseled to avoid having intercourse for the remainder of the cycle. A return visit 2 to 3 weeks later should be arranged for teens to obtain a pregnancy test and ensure that contraception is addressed for the future. Since the Yuzpe regimen probably does not protect against tubal pregnancy, a prior tubal pregnancy is a cause for extra caution in follow-up. An encouraging study from the

TABLE 20-9. *Pregnancies prevented and pregnancy rate by day from unprotected intercourse for the use of three doses of emergency contraception: Levonorgestrel (LNG) 0.75 for two doses, levonorgestrel 1.5-mg single dose, and Mifepristone 10-mg single dose.*

	% (95% CI) pregnancies prevented		Pregnancy rate	
Time	LNG 0.75 mg × 2	LNG 1.5 mg	LNG 0.75 mg × 2	LNG 1.5 mg
1 to 3 days	79% (66.2 to 86.8)	84% (73 to 90.5)	1.69%	1.34%
4 to 5 days	60% (−5.9 to 84.6)	63% (1.5 to 85.7)	2.44%	2.67%

	Mifepristone 10 mg	
Time	% (95% CI) pregnancies prevented	Pregnancy rate
1 to 3 days	82% (70.5 to 89)	1.48%
4 to 5 days	58% (−23.8 to 86)	2.19%

Adapted from: von Hertzen H, Piaggio G, Ding J, et al. Low dose mifepristone and two regimens of levonorgestrel for emergency contraception: a WHO multicentre randomised trial. *Lancet* 2002;360:1803.

United Kingdom found that only 4% of women 14 to 29 years of age received EC more than once in any year and the 70% who had not previously used regular contraception initiated use (421). Patients can start their hormonal method of contraception such as OCs the day after the EC and use back-up for 7 days. The directory of sites providing emergency contraception in the United States is available through 1-800-584-9911 and 1-888-NOT-2-LATE or on the World Wide Web (http://opr.princeton.edu/ec). Information on Plan B can be obtained through www.youngwomenshealth.org and www.go2planb.com. Emergency contraception with multiload Cu-375 SL IUD inserted within 120 hours led to a 98% prevention of pregnancy in the parous group and 92% in the nulliparous group (422). The LNG IUS cannot be used for EC.

STERILIZATION

Sterilization is rarely chosen by adolescent patients, with the exception of those with chronic diseases in whom pregnancy is contraindicated. A number of options are available including clips, rings, and interruptive and destructive surgical methods of tubal ligation. Transcervical methods are the latest advance. The Essure micro-inserts (coil-like devices) are inserted into the proximal fallopian tube under hysteroscopic visualization; they appear to be safe and effective (423). Contraindications include pregnancy, recent (<6 weeks) abortion, miscarriage, or birth, uterine malformation, known allergy to contrast dye or nickel, unwillingness to use another method of contraception for 3 months or to undergo a hysterosalpingogram to assure that the tubes are blocked, or a prior tubal ligation. Other methods under study include quinacrine pellets, intratubal ligation, and nonbiodegradable implant matrix following creation of a superficial tubal lesion by a catheter.

REFERENCES

1. McCann MF, Potter LS. Progestin-only oral contraception: comprehensive review. *Contraception* 1994;50(Suppl 1):1.
2. *Facts in brief: teenage reproductive health in the United States.* New York: The Alan Guttmacher Institute, 1999.
3. Centers for Disease Control, Youth Risk Behavior Surveillance—United States, 2003. *MMWR* 2004;53(SS-2):1.
4. Abma JC, Chandra A, Mosher WD, et al. Fertility, family planning, and women's health: new data from the 1995 National Survey of Family Growth. National Center for Health Statistics. *Vital Health Stat* 1997;23.
5. Ford K, Sohn W, Lepkowski J. Characteristics of adolescents' sexual partners and their association with use of condoms and other contraceptive methods. *Fam Plan Perspect* 2001;33:100,132.
6. Shrier A, Emans SJ, Woods ER, DuRant RH. The association of sexual risk behaviors and problem drug behaviors in high school students. *J Adolesc Health* 1997;20:377.
7. Arias E, MacDorman MF, Strobino DM, et al. Annual summary of vital statistics—2002. *Pediatrics* 2003:112;1215.
8. Rosenberg MJ, Waugh MS, Long S. Unintended pregnancies and use, misuse and discontinuation of oral contraceptives. *J Reprod Med* 1995;40:355.
9. Blake SM, Simkin L, Ledsky R, et al. Effects of a parent-child communication intervention on young adolescents' risk for early onset of sexual intercourse. *Fam Plan Perspect* 2001;33:52.
10. Emans SJ, Grace E, Woods ER, et al. Adolescents' compliance with the use of oral contraceptives. *JAMA* 1987;257:3377.
11. Ranjit N, Bankole A, Darroch JE, et al. Contraceptive failure in the first two years of use: differences across socioeconomic subgroups. *Fam Plan Perspect* 2001;33:19.
12. Furstenberg FE Shea J, Allison P, et al. Contraceptive continuation among adolescents attending family planning clinics. *Fam Plan Perspect* 1983;15:211.
13. Adler NE, Kegeles SM, Irwin CE, et al. Adolescent contraceptive behavior: an assessment of decision process. *J Pediatr* 1990;116:463.
14. Kegeles SM, Adler NE, Irwin CE. Adolescents and condoms: associations of beliefs with intention to use. *Am J Dis Child* 1989;143:911.
15. Oakley D. Rethinking patient counseling techniques for changing contraceptive behavior. *Am J Obstet Gynecol* 1994:170:1585.
16. Loeb L, Colacurio V, Atkinson E, et al. Concurrent condom use intentions and practice among adolescent users of hormonal contraceptives. Presented at the American Public Health Association (APHA), Nov 1994.
17. Hatcher RA, Zieman M, Cwiak C, et al. *Managing Contraception 2004–2005.* Tiger, Georgia: Bridging the Gap Foundation, 2004.
18. Trussell J, Vaughan B. Contraceptive failure, method-related discontinuation and resumption of use: results from the 1995 National Survey of Family Growth. *Fam Plan Perspect* 1999;31:64,93.
19. Trussell J, Hatcher RA, Cates E, et al. A guide to interpreting contraceptive efficacy studies. *Obstet Gynecol* 1990;76:558.
20. Trussell J, Kost K. Contraceptive failure in the United States: a critical review of the literature. *Stud Fam Plan* 1987;18:237.
21. Mishell DR, Burkman RT, Shulman LP, et al. Understanding contraceptive effectiveness. *Dialog-Contracept* 2002;7:1.
22. Audet M-C, Moreau M, Koltun WD, et al. Evaluation of contraceptive efficacy and cycle control of a transdermal contraceptive patch vs an oral contraceptive: a randomized trial. *JAMA* 2001; 285:2347.
23. Woutersz TB, Korba VD. Five-year multicenter study of a triphasic, low-dose, combination oral contraceptive. *Inter J Fertil* 1988;33:406.
24. Potter L, Oakley D, Leon-Wong E, et al. Measuring compliance among oral contraceptive users. *Fam Plan Perspect* 1996;28:154.
25. Grady WR, Billy JOG, Klepinger DH. Contraceptive method switching in the United States. *Perspect Sexual Reprod Health* 2002;34:135.
26. Gazmararian JA, Parker RM, Baker DW. Reading skills and family planning knowledge and practices in a low-income managed-care population. *Obstet Gynecol* 1999;93:239.

27. WHO website for medical eligibility criteria 2004: http//www.who.int/reproductive-health/publications/RHR_00_2_medical_eligibility_criteria_3rd/index.htm 2004 summary tables: http//www.who.int/reproductive-health/publications/MEC_3/mec.pdf.

28. World Health Organization. Medical Eligibility Criteria for Contraceptive Use. 3rd ed, Geneva 2004.

29. Stanback J, Katz K. Methodological quality of WHO medical eligibility criteria for contraceptive use. *Contraception* 2002;66:1.

30. Hannaford P, Webb A. Evidence-guided prescribing of combined oral contraceptives: consensus statement. *Contraception* 1996;54:125.

31. Hannaford P, Webb A. *Evidence-guided prescribing of the pill.* Carnforth, England: Parthenon Publishing, 1996.

32. Cochrane Reviews. http://www.cochrane.org/

33. Paukku M, Quan J, Darney P, et al. Adolescents' contraceptive use and pregnancy history: Is there a pattern? *Obstet Gynecol* 2003:1010:534.

34. Zabin LS, Stark HA, Emerson MR. Reasons for delay in contraceptive clinic utilization. *J Adolesc Health* 1991;12:225.

35. Armstrong KA, Stover MA. Smart start: an option for adolescents to delay the pelvic examination and blood work in family planning clinics. *J Adolesc Health* 1994;15:389.

36. Goldzieher JW. Pharmacokinetics and metabolism of ethynyl estrogens. In: Goldzieher JW, Fotherby K, eds. *Pharmacology of the contraceptive steroids.* Philadelphia: Lippincott-Raven, 1994;127.

37. Brody SA, Turkes A, Goldzieher JW. Pharmacokinetics of three bioequivalent norethindrone/mestranol 50 μg pills and three norethindrone/ethinyl estradiol OC formulations: are "low-dose" pills really lower? *Contraception* 1989:40:269.

38. Fotherby K. Pharmacokinetics and metabolism of progestins in humans. In: Goldzieher JW, Fotherby K, eds. *Pharmacology of the contraceptive steroids.* Philadelphia: Lippincott-Raven, 1994;99.

39. Dorflinger LJ. Relative potency of progestins used in oral contraceptives. *Contraception* 1985; 31:557.

40. Krattenmacher R. Drospirenone: pharmacology and pharmacokinetics of a unique progestogen. *Contraception* 2000;62:29.

41. Ludicke F, Johannisson E, Helmerhorst FM, et al. Effect of a combined oral contraceptive containing 3 mg of drospirenone and 30 μg of ethinyl estradiol on the human endometrium. *Fertil Steril* 2001;76: 102.

42. Blode H, Wuttke W, Loock W, et al. A 1-year pharmacokinetic investigation of a novel oral contraceptive containing drospirenone in healthy female volunteers. *Eur J Contracept Reprod Health Care* 2000;5:256.

43. Parsey KS, Pong A. An open-label, multicenter study to evaluate Yasmin, a low-dose combination oral contraceptive containing drospirenone, a new progestogen. *Contraception* 2000;61:105.

44. Letterie GS, Chow GE. Effect of "missed" pills on oral contraceptive effectiveness. *Obstet Gynecol* 1992;79:979.

45. Grimes DA, Godwin AJ, Rubin A, et al. Ovulation and follicular development associated with three low-dose oral contraceptives: a randomized controlled trial. *Obstet Gynecol* 1994;83:29.

46. Creinin MD, Lippman JS, Eder SE, et al. The effect of extending the pill-free interval on follicular activity: triphasic norgestimate/35 μg ethinyl estradiol versus monophasic levonogestrel/20 μg ethinyl estradiol. *Contraception* 2002;66:147.

47. Holt VL, Cushing-Haugen KL, Daling JR. Body weight and risk of oral contraceptive failure. *Obstet Gynecol* 2002;99:820.

48. Rosenberg MJ, Meters A, Roy V. Efficacy, cycle control, and side effects of low- and lower-dose oral contraceptives. *Contraception* 1999;60:321.

49. Van Vliet H, Grimes D, Helmerhorst F, et al. Biphasic versus triphasic oral contraceptives for contraception. *Cochrane Database Syst Rev* 2001:CD003283.

50. Van Vliet H, Grimes D, Helmerhorst F, et al. Biphasic versus monophasic oral contraceptives for contraception.[update of Cochrane Database Syst Rev. 2001;(2):CD002032; PMID: 11406026]. *Cochrane Database Syst Rev* 2001:CD002032.

51. Sulak P, Lippman J, Siu C, et al. Clinical comparison of triphasic norgestimate/35 micrograms ethinyl estradiol and monophasic norethindrone acetate/20 micrograms ethinyl estradiol. Cycle control, lipid effects, and user satisfaction. *Contraception* 1999;59:161.

52. Woods ER, Grace E, Havens KK, et al. Contraceptive compliance with a levonorgestrel triphasic and a norethindrone monophasic oral contraceptive pill in adolescent patients. *Am J Obstet Gynecol* 1992;166:901.

53. Miller L, Notter KM. Menstrual reduction with extended use of combination oral contraceptive pill: randomized controlled trial. *Obstet Gynecol* 2001;98:771.
54. Anderson FD, Hait H. A multicenter randomized study of an extended cycle oral contraceptive. *Contraception* 2003:68:89.
55. Miller L, Hughes J. Continuous combination oral contraceptive pills to eliminate withdrawal bleeding: A randomized trial. *Obstet Gynecol* 2003;101:653.
56. Corson SL. Efficacy and clinical profile of a new oral contraceptive containing norgestimate. U.S. clinical trials. *Acta Obstet Gynecol Suppl* 1990:152:25.
57. Moore PJ, Adler NE, Kegeles SM. Adolescents and the contraceptive pill: the impact of beliefs on intentions and use. *Obstet Gynecol* 1996;88:485.
58. Robinson TC, Plichta S. Weisman CS, et al. Dysmenorrhea and use of oral contraceptives in adolescent women attending a family planning clinic. *Am J Obstet Gynecol* 1992;166:578.
59. Westhoff C, Kerns J, Morroni C. Quick Start: a novel oral contraceptive method. *Contraception* 2002; 66:141.
60. Lara-Torre E, Schroeder B. Adolescent compliance and side effects with Quick Start initiation of oral contraceptive pills. *Contraception* 2002;66:81.
61. Westhoff C, Morroni C, Kerns J, et al. Bleeding patterns after immediate vs conventional oral contraceptive initiation: A randomized trial. *Fertil Steril* 2003;79:322.
62. Gallo MF, Grimes DA, Shulz KF, Helmerhorst FM. Combination contraceptives: effects on weight. *Cochrane Database Syst Rev* 2003;(2):CD003987.
63. Carpenter S, Neinstein LS. Weight gain in adolescent and young adult oral contraceptive users. *J Adolesc Health Care* 1986;7:342.
64. Reubinoff BE, Grubstein A, Meirow D, et al. Effects of low-dose estrogen oral contraceptives on weight, body composition, and fat distribution in young women. *Fertil Steril* 1995;63:516.
65. Lloyd T, Lin HM, Matthews AE, et al. Oral contraceptive use by teenage women does not affect body composition. *Obstet Gynecol* 2002;100:235.
66. Oelkers W, Foidart JM, Dombrovicz N, et al. Effects of a new oral contraceptive containing an antimineralocorticoid progestogen, drospirenone, on the renin-aldosterone system, body weight, blood pressure, glucose tolerance, and lipid metabolism. *J Clin Endocrinol Metabol* 1995;80: 1816.
67. Oelkers W, Helmerhorst FM, Wuttke W, et al. Effect of an oral contraceptive containing drospirenone on the renin–angiotensin–aldosterone system in healthy female volunteers. *Gynecol Endocrinol* 2000;14:204.
68. Huber J, Foidart JM, Wuttke W, et al. Efficacy and tolerability of a monophasic oral contraceptive containing ethinylestradiol and drospirenone. *Eur J Contracept Reprod Health Care* 2000;5(1):25.
69. Rosenberg MJ, Waugh MD, Stevens CM. Smoking and cycle control among oral contraceptive users. *Am J Obstet Gynecol* 1996;174:628.
70. Krettek JE, Arkin SI, Chaisilwattana P, et al. *Chlamydia trachomatis* in patients who used oral contraceptives and had intermenstrual spotting. *Obstet Gynecol* 1993;81:728.
71. Darney PD, Klaisle CM. Contraception-associated menstrual problems: Etiology and management. *Dialog Contracept* 1998;5(5):1.
72. Speroff L, Darney PD. *A clinical guide for contraception.* Philadelphia: Lippincott Williams & Wilkins, 2001.
73. Mattson RH, Rebar RW. Contraceptive methods for women with neurologic disorders. *Am J Obstet Gynecol* 1993;168:2027.
74. Chang CL, Donaghy M, Poulter N, et al. Migraine and stroke in young women: case-control study. *BMJ* 1999;318:13.
75. Curtis KM, Chrisman CE, Peterson HB. Contraception for women in selected circumstances. *Obstet Gynecol* 2002;99:1100.
76. Donaghy M, Chang CL, Poulter N, European Collaborators of The World Health Organization Collaborative Study of Cardiovascular D, Steroid Hormone C. Duration, frequency, recency, and type of migraine and the risk of ischaemic stroke in women of childbearing age. *J Neurology Neurosurg Psych* 2002;73:747.
77. Bousser MG, Conard J, Kittner S, et al. Recommendations on the risk of ischaemic stroke associated with use of combined oral contraceptives and hormone replacement therapy in women with migraine. The International Headache Society Task Force on Combined Oral Contraceptives & Hormone Replacement Therapy. *Cephalalgia* 2000;20:155.

78. Sulak PJ, Scow RD, Preece C, et al. Hormone withdrawal symptoms in oral contraceptive users. *Obstet Gynecol* 2000;95:261.

79. Schwartz SM, Petitti DB, Siscovick DS, et al. Stroke and use of low-dose oral contraceptives in young women: A pooled analysis of two US studies. *Stroke* 1998;29:2277.

80. Headache Classification Committee of the International Headache Society. Classification and diagnostic criteria for headache disorders, cranial neuralgias and facial pain. *Cephalalgia* (Suppl 8);1988;7:1.

81. De Leo V, la Marca A, Morgante G, et al. Evaluation of plasma levels of renin-aldosterone and blood pressure in women over 35 years treated with new oral contraceptives. *Contraception* 2001; 64: 145.

82. Update on the 1987 Task Force report on high blood pressure in children and adolescents: a working group report from the National High Blood Pressure Education Program. *Pediatrics* 1996;98: 649.

83. Porter JB, Hunter JR, Jick H, et al. Oral contraceptives and nonfatal vascular disease. *Obstet Gynecol* 1985;66:1.

84. Ramcharan S, Pellegrin FA, Ray RM, et al. The Walnut Creek contraceptive drug study: a prospective study of the side effects of oral contraceptives. *J Reprod Med* 1980;25(Suppl 6):345.

85. Hirvonen E, Idanpaan-Heikkila JI. Cardiovascular death among women under 40 years of age using low-estrogen oral contraceptives and intrauterine devices in Finland from 1975. *Am J Obstet Gynecol* 1990;163:281.

86. Gerstman BB, Piper JM, Freiman JP, et al. Oral contraceptive oestrogen and progestin potencies and the incidence of deep venous thromboembolism. *Int J Epidemiol* 1990;19:931.

87. Gerstman BB, Piper JM, Tomita DK, et al. Oral contraceptive estrogen dose and the risk of deep venous thromboembolic disease. *Am J Epidemiol* 1991;133:32.

88. Beller FK. Cardiovascular system: coagulation, thrombosis, and contraceptive steroids—is there a link? In: Goldzieher JW, Fotherby K, eds. *Pharmacology of the contraceptive steroids*. Philadelphia: Lippincott-Raven, 1994;301.

89. Vandenbroucke JP, Rosing J, Bloemenkamp KW, et al. Oral contraceptives and the risk of venous thrombosis. *N Engl J Med* 2001;344:1527.

90. Aznar J, Vaya A, Estelles A, et al. Risk of venous thrombosis in carriers of the prothrombin G20210A variant and factor V Leiden and their interaction with oral contraceptives. *Haematologica* 2000;85:1271.

91. Chan HH, Douketis JD, Nowaczyk MJ. Acute renal vein thrombosis, oral contraceptive use, and hyperhomocysteinemia. *Mayo Clin Proc* 2001;76:212.

92. Bloemenkamp KW, Helmerhorst FM, Rosendaal FR, et al. Venous thrombosis, oral contraceptives and high factor VIII levels. *Thromb Haemost* 1999;82:1024.

93. Farmer RD, Lawrenson RA, Todd JC, et al. A comparison of the risks of venous thromboembolic disease in association with different combined oral contraceptives. *Br J Clin Pharmacol* 2000; 49:580.

94. Black C, Kaye JA, Jick H. Clinical risk factors for venous thromboembolus in users of the combined oral contraceptive pill. *Br J Clin Pharmacol* 2002;53:637.

95. World Health Organization Collaborative Study of Cardiovascular Disease and Steroid Hormone Contraception. Venous thromboembolic disease and combined oral contraceptives: results of an international multicentre case-control study. *Lancet* 1995;346;1575.

96. World Health Organization Collaborative Study of Cardiovascular Disease and Steroid Hormone Contraception. Effect of different progestagens in low-oestrogen oral contraceptives on venous thromboembolic disease. *Lancet* 1995;346;1582.

97. Jick H, Eck SS, Gurewich V, et al. Risk of idiopathic cardiovascular death and nonfatal venous thromboembolism in women using oral contraceptives with differing progestagen components. *Lancet* 1995;346;1589.

98. Bloemenkamp KW, Rosendaal FR, Helmerhorst FM, et al. Enhancement of factor V Leiden mutation of risk of deep-vein thrombosis associated with oral contraceptives containing a third-generation progestagen. *Lancet* 1995;346;1593.

99. Vasilakis C, Jick SS, Jick H. The risk of venous thromboembolism in users of postcoital contraceptive pills. *Contraception* 1999;59:79.

100. Lawrenson R, Farmer R. Venous thromboembolism and combined oral contraceptives: does the type of progestogen make a difference? *Contraception* 2000;62(2 Suppl):21S; discussion 37S.

101. Lewis MA. The Transnational Study on Oral Contraceptives and the Health of Young Women. Methods, results, new analyses and the healthy user effect. *Hum Reprod Update* 1999;5:707.
102. Farmer RD, Williams TJ, Simpson EL, et al. Effect of 1995 pill scare on rates of venous thromboembolism among women taking combined oral contraceptives: analysis of general practice research database. *BMJ* 2000;321:477.
103. Speroff L, DeCherney A. Evaluation of a new generation of oral contraceptives. *Obstet Gynecol* 1993;81:1034.
104. Burnhill MS. The use of a large-scale surveillance system in Planned Parenthood Federation of America clinics to monitor cardiovascular events in users of combination oral contraceptives. *Int J Fertil Womens Med* 1999;44:19.
105. Hennessy S, Berlin JA, Kinman JL, et al. Risk of venous thromboembolism from oral contraceptives containing gestodene and desogestrel versus levonorgestrel: a meta-analysis and formal sensitivity analysis. *Contraception* 2001;64:125.
106. Kemmeren JM, Algra A, Grobbee DE. Third generation oral contraceptives and risk of venous thrombosis: meta-analysis. *BMJ* 2001;323:131.
107. Bloemenkamp KW, Rosendaal FR, Helmerhorst FM, et al. Higher risk of venous thrombosis during early use of oral contraceptives in women with inherited clotting defects. *Arch Int Med* 2000; 160:49.
108. Lidegaard O, Edstrom B, Kreiner S. Oral contraceptives and venous thromboembolism: a five-year national case-control study. *Contraception* 2002;65:187.
109. Sheldon T. Dutch GPs warned against new contraceptive pill. *BMJ* 2002;324(7342):869.
110. Ridker PM, Miletich J, Hennekens CH, et al. Ethnic distribution of factor V Leiden in 4,047 men and women. *JAMA* 1997;277:1305.
111. Creinin MD, Lisman R, Strickler RC. Screening for factor V Leiden mutation before prescribing combination oral contraceptives. *Feril Steril* 1999;72: 646.
112. Spannagl M, Heinemann LA, Schramm W. Are factor V Leiden carriers who use oral contraceptives at extreme risk for venous thromboembolism. *Eur J Contracept Reprod Health Care* 2000;5:105.
113. ACOG Practice Bulletin. The use of hormonal contraception in women with coexisting medical conditions. *Int J Gynecol Obstet* 2001:75:93.
114. Heinemann LA. Emerging evidence on oral contraceptives and arterial disease. *Contraception* 2000;62(2 Suppl):29S; discussion 37S.
115. Kittner SJ, Stern BJ, Wozniak M, et al. Cerebral infarction in young adults: the Baltimore-Washington Cooperative Young Stroke Study. *Neurology* 1998;50:890.
116. Kemmeren JM, Tanis BC, van den Bosch MA, et al. Risk of Arterial Thrombosis in Relation to Oral Contraceptives (RATIO) study: oral contraceptives and the risk of ischemic stroke. *Stroke* 2002;33:1202.
117. Lidegaard O, Kreiner S. Contraceptives and cerebral thrombosis: a five-year national case-control study. *Contraception* 2002;65:197.
118. Gillum LA, Mamidipudi SK, Johnston SC. Ischemic stroke risk with oral contraceptives: A meta-analysis. *JAMA* 2000;284:72.
119. Vessey M, Villard-Mackintosh L, McPherson K, et al. Mortality among oral contraceptive users: 20 year followup of women in a cohort study. *BMJ* 1989;299:1487.
120. Colditz GA. Oral contraceptive use and mortality during 12 years of follow-up: the Nurses Health Study. *Ann Intern Med* 1994;120:821.
121. WHO Collaborative Study of Cardiovascular Disease and Steroid Hormone Contraception. Ischaemic stroke and combined oral contraceptives: results of an international, multicentre, case-control study. *Lancet* 1996;348:498.
122. WHO Collaborative Study of Cardiovascular Disease and Steroid Hormone Contraception. Hemorrhagic stroke, overall stroke risk, and combined oral contraceptives: results of an international, multicentre, case-control study. *Lancet* 1996;348:505.
123. Petitti DB, Sidney S, Bernstein A, et al. Stroke in the users of low-dose oral contraceptives. *N Engl J Med* 1996;335:8.
124. Schwartz SM, Siscovick DS, Longstreth WT, et al. Use of low-dose oral contraceptives and stroke in young women. *Ann Intern Med* 1997;127(8):596.
125. Thorogood M, Vessey MP. An epidemiologic survey of cardiovascular disease in women taking oral contraceptives. *Am J Obstet Gynecol* 1990;163:274.
126. Stampfer MJ, Willett WC, Colditz GA. A prospective study of past use of oral contraceptive agents and risk of cardiovascular diseases. *N Engl J Med* 1988;319:1313.

127. Goldbaum GM, Kendrick JS, Hogelin GC, et al. The relative impact of smoking and oral contraceptive use on women in the United States. *JAMA* 1987;258:1339.
128. Tanis BC, van den Bosch MA, Kemmeren JM, et al. Oral contraceptives and the risk of myocardial infarction. *N Engl J Med* 2001;345:1787.
129. Lewis MA, Spitzer WO, Heinemann LAJ, et al. Third-generation oral contraceptives and risk of myocardial infarction: an international case-control study. *BMJ* 1996;312:88.
130. Dunn NR, Arscott A, Thorogood M. The relationship between use of oral contraceptives and myocardial infarction in young women with fatal outcome, compared to those who survive: results from the MICA case-control study. *Contraception* 2001;63:65.
131. Hoyle M. Small bowel ischaemia and infarction in young women taking oral contraceptives and progestromal agents. *Br J Surg* 1977;64:533.
132. Hassan HA. Oral contraceptive-induced mesenteric venous thrombosis with resultant intestinal ischemia. *J Clin Gastroenterol* 1999;29:90.
133. Minnema MC, Janssen HL, Niermeijer P, et al. Budd-Chiari syndrome: combination of genetic defects and the use of oral contraceptives leading to hypercoagulability. *J Hepatol* 2000;33:509.
134. Krauss R, Burkman RT. The metabolic impact of oral contraceptives. *Am J Obstet Gynecol* 1992;167:1177.
135. Ludicke F, Gaspard UJ, Demeyer F, et al. Randomized controlled study of the influence of two low estrogen dose oral contraceptives containing gestodene or desogestrel on carbohydrate metabolism. *Contraception* 2002;66:411.
136. Crook D, Godsland IF, Worthington M, et al. A comparative metabolic study of two low-estrogen-dose oral contraceptives containing desogestrel or gestodene progestins. *Am J Obstet Gynecol* 1993: 169:1183.
137. Endrikat J, Klipping C, Cronin M, et al. An open label, comparative study of the effects of a dose-reduced oral contraceptive containing 20 μg ethinyl estradiol and 100 μg levonorgestrel on hemostatic, lipid, and carbohydrate metabolism variables. *Contraception* 2002;65:215.
138. Garg SK, Chase HP, Marshall G. Oral contraceptives and renal and retinal complications in young women with insulin-dependent diabetes mellitus. *JAMA* 1994;271:1099.
139. Foulon T, Payen N, Laporte F, et al. Effects of two low-dose oral contraceptives containing ethinylestradiol and either desogestrel or levonorgestrel on serum lipids and lipoproteins with particular regard to LDL size. *Contraception* 2001;64:11.
140. van Rooijen M, von Schoultz B, Silveira A, et al. Different effects of oral contraceptives containing levonorgestrel or desogestrel on plasma lipoproteins and coagulation factor VII. *Am J Obstet Gynecol* 2002;186:44.
141. Young RL, DelConte A. Effects of low-dose monophasic levonorgestrel with ethinyl estradiol preparation on serum lipid levels: A twenty-four month clinical trial. *Am J Obstet Gynecol* 1999; 181:59.
142. Adams MR, Clarkson TB, Koritnik DR, et al. Contraceptive steroids and coronary artery disease in *Cynomolgus* macaques. *Fertil Steril* 1987;47:1010.
143. Davidoff F, Tishler S, Rosoff C. Hyperlipidemia and pancreatitis associated with oral contraceptive therapy. *N Engl J Med* 1973;289:552.
144. Miale JB, Kent JW. The effects of oral contraceptives on the results of laboratory tests. *Am J Obstet Gynecol* 1974;120:264.
145. Grace EA, Emans SJ, Drum D. Hematologic abnormalities in adolescents on birth control pills. *J Pediatr* 1982;101:771.
146. Amatayakul K. Metabolism: vitamins and trace elements. In: Goldzieher JW, Fotherby K, eds. *Pharmacology of the contraceptive steroids*. Philadelphia: Lippincott-Raven, 1994;363.
147. Thijs C, Knipschild E. Oral contraceptives and the risk of gallbladder disease: a meta-analysis. *Am J Public Health* 1993;83:1113.
148. Vessey M, Painter R. Oral contraceptive use and benign gallbladder disease; revisited. *Contraception* 1994;50:167.
149. Grodstein F, Colditz GA, Hunter DJ, et al. A prospective study of symptomatic gallstones in women: relation with oral contraceptives and other risk factors. *Obstet Gynecol* 1994;84:207.
150. Logan RFA, Kay CR. Oral contraception, smoking and inflammatory bowel disease—findings in the Royal College of General Practitioners' oral contraception study. *Int J Epidemiol* 1989;18:105.
151. Vessey MP, Jewell D, Smith A, et al. Chronic inflammatory bowel disease, cigarette smoking and the use of oral contraceptives: findings in a large cohort study of women of childbearing age. *BMJ* 1986;292:1101.

152. Boyko EJ, Theis MK, Vaughan TL, et al. Increased risk of inflammatory bowel disease associated with oral contraceptive use. *Am J Epidemiol* 1994;140:269.
153. Corrao G, Tragnone A, Caprilli R, et al. Risk of inflammatory bowel disease attributable to smoking, oral contraception and breastfeeding in Italy: a nationwide case-control study. Cooperative Investigators of the Italian Group for the Study of the Colon and the Rectum (GISC). *Int J Epidemiol* 1998;27:397.
154. Cosnes J, Carbonnel F, Carrat F, et al. Oral contraceptive use and the clinical course of Crohn's disease: a prospective cohort study. *Gut* 1999;45:218.
155. Timmer A, Sutherland LR, Martin F. Oral contraceptive use and smoking are risk factors for relapse in Crohn's disease. The Canadian Mesalamine for Remission of Crohn's Disease Study Group. *Gastroenterology* 1998;114:1143.
156. Sillem MH, Teichmann AT. The liver. In: Goldzieher JW, Fotherby K, eds. *Pharmacology of the contraceptive steroids.* Philadelphia: Lippincott-Raven, 1994;247.
157. De Block CE, Leeuw IH, Gaal LF. Premenstrual attacks of acute intermittent porphyria: hormonal and metabolic aspects—a case report. *Eur J Endocrinol* 1999;141:50.
158. Julkunen HA, Kaaja R, Friman C. Contraceptive practice in women with systemic lupus erythematosus. *Br J Rheumatol* 1993;32:227.
159. Julkunen HA. Oral contraceptives in systemic lupus erythematosus: side-effects and influence on the activity of SLE. *Scand J Rheumatol* 1991;20:427.
160. Mok CC, Lau CS, Wong RW. Use of exogenous estrogens in systemic lupus erythematosus. *Seminars Arthritis Rheum* 2001;30:426.
161. Cooper GS, Dooley MA, Treadwell EL, et al. Hormonal and reproductive risk factors for development of systemic lupus erythematosus: results of a population-based, case-control study. *Arthritis Rheum* 2002;46:1830.
162. Drossaers-Bakker KW, Zwinderman AH, van Zeben D, et al. Pregnancy and oral contraceptive use do not significantly influence outcome in long term rheumatoid arthritis. *Ann Rheum Dis* 2002;61:405.
163. Brennan P, Bankhead C, Silman A, et al. Oral contraceptives and rheumatoid arthritis: results from a primary care-based incident case-control study. *Seminars Arthritis Rheum* 1997;26:817.
164. Pladevall-Vila M, Delclos GL, Varas C, et al. Controversy of oral contraceptives and risk of rheumatoid arthritis: meta-analysis of conflicting studies and review of conflicting meta-analyses with special emphasis on analysis of heterogeneity. *Am J Epidemiol* 1996;144:1.
165. Mattson RE, Cramer JA, Darney PD, et al. Use of oral contraceptives by women with epilepsy. *JAMA* 1986;256:238.
166. Vessey M, Painter R, Yeates D. Oral contraception and epilepsy: finding in a large cohort study. *Contraception* 2002;66:77.
167. Fattore C, Cipolla G, Gatti G, et al. Induction of ethinylestradiol and levonorgestrel metabolism by oxcarbazepine in healthy women. *Epilepsia* 1999;40:783.
168. Sabers A, Buchholt JM, Uldall P, et al. Lamotrigine plasma levels reduced by oral contraceptives. *Epilepsy Research* 2001;47:151.
169. Crawford P, Chadwick DJ, Martin C, et al. The interaction of phenytoin and carbamazepine with combined oral contraceptive steroids. *Br J Clin Pharmacol* 1990;30:892.
170. Back DJ, Orme ML. Drug interactions. In: Goldzieher JW, Fotherby K, eds. *Pharmacology of the contraceptive steroids.* Philadelphia: Lippincott-Raven, 1994;407.
171. Crawford P. Interactions between antiepileptic drugs and hormonal contraception. *CNS Drugs* 2002;16:263.
172. Wilbur K, Ensom MH. Pharmacokinetic drug interactions between oral contraceptives and second-generation anticonvulsants. *Clinical Pharmacokinetics* 2000;38:355.
173. Crawford P, Chadwick D, Cleland P, et al. The lack of effect of sodium valproate on the pharmacokinetics of oral contraceptive steroids. *Contraception* 1986;33:23.
174. Ragueneau-Majlessi I, Levy RH, Janik F. Levetiracetam does not alter the pharmacokinetics of an oral contraceptive in healthy women. *Epilepsia* 2002;43:697.
175. Sparrow MJ. Pregnancies in reliable pill takers. *N Z Med J* 1989;102:575.
176. Weaver K, Glasier A. Interaction between broad-spectrum antibiotics and the combined oral contraceptive pill: a literature review. *Contraception* 1999;59:71.
177. Dickinson BD, Altman RD, Nielsen NH, et al. Drug interactions between oral contraceptives and antibiotics. *Obstet Gynecol* 2001;98:853.

178. Henney J. Risk of drug interactions with St. John's wort. *JAMA* 2000;283:1679.
179. Koke SC, Brown EB, Miner CM. Safety and efficacy of fluoxetine in patients who receive oral contraceptive therapy. *Am J Obstet Gynecol* 2002;187:551.
180. Back DJ, Breckenridge AM, Crawford FE, et al. The effects of rifampicin on the pharmacokinetics of ethinyl estradiol in women. *Contraception* 1980;21:135.
181. Szoka PR, Edgren RA. Drug interactions with oral contraceptives: compilation and analysis of an adverse experience report database. *Fertil Steril* 1988;49:318.
182. Van Puijenbroek EP, Egberts AC, Meyboom RH, et al. Signalling possible drug-drug interactions in a spontaneous reporting system: Delay of withdrawal bleeding during concomitant use of oral contraceptives and itraconazole. *Br J Clin Pharmacol* 1999;47:689.
183. Sinofsky FE, Pasquale SA. The effect of fluconazole on circulating ethinyl estradiol levels in women taking oral contraceptives. *Am J Obstet Gynecol* 1998;178:300.
184. Murphy AA, Zacur HA, Chararche P, et al. The effect of tetracycline on levels of oral contraceptives. *Am J Obstet Gynecol* 1991;164:28.
185. Friedman CI, Huneke AL, Kim MH, et al. The effect of ampicillin on oral contraceptive effectiveness. *Obstet Gynecol* 1980;55:33.
186. Archer JS, Archer DF. Oral contraceptive efficacy and antibiotic interaction: a myth debunked. *J Am Acad Dermatol* 2002;46:917.
187. Helms SE, Bredle DL, Zajic J, et al. Oral contraceptive failure rates and oral antibiotics. *J Am Acad Dermatol* 1997;36:705.
188. Zamah NM, Humepl M, Kuhnz W, et al. Absence of an effect of high vitamin C dosage on the systemic availability of ethinyl estradiol in women using a combination oral contraceptive. *Contraception* 1993;48:377.
189. Hull MG. Normal fertility in women with post-pill amenorrhea. *Lancet* 1981;1:1329.
190. Oinonen KA, Mazmanian D. To what extent do oral contraceptives influence mood and affect? *J Affect Disord* 2002;70:229.
191. Freeman MP. Depression and hormonal contraception. *JAMA* 2001;286:671.
192. Burdick RS, Hoffmann R, Armitage R. Short note: oral contraceptives and sleep in depressed and healthy women. *Sleep* 2002;25:347.
193. Freeman EW, Kroll R, Rapkin A, et al. Evaluation of a unique oral contraceptive in the treatment of premenstrual dysphoric disorder. *J Womens Health Gender-Based Med* 2001;10:561.
194. Brown C, Ling F, Wan J. A new monophasic oral contraceptive containing drospirenone. Effect on premenstrual symptoms. *J Reprod Med* 2002;47:14.
195. American College of Obstetricians and Gynecologists. Committee Opinion: Committee on Gynecologic Practice. Contraceptives and congenital anomalies. *Int J Gynaecol Obstet* 1993;42:316.
196. Holt VL, Daling JR, McKnight B, et al. Functional ovarian cysts in relation to the use of monophasic and triphasic oral contraceptives. *Obstet Gynecol* 1992;79:529.
197. Lanes SF, Birmann B, Walker AM, et al. Oral contraceptive type and functional ovarian cysts. *Am J Obstet Gynecol* 1992;166:956.
198. Christensen JT, Boldsen JL, Westergaard JG. Functional ovarian cysts in premenopausal and gynecologically healthy women. *Contraception* 2002;66:153.
199. Grimes DA, Godwin AJ, Rubin A, et al. Ovulation and follicular development associated with three low-dose oral contraceptives: a randomized controlled trial. *Obstet Gynecol* 1994;83:29.
200. Steinkampf MP, Hammond KR, Blackwell RE. Hormonal treatment of functional ovarian cysts: a randomized, prospective study. *Fertil Steril* 1990;54: 775.
201. The Cancer and Steroid Hormone Study of the Centers for Disease Control and the National Institute of Child Health and Human Development. Oral-contraceptive use and the risk of breast cancer. *N Engl J Med* 1986;315:405.
202. Collaborative Group on Hormonal Factors in Breast Cancer. Breast cancer and hormonal contraceptives: collaborative reanalysis of individual data on 53,297 women with breast cancer and 100,239 women without breast cancer from 54 epidemiological studies. *Lancet* 1996;347: 1713.
203. Collaborative Group on Hormonal Factors in Breast Cancer. Breast cancer and hormonal contraceptives: further results. *Contraception* 1996;54:1S.
204. Marchbanks PA, McDonald JA, Wilson HG, et al. Oral contraceptives and the risk of breast cancer. *N Engl J Med* 2002;346:2025.
205. Westhoff CL. Breast cancer risk: perception versus reality. *Contraception* 1999;59(1 Suppl):25S.

206. Narod SA, Dube MP, Klijn J, et al. Oral contraceptives and the risk of breast cancer in BRCA1 and BRCA2 mutation carriers. *J Natl Cancer Inst* 2002;94:1773.
207. Heimdal K, Skovlund E, Moller P. Oral contraceptives and risk of familial breast cancer. *Cancer Detect Prevent* 2002;26:23.
208. Rohan TE, Miller AB. A cohort study of oral contraceptive use and risk of benign breast disease. *Int J Cancer* 1999:82:191.
209. Ye Z, Thomas DB, Ray RM, et al. Combined oral contraceptives and risk of cervical carcinoma in situ. *Int J Epidemiol* 1995;24:19.
210. Smith JS, Green J, Berrington de Gonzalez A, et al. Cervical cancer and use of hormonal contraceptives: a systematic review. *Lancet* 2003;361:1159.
211. Moreno V, Bosch FX, Munoz N, et al. International Agency for Research on Cancer. Multicentric Cervical Cancer Study G. Effect of oral contraceptives on risk of cervical cancer in women with human papillomavirus infection: the IARC multicentric case-control study. *Lancet* 2002;359:1085.
212. Kjellberg L, Hallmans G, Ahren AM, et al. Smoking, diet, pregnancy and oral contraceptive use as risk factors for cervical intra-epithelial neoplasia in relation to human papillomavirus infection. *Br J Cancer* 2000;82:1332.
213. Kaufman DW, Shapiro S, Slone D, et al. Decreased risk of endometrial cancer among oral-contraceptive users. *N Engl J Med* 1980;303:1045.
214. Centers for Disease Control. Oral contraceptive use and the risk of endometrial cancer. *JAMA* 1983;249:1600.
215. CASH, Cancer and Steroid Hormone Study of the Centers for Disease Control and the National Institute of Child Health and Human Development. Combination oral contraceptive use and the risk of endometrial cancer. *JAMA* 1987;257:796.
216. Jick SS, Walker AM, Jick H. Oral contraceptives and endometrial cancer. *Obstet Gynecol* 1993;82:931.
217. Weiderpass E, Adami HO, Baron JA, et al. Use of oral contraceptives and endometrial cancer risk (Sweden). *Cancer Causes Control* 1999;10:277.
218. The Cancer and Steroid Hormone Study of the Centers for Disease Control and the National Institute of Child Health and Human Development. The reduction in risk of ovarian cancer associated with oral contraceptive use. *N Engl J Med* 1987;316:650.
219. Hankinson SE, Colditz, GA, Hunter DJ, et al. A quantitative assessment of oral contraceptive use and risk of ovarian cancer. *Obstet Gynecol* 1992;80:708.
220. Gross TP, Schlesselman JJ. The estimated effect of oral contraceptive use on the cumulative risk of epithelial ovarian cancer. *Obstet Gynecol* 1994;83:419.
221. Prentice RL. Epidemiologic data on exogenous hormones and hepatocellular carcinoma and selected other cancers. *Prev Med* 1991;20:38.
222. Ness RB, Grisso JA, Klapper J, et al, and the SHARE Study Group. Risk of ovarian cancer in relation to estrogen and progestin dose and use characteristics of oral contraceptives. *Am J Epidemiol* 2000;152:233.
223. Schildkraut JM, Calingaert B, Marchbank PA, et al. Impact of progestin and estrogen potency in oral contraceptives on ovarian cancer risk. *J Natl Cancer Inst* 2002;94:32.
224. Walker GR Schlesselman JJ. Ness RB. Family history of cancer, oral contraceptive use, and ovarian cancer risk. *Am J Obstet Gynecol* 2002;186:8.
225. Narod SA, Risch H, Moslehi R, et al. Oral contraceptives and the risk of hereditary ovarian cancer. *N Engl J Med* 1998;339:424.
226. Schlesselman, JJ. Net effect of oral contraceptive use on the risk of cancer in women in the United States. *Obstet Gynecol* 1995;85:793.
227. Coker AL, Harlap S, Fortney JA. Oral contraceptives and reproductive cancers: weighing the risks and benefits. *Fam Plan Perspect* 1993;25:17.
228. Schlesselman J, Neoplastic effects of hormonal contraception. Scientific Conference of the NICHD, "Preventing Unintended Pregnancy: Advances in Hormonal Contraception." Bethesda June 11–12, 2001.
229. World Health Organization Collaborative Study of Neoplasia and Steroid Contraceptives. Combined oral contraceptives and liver cancer. *Int J Cancer* 1989;43:254.
230. Heinemann LA, Weimann A, Gerken G, et al. Modern oral contraceptive use and benign liver tumors: the German Benign Liver Tumor Case-Control Study. *Eur J Contraception Reprod Health Care* 1998;3:194.
231. Goodman ZD, Ishak KG. Hepatocellular carcinoma in women: probable lack of etiologic association with oral contraceptive steroids. *Hepatology* 1982;2:440.

232. Aseni P, Sansalone CV, Sammartino C, et al. Rapid disappearance of hepatic adenoma after contraceptive withdrawal. *J Clin Gastroenterol* 2001;33:234.
233. Troisi R, Schairer C, Chow WH et al. Reproductive factors, oral contraceptive use, and risk of colorectal cancer. *Epidemiology* 1997;8:75.
234. Fernandez E, La Vecchia C, Franceschi S, et al. Oral contraceptive use and risk of colorectal cancer. *Epidemiology* 1998;9:295.
235. Potter JD, McMichael AJ. Large bowel cancer in women in relation to reproductive and hormonal factors: a case-control study. JNCIO 1983;71:703.
236. Martinez ME, Grodstein F, Giovannucci E, et al. A prospective study of reproductive factors, oral contraceptive use, and risk of colorectal cancer. *Can Epidemiol Biomarkers Prev* 1997;6:1.
237. Fernandez E, LaVecchia C, D'Avanzo B, et al. Oral contraceptives, hormone replacement therapy and the risk of colorectal cancer. *Br J Cancer* 1996;73:1431.
238. Berel V, Hermon C, Kay C, et al. Mortality associated with oral contraceptive use: 25 year follow-up of cohort of 46,000 women from Royal College of General Pracititoners' oral contraceptive study. *Br Med J* 1999;918:96.
239. Rabe T, Kowald A, Ortmann J, et al. Inhibition of skin 5α-reductase by oral contraceptive progestins *in vitro. Gynecol Endocrinol* 2000;14:223.
240. Goldzieher JW Effects on the skin. In: Goldzieher JW, Fotherby K, eds. *Pharmacology of the contraceptive steroids.* Philadelphia: Lippincott-Raven, 1994;271.
241. Murphy AA, Cropp CS, Smith BS, et al. Effect of low-dose oral contraceptive on gonadotropins, androgens, and sex hormone binding globulin in nonhirsute women. *Fertil Steril* 1990;53:35.
242. Lucky AW, Henderson TA, Olson WH et al. The effectiveness of norgestimate and ethinyl estradiol in treating moderate acne vulgaris. *J Am Acad Dermatol* 1997;37:746.
243. Redmond GP, Olson WH, Lippman JS et al. Norgestimate and ethinyl estradiol in the treatment of acne vulgaris: a randomized, placebo-controlled trial. *Obstet Gyncol* 1997;89:615.
244. Leyden J, Shalita A, Hordinsky M, et al. Efficacy of a low-dose oral contraceptive containing 20 microg of ethinyl estradiol and 100 microg of levonorgestrel for the treatment of moderate acne: A randomized, placebo-controlled trial. *J Am Acad Dermatol* 2002;47:399.
245. Rosen MP, Breitkopf DM, Nagamani M. A randomized controlled trial of second- versus third-generation oral contraceptives in the treatment of acne vulgaris. Am J Obstet Gynecol 2003;188:1158.
246. Thiboutot D, Archer DF, Lemay A, et al. A randomized, controlled trial of a low-dose contraceptive containing 20 microg of ethinyl estradiol and 100 microg of levonorgestrel for acne treatment. *Fertil Steril* 2001;76:461.
247. Vree ML, Schmidt J. A large observational clinical evaluation of a desogestrel-containing combiphasic oral contraceptive in Germany. *Eur J Contraception Reprod Health Care* 2001;6:108.
248. Vartiainen M, de Gezelle H, Broekmeulen CJ. Comparison of the effect on acne with a combiphasic desogestrel-containing oral contraceptive and a preparation containing cyproterone acetate. *Eur J Contraception Reprod Health Care* 2001;6):46.
249. van Vloten WA, van Haselen CW, van Zuuren EJ, et al. The effect of 2 combined oral contraceptives containing either drospirenone or cyproterone acetate on acne and seborrhea. *Cutis* 2002;69(4 Suppl):2.
250. Cibula D, Hill M, Fanta M, et al. Does obesity diminish the positive effect of oral contraceptive treatment on hyperandrogenism in women with polycystic ovarian syndrome? *Hum Reprod* 2001; 16:940.
251. Petursson GJ, Fraunfelder FT, Meyer SM. Oral contraceptives. *Ophthalmology* 1981;88:368.
252. Corson SL. Oral contraceptives for the prevention of osteoporosis. *J Reprod Med* 1993;38;1015.
253. Nappi C, DiSpiezo Sardo A, Acunzo G, et al. Effects of a low-dose and ultra-low-dose combined oral contraceptive use on bone turnover and bone mineral density in young fertile women: a prospective controlled randomized study. *Contraception* 2003;67:355.
254. Recker RR, Davies M, Hinders SM, et al. Bone gain in young adult women. *JAMA* 1992;268:2403.
255. Reed SD, Scholes D, LaCroix AZ, et al. Longitudinal changes in bone density in relation to oral contraceptive use. *Contraception* 2003;68:177.
256. Kuohung W, Borgatta L, Stubblefield P. Low-dose oral contraceptives and bone mineral density: an evidence-based analysis. *Contraception* 2000;95:87.
257. Berenson AB, Radecki, CM, Grady JJ, et al. A prospective controlled study of effects of hormonal contraception on bone mineral density. *Obstet Gynecol* 2001;98:576.
258. DeCherney A. Bone-sparing properties of oral contraceptives. *Am J Obstet Gynecol* 1996;174:15.

259. Pinter B, Kocijancic A, Marc J, et al. Vitamin D receptor gene polymorphism and bone metabolism during low-dose oral contraceptive use in young women. *Contraception* 2003;67:33.

260. Polatti F, Perotti F, Filippa N, et al. Bone mass and long-term monophasic oral contraceptive treatment in young women. *Contraception* 1995:51:221.

261. Cromer B, Stager P, Bonny A, et al. A longitudinal study of bone mineral density in adolescent girls using either depot medroxyprogesterone acetate or oral contraceptives. Society for Adolescent Medicine, 2003. (Abstracts)

262. Eschenbach DA, Patton DL, Meier A, et al. Effect of oral contraceptive pill use on vaginal flora and vaginal epithelium. *Contraception* 2000;62:107.

263. Wolner-Hanssen P, Eschenbach DA, Paavonen J, et al. Decreased risk of symptomatic chlamydial pelvic inflammatory disease associated with oral contraceptive use. *JAMA* 1990;263:54.

264. Ness RB, Soper DE, Holley RL, et al. Hormonal and barrier contraception and risk of upper genital tract disease in the PID evaluation and clinical health (PEACH) study. *Am J Obstet Gynecol* 2001:185:121.

265. Bjarnadottir RI, Gottfredsdottir H, Sigurdardottir K, et al. Comparative study of the effects of a progestogen-only pill containing desogestrel and an intrauterine contraceptive device in lactating women. *BJOG: Int J Obstet Gynecol* 2001;108:1174.

266. Halderman LD, Nelson AL. Impact of early postpartum administration of progestin-only hormonal contraception compared with nonhormonal contraceptives on short-term breast-feeding patterns. *Am J Obstet Gynecol* 2002;186:1250.

267. World Health Organization. A multicentered phase III comparative clinical trial of depotmedroxy progesterone acetate given three monthly at doses of 100 mg or 150 mg: contraceptive efficacy and side effects. *Contraception* 1986;34:223.

268. Jeppson S, Gerhagen S, Johansson EDB, et al. Plasma levels of medroxyprogesterone acetate (MPA), sex hormone binding globulin, gonadal steroids, gonadotropins and prolactin in women during long-term use of depo-MPA (Depo-Provera) as a contraceptive agent. *Acta Endocrinol* 1982; 99:339.

269. Borgatta L, Murthy A, Chuang C, et al. Pregnancies diagnosed during Depo-Provera use. *Contraception* 2002;66:169.

270. Risser WI, Gefter LR, Barratt MS, et al. Weight changes in adolescents who use hormonal contraception. *J Adolesc Health* 1999;24:433.

271. Polaneczky M, Guarnaccia M, Alon J, et al. Early experience with the contraceptive use of depot medroxyprogesterone acetate in an inner-city population. *Fam Plan Perspect* 1996;28:174.

272. Amatayakul K, Sirassomboom B, Singkamani R. Effects of MPA in serum lipids, protein, glucose tolerance and liver function in Thai women. *Contraception* 1980;21:283.

273. Gupta N, O'Brien R, Jacobsen LJ, et al. Mood changes in adolescents using depot-medroxyprogesterone acetate for contraception: a prospective study. *J Pediatr Adolesc Gynecol* 2001;14:71.

274. Skegg DCG, Noonan EA, Paul C, et al. Depot-medroxyprogesterone acetate and breast cancer. *JAMA* 1995;273:799.

275. Shapiro S, Rosenberg L, Hoffman M, et al. Risk of breast cancer in relation to the use of injectable progestogen contraceptives and combined estrogen/progestogen contraceptives. *Am J Epidemiol* 2000;151:396.

276. Cundy T, Evans M, Roberts H, et al. Bone density in women receiving depot-medroxyprogesterone acetate for contraception. *BMJ* 1991;303:13.

277. Scholes D, LaCroix AZ, Ichikawa LE, et al. The association between depot medroxyprogesterone acetate contraception and bone mineral density in adolescent women. *Contraception* 2004;69:99.

278. Merki-Feld GS, Neff M, Keller PJ. A 2-year prospective study in the effects of depot medroxyprogesterone acetate on bone mass—response to estrogen and calcium therapy in individual users. *Contraception* 2003;67:79.

279. Cundy T, Cornish J, Roberts H, et al. Spinal bone density in women using depot medroxyprogesterone contraception. *Obstet Gynecol* 1998; 92:569.

280. Cromer BA, Blair JM, Mahan JD, et al. A prospective comparison of bone density in adolescent girls receiving depot medroxyprogesterone acetate (Depo-Provera), levonorgestrel (Norplant), or oral contraceptives. *J Pediatr* 1996;129:671.

281. Scholes D, LaCroix AZ, Ichikawa LE, et al. Injectable hormone contraception and bone density: results from a prospective study. *Epidemiology* 2002;13:581.

282. De Ceulaer K, Hayes R, Gruber C, et al. Medroxyprogesterone acetate and homozygous sickle cell disease. *Lancet* 1982;2:229.

283. Smith RD, Cromer BA, Hayes JR, et al. Medroxyprogesterone (Depo-Provera) use in adolescents: uterine bleeding and blood pressure patterns, patient satisfaction, and continuation rates. *Adolesc Pediatr Gynecol* 1995;8:24.

284. World Health Organization. Multinational comparative trial of long-active injectable contraceptives: norethisterone enanthate given in two dosage regimens and depot-medroxyprogesterone acetate: final report. *Contraception* 1983;28:1.

285. Kaunitz AM, Garceau RJ, Cromie MA. Comparative safety, efficacy, and cycle control of Lunelle monthly contraceptive injection (medroxyprogesterone acetate and estradiol cypionate injectable suspension) and Ortho-Novum 7/7/7 oral contraceptive (norethindrone/ethinyl estradiol triphasic). Lunelle Study Group. *Contraception* 1999;60:179.

286. Anonymous. A multicentred phase III comparative study of two hormonal contraceptive preparations given once-a-month by intramuscular injection: I. Contraceptive efficacy and side effects. World Health Organization. Task Force on Long-Acting Systemic Agents for Fertility Regulation. *Contraception* 1988;37:1.

287. Newton JR, D'Arcangues C, Hall PE. A review of "once-a-month" combined injectable contraceptives. *J Obstet Gynecol* 1994;4 Suppl:S1.

288. Sang GW, Shao QX, Ge RS, et al. A multicentred phase III comparative clinical trial of Mesigyna, Cyclofem and Injectable No. 1 given monthly by intramuscular injection to Chinese women. I. Contraceptive efficacy and side effects. *Contraception* 1995;51:167.

289. Garceau RJ, Wajszczuk CJ, Kaunitz AM, and Lunelle Study Group. Bleeding patterns of women using Lunelle monthly contraceptive injections (medroxyprogesterone acetate and estradiol cypionate injectable suspension) compared with those of women using Ortho-Novum 7/7/7 (norethindrone/ethinyl estradiol triphasic) or other oral contraceptives. *Contraception* 2000;62:289.

290. Rahimy MH, Cromie MA, Hopkins NK, Tong DM. Lunelle monthly contraceptive injection (medroxyprogesterone acetate and estradiol cypionate injectable suspension): effects of body weight and injection sites on pharmacokinetics. *Contraception* 1999;60:201.

291. Cromie MA, Maile MH, Wajszczuk CP. Comparative effects of Lunelle monthly contraceptive injection (medroxyprogesterone acetate and estradiol cypionate injectable suspension) and Ortho-Novum 7/7/7 oral contraceptive (norethindrone/ethinyl estradiol triphasic) on lipid profiles. Investigators from the Lunelle Study Group. *Contraception* 2000;61:51.

292. Jain JK, Ota F, Mishell DR. Comparison of ovarian follicular activity during treatment with a monthly injectable contraceptive and a low-dose oral contraceptive. *Contraception* 2000; 61:195.

293. Rahimy MH, Ryan KK. Lunelle monthly contraceptive injection (medroxyprogesterone acetate and estradiol cypionate injectable suspension): assessment of return of ovulation after three monthly injections in surgically sterile women. *Contraception* 1999;60:189.

294. Shulman LP, Oleen-Burkey M, Willke RJ. Patient acceptability and satisfaction with Lunelle monthly contraceptive injection (medroxyprogesterone acetate and estradiol cypionate injectable suspension). *Contraception* 1999;60:215.

295. International Collaborative Post-Marketing Surveillance of Norplant. Post-marketing surveillance of Norplant (R) contraceptive implants: II. Non-reproductive health. *Contraception* 2001;63:187.

296. Singh K, Viegas OAC, Loke DFM, et al. Effect of Norplant implants on liver, lipid, and carbohydrate metabolism. *Contraception* 1992;45:141.

297. Anonymous. Study of the effects of the implantable contraceptive Norplant on lipid and lipoprotein metabolism. UN Development Programme/UN Population Fund/WHO/World Bank, Special Programme of Research, Development and Research Training in Human Reproduction, Task Force on Long-Acting Systemic Agents for Fertility Regulation. *Contraception* 1999;59:31.

298. Darney PD, Atkinson E, Tanner S, et al. Acceptance and perceptions of Norplant among users in San Francisco, USA. *Stud Fam Plan* 1990;21:152.

299. Diaz S, Pavez M, Cardenas H, et al. Recovery of fertility and outcome of planned pregnancies after removal of Norplant subdermal implants or copper-T IUDs. *Contraception* 1987;35:569.

300. Meirik O, Farley TM, Sivin I. Safety and efficacy of levonorgestrel implant, intrauterine device, and sterilization. *Obstet Gynecol* 2001;97:539.

301. Cromer BA, Smith RD, Blair JA, et al. A prospective study of adolescents who choose among levonorgestrel implant (Norplant), medroxyprogesterone acetate (Depo-Provera), or the combined oral contraceptive pill as contraception. *Pediatrics* 1994;94:687.

302. Polaneczky M, Slap G, Forke C, et al. The use of levonorgestrel implants (Norplant) for contraception in adolescent mothers. *N Engl J Med* 1994;331:1201.

303. Rickert VI, Hendon AE, Davis P, et al. Maternal influence on the decision to adopt Norplant. *J Adolesc Health* 1995;16:354.
304. Kozlowski KJ, Rickert VI, Hendon AE, Davis P. Adolescents and Norplant: preliminary findings of side effects. *J Adolesc Health* 1995;16:373.
305. Stevens-Simon C, Kelly L, Wallis J. The timing of Norplant insertion and postpartum depression in teenagers. *J Adolesc Health* 2000;26:408.
306. Jordan A. Toxicology of progestogens of implantable contraceptives for women. *Contraception* 2002;65:3.
307. Meirik O. Implantable contraceptives for women. *Contraception* 2002;65:1.
308. Buckshee K, Chatterjee P, Dhall GI, et al. Phase III clinical trial with Norplant II (two covered rods): report on five years of use. *Contraception* 1993;48:120.
309. Sivin I, Alvarez F, Mishell DR, et al. Contraception with two levonorgestrel rod implants: a 5-year study in the United States and Dominican Republic. *Contraception* 1998;58:275.
310. Croxatto HB. Progestin implants for female contraception. *Contraception* 2002;65:15.
311. Hickey M, d'Arcangues C. Vaginal bleeding disturbances and implantable contraceptives. *Contraception* 2002;65:75.
312. Suherman SK, Affandi B, Korver T. The effects of Implanon on lipid metabolism in comparison with Norplant. *Contraception* 1999;60:281.
313. Glasier A. Implantable contraceptives for women: effectiveness, discontinuation rates, return of fertility, and outcome of pregnancies. *Contraception* 2002;65:29.
314. Abrams LS, Skee DM, Natarajan J, et al. Multiple-dose pharmacokinetics of a contraceptive patch in health women participants. *Contraception* 2001;64:287.
315. Abrams LS, Skee D, Natarajan J, et al. Pharmacokinetic overview of Ortho Evra/Evra. *Fertil Steril* 2002;77[Suppl 2]:S3.
316. Abrams LS, Skee DM, Natarajan J, et al, Anderson GD. Pharmacokinetics of a contraceptive patch (Evra/Ortho Evra) containing norelgestromin and ethinyloestradiol at four application sites. *Br J Clin Pharmacol.* 2002;53:141.
317. Zacur HA, Hedon B, Mansour D, et al. Integrated summary of Ortho Evra/Evra contraceptive patch adhesion in varied climates and conditions. *Fertil Steril* 2002;77[Suppl 2]:S32.
318. Zieman M, Guillebaud J, Weisberg E, Shangold GA, Fisher AC, Creasy GW. Contraceptive efficacy and cycle control with the Ortho Evra/Evra transdermal system: the analysis of pooled data. *Fertil Steril* 2002;77[Suppl 2]:S13.
319. Sibai BM, Odlind V, Meador ML, et al. A comparative and pooled analysis of the safety and tolerability of the contraceptive patch (Ortho Evra/Evra). *Fertil Steril* 2002;77[Suppl 2]:S19.
320. Archer DF, Bigrigg A, Smallwood GH, et al. Assessment of compliance with a weekly contraceptive patch (Ortho Evra/Evra) among North American women. *Fertil Steril* 2002;77[Suppl 2]:S27.
321. FDA approves NuvaRing contraceptive implant. *J Gender Specific Med* 2002;5:6.
322. Mulders TM, Dieben TO, Bennink HJ. Ovarian function with a novel combined contraceptive vaginal ring. *Hum Reprod* 2002;17:2594.
323. Timmer CJ, Mulders TM. Pharmacokinetics of etonogestrel and ethinylestradiol released from a combined contraceptive vaginal ring. *Clin Pharmacokinetics.* 2000;39:233.
324. Davies GC, Feng LX, Newton JR, et al. Ovarian activity and bleeding patterns during extended continuous use of a combined contraceptive vaginal ring. *Contraception* 1992;46:269.
325. Bjarnadottir RI, Tuppurainen M, Killick SR. Comparison of cycle control with a combined contraceptive vaginal ring and oral levonorgestrel/ethinyl estradiol. *Am J Obstet Gynecol* 2002;186:389.
326. Roumen FJ, Apter D, Mulders TM, Dieben TO. Efficacy, tolerability and acceptability of a novel contraceptive vaginal ring releasing etonogestrel and ethinyl oestradiol. *Hum Reprod* 2001; 16:469.
327. Dieben TO, Roumen FJ, Apter D. Efficacy, cycle control, and user acceptability of a novel combined contraceptive vaginal ring. *Obstet Gynecol* 2002;100:585.
328. Mulders TM, Dieben TO. Use of the novel combined contraceptive vaginal ring NuvaRing for ovulation inhibition. *Fertil Steril* 2001;75:865.
329. Davies GC, Feng LX, Newton JR, et al. The effects of a combined contraceptive vaginal ring releasing ethinyloestradiol and 3-ketodesogestrel on vaginal flora. *Contraception* 1992;45:511.
330. Weisberg E, Fraser IS, Baker J, et al. A randomized comparison of the effects on vaginal and cervical epithelium of a placebo vaginal ring with non-use of a ring. *Contraception* 2000;62(2):83.
331. Fraser IS, Lacarra M, Mishell DR, et al. Vaginal epithelial surface appearances in women using vaginal rings for contraception. *Contraception* 2000;61:131.

332. Harwood B, Mishell DR, Jr. Contraceptive vaginal rings. *Seminars Reprod Med* 2001;19(4):381.
333. Brache V, Mishell DR, Lahteenmaki P, et al. Ovarian function during use of vaginal rings delivering three different doses of Nestorone. *Contraception* 2001;63:257.
334. Weisberg E, Fraser IS, Lacarra M, et al. Efficacy, bleeding patterns, and side effects of a 1-year contraceptive vaginal ring. *Contraception* 1999;59:311.
335. Weisberg E, Fraser IS, Mishell DR, Jr., et al, A comparative study of two contraceptive vaginal rings releasing norethindrone acetate and differing doses of ethinyl estradiol. *Contraception* 1999;59:305.
336. Sivin I, Stern J. Health during prolonged use of levonorgestrel 20 µg/d and the copper TCU 380 Ag intrauterine contraceptive devices: a multicenter study. International Committee for Contraception Research. *Fertil Steril* 1994;61:70.
337. Hodoglugil NN, Aslan D, Bertan M. Intrauterine device use and some issues related to sexually transmitted disease screening and occurrence. *Contraception* 2000;61:359.
338. Rossing MA, Daling JR, Voigt LF, et al. Current use of an intrauterine device and risk of tubal pregnancy. *Epidemiology* 1993;4:252.
339. Stanwood NL, Grimes DA, Schulz KF. Insertion of an intrauterine contraceptive device after induced or spontaneous abortion: a review of the evidence. *BJOG: Int J Obstet Gynecol* 2001;108:1168.
340. Grimes D, Schulz K, van Vliet H, et al. Immediate post-partum insertion of intrauterine devices. *Cochrane Database Syst Rev* 2001:CD003036.
341. Lahteenmaki P, Rauramo I, Backman T. The levonorgestrel intrauterine system in contraception. *Steroids* 2000;65:693.
342. Jonsson B, Landgren BM, Eneroth P. Effects of various IUDs on the composition of cervical mucus. *Contraception* 1991;43:447.
343. Silverberg SG, Haukkamaa M, Arko H, et al. Endometrial morphology during long-term use of levonorgestrel-releasing intrauterine devices. *Int J Gynecol Path* 1986;5:235.
344. Andersson K, Odlind V, Rybo G. Levonorgestrel-releasing and copper-releasing (Nova T) IUDs during five years of use: a randomized comparative trial. *Contraception* 1994;49:56.
345. Cox M, Blacksell S. Clinical performance of the levonorgestrel intra-uterine system in routine use by the UK Family Planning and Reproductive Health Research Network: 12-month report. *Br J Fam Plan* 2000;26:143.
346. Lahteenmaki P, Rauramo I, Backman T. The levonorgestrel intrauterine system in contraception. *Steroids* 2000;65:693.
347. Diaz J, Faundes A, Diaz M, et al. Evaluation of the clinical performance of a levonorgestrel-releasing IUD, up to seven years of use, in Campinas, Brazil. *Contraception* 1993;47:169.
348. Dubuisson JB, Mugnier E. Acceptability of the levonorgestrel-releasing intrauterine system after discontinuation of previous contraception: results of a French clinical study in women aged 35 to 45 years. *Contraception* 2002;66:121.
349. Monteiro I, Bahamondes L, Diaz J, et al. Therapeutic use of levonorgestrel-releasing intrauterine system in women with menorrhagia: a pilot study (1). *Contraception* 2002;65:325.
350. Stewart A, Cummins C, Gold L, et al. The effectiveness of the levonorgestrel-releasing intrauterine system in menorrhagia: a systematic review. *BJOG: Int J Obstet Gynecol* 2001;108:74.
351. Fedele L, Gammaro L, Bianchi S. Levonorgestrel-releasing intrauterine device for the treatment of menometrorrhagia in a woman on hemodialysis. *N Engl J Med* 1999;341:541.
352. Hidalgo M, Bahamondes L, Perrotti M, et al. Bleeding patterns and clinical performance of the levonorgestrel-releasing intrauterine system (Mirena) up to two years. *Contraception* 2002; 65(2):129.
353. Backman T, Huhtala S, Luoto R, et al. Advance information improves user satisfaction with the levonorgestrel intrauterine system. *Obstet Gynecol* 2002;99:608.
354. French R, Cowan F, Mansour D, et al. Hormonally impregnated intrauterine systems (IUSs), versus other forms of reversible contraceptives as effective methods of preventing pregnancy. *Cochrane Database Syst Rev* 2001:CD001776.
355. Farley TM, Rosenberg MJ, Rowe PJ, et al. Intrauterine devices and pelvic inflammatory disease: an international perspective. *Lancet* 1992;339:785
356. Grimes DA. Intrauterine device and upper-genital-tract infection. *Lancet* 2000;356:1013.
357. Shelton JD. Risk of clinical pelvic inflammatory disease attributable to an intrauterine device. *Lancet* 2001;357:443.
358. Walsh, T, Grimes D, Frezieres R, et al. Randomized controlled trial of prophylactic antibiotics before insertion of intrauterine devices. *Lancet* 1998;351:1005.

359. Grimes DA, Schulz KF. Antibiotic prophylaxis for intrauterine contraceptive device insertion. *Cochrane Database Syst Rev* 2001:CD001327.

360. Hubacher D, Lara-Ricalde R, Taylor DJ, et al. Use of copper intrauterine devices and the risk of tubal infertility among nulligravid women. *N Engl J Med* 2001;345:561.

361. Ronnerdag M, Odlind V. Health effects of long-term use of the intrauterine levonorgestrel-releasing system. A follow-up study over 12 years of continuous use. *Acta Obstet Gynecol Scand* 1999; 78:716.

362. Curtis KM, Chrisman CE, Peterson HB. Contraception for women in selected circumstances. *Obstet Gynecol* 2002;99:1100.

363. O'Brien PA, Marfleet C. Frameless versus classical intrauterine device for contraception. *Cochrane Database Syst Rev.* 2001:CD003282.

364. Wildemeersch D, Schacht E. Treatment of menorrhagia with a novel 'frameless' intrauterine levonorgestrel-releasing drug delivery system: a pilot study. *Eur J Contraception Reprod Health Care* 2001;6:93.

365. Miller L, Nielson C. Internet availability of contraceptives. *Obstet Gynecol* 2001;97:121.

366. Trussell J, Strickler J, Vaughan B. Contraceptive efficacy of the diaphragm, the sponge, and the cervical cap. *Fam Plan Perspect* 1993;25:100.

367. Film SD, Lathan RH, Roberts P, et al. Association between diaphragm use and the urinary tract infection. *JAMA* 1985;254:240.

368. Hooten TM, Hillier S, Johnson C, et al. *Escherichia c*oli bacteremia and contraceptive method. *JAMA* 1991;265:64.

369. Gallagher DM, Richwald GA. *Fitting the cervical cap: a handbook for clinicians.* Los Gatos, CA: Cervical Cap Ltd, 1989.

370. Richwald GA, Greenland S, Gerber M, et al. Effectiveness of the cavity rim cervical cap: results of a large clinical study. *Obstet Gynecol* 1979;74:143.

371. Koch JP. The Prentif cervical cap: a contemporary study of its clinical safety and effectiveness. *Contraception* 1982;25:135.

372. Bounds W, Guillebaud J. Lea's Shield contraceptive device: pilot study of its short-term patient acceptability and aspects of use. *Br J Fam Plan* 1999;24:117.

373. Mauck C, Glover LH, Miller E, et al. Lea's Shield: a study of the safety and efficacy of a new vaginal barrier contraceptive used with and without spermicide. *Contraception* 1996;53:329.

374. Mauck C, Callahan M, Weiner DH, et al. A comparative study of the safety and efficacy of FemCap, a new vaginal barrier contraceptive, and the Ortho All-Flex diaphragm. The FemCap Investigators' Group. *Contraception* 1999;60:71.

375. World Health Organization. WHO/CONRAD Technical Consultation on Nonoxynol-9. Summary Report. Oct. 9–10, 2001. Http://www.who.int/reproductive-health/rtis/N9_meeting-report.

376. Van Damme L, Ramjee G, Alary M, et al. Effectiveness of COL-1492, a nonoxynol-9 vaginal gel, on HIV-1 transmission in female sex workers: a randomized controlled trial. *Lancet* 2002;360:971.

377. Squire JJ, Berger GS, Keith L. A retrospective clinical study of a vaginal contraceptive suppository. *J Reprod Med* 1977;22:319.

378. Gupta K, Hillier SL, Hooton TM, et al. Effects of contraceptive method on the vaginal microbial flora: a prospective evaluation. *J Infect Dis* 2000;181:595.

379. Warburton D, Neugut RH, Lustenberger A, et al. Lack of association between spermicide use and trisomy. *N Engl J Med* 1987;317:478.

380. Louik C, Mitchell AA, Werler MM, et al. Maternal exposure to spermicides in relation to certain birth defects. *N Engl J Med* 1987;317:474.

381. Kuyoh MA, Toroitich-Ruto C, Grimes DA, et al. Sponge versus diaphragm for contraception. *Cochrane Database Syst Rev.* 2002:CD003172.

382. Creatsas G, Guerrero E, Guilbert E, et al. A multinational evaluation of the efficacy, safety and acceptability of the Protectaid contraceptive sponge. *Eur J Contraception Reprod Health Care* 2001;6:172.

383. Farr G, Gabelnick H, Sturgen K, et al. Contraceptive efficacy and acceptability of the female condom. *Am J Public Health* 1994;84:1960.

384. Trussell J, Sturgen K, Strickler J, et al. Comparative contraceptive efficacy of the female condom and other barrier methods. *Fam Plan Perspect* 1994;26:66.

385. Soper DE, Brockwell NJ, Dalton HP. Evaluation of the effects of a female condom in the female lower genital tract. *Contraception* 1991;44:21.

386. Haignere CS, Gold R, Maskovsky J, et al. High-risk adolescents and female condoms: knowledge, attitudes, and use patterns. *J Adolesc Health* 2000;26:392.
387. Macaluso M, Demand M, Artz L, et al. Female condom use among women at high risk of sexually transmitted disease. *Fam Plan Perspect* 2000;32:138.
388. Artz L, Demand M, Pulley L, et al. Predictors of difficulty inserting the female condom. *Contraception* 2002;65:151.
389. Beksinska ME, Rees HV, Dickson-Tetteh KE, et al. Structural integrity of the female condom after multiple uses, washing, drying, and re-lubrication. *Contraception* 2001;63:33.
390. Grady WR, Tanfer K. Condom breakage and slippage among men in the United States. *Fam Plan Perspect* 1994;26:107.
391. Sparrow MJ, Lavill K. Breakage and slippage of condoms in family planning patients. *Contraception* 1994;50:117.
392. Steiner M, Piedrahita C, Glover L, et al. Can condom users likely to experience condom failure be identified? *Fam Plan Perspect* 1993;25:220.
393. CDC, Male Latex Condoms and Sexually Transmitted Diseases. Retrieved June 13, 2003, from http://www.cdc.gov/nchstp/od/latex.htm.
394. National Institute of Allergy and Infectious Diseases, National Institutes of Health, Department of Health and Human Services. Workshop summary: Scientific evidence on condom effectiveness for sexually transmitted disease (STD) prevention. June 12–13, 2000. Retrieved June 20, 2003, from http://www.niaid.nih.gov/dmid/stds/condomreport.pdf.
395. Davis KR, Weller SC. The effectiveness of condoms in reducing heterosexual transmission of HIV. *Fam Plan Perspect* 1999;31:272.
396. Handley MA. Incidence of acute urinary tract infection in young women and use of male condoms with and without nonoxynol-9 spermicides. *Epidemiology* 2002;13:431.
397. Frezieres RG, Walsh TL, Nelson AL, et al. Evaluation of the efficacy of a polyurethane condom: results from a randomized, controlled clinical trial. *Fam Plan Perspect* 1999;31:81.
398. Callahan M, Mauck C, Taylor D, et al. Comparative evaluation of three Tactylon condoms and a latex condom during vaginal intercourse: breakage and slippage. *Contraception* 2000;61:205.
399. Macaluso M, Blackwell R, Carr B, et al. Safety and acceptability of a baggy latex condom. *Contraception* 2000;61:217.
400. Arevalo M, Jennings V, Sinai I. Efficacy of a new method of family planning: the Standard Days Method. *Contraception* 2002;65:333.
401. Wade ME, McCarthy P, Braunstein GD, et al. A randomized prospective study of the use-effectiveness of two methods of natural family planning. *Am J Obstet Gynecol* 1981;141:368.
402. Rice FJ, Lanctot CA, Garcia-Deversa C. Effectiveness of the symptothermal method of natural family planning: an international study. *Int J Fertil* 1981;26:222.
403. Kennedy K, Rivera R, McNeilly A. Consensus statement on the use of breastfeeding as a family planning method. *Contraception* 1989;39:477.
404. Peterson AE, Perez-Escamilla R, Labboka MH, et al. Multicenter study of the lactational amenorrhea method (LAM) III: effectiveness, duration, and satisfaction with reduced client-provider contact. *Contraception* 2000;62:221.
405. Grimes DA, Raymond EG. Emergency Contraception. *Ann Int Med* 2002;137(3):E180.
406. Trussell J, Ellertson C, von Hertzen H, et al. Estimating the effectiveness of emergency contraceptive pills. *Contraception* 2003;67:259.
407. Yuzpe AA, Thurlow HJ, Ramzy I, et al. Postcoital contraception: a pilot study. *J Reprod Med* 1974; 13:53.
408. Yuzpe AA, Lancee WJ. Ethinyl estradiol and *dl*-norgestrel as a postcoital contraceptive. *Fertil Steril* 1977;28:932.
409. Ho PC, Kwan MSW. A prospective randomized comparison of levonorgestrel with the Yuzpe regimen in post-coital contraception. *Hum Reprod* 1993;8:389.
410. Hatcher RA, Trussell J, Stewart F, et al. *Emergency contraception: the nation's best-kept secret.* Atlanta GA: Bridging the GAP Communications, 1995.
411. Westhoff C. Emergency contraception. *N Engl J Med* 2003;349:1830.
412. Trussell J, Ellertson C, Stewart E The effectiveness of the Yuzpe regimen of emergency contraception. *Fam Plan Perspect* 1996;28:58.
413. Trussell J, Ellertson C, Rodriquez G. The Yuzpe regimen of emergency contraception: how long after the morning after? *Obstet Gynecol* 1996;88:151.

414. Vasilakis C, Jick SS, Jick H. The risk of venous thromboembolism in users of postcoital contraceptive pills. *Contraception* 1999;59:79.
415. FDA prescription drug products: certain combined oral contraceptives for use as postcoital emergency contraception. *Federal Register* 1997;62:8610.
416. Taskforce on postovulatory methods of fertility regulation. Randomised controlled trial of levonorgestrel versus the Yuzpe regimen of combined oral contraceptives for emergency contraception. *Lancet* 1998;352:428.
417. von Hertzen H, Piaggio G, Ding, J et al. Low dose mifepristone and two regimens of levonorgestrel for emergency contraception: a WHO multicentre randomised trial. *Lancet* 2002;360:1803.
418. Trussell J, Raymond EG. Statistical evidence about the mechanism of action of the Yuzpe regimen of emergency contraception. *Obstet Gynecol* 1999;93:872.
419. Raymond EG, Lovely LP, Chen-Mok M, et al. Effect of the Yuzpe regimen of emergency contraception on markers of endometrial receptivity. *Hum Reprod* 2000;15:2351.
420. Durand M, del Carmen Cravioto M, Raymond EG, et al. On the mechanisms of action of short-term levonorgestrel administration in emergency contraception. *Contraception* 2001;64:227.
421. Rowlands S, Devalia H, Lawrenson R, et al. Repeated use of hormonal emergency contraception by younger women in the UK. *Br J Fam Plan* 2000;26:138.
422. Zhou L, Xiao B. Emergency contraception with Multiload Cu-375 SL IUD: a multicenter clinical trial. *Contraception* 2001;64:107.
423. Kerin JF, Carignan CS, Cher D. The safety and effectiveness of a new hysteroscopic method for permanent birth control: results of the first Essure pbc clinical study. *Austral NZJ Obstet Gynecol* 2001;41:364.

Additional Reading

Hatcher RA, Zieman M, Cmiak C, et al. Managing Contraception 2004–2005. Tiger, Georgia: Bridging the Gap Foundation, 2004

Hatcher RA, Trussell J, Stewart F, et al. *Contraceptive Technology,* 18th ed. Tiger, Georgia: Bridge the Gap Foundation, 2004.

Pettiti DB. Combination estrogen-progestin oral contraceptives. *N Engl J Med* 2003;349:1443.

Westhoff C. Depot-medroxyprogesterone acetate injection (Depo-Provera): a highly effective contraceptive option with proven long-term safety. *Contraception* 2003;68:75.

WHO. Selected practice recommendations for contraceptive use. WHO Publications, 2002.

Websites

See Appendix 1 for patient sites.
www.youngwomenshealth.org

For providers:
www.managingcontraception.com
www.contraceptiononline.org/contrareport
www.arhp.org

21

Teen Pregnancy

Angela Maida Nicoletti

INCIDENCE OF TEEN PREGNANCY

The United States has the dubious distinction of having the highest teen pregnancy, birth, and abortion rates in the developed world (1–5) (see Fig. 21-1). Adolescent pregnancy rates vary across developed countries, from a very low rate in the Netherlands (12 per 1,000 women aged 15 to 19 per year), to a very high rate in the Russian Federation (102 per 1,000) (1). Japan and most western European countries have low teen pregnancy rates, less than 40 per 1,000. Five countries have teen pregnancy rates of 70 or more per 1,000 per year: Belarus, Bulgaria, Romania, the Russian Federation, and the United States. The majority of young women in the developed world become sexually active during their teenage years (1). Levels of sexual activity and the age at which teenagers become sexually active do not vary much across comparable developed countries, such as Canada, Great Britain, France, Sweden, and the United States (see Fig. 21-2.). Differences in sexual activity and the age at which teenagers become sexually active do not account for the wide variation in pregnancy rates among developed countries. Cross-national studies suggest a number of important factors for the observed differences. Strong public support and expectations for the transition to adult economic roles, and for parenthood, provide young people with greater incentives and means to delay childbearing. Countries with low levels of adolescent pregnancy, childbearing, and STDs are characterized by societal acceptance of adolescent sexual relationships, combined with comprehensive and balanced information about sexuality and clear expectations about commitment and prevention of pregnancy within these relationships. Easy access to contraceptives and other reproductive health services contributes to better contraceptive use and low teen pregnancy rates (1,6,7).

In the past 25 years, adolescent pregnancy rates have decreased in the developed world (1). Reasons for the decline in pregnancy rates include increased motivation of youth to achieve higher levels of education, employment training, and goals in

U.S. teenagers have higher pregnancy rates, birthrates and abortion rates than adolescents in other developed countries.

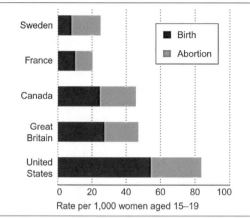

FIG. 21-1. From: Alan Guttmacher Institute [AGI], Teenagers' sexual and reproductive health. *Facts in Brief.* New York: AGI, 2001; with permission.

Note: Data are for mid-1990s.

addition to motherhood and family formation; provision of comprehensive sexuality education leading to greater knowledge about contraception among youth; more effective contraception use especially of long-acting methods and improved ability to negotiate contraceptive practice; and greater social support for services related to both pregnancy and disease prevention among adolescents (1).

Differences in levels of teenage sexual activity across developed countries are small.

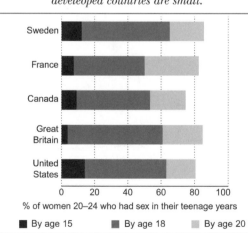

FIG. 21-2. From: Alan Guttmacher Institute [AGI], Teenagers sexual and reproductive health. *Facts in Brief.* New York: AGI, 2001; with permission.

Note: Data are for mid-1990s.

In the United States, rates of sexual activity, pregnancies, and births have declined and contraceptive use has increased (1,3,8,9). The birth rate for teenagers in 2002 was 42.9 births per 1,000 women aged 15 to 19 years, a record low for the nation (10). The birth rate for young teens ages 15 to 17 years in 2002 was also at an all time low at 24.7, a decline of more than 35% below the 1991 peak. The rate for older teens has declined 20% since 1991. Reductions in teenage birth rates have been particularly large for young black teenagers (down 40% since 1991) (Fig. 21-3). The teenage pregnancy rate has declined 19% in the 1990s to 94.3 per 1,000 teenagers 15 to 19 years in 1997, reflecting concurrent declines in birth and abortion rates (11). Non-marital births to teens have declined although they have risen in older women (9).

During the period 1991 to 2001, the percentage of U.S. high school students who ever had sexual intercourse and the percentage who had multiple sexual partners decreased (12). The decrease in sexual activity and the increased contraceptive use are attributed, at least in part, to fear of contracting HIV/AIDS. Other contributing factors may be health education programs, a changing moral climate, new contraceptives, and the strength of the economy (2). Improved contraceptive use may be a reflection of the fact that some of the newer methods do not require remembering to take a pill every day. The significantly higher rates of teen pregnancy and early childbearing in the United States compared with other developed countries with equally high rates of adolescent sexual activity, but lower rates of pregnancy and STDs, seem to be due to multiple factors. U.S. parents seem to be caught in the middle of societal ambivalence regarding sexuality, especially teen sexuality. They are uncomfortable with the changing sexual mores and yet often unable or

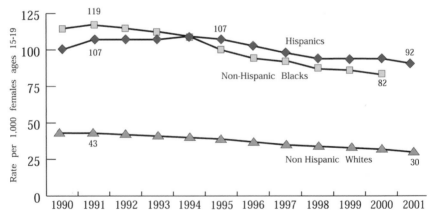

FIG. 21-3. US teen birthrate by race/ethnicity, 1990 to 2001. (From: Compiled by Child Trends [2003] from National Center for Health Statistics, National Vital Statistics Reports, 2002 and 2003; with permission.)

unwilling to initiate the necessary discussion about either abstinence or contraception. Failure to provide age-appropriate education, both in home and in school, has resulted from the continuing controversy regarding sex education in the United States. There continues to be limited access to effective birth control methods and to systems of care that monitor and support sexual decision making. Sex continues to be portrayed irresponsibly in the media. In addition, poverty is a significant contributor to a high U.S. teen pregnancy rate (13). Emergency contraception, sometimes known as postcoital contraception, is much less frequently prescribed in the United States compared to other countries (14).

Another factor that has affected our ability to address the problem of teen pregnancy, is our acceptance of "unintended" as meaning a contraceptive failure or lack of access to or knowledge of contraception. Most teenagers report their births as unintended (15). It may be more productive clinically to explore a teen's motivation to avoid pregnancy and ask how they intend to remain nonpregnant. This line of questioning will often expose the teen's ambivalence about pregnancy and about contraceptive use (16). Frequently there is an unconscious desire to become pregnant (17). Recent findings reveal that for many teen's mothering makes sense of the limited life options that precede pregnancy (18). A strong desire to avoid pregnancy has been shown to correlate significantly with dual method contraceptive use (19).

RISK FACTORS ASSOCIATED WITH TEEN PREGNANCY

In spite of the above issues, most teens do not become early childbearers. Multiple factors are associated with those who do engage in high risk behaviors and become pregnant (20). They are intrafamilial, sociocultural, intrapersonal, and biologic. Factors within the family include low parental monitoring (21,22,23), having a sibling who is a teenage parent (24,25,26), and a family history of teenage parenting (27) (Fig. 21-4). Low parental monitoring can be associated with parental mental illness and/or parental abuse of drugs and/or alcohol.

The physical and social environment are powerful factors that shape the teen's perception of the world and its potential. Surrounded by poverty and unemployment and families who have been unable to surmount it, teens often internalize a feeling of hopelessness and despair. Eighty percent of all adolescents who give birth are poor or low income (28). They perceive little value in education and do not develop the motivation necessary to use contraception and avoid pregnancy. Often parenthood is viewed as the only viable rite of passage to adulthood (29). It takes an extraordinarily determined young woman to separate herself from her family, friends and neighbors and say, "I am going to live differently" (30). That kind of resilience and empowerment is fostered by parents or parental figures who effectively communicate positive messages about self-worth and ability to achieve (31). Some recent evidence suggests that adolescents whose families receive welfare benefits may be more vigilant in their pregnancy prevention (32).

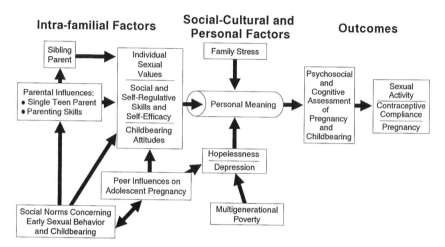

FIG. 21-4. Early parenthood for the sisters of adolescent mothers: a proposed conceptual model of decision making. (From: Cox JE, et al. *J Adolesc Pediatr Gynecol* 1995;8:188; with permission.)

Intrapersonal qualities are the filter through which teens perceive their world. A poorer sense of personal efficacy and an external locus of control are associated with early childbearing (33). Depression (34), physical and sexual abuse (35–37), academic underachievement, and substance use (13,35) have all been associated with pregnancy in adolescence.

Up to 66% of pregnant teens report histories of past sexual abuse (38). Conversely, sexually abused adolescent girls are significantly more likely to become pregnant than teens without abuse histories (36). A history of sexual abuse has been linked to high-risk behaviors that may account for early unplanned pregnancy, including young age at initiation of sexual intercourse, failure to use contraception, prostitution, physically assaultive relationships, and abuse of alcohol and other drugs (36,39–41). Seventy-four percent of women who had sex before age 14 and 60% of those who had sex before age 15 report having had sex involuntarily (28). Perceived emotional deprivation may cause adolescents to engage in sexual activity in search of emotional closeness (42,43). Shearer and colleagues, using data from the National Longitudinal Survey of Youth, found that young women with low cognitive ability are at increased risk for early initiation of sexual activity and early pregnancy (44).

Adverse childhood experiences have an important relationship to male involvement in teen pregnancy., In a retrospective study of 7,399 males visiting a primary care clinic, Anda and colleagues collected data through a questionnaire about the age of the youngest female ever impregnated; the man's own age at the time; his history of childhood emotional, physical, or sexual abuse; having a battered mother; parental separation or divorce; and having household members who were substance abusers, mentally ill, or criminals. They found strong graded relationships between the number of adverse childhood experiences and the risk of involvement in a teen pregnancy for each of the four birth cohorts during the last century (45). This suggests that adverse male childhood experiences transcend changing sexual mores and contraceptive methods.

The majority of pregnant teens have partners who are considerably older (46–48). Over half of all infants born to teens younger than 18 are fathered by adult men (46). Although some states have taken steps to punish these "male predators" (49), it is not at all clear that these steps are effective in reducing the teen pregnancy rate. Many of these relationships are consensual. Fear of having to reveal the age and identity of their partner may actually deter sexually active or pregnant girls from seeking timely medical care or social services (49,50).

Biologic and physical developmental factors are also influential. Many teens are not future oriented but are at a concrete cognitive level. An earlier menarche and younger age at first intercourse often coincide with unsophisticated cognitive skills. These teens do not consider the consequences of their behavior (51), nor do they have the skills to negotiate especially if their partner is older (52). Adolescents' perception of their boyfriends' desire for conception may also be an important predictor of pregnancy risk (32). Young adolescent females with substantially older partners are much more likely than their peers to have sex with their partner, which exposes them to the risk of pregnancy (15,53). Unequal gender relations and cultural and ethnic expectations of gender roles may contribute to the difficulty some teens face discussing contraception or saying "no" to sexual intercourse. The personal fable of omnipotence, characteristic of middle adolescence, allows those teens who perceive parenthood to be attractive to overlook the negative aspects of parenting as a teen (54).

Many teens deny their own risk of pregnancy and hold misconceptions, such as believing that only frequent sexual activity can lead to pregnancy. For some adolescents their reluctance to acknowledge their sexuality results in improper contraceptive usage. Denial of fertility is a common theme; statements such as "I didn't think it would happen to me," or "I had sex for 2 years and didn't get pregnant," or "I never thought I would get pregnant" are frequently expressed. Often the longer that adolescents are sexually active without experiencing pregnancy, the more the risk-taking behavior is reinforced. Adolescents are usually unaware that with increasing gynecologic age, the chance of regular ovulatory cycles and thus fertility is greater. They are also often unable to identify the time of greatest risk for fertility in their menstrual cycle or to understand the impact of irregular cycles on ovulation. Including a simple factual explanation of the menstrual cycle in sexuality courses in schools and office-based interventions is important.

Frequent office visits for pregnancy tests that are negative have also been labeled a risk marker for teenage pregnancy (55–57). Fifty-six percent of teens with a negative pregnancy test are pregnant within 18 months (57). Adolescents with negative pregnancy tests are good candidates for counseling and interventions aimed at addressing their motivation to become pregnant. Health care providers should begin addressing sexual issues early—at 10 to 12 years of age in some patients (58).

TEEN PREGNANCY PREVENTION

Research attempting to identify effective primary pregnancy prevention among teens points to the need for a multifaceted approach and the need to begin early (59–61). Sabo and colleagues found that female adolescents who participated in sports were less likely than their nonathletic peers to engage in sexual activity and/or report a pregnancy. Among male adolescents, athletic participation was unrelated to sexual behavior and pregnancy involvement (62). Other protective factors against early initiation of sexual activity include dual-parent families, higher socioeconomic status, better school performance, greater religiosity, absence of suicidal thoughts, feeling adults or parents cared, and high parental expectations (63).

The most comprehensive evaluation of pregnancy prevention programs has been reported by Kirby (64). To be included in his study, called Emerging Answers, a program evaluation had to meet multiple criteria, the most important of which were: completed in 1980 or later; conducted in the United States or Canada; targeted at adolescents of middle school or high school age (roughly 12 to 18); employed an experimental or quasi-experimental design; had a sample size of at least 100 in the combined treatment and control group; and measured impact on sexual or contraceptive behavior, pregnancy, or childbearing. There were several programs with strong evidence of success (Table 21-1). Only three abstinence-only programs met Kirby's rigorous evaluation criteria and they did not show an overall positive effect on sexual behavior, nor did they affect contraceptive use among sexually active teenagers. However, given the paucity of research, it is unwise to draw conclusions about abstinence-only programs. Results from a well-designed, federally sponsored evaluation of Title V–funded abstinence programs should be available shortly.

Among the programs that focus on sexual antecedents, several sexuality and HIV education programs were shown to delay the onset of sex, reduce the frequency of sex, reduce the number of sexual partners among teens, or increase the use of condom or other forms of contraception (Table 21-2).

Among the programs that focus on non-sexual antecedents, certain service learning programs, which do not focus on sexual issues at all, have the strongest evidence that they actually reduce teen pregnancy rates (61). The success of these programs may be that they contribute to developing the personal resilience and internal locus of control that characterize those who do not become pregnant as teens. Vocational education programs such as the Summer Training and Education Program (STEP) and Job Corps, which are intensive and offer academic and vocation education and a few support services, were shown not to decrease pregnancy or birth rates among disadvantaged teens (65). High-risk teens may need considerably more intervention time and more intensive services than programs normally provide. The Children's Aid Society–Carrera Program, which includes both youth development and reproductive health components has been demonstrated to substantially reduce teen pregnancy and birth rates over a long period of time. This program did not, however, reduce risk-taking behavior among boys (64). Gender differences must be addressed in

TABLE 21-1. *Programs with strong evidence of success*

I. Programs that Focus Primarily on Sexual Antecedents
    Sex education programs covering both pregnancy and STDs/HIV[1]
    - *Reducing the Risk*
    - *Safe Choices*

    HIV education programs[1]
    - *Becoming a Responsible Teen: An HIV Risk Reduction Intervention for African-American Adolescents*
    - *Making a Difference: An Abstinence Approach to STD, Teen Pregnancy, and HIV/AIDS Prevention*
    - *Making a Difference: A Safer Sex Approach to STD, Teen Pregnancy, and HIV/AIDS Prevention*

II. Programs that Focus Primarily on Non-Sexual Antecedents
    Service learning[2]
    - *Teen Outreach Program (TOP)*
    - *Reach for Health Community Youth Service Learning*

III. Programs that Focus Upon Both Sexual and Non-Sexual Antecedents
    Multi-component programs with intensive sexuality and youth development component
    - *Children's Aid Society-Carrera Programs*[3]

---

[1] While the sex and HIV education programs identified in this table demonstrated a positive impact upon sexual behavior and condom and contraceptive use, some other sex and HIV education programs did not have positive effects. Studies indicated that the sex and HIV education programs in this table reduced sexual risk-taking, but they did not provide evidence they reduced teen pregnancy.

[2] All the service learning programs that have been evaluated, including the *Learn and Serve* programs, have found results suggesting a positive impact upon either sexual behavior or pregnancy. The *Learn and Serve* study is not included on this list because it did not meet the criteria for being on this list, but it did confirm the efficacy of service learning. According to the analysis of TOP, the particular curriculum used in the small group component did not appear to be critical to the success of service learning.

[3] This program has provided the strongest evidence for a three-year impact upon pregnancy.

Source: Kirby, D. Emerging Answers: research findings on programs to reduce teen pregnancy (Summary). Washington, DC: National Campaign to Prevent Teen Pregnancy, 2001.

order to create effective programs for adolescent males (66). It is encouraging that a variety of types of pregnancy prevention program were shown to be effective. Kirby's summary offers guidance on how communities may use this information. Additionally, there is some evidence that zip codes might be used to more effectively target pregnancy prevention efforts (67).

PREGNANCY DIAGNOSIS AND COUNSELING

Pregnancy should be excluded as a cause of one or more missed periods in any adolescent who has achieved menarche. Though rare, pregnancies have been seen in teens before the appearance of their first menstrual period. Pregnancy is the most common cause of secondary amenorrhea. In adolescent health care, the denial of sexual activity is not reliable enough to exclude pregnancy (68). Common presenting

TABLE 21-2. *10 Characteristics of effective sex and HIV educations programs*

The curricula of the most effective sex and HIV education programs share ten common characteristics. These programs:

1. Focus on reducing one or more sexual behaviors that lead to unintended pregnancy or HIV/STD infection.
2. Are based on theoretical approaches that have been demonstrated to influence other health-related behavior and identify specific important sexual antecedents to be targeted.
3. Deliver and consistently reinforce a clear message about abstaining from sexual activity and/or using condoms or other forms of contraception. This appears to be one of the most important characteristics that distinguishes effective from ineffective programs.
4. Provide basic, accurate information about the risks of teen sexual activity and about ways to avoid intercourse or use methods of protection against pregnancy and STDs.
5. Include activities that address social pressures that influence sexual behavior.
6. Provide examples of and practice with communication, negotiation, and refusal skills.
7. Employ teaching methods designed to involve participants and have them personalize the information.
8. Incorporate behavioral goals, teaching methods, and materials that are appropriate to the age, sexual experience, and culture of the students.
9. Last a sufficient length of time (i.e., more than a few hours).
10. Select teachers or peer leaders who believe in the program and then provide them with adequate training.

Generally speaking, short-term curricula—whether abstinence-only or sexuality education programs—do not have measurable impact on the behavior of teens.

Source: Kirby, D. Emerging Answers: research findings on programs to prevent teen pregnancy (Summary). Washington, DC: National Campaign to Prevent Teen Pregnancy, 2001.

complaints of teens with undiagnosed pregnancies are vaginal and urinary symptoms, abdominal pain, syncope, nausea, and vomiting. A urine sample should be screened for human chorionic gonadotropin (HCG). Teens who present requesting pregnancy testing may or may not be pregnant but a valid assumption is they have initiated sexual activity and should have contraceptive counseling.

Some teens deny the possibility of pregnancy after a missed period. They are subsequently falsely reassured by light bleeding in the first trimester commonly caused by implantation of the blastocyst in the uterus or rupture of a corpus luteum cyst. Many teens make an appointment hoping the clinician will accidentally discover the pregnancy. More concerning are those teens who deliberately avoid an early diagnosis of their pregnancy because they want a baby and fear their family will insist they abort the pregnancy. Some express fear of physical harm. These teens will need the services of a social worker or social service agency to ensure their safety and appropriate follow-up.

Pregnancy Dating and Sizing

Pregnancies are usually dated from the first day of the last menstrual period, even though ovulation usually occurs about 2 weeks later. Assuming an accurate LMP, an estimated due date can be arrived at using the Nägele rule: to the first day of the LMP add 7 days, subtract 3 months, and add 1 year (69). Calculation of dates from the last menstrual period along with a uterine sizing is necessary to estimate gestational age and offer appropriate counseling. Options are to terminate the pregnancy, continue the pregnancy and either place the baby for adoption, or parent the baby. In 2000, about 25% of pregnant teens had elective abortions (70). The proportion of pregnant teens placing infants for adoption has declined sharply over the decade. In 1995 less than 1% chose adoption (71). Teens choosing adoption should be referred to an agency that will provide both preadoption and postadoption counseling. There are inevitably significant issues of grief and loss when a teen relinquishes an infant. She will need some ongoing support in order to integrate the experience into her life in a healthy manner. Many adoption agencies provide scant postadoption services.

By rectal or vaginal examination the 8-week uterus feels about the size of an orange; the 12-week uterus is approximately the size of a grapefruit. Since the uterus rises out of the pelvis in later gestations, a pregnancy can be missed on pelvic examination especially if the index of suspicion is low. An abdominal examination with the patient supine helps in staging a later pregnancy. A 12-week uterus is just palpable at the symphysis pubis; a 20-week uterus, at the level of the umbilicus; and a 16-week uterus, midway between (Fig. 21-5).

Pregnancy Hormone Testing

Sensitive serum pregnancy tests have made the diagnosis of early pregnancy much easier. HCG is a glycoprotein hormone secreted by the trophoblast. It is composed of an α and a β subunit. The β subunit is specific to HCG (72). The most accurate measure of serum HCG levels is a radioimmunoassay using highly specific antiserum to the β subunit of HCG. Radioimmunoassay can detect HCG levels as low as 2 to 7 mIU/ml in maternal serum. In general, results of less than 5 mIU/ml are considered negative.

About 7 days after fertilization, the implanted trophoblast begins to secrete HCG. In normal pregnancy, the HCG levels then rise rapidly, reaching approximately 100 mIU/ml in maternal serum by the expected date of the missed menses (73). An estimate of gestational age can be established because HCG levels double approximately every 2 days in the first 6 to 7 weeks of pregnancy and a gestational sac is identifiable using vaginal sonography at HCG levels of 1,000 to 2,000 mIU/ml (73). In both ectopic gestations and spontaneous abortions, HCG levels are usually lower than normal and increase at less-than-normal rates during early pregnancy (see Ectopic Pregnancy, p. 866). Multiple gestations and molar pregnancies are both associated with higher-than-normal HCG levels.

In the absence of an accurate LMP, sonographic dating may be more reliable. In the first trimester, sonographic dating is correct within 3 to 5 days. The margin of error is about 1 week in the second trimester and 2 to 3 weeks in the third trimester (73). Patient management should not be based on the results of a home pregnancy test. In

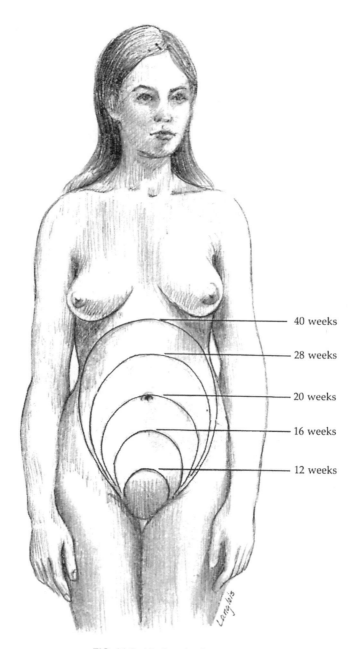

FIG. 21-5. Uterine size in pregnancy.

general, pregnancy tests done at home have been shown to be of considerably lower sensitivity and specificity than office-based testing (74). This is most likely because patients incorrectly perform them or misread correctly performed tests. Repeat testing should be done in the office.

Because of the high prevalence of sexually transmitted diseases (STDs) in pregnant teenagers, the Centers for Disease Control (CDC) recommends that endocervical tests for *Neisseria gonorrhoeae* and *Chlamydia trachomatis* should be obtained at the time of the examination (75). Routine prenatal tests include Papanicolaou (Pap) tests and serology for syphilis, rubella, blood type and Rh factor, complete blood count, and hepatitis B surface antigen. Varicella antibody screening is indicated in the absence of a positive history of varicella. Hemoglobin electrophoresis is recommended in populations at risk for sickle cell anemia and thalassemia. HIV testing is strongly recommended but not required in most states. Transmission of HIV from mother to infant can be dramatically reduced with medication (76–78) and operative delivery (79–81).

After diagnosing a pregnancy in a teen, the clinician should provide appropriate options counseling and referral and assist the teen in keeping the appointment to the referral service. Although adolescents can be quite uncertain about the date of their last menstrual period, other diagnoses need to be entertained if the uterus is small or large for dates given. If the uterus is smaller than expected, possible diagnoses include inaccurate dates (or oligomenorrhea and irregular ovulation), lab error, incomplete or missed abortion, ectopic pregnancy or, rarely, other sources of HCG (tumors). A uterus felt to be larger than expected may be caused by inaccurate dates, twin pregnancy, leiomyomata, molar pregnancy, or a corpus luteum cyst of pregnancy, which may be mistaken initially as part of the enlarged uterus. Ultrasonography (including the use of a vaginal probe) and, if indicated, serial quantitative HCG measures are important in making the correct diagnosis. Vitamins with 1 mg of folic acid should be provided to teens if they are ambivalent or plan to continue the pregnancy to term to reduce the chances of having an infant with a neural tube defect (82). A prescription of a small number (perhaps 30 tablets) increases the chances that they will buy the medication. Many teens at this early stage are not ready to inform their parents and therefore will not have access to insurance. Folic acid is most effective if adequate levels are achieved prior to conception. For this reason, clinicians should consider advising all sexually active girls to take a multivitamin with 0.4 mg of folic acid every day.

Medications/Toxins During Pregnancy

Pregnant teens should also be cautioned about drug use, alcohol intake, and smoking. They should avoid over-the-counter medications and herbal substances and should be encouraged to inform anyone who prescribes medications to them of their pregnancy. Some drugs with known or suspected teratogenicity include anticonvulsants such as hydantoin and valproate sodium, anticoagulants, alcohol, folic acid antagonists (methotrexate, aminopterin), diethylstilbestrol, isotretinoin, thalidomide, alkylating agents, and lithium carbonate (83). Up-to-date information regarding the risks of medications in pregnancy can be found at www.otispregnancy.org; www.reprotox.org; http://toxnet.nlm.nih.gov.

Radiation Exposure During Pregnancy

Teratogenic effects, including growth restriction, microcephaly and mental retardation, can also occur in patients exposed to high-dose radiation (100 to 200 rad) (84). The greatest risk of central nervous system effects appears to be with exposure to more than 20 rad between 8 and 15 weeks of gestation with no proven risk at less than 8 weeks or more than 25 weeks (84). Fetal risks do not appear to increase with radiation less than 5 rad, a level above the range of fetal exposure in common diagnostic procedures (e.g., 0.02 to 0.07 mrad from a chest x-ray or 200 mrad from a hip x-ray); however, certain procedures do give higher doses (e.g., 2 to 4 rad from a barium enema or a small bowel series or 3.5 rad from computed tomography of the abdomen and lumbar spine) (84). Routine ultrasound in pregnancy has not been associated with any adverse outcomes for the fetus (85). Magnetic resonance imaging (MRI) appears to be safe in pregnancy, although it is usually reserved for use after 18 weeks of gestation (85).

Emotional Support Around the Time of Teen Pregnancy Diagnosis

A diagnosis of pregnancy may be initially received by a teen with shock, ambivalence, fear, anxiety, happiness, or a combination of emotions. The teen's perception of the implications of a pregnancy frequently bear little resemblance to reality. At this point, she is unlikely to be able to make a firm decision about whether to continue the pregnancy to term and raise the child or place it for adoption or to terminate the pregnancy, but issues to consider should be raised. Counseling is most therapeutic if it is unbiased and unhurried. If a health care provider is unable to be objective, it is in the teen's best interests to refer her to a social service agency reputed to be unbiased.

It is essential to ascertain the teen's safety. What does she anticipate the reaction to her pregnancy will be by her parent(s)/family/guardian/boyfriend/father of her pregnancy? Social service agencies may need to be involved if she fears for her personal safety. Offer to help her tell whomever she is anxious about informing of her pregnancy or to identify a family member, teacher, or faith-based counselor to help her tell her parent(s). Frequently anger and/or tension can be defused this way. Many teens will choose not to reveal their pregnancy at first for reasons other than safety. Depressed teens often view having a baby as a positive event. Other teens believe a baby will cement the relationship with their boyfriend. They don't want to be dissuaded or forced to terminate the pregnancy.

There are a number of issues to be considered in counseling the pregnant teen (Table 21-3). Family structure and communication will influence whom she tells of

TABLE 21-3. *Assessment and counseling of the pregnant teenager*

Personal history
   Social situation
      Who currently lives with you?
      Who is in your family?
      In whom do you confide?
      Who knows about the possible pregnancy?
   Educational/life goals
      Are you currently in school? How are you doing?
      What do you want to do in 1 year? In 5 years?
   Self-esteem/self-efficacy
      What kinds of decisions have you made before?
   Psychiatric history
      Previous coping skills, counseling
      Suicide attempts
   Financial status/insurance
      Do you have insurance? Can you access it without loss of confidentiality?
      Are there resources for parenting or termination?

Medical/gynecologic/sexual history
   Current/prior medical problems and medications
   Information level about conception and contraception
   Previous contraceptive use
   Previous pregnancies and outcomes
   Previous sexually transmitted diseases

Personal beliefs about parenting, abortion, adoption
   Experiences with sisters, relatives, or friends who have been pregnant
   What do you think is the best age to be pregnant?
   What do you think is the best age to parent?
   Religious/cultural beliefs

Family/friend/partner influences and beliefs
   Which adult can be supportive—i.e., parent, teacher, counselor, relative, partner
   Whom do you plan to tell?
   Attitudes/beliefs of others toward pregnancy, parenting, abortion, adoption

Current pregnancy
   Intended or unintended?
   Who wants to continue to term?
   Who wants an abortion?
   Has adoption/ placement been considered?

Information about options
   Concrete issues about termination and parenting
   Health risks and costs

Postpregnancy
   Anticipatory guidance
   Anticipation of feelings
   Contraception
   Health care options

her pregnancy and when. Educational achievement and career goals are associated more often with a choice to terminate, whereas academic underachievement is associated with a decision to continue the pregnancy and raise the child. It is important to assess for emotional instability. If the pregnancy is unintended, was coercion or force used? Many teens do not recognize or are afraid to admit to an abusive relationship. Young age is a red flag for a coercive/abusive and/or incestuous relationship. The younger teen, <16 years old, who has not begun to think abstractly may be unable to understand the symptoms of pregnancy, the concept of gestational age, and the need to make a decision. She is likely to have difficulty connecting the pregnancy to the responsibilities of motherhood. Contraceptive counseling at this point is important. The event of conception is recent enough to determine if the pregnancy occurred as the result of the misuse of a birth control method or if birth control was not used because of misinformation about risks and side effects. If the teen is not ready/able to make a decision, a follow-up appointment should be made, with instructions to return promptly with any bleeding or pain. Identify a phone number where she can be reached. Often reaching her at school through the school nurse is preferable. It may be of some consolation to the teen to learn from the health care provider that experience has shown that most parents, though they may be angry initially, want to help their adolescent and are supportive.

A decision to continue the pregnancy or to terminate needs to be reality tested. Many teens will elect to continue a pregnancy to term and raise the baby assuming child care help from family, friends, and the baby's father that is unrealistic. Pledges of support from family and friends who say they will "help", very often are not dependable, resulting in an interrupted school career and isolation for the young mother. Relationships with the baby's father, tenuous to begin with, often wither in the face of parental responsibilities for which he is unprepared.

Teens who choose to have an abortion need to be counseled around how they will pay for it, issues of parental consent, what agency they can go to for the abortion, an explanation of the procedure, and how to cope with the loss they may experience after the procedure. It is wise to prepare them for the possibility of antiabortion protestors outside of the facility. Postabortion follow-up is critical to help the teen come to terms with any loss issues and for contraception.

A list of the pros and cons of each decision can sometimes help the teen look more realistically at the potential consequences. Most teens who terminate their pregnancies do so with the support of their parents (86). Teens in low density population areas tend not to choose pregnancy termination, however low density population areas tend to have fewer abortion facilities/services (87). Some states provide a judicial bypassing process that allows minors (<18 years old) to terminate a pregnancy without parental permission. It remains to be seen how the implementation of the Health Insurance Accountability and Portability Act (HIPAA), Public Law 104, regulations will affect the issue of parental involvement versus adolescent privacy rights (88). HIPAA does not preempt current state laws that allow minors to obtain care and have control of confidential health information. However, HIPAA also does not preempt existing parental notification laws (89). Teens often find it easier to have a health care provider help them tell their parents of the pregnancy and their decision whether to continue the pregnancy or terminate the pregnancy. Parents may respond in anger at first and demand the teen do whatever the parent thinks is best. In reality, such demands often push the teen in the opposite direction. Both the parent and the teen need to hear in an understanding manner that poor decisions are made that way and the consequences will have to be lived with for a long time. For example, teens forced to terminate a pregnancy frequently get pregnant again fairly soon.

CONTINUING THE PREGNANCY

Teens who plan to continue their pregnancy to term should be given an appointment with a prenatal provider within 1 to 2 weeks. When possible, referral to a comprehensive, multidisciplinary service specifically for adolescents is preferable. There is strong evidence in the literature that the outcomes of teen births are better when the services are tailored to the teen's medical, psychosocial, and nutritional needs (90–93). Those better outcomes can also result in reduced costs (94–96). Adherence to medical regimens and appointments is increased with nonjudgmental and developmentally appropriate interactions between teen and caregivers. Adolescent-specific services tend to see the teen more frequently, provide follow-up for missed appointments, and include nutritional and social services that address financial, home, school and mental health problems. They provide education and support specific to the adolescent's needs.

Young maternal age (<16 years old) does not seem to be an independent risk factor for poor birth outcomes (97,98); however, the post-neonatal mortality rates for the infants of young adolescent mothers is substantially higher (99). There is unanimity that teens are at increased risk for preterm births and low-birth-weight babies (100); however, these outcomes seem to be more closely related to inadequate prenatal care and nutrition (101–103) and poverty (104,105) than to age.

Nutrition

Nutritional counseling is a most important component of teen prenatal care. To be effective, it must be tailored to the teen's developmental level and lifestyle. Poor dietary habits are common among the general population of adolescent girls; thus pregnant adolescents often enter pregnancy with reduced nutritional stores, marginal diets, and increased risk for poor nutritional status (106). Low maternal weight gain has been consistently linked to poor fetal growth. Iron deficiency anemia is associated with an increased risk of low birth weight and preterm delivery (106). Teens need specific education as to why they should gain 30 to 40 lb if the baby will only weigh 7 to 8 lb and why they should try to have a baby of about 7 lb when a 5-lb baby would be much easier to deliver! Every teen should be referred to the Women, Infants and

Children's (WIC) supplemental food program as soon as possible. WIC provides vouchers for some of the nutritious foods needed in pregnancy and education about pregnancy and breastfeeding.

Substance Abuse

Substance use and abuse should be addressed as soon as a pregnancy is realized. Many teens reduce drug use during pregnancy but resume use within the first 6 months postpartum (107). Caregivers should be mindful that underreporting of substance use is likely (108). Smoking and the use of drugs and alcohol increase the teen's risk for health problems during pregnancy and are associated with poorer birth outcomes (109), as well as negative effects on child health and development (110). Tobacco use in pregnancy is associated with a number of adverse pregnancy outcomes including low birth weight (LBW), intrauterine growth restriction (IUGR), miscarriage, and infant mortality (111,112). Increased rates of childhood asthma and behavioral problems are seen in children exposed to tobacco in utero (110,113). In 2000, as in previous years, smoking rates were highest for older teenagers, 18 to 19 years (19.2%), although large disparities were seen in certain teenage population subgroups. Rates ranged from 3.2% among Mexican teenagers to 30.8% for non-Hispanic white teens (111). Interventions that have shown promise in increasing quit rates among pregnant teens are the Teen FreshStart program and Teen FreshStart with a Buddy program (114) and voucher-based incentives (115). There is evidence that the risk of stillbirth and infant death can be significantly reduced if pregnant smokers stop smoking by week 16 of pregnancy (116).

Alcohol use by pregnant teens can have serious adverse effects on the fetus (117). Teens are often unaware that there is no well-established quantity that is safe in pregnancy. They need to be educated to read the labels of beverages, such as wine coolers, which may seem nonalcoholic but in fact do contain alcohol.

Marijuana is the most commonly used illicit substance after alcohol and tobacco (118). Studies on the effect of prenatal marijuana exposure on birth and neonatal outcomes have been contradictory (119). However, a prospective study on the effects on children of prenatal exposure to marijuana has shown a significant relationship to increased hyperactivity, impulsivity, increased delinquency, and externalizing problems (118–120). Teens find it difficult to make the connection between their prenatal marijuana use and subsequent behavioral problems in their children.

It is well-established that cocaine use in pregnancy results in increased rates of placental abruption, premature rupture of membranes, increased rates of spontaneous abortions, poor pregnancy weight gain, and undernutrition secondary to appetite suppression (121,122). Long-term effects on the child are not certain, but there is increasing evidence that prenatal exposure to cocaine has adverse effects on language functioning (123).

A number of factors including substance use/abuse by the pregnant teen and/or those in her social and/or support network are responsible for increased rates of violence in pregnant teens as compared with adult pregnant women (124,125). In a multicenter prospective cohort study of 537 pregnant teens, Quinlivan and Evans found that 29.2% were victims of domestic violence (126). Pregnant teens who are in abusive relationships have been shown to have a reduced ability to take care of themselves and to utilize the therapeutic behaviors that promote healthy pregnancies (127). They are often ashamed or afraid to admit to abusive or controlling behavior by their partner. Often their life experience has led them to believe that this is the normal nature of male–female relationships. Some indicators of unhealthy relationships are frequent missed appointments, flat and/or guarded affect, reluctance to accept home visiting, deferment to partner when he is present, reluctance of partner to leave the exam room when asked, and reluctance of the teen to make an appointment at a time her partner cannot also come. Counseling should be offered these teens. If they are not ready to admit to the abusive nature of their relationship with their partner, they can at least be given information about where to get help if they need it, especially safety planning. Sometimes counseling that focuses on the nature of what a healthy relationship looks like is a constructive first step. Violence is one of several factors that contribute to the high rates of preterm labor and low-birth-weight babies among pregnant teens (100,128,129). Pregnant teens need education tailored to their developmental level about how to recognize the signs and symptoms of preterm labor, and how to avoid or treat some of other contributing factors such as urinary tract infections, sexually transmitted infections, and anemia.

Depression

Depression has been reported in 16% to 44% of teenage pregnancies (130), almost twice as high as the incidence in adult women (131). Longitudinal studies have shown that depressive symptoms become more severe in the second and third trimesters (132), possibly related to such stressors as conflicts with the baby's father, lack of social support, and concerns about caring for an infant (133). Developmental delays are often seen in the infants of adolescent mothers if the depression persists beyond 6 months of age (134). Depression in adolescent mothers has been shown to be associated with behavioral problems in their children (135).

Programs tailored to the pregnant and parenting teen, such as the Adolescent Reproductive Health Service at Brigham and Women's Hospital and the Young Parents Program at Children's Hospital Boston, work closely with maternal-child home visiting programs, social service agencies, and schools. Staff of home visiting programs may be nurses and/or trained paraprofessionals who can educate teens about pregnancy and preparing for the baby and provide support and resources. They also can assess the safety and adequacy of the teen's living situation. Many teens live a surprisingly transient existence that is inimical to the nurture and stability that an infant needs. Postpartum home visiting can provide critical support and education about parenting and has been shown to reduce adverse neonatal outcomes and promote healthy maternal behaviors (136,137).

PREGNANCY TERMINATION

In 2000, the elective abortion rate for teens ages 15 to 19 was 25/1,000 (138), a significant decline from 43.5 in 1985 (139). The rate increased from 6 per 1,000 for 15-year-olds to 29 per 1,000 for 19-year-olds (140). Teen abortions accounted for about 18.7% of the total number of abortions. The decrease in the abortion rate for teens may reflect multiple factors: a decrease in the number of unintended pregnancies, reduced access to abortion services, including the passage of abortion laws that affect adolescents (e.g., parental consent or notification laws and mandatory waiting periods); and changes in contraceptive practices, including increased use of long acting contraceptive methods (140).

In 2000, approximately 88% of all abortions were obtained during the first 12 weeks of gestation, and 58% were performed during the first 8 weeks of pregnancy (140). Curettage (suction and sharp) was reported to be the procedure used in 99.4% of abortions (140). Medical (nonsurgical) abortions represented about 1.0% of all abortions done at ≤8 weeks gestation (140). It is likely that medical abortions are underreported due to differences between reporting areas in how the data is collected.

Teenagers are more likely to have abortions in the second 3 months of pregnancy than are older women (140). Reasons for delay in seeking abortion services include young age, irregular menses, failure to recognize pregnancy symptoms, ambivalence about pregnancy, low educational level, and lack of awareness and availability of a clinic. With legalization, abortion has become remarkably safe over the past 3 decades (140). In 1972, 24 women died from causes known to be associated with legal abortions and 39 died as a result of known illegal abortions. In 1999, four died as a result of legal induced abortion, and none died as a result of illegal induced abortion (140). The risk of death associated with abortion increases with the length of the pregnancy (141).

Preabortion counseling is critical to how the adolescent incorporates the experience into her life. It is important to discuss the reasons for her decision, who in her family and social network will support her, and how local legislation regarding minors' rights and abortion may affect her. A contraceptive plan should be established. Zabin and colleagues followed 360 black teenage women for 2 years after a positive pregnancy test and found that those who terminated their pregnancies were no more likely to have psychological problems 2 years later and were better off economically (142). Postabortion support helps them to integrate the experience in a healthy manner. A phone call a day or two later to ask a few brief questions can be therapeutic; "How did it go? How are you doing? How are you feeling?" This contact with an understanding health care provider may provide the teen with a needed opportunity to express some feelings. Family and friends are often reluctant to raise the subject. It is also an opportunity to discuss again contraceptive plans, such as when to start hormonal methods. A 2-week-postabortion exam provides another chance to review the experience and contraception. Subsequent regular visits are advisable particularly for the teen who has chosen condoms or no method of birth control. Certainly abstinence should be encouraged but condoms or no method may reflect some ambivalence about the abortion and portend another unplanned pregnancy.

The evaluation of adolescents planning to have an elective pregnancy termination should include a history and physical examination. An accurate assessment and correlation of gestational age and uterine size are necessary, as many adolescents have irregular cycles, making dating difficult. If an adequate uterine sizing cannot be obtained, an ultrasound is necessary so that patients can be offered safe options prior to initiating a surgical procedure. Laboratory tests should include a documented pregnancy test, a Pap smear (within 1 year), endocervical tests for *N. gonorrhoeae* and *C. trachomatis,* hematocrit, urinalysis, Rh determination, and in most adolescents, a serology for syphilis. HIV testing should be offered. If cultures are done with sufficient time to obtain results before the procedure, treatment with antibiotics can be instituted for positive results. Many clinics prefer to give prophylactic tetracycline or doxycycline for 4 to 7 days in high-risk patients, including adolescents and those with a history of previous pelvic inflammatory disease (PID). In a randomized clinical trial of 800 first-trimester abortions, Lichtenberg and Shott found that shortening oral doxycycline prophylaxis from 7 to 3 days had no adverse effect on the incidence of postabortion infection (143). In a study in Sweden, a single dose of doxycycline 10 to 12 hours before a first-trimester abortion resulted in a lower rate of postabortion endometritis/PID (2.1% vs. 6.2% for placebo; $p < 0.01$) but more nausea and vomiting (144). All Rh negative women should receive immune globulin at the time of the abortion to prevent possible sensitization and resulting erythroblastosis fetalis with future pregnancies (see section on Rh(D) Immune Globulin).

In the first 12 weeks of gestation, the most commonly used method for abortion in the United States is suction curettage. Suction curettage or dilatation and evacuation (D&E) involves mechanical dilatation of the cervix. Clinicians follow their individual preference as to the use or nonuse of laminaria, since controlled studies of complications and morbidity are conflicting. Laminaria are seaweed or synthetic sticks that are hydrophilic, absorb water, and thus result in mechanical dilatation of the uterine cervix. They must be put in place in the endocervical canal 3 to 24 hours before the procedure, and thus cause delay and an added procedure for the patient. Use of laminaria may lessen the risk of cervical lacerations and uterine perforation, as these complications are most likely to occur during the dilatation portion of the procedure.

Patients are instructed that a D&E feels like a very intense and severe menstrual cramp. The suction procedure itself lasts only a few minutes, but the uterine cramping, although brief, may be severe. The procedure can be performed with a local paracervical block and/or intravenous sedation in a freestanding clinic or a hospital-based ambulatory setting. It is essential that patients be calm so that movement is limited during the procedure in order to decrease the risk of uterine perforation. Very young adolescents or victims of rape may prefer general anesthesia, as the pelvic exam alone may be difficult. General anesthesia is associated with a two- to fourfold increase in the risk of death compared with local anesthesia and a higher rate of uterine perforation and hemorrhage, intraabdominal hemorrhage, and cervical trauma (145). Inhalation anesthetics relax the uterus, which may cause a larger blood loss.

After the procedure, patients should be informed that they may have bleeding like a "heavy period" that may continue for several days and up to 2 weeks after the procedure. They are encouraged to start hormonal methods such as the birth control pills, the transdermal contraceptive patch, or the intravaginal contraceptive ring, within 3 days of the procedure or the following Sunday. An injection of depot medroxyprogesterone 150 mg IM may be given before they are discharged home. The products of conception should always be carefully examined (and optimally sent to pathology) to make sure that a pregnancy has been completely terminated and to rule out a molar gestation (gestational trophoblastic disease). Failure to detect fetal parts or villi and an implantation site should prompt the clinician to consider diagnoses such as ectopic pregnancy, a false-positive pregnancy test (rare with the new kits), unrecognized early spontaneous abortion, interrupted uterine pregnancy, uterine anomaly with a continued pregnancy, or incomplete evacuation of the uterus. Repeat pregnancy test, curettage, ultrasonography, and laparoscopy are tools for making the correct diagnosis. When an early pregnancy (5 to 6 weeks) is terminated by menstrual extraction, it is especially important to consider the possibility of a failed abortion. No matter what type of abortion is performed, the patient must be seen in 2 weeks for follow-up to avoid missing a failed abortion with ongoing pregnancy, ectopic pregnancy, pathologic identification of trophoblastic disease, or other complications.

Complications of first-trimester abortion include excessive blood loss resulting in transfusion, perforation of the uterus, postabortion hematometra, cervical trauma, infection, retained products of conception, and failed abortion (144). Immediately after the procedure, oxytocic agents may decrease blood loss and are used primarily in second-trimester abortions and with general anesthesia. Women with retained products of conception usually complain of heavy bleeding and cramps, with or without fever, in the first week after the abortion and require repeat curettage. Pelvic infection (PID) following abortion is a potentially serious problem because it is a factor in the development of tubal disease, Asherman syndrome (intrauterine adhesions), and infertility. Risk factors for postabortion endometritis or PID include late gestational age, endocervical gonorrhea or chlamydial infection, and intraamniotic instillations for induction of abortion. Patients with infections typically complain of fever and bleeding 3 to 7 days after the abortion and have uterine tenderness and sometimes adnexal tenderness on examination. Antibiotics for the treatment of PID (see Chapter 15) should be instituted, and if retained products of conception are present, repeat curettage should be performed.

The data on long-term medical and psychological effects of first-trimester abortion are reassuring. There is no conclusive evidence of an increase in miscarriages, ectopic pregnancy, or adverse late pregnancy outcomes in patients with one previous induced abortion (146). Two or more induced abortions may increase the risk of a preterm delivery (147). The most common emotional reactions after pregnancy termination are relief, transient guilt, sadness, and a sense of loss (148). Risk factors for postabortal psychosocial problems include previous or concurrent psychiatric illness, coercion, medical indications requiring termination of a wanted pregnancy, increasing length of gestation, ambivalence, and lack of social support (149).

In 2000, about 1% of abortions were nonsurgical procedures (140). Medical terminations of pregnancies offer the advantage of some anonymity since they do not require a visit to an abortion service; however, teens may have more difficulty dealing with some of the side effects. The mean duration of vaginal bleeding ranges from 8 to 17 days (150). Other side effects reported are abdominal pain and uterine cramping requiring medication, and nausea and vomiting (150). The side effects plus the need to return for follow-up to confirm complete termination of the pregnancy may be less well-tolerated by teens than the one-time visit required by the surgical method. Home support may make the difference between a negative and a positive experience with medical pregnancy termination for adolescents.

The combination of a synthetic progesterone antagonist mifepristone (RU 486) and the prostaglandin misoprostol administered vaginally has a success rate of 94% to 97% among women with pregnancies of 49 days duration or less (150). Recent studies are suggesting equal efficacy in pregnancies up to 63 days (151–153). The progesterone antagonist methotrexate used with misoprostol is equally effective and was used in the United States before the FDA approval of mifepristone. However, the methotrexate/misoprostol regimen takes longer to effect abortion than those using mifepristone and misoprostol (or another prostaglandin analog) (154). Sublingual administration of the misoprostol has shown some promise (155). Vaginal misoprostol as a single agent for abortion has been shown to be less effective and may be clinically acceptable when a progesterone antagonist is not available (156).

Second-trimester abortions (≥13 weeks) account for only about 12% of abortions in the United States (140). These later abortions carry higher risks to the patient and have more ethical issues and emotional consequences. Due to normally irregular menstrual cycles, an adolescent may not be concerned about a late period and thus lengthen the time to confirmation of the pregnancy. Unfortunately, the political climate, the restriction of funding for indigent patients, the lack of convenient access to first-trimester abortion in some communities, and legislation related to parental consent in some states may delay adolescents' decisions and result in more late abortions. For one or more of these reasons, teens are more likely than older women to delay having an abortion until after 15 weeks of pregnancy (140).

Techniques of performing second-trimester abortions have significantly evolved since studies in the 1970s revealed that D&E was significantly safer than intrauterine instillation. From 1974 to 2000, the percentage of second-trimester abortions performed by D&E increased from 31% to 96% and the percentage performed by intrauterine instillation decreased from 57% to 1.7% (140). The risks of cervical injury are lessened if laminaria are used before dilatation, and new materials continue to be investigated. Prostaglandins such as mifepristone are being explored to facilitate cervical softening prior to laminaria insertion (157). Placement of laminaria overnight followed by D&E can be used up to 21 weeks (depending on state laws) by an appropriately skilled surgeon. A combination of urea and prostaglandin appears to be particularly useful when D&E is not available. Most clinicians feel that intravenous sedation with local anesthesia is the safest for patients to lessen the chance of uterine perforation. Ultrasound determination of gestational age is extremely useful in pregnancies of at least 13 weeks and should be done in all gestations of over 20 weeks to prevent ethical, legal, and medical complications. Intraoperative ultrasound, particularly in terminations at ≥18 weeks, has proved invaluable to ensure that the uterine cavity is empty.

The major complication of second trimester extraction is hemorrhage due to uterine perforation. Infection is another serious complication that can occur and can be significantly reduced with antibiotic prophylaxis. Symptoms of infection include fever, prolonged vaginal bleeding, and pelvic pain. Most studies indicate that complications are more frequent at later gestational age (158). Cervical incompetence and later spontaneous losses may be associated with forceful dilatation of the cervix.

Health care providers need to know in detail the medical procedures that are available in their community (including the availability and type of abortion done between 16 and 20 weeks of gestation) in order to counsel and refer appropriately. The telephone numbers and fees (and type of insurance accepted) should be updated once a year. The Abortion Access Project and the Planned Parenthood Federation of America both have web sites that provide information and clinic locations.

Disorders of Early Pregnancy

Adolescents can present with some of the same disorders of early pregnancy as adults, including ectopic pregnancy (EP), molar pregnancy, and threatened, missed, or incomplete abortion. Adolescents often differ, however, in that they may be unaware of or in complete denial that they could be pregnant when they present to an emergency room with pain and/or bleeding. A positive pregnancy test makes PID unlikely but possible.

Ectopic Pregnancy

The incidence of ectopic pregnancy (EP) has increased over the past three decades, plateauing at approximately 19 per 1,000 pregnancies in the past few years (159). The mortality rate has decreased due in large part to earlier pregnancy detection with more sensitive pregnancy testing methods (160). The pregnancy-related mortality rate due to EP is higher in blacks (8%) than in whites (4%)(161). Teens are at risk for EP because of the high incidence among teens of STDs, particularly chlamydia (162).

Disruption of normal tubal anatomy such as that caused by infection is a major cause of EP (163). Therefore, in the setting of pain and vaginal bleeding in an adolescent, a history should include risk factors for EP: previous EP, history of PID, STDs, previous intraabdominal or pelvic surgery, and reproductive tract congenital anomalies. The intrauterine device has traditionally been listed as a risk factor for ectopic pregnancy; however, more recent information indicates neither past nor current use of a modern copper-bearing device such as the TCu-380A increases the risk of a subsequent ectopic pregnancy (164).

Although the classic picture of EP is pain, vaginal bleeding, and a missed menstrual period, ectopic pregnancy is the great masquerader. The clinical presentation can vary from vaginal spotting to vasomotor shock (164). Physical exam may include adnexal tenderness and/or abdominal tenderness, an adnexal mass, and uterine enlargement. An early intrauterine pregnancy is identified sonographically by the presence of a true gestational sac, which has double echogenic rings. However, fluid accumulation inside the uterine cavity occasionally produces a pseudosac that can be mistaken for a gestational sac. Using transvaginal ultrasound (TVS), the gestational sac is usually visible at 4.5 to 5 weeks of gestation. The yolk sac appears at 5 to 6 weeks and remains until approximately 10 weeks. A fetal pole with cardiac activity is first detected at 5.5 to 6 weeks. The discriminatory zone is that HCG titer above which a gestational sac can be identified with ultrasonography. Previously, with abdominal ultrasonography, this level was approximately 6,000 mIU/ml (164). Using TVS, the discriminatory zone is now 1,000 to 1,500 mIU/ml with some variation related to sonographic expertise and resources available (164). The gestational sac may be observed by TVS in patients with β-HCG concentrations as low as 800 mIU/ml and is usually identified by expert ultrasonographers at concentrations above 1,500 to 2,000 mIU/ml (165).

The absence of an intrauterine gestational sac at β-HCG levels above 2,000 mIU/ml strongly suggests an EP, although a single value below this level is consistent with either an early EP or an early intrauterine pregnancy. Beta-HCG can be detected as early as 8 days after the LH surge if pregnancy has occurred. The β-HCG concentration in a normal intrauterine pregnancy rises in a curvilinear fashion until 41 days of gestation at which time it plateaus at approximately 100,000 mIU/ml and the mean doubling time for the hormone is from 1.4 to 2.1 days (166). The rate of rise normally slows after 40 days of gestation, but by this time an intrauterine pregnancy should be visible on TVS. The β-HCG concentration rises at a much slower rate in most, but not all, ectopic and nonviable intrauterine pregnancies. There is a 10% to 15% interassay variability in these measurements as well as variability between laboratories. Interpretation of serial tests is more reliable if the tests are performed in the same laboratory.

Serum progesterone levels are higher in intrauterine pregnancies than in ectopic pregnancies. A level of more than 25 ng/ml is usually (98% to 99%) associated with a viable intrauterine pregnancy. Lower levels are seen in ectopic pregnancies and pregnancies that are destined to abort. A concentration less than 5 ng/ml almost always (99.8%) means the pregnancy is nonviable. The serum progesterone measurement is of questionable diagnostic value because it does not distinguish between an EP and a threatened abortion (167).

The diagnostic mainstay of EP is serial serum β-HCG testing and TVS. If the β-HCG level is greater than 1,500 mIU/ml, the interpretation depends on the transvaginal ultrasound (TVS):

A TVS positive for an intrauterine pregnancy almost always excludes an EP.

A TVS negative for an intrauterine pregnancy strongly suggests an EP. A serum β-HCG should be repeated 2 days later along with TVS. The EP diagnosis is certain if no intrauterine pregnancy is seen and the serum β-HCG level is increasing or plateauing. A falling β-HCG level is most consistent with a failed pregnancy such as a missed abortion, a blighted ovum, a tubal abortion, or a spontaneously resolving EP. The rate of fall is slower with an EP than a complete abortion. Weekly β-HCG levels should be monitored until they are negative.

An EP is almost certain if a nonspecific adnexal mass is noted and no intrauterine pregnancy is seen with TVS.

If the serum β-HCG is lesss than 1,500 mIU/ml:

With a negative TVS, an EP or an early intrauterine pregnancy may be present. Serial β-HCGs should be instituted. A β-HCG that does not double over 72 hours with a repeat TVS that is negative for an intrauterine pregnancy means that the pregnancy is nonviable.

During the diagnostic evaluation, it is essential that the teen be made to understand the life-threatening nature of a tubal pregnancy and signs and symptoms for which she should seek immediate medical help. A quick illustration of the size of a fallopian tube lumen, the significant blood supply involved, and the possibility of death in the event of rupture may be necessary to help the teen to understand the importance of compliance. The clinician should always have the teen give a phone number where she can be reached. Phone numbers can change frequently for this population.

Clinical management depends on the status of the patient, the β-HCG levels, the desire to continue an intrauterine pregnancy, and the ultrasound results. If the teen is without symptoms and has falling HCG levels, the health care provider should follow the HCG levels to zero to confirm the resolution of pregnancy (tubal, missed abortion, or abortion). If the HCG level either plateaus or does not increase appropriately, the management depends in part on whether the pregnancy is desired. If an EP is strongly suspected (β-HCG >1,500 mIU/ml, increasing subnormally and a negative TVS), intervention should be initiated. If the pregnancy is desired, a laparoscopy is done first. If the pregnancy is not desired, a D&E is done first. If no villi from an intrauterine pregnancy are identified grossly or by pathology at the time of the D&E, then treatment for an EP must be undertaken.

Management of EP has dramatically changed from a primarily surgical approach to the medical therapies that currently predominate (168), although in some settings the success rate is higher with surgical therapy (169). The aim of either treatment is to successfully eliminate the EP and preserve future fertility.

Surgical treatment is indicated if (a) the ectopic has ruptured, especially in a hemodynamically unstable woman, (b) the woman is unwilling or unable to comply with posttreatment monitoring after medical therapy, (c) access is lacking to a medical institution for management of a tubal rupture, which can occur during conservative therapy. Surgery tends to be more successful if the β-HCG level is greater than 5,000 mIU/ml before treatment; the tubal size is larger than 3 cm; fetal cardiac activity is seen on ultrasonographic examination. In the setting where surgical treatment is indicated, laparoscopic linear salpingostomy with preservation of the fallopian tube is the gold standard for management of EP in women who wish to preserve their future fertility (170). Laparoscopic salpingectomy is reserved for the fallopian tube that is felt to be irreversibly destroyed by the EP or for cases in which hemostasis cannot be achieved with salpingostomy. Free fluid or blood in the pelvis is not a contraindication to a laparoscopic approach, unless the patient is hypotensive. Many young women will be orthostatic, but not hypotensive. And thus a laparoscopic approach is not contraindicated.

Medical treatment of EP with methotrexate has supplanted surgical therapy in most cases (170). Methotrexate is a folic acid antagonist that interferes with DNA synthesis and has a long history of effectiveness against trophoblastic tissue, derived from experience in the treatment of hydatidiform moles and choriocarcinoma (164). Medical treatment success rates for treatment of EP have improved as definitive protocols for use have been developed and the best route of methotrexate administration has been identified. To date, systemic, multiple-dose methotrexate compares most favorably with salpingostomy (171). However, single-dose therapy with a repeat dose on day 7 if the β-HCG has not declined by at least 25% from day 0 level is increasingly used (172).

Success rates vary widely, from 71% to 100%. The highest success rates are reported to be from institutions that have detailed diagnostic and therapeutic protocols, readily available assays for serum HCG levels, high resolution vaginal probe ultrasound, and support staff that can closely monitor clinical response (170). Most protocols have found that the highest success rates occur in cases in which the EP is less than 3 to 5 cm on ultrasound, no evidence of tubal rupture exists, and no fetal cardiac activity is found within the fallopian tube. The intramuscular methotrexate dose is calculated according to estimated body surface area (50 mg/m^2 of body surface area) (173). A recent meta-analysis found that the multidose regimen of methotrexate is more effective than the single dose (174); however, single dose therapy has the advantage of fewer side effects and shorter treatment time since the citrovorum factor rescue is unnecessary (164). Medical treatment for EP can result in significant cost savings; however, there are adverse quality of life issues to consider because of the significant side effects of the methotrexate and lengthy treatment time (171). New evidence suggests that combining methotrexate and mifepristone can shorten the time needed for resolution of the EP (175). Many adolescents may not be appropriate candidates for medical management of an EP due to compliance issues and the need to adhere to a rigid protocol.

Expectant management is a reasonable option if (a) the HCG titer is falling, (b) the EP is definitely in the tube, (c) there is no significant bleeding and there is no evidence of rupture, and (d) the ectopic mass is not larger than 4 cm in greatest diameter (166). In all cases, β-HCG levels should be followed until they have fallen to zero. A salpingectomy should be avoided whenever possible to preserve future fertility options, since the patient is at increased risk for another EP.

Nonviable Intrauterine Pregnancy

The treatment of the nonviable intrauterine pregnancy depends on several factors. As with the management of ectopic pregnancies, declining or plateauing HCG levels must be from the same laboratory in order to establish that the pregnancy is nonviable. Patients without significant trophoblastic tissue and low levels of HCG can be followed with expectant management, provided that heavy bleeding does not occur and the HCG declines to zero. Rh status should be established at initial presentation, and Rh(D) immune globulin administered when indicated. In spontaneous abortion, the HCG is usually near zero by 19 days. In contrast, following elective first-trimester abortion, patients will have slower decline of HCG to zero because of higher initial levels; HCG is detectable for 16 to 60 days after D&E, with a mean of 30 days.

Two treatment options may be considered for adolescents with a nonviable pregnancy, intrauterine products of conception, a closed cervix, and declining HCG levels: observation or D&E. If observation is chosen, patients must be followed closely and be able to return promptly for curettage if there is excessive bleeding with the spontaneous passage of tissue. The open os makes the procedure less risky, but adolescents may have difficulty arranging transportation to the hospital. Electively scheduled D&E avoids adolescents' having to carry a nonviable pregnancy and having to return to the emergency department for sudden profuse bleeding. Many hospital emergency departments are able to offer immediate suction and curettage. Cultures for *N. gonorrhoeae* and *C. trachomatis* should be done at the time of the examination, and antibiotic prophylaxis considered with doxycycline 100 mg twice daily for 5 to 7 days following D&E.

Adolescents seen for irregular bleeding at follow-up after a spontaneous abortion, term pregnancy, or elective termination of pregnancy should always have a pregnancy test done at the appropriate interval when it would be expected to be negative. Irregular bleeding should not be assumed to be due to oral contraceptive breakthrough bleeding. A positive pregnancy test should raise the possibility of a new pregnancy (normal or abnormal), retained products of conception, or gestational neoplasia.

Gestational Trophoblastic Disease

Gestational trophoblastic disease (GTD) is a spectrum of disease processes involving abnormal placental tissue from an aberrant fertilization event (176). It may occur after any gestational experience. The term includes hydatidiform mole (complete or partial); persistent/invasive gestational trophoblastic disease; choriocarcinoma; and placental site trophoblastic tumors.

The incidence varies throughout the world. The rate in the United States is about one per 1,000 pregnancies. In Japan, which has the highest incidence, the rate is about two per 1,000 pregnancies (177). The risk is greatest in women older than 35 (177,178) and slightly increased in women under age 20 (177–179). Complete and partial moles are differentiated by their karyotype, gross morphology, histologic appearance, and clinical features (180). A complete mole is characterized by hydropic (swollen) chorionic villi, diffuse trophoblastic hyperplasia, and no identifiable embryonic or fetal tissue. Complete moles have a diploid karyotype, and all chromosomes are of paternal origin. Most often, a haploid (23,X) sperm fertilizes an anuclear ovum and then replicates its own chromosomes. A partial mole is characterized by focal swelling of the chorionic villi, focal trophoblastic hyperplasia, and the presence of embryonic or fetal tissues. Partial moles are karyotypically distinct in that they are usually triploid due to the fertilization of an ovum (one set of haploid maternal chromosomes) by two sperm (two sets of haploid paternal chromosomes). Surveillance is essential after the evacuation of a molar pregnancy, since persistent/invasive gestational trophoblastic neoplasia develops in about 20% of patients (181).

Vaginal bleeding and excessive uterine size in the first trimester are the most common presenting symptoms of a complete molar pregnancy associated with abnormally high β-HCG levels (181). The classic ultrasound picture is the snowstorm appearance of cystic tissue. Uterine evacuation is the treatment, and Rh(D) immune globulin should be given to Rh negative patients. Prior to evacuation, a chest x-ray should be obtained and a complete blood cell count including a platelet count, clotting function tests, renal and liver function tests, blood type and antibody screen, and a sensitive quantitative β-HCG. A quantitative β-HCG should be obtained 48 hours after evacuation and every 1 to 2 weeks until the levels are normal, and then at 1- to 2-month intervals for an additional six months. If the β-HCG level rises, additional evaluation and therapy will be initiated by a gynecologist–oncologist. A physician familiar with this disease should manage the patient. Contraception for 1 year after remission is recommended. With medical advances in diagnosis and treatment, most women can be successfully treated for GTD and maintain reproductive function.

Rh(D) Immune Globulin

Rh negative women are at risk for hemolytic disease unless they receive Rh(D) immune globulin in the following clinical scenarios: bleeding in pregnancy, spontaneous abortion, therapeutic abortion, ectopic pregnancy, molar pregnancy, at the time of amniocentesis, chorionic villus sampling, percutaneous umbilical cord blood sampling, or fetal surgery or manipulation; at 28 to 29 weeks of gestation; and at delivery (182). Therapy is always indicated unless the father's blood type has been documented to be Rh negative also. The standard therapy is intramuscular administration of 300 μg Rh(D) immune globulin. In pregnancies under 12 weeks gestation 50 μg is effective due to the small volume of red cells in the fetoplacental circulation, although there is no harm giving the standard 300 μg dose (182).

The pregnant teen presents a multitude of challenges to the health care provider and society. Sensitive, caring programs and providers can help to reduce adverse birth outcomes and support healthy parenting. A national commitment to address the antecedents of teen pregnancy and other high-risk behaviors is necessary to continue to reduce the ranks of adolescent mothers further.

REFERENCES

1. Teenager's sexual and reproductive health: developed countries. *Facts in Brief,* 2002, http://www. agi-usa.org/pubs/fbteens.html.
2. Klerman LV. Adolescent pregnancy in the United States. *Int J Adolesc Med Health* 2002;14:91.
3. Spitz AM. Pregnancy, abortion and birthrates among US adolescents. *JAMA* 1996; 275:989.
4. Darroch JE. Adolescent pregnancy trends and demographics. *Curr Wom Health Rep* 2001;1:102.
5. Cockey CD. Preventing teen pregnancy: it's time to stop fooling around: *AWOHNN Lifelines* 1997;1:32.
6. Franklin C, Corcoran J. Preventing adolescent pregnancy: a review of programs and practices. *Social Work* 2000;45:40.
7. Ruusuvaara L, Johansson ED. Contraceptive strategies for young women in the 21st century. *Eur J Contrac Reprod Health Care* 1999;4:255.
8. Facts At A Glance. Child Trends, Inc. Data from National Center for Health Statistics, Sept. 2001. http://www.childtrends.org.
9. HHS report shows teen birth rate falls to new record low in 2001. CDC National Center for Health Statistics, Division of Data Services. June 6 2000. http://www.cdc.gov/nchs/datawh/statab/upubd/ natality/natab98.htm.
10. Arias E, MacDorman MF, Strobino DM, et al. Annual summary of vital statistics—2002. *Pediatrics* 2003;112:1215.
11. Martin JA, Hamilton BE, Ventura, SJ, et al. National Vital Statistics Report, Births: Final Data for 2000, Division of Vital Statistics, *CDC* 2002;5:6.
12. Centers for Disease Control and Prevention (CDC) Trends in sexual risk behaviors among high school students–US, 1991–2001. *MMWR* 2002;51:856.
13. Litt IF. Pregnancy in adolescence. *JAMA* 1996;275:1030.
14. Schein AB. Pregnancy prevention using emergency contraception: efficacy, attitudes, and limitations to use. *J Pediatr Adolesc Gynecol* 1999;12:3.
15. Henshaw SK. Unintended pregnancy in the United States. *Fam Plann Perspect* 1998;30:24.
16. Stevens-Simons C, Beach RK, Klerman LV. To be rather than not to be—that is the problem with the questions we ask adolescents about their childbearing intentions. *Arch Pediatr Adolesc Med* 2001;155:1298.
17. Pinto E, Silva JL. Pregnancy during adolescence: wanted vs. unwanted. *Int J Obstet Gynecol* 1998;63:151.
18. Smith Battle L. The vulnerabilities of teenage mothers: challenging prevailing assumptions. *Adv Nurs Sci* 2000;23:29.

19. Crosby RA, DiClemente RJ, Wingood GM, et al. Correlates of using dual methods for sexually transmitted diseases and pregnancy prevention among high-risk African-American female teens. *J Adolesc Health* 2001;28:410.

20. Kirby D. Antecedents of adolescent initiation of sex, contraceptive use, and pregnancy. Proceedings of the 2nd Scientific Meeting of the American Academy of Health Behavior, March 24–27, 2002, Napa Valley, CA. *Am J Health Behav* 2002;26:473.

21. Baker JG, Rosenthal SL, Leonhardt D, et al. Relationship between perceived parental monitoring and young adolescent girls' sexual and substance abuse behaviors. *J Pediatr Adolesc Gynecol* 1999;12:17.

22. Crosby RA, DiClemente RJ, Wingood GM, et al. Low parental monitoring predicts subsequent pregnancy among African-American adolescent females. *J Pediatr Adolesc Gynecol* 2002; 15:43.

23. Crosby RA, DiClemente RJ, Wingood GM, et al. Correlates of continued risky sex among pregnant African American teens: implications for STD prevention. *Sex Transm Dis* 2003;30:57.

24. East PL. Do adolescent pregnancy and childbearing affect younger siblings? *Fam Plann Perspect* 1996;28:148.

25. Cox J, Emans SJ, Bithoney W. Sisters of teen mothers: increased risk for adolescent parenthood, *J Pediatr Adolesc Gynecol* 1993;6:138.

26. Cox JE, DuRant RH, Emans SJ, et al. Early parenthood for the sisters of adolescent mothers: a proposed conceptual model of decision making. *J Pediatr Adolesc Gynecol* 1995;8:188.

27. Furstenberg FF, Levine JA, Brooks-Gunn J. The children of teenage mothers: patterns of early childbearing in two generations. *Fam Plann Perspect* 1990;22:54.

28. Sex and America's Teenagers. New York, Washington: The Alan Guttmacher Institute, 1994.

29. Mims B. Afrocentric perspective of adolescent pregnancy in African American families: a literature review. *Afr Black Nurs Found J* 1998;9:80.

30. Klerman LV. Adolescent pregnancy and parenting: controversies of the past and lessons for the future. *J Adolesc Health* 1993;14:553.

31. Martyn KK, Hutchinson SA. Low-income African American adolescents who avoid pregnancy: tough girls who rewrite negative scripts. *Qual Health Res* 2001;11:238.

32. Crosby RA, DiClemente RJ, Wingood GM, et al. Psychosocial predictors of pregnancy among low-income African-American adolescent females. *J Pediatric Adolesc Gynecol* 2002; 15:293.

33. Young TM, Martin SS, Young ME, et al. Internal poverty and teen pregnancy. *Adolescence* 2001;36:289.

34. Omar HA, Martin C, McElderry D, et al. Screening for depression in adolescents: association with teen pregnancy. *J Pediatr Adolesc Gynecol* 2001;14:129.

35. Adams JA, East PL. Past physical abuse is significantly correlated with pregnancy as an adolescent. *J Pediatr Adolesc Gynecol* 1999;12:133.

36. Elders MJ, Albert AE. Adolescent pregnancy and sexual abuse. Commentary. *JAMA* 1998;80:648.

37. Stevens-Simon C, Reichert S. Sexual abuse, adolescent pregnancy and child abuse: a developmental approach to an intergenerational cycle. *Arch Pediatr Adolesc Med* 1994;148:26.

38. Boyer D, Fine D. Sexual abuse as a factor in adolescent pregnancy and child maltreatment. *Fam Plann Perspect* 1992;24:4.

39. Nagy S, DiClemente R, Adcock AG. Adverse factors associated with forced sex among Southern adolescent girls. *Pediatrics* 1995;96:944.

40. Stock JL, Bell MA, Boyer DK. Adolescent pregnancy and sexual risk taking among sexually abused girls. *Fam Plann Perspect* 1997;29:200.

41. Widom CS, Kuhns JB. Childhood victimization and subsequent risk for promiscuity, prostitution, and teenage pregnancy: a prospective study. *Am J Public Health* 1996;86:1607.

42. Montgomery KS. Planned adolescent pregnancy: what they wanted. *J Pediatr Health Care* 2002; 16:282.

43. Kegler MC, Bird ST, Kyle-Moon K, et al. Understanding teen pregnancy from the perspective of young adolescents in Oklahoma City. *Health Promot Pract* 2001;2:242.

44. Shearer DL, Mulvihill BA, Klerman LV, et al. Association of early childbearing and low cognitive ability. *Perspect Sex Reprod Health* 2002;34:236.

45. Anda RF, Chapman DP, Felitti VJ, et al. Adverse childhood experiences and risk of paternity in teen pregnancy. *Obstet Gynecol* 2002;100:37.

46. Landry DJ, Forrest JD. How old are US fathers? *Fam Plann Perspect* 1995;27:159.

47. Males M, Chew KSY. The ages of fathers in California adolescent births. *Am J Public Health* 1996;86:565.
48. Males MA. Adult involvment in teenage childbearing and STD, *Lancet* 1995;346:64.
49. Donovan P. Can statutory rape laws be effective in preventing adolescent pregnancy? *Fam Plann Perspect* 1997;29:30.
50. Elstein SG, Davis N. Sexual relationships between adult males and young teen girls: exploring the legal and social responses. Washington, DC. American Bar Association Center on Children and the Law; 1997.
51. Drake P. Assessing developmental needs of pregnant adolescents. *J Obstet Gynecol Neonatal Nurs* 1996;25:518.
52. Doswell WM, Braxter B. Risk-taking behaviors in early adolescent minority women: implications for research. *J Obstet Gynecol Neonatal Nurs* 2002;31:454.
53. Kaestle CE, Moriskey DE, Wiley DJ. Sexual intercourse and the age difference between adolescent females and their romantic partners. *Perspect Sex Adolesc Health* 2002;34:1.
54. Stevens-Simon C. Does mothering a doll change teens' thoughts about pregnancy. *Pediatrics* 2002;105:625.
55. Sadler LS, Daley AM. A model of teen-friendly care for young women with negative pregnancy test results. *Nurs Clin North Am* 2002;37:523.
56. Zabin LS, Emerson MR, Ringers PA, et al. Adolescents with negative pregnancy test results. *JAMA* 1996;275:113.
57. Zabin LS, Hirsch MB, Boscia JAB. Differential characteristics of adolescent pregnancy test patients: abortion, childbearing and negative test groups. *Fam Plann Perspect* 1994;26:212.
58. Rhinehart SN, Gabel LL. Teenage pregnancy: an update on impact and preventive measures. *Fam Prac Recertif* 1998;20:61.
59. Zoritch B, Roberts I, Oakley A. Day care for preschool children. *Cochrane Data Syst Rev* 2000;(2):CD000564.
60. Manning MD, Longmore MA, Giordano PC. The relationship context of contraceptive use at first intercourse. *Fam Plann Perspect* 2002;32:104.
61. Franklin C, Corcoran J. Preventing adolescent pregnancy: a review of programs and practices. *Social Work* 2000;45:40.
62. Sabo DF, Miller KE, Farrell MP, et al. High school athletic participation, sexual behavior and adolescent pregnancy: a regional study. *J Adolesc Health* 1999;25:207.
63. Lammers C, Ireland M, Resnick M, et al. Influences on adolescents' decision to postpone onset of sexual intercourse: a survival analysis of virginity among youths ages 13–18 years. *J Adolesc Health* 2000;26:42.
64. Kirby D. Emerging answers: research findings on programs to reduce teen pregnancy (summary). Washington, DC: National Campaign to Prevent Teen Pregnancy, 2001. http://www.teen prenancy.org/resources/data/pdf/emeranswsum.pdf.
65. McBride D, Gienapp A. Using randomized designs to evaluate client-centered programs to prevent adolescent pregnancy. *Fam Plann Perspect* 2000;32:227.
66. Watt LD. Pregnancy prevention in primary care for adolescent males. *J Pediatr Health Care* 2001;15:223.
67. Gould JB, Herrchen B, Pham T, et al. Small-area analysis: targeting high-risk areas for adolescent pregnancy prevention programs. *Fam Plann Perspect* 1998;30:173.
68. Causey AI, Seago K, Wahl NG, et al. Pregnant adolescents in the emergency department: diagnosed and undiagnosed. *Am J Emerg Med* 1997;15:125.
69. Cunningham FG, Macdonald PC, Gant NF, et al. *Williams Obstetrics, 20th ed.* Stamford, CT: Appleton and Lange 1997;229.
70. Finer LB, Henshaw SK. Abortion incidence and services in the United States in 2000. *Perspect Sex Reprod Health* 2003;35:6, Table 1.
71. Moore KA, Miller BC, Sugland BW, et al. Beginning too soon: adolescent sexual behavior, pregnancy and parenthood. Executive Summary.1995, Child Trends: Washington DC.
72. Speroff L, Glass RH, Kase NG. The endocrinology of pregnancy. In: Speroff L, Glass RH, Kase NG, eds. *Clinical gynecologic endocrinology and infertility, 6th ed.* Baltimore: Lippincott Williams & Wilkins, 1999:Chap 8.
73. Polaneczky M, O'Connor K. Pregnancy in the adolescent patient: screening, diagnosis and management. *Pediatr Clin North Am* 1999;46:649.

74. Bastian LA, Nanda K, Hasselblad V, et al. Diagnostic efficiency of home pregnancy test kits: A meta analysis. *Arch Fam Med* 1998;7:465.
75. Centers for Disease Control and Prevention. Sexually transmitted diseases treatment guidelines 2002. *MMWR* 2002;51(RR-6): 5.
76. Cooper ER, Charurat M, Burns DN, et al. The Women and Infants Transmission Study Group. Trends in antiretroviral therapy and mother-infant transmission of HIV. *J Acquir Immun Defici Synd* 2000;24:45.
77. The Italian Register for Human Immunodeficiency Virus Infection in Children. Determinants of mother-to-infant transmission. *Arch Pediatr Adolesc Med* 2002;156:915.
78. Perinatal HIV Guidelines Working Group. Public Health Service Task Force Recommendations for use of antiretroviral drugs in pregnant HIV-1 infected women for maternal health and Interventions to reduce perinatal HIV-1 transmission in the United States; 2004: 6/23/2004.
79. International Perinatal HIV Group. The mode of delivery and the risk of vertical transmission of human immunodeficiency virus type 1: a meta analysis of 15 prospective cohort studies. *N Engl J Med* 1999;340:977.
80. European Mode of Delivery Collaboration. Elective caesarean section versus vaginal delivery in prevention of vertical HIV-1 transmission: a randomized clinical trial. *Lancet* 1999;353:1035.
81. Scheduled Cesarean delivery and the prevention of HIV infection. *ACOG Committee Opinion, Committee on Practice* 2000;234:130.
82. Czeizel AE, Dudas I. Prevention of the first occurrence of neural-tube defects by periconceptual vitamin supplementation. *N Engl J Med* 1992;237:1832.
83. Preconceptual care, *American College of Obstetricians and Gynecologists Technical Bulletin* 1995;205:701.
84. Guidelines for diagnostic imaging during pregnancy. *American College of Obstetricians and Gynecologists Committee Opinion* 1995;158:1.
85. Bianchi DW, Crombeholme TM, D'Alton ME. Eds. *Fetology: diagnosis and management of the fetal patient prenatal imaging,* New York: McGraw-Hill, 2000: Chap. 1.
86. Henshaw SK, Kost K. Parental involvement in minors' abortion decisions. *Fam Plann Perspect* 1992;24:196.
87. Barbieri RL. Population density and teen pregnancy. *Obstet Gynecol* 2004; in press.
88. Administraive simplification under HIPPA: national standards for transactions, security and privacy. Fact Sheet, USDHHS, Mar 3 2003. http://www.hhs.gov/news/press/2002pres/hippa.html.
89. Maradiegue A. The health insurance portability and accountability act and adolescents. *Pediatr Nurs* 2002;28:417.
90. Hoyer PJ. Prenatal and parenting programs for adolescent mothers. *Ann Rev Nurs Res* 1998;16:221.
91. Stevens-Simons C, Fullar S, McAnarney ER. Tangible differences between adolescent-oriented and adult-oriented prenatal care. *J Adolesc Health* 1992;33:298.
92. Scholl TO, Hediger ML, Belsky HB. Prenatal care and maternal health during adolescent pregnancy: a review and meta-analysis. *J Adolesc Health* 1994;15:444.
93. Koniak-Griffin D, Turner-Pluta C. Health risks and psychosocial outcomes of early childbearing: a review of the literature. *J Perinat Neonatal Nurs* 2001;15:1.
94. Benussen-Walls W. Saewyc EM. Teen-focused care versus adult-focused care for the high-risk pregnant adolescent: an outcomes evaluation. *Public Health Nurs* 2001;18:424.
95. Blackhurst DW, Gailey TA, Bagwell VC, et al. Benefits from a teen pregnancy program: neonatal outcomes potential cost savings. *J S Carol Med Assoc* 1996;92:209.
96. Martin RD, MacDowell NM, MacMann JM. Effectiveness of a teen pregnancy clinic in a managed care setting. *Manag Care Quart* 1997;5:20.
97. Yoder BA. Young MK. Neonatal outcomes of teenage pregnancy in a military population. *Obstet Gynecol* 1997;90:500.
98. Berenson AB, Wiemann CM, McCombs SL. Adverse perinatal outcomes in young adolescents. *J Reprod Med* 1997;42:559.
99. Phipps MG, Blume JD, DeMonner SM. Young maternal age associated with increased risk of post-neonatal death. *Obstet Gynecol* 2002;100:481.
100. Jolly MC, Sebire N, Harris J, et al. Obstetric risks in women less than 18 years old. *Obstet Gynecol* 2000;6:962.
101. Phipps MG, Sowers MF. Defining early adolescent childbearing. *Am J Public Health* 2002;92:125.

102. Treffers PE, Olukoya AA, Ferguson BJ, et al. Care for adolescent pregnancy and childbirth. *Int J Gynaecol Obstet* 2001;75:111.
103. Gortzak-Uzan L, Hallak M, Press F, et al. Teenage pregnancy: risk factors for adverse perinatal outcome. *J Mat-Fetal Med* 2001;10:393.
104. Foster HW, Bond T, Ivery DG, et al. Teen pregnancy-problems and approaches: panel presentations. *Am J Obstet Gynecol* 1999;181:32S.
105. Bennett TA, Kotelchuck M, Cox CE, et al. Pregnancy–associated hospitalizations in the United States in 1991–1992: a comprehensive review of maternal morbidity. *Am J Obstet Gynecol* 1998;178:346.
106. Story M. Promoting healthy eating and ensuring adequate weight gain in pregnant adolescents: issues and strategies. *Annals N Y Acad Sci* 1997;817:321.
107. Gilchrist LD, Hussey JM, Gillmore MR, et al. Drug use among adolescent mothers: prepregnancy to 18 months postpartum. *J Adolesc Health* 1996;19:337.
108. Markovic N, Bess RB, Cefilli D, et al. Substance use measures among women in early pregnancy. *Am J Obstet Gynecol* 2000;183:627.
109. Richardson KK. Adolescent pregnancy and substance abuse. *J Obstet Gynecol Neonatal Nurs* 1999;28:623.
110. Faben VB. Graubard BI. Maternal substance use in pregnancy and developmental outcome at age 3. *J Subst Abuse* 2000;12:329.
111. Martin JA, Hamilton BE, Ventura SJ, et al. Births: final data for 2000, *National Vital Statistcs Report, CDC* 2002;50:1.
112. Andres RL, Day MC. Perinatal complications associated with maternal tobacco use. *Sem Neonatal* 2000;5:231.
113. Gilliland FD, Li YF, Peters JM. Effects of maternal smoking during pregnancy and environmental tobacco smoke on asthma and wheezing in children. *Am J Resp Crit Care Med* 2001;163:429.
114. Albrecht SA, Higgins LW, Lebow H. Knowledge about the deleterious effects of smoking and its relationship to smoking cessation among pregnant adolescents. *Adolesc* 2000;35:709.
115. Higgins ST, Alessi SM, Dantona RL. Voucher-based incentives: a substance abuse treatment innovation. *Addict Behav* 2002;27,887.
116. Wisborg K, Kesmodel U, Henriksen TB, et al. Exposure to tobacco smoke in utero and the risk of stillbirth and death in the first year of life. *Am J Epidemiol* 2001;154:322.
117. Cornelius MD, Goldschmidt L, Taylor PM, et al. Prenatal alcohol use among teenagers: effects on fetal outcomes. *Alcohol Clin Exp Res* 1999;23:1238.
118. Fried PA, Smith AM. A literature review of the consequences of prenatal marihuana exposure: an emerging theme of a deficiency in aspects of executive functions. *Neurotoxicol Teratol* 2001;23:1.
119. Day NL, Richardson GA. Prenatal marijuana use: epidemiology, methodologic issues and infant outcome. *Clin Perinat* 1991;18:77.
120. Goldschmidt L, Day NL, Richardson GA. Effects of prenatal marijuana exposure on child behavior problems at age 10. *Neurotoxical Teratol* 2000;22:325.
121. Addia A, Moretti ME, Ahmed SF, et al. Fetal effects of cocaine: an updated meta-analysis. *Reprod Toxicol* 2001;15:341.
122. Church MW, Crossland WJ, Holmes PA, et al. Effects of prenatal cocaine on hearing, vision, growth, and behavior. *Ann N Y Acad Sci* 1998;846:12.
123. Bandstra ES, Morrow CE, Vogel AL, et al. Longitudinal influence of prenatal cocaine exposure and child language functioning. *Neurotoxicol Teratol* 2002;243:297.
124. Parker B, McFarlane J, Soeken K, et al. Physical and emotional abuse in pregnancy: A comparison od adult and teenage women. *Nurs Res* 1999;42:173.
125. Martin SL, Clark KA, Lynch SR, et al. Violence in the lives of pregnant teenage women: associations with multiple substance use. *Am J Drug Alcohol Abuse* 1999;25:425.
126. Quinlivan JA, Evans SF. A prospective cohort study of the impact of domestic violence on young teenage pregnancy outcomes. *J Pediat Adolesc Gynecol* 2001;141:17.
127. Renker PR. Physical abuse, social support, self-care agency, self-care practices and pregnancy outcomes of older adolescents. *J Obstet Gynecol Neonatal Nurs* 1999;28:377.
128. Cokkinidies VE, Coker AL, Sanderson M, et al. Physical violence during pregnancy: maternal complications and birth outcomes. *Obstet Gynecol* 1999;93:661.
129. Murphy CC, Schei B, Mythr TL, et al. Abuse: a factor for low birth weight? A systematic review and meta-analysis. *Can Med Assoc J* 2001;164:1567.

130. Miller L. Depression among pregnant adolescents (letter). *Psychiatr Serv* 1998;49:970.
131. Deal LW, Holt VL. Young maternal age and depressive symptoms: results from the 1998 National Maternal and Infant Health Survey. *Am J Public Health* 1998;88:266.
132. Szigethy EM, Ruiz P. Treatment of depression during adolescent pregnancy. *J Pract Psychiatr Behav Health* 1999;5:256.
133. Barnet B, Joffe A, Duggan AK, et al. Depressive symptoms, stress, and social support in pregnant and parenting adolescents. *Arch Pediatr Adolesc Med* 1996;150:64.
134. Field T, Pickens J, Prodromidis M, et al. Targeting adolescent mothers with depressive symptoms for early intervention. *Adolescence* 2000;35:381.
135. Black MM, Papas MA, Hussey JM, et al. Behavior problems among preschool children born to adolescent mothers: effects of maternal depression and perceptions of partner relationships. *J Clin Child Adolesc Psychol* 2002;31:16.
136. Koniak-Griffin D, Verzemnieks IL, Anderson NL, et al. Nurse visitation for adolescent mothers: two-year infant and maternal outcomes. *Nurs Res* 2003;52:127.
137. Quinlivan JA, Box H, Evans SF. Postnatal home visits in teenage mothers: a randomized controlled trial. *Lancet* 2003;361:893.
138. Jones RK. Darroch JE. Henshaw SK. Patterns in the socioeconomic characteristics of women obtaining abortions in 2000–2001. *Perspect Sex Reprod Health* 2002;226.
139. Teen pregnancy statistics and national trends. Alan Guttmacher Institute. http://www.agi-usa.org/.
140. Abortion surveillance–United States, 2000. Centers for Disease Control, *MMWR* 2003;52(SS-12):1.
141. Abortion and women's health: a turning point for America? Alan Guttmacher Institute (AGI), New York: AGI, 1990.
142. Zabin LS, Hirsch MB, Emerson MR. When urban adolescents choose abortion: effects on education, psychological status and subsequent pregnancy. *Fam Plann Perspect* 1989;21:248.
143. Lichtenberg ES, Shott S. A randomized clinical trial of prophylaxis for vacuum abortion: 3 versus 7 days of doxycycline. *Obstet Gynecol* 2003;101:726.
144. Darj E, Stralin EB. The prophylactic effect of doxycycline on postoperative infection rate after first trimester abortion. *Obstet Gynecol* 1987;70:755.
145. Kaunitz AM, Grimes DA. First trimester abortion technology. In: Corson SL. Derman RJ, Tyrer LB, eds. *Fertility control,* Boston: Little, Brown and Company, 1985;63.
146. Atrash HK, Strauss LT, Kendrick JS. The relation between induced abortion and ectopic pregnancy. *Obstet Gynecol* 1997;89:512.
147. Henriet L, Kaminski M. Impact of induced abortions on subsequent pregnancy outcome: the 1995 French national perinatal survey. *BJOG: Int J Obstet Gynaecol* 2001;108:1036.
148. Stotland NL. The myth of the abortion trauma syndrome. *JAMA* 1992;268:2078.
149. Stotland NL. Psychosocial aspects of induced abortion. *Clin Obstet Gynecol* 1997;40:673.
150. Christin-Maitre S, Bouchard P, Spitz IM. Drug therapy: medical termination of pregnancy. *N Engl J Med* 2000;324:946.
151. Fox MC, Creinin MD, Harwood B. Mifepristone and vaginal misoprostol on the same day for abortion from 50 to 63 days' gestation. *Contraception* 2002;66:225.
152. Schaff EA, Fielding SL, Westhoff C. Randomised trial of oral versus vaginal misoprostol 2 days after mifepristone 200 mg for abortion up to 63 days of pregnancy. *Contraception* 2002;66:247.
153. Creinin MD, Potter C, Holovanisin M, et al. Mifepristone and misoprostol and methotrexate/misoprostol in clinical practice for abortion. *Am J Obstet Gynecol* 2003;188:664.
154. American College of Obstetricians and Gynecologists, Practice Bulletin. Medical management of abortion 2001;26.
155. Tang OS, Xu J, Cheng L, et al. Pilot study on the use of sublingual misoprostol with mifepristone in termination of first trimester pregnancy up to 9 weeks gestation. *Hum Reprod.* 2002;17:1738.
156. Jain JK, Dutton C, Harwood B, et al. A prospective, randomized, double-blinded, placebo-controlled trial comparing mifepristone and vaginal misoprostol to vaginal misoprostol alone for elective termination of early pregnancy. *Hum Reprod* 2002;17:1477.

157. Ekerhovd E, Radulovic N, Norstrom A. Gemeprost versus misoprostol for cervical ripening before first-trimester abortion: a randomized controlled trial. *Obstet Gynecol* 2003;101:722.
158. Peterson WF, Berry FN, Grace MR, et al. Second trimester abortion by dilatation and evacuation: an analysis of 11,747 cases. *Obstet Gynecol* 1983;62:185.
159. Centers for Disease Control. Ectopic pregnancy-United States, 1990–1992. *MMWR* 1995;44:46.
160. Luciano AA, Roy G, Solima E. Ectopic pregnancy from surgical emergency to medical management. *Ann Am Acad Sci* 2001;943:235.
161. Center for Disease Control. Pregnancy-related mortality surveillance, United States 1991–1999. *MMWR* 2003;52(SS–02)1. http://www.cdc.gov/mmwr/mmwrsrch.htm.
162. Cates Willard Jr. Chlamydial infections and the risk of ectopic pregnancy. *JAMA* 1999;281:117.
163. Ankum WM, Mol BWJ, Van Der Veen F, et al. Risk factors for ectopic pregnancy: a meta-analysis. *Fertil Steril* 1996;65:1093.
164. Speroff L, Glass RH, Kase NG. Ectopic pregnancy. In Speroff L. Glass RH. Kase NG. *Clinical gynecological endocrinology and infertility.* 6th ed. Baltimore: Lippincott Williams & Wilkins, 1999.
165. Paul M, Schaff E, Nichols M. The roles of clinical assessment, human chorionic gonadotropin assays, and ultrasonography in medical abortion practice. *Am J Obstet Gynecol* 2000;183:S34.
166. Daya S. Human chorionic gonadotropin increase in normal early pregnancy. *Am J Obstet Gynecol* 1987;156:286.
167. Mol BW, Lijmer JG, Ankum WM, et al. Single serum progesterone as a screen for ectopic pregnancy: a meta-analysis. *Hum Reprod* 1998;13:3220.
168. Tulandi T. Current protocol for ectopic pregnancy. *Contemp Obstet Gynecol* 1999;44:42.
169. Lewis-Bliehall C, Rogers RG, Kammerer-Doak DN, et al. Medical vs. surgical treatment of ectopic pregnancy. The University of New Mexico's six-year experience. *J Reprod Med* 2001;46:983.
170. Tulandi T. Surgical treatment of ectopic pregnancy and prognosis for future fertility. UpToDate, 2003. http://www.uptodate.com.
171. Hajenius PJ, Mol BW, Bossuyt PM, et al. Interventions for ectopic pregnancy. *Cochrane Data Syst Rev* (2)CD000324, 2000.
172. Lipscomb GH, Bran D, McCord ML, et al. Analysis of three hundred fifteen ectopic pregnancies treated with single-does methotrexate. *Am J Obstet Gynecol* 1998;178:1354.
173. ACOG Practice Bulletin. Clinical Management Guidelines for Obstetrician-Gynecologists. No. 3, Dec 1998.
174. Barnhart KT, Gosman G, Ashby R, et al. The medical management of ectopic pregnancy: a meta-analysis comparing "single dose" and "multidose" regimens. *Obstet Gynecol* 2003;101:778.
175. Tulandi T, Sammour A. Evidence-based management of ectopic pregnancy. *Curr Opin Obstet Gynecol* 2000;12:289.
176. Berkowitz RS, Goldstein DP. Chorionic tumors. *N Engl J Med* 1996;335.
177. Palmer JR. Advances in the epidemiology of gestational trophoblastic disease. *J Reprod Med* 1994;39:155.
178. Martin BH, Kim JH. Changes in gestational trophoblastic tumors over four decades. A Korean experience. *J Reprod Med* 1998;43:60.
179. Di Cintio E, Parazzini F, Rosa C, et al. The epidemiology of gestational trophoblastic disease. *Gen Diagn Pathol* 1997;143:103.
180. Lurain JR. Gestational triophoblastic tumors. *Semin Surg Oncol* 1990;6:347.
181. Ainbinder MD, Berek KS. Epidemiology and pathology of gestational trophoblastic disease. UpToDate, July 16, 2002.
182. Prevention of Rh(D) alloimmunization. *American College of Obstetricians and Gynecologists Practice Bulletin No. 4.* American College of Obstetricians and Gynecologists, Washington, DC, 1999.

22

Adolescent Sexuality

Amy B. Middleman and Maurice Melchiono

When most people think and talk about adolescent sexuality, they often focus on the sexual behaviors and outcomes of adolescents. While this represents an important component of sexuality, it does not describe sexuality in its most comprehensive terms. Sexuality, as explained by the Sex Information and Education Council of the United States (SIECUS), refers to the totality of being a person. Sexuality reflects human character, the way in which people interact. Sexuality education is the lifelong process of acquiring information and developing values about one's identity, relationships, and intimacy. It includes learning about sexual development, reproductive health, interpersonal relationships, affection, body image, and gender roles. Sexuality is a multidimensional concept with ethical, psychological, biological, and cultural dimensions (1). In this chapter, we will first discuss the adolescent sexual behaviors and outcomes as they exist today. We will then look more closely at the more complex factors that shape those behaviors, and we will investigate ways in which we can all potentially impact adolescent sexual behaviors and outcomes for the future.

CURRENT TEEN SEXUAL BEHAVIORS AND OUTCOMES

Although coital sexual behaviors are the primary behaviors focused upon in most studies of adolescent sexual behavior, noncoital behaviors may be on the rise as teens learn more about the risks of sexual intercourse. Many teens are not aware that some noncoital behaviors are also associated with risk of sexually transmitted infections (STI).

Experimentation and exploration of sexuality often begins with masturbation. Although few United States data are available, Australian data indicate that among high school students, 58.2% of male and 42.7% of female students report having masturbated; 38.2% of male and 8.7% of female students report masturbating three or more times per week (2). The taboo associated with the topic of masturbation in the United States has hindered open discussion and may limit providers' ability to counsel teens about this expression of sexuality (2). Data from the Australian study suggested a possible association between masturbation and increased sexual self-esteem (2).

Although the majority of sexuality data on adolescents focuses on vaginal intercourse, it is also important to look at what "virgin" youth are doing to express their sexuality. In one study of urban youth in grades 9 through 12 (3), 47% had not had vaginal intercourse. Twenty-nine percent of virgins had masturbated a partner of the other gender, while 31% had been masturbated by the other gender. Nine percent had been involved in fellatio with ejaculation with a partner of the other gender; 10% had engaged in cunnilingus with a partner of the other gender. Only 1% of virgins report having had anal intercourse with a partner of the other gender in the past year. While we know that rates of vaginal intercourse among youth age 15 to 19 years is declining, there is concern that rates of other sexual behaviors that include risk of STI transmission may be on the rise. The National Survey of Adolescent Males also reported figures on the prevalence of oral sex in its 1995 survey; 49% of males 15 to 19 years of age had received oral sex, 39% had performed oral sex on a female, and 11% reported having engaged in anal sex (4). Rates of oral sex among black youth more than doubled between 1988 and 1995, bringing rates close to those among Hispanic and white youth (4).

According to data collected every 2 years by the Centers for Disease Control and Prevention in the form of the Youth Risk Behavior Survey, the rates of sexual intercourse among in-school youth grades 9 to 12 have declined significantly between 1991 and 2003 (5) (see also Chapter 20). It is estimated that the mean age of first sexual intercourse in the United States is 16.5 years, however, in many urban communities among minority youth, this mean is clearly younger (6). Of concern is that nearly one in five youth have had sex before the age of 15 years. Although the proportion of 15-to-19 year old unmarried teens who had had sexual intercourse declined between 1988 and 1995, the rates among unmarried teens 14 years of age and younger unfortunately increased during the same time period (7). This is especially concerning when considering normal adolescent development. Most adolescents, especially younger teens, have not developed the ability to think abstractly in a way that helps them anticipate unexpected situations, thus making refusal skills difficult for them to access. In addition, their behaviors are often guided by their feelings of invincibility and adherence to peer pressure in order to reap the resulting perceived social benefits. This cognitive stage of development makes teens particularly vulnerable to negative outcomes of early sexual behaviors including pregnancy and STI acquisition. One encouraging statistic is that among younger teens, sexual activity is often sporadic; the National Longitudinal Survey of Youth 1997 data indicate that half of sexually active 14 year olds had had sex only zero to two times in the past 12 months (7).

The majority of teens are having relationships with partners of a similar age; 63% of sexually active females have partners within 2 years of their age but 28% have partners 3 to 5 years older (8). Among 12- to 14-year-olds, 12% have relationships with partners more than 3 years older, and relationships with older partners are more likely to involve sexual intercourse (7). Girls are more likely than boys to have older partners, and the rates of intercourse for these younger females rise in conjunction with the age of their partners; 13% of relationships with same age partners included intercourse, 26% when the partner was 2 years older, 33% when the partner was 3 years older, and 47% when the partner was 4 or more years older (7).

Pregnancy rates, as noted in Chapter 21, have declined for teen females over the past 10 years (7,9,10). However, one in seven sexually active teens 14 years old and younger and one in five of sexually active 15- to 19-year-olds reported having been pregnant (7). There are 3 million STIs reported for teens every year; approximately one in four sexually active teens acquire an STI each year (9). US rates of *chlamydia* are highest among sexually active females with a median state specific prevalence of 10.6% among approximately 20,000 16- to 24-year-old women entering the National Job Training Program in 1990 (11). Teens have significantly higher rates of STIs than adults; gonorrhea rates among 15- to 19-year-old females in 2000 was 699.3 cases per 100,000 compared to the overall US rate that same year of 131.6 per 100,000 (11). The reasons for this are multifactorial and include social as well as biological components (see Chapter 15).

Perhaps most concerning is that many teens, and younger teens in particular, report that their first sexual experiences, if not forced, were "unwanted." The National Survey of Family Growth (1995) found that 13% of those who had sex at age 14 years or younger described the experience as "involuntary"(7). Among females age 15 to 19 years who have had sex, 7% report their first experience as "involuntary," 24% as "voluntary but unwanted," and 69% as "voluntary and wanted" (12). Alcohol and drugs also play a role in sexual activity. Data from a Kaiser Family Foundation (KFF) survey of 1,800 teens in 3 key age groups indicate that four of five teens believe that people their age usually drink or use drugs before having sex (13). Twenty-five percent of sexually active youth grades 9 to 12 report having had alcohol or drugs prior to their last sexual encounter (males > females) (5). The use of drugs and alcohol also affects a teen's judgment and makes it more likely that an adolescent or young adult under the influence may be coerced or forced into having sex. Almost a third of young adults report having "done more" sexually than they had planned while under the influence of drugs and/or alcohol (13). According to data from the National Longitudinal Study of Adolescent Health (Add Health data), 17% of girls and 11% of boys up to 14 years old report alcohol as a cause for a sexual situation they regret (7). The use of alcohol and drugs decreases the use of contraception and condoms during sexual intercourse; of sexually active teens, 62% of those who did not drink alcohol prior to their last intercourse report using contraception, and only 45% of those who did drink prior to their last intercourse used contraception (7).

It is important to be aware that sexual minority youth encounter risk of STIs and pregnancy as well. In a study by Remafedi, at least 10.7% of students in high school were "unsure" of their sexual orientation with 5.2% of males and 8.5% of females identifying as homosexual by the 12th grade (14). In comparison to their heterosexual peers, lesbian, gay, bisexual, and transgender (LGBT) youth are more likely to experience depression, substance abuse, social isolation, rejection by family and peers, harassment, violence, school dropout, suicidal ideation, running away, and sexual risks such as exposure to human immunodeficiency virus (HIV) infection (15,16). In addition, as youth struggle to identify their orientation, GLB youth are more likely to report a greater number of lifetime and recent sexual partners, earlier age at sexual debut, and higher pregnancy rates, yet they were no more likely to use condoms than their heterosexual peers (16). Encouragingly, gay-sensitive HIV education can decrease the prevalence of these high-risk behaviors.

FACTORS INFLUENCING BEHAVIORS

As young children and adolescents grow and develop physically and cognitively, they are exposed to and receive sexuality education from multiple sources. More than three in four adolescents and young adults report a clear desire to learn more information pertaining to sexual health topics; specifically, one in four report the need for more information regarding how to use condoms, and two in five want more information about communicating effectively with partners about sensitive sexual concerns (13). Currently, youth list their top three sources of information as sex education through school, friends, and parents. Various media sources also play a clear role including television, movies, videos, and magazines. Health care providers are not on many teens' lists; however, health care providers can impact teen sexuality behaviors and outcomes as advocates and sources of information for parents and friends.

SEXUALITY EDUCATION IN SCHOOL

Organized sexuality education in the schools and/or community groups represents an important part of a child's education. Despite some controversy about specific course content, 87% to 90% of parents, both urban and rural, have approved of school-based sexuality education, and a significant proportion endorse starting such education in the elementary grades (17,18). Eighty-one percent of Americans feel schools should teach abstinence *and* information to prevent pregnancy and STIs; only 18% support teaching abstinence-only until marriage (19). A nationwide survey of principals of public secondary schools conducted by the KFF in 1999 reveals that 95% of those surveyed state that sex education in some form is taught in their schools. Fifty-eight percent describe their curricula as "comprehensive," including the idea of waiting to have sex but providing information regarding birth control and safer sexual practices. Thirty-four percent say they teach abstinence-only (19). Schools also teach HIV education and have been funded in that endeavor by the CDC since 1988; Ohio and Utah are the only states that do not accept HIV education funding from the CDC (19). Indeed, the YRBS data from 2003 confirm that 88% of teens do claim to have received AIDS or HIV education in school (5). Despite federal efforts, most states determine their own sex education requirements. All states differ in their mandates. For example, as of September, 2002, 22 states required students to receive sex education and 39 required HIV/STD instruction (19). Some states include specific requirements about what should be taught: eight states require abstinence education be covered, and 22 states require that abstinence be stressed, while 13 of these states require local school districts to cover contraception information. Thirty-four states allow parents to opt their child out of sex education or STD instruction—three of which require active consent before instruction can begin (AZ, NV, UT) (19).

The content of traditional sex education is controversial, and the goals and means of evaluating this education are still less than optimal. Teaching healthy attitudes, feelings, and behaviors about sex and sexuality is not a universal goal, and achievement of healthy feelings about sexuality is an ambiguous measure to evaluate. Articles evaluating sex education programs frequently focus on statistics about the high rates of teen sexually transmitted disease and sexual activity, early age of sexual debut, and high rates of pregnancies and abortions. This creates a difficult standard by which to evaluate sex education programs in the schools. Sexual behavior and the consequences of such behavior have multifactorial causes in this country, including the biological urges, cognitive developmental stage, and natural desire for experimentation among teens, as well as more pervasive political, socioeconomic, moral, and financial concerns. These latter concerns are inextricably intertwined with the type of formal education provided to youth, and they affect the way parents teach children at home. Although it is difficult to evaluate the efficacy of sexuality education without examining behavioral outcomes, it is critical when discussing traditional educational programs to understand the shortcomings of this means of evaluation.

Approaches to sex education have evolved through several "generations" (20). First-generation programs imparted knowledge about sexuality, pregnancy, and birth control. Second-generation programs continued to focus on knowledge but also included values clarification, decision making, and communication-skills building. Evaluations of both first- and second-generation programs demonstrated that they had no effect, positive or negative, on adolescent sexual behavior (20). Third-generation programs were a departure from the path of program development and arose in part from opposition to traditional sex education, often eliminating "conflictual" information from the curriculum about contraception and "safe sex." The limited evaluation of these programs that has been done reveals that they do not reduce the age of sexual debut or the frequency of intercourse among youth (20). A study of an abstinence-based program, Sex Respect, found that the program had significant limitations in content (21). It is important to note that evaluative studies of all three of these early generations of sex education programs were not always methodologically sound (20), and this limitation may have contributed to some of the null findings. The methodology within this field of research has been found to be weak in several areas, most notable being the lack of control groups and failure to present pre- and postintervention data (20,22). Oakley and colleagues (22) reported that only 18% of the educational outcome evaluation studies published between 1982 and approximately 1995 were methodologically sound. In a May 2001 report, the National Campaign to Prevent Teen Pregnancy found that only three published evaluations of abstinence-only programs in particular were rigorous enough to be included in an analysis of efficacy; none of the three evaluations found any impact on sexual behavior or on contraceptive use behavior among sexually active participants (19). More rigorous evaluation of a variety of abstinence based curricula are underway and should better inform future efforts.

The fourth-generation educational programs were based initially on the health-belief model, which emphasizes the importance of the perceived risk/benefit ratio to young persons in health decision making, and more recently on social learning theory, which includes the concept that societal pressures and interaction play a role in the young person's health decisions. These educational programs acknowledge and address the adolescent developmental and motivational framework (20). They emphasize delaying intercourse as a safe and wise decision yet also provide information about contraception and safe sex. There is a strong component of experiential skills building within the curriculum for teens to learn how to avoid unwanted or unprotected intercourse. This format allows adolescents to practice and develop confidence with these skills. Learning and practicing these skills via various media (i.e., role playing, computer simulation games) not only teach decision-making skills but stimulate discussion of these issues with peers and parents, an important advantage of such exercises. Several of these programs have been rigorously evaluated and have been found to be effective in decreasing pregnancy rates and in increasing the rates of contraception use; the programs did not lower the age at which adolescents initiate sexual activity or increase frequency of intercourse or number of partners (19,23–25). The most successful programs incorporate many of the educational strategies found to be most effective in the evaluation literature (23–25):

1. They provide a narrow focus on reducing sexual risk-taking behaviors, including behaviors increasing the likelihood of pregnancy or sexually transmitted diseases including human immunodeficiency virus (HIV) infection, although some broad-based programs have been effective.
2. They are based on theoretical approaches demonstrated to be effective in changing behavior and norms and on research studies of efficacy.
3. They reinforce clear values and group attitudes about unsafe sexual practices and about sexuality and contraceptive use.
4. They include accurate information as well as experiential activities to personalize and reinforce information about risk and methods to avoid intercourse and protect against pregnancy and STDs.
5. They address the social and media influences on sexual behavior.
6. They use a variety of teaching methods to involve participants.
7. They provide modeling of and practice in communication and negotiation skills (i.e., role-play activities, refusal skills).
8. They are of sufficient length to complete essential activities.
9. Teachers and peers implementing the program have been well trained, and believe in the program, and replicate with fidelity.

Although few studies have been done, it appears that linking these educational programs to a school-based clinic that may or may not distribute contraception does not increase the frequency of risky sexual behaviors. In fact, the presence of school-based clinics may increase the use of condoms and other forms of contraception (26).

In addition, one of the most successful (and expensive) and broad-based programs is the Children's Aid Society-Carrera Program, an extremely comprehensive program including sex education as one of many components including individual tutoring, sports and art activities, work-related activities, and health care services (19). This finding emphasizes the integral role sexuality plays in a person's total expression of individuality and indicates the complex relationships between sexuality, school, parental and peer influences, and society as a whole. Additionally several programs focusing on positive youth development among children in elementary school, such as the Seattle Social Development Project, have shown promising outcomes in sexual risk behaviors among teens, years later (26).

SEXUALITY EDUCATION FOR ALL

This same structured educational process must be available for youth with both mental and physical disabilities. People with emotional and mental disabilities are also sexual beings and often have unmet needs for sexuality education; programs that address this special population's needs are important to protect the rights of this group in our society and help them function to achieve their highest potential for social interaction (27). Materials need to be taught more slowly and graphically, but in general the same topics are appropriate for this special group of students (28). Young people with physical disabilities and chronic illnesses have sometimes been seen as asexual; their disability may be the focus during health care interactions and their need for sexuality education ignored (29–31). Young people with sensory impairments may require specialized teaching techniques.

It is also critical to be sensitive to cultural diversity among sexuality education students and encourage community participation (32,33). It is important for programs to:

1. Use appropriate and understandable language.
2. Choose appropriate staff who are familiar with the culture of the student.
3. Choose the goals of prevention based on the culture.
4. Try to reflect the given culture in the activities and materials chosen for the program.
5. Promote positive self-images and relationships with others.
6. Examine the expectations for the intervention (program directors should expect equal learning from all groups, and programs may need adjustment to attain such a goal in various situations).

Bias can plague a sexuality education curriculum, especially heterosexual bias that alienates adolescents who are questioning their sexual orientation (14). Issues of sexual orientation (the physical/emotional attraction to members of the same or other sex) and gender identity (one's feelings of maleness or femaleness) surface during adolescence and should be addressed in a sexuality education curriculum. As children enter adolescence, they begin to experiment with their sexual roles in society. This experimentation does not necessarily predict their sexual preferences in the future, and experimentation is thought by most experts to represent normative adolescent behavior and sexual-identity formation. Gender identity disorders range from transvestitism (cross-dressing that is linked to sexual excitement) to transgenderism (a profound discomfort with one's anatomic body to the point of seeking surgical/hormonal gender reassignment), and these behaviors and feelings evolve during the adolescent years. This group of teens needs support during this time of change in their lives. It has been estimated that teens questioning their sexual identity or sexual orientation are two to seven times more likely to attempt suicide (34), and despair can also lead to acting out or involvement in high-risk behaviors.

One final, critical element to include in a sexuality education curriculum is the element of eroticism. Given the dangers of unsafe sex, information about sex and sexuality has necessarily become medicalized. Relationship "instructions" include quizzing partners about their sexual histories and maintaining safe behaviors (35). The elements of desire and intimacy can easily get lost, and examining these topics and promoting interpersonal communication may help students foster the elements of healthy decision making in their sexual relationships.

SEXUALITY AND PEER INFLUENCES

Adolescent males and females report being most comfortable talking about sexual issues with their friends (36). This is a concerning finding given the effect of peer pressure on adolescent behaviors. Studies have shown that, especially at younger ages, whether friends are having sexual intercourse can have a significant effect on whether a young teen decides to have sex as well (37,38). Unfortunately, the perception of friends' sexual activity is often incorrect and exaggerated; in one study, 40% of 14 year olds report that "most teens your age are having sex," when, in fact, the numbers of 14 years olds having sex are relatively smaller (7).

In a study conducted by KFF and *Seventeen* magazine, five hundred twelve 15 to 17 year olds were interviewed by random national phone survey in the fall of 2002. The majority of teens surveyed report at least "some" or "a lot" of pressure from peers about sex (39). Although the largest amount of reported pressure stems from pressure that girls feel from boys, it is important to note that a significant number of boys feel pressure as well, not only from other boys but from girls as well. Peer pressures also affect safe sex behaviors. In the same survey, if a boy carries a condom, 43% of boys and 36% of girls feel that "people will think he is easy;" if a girl carries a condom, 70% of boys and 75% of girls report that "people will think she is easy." A clear double standard of pressure exists among the genders (39). Further, nine in 10 teens believe that girls get a bad reputation if they have sex, while four in 10 teens believe that boys get a bad reputation if they have sex (39). In a separate survey, as noted previously, the KFF found that four in five teens believe that people their age usually drink or use drugs before having sex (13). This belief may have an impact on the number of teens willing to drink or use drugs prior to intercourse.

SEXUALITY EDUCATION AT HOME: THE ROLE OF PARENTS

True sexuality education begins much earlier than school programs, and the primary instructors are parents. As children grow, become curious about their bodies and sexual issues, and develop relationships within and outside of the family, they glean information with which to develop their belief systems and patterns of behavior from their most valued role models. When parents are uncomfortable discussing sex and sexuality, either the physical or more emotional dimensions, this discomfort may be transmitted and incorporated by the child. Children who are uncomfortable with sexuality topics may be less tolerant of sexuality differences among others and may be less likely to discuss and seek help for concerns about sexuality. Family values and communication about sex and sexuality can have a significant impact on the initiation of sex and use of contraception among youths (40).

The parental responses to children's early questions can establish the tone of future interactions and discussions about sexuality. Educational programs for parents have been shown to facilitate parent-child communication about sex (41). Parents should be encouraged to know the facts about sex, develop comfort with issues of sexuality, be honest and open with children on an age-appropriate level (i.e., use appropriate names for body parts in lieu of made-up names that may relay a message of discomfort with the facts), and avoid judgmental or argumentative discussions about sex. It is helpful for parents to anticipate the role that the media will play in their children's attitudes about sex; parents may want to watch some of those messages with children and use the media as a means to discuss sex within a context in which parents can introduce their own values and attitudes. As children develop physically, it is important to provide them with communication skills. Children are not cognitively able to anticipate situations, including sexual situations, in which they might be placed; one skills-building strategy is to role-play various age-appropriate scenarios. Five year olds might benefit from role-playing a scenario of what to say to someone who wanted to touch them where they did not want to be touched, and adolescents might learn from a scenario where they want to say no to sex or a partner refuses to wear a condom. By thinking about possible responses to such situations, youth can be prepared to react nonimpulsively, incorporating cultural or family values in ways consistent with their own developing belief systems to any unanticipated predicaments.

Parental influence on teen sexual behaviors is becoming clearer with recent research. Females with greater parental supervision have been found to have older age of sexual initiation (37). Other factors associated with later sexual debut include higher SES as measured by maternal education level, moral or religious emphasis in upbringing, and later menarche (37). In addition, girls with less perceived parental monitoring were more likely to test positive for an STI, have multiple sexual partners and a new partner in the past 6 months, and not use contraception during the last episode of intercourse (42). DiIorio and colleagues found that adolescents who spoke to their mothers about a greater number of sexuality topics were more likely not to have initiated sexual intercourse and to have more conservative values than those who discussed more topics with friends (36). Although the importance of parental involvement and communication is becoming more clearly established, recent studies show an element of "disconnect" in terms of adolescent and parental perceptions of communication about sexuality issues. In a study done by the California Wellness Foundation, while 65% of parents state they have spoken to their children about sex or birth control, only 41% of youth report the same; 66% to 74% of 11 to 14 year olds said they could speak to their parents on the subjects of sex, contraception and pregnancy, while 90% of parents thought their teen felt comfortable discussing those issues with them (7). In addition, Add Health data indicate that only 30% of parents of sexually active 14 year olds believed their child had had intercourse (7).

THE MEDIA

The media has a strong influence on the behaviors of teens. Teens have multiple exposures: television, magazines, radio, movies, internet, and chat rooms. These media sources can serve as sources of information regarding sex and sexuality, both positive and informative sources as well as potentially negative sources of information. The advent of internet use and chat rooms has opened up homes to the threat of sexual predators. Studies have revealed that young adults do find sexual partners on the internet, and the sexual behaviors among partners found on the Internet are potentially much more risky than the behaviors among partners found in person (43).

In an effort to determine teens' thoughts regarding television and its effect on teen sexual behaviors, the KFF conducted a telephone survey of 503 15- to 17-year olds in April, 2002. Of those surveyed, 72% feel that sex on television influences the sexual behaviors of others their age "somewhat" or "a lot;" interestingly, only 22% feel that television influences their own behavior (44). Forty-three percent of teens surveyed felt that television had actually been beneficial in teaching them how to talk to a partner about safer sex, 60% say they learned how to say no to a sexual situation that makes them uncomfortable, and 33% say that something they saw on television caused them to talk to their parents about a sexual issue (44).

THE ROLE OF CULTURE

Culture plays a significant yet often underestimated role in the sexual behaviors and outcomes of our youth. It is an important factor to consider when counseling parents and youth. Some cultures view sex as a natural part of being a human being, accept teen sexuality, and provide comprehensive and balanced information along with clear expectations about commitment and prevention of pregnancy and STIs within these relationships. Cultures that embrace this attitude toward sexuality have lower teen pregnancy rates. For example, teen sexual debut and sexual activity data do not differ significantly among many Western cultures (Sweden, France, Canada, Great Britain); however, US birth and abortion rates are much higher than those in these other countries (45). Teens in the United States are less likely to use contraception, face more negative societal views regarding teen sexual relationships, deal with restricted access to and higher cost of reproductive health services, and are less able to avoid pregnancy (45). Only five countries have teen pregnancy rates greater than 70 per 1000 per year: the United States, the Russian Federation, Romania, Bulgaria, and Belarus (45).

ROLE OF THE HEALTH CARE PROVIDER

The health care provider plays an important role in the sexuality education of youth, giving children, teens, and young adults correct information, the opportunity to develop their own values, attitudes, and insights, and the skills with which to effectively communicate and make decisions. Health care providers are seen as the logical choice of professionals to discuss these health issues with parents, children, and teens. Parents, however, may perceive that some health care providers have varying degrees of comfort with sexuality issues (46). Many professionals use "medicalese" and terms that are unfamiliar to patients and parents when discussing sexual issues, and many adolescent patients do not fully understand the information being imparted to them (46). Discussing sex should be a routine part of a medical assessment. It is critical that health care professionals explore and understand their own feelings about sexuality topics so that they can feel more comfortable counseling parents and patients about sexuality and health.

As children enter adolescence, the patient-provider relationship changes. Patients need to have private and confidential time with a provider. The importance of confidentiality within the context of these discussions with teens has been well established. Major medical associations support confidential care for adolescents including the Society for Adolescent Medicine, American College of Obstetricians and Gynecologists, the American Public Health Association, the American Academy of Pediatrics, and others. Studies have shown that confidentiality policies dramatically increase the number of adolescents willing to disclose sexual information to providers and return for follow-up care (47), and given the rates of STIs among adolescent in particular, disclosure is critical for diagnosis and treatment on a patient as well as a public health level. In fact, in a survey of young females in a private practice setting, 92% reported they would consent to *chlamydia* testing if certain their parents would not be told about the testing versus 38% who would not consent if such confidentiality could not be assured (48).

It is important to establish rapport with a patient prior to asking questions about sexuality. Adolescents may need help broaching these topics; providers need to ask appropriate questions about sexual behaviors, sexual orientation, and history of sexual abuse or coercion. Adolescents may initially feel awkward or be unresponsive, but if clinicians routinely ask questions in a comfortable and nonjudgmental manner, patients sense their interest and concern and receive the message that they are available and willing to discuss those issues. In some cases, it may be helpful to role-play scenarios of sexual decision making (i.e., what would you say if your partner refused to practice safer sex?) with sexually active teens or those contemplating sexual involvement to help them develop communication and refusal shills. The Guidelines for Adolescent Preventive Services and Bright Future Health Supervision Guidelines delineate specific recommendations regarding sexuality screening and anticipatory guidance about responsible sexual behaviors, avoidance of alcohol and other drugs prior to or during sex, sexual orientation, abstinence, the correct use of condoms, contraceptive information, the prevention of sexually transmitted diseases including HIV infection, sexual exploitation, and sexual abuse (see Chapter 1). Heterosexually biased phrasing of questions such as "Do you have a boyfriend/girlfriend?" should be avoided. It is less biased to ask, "Is there someone with whom you are in a sexual relationship? Tell me about your partner." Or if the patient is sexually involved, one can ask, "With males, females, or both?" If some patients laugh or scoff at these questions, this provides clinicians with an opportunity to model tolerance and an appreciation for personal differences. Asking these questions allows teens to seek the support they need. The goal of counseling should be to guide them to appropriate resources.

Given that a primary source of sexuality education for teens is school education, providers can also serve as strong community advocates for sexuality education. Clinicians see the effects of inadequate health education daily; they are well qualified to speak out for the education of our youth. Talking to parents and teens either in a clinical setting or through community groups about the sexuality education needs of the community allows the provider to work in concert with the community for change. This method also empowers parents and teens to organize their own thoughts and campaign for what they would like to see happen in the schools and community. Providers can initiate improvements in sexuality education on multiple levels. Talking to small groups of youth in focus groups or developing peer leadership groups are effective methods to educate young people about how to teach themselves and each other accurate sexuality information, behaviors, and skills. Community organizations such as the neighborhood boys or girls clubs could benefit from a health care provider knowledgeable in sexuality serving as advisor or perhaps sitting on the board. Materials are available for providers to use for their own and their patients' education through several organizations (see Appendix 1 for Internet sites and reading materials).

Providers are also needed at parent-teacher organizations, both as information resources and as advocates for appropriate sexuality education curricula in the schools. Clinicians can offer their services in the media, writing letters and speaking out when misinformation or biased views on sexuality education are expressed. Information is available to aid health care providers discuss sexuality education in communities (28,49,50). Clinicians can have a strong voice in government policy that is rarely heard. Without health care professionals' expert advice, community and state representatives have no guidance on sexuality education issues. Advocacy is a role for which most providers feel untrained, yet health care providers are perhaps the most appropriate experts to speak out about the importance of effective sexuality education. Clinicians need to become more adept at advocacy to help shape sexuality education based on implementation and rigorous evaluation of state-of-the-art curricula.

REFERENCES

1. Sex Information and Education Council for the United States (SIECUS). *Issues and Answers: Fact Sheet on Sexuality Education.* New York: SIECUS Report, 2001;29(6).
2. Smith AM, Rosenthal DA, Reichler H. High schoolers masturbatory practices: their relationship to sexual intercourse and personal characteristics. *Psychol Rep* 1996;79:499.
3. Schuster MA, Bell R, Kanouse DE. The sexual practices of adolescent virgins: genital sexual activities of high school students who have never had vaginal intercourse. *Am J Public Health* 1996;86:1570.
4. Gates GJ, Sonenstein FL. Heterosexual genital activity among adolescent males: 1988 and 1995. *Fam Plann Perspect* 2000;32:295,304.
5. Centers for Disease Control and Prevention. *Youth Risk Behavior Surveillance System, 2003. MMWR* 2004;53:1.
6. O'Donnell L, O'Donnell CR, Stueve A. Early sexual initiation and subsequent sex-related risks among urban minority youth: the Reach for Health study. *Fam Plann Perspect* 2001; 33:268.
7. The National Campaign to Prevent Teen Pregnancy. *Summary Report: 14 and younger: the sexual behavior of young adolescents.* Washington DC: The National Campaign to Prevent Teen Pregnancy, May, 2003.
8. Kaiser Family Foundation. *Fact sheet: Teen sexual activity.* Menlo Park, CA: Kaiser Family Foundation, January, 2003.
9. Alan Guttmacher Institute. *Facts in brief—teen sex and pregnancy.* New York: AGI, September, 1999.
10. Henshaw SK. Unintended pregnancy in the United States. *Fam Plann Perspect* 1998;30:24.
11. Centers for Disease Control and Prevention. *Sexually transmitted disease surveillance report 2001: STDs in adolescents and young adults.* Atlanta: CDC, 2001.
12. Moore KA, Driscoll A, Linderg LD, et al. A statistical portrait of adolescent sex, contraception, and childbearing. Washington, DC: National Campaign to Prevent Teen Pregnancy, 1998:11.
13. Kaiser Family Foundation, Hoff T, Greene L, Davis J. *National Survey of Adolescents and Young Adults: Sexual Health Knowledge, Attitudes, and Experiences.* Menlo Park: KFF, 2003.
14. Remafedi G, Resnick M, Blum R, et al. Demography of sexual orientation in adolescents. *Pediatrics* 1992;89:714.
15. Stevens PE, Morgan S. Health of lesbian, gay, bisexual, and transgender Youth. *J Pediatr Health Care* 2001:15:24
16. Blake SM, Ledsky R, Lehman T, et al. Preventing sexual risk behaviors among gay, lesbian, and bisexual adolescents: the benefits of gay-sensitive HIV instruction in schools. *Am J Public Health* 2001; 91:940.
17. Sex in America. *Gallup Poll Monthly* 1991;56:1.
18. Welshimer KJ, Harris SE. A survey of rural parents' attitudes toward sexuality education. *J Sch Health* 1994;64:347.
19. Kaiser Family Foundation. *Update: sex education in the US: policy and politics.* Menlo Park: KFF, October, 2002.
20. Stout JW, Kirby D. The effects of sexuality education on adolescent sexual activity. *Pediatr Ann* 1993;22:120.

21. Goodson P, Edmondson E. The problematic promotion of abstinence: an overview of Sex Respect. *J Sch Health* 1994; 64:205.
22. Oakley A, Fullerton D, Holland J, et al. Sexual health education interventions for young people: a methodological review. *BMJ* 1995;310:158.
23. Robin L, Dittus P, Whitaker D, et al. Behavioral interventions to reduce incident of HIV, STD, and pregnancy among adolescents: a decade in review. *J Adolesc Health* 2004;34:3.
24. Frost JJ, Forrest JD. Understanding the impact of effective teenage pregnancy prevention programs. *Fam Plann Perspect* 1995;27:188.
25. Kirby D. Risk and protective factors affecting teen pregnancy and the effectiveness of program designed to address them. In: Romer D, ed. *Reducing adolescent risk.* Thousand Oaks, CA: Sage Publications, 2003:265.
26. Hawkins JD, Catalano RF, Kosterman R, et al. Preventing adolescent health-risk behaviors by strengthening protection during childhoood. *Arch Pediatr Adolesc Med* 1999;153:226.
27. McCabe ME. Sex education programs for people with mental retardation. *Ment Retard* 1993;31:377.
28. Bruess CE, Greenberg JS. *Sexuality education: theory and practice.* New York: MacMillan, 1988.
29. Anderson MM. Principles of care for the ill adolescent. *Adolesc Med* 1991;2:441.
30. Cromer BA Enrile B, McCoy K, et al. Knowledge, attitudes and behavior related to sexuality in adolescents with chronic disability. *Dev Med Child Neurol* 1990;32:603.
31. Coupey SM, Alderman EM. Sexual behavior and related health care for adolescents with chronic medical illness. *Adolesc Med State Art Rev* 1992;3:317.
32. Pittman KJ, Wilson PM, Adams-Taylor S, et al. Making sexuality education and prevention programs relevant for African-American youth. *J Sch Health* 1992;62:339.
33. Waiters JL, Canady R, Stein T. Evaluating multicultural approaches in HIV/AIDS educational material. *AIDS Educ Prev* 1994;6:446.
34. Committee on Adolescence. Sexual orientation and adolescents. *Pediatrics* 2004;113:1827.
35. Adelman MB. Sustaining the passion: eroticism and safe-sex talk. *Arch Sex Behav* 1992;21:481.
36. DiIorio C, Kelley M, Hockenberry-Eaton M. Communication about sexual issues: mothers, fathers, and friends. *J Adolesc Health* 1999;24:181.
37. Rosenthal S, Von Ranson KM, Cotton S, et al. Sexual initiation: predictors and developmental trends. *Sex Transm Dis* 2001;28:527.
38. Beal AC, Ausiello J, Perrin JM. Social influences on health-risk behaviors among minority middle school students. *J Adolesc Health 2001*; 28:474.
39. Kaiser Family Foundation and Seventeen Magazine. *SexSmarts.* Menlo Park: KFF, Publication no. 3309, December, 2002.
40. Hofferth SL. Factors affecting the initiation of sexual intercourse. In: *Risking the future: adolescent sexuality, pregnancy, and childbearing,* vol. 2. Washington, DC: National Academy Press, 1987.
41. Huston RL, Martin LJ, Foulds DM. Effect of a program to facilitate parent-child communication about sex. *Clin Pediatr* 1990;29:626.
42. DiClemente RJ, Wingwood GM, Crosby R, et al. Parental monitoring: association with adolescents' risk behaviors. *Pediatrics* 2001; 107:1363.
43. McFarlane M, Bull SS, Rietmeijer CA. Young adults on the Internet. *J Adolesc Health* 2002;31:11. (KFF Teens, Sex, and TV, May, 2002.)
44. Alan Guttmacher Institute. Facts in Brief: Teenager's Sexual and Reproductive Health: Developed Countries. New York: AGI, 2002.
45. Croft CA, Assmussen L. A developmental approach to sexuality education: implications for medical practice. *J Adolesc Health* 1993;14:109.
46. Ammerman SD, Perelli E, Adler N, Irwin CE. Do adolescents understand what physicians say about sexuality and health? *Clin Pediatr* 1992;31:590.
47. Ford CA, Millstein S, Halpern-Felsher BL, et al. Influence of physician confidentiality assurances on adolescents' willingness to disclose information and seek future health care: a randomized controlled trial. *JAMA* 1997;278:1029.
48. Ford CA. Confidentiality and adolescents' willingness to consent to sexually transmitted disease testing. *Arch Pediatr Adolesc Med* 2001;155:1072.
49. HIV *Prevention: looking back, looking ahead: does sex education work?* San Francisco: University of California Center for AIDS Prevention Studies, 1994.
50. Perrin EC. *Sexual orientation in child and adolescent health care.* New York: Kluwer Academics/Plenum Publishers, 2002.

23

Gynecologic Issues in Young Women with Chronic Diseases

Marc R. Laufer and S. Jean Emans

Tremendous medical advances have improved the quality of life of patients with chronic disease as well as their life expectancies. This chapter focuses on gynecologic health issues specific for these young women, including pubertal development, menstrual function, fertility, and pregnancy. Contraception is discussed separately in Chapter 20.

CANCER

Advances in diagnosis and therapies have greatly enhanced the life expectancy of children and adolescents with malignancies (1). For example, children with acute lymphoblastic leukemia who did not receive radiation therapy and who are at least 10 years cancer free can expect a normal long-term survival (2). Information regarding cancer survivorship is available at the National Cancer Institute's Surveillance, Epidemiology, and End Results Web site, which is updated on a regular basis (http://seer.cancer.gov/csr). While the cancers themselves may have an impact on reproductive function, the treatment-specific therapies (surgery, chemotherapy, and/or radiation) may produce long-term adverse reproductive outcomes (3).

Pubertal Development and Menstrual Function

Radiation Therapy

Radiation therapy can result in permanent ovarian damage and ovarian failure. In a study of long-term survivors of childhood malignancies, Stillman and colleagues (4) reported that ovarian failure occurred in 68% of patients with both ovaries within the radiation field, in 14% whose ovaries were at the edge of the treatment beam, and in none with one or both ovaries outside the field. Ovarian function is directly related to the dose of radiation and the age of the patient at the time of treatment (5–7). The median lethal dose (LD_{50}) for the human oocyte has been estimated to be approximately 400 rad. A single dose of 250 to 500 rad results in menstrual irregularities in all women; up to 60% to 70% of women 15 to 40 years of age and 100% of women over 40 years of age will be permanently sterilized (Fig. 23-1). Women aged 20 to 30 years of age can tolerate 2,000 rad fractionated over 5 to 6 weeks with less risk of sterility than women over 40 years of age, in whom 600 rad will induce menopause (8–10). Thus, children and adolescents have a better prognosis for preservation of reproductive function than women over 40 years of age (5,8).

Radiation to areas outside the pelvis can also affect reproductive function. Dysfunction of the hypothalamic-pituitary axis resulting in hypogonadotropic amenorrhea is a common sequela of cranial tumors treated with surgery and/or radiation. Hall and colleagues (11) administered a physiologic replacement regimen of exogenous gonadotropin-releasing hormone (GnRH) to survivors of brain tumors, based on the hypothesis that the defect would be hypothalamic rather than pituitary in origin. Ovulation occurred in 78% of the nine patients. Hyperprolactinemia may also occur secondary to whole-brain irradiation for brain tumors. Early and precocious puberty may occur in girls who received hypothalamic-pituitary radiation for acute lymphoblastic leukemia (12). Radiation to the neck can result in hypothyroidism in as many as one-third to one-half of patients who received doses of over 3,500 cGy, resulting in delayed maturation and poor linear growth if undiagnosed (13) (see Chapters 6 and 7).

Ovarian dose (rads)	Results
60	No deleterious effect
150	No deleterious effect in young women; some risk for sterilization women older than 40
250–500	In women aged 15 to 40, 60% permanently sterilized; remainder may suffer temporary amenorrhea. In women older than 40, 100% permanently sterilized
500–800	In women aged 15 to 40, 60% to 70% permanently sterilized; remainder may experience temporary amenorrhea. No data available for women over 40
>800	100% permanently sterilized

FIG. 23-1. Effects of ionizing radiation on ovarian function. (From: Damewood MD. What factors underlie premature ovarian failure? *Contemp Obstet Gynecol* 1990:31; with permission.)

Chemotherapy

Chemotherapeutic agents affect ovarian function and fertility in a dose-dependent fashion. The marked cytotoxicity of most anticancer drugs, in particular the alkylating agents, can have adverse affects on reproductive potential. Cytotoxic agents produce azoospermia and compromised Leydig cell function in males, and the testicles appear to be more sensitive to these agents than the ovaries (14,15). Cytotoxic agents produce perifollicular agenesis progressing to premature ovarian failure in females (16,17). Chemotherapeutic agents that have been associated with premature ovarian failure in adults include cyclophosphamide, chlorambucil, busulfan, and melphalan (LPAM) and the combination regimens mechlorethamine, vincristine, procarbazine, and prednisone (MOPP); nitrogen mustard, vinblastine, procarbazine, and prednisolone (MVPP); and chlorambucil, vinblastine, prednisolone, procarbazine, doxorubicin, and etoposide (ChlVPP/EVA) (3–5,7,18–20).

The severity of gonadal dysfunction is a function of the chemotherapeutic regimen and total dose in both sexes, as well as the age of the patient at the time of therapy (21,22) (Fig. 23-2). Children and adolescents appear more resistant to the deleterious effects of these agents, although long-term effects have not been fully assessed. In a review of 30 studies that evaluated patients who had received chemotherapy for renal disease (cyclophosphamide), Hodgkin disease, or acute lymphocytic leukemia, Rivkees and Crawford (19) concluded that chemotherapy-induced damage was more likely to occur in sexually mature females and with higher doses of alkylating agents. They found gonadal dysfunction at follow-up in none of the girls given cyclophosphamide during prepuberty and midpuberty compared with 58% of those who were sexually mature. For Hodgkin disease, 7% of those treated in midpuberty and 71% of the sexually mature had gonadal dysfunction. For leukemia, the percentages were 10% for those treated before puberty, 36% for midpuberty, and 22% for those sexually mature. For cyclophosphamide, a dose of 5.2 g is associated with amenorrhea in women over 40 years of age, whereas a dose of 20.4 g is associated with the same effect in women 20 to 29 years of age (23). Even in girls who appear to go through a normal or early puberty, prior chemotherapy for acute lymphocytic leukemia can result in elevated follicle-stimulating hormone levels and decreased plasma inhibin levels, despite normal plasma estradiol levels (24,25).

Combined Chemotherapy and Radiation Therapy

The combination of chemotherapy and radiation therapy, especially in Hodgkin disease, often significantly impairs ovarian function. Patients less than 30 years of age have the best chance for recovery of ovarian function (26). In a long-term follow-up study of 92 girls treated for Hodgkin disease at age 15 years and older, 87% had normal menstrual function: 83% following pelvic irradiation, 94% following chemotherapy, and 67% following combined modality treatment (27). None of the girls who had subtotal lymphoid irradiation alone (mantle or spade field) or those

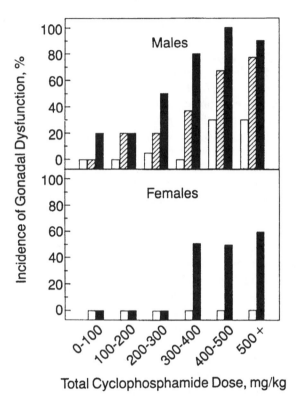

FIG. 23-2. Incidence of chemotherapy-induced gonadal dysfunction as related to pubertal stage during therapy and total dose of cyclophosphamide administered for treatment of renal disease. *Open bars* indicate prepubertal; *slashed bars,* midpubertal; and *solid bars,* sexually mature. Mid-pubertal females are not included due to insufficient data. (From: Rivkees SA, Crawford JD. The relationship of gonadal activity and chemotherapy-induced gonadal damage. *JAMA* 1988;259: 2123; with permission.)

who received three cycles or less of MOPP developed ovarian failure. Among 1,067 5-year cancer survivors with disease diagnosed at 13 to 19 years of age and still menstruating at age 21, Byrne and associates (28) noted the risk of early menopause was four times greater than that of control women 21 to 25 years of age (Fig. 23-3). The relative risk (RR) for early menopause was increased with radiation treatment alone [RR: 3.7; 95% confidence interval (CI): 1.3,10.0], with alkylators alone (RR: 9.2; 95% CI: 2.7, 31.5), and combined modality of radiation below the diaphragm and alkylating agents (RR: 27.4; 95% CI: 12.4, 60.4), when compared to controls. It is thus important to counsel long-term cancer survivors that, even if they have regular menses and ovulatory function, they may undergo a premature menopause and they should consider not delaying pregnancies.

In a long-term follow-up study of girls with acute lymphoblastic leukemia (ALL), menarche occurred in the normal age range in 92% of survivors and 96% of controls (29). In this study, survivors receiving 2,400 cGy of craniospinal radiation with or without abdominal radiation had significantly later menarche than controls.

Bone Marrow Transplantation

Although bone marrow transplantation (BMT) has been life saving in girls with advanced cancer, as well as for those with metabolic and hematologic diseases, significant gonadal damage may result from preconditioning therapies (30–36). Spinelli and colleagues (32) calculated that among 79 females undergoing allogeneic BMT with total body irradiation, the actuarial chance of having a menstrual period at 10 years after BMT was 43%. Four of five girls who received BMT in the premenarcheal age started menses. Immediately after BMT, all adult women had clinical evidence of ovarian insufficiency. Ten (13.5%) of 74 postmenarcheal women showed ovarian recovery ranging from 21 to 87 months. Patients under 18 years of age had a much better prognosis than those over 18 years. Girls undergoing bone marrow transplantation for ALL were found to have normal ovarian function in 50% of cases (37). In a study by Thibaud, of 31 girls treated with BMT only 6 of 31 were reported to have normal ovarian function (36). In a study of 44 postpubertal women after allogeneic BMT,

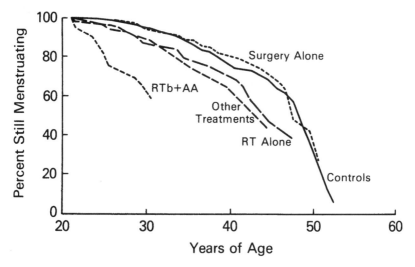

FIG. 23-3. Proportion still menstruating among cancer survivors diagnosed between ages 13 and 19 years grouped by type of treatment received compared with proportion of controls still menstruating (Kaplan-Meier curves). Survivor and control cohorts only (RTb + AA, radiotherapy below diaphragm plus alkylating agents; RT, radiotherapy). (From: Byrne J, Fears TR, Gail MH. Early menopause in long-term survivors of cancer during adolescence. *Am J Obstet Gynecol* 1992;166:788; with permission.)

Schubert and co-workers (34) reported that 80% (35/44) had reduced vaginal elasticity and rugae, small vaginal, uterine, and cervical size, atrophic vulvovaginitis, introital stenosis, and/or loss of pubic hair. Even prepubertal girls treated with BMT for sickle cell disease or thalassemia and given standard preconditioning therapies may have significant gonadal damage (31,35,38).

Suppression of Menstruation during Chemotherapy

Suppression of menstruation (Table 23-1) during chemotherapy can be safely achieved with a number of different medical options as outlined in Table 23-2 (39–43). Oral contraceptive pills can be initiated if there is concern of irregular bleeding during thrombocytopenia or can be initiated to treat the onset of irregular bleeding (see Chapter 8). Oral contraceptive pills have been associated with hyperbilirubinemia in cancer patients and may need to be discontinued if this occurs (44). A vaginal ring or IUD should be avoided in patients with mucositis or immunosuppression.

Use of long-acting GnRH agonist to induce amenorrhea prior to the chemotherapy is an option for controlling irregular menstrual bleeding during cancer therapy (39,40). GnRH agonists produce an initial increase in gonadotropins and gonadal steroids that is followed in approximately 3 weeks by suppression of the gonadotropins and the gonadal steroids. A menstrual period typically occurs 2 to 3 weeks after the first injection. Thus GnRH agonists are initiated at least 3 to 4 weeks before conditioning therapy for BMT (40). We currently utilize the 3 month formulation of leuprolide acetate 3 to 4 weeks prior to BMT induction therapy in order to suppress menses and ovarian function.

TABLE 23-1. *Conditions for possible therapeutic amenorrhea treatment.*

Cancer
Malignancy requiring chemotherapy
Asthma
   Premenstrual or menstrual exacerbations
Hematologic conditions
   Sickle cell disease
   Thalassemia
   Fanconi anemia
   Von Willebrand disease
   Hemophilia
   Thrombocytopenia
   Idiopathic thrombocytopenic purpura
   Fibrinogen disorders
   Other clotting disorders
Neurologic conditions
   Seizures with premenstrual or menstrual exacerbations
   Migraines with premenstrual or menstrual exacerbations
Developmental delay

TABLE 23-2. *Medications used to induce therapeutic amenorrhea.*

Continuous combination monophasic progestin dominant oral contraceptive pills
Continuous transdermal combination contraceptive patch
Continuous vaginal contraceptive ring*
Depot medroxyprogesterone acetate (DMPA)
Continuous oral progestins
Danocrine
Continuous progestin containing intrauterine device*
GnRH agonists
   With add-back therapy (estrogen and progestin, or norethindrone acetate)
GnRH antagonists
   With add-back therapy (estrogen and progestin or norethindrone acetate)

*Not optimal or contraindicated in cases of mucositis or immunosuppression.

Menstrual Function after Chemotherapy

Adolescents with impaired or absent ovarian function may experience no secondary sexual development or may have some development and subsequently present with primary or secondary amenorrhea. Replacement therapy with estrogen and progestin can provide normal secondary sexual development (see Chapters 6 and 7). Hormonal therapy should be provided to young women with premature ovarian failure, as this group is different from postmenopausal women who underwent spontaneous menopause.

Young women newly diagnosed with a malignancy may experience a spectrum of menstrual disorders. Adolescents with leukemia and thrombocytopenia may present with heavy or prolonged menses. Menarcheal females undergoing treatments for active disease may experience significant bone marrow suppression that may also lead to severe dysfunctional uterine bleeding. Once pathology is excluded, combination hormonal therapy [oral contraceptive (OC), or combination hormonal contraceptive patch] can be prescribed in a continuous fashion. When utilizing oral contraceptives (OCs), packages containing 21 days of active pills are prescribed and the young woman takes a hormonal pill daily without breaks or placebos. In a similar fashion, if the patch is used it is changed weekly with a new hormonally active patch and no breaks are taken. The continuous combination hormonal therapy is continued until the platelet count is over $50,000/mm^3$ (39) and it is deemed safe for the patient to have menses. At this point, these girls can be changed to cyclic therapy with a low-dose progestin-dominant OC or the patch. Medroxyprogesterone acetate (10 mg taken once daily tapered to 5 mg) or megace (80 mg taken twice daily) has been used in some centers to induce amenorrhea for months and even years, but breakthrough bleeding is common (36,37). Patients who have weight loss with resultant hypothalamic amenorrhea from radiation or chemotherapy may not require hormonal therapy during the time interval of thrombocytopenia.

Vaginal Graft-Versus-Host Disease

Graft-versus-host disease can affect the vagina (45,46). Women who present with vaginal pain, stenosis, or difficulty with sexual intercourse should be examined to determine if they have GVH of the vagina. In our series of patients with GVH of the vagina, local therapy with immunosuppressive agents was effective, although some required a surgical lysis of the vaginal scar tissue (46).

Options of Preservation of Fertility

Oophoropexy   Because of the problems associated with cancer treatments, investigators have looked toward preventive measures. Several procedures have been proposed to lessen the exposure of the ovaries to radiation, including ovarian suspension (also termed *transposition of the ovaries* or *oophoropexy*). The ovaries are shielded or moved out of the radiation field. In a study of Hodgkin disease, none of the girls treated with pelvic radiation without oophoropexy maintained ovarian function (27). For those with optimal oophoropexy, the ovarian doses ranged between 6% and 14% (47). Thibaud and colleagues (8) studied 18 girls (12 prepubertal and six postmenarcheal) who had ovarian transposition (15 bilateral, three unilateral) before external-beam irradiation (11 patients) or vaginal implants (seven patients). At a mean follow-up of 8.6 ± 0.9 years after ovarian transposition, 16 had menstruated and two remained amenorrheic. Ovulation was documented in seven, and two pregnancies had occurred. Complications of the ovarian transposition in four patients included intestinal occlusion, dyspareunia, and pelvic adhesions with tubal obstruction. The ovary may be pexed to different locations depending on the planned radiation field. Historically, oophoropexy for Hodgkin disease utilized medial transposition, in which the ovary is mobilized on a vascular pedicle and placed medially by suturing it to the serosal surface of the uterus (10,48) (Fig. 23-4). Hadar and Loven (49) reported using the lateral transposition approach for Hodgkin patients, in which the

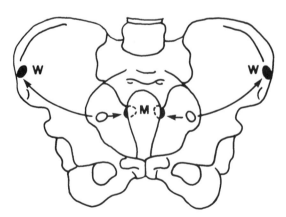

FIG. 23-4. Oophoropexy sites (M, medial displacement; W, wide lateral displacement). (From: Damewood MD. What factors underlie premature ovarian failure? *Contemp Obstet Gynecol* 1990:31; with permission.)

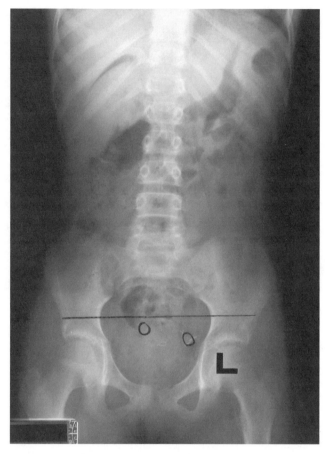

FIG. 23-5. Postoperative KUB film showing the location of the right ovary and the pexed left (*L*) ovary, with demonstration of the radiation beam edge. (From: Laufer MR, Billett AL, Diller L, et al. A new technique for laparoscopic prophylactic oophoropexy before craniospinal irradiation in children with medulloblastoma. *Adolesc Pediatr Gynecol* 1995;8:81; with permission.)

ovary and its vascular pedicle are placed retroperitoneally by suturing the ovary to the peritoneum lateral to the colon and superior to the iliac crest (Fig. 23-4).

Laufer and associates (50) described the first outpatient laparoscopic technique for oophoropexy for girls with brain tumors who are planned to receive craniospinal radiation therapy. The ovary in a young girl is higher out of the pelvis than the ovaries of an adult woman, and thus craniospinal radiation therapy to the level of S2 will put the ovaries at risk for ovarian failure. Studies of girls with brain tumors have shown a 60% risk of ovarian failure (51). Both ovaries are marked with titanium clips in order to calculate the radiation dose to each ovary (Fig. 23-5). The right ovary was marked and the left ovary was attached to the anterior peritoneum (in the initial re-

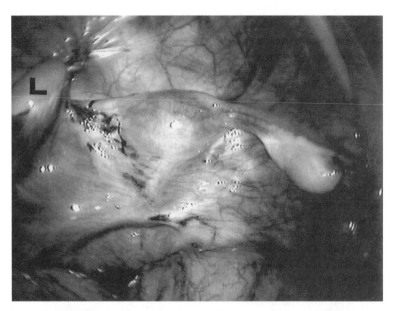

FIG. 23-6. Postoophoropexy showing the location of the right ovary and the pexed left (*L*) ovary. (From: Laufer MR, Billett AL, Diller L, et al. A new technique for laparoscopic prophylactic oophoropexy before craniospinal irradiation in children with medulloblastoma. *Adolesc Pediatr Gynecol* 1995;8:81; with permission.)

port), both with 4.8-mm titanium staples (Fig. 23-6). All patients underwent craniospinal irradiation for medulloblastoma after recovery from the oophoropexy. The authors calculated that if the pexed ovary is moved 2 cm outside of a megavoltage radiation beam, the dosage is reduced to less than 5% of the total exposed dose. Revisions to the technique have been implemented and we now move the ovary and sew it with a free needle and permanent suture to the uterosacral ligament (see Fig. 18-11 A–D). Although there is a report of robotically assisted endoscopic ovarian transposition, it is unclear that this technical modification improves the surgical outcome (52). Long-term follow-up data from 26 patients with brain tumors showed that the rate of ovarian failure was 7.1% in the oophoropexy group compared to 45.5% in the non-oophoropexy group (53). Based on this data, laparoscopic oophoropexy should be considered and offered to all girls undergoing craniospinal radiation therapy.

Oophoropexy has also been described with moving ovarian tissue out of the abdomen to the axillary for girls who are receiving high dose abdominal radiation therapy (54). Others have subsequently described a similar technique for oophoropexy (55,56). Long-term follow-up of these prepubertal girls, who underwent axillary oophoropexy, for over 20 years showed that they had ovarian function lasting for 14 to 15 years with normal pubertal development prior to the onset of premature ovarian failure (54).

Gonadal Suppression   To prevent the detrimental effects of chemotherapy on ovarian function, several hormonal therapies have been investigated. The potential for preserving reproductive function through the suppression of ovarian activity using OCs is not well studied. In 1981 Chapman and Sutcliffe (57) reported ovarian function to be normal in five women treated for Hodgkin disease who were concomitantly treated with OCs. Use of long-acting GnRH agonists to induce a "quiescent state" with the potential for preserving ovarian function has been proposed (58–61). Since it takes GnRH agonists at least 3 to 4 weeks to suppress ovarian function, the medication needs to be initiated with adequate time prior to induction chemotherapy (40). Although the data are scant and inconclusive, we currently offer the utilization of the 3-month formulation of leuprolide acetate in order to suppress menses and ovarian function 3 to 4 weeks prior to BMT induction therapy. Additional studies are needed to determine if this therapy is beneficial.

Assisted Reproductive Technologies and Cryopreservation

Cryopreservation of Embryos   In addition to the utilization of current assisted reproductive techniques, donor- or partner-inseminated oocytes can be cryopreserved as embryos for later implantation and gestation. These techniques are readily available and highly successful but require the fertilization of the oocytes with sperm. The need for fertilization of the oocytes creates an ethical dilemma for many adolescents who do not yet have a life partner and would require donor sperm from a sperm bank.

Cryopreservation of Oocytes   For adolescents who are already pubertal and in whom the potential for permanent gonadal failure from therapy exists, the cryopreservation of nonfertilized oocytes is now a possibility (62–68). Most centers have had poor results thus far with pregnancy rates of less than 1% but some centers have reported higher success rates. At this time we are offering this technique as an option but expense, poor results, and timing have not yet made this an ideal option.

Cryopreservation of Ovarian Tissue   Ovarian tissue cryopreservation has been proposed as a method to preserve fertility in young women with cancer (69–71). Preserved frozen ovarian tissue has been thawed and replaced back into the woman (72). This technique can be applied for women undergoing radiation therapy (73). Alternatively oocytes could be matured in culture and used for assisted reproductive technologies. This option is offered in some parts of the world but is still considered experimental as pregnancy rates have been poor.

Future Options   Additional investigation with such assisted reproductive techniques as ovulation induction, ovum donation, and *in vitro* fertilization needs to be undertaken in this group of patients.

Reproductive Issues

In a large National Cancer Institute study of 2,283 adult survivors of childhood and adolescent cancer (diagnosed in the period 1945 to 1975) that included both sexes and a variety of treatment agents (74), the overall crude relative fertility of survivors of cancer as compared with their sibling controls was 0.88. The male survivors had a greater fertility deficit than the female survivors (relative fertility: 0.83 vs. 0.94, respectively). Treatment effects were pronounced, with increased infertility in those treated with a combination of radiation and alkylating agents (2). Other studies have also found increased infertility (75). After bone marrow transplant there are high rates of menopause, but some reports show that 29% recover ovarian function (76). Younger age predicted return of ovarian function, whereas total body irradiation had a negative effect (76,77).

Lacher and Toner (78) found better fertility rates and better pregnancy outcomes in patients with Hodgkin disease treated with a limited field of radiation and chemotherapy with thiotepa, vinblastine, vincristine, procarbazine, and prednisone, when compared with the results published in the Horning (26) review of 103 women treated with multiple modalities of chemotherapy with or without total body irradiation after oophoropexy.

For women with ovarian function after cancer therapy, ovulation may be irregular. Induction of ovulation for attempts of conception should proceed along routine infertility algorithms. There have been reports of induction of ovulation with cancer survivors with abnormal gonadotropin levels with the use of clomiphene citrate and gonadotropins (79–81).

For those cancer survivors who retain their fertility after treatment excluding those who have received direct pelvic high-dose radiation, complications of pregnancy, spontaneous abortions, or congenital abnormalities are not increased compared to pregnancies in the general population (4,75,82–84). The health of offspring of childhood survivors of cancer is usually normal (2,48,75,85,86). However, in a study of 202 pregnancies in 100 survivors, 2 of 20 offspring born to 8 women treated with dactinomycin had structural cardiac defects: a ventricular septal defect and a tetralogy of Fallot (86). Although these data are not conclusive, given the small numbers, fetal echocardiogram may be useful in screening those mothers who have been treated with dactinomycin.

Iodohippurate sodium (^{131}I) in standard doses of 250 mCi to treat thyroid cancer 1 year or more before conception is not associated with any long-term risks (87). Two children born to mothers treated in pregnancy or 6 months before conception showed fetal brain deformities. Most health care providers now recommend waiting 1 year after therapy before women become pregnant.

Survivors of Wilms tumor who had received abdominal radiation therapy have been noted to have an increase in perinatal mortality and low birth weight in their offspring (88,89). Women survivors of Wilms tumor had more adverse pregnancy outcomes (defined as miscarriage, preterm delivery, or infants with birth defects) than did controls (89,90). Radiation-induced damage of the uterus may impair adequate expansion, possibly leading to premature delivery (89,91). An increased rate of one or more congenital malformations has been observed (89).

Data are limited on pregnancies after BMT. In a series reported by Hinterberger-Fischer and associates (92), three patients who received transplants for severe aplastic anemia (two female, one male) parented four healthy children, but offspring complications included persistence of fetal circulation, erythroblastosis fetalis, and prolonged newborn icterus. Others have reported pregnancies with successful outcomes in women following BMT for acute leukemia (93–95). At our adult Center for Reproductive Medicine at Brigham and Women's Hospital, there are a number of BMT cancer survivors who have conceived either spontaneously or with assisted fertility methods (utilizing either their own or donor oocytes or sperm) and have had successful pregnancies.

Ovum Donation for Cancer Survivors

Cancer survivors who have premature ovarian failure can still achieve a pregnancy with the assistance of an ovum donor. Obtaining an oocyte for fertilization with a partner's sperm or sperm from a donor bank and implantation of the embryo into the uterus has been successful. Oocytes can be obtained from known or unknown donors. Ethical recommendations have been made by the American Society for Reproductive Medicine regarding the use of gametes from family members (96)

Gestational Carriers

Cancer survivors who have had their uterus removed or who have had extensive pelvic radiation therapy, and who maintain ovarian function can opt to utilize a gestational carrier to achieve a genetic offspring. The oocyte is removed from her body and fertilized, and the embryo is carried in the uterus of the gestational carrier. Legal assistance from a lawyer familiar with reproductive law issues is required to adhere to individual state laws and requirements.

Risks of Second Malignancy

Cancer survivors are also at risk for the development of a second malignancy, often 10 years or more after completion of therapy for the primary neoplasm (97–100). The Late Effects Study Group (101) followed a cohort of 1,380 children with Hodgkin disease and found 88 second neoplasms compared with 4.4 expected in the general population: 56 had solid cancers, 26 had leukemia, and six had non-Hodgkin lymphoma. The estimated actuarial incidence of a second neoplasm 15 years after the diagnosis of Hodgkin disease was 7.0% (95% CI: 5.2, 8.8%); the incidence of solid tumors was 3.9% (95% CI: 2.3, 5.5%). Breast cancer was the most common solid tumor, with an estimated actuarial incidence in women that approached 35% (95% CI:

17.4, 52.6%) by age 40 years. Older age (10 to 16 years vs. <10 years) at the time of radiation treatment (RR: 1.9) and a higher dose (2,000 to 4,000 vs. <2,000 cGy) of radiation (RR: 5.9) were associated with a significantly increased risk of breast cancer. High cure rates should continue to be the essential priority in the management of childhood Hodgkin disease; however, better strategies need to be developed to maintain lifelong follow-up of treated patients in order to minimize their risks from any of these treatment modalities (102,103).

ASTHMA

Asthma is one of the most common chronic diseases. By age 18, one in five Americans is diagnosed with asthma (104,105). Asthma is seen three to four times more commonly in boys than in girls prior to puberty, and by age 10 the ratio begins to change such that after puberty asthma is more common in girls and remains so throughout adulthood (104–106). The rise of asthma at the time of puberty has been noted to correspond with the change in sex steroids (107). Some have proposed that the immune system is the link between asthma and sex steroids since estrogen, progesterone, and testosterone all affect levels of components in the inflammatory cascade (106–108).

Up to 33% of women with asthma report an increase in symptoms during the premenstrual period (106). Women with moderate to severe asthma have three to five times more exacerbations premenstrually when compared to women with mild disease (109–111). Exacerbations in the premenstrual and menstrual time periods have been proposed to be due to increased allergic responses due to increases in estrogen and/or progesterone (106,112). The exact etiology of these changes has not been determined but studies have shown premenstrual drops in 1-second forced expiratory volume (FEV_1) in up to 20% of women with asthma (106). These women may also experience other symptoms consistent with premenstrual dysphoric disorder (see Chapter 11).

There are no studies demonstrating effective therapies to decrease the cyclic asthma exacerbations. A trial of continuous combination hormonal (low-dose estrogen and progestin) therapy taken in a noncyclic fashion may be helpful (see Tables 23-1 and 23-2). Optimization of asthma therapies prior to the onset of the regular cyclic exacerbations is also helpful. Asthma treatment guidelines can be obtained from the National Heart, Lung, and Blood Institute (www.nhlbi.nih.gov/guidelines/asthma).

Asthma and Pregnancy

Pregnancy is not associated with an increase in new onset asthma, but approximately 5% of those with preexisting asthma will develop problems during pregnancy (106,107). The severity of the disease during pregnancy may worsen, stay the same, or improve. Pregnant women with asthma should be managed by health care providers familiar with all aspects of asthma and pregnancy conditions. The American College of Obstetricians and Gynecologists and the American College of Allergy, Asthma, and Immunology have a guideline for asthma management and medications during pregnancy (113).

CYSTIC FIBROSIS

Cystic fibrosis is the most common autosomal recessive life-threatening disease among whites and occurs in one in 2,500 live births. It is caused by mutations in the gene encoding for the CF transmembrane conductance regulator located on chromosome 7. In the past 40 years, the life expectancy of persons with cystic fibrosis (CF) has greatly increased. National median survival was 10.6 years in 1966, 20 years in 1981, 29.4 years in 1992, and 33.4 years in 2001 (Cystic Fibrosis Foundation. Annual Data Report 2001. Bethesda MD, 2001). In 1996, the Danish Cystic Fibrosis Center reported that the probability of surviving to age 40 with aggressive treatment was 83% (114). As a result, reproductive health needs have greatly increased for this population.

Pubertal Development and Menstrual Function

In young women with CF, Neinstein and co-workers (115) noted a mean age of menarche of 14.4 years versus 12.9 years for controls. Adolescent girls with CF often have low weight for height and chronic pulmonary infections that may significantly delay pubertal development and menarche (64–66). A recent study (116) of Swedish girls with CF found that pubertal and menarcheal delay was still present even with improved nutritional and clinical status; the mean age of peak height velocity was 12.9 ± 0.8 years and the mean age of menarche was 14.9 ± 1.4 years. Patients who were homozygous for $\Delta F508$ and those with abnormal oral glucose tolerance tests were significantly older at menarche (15.2 ± 1.9 years) compared to those who were not (14.7 ± 0.9 years) (116).

In summary, in spite of improvements in medical treatment of CF and nutritional support, patients often have: subnormal growth; marked delay in the onset and progression of sexual maturation; a 1- to 2-year delay of the mean menarcheal age compared to normal girls; and a delay of puberty even with optimal medical and nutritional status (117).

Reproductive Issues

Young women with CF generally initiate sexual activity at the same age as other healthy young women but may be less likely to use contraception than control subjects (118). Pregnancies in women with CF are frequently unplanned, and some women may assume that they are infertile. Because adolescent and young adult patients with CF often think of their pulmonologist as their "main doctor," they often do not receive adequate clinical preventive services and counseling about sexuality (119). At our hospital patients with CF indicated a desire to spend time alone with their "main doctor" between 13 and 16 years of age and wanted their health care providers to discuss risk behaviors, school, work and finances with them (119).

Although chronic illness and poor nutritional state may lower the fertility of an individual woman with CF (120–122), some have postulated that the thick cervical mucus (lower water content) may also be a barrier to sperm (123). A woman with CF has approximately a 1:40 chance of having an affected offspring if the carrier status of the father is unknown, and a 50% chance if the father is a heterozygote (124). Combining *in vitro* fertilization and preimplantation diagnostic testing for CF has resulted in normal offspring (125).

Successful pregnancies have been reported in women with CF (122,126–131). These studies confirm that pregnancy is well tolerated by women with mild disease but that both maternal and fetal outcomes are more guarded for those with moderate to severe disease. Outcomes for the infant are generally good, and the maternal outcomes depend on the severity of disease. Pregnancy is most likely normal in women with normal lung function; however, pregnancy should be avoided in cases of pulmonary hypertension, cor pulmonale, and when forced expiratory volume is less than 50% of expected (132). Careful medical assessment of the cardiac, pulmonary, and nutritional status is important before patients undertake a planned pregnancy (127).

Other Issues

A pseudopolypoid cervical ectropion has been noted in CF patients, in both users and nonusers of OCs (133,134). There is also increased production of cervical and vaginal mucus, which can present with a bothersome discharge.

GASTROINTESTINAL DISEASE

Pubertal Development and Menstrual Function in Inflammatory Bowel Disease

Adolescents with inflammatory bowel disease (IBD) may experience growth failure and delay of puberty and menarche. Delayed growth may be the first sign of IBD, especially in Crohn disease (Fig. 23-7), and may overshadow symptoms of the gastrointestinal dysfunction (135,136). In girls with IBD, gonadotropin and estrogen levels are low, implying a depressed hypothalamic-pituitary axis. Nutritional and

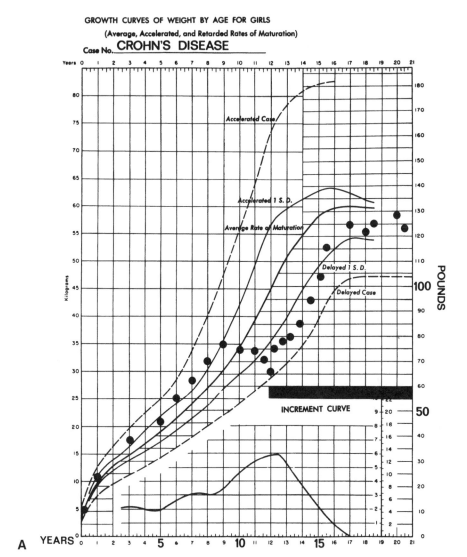

FIG. 23-7. Growth chart of a patient with Crohn's disease; bar represents treatment with pred-nisone., **(A)** Weight.

medical therapy, and sometimes surgery to treat active bowel disease, are important to ensure normal pubertal growth and development and regular menses (135). Al-though excess corticosteroids may impair growth, when the illness is adequately treated, the patient often has a growth spurt.

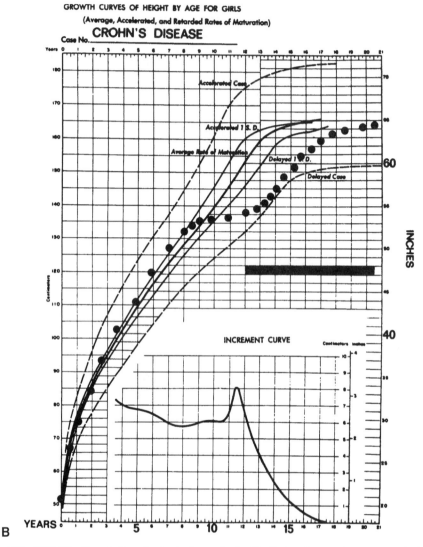

FIG. 23-7 (*Continued*) Growth chart of a patient with Crohn disease; bar represents treatment with prednisone, **(B)** Height.

Reproductive Issues in IBD

Several studies have suggested subfertility in women with IBD (136–138); however, many of these reports failed to adjust for factors such as smoking, age, or whether the patient was attempting to conceive. A woman's fertility does not appear to be affected by the presence of ulcerative colitis; 90% of patients with this disorder will be able to conceive if pregnancy is desired (137,139). There are conflicting data regarding fertility in women with Crohn disease, with factors such as lack of a desire for intercourse, occlusion of fallopian tubes, and perineal fistula affecting conception rates (140,141). Diagnosis during pregnancy or activation of disease during pregnancy may increase the risk of spontaneous abortion (138).

The common medications used to treat IBD, sulfasalazine and corticosteroids, are usually well tolerated in pregnancy (142). According to a study by Francella, the use of 6-mercaptopurine/azathioprine use before or at conception and during pregnancy appears to be safe, and discontinuation of the drug before or during pregnancy is not indicated (143). A differing study by Norgard and colleagues suggest that there is an increased risk of congenital malformations, perinatal mortality, and preterm birth in children born to women treated with azathioprine or mercaptopurine during pregnancy (144). More data are needed to determine if the findings in this study were causal or occurred through cofounding factors. Most specialists feel that active disease is more deleterious to the pregnancy than maintaining medical therapy and thus the medications are continued during pregnancy and breast-feeding (145).

The majority of women with either ulcerative colitis or Crohn disease complete normal full-term pregnancies with healthy offspring. Ninety percent of women with inactive ulcerative colitis complete a full-term pregnancy; those with active colitis do not do as well (146). Successful pregnancy outcome in women with Crohn disease also reflects the predominance of women with inactive disease in these studies (137,139,147). Active Crohn disease probably results in a higher incidence of spontaneous abortion and prematurity (148). It has been estimated that 15% to 40% of patients with Crohn disease will have an exacerbation during their pregnancy and about an equal number will remain unchanged or improved (149). In one large study of 756 pregnant women with IBD, there was an increased risk of preterm birth and low birth weight babies (150). The absence of gastrointestinal problems in a pregnancy does not predict the course of IBD in future pregnancies. Postpartum, the patients usually return to their prepregnancy gastrointestinal disease state.

Other Issues

In Crohn disease, ulcers of the perineum may mimic herpetic lesions but in fact are granulomatous lesions. They may last for weeks to months and can progress to fistula tracts that may require long-term antibiotic therapy (e.g., metronidazole) or even surgery (151). The possible association of IBD and OCs is discussed in Chapter 20.

Peutz-Jeghers syndrome has been found to be associated with an increased risk of malignant neoplasia. The associated gynecologic malignancies that have been reported are ovarian and cervical. The ovarian tumors (see Chapter 18) include Sertoli cell tumors (152), mucinous adenocarcinoma, mucinous cystadenoma (153), and sex cord tumors (154). The associated cervical neoplasia is a specific type of adenocarcinoma termed *adenoma malignum* (154). Breast carcinoma has also been reported (155). Regular yearly gynecologic examinations are essential in this at-risk population.

LIVER DISEASE

Pubertal Development and Menstrual Dysfunction

Women with chronic liver disease may have irregular menses, particularly amenorrhea that resolves if the liver disease improves. Amenorrhea has also been noted to resolve when spironolactone, an androgen inhibitor, was discontinued (156). Women with severe liver disease may also present with severe menorrhagia due to thrombocytopenia and the decreased production of clotting factors. Treatment of menorrhagia should be directed at treating the underlying disease and replacing clotting factors. Patients with this condition may not do well with oral estrogen therapy, as their liver dysfunction precludes adequate metabolism (157). Other possibilities of hormonal control of the bleeding with liver failure include medroxyprogesterone acetate, GnRH analogs, combination hormonal contraceptive, and the estrogen patch with an added oral progestin (157–159). The hormonal patches have an advantage over oral conjugated estrogens, as they avoid the liver "first-pass" effect. In the rare occasion hormonal manipulation fails, a dilatation and curettage with adequate preoperative coagulation factor replacement may be necessary.

Reproductive Issues

Chronic liver disease is associated with anovulation and decreased fertility. Amenorrhea is commonly seen. Pregnancy can be expected only if the liver dysfunction can be reversed.

Wilson disease, a disorder of copper metabolism, is treated with chelation therapy, which should be maintained during the pregnancy (160–165). There has been a report of 26% spontaneous abortion rate in treated and nontreated women with Wilson disease (162). As noted above, chelation therapy during pregnancy is felt to be safe and should be continued, but there are a few cases of congenital anomalies reported with the utilization of penicillamine, or newer chelators such as trientine alone or in combination with zinc (160–165).

SICKLE CELL DISEASE

Pubertal Development and Menstrual Function

Individuals with sickle cell disease and thalassemia can have endocrine complications affecting growth, sexual development, fertility, bone mineral density, diabetes, hypothyroidism, hypoparathyroidism, and hypoadrenalism (166,167). In a study of over 2,000 patients with homozygous SS disease (SS), sickle C disease (SC), sickle β^+-thalassemia (Sβ^+), and sickle β^0-thalassemia (Sβ^0), patients with SS and Sβ^0

were shorter on cross-sectional growth data than those with SC and $S\beta^+$. The weight curves followed a similar but more pronounced pattern than the heights: SS and $S\beta^0$ patients weighed less than SC and $S\beta^+$ patients. Analysis of Tanner staging showed that patients with SS and $S\beta^0$ were less sexually developed than those with $S\beta^+$ and SC disease. When age and weight were included in the statistical model, menarcheal status did not differ among the various hemoglobinopathies (168).

This notable delay in growth in sickle cell disease is associated with a delay in menarche (169–171). Mann (169) reported a mean age of menarche to be 11.6 years versus 15 years for SS disease and 11 years in girls with SC thalassemia. In a sample of Jamaican women with SC disease over 15 years of age (range, 15 to 65 years), Alleyne and co-workers (170) reported a mean age of menarche of 15.4 ± 1.7 years compared to 13.1 ± 1.7 years in a control population.

An analysis of the growth of young children with homozygous β-thalassemia treated for 36 months with deferoxamine (172) concluded that abnormalities occurred in metaphyseal growth plates in 11 of 37 patients in whom a significant decline in mean height percentile was also noted (173).

Reproductive Issues

Although an earlier study reported fetal wastage rates to be 19.7% in sickle cell disease versus 9.5% in the general population (170), maternal and perinatal morbidity and mortality among pregnant patients with sickle cell disease have been decreasing in the past two decades with the coordinated efforts of the obstetric and hematologic teams (174). Despite this effort, women with sickle cell anemia are 2.5 times more likely to bear newborns who are small for gestational age than are women with other types of sickle cell disease, sickle trait, or C trait (175). In a retrospective analysis of records of patients with the sickle hemoglobinopathies (SS and SC diseases), there was a high occurrence of preterm labor, preeclampsia, pain crisis, pulmonary complications, and cesarean sections (176). An average of 2 units of blood was required by 43.1% of the patients. Two patients with SS disease had unpreventable deaths, and there were two intrauterine fetal deaths and two neonatal deaths (perinatal mortality was 10.5% for SS disease and 2.9% for SC disease). In a report of 20 years of experience and 127 deliveries of women with sickle disease (SS or SC), there were increased risks for intrauterine growth restriction, antepartum hospital admission, and postpartum infection (177). In addition, this study found that deliveries among women with SS were more likely to be complicated by low birth weight, prematurity, and preterm labor or premature rupture of membranes as compared with deliveries among women with hemoglobin AA. This study also found no significant differences among groups of women with hemoglobin SS, SC or AA in terms of perinatal or maternal deaths (177).

The role of partial prophylactic red cell exchange transfusion in the management of pregnant patients with major sickle hemoglobinopathies is unclear (178–180). In a series of 131 patients with major sickle hemoglobinopathies studied over a 10-year period, transfusion provided a benefit in terms of lowering the number of preterm deliveries, the prevalence of low-birth-weight infants, and the perinatal death rate (178). However, a smaller series by Howard and colleagues (179) could not demonstrate a direct relationship between uteroplacental circulation (measured by Doppler ultrasound) and the use of prophylactic blood transfusion in these pregnancies. A recent Cochrane review concludes that there is not enough evidence to draw conclusions about the prophylactic use of blood transfusion for sickle cell anemia during pregnancy (180). Contraceptive choices for sickle cell disease are discussed in Chapter 20.

Major problems for women with β-thalassemia major seeking fertility treatment are hypogonadism, diabetes, and cardiomyopathy. In a study of 16 pregnancies in 11 women with β-thalassemia major, Jensen and colleagues (181) found no increased obstetric complications except a high cesarean section rate (10/13) felt to be primarily due to cephalopelvic disproportion. In a review of the literature, however, Savona-Ventura and Bonello (182) felt that pregnant mothers with thalassemia faced deleterious consequences resulting from chronic anemia, including a poor fetal outcome with greater fetal loss, preterm labor, and intrauterine growth retardation. Nonsplenectomized patients had an increased risk of a hypersplenic crisis.

RENAL DISEASE

Pubertal Development and Menstrual Function

Patients with renal disease, as with other chronic diseases, often have a delay in pubertal growth and development and menarche (183). The constellation consisting of uremic syndrome, metabolic acidosis, chronic malnutrition, chronic infection, and interference with bone growth and mineralization contributes to the growth failure.

Patients on chronic dialysis do not usually have regular menses, and most are amenorrheic and do not ovulate (184). In one study of gynecologic issues of women undergoing dialysis, 50% of these adult women were sexually active, only 36% were using contraception, and only 13% reported that their nephrologist discussed possible pregnancy and contraception during dialysis (184). In a survey of 17 premenopausal patients, only one had regular menses, six had irregular menses with occasional spotting to dysfunctional uterine bleeding, and 10 were amenorrheic. Follicle-stimulating hormone (FSH) levels were comparable to those of normal women; luteinizing hormone (LH) levels were normal or increased and showed an absence of cyclicity (185–186). Prolactin levels are often elevated in uremic patients on hemodialysis because of impaired renal clearance, and the hyperprolactinemia may contribute to persistent amenorrhea. Lim and colleagues (185) reported prolactin levels of 41.4 ± 5.8 ng/ml in uremic women versus 11.7 ± 1.1 ng/ml in controls; 7 of 17 women had galactorrhea (185). Administration of bromocriptine to three patients led to resumption of menstruation in only one.

Since the studies indicate that most women on dialysis are anovulatory despite the type of menstrual pattern, a progestin should be administered cyclically. Patients on dialysis with significant menorrhagia often require treatment with an OC.

Reproductive Issues

Most patients with chronic renal failure are anovulatory and therefore subfertile, but dialysis and transplantation may correct this problem (184,186). Sexual dysfunction and decreased libido occur in female patients undergoing dialysis, and thus the quality of sexual function should be addressed with the patient, as well as contraceptive counseling.

Pregnant women with mild renal insufficiency (serum creatinine <1.4 mg/dL) appear to have only mildly reduced fetal survival and experience no effect on the underlying disease, whereas women with moderate to severe renal insufficiency have worse pregnancy outcomes (187–189). Jones and Hayslett (190) reported that among 67 women with moderate or severe renal insufficiency, serum creatinine increased from a mean of 1.9 ± 0.8 mg/dL in early pregnancy to 2.5 ± 1.3 mg/dL in the third trimester, hypertension increased from 28% to 48%, and high-grade proteinuria from 23% to 41%. Pregnancy-related loss of renal function occurred in 43% of women, often irreversibly. For those with initial serum creatinine over 2 mg/dL, 65% had worsening of renal function, and 35% had end-stage renal failure necessitating dialysis. Preterm delivery occurred in 59% and growth retardation in 37%, but infant survival was 93%. Thus, young women with moderate to severe renal disease need sensitive counseling about the risks of undertaking pregnancy (191).

Patients on dialysis rarely conceive, but if they do, special considerations must be undertaken (192,193), including longer and more frequent periods of dialysis and strict adherence to diet. Aggressive blood pressure control and prompt diagnosis and treatment of bleeding episodes are essential, although severe complications may occur. Of dialysis patients who conceive, reports show that up to 60% will have a successful pregnancy (192,193). In a survey of US centers providing women with continuous peritoneal dialysis, 44 pregnancies were identified. Two-thirds of the pregnancies were complicated by hypertension; 48% of pregnancies resulted in surviving infants with all but one premature (194). Erythropoietin is helpful during pregnancy (192,193). Up to 46% of reported pregnancies are delivered by cesarean section, usually for worsening fetal or maternal condition (186,193). Reasons for early delivery include premature labor (often complicated with polyhydramnios), placental abruption, ruptured membranes, fetal distress, growth retardation, worsening maternal hypertension, and preeclampsia (186,192,193).

Many patients after transplantation have the return of ovulation and fertility within 6 months of a successful procedure. Pregnancies should be carefully planned. Patients should have good renal status for a minimum of 1 year after a transplant before attempting pregnancy (195,196).

Pregnancy after renal transplant is followed by the National Transplantation Pregnancy Registry, Philadelphia, PA (197). This registry has demonstrated that the vast majority of renal transplant patients and their babies do well during pregnancy. There is a small percentage of pregnancies complicated by rejection. Women with transplants due to SLE have similar outcomes to women with renal transplant due to other diseases (197). Twin and triplet gestations have been successfully reported in this registry (198).

Among women with autosomal-dominant polycystic kidney disease (ADPKD), normotensive women usually have successful, uncomplicated pregnancies, but hypertensive women are at an increased risk for fetal and maternal complications (199,200). Measures should be taken to prevent the development of preeclampsia in these women. Any patient with ADPKD should be counseled that the disease can be transmitted genetically in an autosomal-dominant pattern leading to a 50% risk of having an affected offspring.

DIABETES MELLITUS

Pubertal Development and Menstrual Function

Girls with insulin-dependent diabetes mellitus (IDDM) may have a later onset of puberty and menarche, although most do not vary from the norm. Insulin resistance develops at the time of puberty, associated with increased production of growth hormone, and thus increases in daily insulin may be required for glucose control (201–205). Puberty accelerates complications of DM, including nephropathy (206). Impaired growth, hepatomegaly, and delayed puberty have been described in children with poorly controlled diabetes (Mauriac syndrome). Other disorders such as hypothyroidism, Addison disease, and celiac disease can cause the same constellation of symptoms and occur with an increased frequency in patients with IDDM. The effect of diabetes on both longitudinal growth and specific growth phases has been studied, with conflicting results. In a longitudinal study, DuCaju and colleagues (207) concluded that diabetic children have a normal height at the onset of the disease, that final height in girls is reduced from target height, and that girls have a tendency to become obese during puberty. While this study did not find a correlation between growth velocity or attainment of final height and metabolic control, other reports have shown improvement of growth with tight control of diabetes (173,208). Tight control of diabetes is often accompanied by excessive weight gain, which may lead to disordered eating behaviors including binge eating and bulimia (209,210). As noted in Chapter 7, disordered eating is associated with menstrual irregularity.

Menstrual function in IDDM is usually normal, but irregular cycles can occur, especially in girls with elevated glycosylated hemoglobin and poor diabetic control (211,212). In a study of 24 type I diabetics, irregular cycles were associated with higher hemoglobin A1c (HbA1c) and body mass index, a lower sex hormone-binding globulin, a higher LH/FSH ratio, and polycystic ovaries on ultrasound (213).

The literature is conflicting on the effect of the menstrual cycle on glucose homeostasis. In the majority of women, there appears to be no change in insulin requirements during the menstrual cycle. However, a subgroup of patients shows worsening premenstrual hyperglycemia and significantly decreased insulin sensitivity during the luteal phase (212,214). Many women also report an increased appetite accompanied by greater food consumption during this phase. Brown and colleagues (215) reported a small series of seven diabetic girls who presented with cyclical disturbance of diabetic control before the menarche, usually hyperglycemia occurring at 21- to 34-day intervals and lasting 2 to 5 days. The precise mechanism for this disturbance is unknown. Contraceptive options for diabetics are discussed in Chapter 20.

Reproductive Issues

In a survey of infertility and pregnancy outcomes in an unselected group of women with IDDM, Kjaer and associates (216) found that the ability to conceive was normal but fewer pregnancies and fewer births per pregnancy occurred than in normal controls. Offspring of women with IDDM have a significantly lower risk of IDDM than the offspring of men with IDDM (217). In a study of 304 offspring of women with IDDM, the risk of IDDM for the offspring by age 20 was 6.0% $\pm$ 2.4% for those born at maternal ages less than 25 years, whereas the risk was significantly lower (0.7% $\pm$ 0.7%) for those born at older maternal ages ($p = 0.03$) (217).

The importance of planning pregnancies in diabetic women cannot be too strongly emphasized (218). Diabetic women need effective diabetic control, reflected in a normal glycosylated hemoglobin level, so that when they become pregnant, good metabolic control will help lessen the risk of fetal congenital malformations and prematurity (219–222). Rosenn and colleagues (223) reported that women with IDDM with initial HbA1c concentrations over 12% or median first-trimester preprandial glucose concentrations over 120 mg/dL have an increased risk of abortion and malformations.

Other Issues

In diabetic adolescents, persistent candidal vulvovaginitis is often associated with poor control. The use of topical antifungal therapy is preferred, and weekly therapy may be indicated. Oral fluconazole should be used only as needed to prevent chronic use (see Chapter 14).

Insulin dependant diabetic adolescent women should be discouraged from shaving their pubic hair. We have seen necrotizing fasciitis of the vulva in an adolescent woman in diabetic ketoacidosis who had a folliculitis after shaving her vulvar hair.

THYROID DISEASE

Pubertal Development and Menstrual Function

Thyroid disease may be associated with delayed development, precocious puberty, amenorrhea, and irregular menses (see Chapters 4 to 8) (224). Patients with acquired hypothyroidism associated with growth deceleration and retarded skeletal maturation during late childhood or early adolescence may experience rapid growth acceleration and pubertal advance when euthyroidism is restored with appropriate doses of levothyroxine (225).

Menstrual irregularities are common in hypothyroid women (226). Amenorrhea can be a consequence of hypothyroidism; prolactin levels may be elevated because of thyrotropin-releasing hormone-induced increases (227). Menstrual changes associated with hyperthyroidism are unpredictable, ranging from amenorrhea to normal cycles to dysfunctional uterine bleeding (226). These menstrual changes usually resolve when the euthyroid state is restored.

Reproductive Issues

In response to the metabolic demands of pregnancy, there are increases in the basal metabolic rate, iodine uptake, and the size of the thyroid gland (caused by hyperplasia and increased vascularity). However, a pregnant woman is euthyroid with normal levels of thyroid-stimulating hormone (TSH), free T_4, and free triiodothyronine (T_3); thyroid nodules or goiter require further evaluation. In normal pregnancies, placental transfer of TSH, T_4, and T_3 is severely limited in both directions (227).

Untreated thyrotoxicosis in pregnancy is associated with a higher risk of preeclampsia, heart failure, intrauterine growth retardation, and stillbirth (228). Heart failure is a consequence of the demands of pregnancy superimposed on the hyperdynamic cardiovascular state induced by the increased thyroid hormone (229). Although the most common cause of thyrotoxicosis in pregnancy is Graves' disease, trophoblastic disease can cause hyperthyroidism due to the cross-reactivity between TSH and human chorionic gonadotropin. The aim of treatment of Graves' disease should be to maintain mild hyperthyroidism in the mother to avoid thyroid dysfunction in the fetus (227). Treatment of maternal hyperthyroidism with propylthiouracil is preferred, as methimazole crosses the placenta more readily (230). Follow-up assessment of children whose mothers received propylthiouracil during pregnancy has indicated normal intellectual development (231). Although small amounts of antithyroid drugs are transmitted in breast milk, the amount has no impact on neonatal thyroid function, and breast-feeding can be encouraged (227). Once the pregnancy and breast-feeding are completed, definitive treatment with radioactive iodine can be undertaken, if indicated.

Preeclampsia and intrauterine growth retardation are more frequent in women with significant hypothyroidism (232). Women being treated for hypothyroidism may require a small increase in levothyroxine during pregnancy, and TSH should be monitored through the pregnancy to keep the level in the normal range (233).

Autoimmune thyroid disease is suppressed to some degree by the immunologic changes of pregnancy (234). Thus, postpartum thyroiditis is not uncommon 3 to 6 months after delivery, manifested by either hyperthyroidism or hypothyroidism (235). Women at risk for postpartum thyroiditis are those with a personal or family history of autoimmune disease or with a previous postpartum episode. The symptoms usually last 1 to 3 months, and most women return to normal thyroid function (227,236).

CONNECTIVE TISSUE DISEASES

Pubertal Development and Menstrual Function

As with other chronic diseases, delayed growth and sexual development may occur in adolescents with systemic lupus erythematosus (SLE), juvenile rheumatoid arthritis, and other connective tissue disorders (237). Rarely is there an autoimmune disorder of the ovary associated with these conditions (see Chapter 6 and 7).

Reproductive Issues

Autoimmune rheumatic diseases (ARDs) are known to occur predominantly in women. Fertility in patients with an ARD does not seem to be impaired. On the other hand, long-term uses of some of the medical treatments, specifically cyclophosphamide, are associated with gonadal dysfunction and infertility (238,239). As discussed above (see Cancer section), cyclophosphamide can adversely affect ovarian function and thus protocols utilizing pretreatment-assisted reproductive technologies and suppressive hormonal therapy should be considered (238).

It is believed that infertile women with SLE can safely undergo ovulation induction and assisted reproductive technologies (189). Spontaneous abortion, premature deliveries, and intrauterine growth retardation are frequently encountered in pregnant women with SLE. The increased incidence of fetal loss in patients with SLE has been attributed to the presence of placental vasculitis and infarctions. Medications used to treat the underlying disease and vasculitis can generally be continued through pregnancy with the exception of methotrexate and leflunamide, which should never be used during pregnancy (240). Other factors that have been associated with fetal loss are maternal autoantibody responses, including immune complex deposition, and the cross-reaction of lymphocytotoxic antibodies with trophoblasts (189,240,241). More recently SLE has not been perceived as an unacceptable high-risk condition of the mother or baby as long as careful monitoring of both is carried out (242). Women with renal lupus have higher risk (see above Renal section) (188). Neonatal lupus syndrome and cardiac conduction defects may occur.

With systemic sclerosis (scleroderma), the reports of pregnancies are few. An increased incidence of maternal complications of hypertension and preeclampsia and perinatal mortality in scleroderma has been reported (243,244).

Neither rheumatoid arthritis nor scleroderma seem to be exacerbated by pregnancy (243–245). Symptoms from ankylosing spondylitis either stay the same or are slightly aggravated during the course of pregnancy. Patients with psoriatic arthritis have been reported to improve or even have remission of symptoms during pregnancy (246).

When evaluating all women with connective tissue disorders, the clinician should be aware that there appears to be an increased risk of premature birth (OR 3.98), low birth weight (OR 5.8), and small for gestational age infants (OR 1.6) (247). Perinatal mortality, including stillbirths and early neonatal deaths, were also increased in infants of women with connective tissue disease (247).

CARDIOVASCULAR DISEASE

Pubertal Development and Menstrual Function

Significant congenital cardiac anomalies commonly lead to decreased height and weight, with weight more often retarded than height. The retardation of growth seems to be more profound in early childhood than in adolescence. Skeletal growth and maturation are also delayed. The more severe and prolonged the cardiac failure, the greater is the effect on growth and puberty.

Reproductive Issues

Women with heart disease on anticoagulation therapy are at increased risk for hemorrhagic corpus luteal cyst formation and for menorrhagia (see Chapters 8 and 18). If there is no contraindication, these individuals may benefit from the utilization of low-dose combination hormonal contraceptive therapy (see Chapter 20). For adolescents on anticoagulants not responding to combination hormonal therapies, GnRH agonists with norethindrone add-back has been an option.

Pregnancy is associated with major hemodynamic changes in the cardiovascular system that can contribute to greater morbidity and mortality in women with underlying heart disease (248). Knowledge of the specific congenital cardiac lesion is essential (249–252).

Pregnancy in Marfan syndrome is associated with several problems, including the potential for catastrophic aortic dissection and the 50% risk for having a child with the syndrome. Gestation seems to be safer in women without preexisting cardiovascular disease; a preconceptual transesophageal echocardiogram is helpful in delineating aortic disease. A preconception aortic diameter of 40 mm or more, progression of dilatation, and decreased cardiac function are risk factors in pregnancy for women with Marfan syndrome (253). However, the absence of any vascular pathology does not preclude complications. The prophylactic use of β-blockers may help in preventing aortic dilatation (254).

Pregnancies complicated by hypertension require a well-formulated management plan. At the onset of pregnancy, women should be classified as having low-risk or high-risk hypertension, with the latter requiring medication. Those classified as low risk should have a favorable perinatal outcome. Both classes of hypertensive disorders are at risk for preeclampsia (255).

COAGULATION DISORDERS

Pubertal Development and Menstrual Function

Rigorous double-blind trials have not been conducted in adolescents with known or potential coagulation disorders to define the best medical management to control menstrual bleeding. For adolescents with von Willebrand disease (vWD) and other factor deficiencies, consultation with a hematologist is critical in making a plan for menarche and subsequent cycles (256–260). In addition to the use of desmopressin and coagulation factors, most girls benefit from the prophylactic management of menses using low-dose cyclic combined OCs or patches. We typically prescribe OCs with moderate progestin potency and low-dose estrogen to lessen the chance of breakthrough bleeding (e.g., 0.3 mg norgestrel [or 0.15 mg levonorgestrel] and 30 μg ethinyl estradiol).

Induction of amenorrhea may be the best option for patients with recurrent heavy bleeding and an underlying hematologic disorder (see Table 23-1) (39,258). For individuals with bleeding refractory to combination estrogen and progestin or progestin therapy, GnRH agonist therapy may be indicated. This therapy requires advanced planning, as suppression with a GnRH agonist takes approximately 3 weeks (40). In the case of acute bleeding, stability can be gained with conventional hormone (OC) therapy, and long-term prevention can be initiated with a GnRH agonist (39). Conventional OC therapy can subsequently be discontinued with a limited, if any, withdrawal bleed (39). The use of long-term GnRH agonist therapy (i.e., >6 months) with estrogen/progestin or norethindrone acetate add-back treatment may be a long-term solution for patients with an underlying coagulopathy and recurrent life-threatening dysfunctional uterine bleeding (DUB). Rau and Muram (261) reported the successful use of medroxyprogesterone and intranasal GnRH agonist in controlling severe DUB in a young woman with thrombotic thrombocytopenic purpura and abnormal liver function tests.

Oral anticoagulation is not a contraindication to OCs. OCs reduce the chance of serious hemorrhage during ovulation and lessen the risk of unplanned pregnancy (262).

Reproductive Issues

In a retrospective review over 30 years (256), the pregnancies of 18 obligate carriers of hemophilia A, five carriers of Christmas disease, and eight patients with vWD were reported. In 14 pregnancies in seven patients with vWD, there were four primary and four secondary postpartum hemorrhages and one perineal hematoma. These problems occurred despite the endogenous rise in coagulation factor VIIIc seen with pregnancy. In 43 pregnancies in the carriers of hemophilia A and Christmas disease, there were five postpartum hemorrhages and one perineal hematoma (256). While there is significant increased risk for postpartum hemorrhage, patients with vWD should not be discouraged from undertaking pregnancy (263).

SEIZURE DISORDERS

Pubertal Development and Menstrual Function

Although epilepsy is a common neurologic disorder that affects 1 in every 100 individuals, studies of gynecologic issues in young women with seizure disorders are few. Although there are some reports of menstrual dysfunction, it is difficult to establish whether the etiology is the neurologic disorder, its treatment, or both. Some antiepileptic drugs will reduce levels of physiologic ovarian sex steroid hormones and may also reduce the efficacy of contraceptive steroids, both of which can cause irregular bleeding (see also Chapter 20) (264). Higher incidences of polycystic ovary disease and hypogonadotropic hypogonadism have been suggested (265–267). Phenytoin has been reported to cause hirsutism, and valproate has been reported to be associated with polycystic ovary disease in some but not all studies (see Chapter 9). Seizure frequency may increase in the luteal or menstrual phase of the cycle (268), and thus suppression of menses and hormonal fluctuations may be helpful (see Tables 23-1 and 23-2).

Reproductive Issues

Women with epilepsy have a reduction in fertility (269–271), the cause of which is felt to be multifactorial. One study suggested that persons with epilepsy were less likely to marry and to have offspring (272). Women with epilepsy account for approximately 0.5% of all pregnancies (273). Clinicians and their female patients with epilepsy face difficult decisions. Antiepileptic drugs, including valproate and carbamazepine, increase the risk of major malformations, minor anomalies, neonatal hemorrhage, and delayed fetal growth and development. The North American Antiepileptic Drug Pregnancy Registry reports a 12% rate of major malformations after first trimester exposure to phenobarbital and an 8.8% rate after first trimester exposure to valproate as compared to 1.62% of pregnancies with no antiepileptic drug exposures

(264,274–276). Updates of the finding from the Antiepileptic Drug Pregnancy Registry can be located at: http://www.massgeneral.org/aed/AED_findings.htm (accessed July 23, 2004).

Maternal seizures also appear to be disadvantageous to the fetus, increasing the risk of miscarriage, premature labor, intracranial hemorrhage, and, perhaps, developmental or learning difficulties. There have been improved pregnancy outcomes in epileptic women with improved medical therapies during pregnancy (277). Clinicians caring for pregnant women with epilepsy are therefore faced with a dilemma and must carefully chart a middle ground, providing effective seizure control while minimizing fetal exposure to antiepileptic drugs (264,278–279).

NEUROLOGIC ABNORMALITIES

Upper and lower urogenital tract dysfunction often occurs in adolescents with neurologic deficits, including those with central nervous system lesions (developmental delay and/or cerebral palsy), spinal cord lesions from congenital anomalies (spina bifida or sacral agenesis), or lesions acquired from trauma or neoplasm.

Pubertal Development and Menstrual Function

Major concerns in adolescents with these disorders include bladder and bowel control, management of menses, and sexual function. In a study of 25 patients with spina bifida, Furman and Mortimer (280) reported an earlier mean age of menarche (10.3 years) for these patients compared to mothers (11.9 years) and unaffected sisters (12.3 years). There was no difference with respect to dysmenorrhea, premenstrual syndrome (PMS) (see Chapter 11), and irregular menses.

If perineal hygiene becomes a problem, induction of amenorrhea may be indicated (see Table 23-1). Although some have suggested endometrial ablation as an alternative to hysterectomy for severe problems with menstrual bleeding or hygiene (281), we recommend medical management before surgical intervention is undertaken.

The gynecologic examination is often frightening to adolescents who is developmentally disabled, as she may not fully understand the importance of such an examination. Presenting the examination in a relaxed setting, as recommended with the prepubertal population, is useful with this group as well. The use of smaller swabs and instruments is also recommended. Rectoabdominal examination, pelvic ultrasound, and occasionally examination under anesthesia may be utilized (see Chapter 1 and Appendix 1 for resources).

Calendars to document menstrual problems, including irregularity and behavioral symptoms (tantrums, crying spells, self-abusive behavior, and seizures) suggestive of PMS or dysmenorrhea, are essential to provide optimal care to developmentally disabled young women. Nonsteroidal antiinflammatory drugs are first-line treatment, followed by the use of therapies for inducing amenorrhea (see Table 23-1 and Chapter 20).

Sexual, Gynecologic, and Reproductive Issues

It is important to address issues of sexual function and sexuality, when appropriate, with adolescents and their parents. For adolescents with mental retardation, special social and sexuality programs have been developed. For example, the Edwards assessment of social–sexual skills has photo cards that allow the student to learn the concepts of private and public places for behaviors (282,283).

In a study of female adolescents with spina bifida in Louisiana, the sexuality dimension of the self-image profile was significantly below normal compared to the other 10 dimensions that were normal (284). In a retrospective interview, 24 of 35 female patients aged 16 years or older with myelomeningocele were sexually active, and 12 had become pregnant (285). In Furman and Mortimer's study (280), only four of 20 young women with spina bifida were offered family planning counseling, although 13 desired it.

Individuals with spina bifida may present with uterine, cervical and/or vaginal prolapse. If the young woman is symptomatic, the pelvic structures can be supported with a pessary. Alternatively a suspension procedure can be performed, sewing the uterus and cervix to the sacrum with a mesh sling.

With more aggressive surgical management, patients with spina bifida may now reach adulthood and achieve pregnancy (285,286). Preconceptual genetic counseling and folic acid high dose (4mg) supplementation should be strongly recommended. Special care is needed during pregnancy in the management of urologic, obstetric, neurologic, and anesthetic problems. Compromise of urologic function may occur, including obstruction of the urinary tract (287). The incidence of preterm labor is increased. Although there is a risk of a contracted pelvis, vaginal delivery should be allowed if the head engages normally and the labor pattern proceeds appropriately.

Cerebral peritoneal shunts may malfunction and cause focal neurologic problems. A pelvic mass or fluid collection may result from pelvic adhesions and loculated collections of CSF. In pregnant patients with a shunt, vaginal delivery is preferable, and pushing during the second stage is not contraindicated (288). Peripartum prophylactic antibiotics may be indicated, and special care is exercised if epidural analgesia and cesarean section are necessary (288).

MENTAL HEALTH DISORDERS

Approximately 22% of Americans will experience a psychiatric disorder within the span of their lifetime. Anxiety disorders will afflict some 14% of the general population, and depression 8% to 10%. These numbers increase when concomitant illicit drug abuse is included.

Pubertal Development and Menstrual Function

Research has suggested that there is an impaired response of FSH secreting pituitary cells in girls with mental retardation going through initial pubertal stages (289). In addition, adolescents and women taking psychotropic drugs such as phenothiazines, tricyclic antidepressants, or risperidone may have elevated prolactin levels, leading to galactorrhea, anovulation, and amenorrhea (see Chapter 7). OCs are beneficial in reversing amenorrhea, irregular anovulatory bleeding, and hypoestrogenization resulting from either medications or from hypothalamic-pituitary dysfunction.

Contraception

Barriers to effective use of contraception by mentally ill patients are sometimes magnified by their inability to establish reliable, long-term approaches to pregnancy prevention. A contraceptive program tailored to the individual needs of patients is essential. Whereas laws vary from state to state, the criteria for informed consent always should include an explanation of risks, benefits, and alternatives, as well as a determination of whether the patient is competent to understand the informed consent. Mental and reproductive health professionals must collaborate with legal professionals in making this determination.

Several factors need to be addressed in choosing a specific hormonal preparation. Hepatic enzyme induction by some antiepileptic agents can result in increased contraceptive failures with OCs, and women taking such agents may do better with an alternative contraceptive method such as depot medroxyprogesterone acetate (Depo-Provera) or a higher dose of OCs (see Chapter 20) (290). In the institutionalized patient, who is accustomed to long-term drug regimens, an OC, patch, or vaginal ring would be an appropriate choice in the absence of risk factors. Compliance is more difficult to ensure in the outpatient psychiatric patient. In these situations, the progestin-only injectables or implants may be considered. However, the side effect of irregular bleeding may be perceived as a sign of "ill health" and less tolerated in these women (291). Some women who use progestin-only preparations may experience depressed mood. To alleviate confusion between an underlying depressive condition and the possible medication effect, we may initiate a trial of a progestin-only pill for a month or longer before using an injectable or implant. The need to take oral medication at the same time every day and the use of condoms must be emphasized.

Reproductive Issues

Areas that should be included in discussions with patients considering pregnancy and, if possible, their partners are heritability of the underlying mental health disorder, risks during pregnancy, and risks during the postpartum period (292). Although women with serious mental illness have normal fertility rates, multiple risk factors and a paucity of emotional and economic support during the initial phases of parenthood may be present (293). These risks are significantly multiplied when one factors in the issues of pregnancy in adolescence (294) (see Chapter 21).

Although pregnancy is often believed to be a time of emotional well-being, many women develop or have a recurrence of psychiatric illness during this time. The risks associated with not treating a woman during pregnancy are potentially substantial and must be weighed against the risks of exposing the fetus to potentially teratogenic medications. Studies have suggested a relative safety of use of tricyclic antidepressants and selective serotonin reuptake inhibitors (SSRIs) during pregnancy (295–297). Data on neuroleptics, lithium, and benzodiazepines are mixed but suggest a small but increased risk of congenital malformations if these drugs are used in the first trimester of pregnancy (295,298–303).

STERILIZATION

Sterilization of young nulliparous women arises on rare occasions as an adjunct to the management of certain chronic conditions such as cardiac, pulmonary, and renal impairment, genetic diseases, and neuromuscular and severe seizure disorders, as well as in women with substantial developmental delays. Use of reversible contraception may become a problem because the choice is limited by numerous contraindications and patient adherence. Consequently, these patients may resort to less than optimal methods of birth control, even though their needs may be as real as those of healthy teenagers. Frequently, these young women develop tremendous anxiety regarding pregnancy because it could result in deterioration of their medical condition or in the birth of a baby affected by a genetically transmitted disease or teratogenic medications.

Involuntary sterilization of mentally retarded individuals should be considered only if they do not retain the capacity for reproductive decision making, the ability to raise a child, or the capacity to provide valid consent to sexual relations and in whom temporary contraceptive management is not an option (304,305). Guidelines for sterilization proposed by Paransky and Zurawin are shown in Table 23-3 (306). It is recommended that a legal consultation be obtained to guide the process. This challenging legal and ethical situation is addressed further in Chapter 26.

In a review of patients undergoing tubal ligation from 1977 to 1984 at Children's Hospital Boston, there were 27 patients ranging in age from 15 to 28 years (mean, 21.8 years) (307). Tubal ligations were carried out by laparoscopy: 19 with Falope rings, six with Hulka clips, and two by electrocoagulation and division. General anesthesia was used in 25 patients and local anesthesia in two patients. There were two major postoperative complications, both of which involved excessive bleeding in patients who were anticoagulated. The first patient had bleeding from the necrosis of the Falope ring. Due to that complication, Hulka clips were substituted for Falope rings in the second patient with a bleeding complication. However, this patient also

TABLE 23-3. *Proposed guidelines for sterilization by Paransky and Zurawin.*[a]

The individual is unable to participate in consensual intercourse.

Intellectual, psychological and physical ability to raise children is irreversibly impaired.

The individual is fertile and postmenarchal.

Pregnancy or preserving reproductive potential will significantly increase the difficulty of caring for the patient.

Pregnancy represents a serious, objective physical and/or psychological risk.

Method of medical treatment is consistent with standard medical practice, including the notion that appropriate reversible alternatives have proven unworkable or inapplicable.

Proponents of sterilization are seeking sterilization in good faith and primary concern is for best interest of the respondent rather than their own convenience or the convenience of the public.

---

[a]From: Paransky OI, Zurawin RK. Management of menstrual problems and contraception in adolescents with mental retardation: A medical, legal, and ethical review with new suggested guidelines. *J Pediatr Adolesc Gynecol* 2003;16:223; with permission.

developed postoperative bleeding that was found to be from the infraumbilical trocar site. Since the report of that study, we predominantly use Falope rings for laparoscopic tubal ligation due to the improved success with pregnancy after tubal reversal if the patient should desire fertility at a future time.

The issue of sterilization of young women may represent an uncomfortable subject for the gynecologist, as well as for patients and their families. With modern medical advances in the treatment of these diseases, as well as in the refinement of the progestin-only injectables, the requests are decreasing. However, in those few situations when a mature young woman unwilling to take the risks or comply with the physical restrictions of a high-risk pregnancy requests sterilization, that request needs to be respected. Consultation with the primary provider who is well acquainted with her medical and emotional status is essential. Even if the physician feels that sterilization is the optimal contraceptive modality, the patient should never be rushed into making this decision. In most instances, it is wise to have the patient seen by a mental health professional who can assist with the evaluation and provide subsequent emotional support (308) (see Chapter 26).

The procedure should be performed when the primary disease is under optimal control. The choice of the technique utilized depends on the gynecologist, who should opt for a method requiring the shortest anesthesia time with which he or she feels comfortable.

SUMMARY

Given recent advances in the health care field, persons with chronic diseases are experiencing improved life expectancies. More young women with chronic diseases are now dealing with gynecologic, sexuality, and fertility issues. These concerns present new challenges to health care providers. Further experience and study are needed to improve long-term reproductive health for this unique group of patients.

REFERENCES

1. Ries LAG, Eisner MP, Kosary CL, et al. *SEER Cancer Statistics Review, 1975–2001,* National Cancer Institute, Bethesda, MD, http://seer.cancer.gov/csr/1975_2001/, 2004.
2. Pui CH, Cheng C, Leung W, et al. Extended follow-up of long-term survivors of childhood acute lymphoblastic leukemia. *N Engl J Med* 2003;349:640.
3. Nicholson HS, Byrne J. Fertility and pregnancy after treatment for cancer during childhood or adolescence. *Cancer* 1993;71:3392.
4. Stillman RJ, Schinfeld JS, Schiff I, et al. Ovarian failure in long-term survivors of childhood malignancy. *Am J Obstet Gynecol* 1981;139:62.
5. Damewood MD, Grochow LB. Prospects for fertility after chemotherapy or radiation for neoplastic disease. *Fertil Steril* 1986;45:443.
6. Bookman MA, Longo DL, Young RC. Late complications of curative treatment in Hodgkin's disease. *JAMA* 1988;260:680.
7. Cicognani A, Pasini A, Pession A, et al. Gonadal function and pubertal development after treatment of a childhood malignancy. *J Pediatr Endocrinol Metab* 2003;16:321–326.
8. Thibaud E, Ramirez M, Brauner R, et al. Preservation of ovarian function by ovarian transposition performed before pelvic irradiation during childhood *J Pediatr* 1992;121:880.
9. Gradishar WJ, Schilsky RL. Ovarian function following radiation and chemotherapy for cancer. *Semin Oncol* 1989;16:425.
10. Damewood MD. What factors underlie premature ovarian failure? *Contemp Obstet Gynecol* 1990:31.
11. Hall JE, Martin KA, Whitney HA, et al. Potential for gonadotropin-releasing hormone in long-term female survivors of cranial tumors. *J Clin Endocrinol Metab* 1994;79:1166.
12. Oberfield SE, Soranno D, Nirenberg A, et al. Age at onset of puberty following high-dose central nervous system radiation therapy. *Arch Pediatr Adolesc Med* 1996;150:589.
13. Meadows AT. Follow-up and care of childhood cancer survivors. *Hosp Pract* 1991;26:99.
14. Weil Benarush H, Solt L, Lightman A, et al. Male gonadal function in survivors of childhood Hodgkin and non-Hodgkin lymphoma. *Pediatr Hematol Oncol* 2000;17:239.
15. Kenney LB, Laufer MR, Grant FD, et al. High risk of infertility and long term gonadal damage in males treated with high dose cyclophosphamide for sarcoma during childhood. *Cancer* 2001;91:613.
16. Laufer MR. Reproductive issues for cancer patients/survivors. *J Clin Oncol* 1999;17:2631.
17. Byrne J. Infertility and premature menopause in childhood cancer survivors. *Med Pediatr Oncol* 1999;33:24.
18. Watson AR, Taylor J, Rance CP, et al. Gonadal function in women treated with cyclophosphamide for childhood nephrotic syndromea: a long-term follow-up study. *Fertil Steril* 1986;46:331.
19. Rivkees SA, Crawford JD. The relationship of gonadal activity and chemotherapy-induced gonadal damage. *JAMA* 1988;259:2123.
20. Clark ST, Radford JA, Crowther D, et al. Gonadal function following chemotherapy for Hodgkin's disease: a comparative study of MVPP and a seven-drug hybrid regimen. *J Clin Oncol* 1995;13:134.
21. Schilsky RL, Schering RJ, Hubbard SM. Long-term follow-up of ovarian function in women treated with MOPP chemotherapy for Hodgkin's disease. *Am J Med* 1981;71:552.
22. Whitehead G, Shalet SM, Blackledge G, et al. The effect of combination chemotherapy on ovarian function in women treated for Hodgkin's disease. *Cancer* 1983;52:988.
23. Shalet SM. Effects of cancer chemotherapy on gonadal function of patients. *Cancer Treat* 1980;7:141.
24. Quigley C, Cowell C, Jimenez M, et al. Normal or early development of puberty despite gonadal damage in children treated for acute lymphoblastic leukemia. *N Engl J Med* 1989;321:143.
25. Dacou-Voutetakis C, Kitra V, Grafakos S, et al. Auxologic data and hormonal profile in long-term survivors of childhood acute lymphoid leukemia. *Am J Pediatr Hematol Oncol* 1993;15:227.
26. Horning SJ, Hoppe RT, Kaplan HS, et al. Female reproductive potential after treatment for Hodgkin's disease. *N Engl J Med* 1981;304:1377.

27. Orrin TTS, Shostak CA, Donaldson SS. Gonadal status and reproductive function following treatment for Hodgkin's disease in childhood: the Stanford experience. *Int J Radiat Oncol Biol Phys* 1990;19:873.
28. Byrne J, Fears TR, Gail MH. Early menopause in long-term survivors of cancer during adolescence. *Am J Obstet Gynecol* 1992;166:788.
29. Mills JL, Fears TR, Robinson LL, et al. Menarche in a cohort of 188 long-term survivors of acute lymphoblastic leukemia. *J Pediatr* 1997;131:598.
30. Sanders JE, Buckner CD, Leonard JM, et al. Late effects on gonadal function of cyclophosphamide, total body irradiation and marrow transplantation. *Transplantation* 1983;36:252.
31. Cohen MT, Van-Lint A, Lavagetto S, et al. Pubertal development and fertility in children after bone marrow transplantation. *Bone Marrow Transplant* 1991;8[Suppl]:16.
32. Spinelli S, Chiodi S, Bacigalupo A, et al. Ovarian recovery after total body irradiation and allogeneic bone marrow transplantation: long-term follow up of 79 females. *Bone Marrow Transplant.* 1994;14:373.
33. Ogilby-Stuart AL, Clark DJ, Wallace WHB, et al. Endocrine deficit after fractionated total body irradiation. *Arch Dis Child* 1992;67:1107.
34. Schubert MA, Sullivan KM, Schubert MM, et al. Gynecological abnormalities following allogenic bone marrow transplantation. *Bone Marrow Transplant* 1990;5:425.
35. Vergauwen P, Ferster A, Valsamis J, et al. Primary ovarian failure after prepubertal marrow transplant in a girl. *Lancet* 1994;343:125.
36. Thibaud E, Rodriguez-Macias K, Trivin C, et al. Ovarian function after bone marrow transplantation during childhood. *Bone Marrow Transplant* 1998;21:287.
37. Sarafoglou K, Boulad F, Gillio A, et al. Gonadal function after bone marrow transplanation for acute leukemia during childhood. *J Pediatr* 1997;130:210.
38. DeSanctis V, Galimberti M, Lucarelli G, et al. Gonadal function after allogenic bone marrow transplantation for thalassemia. *Arch Dis Child* 1991;66:517.
39. Laufer MR, Rein MS. Treatment of abnormal uterine bleeding with gonadotropin-releasing hormone analogues. *Clin Obstet Gynecol* 1993;36:678.
40. Laufer, MR, Townsend NL, Parsons KE, et al. Inducing amenorrhea during bone marrow transplantation: A pilot study of leuprolide acetate. *J Reprod Med* 1997;42:537.
41. Hillard PJ. Therapeutic amenorrhea. *J Pediatr Hematol Oncol* 1999;21:350.
42. Thomas SL, Ellertson C. Nuisance or natural and healthy: should monthly menstruation be optimal for women? *Lancet* 2000;355:922.
43. Sulak PJ, Kuehl TJ, Ortiz M, et al. Acceptance of altering the standard 21-day/7-day oral contraceptive regimen to delay menses and reduce hormone withdrawal symptoms. *Am J Obstet Gynecol* 2002;186:1142.
44. Kline RM, Fennewald L, Vore M, et al. Oral contraceptives: a cause of huperbilirubinemia in stem cell transplant patients. *J Pediatr Hematol Oncol* 1999;21:436.
45. Hayes E, Rock JA. Treatment of vaginal agglutination associated with chronic graft-versus-host disease. *Fertil Steril* 2002;78:1125.
46. Spiryda LB, Laufer MR, Soiffer RJ, et al. Graft-versus-host disease of the vulva and/or vagina: diagnosis and treatment. *Biol Blood Marrow Transplantation* 2003;9:760.
47. Lefloch O, Conaldson SS, Kaplan HS. Pregnancy following oophoropexy and total nodal irradiation in women with Hodgkin's disease. *Cancer* 1976;38:2263.
48. Byrne J, Mulvihill JJ. Long-term survivors of childhood and adolescent cancer: their fertility and the health of their offspring. In: Plowman PN, McElwain IT, Meadows AT, eds. *Complications of cancer management.* Gunford, UK: Butterworth Scientific Ltd, 1991.
49. Hadar H, Loven D. An evaluation of lateral and medial transposition of the ovaries out of radiation fields. *Cancer* 1994;74:779.
50. Laufer MR, Billett AL, Diller L, et al. A new technique for laparoscopic prophylactic oophoropexy before craniospinal irradiation in children with medulloblastoma. *Adolesc Pediatr Gynecol* 1995;8:77.
51. Livesey EA, Brook CGD. Gonadal dysfunction after treatment of intracranial tumours. *Arch Dis Child* 1988;63:495.
52. Molpus K, Wedergren J, Carlson M. Robotically assisted endoscopic ovarian transposition. *JSLS* 2003;7:59.
53. Kuohung W, Laufer MR, Marcus KJ, et al. Ovarian function in pediatric brain cancer survivors after laparoscopic oophoropexy. *Fertil Steril* 2003;80:S90.

54. Laufer MR, Upton J, Schuster S, et al. Axillary oophoropexy for girls receiving abdominal /pelvic radiation with over 20 year follow-up. *Fertil Steril* 2001;76:S253.
55. Oktay K, Economos K, Kan M, et al. Endocrine function and oocyte retrieval after autologous transplantation of ovarian cortical strips to the forearm. *JAMA* 2001;286:1490.
56. Oktay K, Buyuk E, Rosenwaks Z, et al. A technique for transplantation of ovarian cortical strips to the forearm. *Fertil Steril* 2003;80:193.
57. Chapman RM, Sutcliffe SB. Protection of ovarian function by oral contraceptive use in women receiving chemotherapy for Hodgkin's disease. *Blood* 1981;58:851.
58. Blumenfeld Z, Avivi I, Linn S, et al. Prevention of irreversible chemotherapy-induced ovarian damage in young women with lymphoma by gonadotropin-releasing hormone agonist in parallel to chemotherapy. *Hum Reprod* 1996;19:1620.
59. Blumenfeld Z, Avivi I, Ritter M, et al. Preservation of fertility and ovarian function and minimizing chemotherapy-induced gonadotoxicity in young women. *J Soc Gynecol Invest* 1999;6:229.
60. Blumenfeld Z. Ovarian rescue/protection from chemotherapeutic agents. *J Soc Gynecol Investig* 2001;8:S60.
61. Pereyra Pancheco B, Mendez Ribas JM, Milone G, et al. Use of GnRH analogs for functional protection of the ovary and preservation of fertility during cancer treatment in adolescents: a preliminary report. *Gynecol Oncol* 2001;81:391.
62. Gook DA, Osborn SM, Bourne H, et al. Fertilization of human oocytes following cryopreservation; normal karyotypes and absence of stray chromosomes. *Hum Reprod* 1994;9:684.
63. Gook DA, Scheiwe MC, Osborn SM, et al. Intracytoplasmic sperm injection and embryo development of human oocytes cryopreserved using 1,2-propanediol. *Hum Reprod* 1995;10:2637.
64. Toth TL, Lanzendorf SE, Sandow BA, et al. Cryopreservation of human prophase I oocytes collected from unstimulated follicles. Fertilization and *in vitro* development of cryopreserved human prophase I oocytes. *Fertil Steril* 1994;61:896.
65. Porcu E, Fabbri R, Seracchioli R, et al. Birth of a healthy female after intracytoplasmic sperm injection of cryopreserved human oocytes. *Fertil Steril* 1997;68:724.
66. Polak de Fried E, Notrica J, Rubinstein M, et al. Pregnancy after human donor oocyte cryopreservation and thaw in association with intracytoplasmic sperm injection in a patient with ovarian failure. *Fertil Steril* 1998;69:555.
67. Fabbri R, Porcu E, Marsella T, et al. Human oocyte cryopreservation: new perspectives regarding oocyte survival. *Hum Reprod* 2001;16:411.
68. Porcu E. Oocyte freezing. *Semin Reprod Med* 2001;19:221.
69. Oktay K, Newton H, Aubard Y, et al. Cryopreservation of immature human oocytes and ovarian tissue: an emerging technology? *Fertil Steril* 1998;69:1.
70. Gosden RG. Low temperature storage and grafting of human ovarian tissue. *Mol Cell Endcrinol* 2000;163:125.
71. Revel A, Koler M, Simon A, et al. Oocyte collection during cryopreservation of the ovarian cortex. *Fertil Steril* 2003;79:1237.
72. Oktay K, Karlikaya G. Ovarian function after transplantation of frozen, banked autologous ovarian tissue. *N Engl J Med* 2000;342:1919.
73. Oktay K. Ovarian tissue cryopreservation and transplantation: preliminary findings and implications for cancer patients. *Hum Reprod Update* 2001;7:526.
74. Byrne J, Mulvihill JJ, Myers MIL et al. Effects of treatment of fertility in long-term survivors of childhood or adolescent cancer. *N Engl J Med* 1987;317:1315.
75. Aisner J, Wiernik PH, Pearl E. Pregnancy outcome in patients treated for Hodgkin's disease. *J Clin Oncol* 1993;1:507.
76. Schimmer A, Quatermain M, Imrie K, et al. Ovarian function after autologous bone marrow transplantation. *J Clin Oncol* 1998;16:2359.
77. Salooja N, Szydlo RM, Socie G, et al. Pregnancy outcomes after peripheral blood or bone marrow transplantation: a retrospective survey. *Lancet* 2001;358:271.
78. Lacher MJ, Toner K. Pregnancies and menstrual function before and after combined radiation (RT) and chemotherapy (TVPP) for Hodgkin's disease. *Cancer Invest* 1986;4:93.
79. Check JH, Chase JS. Ovulation induction in hypergonadotropic amenorrhea with estrogen and human menopausal gonadotropin therapy. *Fertil Steril* 1984;42:919.
80. Davis OK, Ravnikar VA. Ovulation induction with clomiphene citrate in a woman with premature ovarian failure: A case report. *J Reprod Med* 1988;33:559.

81. Chatterjee R, Mills W, Katz M, et al. Induction of ovarian function by using short-term human menopausal gonadotrophin in patients with ovarian failure following cytotoxic chemotherapy for haematological malignancy. *Leuk Lymph* 1993;10:383.
82. Dein RA, Mennuti M, Kovach P, et al. The reproductive potential of young men and women with Hodgkin's disease. *Obstet Gynecol Surv* 1984;39:474.
83. Dodds L, Marrett ED, Tomkins DJ, et al. Case-control study of congenital anomalies in children of cancer patients. *BMJ* 1993;307:164.
84. Byrne J, Rasmussen SA, Steinhorn SC, et al. Genetic disease in offspring of long-term survivors of childhood and adolescent cancer. *Am J Hum Genet* 1998;62:45.
85. Green DM, Fiorello A, Zevon MA, et al. Birth defects and childhood cancer. *Arch Pediatr Adolesc Med* 1997;151:379.
86. Green DM, Aevon MA, Lowrie G, et al. Congenital anomalies in children of patients who received chemotherapy for cancer in childhood and adolescence. *N Engl J Med* 1991;325:141.
87. Smith MB, Xue H, Takahashi H, et al. Iodine 131 thyroid ablation in female children and adolescents: long-term risks of infertility and birth defects. *Ann Surg Oncol* 1994;1:128.
88. Li FP, Gimbrere K, Gelber RD, et al. Outcome of pregnancy in survivors of Wilms' tumor. *JAMA* 1987;257:216.
89. Green D, Peabody E, Nan B, et al. Pregnancy outcome after treatment for Wilms' tumor: a report from the National Wilms Tumor Study Group. *J Clin Oncol* 2002;20:2506.
90. Byrne J, Mulvihill JJ, Connelly RR, et al. Reproductive problems and birth defects in survivors of Wilms' tumor and their relatives. *Med Pediatr Oncol* 1988;16:233.
91. Hawkins MM, Smith FA. Pregnancy outcomes in childhood cancer survivors: probable effects of abdominal irradiation. *Int J Cancer* 1989;43:399.
92. Hinterberger-Fisher M, Kier P, Kahls P. Fertility, pregnancies and offspring complications after bone marrow transplantation. *Bone Marrow Transplant* 1991;7:5.
93. Russell JA, Hanley DA. Full-term pregnancy after allogeneic transplantation for leukemia in a patient with oligomenorrhea. *Bone Marrow Transplant* 1989;4:579.
94. Miliken S, Powles R, Parikh M, et al. Successful pregnancy following bone marrow transplantation for leukemia. *Bone Marrow Transplant* 1990;5:135.
95. Chao HT, Wang PH, Yuan CC, et al. Successful pregnancy in a woman with acute myeloid leukemia treated with high-dose whole-body irradiation. *J Reprod Med* 1998;43:703.
96. The Ethics Committee, American Society for Reproductive Medicine, Birmingham, Alabama. Family members as gamete donors and surrogates. *Fertil Steril* 2003;80:1124.
97. Mike V, Meadows AT, D'Angio GJ. Incidence of second malignant neoplasms in children: results of an international study. *Lancet* 1982;2:1326.
98. Coleman CN, Kaplan HS, Cox R, et al. Leukaemias, non-Hodgkin's lymphoma and solid tumours in patients treated for Hodgkin's disease. *Cancer Surv* 1982;1:733.
99. Boivin IF, Hutchison GB, Lyden M, et al. Second primary cancers following treatment of Hodgkin's disease. *J Natl Cancer Inst* 1984;72:233.
100. Tucker MA, Meadows AT, Boice JD Jr, et al. Leukemia after therapy with alkylating agents for childhood cancer. *J Natl Cancer Inst* 1987;78:459.
101. Bhatia S, Robison LL, Oberlin O, et al. Breast cancer and other second neoplasms after childhood Hodgkin's disease. *N Engl J Med* 1996;334:745.
102. Diller L, Medeiros Nancarrow C, Shaffer K, et al. Breast cancer screening in women previously treated for Hodgkin's disease: a prospective cohort study. *J Clin Oncol* 2002;20:2085.
103. Travis LB, Hill DA, Dores GM, et al. Breast cancer following radiotherapy and chemotherapy among young women with Hodgkin Disease. *JAMA* 2003;290:465.
104. Yawn BP, Wollan P, Kurland MJ, et al. Longitudinal study of asthma prevalence in a community population of school age children. *J Pediatr* 2002;140:576.
105. Mannino DM, Homa DM, Akinbami LJ, et al. Surveillance for asthma—United States, 1980–1999. *MMWR Surveil Summ* 2002;51:1.
106. Tan KS. Premenstrual asthma. Epidemiology, pathogenesis and treatment. *Drugs* 2001;61:2079.
107. Balzano G, Fuschillo S, Melillo G, et al. Asthma and sex hormones. *Allergy* 2001;56:13.
108. Busse WW, Lemanske RF Jr. Asthma. *N Engl J Med* 2001;344:350.
109. Agarwal AK, Shah A. Menstrual-linked asthma. *J Asthma* 1997;34:539.
110. Shames RS, Heilbron DC, Janson SL, et al. Clinical differences among women with and without self-reported perimenstrual asthma. *Ann Allergy Asthma Immunol* 1998;81:65.

111. Forbes L, Jarvis D, Bumey P. Is pre-menstrual asthma related to use of aspirin or non-steroidal anti-inflammatory drugs? *Respir Med* 2000;94:828.
112. Beynon HL, Garbett ND, Barnes PJ. Severe premenstrual exacerbations of asthma: effect of intra-muscular progesterone. *Lancet* 1988;2:370.
113. American College of Obstetricians and Gynecologists and The American College of Allergy, Asthma, and Immunology. The use of newer asthma and allergy medications during pregnancy. *Ann Allergy Asthma Immunol* 2001;84:475.
114. Frederiksen B, Lanng S, Koch C, et al. Improved survival in the Danish center-treated cystic fibro-sis patients: results of aggressive treatment. *Pediatr Pulm* 1996;21:153.
115. Neinstein LS, Stewart D, Wang C, et al. Menstrual dysfunction in cystic fibrosis. *J Adolesc Health Care* 1983;4:153.
116. Johannesson M, Gottlieb C, Hjelte L. Delayed puberty in girls with cystic fibrosis despite good clin-ical status. *J Pediatr* 1997;99:29.
117. Arrigo T, Rulli I, Sferlazzas C, et al. Pubertal developmemt in cystic fibrosis: an overview. J *Pedi-atr Endocrinol Metab* 2003;16:267.
118. Sawyer SM, Phelan PD, Bowles G. Reproductive health in young women with cystic fibrosis: knowledge, attitudes and behavior. *J Adolesc Health* 1995;17:46.
119. Zack J, Jacobs CP, Keenan PM, et al. Perspectives of patients with cystic fibrosis on preventive counseling and transition to adult care. *Pediatr Pulm* 2003;36:376.
120. Sawyer SM. Reproductive health in young people with cystic fibrosis. *Curr Opin Pediatr* 1995;7:376.
121. Stern RC. Cystic fibrosis and the reproductive systems. In: Davis PB, ed. *Cystic fibrosis.* New York: Marcel Dekker, 1993.
122. Lyon A. Bilton D. Fertility issues in cystic fibrosis. *Paedieatr Respir Rev* 2002;3:236.
123. Kopito LE, Losasky HJ, Shwachman H. Water and electrolytes in cervical mucus from patients with cystic fibrosis. *Fertil Steril* 1973;24:512.
124. diSant'Agnese PA, Davis DB. Cystic fibrosis in adults. *Am J Med* 1979;66:121.
125. Handyside AIL, Lesko JG, Tarin JJ, et al. Birth of a normal girl after *in vitro* fertilization and preim-plantation diagnostic testing for cystic fibrosis. *N Engl J Med* 1992;327:905.
126. Kent NE, Farquharson DE. Cystic fibrosis in pregnancy. *Can Med Assoc J* 1993;149:809.
127. Kotloff RM, FitzSimmons SC, Fiel SB. Fertility and pregnancy in patients with cystic fibrosis. *Clin Chest Med* 1992;13:623.
128. Canny GL, Corey M, Livingstone RA, et al. Pregnancy and cystic fibrosis. *Obstet Gynecol* 1991;77:850.
129. Edenborough FP, Stableforth DE, Webb AK, et al. Outcome of pregnancy in women with cystic fi-brosis. *Thorax* 1995;50:170.
130. Olson GL. Cystic fribrosis in pregnancy. *Semin Perinatol* 1997;21:307.
131. Gillet D, de Braekeleer M, Bellis G, et al. Cystic fibrosis and pregnancy. Report from French data (1980–1999). *BJOG* 2002;109:912.
132. Edenborough FP, Mackenzie WE, Stableforth DE. The outcomes of 72 pregnancies in 55 women with cystic fibrosis in the United Kingdom 1977–1996. *BJOG* 2000;107:254.
133. Dooley RR, Braunstein H, Osher AB. Polypoid cervicitis in cystic fibrosis patients receiving oral contraceptives. *Am J Obstet Gynecol* 1974;118:971.
134. Fitzpatirick SB, Stokes DC, Rosenstein BJ, et al. Use of oral contraceptives in women with cystic fi-brosis. *Chest* 1984;86:863.
135. Savage MO, Beattie RM, Camacho-Hübner C, et al. Growth in Crohn's disease. *Acta Paediatr Suppl* 1999;88:89.
136. Simon D. Puberty in chronically diseased patients. *Horm Res* 2002;57:53.
137. Banks BM, Korelitz BI, Zetzel L. The course of nonspecific ulcerative colitis: Review of twenty years' experience and late results. *Gastroenterology* 1980;32:983–1012.
138. Hudson M, Flett G. Sinclair TS, et al. Fertility and pregnancy in inflammatory bowel disease. *Int J Gynaecol Obstet* 1997;58:229.
139. Korelitz BI. Inflammatory bowel disease in pregnancy. *Gastroenterol Clin North Am* 1992;21:827.
140. Khosia R, Willoughby CF, Jewell DP. Crohn's disease and pregnancy. *Gut* 1984;25:52.
141. Mayberry IF, Weterman IT. European survey of fertility and pregnancy in women with Crohn's dis-ease: a case-control study by European collaborative group. *Gut* 1986;27:821.
142. Alstead EM, Nelson-Piercy C. Inflammatory bowel disease in pregnancy. *Gut* 2003;52:159.

143. Francella A, Dyan A, Bodian C, et al. The safety of 6-mercaptopurine for childbearing patients with inflammatory bowel disease: a retrospective cohort study. *Gastroenterology* 2003;124:9.

144. Norgard B, Pedersen L, Fonager K, et al. Azathioprine, mercaptopurine and birth outcome: a population-based cohort study. *Aliment Pharmacol Ther* 2003;17:827.

145. Kane S. Inflammatory bowel disease in pregnancy. *Gastrogenterol Clin North Am* 2003;32:323.

146. Nielsen OH, Andreasson B, Bondesen S, et al. Pregnancy in ulcerative colitis. *Scand J Gastroenterol* 1983;18:735.

147. Baiocco PJ, Korelitz BI. The influence of inflammatory bowel disease and its treatment on pregnancy and fetal outcome. *J Clin Gastroenterol* 1984;6:211.

148. Federkow DM, Persaud D, Nimrod MB. Inflammatory bowel disease: a controlled study of late pregnancy outcome. *Am J Obstet Gynecol* 1989;160:998.

149. Vender FJ, Spiro HM. Inflammatory bowel disease and pregnancy. *J Clin Gastroenterol* 1982;4:231.

150. Kornfeld D, Cnattingius S, Ekborm A. Pregnancy outcomes in women with inflammatory bowel disease. A population-based cohort study. *Am J Obstet Gynecol* 1997;177:942.

151. Kremer M, Nussenson E, Steinfeld M, et al. Crohn's disease of the vulva. *Am J Gastroenterol* 1984; 79:376.

152. Ferry JA, Young RH, Engel G, et al. Oxyphilic Sertoli cell tumor of the ovary: a report of three cases, two patients with the Peutz-Jeghers syndrome. *Int J Gynecol Pathol* 1994;13:259.

153. Young RH, Scully RE. Mucinous ovarian tumors associated with mucinous adenocarcinomas of the cervix: a clinicopathological analysis of 16 cases. *Int J Gynecol Pathol* 1988;7:99.

154. Srivatsa PJ, Keeney GL, Podratz KC. Disseminated cervical adenoma malignum and bilateral ovarian sex cord tumors with annular tubules associated with Peutz-Jeghers syndrome. *Gynecol Oncol* 1994;53:256.

155. Martin-Odegard B, Svane S. Peutz-Jeghers syndrome associated with bilateral synchronous breast carcinoma in a 30-year-old woman. *Eur J Surg* 1994;160:511.

156. Potter C, Willis D, Sharp HL, et al. Primary and secondary amenorrhea associated with spironolactone therapy in chronic liver disease. *J Pediatr* 1992;121:141.

157. Nicholas SL, Rulin MC. Acute vaginal bleeding in women undergoing liver transplantation. *Am J Obstet Gynecol* 1994;170:733.

158. Chetkowski RJ, Meldrum DR, Steingold KA, et al. Biologic effects of transdermal estradiol. *N Engl J Med* 1986;314:1615.

159. Blumenfeld Z, Enat R, Brandes JM, et al. Gonadotropin-releasing hormone analogues for dysfunctional bleeding in women after liver transplantation: a new application. *Fertil Steril* 1992; 57:1121.

160. Brewer GJ, Johnson VD, Dick RD, et al. Treatment of Wilson's disease with zinc. XVII: treatment during pregnancy. *Hepatology* 2000;31:364.

161. Sternlieb I. Wilson's disease and pregnancy. *Hepatology* 2000;31:531.

162. Tarnacka B, Rodo M, Cichy S, et al. Procreation ability in Wilson's disease. *Acta Neurol Scand* 2000;101:395.

163. Schilsky ML. Treatment of Wilson's disease: what are the relative roles of penicillamine, trientine, and zinc supplementation?. *Curr Gastroenterol Rep* 2001;3:54.

164. Furman B, Bashiri A, Wiznitzer A, et al. Wilson's disease in pregnancy: five successful consecutive pregnancies of the same woman. *Eur J Obstet Gynecol Reprod Biol* 2001;96:232.

165. Pellecchia MT, Criscuolo C, Longo K, et al. Clinical presentation and treatment of Wilson's disease: a single-centre experience. *Eur Neurol* 2003;50:48.

166. Zeitler PS, Travers S, Kappy MS. Advances in the recognition and treatment of endocrine complications in children with chronic illness. *Adv Pediatr* 1999;46:101.

167. Tiosano D, Hochberg Z. Endocrine complications of thalassemia. *J Endocrinol Invest* 2001;24:716.

168. Platt OS, Rosenstock W, Espeland MA. Influence of sickle hemoglobinopathies on growth and development. *N Engl J Med* 1984;311:7.

169. Mann J. Sickle cell haemoglobinopathies in England. *Arch Dis Child* 1981;56:676.

170. Alleyne R, Rauseo R, Serjeant G. Sexual development and fertility of Jamaican female patients with homozygous sickle cell disease. *Arch Intern Med* 1981;141:1295.

171. Balgir RS. Age at menarche and first conception in sickle cell hemoglobinopathy. *Ind Pediatr* 1994; 31:827.

172. Olivieri NF, Koren G, Harris J, et al. Growth failure and bony changes induced by deferoxamine. *Am J Pediatr Hematol Oncol* 1992;14:48.

173. Jackson RL. Growth and maturation of children with insulin-dependent diabetes mellitus. *Pediatr Clin North Am* 1984;31:545.

174. Koshy M, Bard L. Management of pregnancy in sickle cell syndromes. *Hematol Oncol Clin North Am* 1991;5:585.

175. Brown AK, Sleeper LA, Peglow CH, et al. The influence of infant and maternal sickle disease on birth outcome and neonatal course. *Arch Pediatr Adolesc Med* 1994;148:1156.

176. Seoud MA, Cantwell D, Nobles G, et al. Outcome of pregnancies complicated by sickle cell and sickle-C hemoglobinopathies. *Am J Perinatol* 1994;11:187.

177. Sun PM, Wilburn W, Raynor BD, Jamieson D. Sickle cell disease in pregnancy: twenty years of experience at Grady Memorial Hospital, Atlanta, Georgia. *Am J Obstet Gynecol* 2001;184:1127.

178. Morrison JC, Morrison FS, Floyd RC, et al. Use of continuous flow erythrocytapheresis in pregnant patients with sickle cell disease. *J Clin Apheresis* 1991;6:224.

179. Howard RJ, Tuck SM, Pearson TC. Blood transfusion in pregnancies complicated by maternal sickle cell disease: effects on blood rheology and uteroplacental Doppler velocimetry. *Clin Lab Hematol* 1994;16:253.

180. Mahomed K. Prophylactic versus selective blood transfusion for sickle cell anaemia during pregnancy. *Cochrane Database Syst Rev* (2):CD000040, 2000.

181. Jensen CE, Tuck SM, Wonke B. Fertility in beta-thalassemia major: a report of 16 pregnancies, preconceptual evaluation and a review of the literature. *Br J Obstet Gynaecol* 1995;102:625.

182. Savona-Ventura C, Bonello F. Beta-thalassemia syndromes and pregnancy. *Obstet Gynecol Surv* 1994;49:129.

183. Hokken-Koelega AC, Saenger P, Cappa M, et al. Unresolved problems concerning optimal therapy of puberty in children with chronic renal diseases. *J Pediatr Endocrinol Metab* 2001;14:945.

184. Holley JL, Schmidt RJ, Bender FH, et al. Gynecologic and reproductive issues in women on dialysis. *Am J Kidney Dis* 1997;29:685.

185. Lim VS, Henriquez C, Stevertson G, et al. Ovarian function in chronic renal failure: evidence suggesting hypothalamic anovulation. *Ann Intern Med* 1980;93:21.

186. Ginsburg ES, Owen WE. Reproductive endocrinology and pregnancy in women on hemodialysis. *Semin Dial* 1993;6:105.

187. Bar J, Ben-Rafael Z, Padoa A, et al. Prediction of pregnancy outcome in subgroups of women with renal disease. *Clin Nephrol* 2000;53:437.

188. Moroni G, Ponticelli C. The risk of pregnancy in patients with lupus nephritis. *J Nephrol* 2003;16:161.

189. Lockshin MD, Sammaritano LR. Lupus pregnancy. *Autoimmunity* 2003;36:33.

190. Jones DC, Hayslett JP. Outcome of pregnancy in women with moderate or severe renal insufficiency. *N Engl J Med* 1996;335:226.

191. Brown MA, Whitworth JA. The kidney in hypertensive pregnancies—victim and villain. *Am J Kidney Dis* 1992;20:427.

192. Luciani G, Bossola M, Tazza L, et al. Pregnancy during chronic hemodialysis: a single dialysis-unit experience with five cases. *Ren Fail* 2002;24:853.

193. Chao AS, Huang JY, Lien R, et al. Pregnancy in women who undergo long-term hemodialysis. *Am J Obstet Gynecol* 2002;187:152.

194. Okundaye I, Hou S. Management of pregnancy in women undergoing continuous ambulatory peritoneal dialysis. *Adv Perit Dial* 1996;12:151.

195. Dafnis E, Sabatini S. The effect of pregnancy on renal function: physiology and pathology. *Am J Med Sci* 1992;303:184.

196. Sgro MD, Barozzino T, Mirghani HM, et al. Pregnancy outcome post renal transplantation. *Teratology* 2002;65:5.

197. McGrory CH, McCloskey LJ, DeHoratius RJ, et al. Pregnancy outcomes in female renal recipients: a comparison of systemic lupus erythematosus with other diagnoses. *Am J Transplant* 2003;3:35.

198. Armenti VT, Radomski JS, Moritz MJ, et al. Report from the National Transplantation Pregnancy Registry (NTPR): outcomes of pregnancy after transplantation. *Clin Transpl* 2002;121.

199. Chapman AB, Johnson AM, Gabow PA. Pregnancy outcome and its relationship to progression of renal failure in autosomal-dominant polycystic kidney disease. *J Am Soc Nephrol* 1994;5:1178.

200. Alcalay M, Blau A, Barkai G, et al. Successful pregnancy in a patient with polycystic kidney disease and advanced renal failure: the use of prophylactic dialysis. *Am J Kidney Dis* 1992;19:382.

201. Caprio S, Cline G, Boulware SD, et al. Effects of puberty and diabetes on insulin-sensitive fuels. *Am J Physiol* 1994;266:885.
202. Rother KI, Levitsky LL. Diabetes mellitus during adolescence. *Endocrinol Metab Clin North Am* 1993;22:553.
203. Amiel SA, Sherwin RS, Cimonson DC, et al. Impaired insulin action in puberty: a contributing factor to poor glycemic control in adolescents. *N Engl J Med* 1986;31:215.
204. Vanelli M, Chiari G, Adinolfi B, et al. Management of insulin-dependent diabetes mellitus in adolescents. *Horm Res* 1997;48:71.
205. Chase HP. Glycemic control in prepubertal years. *Diabetes Care* 2003;26:1304.
206. Lane P. Diabetic kidney disease: impact of puberty. *Am J Physiol Renal Physiol* 2002;283:589.
207. DuCaju MVL, Rooman RP, DeBeeck LO. Longitudinal data on growth and final height in diabetic children. *Pediatr Res* 1995;38:607.
208. Wise J, Kolb E, Sander S. Effect of glycemic control on growth velocity in children with IDDM. *Diabetes Care* 1992;15:826.
209. Rydall AC, Rodin GM, Olmsted MP, et al. Disordered eating behavior and microvascular complications in young women with insulin-dependent diabetes mellitus. *N Engl J Med* 1997;336:1849.
210. Delahanty LM, Meigs JB, Harden D. Psychological and behavioral correlates of baseline BMI in the diabetes prevention program (DPP). *Diabetes Care* 2002;25:1992.
211. Kjaer K, Hagen C, Sando SH, et al. Epidemiology of menarche and menstrual disturbances in an unselected group of women with insulin-dependent diabetes mellitus compared to controls. *J Clin Endocrinol Metab* 1992;75:524.
212. Widom B, Diamond MP, Simonson DC. Alterations in glucose metabolism during menstrual cycle in women with IDDM. *Diabetes Care* 1992;15:213.
213. Adcock CJ, Perry LA, Lindsell DR, et al. Menstrual irregularities are more common in adolescents with type 1 diabetes: association with poor glycemic control and weight gain. *Diabet Med* 1994;11:465.
214. Cawood EH, Bancroft J, Steel JM. Perimenstrual symptoms in women with diabetes mellitus and the relationship to diabetic control. *Diabet Med* 1993;10:444.
215. Brown KC, Darby CW, Ng SH. Cyclical disturbance of diabetic central injuries before the menarche. *Arch Dis Child* 1991;66:1279.
216. Kjaer K, Hagen C, Sando SH, et al. Infertility and pregnancy outcome in an unselected group of women with insulin dependent diabetes mellitus. *Am J Obstet Gynecol* 1992;166:1412.
217. Warram JH, Martin BC, Krolewski AS. Risk of IDDM in children of diabetic mothers decreases with increasing maternal age at pregnancy. *Diabetes* 1991;40:1679.
218. Reece EA, Homko C, Miodovnik M, et al. A consensus report of the Diabetes in Pregnancy Study Group of North America Conference, Little Rock, Arkansas. *J Matern Fetal Neonatal Med* 2002;12:362.
219. Reece EA, Homko CJ. Assessment and management of pregnancies complicated by pregestational and gestational diabetes mellitus. *J Assoc Acad Minor Phys* 1994;5:87.
220. Kappy MS. Diabetes in pregnancy: rationale and guidelines for care. *Compr Ther* 1991;17:50.
221. Aberg A, Westbom L, Kallen B. Congenital malformations among infants whose mothers had gestational diabetes or pre-existing diabetes. *Early Hum Dev* 2001;61:85.
222. Eriksson UJ, Cederberg J, Wentzel P. Congenital malformations in offspring of diabetic mothers—animal and human studies. *Rev Endocr Metab Disord* 2003;4:79–93.
223. Rosenn B, Miodovnik M, Combs CA, et al. Glycemic thresholds for spontaneous abortion and congenital malformations in insulin-dependent diabetes mellitus. *Obstet Gynecol* 1994;84:515.
224. Krassas GE. Thyroid disease and female reproduction. *Fertil Steril* 2000;74:1063–1070.
225. Rivkees SA, Bode HH, Crawford JD. Long-term growth in juvenile acquired hypothyroidism: the failure to achieve normal adult stature. *N Engl J Med* 1988;318:599.
226. Weber G, Vigone MC, Stroppa L, et al. Thyroid function and puberty. *J Pediatr Endocrinol Metab* 2003;16:253.
227. Speroff L, Glass RH, Kase NG. *Clinical gynecologic endocrinology and infertility,* 6th ed. Baltimore, MD: Williams & Wilkins, 1999.
228. Davis LE, Lucas MJ, Hankins GV, et al. Thyrotoxicosis complicating pregnancy. *Am J Obstet Gynecol* 1989;160:63.
229. Easterling TR, Chmucker BC, Carlson KL, et al. Maternal hemodynamics in pregnancies complicated by hyperthyroidism. *Obstet Gynecol* 1991;78:348.

230. Cheron RG, Kaplan MM, Larsen PR, et al. Neonatal thyroid function after propylthiouracil therapy for maternal Graves' disease. *N Engl J Med* 1981;304:525.
231. Mitsuda N, Tamaki H, Amino N, et al. Risk factors for developmental disorders in infants born to women with Graves' disease. *Obstet Gynecol* 1992;80:359.
232. Leung AS, Millar LK, Koonings PP, et al. Perinatal outcome in hypothyroid pregnancies. *Obstet Gynecol* 1993;8:349.
233. Mandel SJ, Larsen PR, Seely EW, et al. Increased need for thyroxine during pregnancy in women with primary hypothyroidism. *N Engl J Med* 1990;323:91.
234. Roti E, Emerson CH. Clinical review 29: postpartum thyroiditis. *J Clin Endocrinol Metab* 1992;74:3.
235. Vargas MT, Bariones-Urbina R, Bladman D, et al. Antithyroid microsomal autoantibodies and HLA-DR5 are associated with postpartum thyroid dysfunction: evidence supporting an autoimmune pathogenesis. *J Clin Endocrinol Metab* 1988;67:327.
236. Walfish PG, Chan YYC. Postpartum hyperthyroidism. *Clin Endocrinol Metab* 1985;14:417.
237. Silva CA, Leal MM, Leone C, et al. Gonadal function in adolescents and young women with juvenile systemic lupus erythematosus. *Lupus* 2002;11:419.
238. Slater CA, Liang MH, McCune JW, et al. Preserving ovarian function in patients receiving cyclophosphamide. *Lupus* 1999; 8:3.
239. Huong du L, Amoura Z, Duhaut P, et al. Risk of ovarian failure and fertility after intravenous cyclophosphamide. A study of 84 patients. *J Rheumatol* 2002;29:2571.
240. Petri M. Immunosuppressive drug use in pregnancy. *Autoimmunity* 2003;36:51.
241. Siamopoulou-Mavridou A, Manoussakis MN, Mavridis AK, et al. Outcome of pregnancy in patients with autoimmune rheumatic disease before the disease onset. *Ann Rheum Dis* 1988;47:982.
242. Cervera R, Font J, Carmona F, et al. Pregnancy outcome in systemic lupus erythematosus: good news for the new millennium. *Autoimmun Rev* 2002;1:354.
243. Gimovsky ML, Montoro M. Systemic lupus erythematosus and other connective tissue disease in pregnancy. *Clin Obstet Gynecol* 1991;34:35.
244. Pisa FE, Bovenzi M, Romeo L, et al. Reproductive factors and the risk of scleroderma: an Italian case-control study. *Arthritis Rheum* 2002;46:451.
245. Ostensen M. Pregnancy in patients with a history of juvenile rheumatoid arthritis. *Arthritis Rheum* 1991;34:881.
246. Ostensen M. The effect of pregnancy on ankylosing spondylitis, psoriatic arthritis and juvenile rheumatoid arthritis. *Am J Reprod Immunol* 1992;28:235.
247. Ostensen M, Skomsvoll JF. Perinatal outcome of pregnancies in women with connective tissue disease. *Lupus* 2002;11:661.
248. Bhagwat AR, Engel PJ. Heart disease and pregnancy. *Cardiol Clin* 1995;13:163.
249. Mendelson MA. Pregnancy in the woman with congenital heart disease. *Am J Card Imaging* 1995;9:44.
250. Perloff JK. Congenital heart disease and pregnancy. *Clin Cardiol* 1994;17:579.
251. Hess DB, Hess LW. Management of cardiovascular disease in pregnancy. *Obstet Gynecol Clin North Am* 1991;18:237.
252. Clark SL. Cardiac disease in pregnancy. *Crit Care Clin* 1991;7:777.
253. Lind J, Wallenburg HC. The Marfan syndrome and pregnancy: a retrospective study in a Dutch population. *Eur J Obstet Gynecol Reprod Biol* 2001;98:28.
254. Elkayam U, Ostrzega E, Shotan A, et al. Cardiovascular problems in pregnant women with the Marfan syndrome. *Ann Intern Med* 1995;123:117.
255. Sibai BM. Hypertension in pregnancy. *Obstet Gynecol Clin North Am* 1992;19:615.
256. Greer IA, Lowe GD, Walker JJ, et al. Haemorrhagic problems in obstetrics and gynaecology inpatients with congenital coagulopathies. *Br J Obstet Gynaecol* 1991;98:909.
257. Kouides PA. Females with von Willebrand disease: 72 years as the silent majority. *Haemophilia* 1998;4:665.
258. Kadir RA, Sabin CA, Pollard D, et al. Quality of life during menstruation in patients with inherited bleeding disorders. *Haemophilia* 1998;4:836.
259. Kouides PA. Obstetrics and gynaecological aspects of von Willebrand disease. *Best Pract Res Clin Haematol* 2001;14:381.
260. Batlle J, Noya MS, Giangrande P, et al. Advances in the therapy of von Willebrand disease. *Haemophilia* 2002;8:301.

261. Rau FJ, Muram D. Control of uterine bleeding in a patient with gonadotropin-releasing hormone agonists. *Adolesc Pediatr Gynecol* 1992;5:256.
262. Comp PC, Zacur HA. Contraceptive choices in women with coagulation disorders. *Am J Obstet Gynecol* 1993;168:1990.
263. Roque H, Funai E, Lockwood CJ. von Willebrand disease and pregnancy. *J Matern Fetal Med* 2000;9:257.
264. Morrell M. Reproductive and metabolic disorders in women with epilepsy. *Epilepsia* 2003;44:11.
265. Herzog AG, Seibel MM, Schomer DL, et al. Reproductive endocrine disorders in women with partial seizures of temporal lobe origin. *Arch Neurol* 1986;43:341.
266. Bilo L, Meo R, Nappi C, et al. Reproductive endocrine disorders in women with primary generalized epilepsy. *Epilepsia* 1988;29:612.
267. Isojarvi JI, Laatikainen TJ, Pakarinen AJ, et al. Menstrual disorders in women with epilepsy receiving carbamazepine. *Epilepsia* 1995;36:676.
268. Herzog AG. Reproductive endocrine considerations and hormonal therapy for women with epilepsy *Epilepsia* 1991;32(suppl):S27.
269. Wallace H, Shorvon S, Tallis R. Age-specific incidence and prevalence rates of treated epilepsy in an unselected population of 2,052,922 and age-specific fertility rates of women with epilepsy. *Lancet* 1998;352:1970.
270. Schupf N, Ottman R. Reproduction among individuals with idiopathic/cryptogenic epilepsy: risk factors for spontaneous abortion. *Epilepsia* 1997;38:824.
271. Morrell MJ, Giudice L, Flynn KL, et al. Predictors of ovulatory failure in women with epilepsy. *Ann Neurol* 2002;52:704.
272. Jalava M, Sillanpaa M. Reproductive activity and offspring health of young adults with childhood-onset epilepsy: a controlled study. *Epilepsia* 1997;38:532.
273. Yerby MS. Pregnancy and epilepsy. *Epilepsia* 1991;32(suppl):S51.
274. Holmes LB, Harvey EA, Coull BA, et al. The teratogenicity of anticonvulsant drugs. *N Engl J Med* 2001;344:1132.
275. Morrow JI, Russell A, Craig JJ, et al. Major malformations in the offspring of women with epilepsy: a comprehensive prospective study. *Epilepsia* 2001;42:125.
276. Masssachusetts General Hospital. Antiepileptic Drug Pregnancy Registry. Findings. available at http://www.massgeneral.org/aed/AED_findings.htm. (Accessed July 27, 2004.)
277. Oguni M, Dansky L, Andermann E, et al. Improved pregnancy outcome in epileptic women in the last decade: relationship to maternal anticonvulsant therapy. *Brain Dev* 1992;14:371.
278. Yerby MS. Epilepsy and pregnancy. New issues for an old disorder. *Neurol Clin* 1993;11:777.
279. Hiilesmaa VK. Pregnancy and birth in women with epilepsy. *Neurology* 1992;42[Suppl]:8.
280. Furman L, Mortimer JC. Menarche and menstrual function in patients with myelomeningoccle. *Dev Med Child Neurol* 1994;36:910.
281. Wingfield M, McClure N, Mamers P, et al. Endometrial ablation: an option for the management of menstrual problems in the intellectually disabled. *Med J Aust* 1994;160:533.
282. Edwards J, Wapnick S. *Being me: a social/sexual training program for the developmentally disabled.* Austin, TX: Pro-ed, 1988.
283. Edwards JP, Elkins TE. *Just between us: a social sexual training guide for parents and professionals with concerns for persons with developmental disabilities.* Austin, TX: Pro-ed, 1988.
284. Cartright DB, Joseph AS, Grenier CE. A self-image profile analysis of spina bifida adolescents in Louisiana. *J La State Med Soc* 1993;145:399.
285. Cass AS, Bloom BA, Luxenberg M. Sexual function in adults with myelomeningocele. *J Urol* 1986;136:425.
286. Rietberg CC, Lindhout D. Adult patients with spina bifida cystica: genetic counselling, pregnancy and delivery. *J Obstet Gynecol Reprod Biol* 1993;52:63.
287. Farine D, Jackson U, Portale A, et al. Pregnancy complicated by maternal spina bifida: a report of two cases. *J Reprod Med* 1988;33:323.
288. Cusimano MD, Meffe FM, Gentili F, et al. Management of pregnant women with cerebrospinal shunts. *Pediatr Neurosurg* 1991;17:10.
289. Cento RM, Ciampelli M, Proto C, et al. Neuroendocrine features of pubertal development in females with mental retardation. *Gynecol Endocrinol* 2001;15:178.
290. Wallach M, Grimes M. Modern Oral Contraception: Updates from the contraception report. Totowa, NJ: Emron 2000.

291. Hankoff LD, Darney PD. Contraceptive choices for behaviorally disordered women. *Am J Obstet Gynecol* 1993;168:1986.
292. Packer S. Family planning for women with bipolar disorder. *Hosp Community Psychiatry* 1992;43:479.
293. Mowbray CT, Oyserman D, Zemencuk TK, et al. Motherhood for women with serious mental illness: pregnancy, childbirth, and the postpartum period. *Am J Orthopsychiatry* 1995;65:21.
294. Trad PV. Mental health of adolescent mothers. *J Am Acad Child Adolesc Psychiatry* 1995;34:130.
295. Altshuler LL, Szuba MP. Course of psychiatric disorders in pregnancy: dilemmas in pharmacologic management. *Neurol Clin* 1994;12:613.
296. Hendrick V, Smith LM, Suri R, et al. Birth outcomes after prenatal exposure to antidepressant medications. *Am J Obstet Gynecol* 2003;188:812.
297. Kulin NA, Pastuszak A, Sage SR, et al. Pregnancy outcome following maternal use of the new selective serotonin reuptake inhibitors: a prospective controlled multicenter study. *JAMA* 1998;279:609.
298. Shepard TH, Brent RL, Friedman JM. Update on new developments in the study of human teratogens. *Teratology* 2002;65:153.
299. Iqbal MM, Sobhan T, Aftab SR, et al. Diazepam use during pregnancy: a review of the literature. *Del Med J* 2002;74:127.
300. Yingling DR, Utter G, Vengalil S, et al. Calcium channel blocker, nimodipine, for the treatment of bipolar disorder during pregnancy. *Am J Obstet Gynecol* 2002;187:1711.
301. Boyle RJ. Effects of certain prenatal drugs on the fetus and newborn. *Pediatr Rev* 2002;23:17.
302. Zegers B, Andriessen P. Maternal lithium therapy and neonatal morbidity. *Eur J Pediatr* 2003;162:348.
303. Bowden CL. Bipolar disorders. *Valproate* 2003;5:189.
304. Diekema DS. Involuntary sterilization of persons with mental retardation: an ethical analysis. *Ment Retard Dev Disabil Res Rev* 2003;9:21.
305. Wehmeyer ML. Eugenics and sterilization in the heartland. *Ment Retard* 2003;41:57.
306. Paransky OI, Zurawin RK. Management of menstrual problems and contraception in adolescents with mental retardation: A medical, legal, and ethical review with new suggested guidelines. *J Pediatr Adolesc Gynecol* 2003;16:223.
307. Goldstein DP, Pinsonneault O. Sterilization of the unusual adolescent female. In: Goldstein DP, ed. *Gynecologic disorders of children and adolescents* 1989;1:167.
308. Peterson K. The family v. the family court: sterilization. *Aust J Public Health* 1992;16:196.

24

Sexual Abuse in the Child and Adolescent

M. Ranee Leder and S. Jean Emans

The past three decades have witnessed an increasing awareness of the broad spectrum of problems that are seen under the term *sexual abuse*. The health care provider may be involved in the diagnosis of sexual abuse cases, the evaluation of adolescents who are victims of sexual assault, and the follow-up of children and adolescents with psychological sequelae. In 1999, there were an estimated 92,000 substantiated cases of sexual abuse (1). Adolescents have the highest rates of sexual assault of any age group. In one study of 7,884 sexually active 8th- to 12th-grade students, 30% of girls and almost 10% of boys reported ever being forced or pressured to have sexual intercourse (2). In a more recent survey of 1,040 adolescents in New York, 20% of sexually active adolescent females and 7% of sexually active adolescent males reported unwanted intercourse (3). In 2001, the National Crime Victimization Survey reported 225,320 rapes and sexual assaults in females 12 years or older and 22,930 rapes and sexual assaults in males 12 years or older (4). The percentage of adult women disclosing histories of sexual abuse ranges from 2% to 62%, with most estimates at 20% or more; for adult men, 3% to 16% have a history of abuse, with most estimates at 5% to 10% (5).

Sexual abuse is generally defined as the involvement of developmentally immature children or adolescents in sexual activities that they do not fully comprehend, to which they are unable to give informed consent, or that violate taboos of family relationships. Sexual abuse may include exhibitionism, fondling, genital viewing, oral–genital contact, insertion of objects, or vaginal or rectal penetration. The contact may be a single event between the child and a stranger occurring with or without the use of force, or it may be a long-standing sexualized relationship with a parent, stepparent, or other known individual and may involve repeated encounters over months to years. The sexual interaction may start with fondling and progress over the course of months to vulvar coitus and penetration. The assailant is known to the child in 70% to 90% of cases, and in half of cases a relative is involved (5–7).

Sexual assault is defined as any sexual act performed by one person on another without that person's consent. The use or threat of force may be involved, or the person may not be able to give consent because of age, mental or physical capacity, or impairment with drugs or alcohol. A child who is unconscious or intoxicated cannot give consent. Different states have varying legal definitions of sexual assault and sexual abuse.

Reported cases of sexual abuse represent a small percentage of actual events. Clinicians should ask questions that would reveal the possibility of sexual abuse at the routine physical examination, especially in children and adolescents with somatic complaints or behavioral changes such as regression, nightmares, running away, school failure, or pregnancy. Patients should be reassured that the questions posed to them are the same as asked of all patients. For adolescents, these questions can be included in the menstrual and sexual history: "Have you ever been touched in your private parts or sexually when you did not want to be touched?", "Have you ever been forced to have sex?", or "Have you ever felt that someone older than you made inappropriate sexual advances?" Acknowledging that some youngsters have felt embarrassed or unable to tell another person in the past can relieve anxiety. Younger children with unexplained somatic symptoms or any evidence of genital infection, pain, or bleeding can be asked: "Has an adult or someone you know ever touched the vaginal area or your private parts?" "If you were ever touched, whom would you tell?" If a child can mention her parent or other trusted adult without hesitation, clinicians can feel at least some reassurance that lines of communication are available.

The recognition of sexual abuse is frequently prompted by a child's disclosure to a parent, friend, teacher, or health professional. The disclosure may be intentional or accidental. For example, a child may have told a peer about abuse, and the peer may subsequently tell her own parent, who reports the case. In most cases, the child does not anticipate the sequelae of the allegation. Sexual abuse may become evident during an evaluation for somatic symptoms or behavioral difficulties. Girls with vaginal bleeding, foreign bodies in the vagina (8), condylomata acuminata, genital herpes, *Trichomonas vaginalis* or *Chlamydia trachomatis* infection, or gonococcal vulvovaginitis need an especially careful history for sexual abuse, and the history is often best obtained without the parents present. Occasionally, a pregnancy in a young adolescent is the first sign of long-standing incest.

Because clinicians frequently feel uncomfortable about making the diagnosis of sexual abuse, even obvious problems are sometimes overlooked (9). Most children who disclose sexual abuse are telling the truth, and it is highly unlikely for a child to make up the concrete details of sexual involvement unless a sexually stimulating experience has occurred. Even if one encounters the rare circumstance in which a child has not had the sexual experience alleged, most likely something sexually stimulating occurred that is unhealthy for the child's development. In cases of incest, there is a great deal of pressure from families to have the child retract the story to prevent disruption of the family unit and possible incarceration of the parent. Thus, clinicians must be prepared to file the necessary report with child protective services, support the youngster in her original story, and proceed with an appropriate referral to a mental health facility capable of dealing with the issues of sexual abuse or to a sexual abuse treatment team in a hospital setting (10). Multidisciplinary teams that include a social worker, psychologist, psychiatrist, nurse, and physician are extremely helpful in sorting out the complex issues involved in child sexual abuse cases, including decreasing the number of interviews for the child, identifying the perpetrator, and pressing charges (7,10,11). Custody battles may be particularly problematic (12).

In all cases of sexual abuse, it is extremely important that patients be given sympathetic medical care. All patients with an episode of sexual abuse should be seen promptly by their primary care clinician and possibly referred to an expert in the medical diagnosis of child sexual abuse. If a sexual assault has occurred within the preceding 72 hours, the clinician should refer to an emergency department setting or forensic center with protocols and special equipment to collect the necessary forensic evidence in the event that prosecution is undertaken.

PATTERNS OF SEXUAL ABUSE

It is important for physicians to understand some of the patterns of sexual abuse of children and to realize that all cases cannot be considered in the same way. Becker (13) used the term *child molester* to refer to perpetrators who choose child victims and the term *sex offender* more broadly to refer to those who offend against adults, children, or both. *Pedophilia* is the preference of an adult for sexual contact with a child. The onset of deviant sexual interest often begins in adolescence, predating any family disruption or dysfunction in adult life. In addition, many apprehended sex offenders are adolescents, and they may offend against peers, younger children, and adults. Few studies have been done of these individuals, although many have histories of depression and of having been sexually abused themselves. Many lack social skills and impulse control.

In its broadest definition, *incest* means a sexual relationship between people who are related and cannot legally marry. It generally refers to relationships between members of the immediate nuclear family, such as between father and daughter, mother and son, father and son, mother and daughter, or between siblings. Although sexual involvement between a stepparent and child is not traditional incest, it has many of the same psychodynamics and problems for treatment as do other forms of incest. A sexual relationship between a stepparent and child or between a parent's partner and child is sometimes called *functional parent incest.* In parental incest, there is some form of major family dysfunction. Isolation and depression are frequently present. The child learns to adapt to the sexual expectations of the relationship. The nonoffending parent may be involved in conscious or unconscious complicity.

Incestuous relationships may start in the early childhood years and continue through adolescence. Often, the child feels the threat of family disruption if she were to tell the secret. A crisis may occur if there is sudden disclosure of the situation when the child is in late puberty or adolescence; the youngster may begin to feel that her involvement is no longer age appropriate and may wish to have more meaningful relationships with her peer group. Clearly, incest occurs in all socioeconomic groups. The secret may remain within the family for years, and it may be disclosed only when a young adult is in psychotherapy.

Little research has been done on recidivism, but rates appear to be 30% to 40% for perpetrators overall and 10% for perpetrators involved in incest (13). Those who target both males and females and pre- and postpubertal victims appear to have the highest recidivism rate (75%). A prior criminal record is a strong predictor of repeat offenses.

PATIENT ASSESSMENT

Due to the legal implications, medical data should be carefully collected and recorded in all cases of alleged rape or sexual abuse (10,14,15). The aim of the evaluation is to document what has happened, obtain adequate medicolegal evidence, and provide patients with medical and psychological follow-up. Clinicians should avoid trying to decide whether rape actually occurred or whether there is sufficient evidence for a verdict.

The timing and the extent of the physical examination depend on the history. Any child who has pain, vaginitis, bleeding, dysuria, a history of trauma, or has been abused within the past 72 hours should be seen immediately for an assessment. Children who may not be safe should also be seen urgently. Physical findings that may corroborate a sexual assault must be documented. Since children often have difficulty disclosing a full history of the nature of the abuse, a complete physical examination is always indicated. Referral to one of many forensic centers that specialize in the multidisciplinary assessment of child sexual abuse may be indicated. If they are unavailable, a standard protocol is available in most emergency departments and should be followed so that forensic evidence can be passed directly to a police officer to maintain a legal "chain of evidence" (16). Protocols that include drawings of male and female genitalia are excellent for documenting abnormalities (Appendix 5).

Patients who were abused weeks to months before seeking help should be interviewed as soon as is practical provided that the child is safe. The physical examination is done at the completion of the initial assessment. Medical providers who evaluate and treat victims of sexual abuse and assault should be aware that DNA amplification technology used to identify assailants allows performance of forensic testing beyond 72 hours, which had previously been considered the cutoff for such testing (16); late positive tests typically come from the environment (clothes, sheets, etc).

Sexually Transmitted Diseases and Sexual Assault

Parents and health care providers often ask about the risk of acquiring a sexually transmitted disease (STD) in the context of sexual abuse. The estimate of the risk determines which, if any, infections should be treated with prophylactic medications at the time of the initial evaluation. The implications of commonly encountered STDs from the 1999 American Academy of Pediatrics statement are shown in Table 24-1.

Previous studies (17–21) have reviewed the risk of STDs in children and adults with histories of sexual abuse. A recent study (22) found an overall prevalence rate of sexually transmitted organisms of 3.7% in child victims of sexual assault. Importantly, Jenny has distinguished between infections noted at the initial evaluation and those found at follow-up visits. This distinction is particularly relevant in the care of adolescents, since adolescent assault victims who come to medical attention in hospital settings may have a preexisting STD (17,18,23–25). It should be noted that not all infections noted at baseline are necessarily preexisting infections since it is possible that a culture could be positive as a result of exposure to the male ejaculate (26). At least one STD is present at the time of evaluation in 29% to 43% of patients (21,27).

Studies of sexual assault victims have found *Neisseria gonorrhoeae* to be present in 2.4% to 12.0% of patients at initial evaluation; studies of patients who are negative at the initial visit have noted positive gonorrhea cultures in 2.6% to 4% of patients at follow-up (17,21,24). The Centers for Disease Control and Prevention (CDC) have estimated the risk of acquiring gonorrhea to be 6% to 12% (28). In sexually abused children, a positive culture for gonorrhea has been reported in 0% to 26.7%, with a usual rate of 1% to 5%. A positive gonorrhea culture in prepubertal girls is almost always associated with vaginal discharge at presentation or by history (29–31). In one series (32), 1.4% (12/865) of prepubertal girls seen within 72 hours of assault were positive, and all had signs of acute vulvovaginitis.

TABLE 24-1. *Implications of commonly encountered sexually transmitted diseases (STDs) for the diagnosis and reporting of sexual abuse of infants and prepubertal children.*

STD confirmed	Sexual abuse	Suggested Action
Gonorrhea*	Diagnostic†	Report‡
Syphilis*	Diagnostic	Report
HIV§	Diagnostic	Report
*Chlamydia**	Diagnostic†	Report
*Trichomonas vaginalis**	Highly suspicious	Report
Condylomata acuminata* (anogenital warts)	Suspicious	Report
Herpes (genital location)	Suspicious	Report‖
Bacterial vaginosis	Inconclusive	Medical follow-up

* If not perinatally acquired.
† Use definitive diagnostic methods such as culture or DNA probes.
‡ To agency mandated in community to receive reports of suspected sexual abuse.
§ If not perinatally or transfusion acquired.
‖ Unless there is a clear history of autoinoculation. Herpes 1 and 2 are difficult to differentiate by current techniques.
(From: American Academy of Pediatrics Committee on Child Abuse and Neglect. Guidelines for the evaluation of sexual abuse of children: subject review. *Pediatrics* 1999;103:186–191; with permission.)

Jenny and colleagues (21) reported that 10% of women were positive for *C. trachomatis* at the initial visit for evaluation of a sexual assault; at follow-up, 2% of women with initially negative cultures who had not been given antibiotics were positive. The risk of acquiring chlamydial infection has been estimated to be 4% to 17% (28). *C. trachomatis* has been reported in 2% to 17% of prepubertal girls, depending on the population studied. *C. trachomatis* may persist after birth for a number of months. Rectal or genital chlamydial infection in young children may be the result of perinatally acquired infection; and perinatal infection has persisted for 2 to 3 years in some cases (33). Because the majority of children will have been treated with antibiotics to which the organism is sensitive by 1 to 3 years of age, the issue of persistence in older children becomes less likely, and the potential for sexual transmission as the source of infection becomes much greater.

The risk of syphilis appears to be low and is estimated by the CDC at 0.5% to 3% (28), although in patients with other STDs the risk is increased (34). A serologic test for syphilis can be done initially and then 8 to 12 weeks later if prophylactic antibiotics are not administered. Because of the low risk of acquiring this infection, many centers do selective testing.

Bacterial vaginosis and *T. vaginalis* infection have been found in 5% to 42% and 6% to 20%, respectively, of postpubertal assault victims (26). *Trichomonas* was found in 17 women (22%), with 29% (5/17) having acquired it during the assault. Data on prepubertal girls are sparse. *Trichomonas* can be transmitted at the time of birth and cause vaginitis and nasal discharge, but the organism usually disappears spontaneously with waning estrogen effects on the vaginal mucosa or with treatment. Trichomoniasis can rarely occur in the vagina of prepubertal girls and is usually associated with sexual abuse (34). Bacterial vaginosis has also been noted at follow-up in children with a history of acute vaginal assault. Conflicting studies have provided data on the prevalence of *Gardnerella vaginalis* in prepubertal girls. The presence of bacterial vaginosis alone in children does not prove sexual abuse (33).

Positive herpes simplex virus (HSV) cultures have been reported in 2% of adolescents at the initial visit for sexual assault and none at follow-up (21). Studies in children have noted that genital herpes can be acquired through self-inoculation from oral–genital contact (HSV type 1 gingivostomatitis occurring simultaneously with genital lesions), but sexual abuse may result in infections with either HSV type 1 or type 2.

The risk of acquiring HPV from sexual abuse is unknown, but adolescents with a single rape episode have been observed to develop cervical dysplasia associated with HPV infection (35). A recent study of 40 girls ages 5 to 12 years who were evaluated for sexual abuse compared the prevalence of genital HPV DNA in girls where sexual abuse was confirmed or suspected with that of girls where sexual abuse was ruled out (36). HPV DNA was detected in 16% of girls with confirmed or suspected sexual abuse and in none of the nonabused girls. None of the girls in the study had genital warts or abnormal colposcopic findings. The authors concluded that genital HPV infection is more common among abused than nonabused girls and that the majority of infections are not clinically apparent.

Condylomata have been reported in 1% to 2% of abused children, and it has been suggested that 50% to 75% of cases of genital warts in children are due to abuse (37). HPV can be acquired perinatally; however, data on the risk of transmission are limited. A recent prospective study of HPV-positive pregnant women found that perinatal transmission was rare; 74% of 151 women had clinical or DNA evidence of HPV infection, but among 479 infant visits for 34 infants, HPV DNA was detected from only five (1.5%) of 335 genital, four (1.2%) of 324 anal, and none of the 372 oral specimens (38). The HPV detected in the infants were all unclassified DNA types. The period of latency for the development of clinically apparent warts has not been definitively determined but none were seen in the perinatal study at 2 years. Thus further research is needed to support the presumption that most genital warts in children less than 3 years of age are due to perinatal acquisition. Genital warts have been diagnosed in children who have been sexually abused but also in children who have no other evidence of sexual abuse (33).

Hepatitis B is caused by infection with hepatitis B virus (HBV). In the United States, approximately 181,000 persons were infected with HBV in 1998 (33). The time from exposure to onset of symptoms ranges from 6 weeks to 6 months. HBV is transmitted percutaneously or by mucous membrane exposure to infected body fluids. Among adults, sexual transmission accounts for most HBV infection in the United States. The frequency with which HBV infection occurs following sexual abuse or rape has not been determined. Fully vaccinated individuals do not need further doses of HBV vaccine. Unvaccinated victims of sexual assault should receive HBV vaccine series (see CDC recommendations for regimens). If the perpetrator is known to have acute hepatitis B, then HBIG should be also administered. The recommended dose of HBIG for children and adults is 0.06 ml/kg.

The potential transmission of HIV to victims of sexual abuse and assault has received increasing attention. A recent survey of all reports by state and local health departments to the national HIV/AIDS surveillance system found 26 children with HIV or AIDS who were sexually abused with confirmed or suspected exposure to HIV infection (39). In a previous survey (40), 28 HIV infected children with sexual abuse as their exclusive risk factor were detected from 5,622 HIV antibody tests during 113,198 sexual abuse assessments (a total of 41 HIV infected children were identified). Another STD was present in 33%. The reasons for HIV testing were physical findings suggestive of HIV infection in 32%, HIV-seropositive or high-risk perpetrator in 21%, and another STD in 14%. Penile–vaginal and/or rectal penetration was reported in only 50%. Fifty-eight percent of perpetrators had behavioral risk factors or signs and symptoms of HIV infection, and the serostatus was known in 67% of cases. Although the authors estimated the prevalence risk at 3.55 per 1,000 HIV antibody tests and 0.25 per 1,000 sexual abuse assessments conducted (41), the children who were tested in the survey were not randomly selected.

Guidelines for HIV counseling and testing children who have a history of sexual abuse continue to be debated (40–44). Recommendations have varied from testing no one, because the risk is small, to universal testing. The low risk of HIV infection should be discussed with parents and child (if old enough), and the benefits and risks of testing made clear. Patients and families may wish to make use of confidential or anonymous counseling and testing centers. Experts generally agree that victims who have been involved in behaviors that place them at risk, have symptoms of HIV infection, have been abused by a perpetrator who is HIV positive, or have another STD should have HIV counseling and testing (40,43,44). Children who have had exposure, particularly of long duration, to semen through oral, genital, or anal sex acts are at increased risk of acquiring HIV. One review suggested that the estimated probability of HIV transmission associated with unprotected receptive anal intercourse with an HIV infected person is 0.008 to 0.032 and with vaginal intercourse is 0.0005 to 0.0015 (45).

Although recognizing constraints within the legal system, Gutman, Rimsza, and others (43,46,47) have advocated the importance of testing the perpetrator to avoid venipuncture in the child. Not only are prospective studies of HIV risk in sexually abused children needed, but clinicians must remain vigilant in exploring the possibility of sexual abuse in any child who tests positive for HIV and in maintaining surveillance of other children in the households of index cases of HIV infection.

Because of the potential for transmission of HIV during sexual assault, protocols have been developed for postexposure prophylaxis of victims although controversy remains as to who should take this therapy (48). New York, California, and Rhode Island have published guidelines for the use of nonoccupational postexposure HIV prophylaxis. The Rhode Island guidelines recommend the use of prophylaxis after any oral, vaginal, anal, or percutaneous exposure to semen, blood, or vaginal secretions that may contain HIV. Prophylaxis should be started no later than 72 hours after possible exposure. A three-drug regimen (zidovudine and lamivudine with the addition of a protease inhibitor) is recommended when the source is known to be HIV positive or has several risk factors for HIV. A two-drug regimen (zidovudine and lamivudine) is suggested when the alleged perpetrator's HIV status is unknown but is presumed to be of lower risk of HIV. Despite guidelines from these three states, there is a need for a national consensus on this subject (49). (See Chapter 16 for a treatment algorithm.) According to the most recent report from the CDC, a definitive recommendation cannot be made regarding administration of postexposure antiretroviral therapy after sexual exposure to HIV (33). In circumstances where the risk for HIV exposure is likely high, antiretroviral therapy should be considered and initiation of prophylaxis should begin as soon as possible (up to 72 hours following the assault). Consultation with an HIV specialist is recommended.

Given the incubation times of STDs, it is clear that initial cultures may miss many infections depending on the number of hours, days, or months the examination is done after sexual contact. Prepubertal children frequently come for examination weeks to months after the abusive episode(s), and thus a single set of cultures is adequate. In contrast, adolescents often come to medical attention shortly after the assault, and thus follow-up cultures and wet preparations for *Trichomonas* infection and bacterial vaginosis are necessary to detect infections acquired at the time of the assault, unless they are treated at the time of the examination. Whether all prepubertal children need to be tested for STDs continues to be debated. Some infections are asymptomatic, but the cost of testing all victims in multiple sites, the low risk of infection, and the potential discomfort remain barriers to universal culturing (30–33,50). On the other hand, a positive culture finding can be very helpful in confirming the diagnosis of sexual abuse.

Selective criteria to limit unnecessary STD testing in prepubertal children has been suggested (51). Factors such as genital discharge, contact with a person thought to have an STD, presence of suspicious ano-genital findings, and disclosure of genital–genital or genital–rectal contact were associated with increased risk of acquiring either gonorrhea and/or chlamydia. A study of sexual abuse victims in Cincinnati reported that positive cultures for gonorrhea were found in prepubertal girls only when a vaginal discharge was present (30). The prevalence of chlamydia and trichomonas in sexually abused prepubertal girls was found to be so small in the study community that it was felt appropriate to omit routine screening for these organisms. A similar study examined the prevalence of gonorrhea in prepubertal girls (less than 12 years of age) with vaginitis who were not suspected of having been sexually abused (52). Of the girls with cultures that were positive for gonorrhea (4/93), all had a vaginal discharge at presentation.

The CDC recommendations for considering testing are outlined in Table 24-2. It has been argued that prevalence rates of STDs among prepubertal girls are low (3.2% overall, 3.1% with *N. gonorrhoeae,* 0.8% with *C. trachomatis,* and 0% with syphilis, trichomoniasis, or HIV infection), even using the guidelines of testing only prepubertal girls with a history of genital discharge or contact with the perpetrator's genitalia or when an examination finds genital discharge or trauma (30). Hymel and

TABLE 24-2. *Recommendations or testing prepubertal girls for sexually transmitted diseases (STDs).*

The decision to conduct an STD evaluation must be made on an individual basis.
Situations involving a high risk for STDs and constitute and strong indication for testing:
- The child has or has had symptoms or signs of an STD.
- Suspected assailant is known to have an STD or be at high risk for STDs.
- Sibling, another child, or an adult in the household has an STD.
- Patient/parent requests testing.
- Prevalence of STDs in the community is high.
- Evidence of genital, oral, or anal penetration or ejaculation is present.
Recommended laboratory tests, if testing is done:
- Cultures for *Neisseria gonorrhoeae* from pharynx, anus, and vagina.
- Cultures for *Chlamydia trachomatis* from anus and vagina.
- Culture and wet mount for *Trichomonas vaginalis* and bacterial vaginosis.
- Serologic testing for syphilis, HIV, and hepatitis B surface antigen.
- Inspection of genital, perianal, and oral area for human papilloma virus.
- *Herpes simplex* virus culture of any ulcerative lesions.

Adapted from Centers for Disease Control and Prevention. Sexually transmitted diseases treatment guidelines 2002. *MMWR* 2002;51(RR-6).

Jenny (31) have proposed that STD screening be done at the time of the assault in prepubertal girls who have a history or physical examination indicative of penetrating trauma, have been molested by a perpetrator at high risk of STD, or have a vaginal discharge or history of vaginal discharge. In low-risk prepubertal patients, they have suggested deferring the cultures to 2 weeks after an acute assault. Muram and colleagues (32) have suggested that culturing for gonorrhea only those seen at the 2-week visit with symptoms may be a reasonable alternative to initial cultures in low-risk prepubertal girls. In contrast to selective testing of prepubertal girls, it has been suggested that all pubertal girls be cultured because of the high prevalence of STDs in the adolescent population.

According to CDC recommendations, only standard culture procedures for the isolation of *N. gonorrhoeae* should be used for children because of the legal implications of a diagnosis of *N. gonorrhoeae* infection in a child. Nonculture gonococcal tests include Gram-stained smear, DNA probes, enzyme immunoassay (EIA), and nucleic acid amplification tests (NAAT). None of these tests have been FDA approved for use with specimens from the oropharynx, rectum, or genital tract of children. Specimens from children should be placed onto selective media and presumptive isolates should be definitively identified by at least two tests that involve different principles (such as biochemical, enzyme substrate, or serologic) and isolates should be preserved to allow for further testing (33).

Only standard culture systems for the isolation of chlamydia should be employed in children because data are not sufficient to assess the use of NAAT for the diagnosis of chlamydia in the evaluation of children who may have been sexually abused (53). However, if culture is not available, a NAAT can be used if confirmation includes a second FDA-approved NAAT that targets a different nucleic acid sequence from the initial test (33).

NAATs have been FDA approved as a substitute for cultures in adolescents and adults. These tests offer the advantage of increased sensitivity. If such a test is used, a positive result should be similarly confirmed by a second FDA licensed nucleic acid amplification test, which targets a different sequence. EIA, nonamplified probes, and direct fluorescent antibody tests yield more false-negative and false-positive results and therefore are not acceptable alternatives for cultures in adolescents (33).

If tests for STDs are to be obtained, the recommended laboratory tests are given in Table 24-2. Vaginal secretions are examined (including by a "whiff" test) for *Trichomonas* and clue cells. Lesions suggestive of HSV infection should be cultured for this virus.

Forensic Evidence Collection

The American Academy of Pediatrics recommends forensic evidence collection (completion of a rape evidence kit) when sexual abuse has occurred within 72 hours or when there is bleeding or acute injury (14). Evidence collection may include swabs from the genital, anal, and oral areas as well as from areas of stained skin. Swabs are tested for blood, sperm, and chemical evidence of semen in an attempt to identify the perpetrator of a sexual assault. Hair and blood standards as well as clothing and foreign debris may be also collected. These items are labeled and sealed in a designated container and sent to the appropriate state crime laboratory with documentation of the individuals who handled the rape kit in order to maintain a "chain of evidence."

Several tests are available for identifying the presence of semen in assault victims. The methods used vary around the country. Acid phosphatase tests may be negative during the first 3 hours; the test is positive in about 50% of vaginal swabs at 12 hours and can be positive for up to 48 hours (54–57). Acid phosphatase may give false-positive results, and thus the test is presumptive, not diagnostic, evidence of semen. The semen protein antigen p30 of prostatic origin is found in the semen of normal and vasectomized men, but not in body fluids of women, and is thus more sensitive and specific than acid phosphatase (57). p30 is undetectable in the vagina by 48 hours after intercourse. A monoclonal antibody (MHS-5) to seminal vesicle specific protein has been devised for use in an ELISA. This assay is highly sensitive and specific for seminal fluid (56) and can be detected in dry semen stains at room temperature for up to 6 months.

Blood group antigens can also be evaluated by many forensic laboratories. DNA mapping of semen, blood, and other biologic material is now commonly used in forensic medicine. DNA typing is potentially the most useful form of forensic evidence due to the high specificity and biochemical stability of DNA making possible the analysis of extremely small samples. DNA evidence can exonerate a person who is falsely accused and can provide courts with a more precise estimation of the odds for a particular perpetrator (56,58,59).

Data vary on the length of time that motile and nonmotile sperm may be found in the vagina or cervical mucus. One study (54) found that in adults with voluntary intercourse only 50% of the specimens examined had motile sperm 3 hours after intercourse, whereas at 72 hours nonmotile sperm could be detected on a fixed preparation in nearly 50%. All specimens contained whole sperm up to 18 hours after intercourse and sperm heads up to 24 hours. A previous study (55) found motile sperm in 31.7% of the victims within 6 hours of the alleged sexual assault and in 18% of those examined 7 to 24 hours after the incident. However, the latter group contained three patients in whom the sperm were detected in cervical mucus, where sperm may remain motile longer (up to 2 to 5 days). Nonmotile sperm may be present in the vagina for 3 to 5 days and in the endocervical canal for up to 17 days (60,61). It should be remembered that the absence of sperm is not evidence against a sexual assault. Up to 50% of specimens obtained from victims of acute rape may have no motile sperm either because the offender has had a vasectomy, sexual dysfunction, oligospermia or because detection techniques are insensitive (62).

Despite the history of using Wood's lamps for the detection of semen, Santucci and colleagues (63) have shown that the four models they tested did not cause semen to fluoresce and other substances such as creams and ointments fluoresced nonspecifically. An alternate light source, Bluemaxx BM 500 (Sirche Finger Print Laboratories, Raleigh, NC), has the correct wavelength for semen fluorescence and can aid trained clinicians in detection of evidence. However, for forensic evaluation, swabs of the umbilical area, perineal area, inner thighs, and buttocks should be obtained for definitive confirmatory studies (DNA analysis) regardless of the light source examination.

Selective completion of the sexual assault kit in the child has been advocated thereby allowing submission of those parts of the evidence collection kit that are pertinent to the history and physical exam. One study found that swabbing a prepubertal child's body for evidence is unnecessary after 24 hours and that clothing and linens yield the majority of evidence in children less than 10 years old (64). After 72 hours, new technology may identify the perpetrator in cases in which evidence is present in vagina in adolescents and adults for 3 weeks or more or on clothing for years; therefore, in certain cases, the kit may be completed after 72 hours (16).

Normal and Abnormal Anogenital Findings in Children and Adolescents

The percentage of sexually abused children with a normal examination has been found to be as high as 90%, depending on the case mix, age of patients, definition of normal versus abnormal, and examiners (65–73). Volumes with photographs and an American Academy of Pediatrics (AAP) slide set are available to clinicians (74,75). The American Professional Society on the Abuse of Children (APSAC) (www.apsac.org) has worked in consensus groups to refine the definitions that can be useful to practicing clinicians. Accurate descriptions of genital findings are essential (Appendix 4).

The use of the colposcope has greatly increased knowledge of normal anatomy (76). The advantages of the colposcope are that the hymen and vulva can be magnified and photographs can be taken at the time of the examination to provide future documentation. Photographs taken with a colposcope or directly with a camera may prevent the need for repeated examinations when the presence of positive physical findings is disputed in court. Photographs are also important for education and for peer review (77). Knowledge of normal anatomy is critical (see chapter 1 and Figs. 24-1 and 24-2).

Cross-sectional data and observations on anogenital anatomy have improved substantially in the last several years (66,78–83). Longitudinal studies of girls with changes in hymenal anatomy have also been reported (84–90). An early study (91) confirmed that all of 1,131 newborn female infants examined were born with hymens. This observation was extended in a study (79) of the hymens of 468 neonates. Most infants had an annular hymen. Complete clefts (noted in 34%) were observed only on the ventral half of the hymen. In a longitudinal study of girls examined at birth and 1 year of age (88), 8% developed labial adhesions, 58% had a decrease in the amount of hymenal tissue, and more infants at 1 year had crescentic configurations. Complete clefts between 4 and 8 o'clock were not observed at either age. In a second longitudinal study of girls examined at 2 months and again at 3 years (87), the

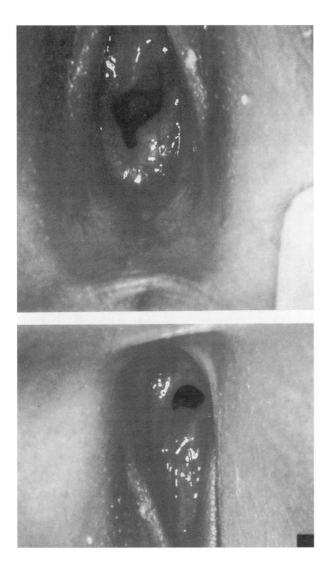

FIG. 24-1. Normal examination. In the supine position (**top**), crescentic hymen with mound of tissue (bump) between 3 and 6 o'clock positions. **Bottom:** In the prone position (knee–chest) the mound of tissue disappears as gravity pulls smooth edge of the hymen ventrally. A normal hymenal border is observed. (From: Heger A, Emans S, Muram D, eds. *Evaluation of the sexually abused child: a medical textbook and photographic atlas.* New York: Oxford University Press, 2000; with permission.)

hymenal configuration changed in 65% of subjects, usually from annular or fimbriated to crescentic. Intravaginal ridges were observed more often at age 3, perhaps in part because observation was easier in the 3-year-old with an unestrogenized hymen. No complete clefts were noted between 5 and 7 o'clock at initial or follow-up study in any of the girls.

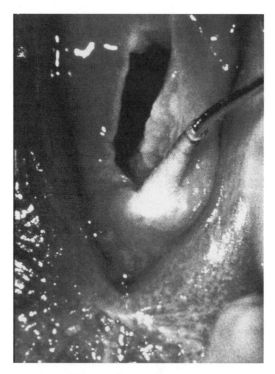

FIG. 24-2. A normal adolescent. The smooth-edged, estrogenized hymen of early adolescence. The cotton swab demonstrates a technique for evaluating the hymen for the presence of transections. (From: Heger A, Emans S, Muram D, eds. *Evaluation of the sexually abused child: a medical textbook and photographic atlas.* New York: Oxford University Press, 2000; with permission.)

A recent cross sectional study was completed that confirmed the findings of earlier research (78,80). A group of 147 premenarchal girls (mean age 63 ± 38 months) selected for nonabuse were studied (Table 24-3) and demonstrated a variety of nonspecific findings (83). The authors concluded that improved techniques and photodocumentation have provided a better understanding of hymenal morphology and that care should be taken not to misinterpret nonspecific findings as posttraumatic changes.

Another study compared the physical findings of a group of abused and nonabused children aged 3 to 8 years (72). Vaginal discharge was more often observed in the abused group. No difference was noted in the numbers of abused versus nonabused children with labial agglutination, increased vascularity, linea vestibularis, friability, a perineal depression, or a hymenal bump, tag, longitudinal intravaginal ridge, external ridge, band, or superficial notch. A hymenal transection, perforation, or deep notch (through more than 50% of the posterior hymenal rim) was observed only in a small number of abused children (4/192). The authors concluded that the genital ex-

TABLE 24-3. *Appearance of the genitalia in 147 premenarchal girls selected for nonabuse (mean age 63 ± 38 mo).*

Hymenal configuration	Nonspecific findings
53% annular	92% perihymenal bands
29% crescentic	94% intravaginal ridges
15% redundant	3% hymenal tags
2% septate	34% hymenal bumps
<1% other	19% linea vestibularis
	79% ventral cleft at 12 o'clock
	19% ventral cleft not at 12 o'clock
	0.6% failure of midline fusion
	49% erythema
	37% change in vascularity
	16% labial adhesions
	18% partial posterior hymenal cleft
	30% posterior hymenal concavity
	22% narrowed hymenal edge

Adapted from: Heger A, Ticson L, Guerra L, et al. Appearance of the genitalia in girls selected for nonabuse: Review of hymenal morphology and nonspecific findings. *J Pediatr Adolesc Gynecol* 2002;15:27.

amination of the abused child rarely differs from that of the nonabused child and that focus should be placed on the child's history as the primary evidence of abuse. Similar results were found in an earlier study of abused and nonabused prepubertal girls (65). A second recent study also arrived at the same conclusion (73). Only 4% of 2,384 children referred for medical evaluation of sexual abuse had abnormal examinations at the time of evaluation. Even with a history of vaginal or anal penetration, the rate of abnormal medical findings was only 5.5%.

Although the term *attenuated* was originally used to describe hymens with narrow rims, this terminology has been replaced with more descriptive terminology to denote whether the rim appears sharply defined or thickened and rounded. A narrow rim hymen that is rounded, thickened, absent, and/or blends into the vagina has been associated with sexual abuse. In contrast, narrow, sharply defined posterior rim hymens can occur in both nonabused populations and in sexually abused girls. Therefore, the significance of this finding is controversial (92). More data on the prevalence of this variant in nonabused populations followed prospectively are needed.

Questions have been raised about the effect of tampon use, sports participation, and prior pelvic examination on hymenal morphology (93,94). In a study (93) of 300 adolescent girls (100 who denied sexual activity and had never used tampons, 100 who denied sexual activity and had used tampons, and 100 consensually active adolescent girls), sexually active girls were significantly more likely to have complete clefts between the 2 and 10 o'clock positions than nonsexually active girls (Table 24-4). Among the nonsexually active girls, only 3% had a complete cleft between 4 and 8 o'clock and only one had a complete cleft at 6 o'clock (0.5%; 95%CI: 0.01, 2.75). The few girls with complete clefts between 4 and 8 o'clock likely had unreported

TABLE 24-4. Genital findings observed in 300 female patients in two adolescent medicine practices: 200 subjects not sexually active, by choice of menstrual hygiene product, and 100 sexually active subjects.

| | Not sexually active | | | |
	Pad users (n = 100)	Tampon users (n = 100)	Sexually active (n = 100)	p*
Subjects with complete clefts (no.)	6	14	84[a]	<0.001[b]
Subjects with complete clefts (2–10 o'clock) (no.)	5	11	81[a]	0.001[b]
Complete hymenal clefts per patient (no.)	0 (0–2)	0(0–2)	2 (0–4)[a]	0.0001[c]
Median hymenal diameter (cm) (range)	1.2 (0.2–2.0)[a]	1.5 (0.3–0.25)[a]	2.5 (1.5–3.5)[a]	<0.0001[c]

*p < 0.01
Ranges are shown in parentheses.
[a] Different from others at p < 0.05 (Duncan, chi-square test).
[b] Chi-square test.
[c] Kruskal-Wallis test.
(From: Emans SJ, Woods ER, Allred EN, Grace E. Hymenal findings in adolescent women: Impact of tampon use and consensual sexual activity. *J Pediatr* 1994;125:153; with permission.)

consensual or nonconsensual sexual intercourse. Tampon use, sports participation (including gymnastics), and prior pelvic examination did not increase the number of complete clefts observed. Among the sexually active group, 74% had complete clefts on the lower half of the hymen between 3 and 9 o'clock. Only sexually active girls had evidence of attenuation or *myrtiform caruncles* (rounded hymenal remnants separated on both sides by complete clefts) (Table 24-5). Adams and colleagues (94) reported posterior notches and clefts in 48% of girls admitting past intercourse compared to 3% of girls who denied intercourse. Two girls who denied intercourse and had a posterior cleft had a history of painful tampon insertion.

TABLE 24-5. Genital findings observed in 300 female patients in two adolescent medicine practices.

	Not sexually active (n = 200)	Sexually active (SA) (n = 100)	p*
Attenuation	0	37%	<0.001
SA ≤3 yr		19/63 (30%)	
SA >3 yr		18/37 (49%)	0.09
Myrtiform caruncles	0	21%	<0.001
SA ≤3 yr		8/63 (13%)	
SA >3 yr		13/37 (35%)	0.009
Age ≤20 yr old		9/61 (15%)	
Age >20 yr old		12/39 (31%)	0.049

*Chi-square test; SA, sexually active.
(From: Emans SJ, Woods ER, Allred EN, Grace E. Hymenal findings in adolescent women: Impact of tampon use and consensual sexual activity. *J Pediatrics* 1994;125:153; with permission.)

Dermatoses, other genital conditions, and accidental genital trauma offer a challenge to the clinician who is called upon to assess whether the genital findings noted are the result of child sexual abuse. Conditions such as lichen sclerosus, urethral prolapse, failure of midline fusion from the anus to the posterior fourchette, localized vulvar pemphigoid, phytophotodermatitis, linear IgA dermatosis, Crohn disease, herpes zoster, allergic contact dermatitis, psoriasis, Ehlers-Danlos syndrome, and ulcerating hemangioma have been confused with trauma from physical and sexual abuse (95).

Genital trauma may be accidental or secondary to sexual abuse (95–99). Straddle injuries may cause trauma to the soft tissues over the symphysis pubis, the ischiopubic ramus, or adductor longus tendon as well as to the posterior fourchette and perineum. These injuries are usually unilateral and anterior and cause damage to the external rather than internal genital structures. The history is usually striking for a fall or other accidental trauma. Vaginal lacerations and rectovaginal injuries can occur in girls who fall astride sharp objects (95). In a large study on unintentional perineal injury in 56 prepubertal girls (ages 1 to 12 years), the labia minora were most commonly involved, and the majority of the injuries were anterior or lateral to the hymen (97). The injuries involved areas posterior to the hymen in 34%. In only one patient was the hymen involved; the patient was 2 years old and fell at a park, abducting her legs in a splits-type mechanism. Among 72 females seen for straddle injuries, 79% had minor lacerations or abrasions of the labia majora or minora, 16% had injuries to the posterior fourchette, and 9% had vulvar hematomas (97). Vaginal injury occurred in 7 patients, and 2 had hymenal injuries (3 had penetrating injuries and 2 others fell on a crossbar or curb). Thus in cases of penetrating trauma, sexual abuse needs to be strongly considered in the presence of a posterior hymenal transection and absence of a convincing history of accidental trauma.

Over the past decade, several classification systems have been proposed for child sexual abuse (Table 24-6) (66–69,92). It is important to remember that a normal examination does not confirm or disprove a history of sexual abuse (68). More than 90% of girls ages 3 to 8 years who described digital or penile-vaginal penetration had no signs of genital injury (72). Definitive and specific findings are more common in those who reported genitogenital assault (86%) than in those who reported digital assault (16%) (69). In a study of physical findings in 31 sexual assault victims (1 to 17 years old) based on offenders' confessions, Muram (67) noted that specific findings suggesting sexual abuse occurred in only 45% of the patients; findings occurred in 11 (61%) of 18 girls when the perpetrator confessed to penetration, compared to three (23%) of 13 when penetration was denied. Thus, seven (39%) of 18 girls in whom the perpetrator confessed to penetration had a normal examination or nonspecific findings. However, both perpetrators and victims may report "vaginal penetration" when vulvar coitus has occurred.

A subsequent study examined the genital and anal findings in children (mean age 9.0 years; range, 8 months to 17 years, 11 months) who were victims of child sexual abuse and whose abusers were convicted (68). The type of molestation described by

A. Muram Classification System

Category 1   Normal-appearing genitalia

Category 2   Nonspecific findings: abnormalities of the genitalia that could have been caused by sexual abuse, but also often seen in girls who are not victims of sexual abuse (e.g. inflammation and scratching). These findings may be the sequelae of poor perineal hygiene or nonspecfic infection. Included in this category are redness of the external genitalia, increased vascular pattern of the vestibular and labial mucosa, presence of purulent discharge from the vagina, small skin fissures or lacerations in the area of the posterior fourchette, and agglutination of the labia minor.

Category 3   Specific findings: the presence of one or more abnormalities strongly suggesting sexual abuse. Such findings include recent or healed lacerations of the hymen and vaginal mucosa, enlarged hymenal opening of ≥1 cm*, procto-episiotomy (a laceration of the vaginal mucosa extending to the rectal mucosa), and indentations in the skin indicating teeth marks (bite marks). The category also includes patients with laboratory confirmation of a venereal disease.

Category 4   Definitive findings: any presence of sperm

* The enlarged opening is not a criteria for the 1997 revision.
From Muram D. Classification of genital findings in prepubertal girls who are victims of sexual abuse. Adolesc Pediatr Gynecol 1988:1:151, with permission.

B. Adams' Classification System

I. Findings documented in newborns or commonly seen in non-abused children

A. Normal variants
Periurethral/vestibular bands
Intravaginal ridges/columns
Hymenal bump/mound
Hymenal tags/septal remnants
Linea vestibularis
Hymenal notch/cleft in anterior half of
    hymenal rim, on/above 3–9 o'clock
    line
External hymenal ridge
Septate hymen
Diastasis ani
Perianal skin tag
Hyperpigmentation of labia minora/
    peri-anal tissues in Mexican-
    American/African-American children
Urethral dilation with labial traction
Thickened hymen
Shallows/superficial notch/cleft in inferior
    rim of hymen, below 3–9 o'clock line

B. Findings caused by other medical conditions
Erythema of vestibule, penis, scrotum,
    or peri-anal tissues
Increased vascularity of vestibule and
    hymen
Labial adhesion
Vaginal discharge
Friability of posterior fourchette or
    commissure
Excoriations/bleeding/vascular lesions
Anal fissures
Venous congestion/pooling
Flattened anal folds
Partial/complete anal dilation to less
    than 2 cm with/without stool present

II. Indeterminate Findings: Findings which, in absence of history of abuse, require further diagnostic studies or careful questioning of child. Consider report to protective services

A. Findings
Deep notches/clefts in posterior/ inferior
    rim of hymen
Posterior rim of hymen which appears to
    be less than 1 mm wide in prone-knee
    chest position or using water to float
    hymen edge when child is supine
Apparent genital warts
Vesicular lesions/ulcers in ano-genital area
Marked, immediate anal dilation to a diame-
    ter of 2 cm or more in absence of chronic
    constipation, sedation, anesthesia,
    neuromuscular conditions.

B. Lesions with confirmed etiology which have indeterminate specificity for sexual transmission
Ano-genital condyloma accuminata
    first appearing in a child older than
    3–5 years of age in absence of
    other abuse indicators
Ano-genital herpes 1 or 2 in child with
    no other indicators of abuse

continues

TABLE 24-6. *(continued)*

III. Findings diagnostic of trauma/sexual contact: Findings which in absence of clear, timely, plausible history of accidental injury or non-sexual transmission, should be reported to child protective services

A. Moderate specificity for abuse
Acute lacerations/extensive bruising of labia, peri-hymenal tissues, penis, scrotum, or perineum
Posterior fourchette scar, not involving hymen
Fresh laceration of posterior fourchette
Peri-anal scar

B. High specificity for abuse/diagnostic of blunt force penetrating trauma
Acute laceration (partial or complete) of hymen
Ecchymosis on hymen
Peri-anal laceration extending deep to external anal sphincter
Healed hymenal transaction
Absence of hymenal tissue in posterior half of hymenal rim

C. Presence of infection confirms mucosal contact with infected genital secretions, contact most likely to have been sexual in nature
Positive confirmed culture for gonorrhea from genitalia, anus, throat outside neonatal period
Confirmed diagnosis of syphilis, if perinatal transmission ruled out
Trichomonas vaginalis infection in child older than 1 year of age
Positive culture from genitalia or anus for Chlamydia in child older than 3 years of age
Positive serology for HIV, if neonatal/blood products transmission ruled out

D. Diagnostic of sexual contact
Pregnancy
Sperm identified in specimens taken by directly from child's body

---

Adapted from: Adams J. Medical evaluation of child sexual abuse. *J Pediatr Adolesc Gynecol* 2004;17:191.

children was fondling in 36%, oral-genital contact in 31%, digital vaginal penetration in 44%, and penile–vaginal contact in 63%. Using their classification schema for genital examination, the authors considered the findings normal in 28%, nonspecific in 49%, suspicious in 9%, and abnormal in 14%. Abnormal anal findings were present in only 1% of patients.

Healing of genital injuries from sexual abuse can occur promptly and thus residua may not be present (71,85,86). In a complete follow-up with photographs of three girls (85), signs of acute injuries disappeared rapidly but some changes, including hymenal transection, persisted throughout the pubertal years. The most persistent findings were irregular hymenal edges and narrow rims at the point of injury. The jagged angular margins smoothed off. Injuries to the posterior fourchette healed with minimal scar tissue and left only the slightest evidence of trauma. Another study noted that wound healing by the process of regeneration might be complete in 48 to 72 hours (86). Complete restoration of epithelial tissues can take 6 weeks (89). Children with epithelial healing had no residua apparent to the naked eye or at 10-fold magnification at follow-up. When injuries are more serious, healing involves repair with formation of granulation tissue and a subsequent scar. Since the linear scar may be only a fraction of the width of the original injury, this too may be difficult for clinicians to detect at follow-up (86). In a 10-year follow-up of 13 boys and 81 girls referred for sexual assault or anogenital trauma, Heppenstall-Heger and colleagues (71) found significant healing in partial tears of the hymen, abrasions, labial trauma, and anal trauma. Those with surgery were more likely to have visible residua. Among the 37 hymenal injuries, two healed after surgery and 15 were unchanged at follow-up.

In the past, hymenal measurements were felt to possibly be of some use in the diagnosis of sexual abuse (78,80,100–102). Subsequent studies have discounted this notion. A recent study (103) compared transhymenal diameters and hymenal measurements of 189 prepubertal children with a history of digital or penile penetration with those of 197 children who denied previous sexual abuse. The authors concluded that most hymenal measurements lack adequate sensitivity and specificity to be used to confirm previous penetration. Less than 1.0 mm of hymenal tissue at the 6 o'clock position was detected only in victims of abuse, but the utility of this measurement was limited by the rarity of this finding. An earlier study arrived at a similar conclusion (104). It is important to remember that several factors affect the diameter of the hymenal orifice, including the position of the child (supine versus knee chest), the amount of labial traction, and the degree of relaxation of the child.

Perianal injuries that result from sexual abuse heal rapidly (71,89). In a follow-up of four children with perianal injuries from sexual abuse documented with photographs, initial findings included erythema, edema of the skin folds, localized venous engorgement, dilatation of the external anal sphincter, and lacerations (89). The superficial lacerations healed in 1 to 11 days; the second-degree wounds in two children healed by the 1- to 5-week return visits, leaving narrow bands of scar tissue. By 12 to 14 months after the assaults, the signs from these two injuries and one surgically repaired injury had virtually disappeared. A skin tag that resulted from the initial injury was persistent, although less evident over time. Importantly, many children with a history of anal assault have no abnormal findings. Specific findings include scars, sphincter tears, and distortion of the anus, although the latter can also occur with inflammatory bowel disease. Fissures can result from sexual abuse and from constipation.

Clinicians should remember that despite the increasing information on associated physical findings, the history is the most important element (105). Table 24-7 provides information for the probability of sexual abuse and the American Academy of Pediatrics guidelines for reporting child sexual abuse combining physical examination, history, and behavioral indicators. It has been noted that in some cases, especially for less experienced examiners, the child's history may influence interpretation of the child's genital findings (106). Physicians should be aware of this potential for bias. In a recent study, physicians self-rated as very experienced in sexual abuse examinations were noted to interpret genital findings that conform more closely to consensus standards (107) than do less experienced physicians. This study underscores the importance of clinician awareness of the most current research findings in the field.

TABLE 24-7. Guidelines for making the decision to report sexual abuse of children.

Data available			Response	
History	Physical examination	Laboratory findings	Level of concern about sexual abuse	Report decision
None	Normal	None	None	No report
Behavioral changes*	Normal	None	Variable depending upon behavior	Possible report†; follow closely (possible mental health referral)
None	Nonspecific findings	None	Low (worry)	Possible report†; follow closely
Nonspecific history by child or history by parent only	Nonspecific findings	None	Intermediate	Possible report†; follow closely
None	Specific findings‡	None	High	Report
Clear statement	Normal	None	High	Report
Clear statement	Specific findings	None	High	Report
None	Normal, nonspecific or specific findings	Positive culture for gonorrhea; positive serologic test for HIV; syphilis; presence of semen, sperm acid phosphatase	Very high	Report
Behavior changes	Nonspecific findings	Other sexually transmitted diseases	High	Report

* Some behavioral changes are nonspecific, and others are more worrisome.
† A report may or may not be indicated. The decision to report should be based on discussion with local or regional experts and/or child protective services agencies.
‡ Other reasons for findings ruled out.
(From American Academy of Pediatrics Committee on Child Abuse and Neglect. Guidelines for the evaluation of sexual abuse of children: Subject review. Pediatrics 1999;103:186–191; with permission)

ASSESSMENT OF THE PREPUBERTAL CHILD

The clinician should take the history from the parents and the child separately, if possible. The physician's interview should not replace a skilled forensic interview. It should be considered a supplement whose purpose is to advocate for the health, well-being, and protection of the child (108). The interview should remain unhurried and calm. It should include the child's past medical history and an assessment of her development as well as family and social history. The clinician should remain non-judgmental and not presuppose that the experience was negative for the child. It may have been neutral or even pleasurable, and the child may not have experienced guilt or anger. In speaking, the clinician should use words that are familiar to the child; it is often helpful to repeat some of the questions during the physical examination to make sure the youngster understands what parts of the anatomy are being questioned. The history, written in the child's words, should include such details as time, place, circumstances, others present, and resistance. Dating the time of the abuse may be easier by referring to a grade in school or a birthday. The child is asked to tell as much about the episode(s) as she remembers. Leading questions should be avoided. Appropriate questions include the following: "Do you know why you are here today?" "Can you tell me what happened?" "How did it begin? What happened?" "Did any other part of his/her body touch you?" "Did you touch any part of his/her body?" "Was the touching over or under your clothes?" "How many times?" Where were you?" "Where was everyone else?" "Who have you told?" "Why tell now?" "Has anybody told you to keep it a secret?" (108). It is important to remember that the first report is almost never the first incident. The interviewer should then ask questions such as "And then what happened?" "What were you wearing?" "What did the room look like?" Older children may be aware of whether ejaculation occurred. The clinician should try to document whether vulvar, vaginal, anal, or oral contact has occurred. The child should be asked about any pain or injuries occurring at the time of the episode. Any symptoms that have occurred following the assault such as sore throat, dysuria, enuresis, vaginal discharge or bleeding, rectal bleeding or pain, abdominal pain, nightmares, or changes in school performance should be recorded.

It is important to establish whether the relationship was prolonged and whether the child has been involved with more than one perpetrator. The child should be asked if she received any gifts and whether she knew the alleged perpetrator. She should also be asked about viewing or taking photographs and about the use of the computer in seducing the child. It is important to know whether she told the parent of the event immediately after its occurrence. Often children have been threatened to keep the abuse a secret. The clinician should make it clear to the child that the abuse is not her fault. It is important to concentrate on what happened rather than why. The child should be told what information needs to be shared, with whom, and why, and she needs an opportunity to ask her own questions.

The child's history is the most important part of the evaluation. To lessen stress in the child and reduce the risk of suggestibility, the number of interviews and interviewers should be minimized, and only interviewers who have skill in eliciting information, are not attached to a particular hypothesis, and are nonjudgmental should be involved (5,109,110). If the initial disclosure can be videotaped, the child may not have to repeatedly relate the story. Children's memories about genital touch have been found to be remarkably accurate, especially with direct questioning (111).

Parents should be allowed to tell their own story separately from the child and to discuss their feelings without the child present. The parental response may greatly influence the reaction of the child to the event (112). The child needs to know that parental anger is directed toward the assailant and not toward her.

The physical examination of the young child should be done in a relaxed setting with a supportive caretaker in the room. Recent studies suggest that adequate preparation of the child for the medical examination may reduce emotional distress during the exam. One study suggests that children with more extensive and aggravated events during the sexual abuse may need more preparation time for the medical assessment (113). A second study found that children viewing a film with a demonstration of the examination reported less fear after film viewing and were less distressed behaviorally, as rated by nurses and mothers, during the exam than children viewing a nonrelevant film (114). A study of 227 children who underwent video colposcopy found that most children were interested in watching their anogenital examination and tolerated the procedure well (115).

An assistant can help in the collection of samples and in reassuring the child. It is extremely important to elicit the cooperation of the child. The steps for evaluation of a victim of an acute assault are outlined here, although most cases seen by clinicians in the office setting will probably involve long-standing cases of abuse often by a known individual. The need to obtain specimens for STD testing is discussed under Sexually Transmitted Diseases and Sexual Assault. Forensic specimens should be collected so that the legal evidence is preserved if the family decides to press charges (see Forensic Evidence Collection).

The physical examination should include the following steps:

1. A description of the patient's general appearance, emotional state, and condition of the clothing should be included. She should be asked if she has changed clothes or bathed since the assault. Clothing worn at the time of the incident should be placed in a paper bag. All debris observed during the gross examination of the patient should be enclosed in a paper container.
2. A general physical examination with notation of any injuries should be completed. The size and color of any hematomas should be recorded on a diagram. Photographs should be taken of any contusions. Bruises may not appear for 24 hours. Any area of dried secretions such as saliva from bite marks, blood, or semen should be scraped or swabbed with a gauze pad or cotton swab slightly moistened with distilled or tap water and retained as evidence after thoroughly air-dried. A Bluemaxx lamp may detect areas of semen by fluorescence (116). Fingernail scrapings should be obtained.

3. A genital examination with careful inspection of the perineum, noting any injuries, signs of sexually transmitted diseases, or evidence of dried secretions should be performed. The hymen and posterior fourchette should be carefully examined using magnification with a handheld lens, otoscope, or colposcope. Acute assaults may be accompanied by extensive hymenal and perineal lacerations or ecchymoses. Dried secretions are collected with a slightly moistened gauze pad. The vagina can be visualized in the frog-leg and/or knee-chest position, and any abnormal hymenal configuration, discharge, bleeding, or foreign bodies should be noted. Abnormal findings in the frog-leg position should be verified using the knee-chest position if at all possible (see Fig. 24-1). In cases where vaginal bleeding is found, the source of the blood should be identified. If the bleeding source is not obvious, a laceration cannot be properly assessed or repaired, or the child has been too traumatized to cooperate, an examination and vaginoscopy under sedation or anesthesia is indicated. One study found that application of toluidine blue to the vulva of girls seen within 48 hours of abuse may aid in the detection of posterior fourchette lacerations (117); many centers use magnified visualization in the green spectrum of the colposcope.

   Specimens to check for the presence of sperm and cultures if indicated can be obtained with a moistened Calgiswab. A wet preparation to look for motile sperm, trichomonads, and clue cells, and a "whiff" test should be done. Any genital or anal discharge should be Gram-stained. Urine can be examined for white cells, trichomonads, and sperm.

4. The perianal area should be inspected. If anal assault is suspected, specimens for detection of semen should be collected from the rectum.

5. Oral swabs are obtained for forensic studies if oral-genital contact within 24 hours is suspected.

6. Blood should be drawn for a serologic test for syphilis [rapid plasma reagin (RPR) test] if indicated.

7. Serum can be collected for testing of HIV and hepatitis B if indicated.

8. Cultures can be individualized in prepubertal children (see Sexually Transmitted Diseases and Sexual Assault). If cultures are obtained, samples for *N. gonorrhoeae* culture are obtained from the vagina, rectum, and throat, and samples for *Chlamydia trachomatis* culture from the vagina and rectum. Genital vesicles and ulcers should be cultured for HSV. (see Table 24-2.)

9. In the asymptomatic prepubertal child involved in chronic or prior abuse, antibiotic treatment is usually prescribed only if a positive culture is found. Presumptive treatment for children who have been sexually abused is not recommended by the CDC because the prevalence of most STDs is low following abuse; prepubertal girls appear to be at less risk for ascending infection than adolescent or adult women; and regular follow-up of children is felt to be better ensured (33). Treatment for gonorrhea and chlamydial infection involves giving ceftriaxone 125 mg followed by erythromycin 50 mg/kg per day for 10

to 14 days, azithromycin 1 gram in a single dose (if the child weighs at least 45 kg), or doxycycline 100 mg BID for 7 days (if the patient is 8 years of age or older). A short course of stool softeners may be prescribed for sodomy cases, and phenazopyridine for girls with vulvar trauma and dysuria. Tetanus toxoid is given according to standard pediatric guidelines following acute injuries. HIV prophylaxis should be individualized (see section on Sexually Transmitted Diseases and Sexual Assault).

The child should be seen for medical follow-up approximately 2 weeks after the evaluation for the acute assault to assess healing of injuries and check the results of the initial cultures. If no prophylactic antibiotics were given at the time of an acute assault, cultures for *N. gonorrhoeae* and *C. trachomatis* can be repeated at the follow-up visit. If, however, 1 to 2 weeks have elapsed between the incident of abuse and the initial evaluation, cultures need not be repeated. Vaginal secretions should be examined for trichomoniasis and bacterial vaginosis. Repeat serology for syphilis and hepatitis B and HIV testing can be obtained 12 weeks after an acute assault (33).

At the conclusion of the examination, it is extremely important to discuss with the child and parents the clinical findings, since many assume the child is "damaged goods." Parents are greatly relieved to be told that their child is normal and healthy. Before the examination, parents often express extreme anxiety over the possible loss of virginity and reproductive potential and are greatly reassured by a careful discussion. When there has been an injury, the treatment and follow-up plan of care should be outlined. Most minor trauma heals without visible sequelae.

The medical record should indicate exactly what was observed as it may be subpoenaed and scrutinized years later. It should describe how the child presented and with whom. The record should clearly indicate who was present for both the interviews of the parent and child. The child's exact words in response to questions should be documented. A clear explanation of the significance of the physical exam findings should be included as well as any recommendations for medical or mental health follow-up.

All cases of sexual abuse in children must be reported to child protective services. The need for long-term psychological support for the child depends on the individual case and the presence of preexisting psychological problems and psychosocial circumstances (118–122). Both a child's stage of development and the nature of the encounter determine the impact on the child. In situations of onetime nonforceful exposure (fondling), a careful history, genital examination, and reassurance for the family are important. Most of the follow-up counseling is directed to the parents since, if they can remain unambiguously supportive, the impact on the child may be minimal. In cases involving a caregiver and/or repetitive abuse, the child and family should receive counseling directed to their needs. Young children may have a high level of anxiety and may manifest somatic and behavioral symptoms. Sorting out good and bad feelings toward the perpetrator, mother, and others involved is important. Children may need to relearn the ability to trust and to display affection; self-esteem needs to be fostered and increased. Allowing the child to make choices can empower her to realize that she can believe in herself and make wise choices in the future.

Cases involving long-standing intrafamilial abuse are particularly problematic. Clinicians need legal and psychological services within the community prepared to deal long-term with these difficult situations. The aim of incest treatment must be to stop the incest and to treat all the family members. The mother must be willing and able to protect her children, and both parents have to admit to the problem and have a desire to remedy it either by improving their marriage or divorcing. The best interests of the child must be foremost. Long-term outcomes are variable, and clearly the inability of parents to provide the necessary protection for the child may cause long-term problems.

Increased court involvement and prosecution have been useful in the resolution of some cases. Children can be helped through the court process by sensitive victim–witness advocates, district attorneys, and mental health professionals. Unfortunately, the long, drawn-out process and the need for the child to confront the defendant directly rather than by videotape have made the judicial process difficult for many (123,124). A not-guilty verdict can be devastating to the victim, who feels she has not been believed. On the other hand, a guilty verdict can be helpful in the child's recovery. Psychotherapy should not await a court verdict but should be ongoing from the time of the disclosure. Physicians and nurse practitioners often find the task of testifying in court problematic because of lack of experience and interruptions to their usual patient schedule. Proper preparation is essential.

ASSESSMENT OF THE ADOLESCENT

In contrast to the pattern of sexual abuse in prepubertal children, sexual abuse during adolescence is more likely to be a one-time assault by either a stranger or acquaintance and involve vaginal intercourse (10). Thus, a rape kit for collection of forensic specimens is more likely to be necessary for this evaluation. Risk-taking behaviors such as alcohol and drug use and hitchhiking may make certain adolescents more vulnerable (125). In fact, more than 40% of adolescent victims and assailants reported using alcohol or drugs immediately before a sexual assault (126). The illegal availability of the sedative, hypnotic "date rape" drug, flunitrazepam (Rohypnol) has contributed to the problem of acquaintance rape (127,128). In other cases, the developmental changes that take place during adolescence may make a long-standing incestuous relationship intolerable; the adolescent may then respond with a sudden disclosure, may seek medical care for somatic symptoms such as abdominal pain or headache, or may become involved in impulsive behavior such as running away. A pregnancy may be the first sign of a previous rape or chronic sexual abuse. It is therefore important to ask the adolescent not only whether she has ever had sexual relations but also whether she has ever been forced into a sexual relationship.

In recording the history of the adolescent with alleged sexual assault, clinicians should follow an outline similar to that described in the above section Assessment of the Prepubertal Child. In acute situations, the patient should be asked if she has bathed, douched, or urinated since the assault. A menstrual and contraceptive history should be obtained. Clinicians should not try to decide whether rape has occurred on the basis of the patient's emotional response to the trauma, for clearly some patients will be tearful, tense, and hysterical, and others will appear controlled or subdued. Questions should focus on what happened and whether vaginal, rectal, or oral penetration occurred. Terms understood by the patient should be used and questions may need to be repeated during the examination when the adolescent is more familiar with the anatomic terms. A rape protocol should be used to collect evidence. It is extremely helpful if a nurse who has experience with adolescent rape victims can be assigned to the adolescent throughout the 2- to 4-hour stay in the emergency department and can be present during the history taking, physical examination, and police interviews.

After the history is obtained, the patient should be told of the need for a thorough physical examination to assess injuries and collect laboratory specimens, including tests for STDs. Each part of the examination should be discussed in advance, and the patient should be given a sense of control over the tempo of the examination. She should be told that the examination is important but that the examiner can stop if the patient wishes and finish at another time. Anatomic pictures or a plastic model (Ortho) can be used to familiarize the adolescent with the type of examination. The following assessment applies to the acute sexual assault.

The physical examination should include the following steps:

1. A description should be recorded of the patient's general appearance, emotional state, and condition of the clothing. Any clothing that might provide evidence in a legal case should be included in the rape evidence bag.
2. A general physical examination should note any evidence of injury. As noted in the examination of the prepubertal child, debris and dried secretions should be properly collected. The Tanner stages of pubertal development should be noted. If the history indicates any attempt by the patient to scratch or fight her assailant, fingernail scrapings should be obtained. Head-hair combings and a head-hair standard are included in many rape kits. The pelvic examination should include a careful inspection of the perineum, noting any evidence of bleeding or lacerations. A gauze pad or cotton swab lightly moistened with nonbacteriostatic sterile saline should be used to wipe the vulva. The location of any dried secretions should be marked on a sketch. A collection paper should be placed under the buttocks of the patient and the pubic hair combed toward the paper to collect any debris, which should be placed in a collection envelope. If any foreign hairs are noted, eight to 25 pubic hairs of the patient should be obtained (preferable plucked) and included in a separate envelope. The hymenal border can be examined for tears by running a saline-moistened cotton-tipped applicator around

the edges (see Fig. 24-2) or by using a Foley bladder catheter. A handheld lens or colposcope can aid in the evaluation. Small abrasions or telangiectasia in the posterior fourchette may be identified with magnification or with toluidine blue (61). Vaginal swabs for semen can be obtained by gently inserting a cotton-tipped applicator through the hymenal ring. A moistened cotton-tipped applicator can be used to obtain further vaginal samples to look for the presence of motile sperm, trichomonads, yeast, and clue cells. A "whiff" test is also done on this specimen. Any genital discharge should be Gram-stained. Genital ulcers suggestive of genital herpes should be cultured.

In most pubertal adolescent girls, a gentle vaginal examination can be done with a water-moistened (Huffman) small speculum. If the hymenal orifice is too small, cultures for *C. trachomatis* and *N. gonorrhoeae* can be obtained from the vagina. It is extremely important to examine the teenager gently so that the examination does not result in further emotional trauma. With the speculum in place, the vagina is inspected for injury and the presence of semen or vaginal discharge, and endocervical specimens for cultures are obtained. A purulent endocervical discharge should be Gram stained to look for white cells and Gram-negative intracellular diplococci. Samples from the vaginal fornices and the cervix are obtained for semen analysis and to check for motile sperm; the wet and dry smears should be appropriately marked. Approximately 1% of victims have moderate or severe genital injuries that require surgical intervention. Upper vaginal lacerations usually require laparotomy.

3. The anus should be inspected, and any discharge swabbed and Gram stained. Specimens for sperm should be obtained if there is a history of rectal assault. Perianal swabs are collected using cotton swabs lightly moistened with saline; anorectal swabs are not moistened prior to collection. Cultures for *N. gonorrhoeae* and *C. trachomatis* are obtained. Anoscopy should be done if rectal bleeding is present or the rectal examination reveals fecal occult blood. Rectal sphincter tone should be assessed since patients subjected to chronic anal abuse may have reflex relaxation.

4. Specimens from the girl's mouth should be obtained, especially if oral-genital contact has occurred. A throat swab should be plated for *N. gonorrhoeae*. Oral swabs are obtained for detection of semen and other foreign matter if oral–genital contact occurred within 24 hours. Dry swabs are wiped on the areas between the lips and gums and along the tooth and gum lines. A saliva sample can also be obtained for secretor status even if no oral contact occurred.

5. Blood should be drawn for a serologic test for syphilis (RPR) and testing for HIV and hepatitis B, if indicated. A blood sample is also frequently included in rape kits for the police laboratory to do ABO blood typing of the victim.

6. A sensitive urine or serum pregnancy test should be done to detect a preexisting pregnancy. A urine sample for toxicology evaluation should be considered up to 72 hours after the assault if drug or alcohol ingestion occurred at the time of the assault (16).

If the patient was unconscious during the assault, samples should be obtained from vagina, rectum, and mouth. All specimens for the pathology laboratory or the police should be delivered personally by the doctor or nurse involved in the case, and properly signed receipts should be obtained. Use of a rape-evidence kit or rape protocol does not imply that the family or patient must proceed with prosecution; however, reporting the rape and using a protocol to collect the evidence ensures that it has been appropriately handled and will be admissible in court if prosecution is to occur.

In cases of acute rape, the decision to prescribe antibiotics should be individualized and based on the risks of acquiring an STD. The benefits of prophylactic treatment for gonorrhea, Chlamydia, and trichomoniasis should be discussed with the patient. In asymptomatic adolescents with long-standing incestuous relationships, clinicians may wait for the results of cultures and blood tests before initiating treatment unless the perpetrator is known to be infected. For the adolescent victim of acute assault, we believe that antibiotics should be given to prevent sequelae, such as pelvic inflammatory disease, and to lessen the need for repeat cultures 2 weeks later, because patients are often lost to follow-up. If prophylactic treatment is given, follow-up cultures do not need to be obtained unless the girl reports having symptoms. The patient should be informed that not all organisms are covered by antibiotics and follow-up within 1 to 2 weeks is essential, especially if antibiotic prophylaxis is not given. For therapy, a single intramuscular dose of ceftriaxone 125 mg, followed by metronidazole 2 g orally in a single dose plus 7 days of doxycycline 100 mg twice a day for 7 days or azithromycin 1 g single dose (33) is recommended. Alternatively, the metronidazole could be given as 500 mg twice a day for 7 days.

If the initial RPR test is negative, a follow-up serologic test at 12 weeks for syphilis is necessary if spectinomycin is chosen as an alternative for gonococcal prophylaxis or no prophylaxis is given. Tetanus toxoid should be given following standard pediatric guidelines for injuries. Hepatitis B vaccine should be administered to victims of sexual assault at the time of the initial examination if they have not been previously vaccinated. Additional doses of vaccine should be given 1 to 2 and 4 to 6 months after the first dose.

Emergency contraception with levonorgestrel 0.75 mg, repeated in 12 hours (Plan B) should be offered to the postpubertal adolescent who was raped within the last 120 hours (see Chapter 20). A sensitive (urine or blood) pregnancy test should be done at the time of the evaluation.

A current telephone number of the patient should be verified, and a follow-up appointment should be arranged for 2 weeks later. A repeat pelvic examination is done to assess healing of injuries and to look for vaginal trichomoniasis and bacterial vaginosis if not treated. It should be remembered that absence of injuries does not preclude the possibility of rape. Repeat cultures for *N. gonorrhoeae* and *C. trachomatis* should be done if initial cultures were positive (and treated) or if prophylaxis was not given. A sensitive pregnancy test should be done 2 to 3 weeks after the rape, regardless of whether emergency contraception was given. Testing for HIV and hepatitis B can be performed at 12 weeks post assault and, if positive, compared with the serum frozen from the initial visit. If HIV testing is negative, it can be repeated 12 months post assault. At long-term follow-up, the patient should be examined for HIV infection and Pap test screening should be initiated.

The patient should be reassured about the findings on genital examination. Patients greatly benefit from drawings, which illustrate normal adolescent genital anatomy. The virginal adolescent who has had a forced episode of sexual intercourse may feel considerably relieved to understand that her external genitalia are not very different from some adolescents who have not had intercourse. She needs to be reassured that the assault in no way changes her ability to have normal sexual intercourse in the future or to have normal, healthy children. Teenagers may have unprotected intercourse because of concern that a rape that occurred when they were 12 or 13 years old markedly diminished their reproductive potential. It is not unusual for a patient to have somatic reactions (muscle soreness, headaches, fatigue, stomach pain, dysuria, sleep disturbances, and nightmares) in the first several weeks following a rape.

The extent of counseling in the aftermath of a sexual assault depends on the initial encounter. For example, in the situation of an isolated episode of exhibitionism or nonforceful genital fondling by a stranger or neighbor, counseling should help integrate the event with a strongly positive view of the future. In the case of a long-standing incestuous relationship, a long-term treatment program may be required. For the victim of acute sexual assault, information about the legal system and the benefits of counseling should be provided. Even if the girl seems nonverbal or appears to be coping well, the counselor can often play an educational and supportive role, reassuring the girl about her intactness and her femininity. Physicians should work with the parents to help them support their daughter. Even when the daughter has been a victim of forced rape, parents may feel that the style of dress, the acceptance of a ride, or other behavior meant the teen was "asking for it." The clinician should make it clear to the parents that the teenager will deal with the crisis considerably better if she has their support.

It is difficult to predict the long-term sequelae of a rape because victims cope with stress in many different ways. However, it is clear that later sexual disturbances are common when the first sexual experience occurs in the context of violence and degradation. The other issues that tend to emerge later include (a) mistrust of men, (b) phobic reactions, and (c) neurotic symptoms of anxiety and depression precipitated by events that remind the victim of the original episode (129). A "rape trauma syndrome" has been described by a number of authors, and the long-term reactions have characteristics of posttraumatic stress disorder (129–133). Patients may have difficulty with pelvic examinations done months to years after the rape episode.

Although improvements are in sight, prosecution may intensify the guilt and shame of the victim. A counselor for the victim should ideally accompany the teenager through the legal process and explain the involvement of prosecutors, judges, and courts.

SEXUAL ABUSE PREVENTION

With the recognition by health care professionals and educators of the widespread problem of sexual abuse, efforts have been made in the area of prevention. The AAP encourages parents to make sure their schools have prevention programs for students and teachers, to discuss the subject with their children, to teach their children about body parts, to be good listeners, and to know with whom their children are spending time. Young children should have sufficient knowledge of their bodies to know what types of behavior from adults to avoid or report. Children need to know that they can refuse demands for physical closeness, even from friends or relatives. They should be told early to avoid accepting rides from strangers or candy or money in exchange for close relationships. Most programs include the following topics: the distinction between good, bad, and questionable touching; the rights of children to control who touches their bodies; the importance of children's telling a responsible adult if someone inappropriately touches them; assertive skills; and support systems. A recent study of 825 women undergraduates at a New England university found that 62% had participated in a "good touch–bad touch" sexual abuse prevention program in childhood. Approximately 8% of respondents who had participated in a prevention program reported subsequent sexual abuse compared with 14% who did not ever participate. This study suggests a reduced incidence of sexual abuse associated with participation in a sexual abuse prevention program in childhood, although confirmation of this observation in a prospective study would provide stronger evidence that school based programs can actually prevent sexual abuse (134).

Most efforts to prevent sexual abuse involve teaching children to resist abuse and to report it promptly to adults. While such programs have been shown to increase children's knowledge and skills (135) and have facilitated disclosures of prior abuse, it is less clear whether this instruction actually decreases the incidence of abuse (136,137). Furthermore, these programs place the burden of stopping and reporting abuse on the children.

A number of other options for preventing sexual abuse have been proposed. A marketing and public education campaign developed in Vermont offers a different approach to prevention. This program asserts that adults, not children, must confront abusers and encourage them to change by offering a toll-free help line with information about referrals to treatment programs and information about the legal system (138). Between 1995 and 1997, 50 individuals who had not entered the legal system sought treatment for sexual offending. State attorney's offices indicated that eight child molesters presented themselves voluntarily to legal authorities (139). It is not possible to know how many of the self-reports by sexual offenders were actually due to the campaign and additional research would be needed to address this question. The value of such a campaign may be its ability to change social attitudes about treatment and control of sexual offenders.

Another method of preventing sexual abuse may be adequate sentencing and treatment of sexual offenders, thereby protecting children who might otherwise have been victimized (140). The sexual offense recidivism rate in a meta-analysis of 61 studies (average follow-up period of 4 to 5 years) was 12% to 20% (141). Evidence suggests that some sexual offenders were also victims of child sexual abuse and that inadequate family support after the abuse may be an important contributing factor in future offending behavior. In the United States, the number of treatment programs for children and adolescents has declined dramatically. There is therefore a desperate need for research, which focuses on the cause of sexually deviant behavior and improvements in treatment for offenders (137).

Programs have been initiated in many communities to help young women deal with rape prevention. Particular risk factors for adolescents who have been victims of sexual assault are voluntarily agreeing to go to the house or apartment or in the car of a young man that they have known for less than 24 hours, impairment with drugs or alcohol, and hitchhiking (125). Adolescents need to be aware of high-risk situations and should be counseled to seek medical care after a rape. Prevention messages should be designed for both males and females. Adolescents should be asked questions regarding past sexual victimization as part of a routine history (10).

Although this chapter has dealt only with girls because the focus of this volume is gynecology, boys, too, may be subject to intrafamilial and stranger homosexual and heterosexual abuse; they need the same type of education and meaningful medical care during childhood as their female counterparts.

REFERENCES

1. Jones L, Finkelhor D, Kopiec K. Why is sexual abuse declining? A survey of state child protection administrators. *Child Abuse Negl* 2001;25:1139.
2. Shrier L, Pierce J, Emans S, et al. Gender differences in risk behaviors associated with forced or pressured sex. *Arch Pediatr Adolesc Med* 1998;152:57.
3. Wilson K, Klein J. Opportunities for appropriate care: health care and contraceptive use among adolescents reporting unwanted sexual intercourse. *Arch Pediatr Adolesc Med* 2002;156:341.
4. Rennison C. Criminal Victimization 2001: Changes 2000–01 with Trends 1993–2001. Washington, DC: Bureau of Justice Statistics; 2002. (Available at: http://www.ojp.usdoj.gov/bjs/.)
5. Finkelhor D. Current information on the scope and nature of child sexual abuse. *Future of Children* 1994;4:31.
6. Orr D, Prietto S. Emergency management of sexually abused children. *Am J Dis Child* 1979;33: 628.
7. Dubowitz H, Black M, Harrington D. The diagnosis of child sexual abuse. *Am J Dis Child* 1992;146: 688.
8. Herman-Giddens M. Vaginal foreign bodies and child sexual abuse. *Arch Pediatr Adolesc Med* 1994;148:195.
9. Leder M, Emans S, Hafler J, et al. Addressing sexual abuse in the primary care setting. *Pediatrics* 1999;104:270.
10. American Academy of Pediatrics Committee on Adolescence. Care of the adolescent sexual assault victim. *Pediatrics* 2001;107:1476.
11. Kienberger Jaudes P, Marione M. Interdisciplinary evaluations of alleged sexual abuse cases *Pediatrics* 1992;89:1164.
12. Paradise J, Rostain A, Nathanson M. Substantiation of sexual abuse charges when parents dispute custody or visitation. *Pediatrics* 1988;81:835.
13. Becker J. Offenders: characteristics and treatment. *Future of Children* 1994;4:176.
14. American Academy of Pediatrics Committee on Child Abuse and Neglect. Guidelines for the evaluation of sexual abuse of children: subject review. *Pediatrics* 1999;103:186–191.

15. Schetsky D, Green A. *Child sexual abuse: a handbook for health care and legal professionals.* New York: Brunner/Mazel, 1988.
16. American College of Emergency Physicians. Evaluation and Management of the Sexually Assaulted or Sexually Abused Patient. Dallas, TX: American College of Emergency Physicians; 1999. (Available at: http://www.acep.org/library/index.cfm/id/2101.)
17. Beck-Sague CM and Jenny C. Sexual assault and STD. In: Holmes KK, Märdh P-A, Sparling PF, et al, eds. *Sexually transmitted diseases,* 3rd ed. New York: McGraw-Hill, 1999.
18. Matson N, Gutman LT. Child sexual abuse and sexually transmitted diseases. In: Holmes KK, Märdh P-A, Sparling PF, et al, eds. *Sexually transmitted diseases,* 3rd ed. New York: McGraw-Hill, 1999.
19. Kellogg N, Huston R, Foulds D. *Chlamydia trachomatis* infections in children evaluated for sexual abuse. *Fam Med* 1991;23:59.
20. Jenny C. Sexually transmitted diseases and child abuse. *Pediatr Ann* 1992;21:497.
21. Jenny C, Hooton T, Bowers B, et al. Sexually transmitted diseases in victims of rape. *N Engl J Med* 1990;322:713.
22. Robinson A, Watkeys J, Ridgway G. Sexually transmitted organisms in sexually abused children. *Arch Dis Child* 1998;79:356.
23. Jones J, Jamauchi T, Lambert B. *Trichomonas vaginalis* infestation in sexually abused girls. *Am J Dis Child* 1985;139:846.
24. Dattel B, Landers D, Coulter K, et al. Isolation of *Chlamydia trachomatis* from sexually abused female adolescents. *Obstet Gynecol* 1988;72:240.
25. Sturm J, Carr M, Luxenberg M, et al. The prevalence of *Neisseria gonorrhoeae* and *Chlamydia trachomatis* in victims of sexual assault. *Ann Emerg Med* 1990;19:597.
26. Glaser J, Schacter J, Benes S, et al. Sexually transmitted diseases in post pubertal female rape victims. *J Infect Dis* 1991;164:726.
27. Estreich S, Forster G, Robinson A. Sexually transmitted diseases in rape victims. *Genitourin Med* 1990;66:433.
28. Schwarcz S, Whittington W. Sexual assault and sexually transmitted diseases: detection and management in adults and children. *Rev Infect Dis* 1990;12[Suppl 6]:5682.
29. Sicoli R, Losek J, Hudlett J, et al. Indications for *Neisseria gonorrhoeae* cultures in children with suspected sexual abuse. *Arch Pediatr Adolesc Med* 1995;149:86.
30. Siegel R, Schubert C, Myers P, et al. The prevalence of sexually transmitted diseases in children and adolescents evaluated for sexual abuse in Cincinnati: rationale for limited STD testing in prepubertal girls. *Pediatrics* 1995;96:1090.
31. Hymel K, Jenny C. Child sexual abuse. *Pediatr Rev* 1996;17:236.
32. Muram D, Speck P, Dockter M. Child sexual abuse examination: Is there a need for routine screening for *N. gonorrhoeae? J Pediatr Adolesc Gynecol* 1996;9:79.
33. Centers for Disease Control and Prevention. Sexually transmitted diseases treatment guidelines 2002. *MMWR* 2002;51(RR-6).
34. Ross J, Scott G, Busuttil A. *Trichomonas vaginalis* infection in pre-pubertal girls. *Med Sci Law* 1993;22:82.
35. Kellogg N, Parro J. The progression of human papillomavirus lesions in sexual assault victims. *Pediatrics* 1995;96:1163.
36. Stevens-Simon C, Nelligan D, Breese P, et al. The prevalence of genital human papillomavirus infections in abused and nonabused preadolescent girls. *Pediatrics* 2000;106:655.
37. Hammerschlag M. The transmissibility of sexually transmitted diseases in sexually abused children. *Child Abuse Negl* 1998;22:623–635.
38. Watts D, Koutsky L, Holmes K, et al. Low risk of perinatal transmission of human papillomavirus: Results of a prospective cohort study. *Am J Obstet Gynecol* 1998;178:365.
39. Lindegren M, Hanson C, Hammett T, et al. Sexual abuse of children: intersection with the HIV epidemic. *Pediatrics* 1998;102:E46. Available at: http://www.pediatrics.org/cgi/content/full/102/4/e46
40. Gellert G, Durfee M, Berkowitz C, et al. Situational and sociodemographic characteristics of children infected with human immunodeficiency virus from pediatric sexual abuse. *Pediatrics* 1993; 91:39.
41. Gellert G. Pediatric acquired immunodeficiency syndrome: testing as a barrier to recognizing the role of child sexual abuse [Editorial]. *Arch Pediatr Adolesc Med* 1994;148:766.
42. Gutman L, Herman-Giddens M, McKinney R. Pediatric acquired immunodeficiency syndrome: barriers to recognizing the role of child sexual abuse. *Am J Dis Child* 1993;147:775.

43. Rimsza M. Words too terrible to hear: sexual transmission of human immunodeficiency virus to children [Editorial]. *Am J Dis Child* 1993;147:711.
44. Gellert G, Durfee M, Berkowitz C. Developing guidelines for HIV antibody testing among victims of pediatric sexual abuse. *Child Abuse Negl* 1990;14:9.
45. Katz M, Gerberding J. Postexposure treatment of people exposed to the human immunodeficiency virus through sexual contact or injection-drug use. *N Engl J Med* 1997;336:1097.
46. Gutman L, St Claire K, Weedy C, et al. Human immunodeficiency virus transmission by child sexual abuse. *Am J Dis Child* 1991;145:137.
47. Gutman L, St Claire K, Weedy C, et al. Sexual abuse of human immunodeficiency virus-positive children: outcomes for perpetrators and evaluation of other household children. *Am J Dis Child* 1992;146:1185.
48. Olshen E, Samples C. Post-exposure prophylaxis: an intervention to prevent HIV in adolescents. *Curr Opin Pediatr* 2003;15:379.
49. Babl F, Cooper E, Kastner B, et al. Prophylaxis against possible human immunodeficiency virus exposure after nonoccupational needlestick injuries or sexual assault in children and adolescents. *Arch Pediatr Adolesc Med* 2001;155:680.
50. Sirotnak A. Testing sexually abused children for sexually transmitted diseases: who to test, when to test, and why. *Pediatr Ann* 1994;23:370.
51. Ingram D, Miller W, Schoenbach V, et al. Risk assessment for gonococcal and chlamydial infections in young children undergoing evaluation for sexual abuse. *Pediatrics* 2001;107:E73. Available at http://www.pediatrics.org/cgi/content;/full/107/5/e73
52. Shapiro R, Schubert C, Siegel R. Neisseria gonorrhea infections in girls younger than 12 years of age evaluted for vaginitis. *Pediatrics* 1999;104:E72. Available at http://www.pediatrics.org/cgi /content/ full/104/6/e72.
53. Hammerschlag, M. Use of nucleic acid amplification tests in investigating child sexual abuse. *Sex Transm Inf* 2001:77:153.
54. Soules M, Pollard A, Brown K, et al. The forensic laboratory evaluation of evidence in alleged rape. *Am J Obstet Gynecol* 1978;130:142.
55. Duenhoelter J, Stone I, Santos-Ramos R, et al. Detection of seminal fluid constituents after alleged sexual assault. *J Forensic Sci* 1978;4:824.
56. Jenny C. Forensic examination: the role of the physician as "medical detective." In: Heger A, Emans S, Muram D eds. *Evaluation of the sexually abused child. a medical textbook and photographic atlas.* New York: Oxford University Press, 2000:79.
57. Graves H, Sensabaugh G, Blake E. Postcoital detection of a male-specific semen protein. *N Engl J Med* 1985;312:330.
58. Annas G. Setting standards for the use of DNA-typing results in the courtroom—the state of the art. *N Engl J Med* 1992;326:1641.
59. Chakroborty R, Kidd K. The utility of DNA typing in forensic work. *Science* 1991;254:1735.
60. Dahlke M, Cooke C, Cunnanne M, et al. Identification of semen in 500 patients seen because of rape. *Am J Clin Pathol* 1977;68:740.
61. Hampton H. Care of the woman who has been raped. *N Engl J Med.* 1995;332:234.
62. Groth A, Burgess A. Sexual dysfunction during rape. *N Engl J Med* 1977;297:764.
63. Santucci K, Nelson D, McQuillen K, et al. Wood's lamp utility in the identification of semen. *Pediatrics* 1999;104:1342.
64. Christian C, Lavelle J, DeJong A, et al. Forensic evidence findings in prepubertal victims of sexual assault. *Pediatrics* 2000;106:100.
65. Emans S, Woods E, Flagg N, et al. Genital findings in sexually abused, symptomatic and asymptomatic girls. *Pediatrics* 1987;79:778.
66. Muram D. Classification of genital findings in prepubertal girls who are victims of sexual abuse. *Adolesc Pediatr Gynecol* 1988;1:151.
67. Muram D. Child sexual abuse: relationship between genital findings and sexual acts. *Child Abuse Negl* 1989;13:211.
68. Adams J, Harper K, Knudson S, et al. Examination findings in legally confirmed child sexual abuse: it's normal to be normal. *Pediatrics* 1994;94:310.
69. Muram D, Speck P, Gold S. Genital abnormalities in female siblings and friends of child victims of sexual abuse. *Child Abuse Negl* 1991;15:105.

70. Adams J, Knudson S. Genital findings in adolescent girls referred for suspected abuse. *Arch Pediatr Adolesc Med* 1996;150:850.
71. Heppenstall-Heger A, McConnell G, Ticson L, et al. Healing patterns in anogenital injuries: A longitudinal study of injuries associated with sexual abuse, accidental injuries, or genital surgery in the preadolescent child. *Pediatrics* 2003;112:829.
72. Berenson A, Chacko M, Wiemann C, et al. A case-control study of anatomic changes resulting from sexual abuse. *Am J Obstet Gynecol* 2000;182:820.
73. Heger A, Ticson L, Velasquez O, et al. Children referred for possible sexual abuse: medical findings in 2384 children. *Child Abuse Negl* 2002;26:645.
74. Finkel, M. Medical findings in child sexual abuse. In: Reece R, ed. *Child abuse.* Baltimore: Williams & Wilkins, 1994.
75. Heger A, Emans S, Muram D, eds. *Evaluation of the sexually abused child: a medical textbook and photographic atlas.* New York: Oxford University Press, 2000.
76. Hobbs C, Wynne J. Use of the colposcope in examination for sexual abuse. *Arch Dis Child* 1996;75:539.
77. Muram D, Arheart K, Jennings S. Diagnostic accuracy of colposcopic photographs in child sexual abuse evaluations. *J Pediatr Adolesc Gynecol* 1999;12:58.
78. McCann J, Wells R, Simon M, et al. Genital findings in prepubertal girls selected for nonabuse: a descriptive study. *Pediatrics* 1990;86:428.
79. Berenson AB, Heger AH, Andrews S. Appearance of the hymen in newborn. *Pediatrics* 1991;87:458.
80. Berenson AB, Heger AH, Hayes JM, et al. Appearance of the hymen in prepubertal girls. *Pediatrics* 1992;89:387.
81. Kellogg N, Parra J. Linea vestibularis: a previously undescribed normal genital structure in female neonates. *Pediatrics* 1991;87:926.
82. Berenson A, Somma-Garcia A, Barnett S. Perianal findings in infants 18 months of age or younger. *Pediatrics* 1993;91;838.
83. Heger A, Ticson L, Guerra L, et al. Appearance of the genitalia in girls selected for nonabuse: Review of hymenal morphology and nonspecific findings. *J Pediatr Adolesc Gynecol* 2002;15:27.
84. Kerns D, Ritter M, Thomas R. Concave hymenal variations in suspected child sexual abuse victims. *Pediatrics* 1992;90:265.
85. McCann J, Voris J, Simon M. Genital injuries resulting from sexual abuse: a longitudinal study. *Pediatrics* 1992;89:307.
86. Finkel M. Anogenital trauma in sexually abused children. *Pediatrics* 1989;84:317.
87. Berenson A. A longitudinal study of hymenal morphology in the first 3 years of life. *Pediatrics* 1995;95:490.
88. Berenson A. Appearance of the hymen at birth and one year of age: a longitudinal study. *Pediatrics* 1993;91:820.
89. McCann J, Voris J. Perianal injuries resulting from sexual abuse: a longitudinal study. *Pediatrics* 1993;91:390.
90. Kellogg N, Parra J. Linea vestibularis: follow-up of a normal genital structure. *Pediatrics* 1993;92:453.
91. Jenny C, Kuhns M, Abrahams E. Hymens in newborn female infants. *Pediatrics* 1987;80:399.
92. Adams J. Evolution of a classification scale: medical evaluation of suspected child sexual abuse. *Child Maltreatment* 2001;6:31.
93. Emans S, Woods E, Allred E, et al. Hymenal findings in adolescent women: impact of tampon use and consensual sexual activity. *J Pediatr* 1994;125:153.
94. Adams JA, Botash A, Kellogg N. Differences in hymenal morphology between adolescent girls with and without a history of consensual sexual intercourse. *Arch Pediatr Adolesc Med* 2004;158:280.
95. Bays J, Jenny C. Genital and anal conditions confused with child sexual abuse trauma. *Am J Dis Child* 1990;144:1319.
96. Bond G, Dowd M, Landsman I, et al. Unintentional perineal injury in prepubescent girls: a multi-center, prospective report of 56 girls. *Pediatrics* 1995;95:628.
97. Dowd M, Fitzmaurice L, Knapp J, et al. The interpretation of urogenital findings in children with straddle injuries. *J Pediatr Surg* 1994;29:7.
98. Pokorny S, Pokorny W, Kramer W. Acute genital injury in the prepubertal girl. *Am J Obstet Gynecol* 1992;166:1461.

99. Hostetler B, Muram D, Jones C. Sharp penetrating injury to the hymen. *J Adolesc Pediatr Gynecol* 1994;7:94.
100. Heger A, Emans S. Introital diameter as the criterion for sexual abuse. *Pediatrics* 1990;85:222.
101. Paradise J. Predictive accuracy and the diagnosis of sexual abuse: a big issue about a little tissue. *Child Abuse Negl* 1989;13:169.
102. McCann J, Voris J, Simon M, et al. Comparison of genital examination techniques in prepubertal girls. *Pediatrics* 1990;85:182.
103. Berenson A, Chacko M, Wiemann C, et al. Use of hymenal measurements in the diagnosis of previous penetration. *Pediatrics* 2002;109:228.
104. Ingram D, Everett V, Ingram D. The relationship between the transverse hymenal orifice diameter by the separation technique and other possible markers of sexual abuse. *Child Abuse Negl* 2001;25;1109.
105. DeJong A, Rose M. Legal proof of child sexual abuse in the absence of physical evidence. *Pediatrics* 1991;88:506.
106. Paradise J, Winter M, Finkel M, et al. Influence of the history on physicians' interpretations of girls' genital findings. *Pediatrics* 1999;103:980.
107. Paradise J, Finkel M, Beiser A, et al. Assessment of girls' genital findings and the likelihood of sexual abuse. *Arch Pediatr Adolesc Med* 1997;151:883.
108. Frasier L. The pediatrician's role in child abuse interviewing. *Pediatric Annals* 1997;26:306.
109. Myers J. Adjudication of child sexual abuse cases. *Future of Children* 1994;4:84.
110. Melton G. Doing justice and doing good: conflicts for mental health professionals. *Future of Children* 1994;4:102.
111. Saywitz K, Goodman G, Nicholas E, et al. Children's memories of a physical examination involving genital touch: implications for reports of child sexual abuse. *J Consult Clin Psychol* 1991; 59:682.
112. DeJong A. Maternal responses to the sexual abuse of their children. *Pediatrics* 1988;81:14.
113. Gully K, Hansen K, Britton H, et al. The child sexual abuse experience and the child sexual abuse medical examination: knowing what correlations exist. *J Child Sexual Abuse* 2000;9:15.
114. Lynch L, Faust J. Reduction of distress in children undergoing sexual abuse medical examination. *J Pediatr* 1998;133:296.
115. Palusci V, Cyrus T. Reaction to videocolposcopy in the assessment of child sexual abuse. *Child Abuse Negl* 2001;25:1535.
116. Nelson DG, Santucci KA. An alternate light source to detect semen. *Acad Emerg Med* 2002;9:1045.
117. McCauley J, German R, Guzinski G. Toluidine blue in the detection of perineal lacerations in pediatric and adolescent sexual abuse victims. *Pediatrics* 1986;78:1039.
118. Paradise J, Rose L, Sleeper L, et al. Behavior, family function, school performance, and predictors of persistent disturbance in sexually abused children. *Pediatrics* 1994;93:452.
119. Bernier L, Williams R, Zetzer H. Efficacy of treatment for victims of child sexual abuse. *Future of Children* 1994;4:156.
120. Briere I, Elliott D. Immediate and long-term impacts of child sexual abuse. *Future of Children* 1994;4:54.
121. Koverola C, Friedrich W. Psychological effects of child sexual abuse. In: Heger A, Emans SJ, Muram D, et al, eds. *Evaluation of the sexually abused child: a medical textbook and photographic atlas.* New York: Oxford University Press, 2000.
122. Wells R, McCann J, Adams J, et al. Emotional, behavioral, and physical symptoms reported by parents of sexually abused, nonabused, and allegedly abused prepubescent females. *Child Abuse Negl* 1995;19:155.
123. Landwirth J. Children as witnesses in child sexual abuse trials. *Pediatrics* 1987;60:585.
124. Berliner L, Barbieri M. The testimony of the child victim of sexual assault. *J Soc Issues* 1984;40:125.
125. Jenny C. Adolescent risk-taking behavior and the occurrence of sexual assault. *Am J Dis Child* 1988; 142:770.
126. Siefert S. Substance use and sexual assault. *Subst Use Misuse* 1999;34:935.
127. Simmons M, Cupp M. Use and abuse of flunitrazepam. *Ann Pharmacother* 1998;32:117.
128. Anglin D, Spears K, Hutson H. Flunitrazepam and its involvement in date or acquaintance rape. *Acad Emerg Med* 1997;4:323.

129. Norman M, Nadelson C. The rape victim: psychodynamic considerations. *Am J Psychiatry* 1976; 133:408.
130. Burgess A, Holmstrom L. Rape trauma syndrome. *Am J Psychiatry* 1974;131:981.
131. Moscarello R. Posttraumatic stress disorder after sexual assault: its psychodynamics and treatment. *J Am Acad Psychoanal* 1991;19:235.
132. Bownes I, O'Gorman E, Sayers A. Assault characteristics and posttraumatic stress disorder in rape victims. *Acta Psychiatr Scand* 1991;83:27.
133. Dahl S. Acute response to rape-a PTSD variant. *Acta Psychiatr Scand Suppl* 1989;80:56.
134. Gibson L, Leitenberg H. Child sexual abuse prevention programs: do they decrease the occurrence of child sexual abuse? *Child Abuse Negl* 2000;24:1115.
135. Hebert M, Lavoie F, Piche C, et al. Proximate effects of child sexual abuse prevention program in elementary school children. *Child Abuse Negl* 2001;25:505.
136. Rispens J, Aleman A, Goudena P. Prevention of child sexual abuse victimization: a meta-analysis of school programs. *Child Abuse Negl* 1997;21:975.
137. Paradise J. Current concepts in preventing sexual abuse. *Curr Opin Pediatrics* 2001;13:402.
138. The Safer Society Foundation Inc. (Available at: http://www.safersociety.org/stopit.html.)
139. Chasan-Taber L, Tabachnick J, McMahon P. Evaluation of a child sexual abuse prevention program-Vermont, 1995–1997. *MMWR* 2001;50:77.
140. Worling J, Curwen T. Adolescent sexual offender recidivism: success of specialized treatment and implications for risk prediction. *Child Abuse Negl* 2000;24:965.
141. Hanson R, Bussiere M. Predicting relapse: A meta-analysis of sexual offender recidivism studies. *J Consult Clin Psychol* 1998;66;348.

Recommended CD ROMs

1. American Academy of Pediatrics. Visual diagnosis of child abuse on CD ROM, 2nd ed. 2003.
2. Muram D, Harrison L, Adams J. (eds). North American Society for Pediatric and Adolescent Gynecology CD-ROM, Sexual abuse: Medical evaluation for the primary care physician. 2002.

25

Complementary and Alternative Medicine for Gynecology Patients

Wendy L. Wornham

DEFINITIONS AND EPIDEMIOLOGY

Complementary and Alternative Medicine (CAM) is defined by the National Center for Complementary and Alternative Medicine (NCCAM) as "a group of diverse medical and health care systems, practices, and products that are not presently considered to be part of conventional medicine" (1). CAM is defined by the Cochranecollaboration as "a broad domain of healing resources that encompasses all health systems, modalities, and practices and their accompanying theories and beliefs, other than those intrinsic to the politically dominant health systems of a particular society or culture in a given historical period" (2). Several therapies once considered to be "alternative," such as acupuncture, massage therapy, and meditative techniques for stress reduction, have become integrated into mainstream medical practice as clinical effectiveness for specific illnesses has been validated by well-designed clinical trials.

In the past decade there has been an increase in the use of CAM therapies by adults in United States, from 33.8% in 1990 to 42.1% in 1997 (3). Worldwide, nearly half of adults living in industrialized countries and a higher percentage of those living in developing countries have used at least one therapy classified as complementary or alternative (4). A study of CAM use by Hispanic, African-American, and white women in New York City found that more than half the sample of 300 women in each group had used a CAM remedy or treatment, and 40% had visited a CAM practitioner. Herbs, medicinal teas, and vitamins were the therapies used most frequently, while chiropractors and nutritionists were the practitioners most often visited. Racial and ethnic differences were minimal (5). A large national survey by Astin concluded that people use CAM therapies "not so much as a result of being dissatisfied with conventional medicine but largely because they find these health care alternatives to be more congruent with their own values, beliefs, and philosophical orientations toward health and life" (6).

Among American adolescents the prevalence of CAM use ranges from 54% in a metropolitan New York county (7) to 70% of homeless youth in Seattle (8). Adolescent patients often seek out CAM therapies for acute and chronic conditions in an effort to self-treat and exert more control and autonomy by choosing therapeutic practices that do not require prescriptions or physician referrals (7). They erroneously believe that "natural" means safe and they use multiple CAM modalities simultaneously and in conjunction with prescription medications (such as oral contraceptives and antidepressants) and over-the-counter analgesics. Most adolescents do not inform their physicians about the CAM therapies they are using unless they are asked specifically by their health care providers, and even then, full disclosure is variable.

In this chapter, several herbs and dietary supplements will be discussed in the context of the clinical conditions in which they are used; these include urinary tract infections (UTIs), dysmenorrhea and premenstrual syndrome (PMS), eating disorders, depression and anxiety, and smoking cessation. Evidence based indications for acupuncture, massage therapy, yoga, and meditation in treating these and other clinical conditions will be presented. A complete review of all CAM modalities is beyond the scope of this chapter; consequently, several modalities, including chiropractic, homeopathy, and energy healing, will not be discussed. Resources for additional clinician and patient information will be provided and suggestions for responsible integration of several beneficial therapies will be proposed.

HERBS AND DIETARY SUPPLEMENTS

Throughout civilizations past and present, plants have been cultivated and utilized for medicinal purposes. Many of our current medications were initially derived from plants, including aspirin, morphine, taxol, and several alkylating agents used in chemotherapy. Ethno-botanists diligently collect and study plants used by traditional healers, hoping to identify active ingredients that can be isolated or synthesized, standardized, and possibly patented. In 1997 Americans spent an estimated $8 billion on herbs and dietary supplements (3), and current estimates are much higher. Most of these products are not standardized, the recommended dosages are variable, and some herbal products, particularly packaged Chinese herbal mixtures, may be contaminated with pesticides, heavy metals, or adulterated with other biologically active chemicals (9,10). At this time, herbal products in the United States are unregulated, although growing concerns of inadvertent overdoses, dangerous drug–herb interactions, and the variability in product quality have prompted policy makers to consider new regulations to protect consumers. When herbal and botanical remedies are recommended and prepared by trained herbalists and experienced practitioners of Chinese traditional medicine and Indian Ayurvedic medicine, the likelihood of quality, safety, and efficacy increases, but well-qualified practitioners can be hard to find and the standards of practice vary. Although an increasing number of randomized controlled trials (RCT), case reports, and meta-analyses of available data have become available for

TABLE 25-1. *Resources for clinicians and patients.*

Internet sites:
  Natural Medicines comprehensive database www.naturaldatabase.com (by subscription)
  National Center for Complementary and Alternative Medicine: http://nccam.nih.org
  NIH Office of Dietary Supplements: http://dietary-supplements.info.nih.gov
  Quackwatch: http://www.quackwatch.com
  ConsumerLab: http://www.consumerlab.com (by subscription)
  Longwood herbal task force: www.mcp.edu/herbal
  HerbMed: http://www.herbmed.org
Books:
  Blumenthal M, ed. *The complete German commission E monographs.* Austin, TX: American Botanical Council, 1998.
  Fugh-Berman, A. *Alternative medicine, what works.* Baltimore: Williams & Wilkins, 1997

clinicians and consumers, much remains to be learned about valid indications, contraindications, potential herb–drug interactions, and the clinical effects of long-term use (11). As more research is done, clinicians will need to keep informed about the products their patients are using. Table 25-1 lists several excellent references and websites for further information about hundreds of herbs and supplements.

Adolescents usually get information about herbal remedies and dietary and performance enhancing supplements from their friends, family members, coaches, sales people in health food stores, magazines, or directly from the Internet. Most herbal products can be ordered via the Internet or obtained at health food stores and pharmacies without a prescription.

It is imperative that clinicians ask patients specifically about their use of herbs, vitamins and supplements, teas, and special diets as part of their standard medical history and preoperative questionnaire. Several popular herbs are now known to inhibit platelet aggregation (garlic and ginseng), inhibit platelet activating factor (gingko), and prolong the sedative effect of anesthesia (kava and valerian); these should be discontinued 7 days before surgery (12). Other herbs, such as St. John's wort (Fig. 25-1) affect the serum drug levels of medications metabolized through the cytochrome P450 enzymes and should be discontinued 5 days before surgery and during treatment with cyclosporine, warfarin, steroids, oral contraceptives, digoxin, and protease inhibitors (12). Many herbs may also interact with analgesic medications and affect the metabolism and efficacy of nonsteroidal antiinflammatory drugs, acetaminophen, and opioids.

URINARY TRACT INFECTION

Cranberry (Vaccinium macrocarpon) has long been recommended by herbalists for the prevention of urinary tract infections. The active ingredient is now known to be proanthocyanidin, which interferes with the adhesion of gram-negative bacteria uropathogens to the bladder epithelium (13). A case-controlled study of sexually active college students showed that regular consumption of cranberry juice was

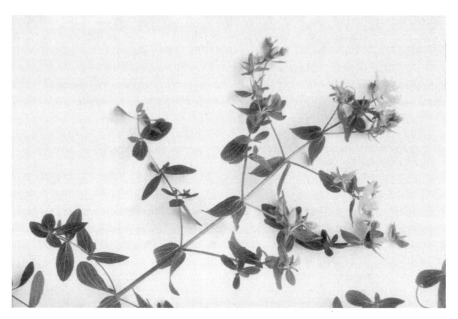

FIG. 25-1. St. John's Wort (Illustration is from THE COMPLETE WOMAN'S HERBAL by Anne McIntyre. Copyright 1995 by Gaia Books, Ltd. Reprinted by permission of Henry Holt and Company, LLC.)

associated with a 50% reduction in the odds of first time UTI (14) and in another small study of women with recurrent UTIs the same women had significantly fewer UTIs during an interval when they took 400 mg of cranberry concentrate daily compared to no therapy (15). Cranberry does not protect against infection with gram-positive bacteria and has not been shown to be helpful in preventing infections in children and adolescents with neurogenic bladder (16).

As antibiotic resistance increases and compliance with antibiotic therapy is variable, patients and medical practitioners seek safe, preventive strategies. Cranberry juice (unsweetened) consumed as 200 ml daily to 250 ml two to three times per day or cranberry extract tablets (greater than 1:30 parts concentrated juice) twice a day are safe and effective (17), and these products can be recommended to adolescent girls with recurrent UTIs and to sexually active young women. Cranberry products are not effective as monotherapy for established UTIs and they should not be used as such.

DYSMENORRHEA, ENDOMETRIOSIS, AND PREMENSTRUAL SYNDROME

An extensive review of randomized controlled trials of CAM therapies in reproductive-age women was published in 2003 by Fugh-Berman and Kronenberg (18).

Herbs that are used to treat menstrual irregularities and/or symptoms of premenstrual syndrome in adult and perimenopausal women have not been adequately studied in adolescents, and the safety of long-term use of these herbal products is not currently known. Three popular botanical products, dong quai (*Angelica sinensis*), evening primrose oil, and chaste tree berry (*Vitex agnus-castus*) are widely marketed remedies, and they are used by adolescents seeking relief from menstrual discomfort and PMS symptoms.

Dong quai (*Angelica sinensis*) is one of several ingredients used in traditional Chinese medicine to create a "female tonic" for menstrual symptoms. Clinical data about its effectiveness for PMS and dysmenorrhea are inconclusive, although one study found that it was "no more efficacious than placebo in relieving menopausal symptoms and does not alter estrogen levels" (19). Dong quai contains coumarins, which potentiate the effects of prescription anticoagulants and have been reported to cause bleeding (11), and photosensitivity and photodermatitis reactions have also been reported (20). Evening primrose oil (EPO), which contains linoleic acid, the prostaglandin E1 precursor, is used as a treatment for premenstrual syndrome and is considered to be safe, although two small trials did not find it to be effective (21,22). Chaste tree berry extract, taken as a single daily tablet of 20 mg dried extract, was found to be beneficial in reducing PMS symptoms of irritability, mood alteration, headache, bloating, and mastalgia in a placebo-controlled study by Schellenberg (23) and seems to be safe, although larger long-term studies will need to be conducted to determine its safety for adolescents.

The effects of several vitamin and mineral supplements on PMS have been studied over the past 20 years. Vitamin B_6, pyridoxine, is used in Western Europe for the reduction of PMS symptoms, although clinical trials have provided conflicting results (24,25). The specific recommended dosages vary, but a daily dose of 100 mg or less is considered safe; neurologic symptoms such as peripheral neuropathy have been observed with prolonged use of excessive daily doses. Calcium supplements (1,000 mg per day) were studied by Thys-Jacobs and colleagues were found to decrease several PMS symptoms in a small sample of adult women (26). Walker and colleagues studied the effect of daily magnesium supplements (200 mg per day) over three consecutive menstrual cycles and found improvement in symptoms of water retention, bloating, and mastalgia after the second cycle (27). Both calcium and magnesium supplements are considered safe when used in the recommended doses.

In many cultures there are traditional dietary recommendations for menstruating women, particularly in cultures influenced by the Chinese medical theories of yin- and yang-containing foods (28). Contemporary studies indicate that a low fat diet may diminish symptoms of PMS and dysmenorrhea (29), and that consumption of fish oil [1,080 mg Eicosapentaenoic acid (EPA), 720 mg docosahexaenoic acid, and 1.5 mg vitamin E in liquid form] ameliorates dysmenorrhea in adolescents, probably through the effects of these polyunsaturated fatty acids on prostaglandins (30). Dietary sources of these omega-3 polyunsaturated acids include flaxseed oil, canola and soybean oil, and fatty fish such as salmon, mackerel, and herring. Soy products contain phytoestrogens and they are sold as "natural" alternatives to hormone replacement therapy for perimenopausal women. The effect of phytoestrogens on the estrogen receptors of breast and endometrial tissue has not been conclusively determined, and the long-term safety for adolescents is not known (31). Regular dietary consumption is considered safe, especially for adolescents who follow a vegetarian–vegan diet, although large quantities of concentrated supplements are not advised.

Acupuncture, the traditional Chinese medical practice of inserting fine needles into specific anatomic points to unblock the flow of chi, the "life energy" through defined but invisible channels, has become widely utilized in American hospitals and clinics for analgesia and the control of perioperative and chemotherapy induced nausea and vomiting (32). A small study done by Helms in 1987 evaluated the effects of acupuncture on dysmenorrhea in adult women and the results showed it was beneficial (33). Additional studies are now underway, and clinical observations suggest that acupuncture may also be useful in ameliorating the dysmenorrhea and pelvic pain caused by endometriosis. (See Fig. 25-2, acupuncture for endometriosis.)

Yoga, the ancient Indian tradition in which the mind and body are said to be united by systematically stretching and balancing the body in a variety of postures, may also be beneficial for PMS, dysmenorrhea, and alleviating pain from endometriosis, although there have been no published RCTs to date. Several specific postures are recommended to treat menstrual discomfort and to enhance "women's health" in

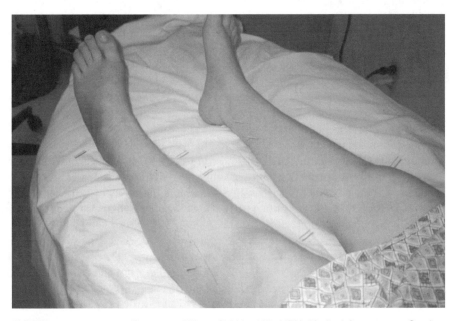

FIG. 25-2. Acupuncture. (Courtesy of Yuan-Chi Lin, MD, MPH; Medical Acupuncture Service, Children's Hospital Boston; with permission.)

general (34,35). For example, for dysmenorrhea "reclining angle bound pose," "child's pose," and "bridge pose" may be beneficial, while "half-moon pose" may help to relieve symptoms of endometriosis (34). According to the Iyengar yoga tradition, inverted poses must be avoided during menstruation. Many women and adolescents find that doing a series of postures for 10 to 30 minutes several times a week brings an improvement in their general sense of well-being and ameliorates distressing menstrual symptoms. There are several different types of yoga, including Hatha, Iyengar, Ashtanga, Kundalini, and "Power" yoga, and they vary in their approach and degree of physical exertion. Classes taught by certified teachers are increasingly available, as are instructive books, video cassettes, and DVDs.

Adolescence is one of the most stressful times in a woman's life. With increasing independence, time demands, and peer pressure, many young women succumb to irregular meals, eat high fat fast and snack foods, skip meals completely, and do not get regular exercise. These factors may also aggravate dysmenorrhea, and merit discussion during the medical evaluation.

WEIGHT LOSS AND EATING DISORDERS

Many adolescent girls and young women use a variety of "natural" products to lose weight by suppressing their appetite and by purging themselves of excess fluids and feces. Some herbal products used for "weight loss" contain ephedra alkaloids, also called *Ma Huang*. Shekelle and colleagues conducted a meta-analysis of controlled trials using ephedra or ephedrine with caffeine for weight loss or enhancement of athletic performance and case reports of adverse events. They found a small short term reduction in weight (0.9 kg per month), insufficient data to support claims that it improves athletic performance, and hundreds of case reports citing significant adverse and life threatening cardiovascular (heart palpitations, hypertension) and neurologic (stroke, seizures, psychiatric symptoms) symptoms (36). Given these concerns and those raised by other investigators (37,38), ephedra was removed from the markets in the U.S., but products may be available over the internets. Caffeine, also an ingredient in "natural weight loss" products and diuretics may cause tachycardia, restlessness, and insomnia when consumed in excessive amounts. Since many "dieting" teens also drink large quantities of caffeinated diet sodas, sports drinks, tea, and coffee, they should also be asked specifically about their daily caffeine consumption.

Many adolescents, especially those with eating disorders, use herbal and botanical products with diuretic and laxative properties to promote weight loss. Roerig and colleagues surveyed 39 consecutive patients with bulimia nervosa and found that 31% had used a diuretic in the past, and 21% in the previous month (39). Of the 25 types of over-the-counter or off-the-shelf diuretics reported several were herbal products such as uva ursi and Burdock root, as well as kola nut and Guarana seed, both of which contain caffeine. Dandelion leaves are also used as diuretics and are consumed fresh in salads or as a tea made from dried leaves (40). Although herbalists recommend these herbs, at this time no controlled clinical trials have validated their diuretic properties. Dandelion is contraindicated for people with gallstones, gastritis, and ulcers; the latex component of fresh leaves may cause an allergic reaction or contact dermatitis. It is unknown whether there is a rebound fluid retention when regular use of these herbs is discontinued.

Senna (*Cassia senna*), the active ingredient in many laxatives, is available in many forms, some of which are classified as over-the-counter "medicines" because they are mixed with synthetic ingredients and others as "natural herbal products." The anthranoid compounds, hydroxyanthracene glycosides (sennosides A and B) are the active ingredient in all forms of senna preparations. These compounds may decrease the absorption of other medications that are absorbed through the intestinal tract (11) and perianal skin irritation and blistering have been reported in young children who accidentally ingested senna containing laxatives (41). When used appropriately, a senna containing tea such as "smooth move herbal stimulant laxative tea" may be beneficial for adolescents with occasional constipation, but when used in excessive quantities, herbal laxatives may cause the same problems with electrolyte imbalance as synthetic laxatives.

Patients with anorexia nervosa and bulimia nervosa often suffer from depression and anxiety disorders (42–44). A 1997–1998 nationally representative survey by Kessler and colleagues they found that 53.6% of adults with severe depression and 56.7% of those with anxiety attacks also used some form of CAM therapy during the previous 12 months. Relaxation techniques, self-hypnosis, imagery, spiritual healing, and herbs were the most frequently utilized treatments (45). In addition to prescription antidepressant and anxiolytic medications, many adolescent patients also self-treat with herbal preparations. The references listed in Table 25-1 provide extensive information about St. John's wort, kava, and other "mood-stabilizing" products adolescent patients are taking.

St. John's wort (*Hypericum perforatum*) (Fig. 25-1) is used to treat depression and although the precise mechanism of action is not yet known it is thought to selectively inhibit serotonin, dopamine, and norepinephrine reuptake. Ernst analyzed 27 randomized double-blind clinical trials, 17 of which were placebo controlled and showed efficacy of St. John's wort superior to placebo in treating mild to moderate depression. The dosage used in most clinical trials is 300 mg three times per day as a standardized extract 0.3% Hypericum content and a clinical effect is observed after 2 to 3 weeks of continuous daily therapy (46). Shelton et al. investigated the efficacy of St. John's wort in the treatment of major depression and found it was no more effective than placebo (47). When used alone in the recommended daily dosage for several months St. John's wort seems to be safe. However, it should *not* be used with other medications such as oral contraceptives, antiviral agents, anticoagulants, digoxin, theophylline, and cyclosporin because it induces the activation of the cytochrome P450 system and alters the metabolism and subsequent serum concentrations of these medications (11,12). When used with prescription selective serotonin re-uptake inhibitors (SSRIs), St. John's wort can cause excessive levels of serotonin and serotonin syndrome. Therefore, it is imperative that patients taking these and possibly other as yet unidentified prescription and analgesic medications be counseled against using St. John's wort and these preparations simultaneously.

Kava (*Piper methysticum*) is marketed and used as an anxiolytic agent; the precise mechanism of action has not yet been identified. In a meta-analysis of seven double blind, placebo-controlled RCTs, Pittler and Ernst concluded that "kava extract is superior compared with placebo and relatively safe as a treatment option for anxiety" (48). The dosages studied have ranged from 70 to 240 mg of standardized kava pyrones in the form of dried root extract preparations, divided into twice or thrice daily doses and taken for 4 weeks. However, in the United States, Germany, and Switzerland there have been at least 11 cases of hepatic toxicity and subsequent liver failure attributed to ingestion of kava products since 1999 (49) and the US Food and Drug Administration has issued a consumer advisory against the use of kava while it continues its investigation. Additional side effects of kava include interactions with alcohol and other central nervous system (CNS) sedatives, which can cause temporary impairment in concentration, attention, and performance. High-dose, long-term use of kava has been associated with dermatitis, anorexia, alopecia, and diminished hearing, all of which are reversible upon discontinuation of kava (50).

Tobacco is frequently used by adolescents who erroneously think that it makes them feel less stressed and more relaxed, increases their concentration, and suppresses their appetite. The biologic effects of nicotine addiction and the social motivations for smoking are complex, and smoking prevention and cessation programs for adolescents have been variably successful. Studies of the effects of acupuncture on smoking cessation have provided conflicting results (51,52). A review of 22 acupuncture smoking-cessation studies by White and colleagues (53) in 2002 concluded that acupuncture was no more effective than sham acupuncture. There was no difference when acupuncture was compared to other antismoking programs, although it was superior to no intervention in the early result phase. Self-massage of specific hand or ear points was found to be effective in reducing smoking-related anxiety, cravings, and withdrawal symptoms in a small study done by Hernandez-Reif (54). Hypnotherapy, though promoted for smoking cessation, was not found to be any more effective after 6 months than other interventions (55). These results raise the complex issues of the effect of placebo phenomenon (56) and the allocation of health insurance dollars for smoking-cessation programs.

Therapies that teach lifelong strategies for stress reduction and impulse control should be investigated further (57). Jon Kabat-Zinn and others have developed stress management programs that teach mindfulness meditation techniques and yoga (58,59). These programs are taught at many hospitals and clinics throughout the United States and are now being developed for adolescents with a variety of chronic illnesses. The combination of yoga and diaphragmatic breathing techniques as well as the ensuing increase in moment-to-moment awareness may also help adolescents to identify and cope with mild anxiety episodes and impulsivity.

Field and colleagues found that bulimic adolescents benefit from massage therapy through reductions in anxiety and depression (60). Acupuncture, especially auricular (ear), has been used to control obesity and binge eating, although a review by Lacey and coworkers indicated inconclusive data on the efficacy and the need for larger, better designed studies (61). Other modalities such as art therapy, psychodrama, and music therapy are becoming integrated into group therapy programs (62) for patients with eating disorders. Finally, it should be acknowledged that spirituality is an important force in the lives of many adolescents (7) and that prayer and faith healing are used by many teens and their families, although this is infrequently disclosed to health care providers (63).

SUMMARY

In this chapter several herbal and dietary remedies and CAM therapies have been discussed in the context of adolescent utilization for a variety of conditions. What can "mainstream" health professions do in response to the widespread use of CAM therapies by their patients?

1. *Always ask* patients specifically if they are taking herbal products, teas, and dietary supplements, and if they are being treated by practitioners of other healing traditions and modalities. *Listen* to their reasons for using specific CAM therapies.
2. *Become informed* about what is known about the products patients have obtained and are using: the correct dosages, drug–herb interactions, clinical efficacy trials and known adverse effects, in an effort to responsibly advise patients about the risks and benefits of the therapies they have selected.
3. *Develop* a referral network of well-trained and respected CAM practitioners (such as acupuncturists, massage therapists, yoga instructors, and herbalists) to whom you can reliably refer appropriate patients.
4. *Communicate,* whenever possible, with the CAM practitioners that your patients are consulting and become informed about the specifics of the "other" therapeutic modalities they are also using. Report adverse outcomes as well as beneficial interventions, for it is through ongoing inquiry, clinical observation, clinical trials, and better communication that effective and therapeutic CAM modalities will be integrated into "mainstream" medical practices and patient safety and well-being will be enhanced.

REFERENCES

1. NCCAM. What is Complementary and Alternative Medicine (CAM)? www.nccam.nih.gov. (Accessed July 26, 2004.)
2. Zollman C, Vickers A. What is complementary medicine? *BMJ* 1999;319:393.

3. Eisenberg DM, Davis RB, Ettner SL, et al. Trends in alternative medicine use in the United States, 1990–1997. *JAMA* 1998;280:1569.
4. Bodecker G, Kronenberg F. A public health agenda for traditional, complementary, and alternative medicine. *Am J Public Health* 2002;92:1582.
5. Factor-Litvak P, Cushman LF, Kronenberg F, et al. Use of complementary and alternative medicine among women in New York City: a pilot study. *J Altern Complement Med* 2001;7:659.
6. Astin J. Why patients use alternative medicine: results of a national study. *JAMA* 1998;279:1548.
7. Wilson KM, Klein JD. Adolescent's use of complementary and alternative medicine. *Ambul Pediatr* 2002;2:104.
8. Breuner C, Barry PJ, Kemper KJ. Alternative medicine use by homeless youth. *Arch Pediatr Adolesc Med* 1998;152:1071.
9. Ko RJ. Adulterants in Asian patent medicines. *N Engl J Med* 1998;339:847.
10. Huang WF, Wen K-C, Hsiao M-L. Adulteration by synthetic therapeutic substances of traditional Chinese medicines in Taiwan. *J Clin Pharmacol* 1997;37:344.
11. Fugh-Berman A. Herb–drug interactions. *Lancet* 2000;355:134.
12. Ang-Lee M, Moss J, Yuan C. *Herbal Med Periop Care* 2001;286:208.
13. Schmidt DR, Sobota AE. An examination of the anti-adherence activity of cranberry juice on urinary and nonurinary bacterial isolates. *Microbios* 1988;55:173.
14. Foxman B, Geiger AM, Palin K, et al. First-time urinary tract infection and sexual behavior. *Epidemiology* 1995;6:162.
15. Walker EB, Barney DP, Mickelson JN, et al. Cranberry concentrate: UTI prophylaxis. *J Fam Pract* 1997;45:167.
16. Schlager TA, Anderson S, Trudell J, et al. Effect of cranberry juice on bacteriuria in children with neurogenic bladder receiving intermittent catheterization. *J Pediatr* 1999;135:698.
17. Kiel RJ, Nashelsky J, Robbins B. Does cranberry juice prevent or treat urinary tract Infections? *J Fam Pract* 2003;52:145.
18. Fugh-Berman A, Kronenberg F. Complementary and alternative medicine in reproductive-age women: a review of randomized controlled trials. *Repro Toxicol* 2003;17;137.
19. Hirata JD, Swiersz LM, Zell LM, et al. Does dong quai have estrogenic effects in postmenopausal women? A double blind, placebo-controlled trial. *Fertil Steril* 1997;68:981.
20. Foster S. *Tyler's honest herbal: a sensible guide to the use of herbs and related remedies,* 3d ed. New York: Hayworth Herbal Press, 1993:20.
21. Khoo SK, Munro C, Battistutta D. Evening primrose oil and treatment of premenstrual syndrome. *Med J Aust* 1990;153:189.
22. Collins A, Cerin A, Coleman G, Landgren BM. Essential fatty acids in the treatment of premenstrual syndrome. *Obstet Gynecol* 1993;81:93.
23. Schellenberg R. Treatment for the premenstrual syndrome with agnus castus fruit extract: a prospective, randomized, placebo controlled study. *Br Med J* 2001;322:134.
24. Bender DA. Non-nutritional uses of vitamin B_6. *Br J Nutr* 1999;81:7.
25. Bendich A. The potential for dietary supplements to reduce premenstrual syndrome (PMS) symptoms. *J Am Coll Nutr* 2000;19:3.
26. Thys-Jacobs S, Starkey P, Bernstein D, et al. Calcium carbonate and the premenstrual syndrome: effects on premenstrual and menstrual symptoms. Premenstrual Syndrome Study Group. *Am J Obstet Gynecol* 1998;179:444.
27. Walker AF, De S, Vickers MF, et al. Magnesium supplementation alleviates premenstrual symptoms of fluid retention. *J Women's Health* 1998;7:1157.
28. Kaptchuck T. *The web that has no weaver: understanding Chinese medicine.* 2nd ed. McGraw-Hill/Contemporary, 2000.
29. Barnard N, Scialli A, Hurlock D, et al. Diet and sex-hormone binding globulin, dysmenorrhea, and premenstrual symptoms. *Obstet Gynecol* 2000;95:245.
30. Harel Z, Biro FM, Kottenhahn RK, et al. Supplementation with omega-3 polyunsaturated fatty acids in the management of dysmenorrhea in adolescents. *Am J Obstet Gynecol* 1996;174:1335.
31. Kurzer MS. Phytoestrogen supplement use by women *J Nutr* 2003;133:1983S.
32. Kaptchuk TJ. Acupuncture: theory, efficacy, and practice. *Ann Intern Med* 2002;136:374.
33. Helms JM. Acupuncture for management of primary dysmenorrhea. *Obstet Gynecol* 1987;69:51.
34. Sparrowe L, Walden P, Martinez D, et al. *The women's book of yoga and health: a lifelong guide to wellness.* Boston: Shambala Publications. 2002.

35. Iyengar BKS. *Yoga: the path to holistic health.* London: Dorling Kindersley, 2001.
36. Shekelle PG, Hardy ML, Morton SC, et al. Efficacy and safety of ephedra and ephedrine for weight loss and athletic performance: a meta analysis. *JAMA* 2003;289:1568.
37. Bent S, Tiedt TN, Odden MC, et al. The relative safety of ephedra compared with other herbal products. *Ann Intern Med* 2003;138:I56.
38. Lawrence ME, Kirby DF. Nutrition and sports supplements: fact or fiction. *J Clin Gastroenterol* 2002;35:299.
39. Roerig JL, Mitchell JE, de Zwaan M, et al. The eating disorders medicine cabinet revisited: a clinician's guide to appetite suppressants and diuretics. *Int J Eat Disord* 2003;33:443.
40. Blumenthal M, Busse WR, Goldberg A, et al., eds. *The complete German commission E monograph guide to herbal medicines.* Austin TX: American Botanical Council, 1998.
41. Spiller HA, Winter ML, Weber JA et al. Skin breakdown and blisters from senna-containing laxatives in young children. *Ann Pharmacol Ther* 2003;37:636.
42. Becker AE, Grinspoon, SK, Klebanski A, et al. Eating disorders. *N Engl J Med* 1999;340:1092.
43. Godart NT, Flament MF, Curt F, et al. Anxiety disorders in subjects seeking treatment for eating disordes: a DSM-IV controlled study. *Psychiatry Res* 2003;117:245.
44. Fairburn CG, Harrison PJ. Eating disorders. *Lancet* 2003;361:407.
45. Kessler R, Soukup J, Davis R, et al. The use of complementary and alternative therapies to treat anxiety and depression in the United States. *Am J Psychiatry* 2001;158:289.
46. Ernst E. The risk-benefit profile of commonly used herbal therapies: ginkgo, St. John's wort, ginseng, echinacea, saw palmetto and kava. *Ann Intern Med* 2002;136:42.
47. Shelton R, Keller M, Gelenberg A, et al. Effectiveness of St. John's wort in major depression. *JAMA* 2001;285:1978.
48. Pittler MH, Ernst E. Kava extract for treating anxiety. *Cochrane Database Syst Rev* 2002;(2):CD003383.
49. Hepatic toxicity possibly associated with kava-containing products—United States, Germany, and Switzerland. 1999–2002. *MMWR Morb Mortal Wkly Rep* 2002;47:1065.
50. Jappe U, Pranke I, Reinhold D, et al. Sebotropic drug reaction resulting from kava-kava extract therapy; a new entity. *J Am Acad Dermatol* 1995;31:89.
51. Linde K, Vickers A, Hondras M et al. Systematic reviews of complementary therapies—an annotated bibliography. Part 1: Acupuncture. *BMC Complement Altern Med* 2001;1:3.
52. Bier ID, Wilson J, Studt P, et al. Auricular acupuncture, education, and smoking cessation: a randomized, sham-controlled trial. *Am J Public Health* 2002;92:1642.
53. White AR, Rampers H, Ernst E. Acupuncture for smoking cessation. *Cochrane Database Syst Rev* 2002;(2):CD000009.
54. Hernandez-Reif M, Field T, Hart S. Smoking cravings are reduced by self-massage. *Prev Med* 1999;28:28.
55. Abbot NC, Stead LF, White AR, et al. Hypnotherapy for smoking cessation. *Cochrane Database Syst Rev* 2000;(2):CD001008.
56. Kaptchuk T. The placebo effect in alternative medicine: Can the performance of a healing ritual have clinical significance? *Ann Intern Med* 2002;136:817.
57. Nichter M, Vuckovic N, Quintero G. Smoking experimentation and initiation among adolescent girls: qualities and quantitative findings. *Tob Control* 1997;6:285.
58. Kabat-Zinn, J. *Full catastrophe living. Using the wisdom of your body and mind to face stress, pain, and illness.* New York: Retta, 1990.
59. Kabat-Zinn, J. *Wherever you go, there you are: mindfulness meditation in everyday life.* New York: Hyperion, 1994.
60. Field T, Schanberg S, Kuhn C et al. Bulimic adolescents benefit from massage therapy. *Adolescence* 1998;33:555.
61. Lacey JM, Tershakovec AM, Foster GD. Acupuncture for the treatment of obesity: a review of the evidence. *Int J Obes Relat Metab Disord* 2003;27:419.
62. Diamond-Raab L, Orrell-Valente JK. Art therapy, psychodrama, and verbal therapy. An integrative model of group therapy in the treatment of adolescents with anorexia nervosa and bulimia nervosa. *Child Adolesc Psychiatr Clin N Am* 2002;2:343.
63. Barnes LL, Plotnikoff GA, Fox K, Spirituality, religion, and pediatrics: intersecting worlds of healing. *Pediatrics (Journal of the Ambulatory Pediatric Association).* 2000;106 [Suppl 4];899.

26

Legal Issues in Pediatric and Adolescent Gynecology

Richard Bourne and the Honorable Susan Ricci

This chapter focuses on legal issues in pediatric and adolescent gynecology. The legal complexity of these issues is compounded by social, psychological, and moral questions (teenage sex); the perceived need for parents to be aware of the behavior of children; the authority to consent to medical intervention; the point at which life begins; the desirability of preventing birth through contraception, abortion, or sterilization; and issues of quality of life.

NATURE AND SOURCES OF LAW

Law emanates from both the state and federal levels of government. In the medical area, state law is generally the more important source of legal guidelines and constraints. It is important to remember that, unlike federal law, state law varies by jurisdiction. Therefore, it is necessary to know the laws of the state in which you practice before making treatment decisions. It is equally important to understand that when state and federal law conflict, federal law under the doctrine of preemption usually takes precedence. Thus, for example, if the federal government permits abortions and state law does not, the federal law controls.

Both state and federal laws have similar sources. The United States Constitution, of course, is interpreted by the federal courts, including the US Supreme Court, while state courts interpret the state constitutions. Constitutional rights may differ between the state and federal levels, with state rights being either broader or narrower when compared with the federal Constitution.

Law that is made or interpreted by judges is called *case law*. Judges, in deciding a particular case, are guided by legal precedents. The process of using decisions of prior courts to decide a case is called *state decisis*. Much legal debate exists as to whether the proper function of judges is to interpret narrowly existing case law and statutes or actually to create law in response to a matter before them. Those who oppose "judicial legislation" argue that courts have as their sole responsibility the interpretation of legislative action, that is, the action of elected representatives.

Laws promulgated by the legislature are called *statutes* and usually appear in bound volumes under various chapters and sections. Generally, when one wishes to clarify the law in a certain area, the first step is to find out whether there is a statute dealing with the issues.

In addition to constitutional law, case law, and statutes there are laws promulgated by the executive branch of government called *executive orders*. There are also laws created by state or federal agencies called *regulations*. State agencies such as a department of public health or a department of mental health and federal agencies such as the Federal Trade Commission enact regulations that serve to clarify and interpret statutes. These regulations of executive agencies have the force and effect of law.

A final distinction of importance is that between civil and criminal law. *Civil law* involves such actions as medical malpractice, where a plaintiff, the alleged victim, brings suit against a defendant, the alleged wrongdoer, seeking monetary damages for harmful acts. In civil actions, the burden of proof is on the plaintiff who must prove his or her case by a preponderance of the evidence, that is, more evidence showing that the plaintiff has been wronged than evidence legally exculpating the defendant. In a *criminal* case, the state acts as the prosecutor and must prove criminal wrongdoing beyond a reasonable doubt. While the primary purpose of a civil suit is to recover damages for an injured plaintiff, the primary purpose of criminal action is to punish a guilty defendant. Such punishment, of course, can range from a fine to death.

CONSENT TO MEDICAL CARE

The general rule regarding consent to medical care is that anyone who has reached the age of majority, usually 18 or 21 years, may consent to treatment. If a patient is under the age of majority, a parent or legal guardian must usually consent to medical intervention. Every legal rule, however, has exceptions. In the case of an emergency, for example, consent is implied, and neither a parent, legal guardian, nor patient need explicitly authorize the medical care. It is important, however, to document that an emergency existed and what efforts were made to notify the parents of a minor patient. It is also necessary to determine how state law defines an emergency. For example, in Massachusetts, an emergency is defined as the following: "When delay in treatment will endanger the life, limb, or mental well-being of the patient" (1). The definition of an emergency may vary from state to state but generally involves the same concept.

In addition to the emergency exception, minors are legally capable of consenting to their own health care if they are emancipated. Emancipation generally has two statutory definitions. The first is a minor fulfilling an adult status. If a patient, for example, is a member of the armed forces, is a parent of a child, is married, widowed, or divorced, or is living separately from and is financially independent of parents, he or she may consent to intervention without informing the parent or guardian.

The second basis of emancipation is where the minor's health may be endangered and the state wishes to encourage the minor to seek help despite possible parental resistance. Such areas where a minor may consent to treatment under state law include pregnancy, diseases dangerous to the public health, and alcohol or drug dependency. Reasoning that getting treatment is more important than obtaining parental consent, the state in these areas encourages the minor to seek intervention on his or her own authority by allowing treatment without parental consent. Unlike minors fulfilling an adult status, who generally may consent to any kind of medical care, minors in the second category generally may only consent to treatment for the specific condition creating emancipation.

The separate concept of mature minor, moreover, has received increasing judicial approval. Courts have recognized that there may be situations not otherwise controlled by statute in which it is in the best interest of the minor not to notify parents of the intended medical treatment. If the minor is able to give informed consent to the intended treatment, the mature minor rule may apply.

The initial determination of whether a minor is mature usually rests with the treating health care provider, who assesses the nature of the procedure, its likely benefit, and the capacity of the particular minor to understand fully what the medical procedure involves. Thus, in a situation where a minor is not emancipated, it may still be possible to enter into a provider–patient relationship with the minor and without parental consent on the basis of the provider's assessment that the minor is mature.

Generally, a health care provider will not be held liable for providing medical treatment without parental consent if he or she relies in good faith on the minor's reasonable representation that he or she is emancipated. Consents obtained from emancipated and mature minors, and any interventions resulting from such consents, moreover, are confidential. Parents should not be informed unless the minor agrees. Such agreements should be documented in the patient's medical record.

Some states require health care providers treating minors to inform the parent if the minor's condition is endangering of life or limb. Under such circumstances, the situation should be discussed with the minor before informing the parent, and this discussion should be documented in the patient's record. Under circumstances not endangering to life or limb, no information should be shared with the parent without the consent of the minor patient, and billings should not be mailed to parents if they undermine or are likely to undermine the confidentiality of the relationship.

In medical management, disagreements may arise among care providers, minor patients, and their parents. For example, an adolescent diagnosed with an ovarian tumor may resist chemotherapy that her parent requests; or both parents and patient may refuse surgery that physicians feel is medically necessary. Hopefully, these conflicts will resolve with ongoing dialogue and the obtaining of second opinions. If consensus does not emerge, however, the legal options vary, depending on such factors as the age of the patient, the seriousness of the underlying condition, the nature and variety of possible interventions, their contraindications, and the probability of their success.

Courts, for example, would likely order treatment in a minor's "best interest" if her parents are unwilling to consent to treatment, the underlying condition is potentially fatal, the recommended treatment is the only one available or is clearly preferred, and the risks of treatment are minimal. However, prior to making an order, the court will generally appoint a Guardian *ad Litem*. A Guardian *ad Litem* (GAL) is generally an attorney or clinician who is appointed to investigate and report to the court regarding the medical necessity of a given procedure and whether it is in the patient's best interest to perform, or not perform, the procedure. The GAL is generally "neutral," and renders a report to the court. The court may also appoint an attorney to represent and advocate for the minor patient in court proceedings (2).

Health care providers should obviously resist the coercive imposition of treatment on a minor. If, however, the patient is not "mature," the underlying condition is serious, and the parents are consenting to its use, the parents' desires can legally "trump" the minor's right to refuse.

Obtaining informed consent is a process that involves four distinct steps. The first step, which has already been discussed, is determining who has the authority to consent. The second step is determining whether the person with the authority to consent is competent to consent. Legally, an adult or mature minor is presumed competent until demonstrated otherwise. Parents of a mentally retarded patient who has reached the age of majority do not automatically become their child's legal guardian. They must be appointed by a court, and without such judicial appointment, they do not have the legal authority to consent to their child's treatment. The provider should be cautious about providing treatment if there is any question regarding a person's capacity to understand the nature and consequences of a proposed procedure. Such reasons may include mental retardation, inebriation, drug usage or mental illness.

The third step in obtaining informed consent involves providing the person who has the authority to consent with all the material information necessary for a reasonable person to make an informed decision. Generally speaking, the patient or parent/guardian must be informed of the nature of the patient's condition, the nature and probability of the risks, the benefits to be reasonably expected, the inability of the treater to predict results, the reversibility of the procedure, the likely result of no treatment, and the alternatives to the proposed treatment, including the risks and benefits of such alternatives. The provider should keep in mind that the more elective a proposed treatment, the more necessary it is to disclose all risks.

The final step in the informed consent process is obtaining the agreement of the person with the authority to consent. The person with legal authority to consent should sign the consent form agreeing to any interventions after such interventions have been fully communicated and understood. It is important to note that merely obtaining the signature of the person with authority to consent, without going through the other steps in the process, does not constitute informed consent. It is advisable therefore to make a note in the medical record documenting the informed consent process.

Finally, it is necessary for the practitioner to be aware of special situations where the general rules of consent may not apply. Such situations include a child's being in the custody of the state or a divorce situation where one parent may have physical care of a child but both parents may have legal custody or decision-making responsibility. Other special situations may include abortion, sterilization, management of child abuse cases, and consent to human immunodeficiency virus (HIV) testing (to be discussed subsequently).

To illustrate a special situation, if the Massachusetts Department of Social Services (DSS) has legal custody of a child, it is authorized to consent to the youngster's routine medical care (e.g., immunizations, preventive health services, and treatment of illnesses). If, however, the required medical interventions are "extraordinary"—for example, "do not resuscitate" orders, the giving or withholding of life-prolonging medical treatment, or the use of antipsychotic medications—the DSS cannot consent but will seek judicial approval before proceeding. If the child is in state custody, the child will have had an attorney appointed to represent the child and that attorney will likely appear at any court hearings and advocate on the child's behalf. Additionally, the court may appoint a GAL to investigate and report to the court.

CONFIDENTIALITY OF PATIENT INFORMATION

As a general rule, medical records and communications between providers and patients and their families are confidential and should not be released without the written authorization of the patient/guardian or a proper judicial order. Even though parents, including noncustodial parents, usually have access to medical information of their minor children, certain situations may mandate a denial of access. As indicated previously, mature minors and emancipated minors who consent to treatment need not reveal either the consent or the treatment to their parents. Later sections will discuss other exceptions to parental notification, including the prescription of contraceptives to unemancipated minors.

Physicians and other care providers should learn whether statutory or common law privileges protect the confidentiality of a patient relationship. In some jurisdictions, for example, statutory privileges exist between psychotherapists and patients, physicians and patients, and social workers and clients. Absent a duty to warn or protect because of a patient's dangerousness, these privileges prevent professionals from revealing any information about their patients without specific authorization. Case law may further prohibit a professional's ability to disclose information without written consent.

Regardless of maturity, emancipation, or privilege, teenagers may hesitate to reveal sensitive information to care providers if it is automatically shared with their parents. At the beginning of the professional relationship, therefore, the physician should consider negotiating ground rules with families: that before any sharing, the older minor will be notified as to what will be communicated and why and that to maintain a teenager's trust, parents will only receive information that is legally or clinically necessary to share—for example, indications of serious illness or potentially life-threatening behavior.

Though all clinical information in a patient's chart is confidential, recorded data concerning such matters as psychiatric history and HIV status are especially sensitive. To facilitate increased protection of these notes, care providers might stamp the word "confidential" on the relevant pages.

On April 14, 2003, federal privacy legislation called the Health Insurance Portability and Accountability Act (HIPAA) went into effect. Covered entities, including health care providers, must implement standards to protect against the misuse of individually identifiable health information. Such protected health information (PHI) may not be used or disclosed except as required or permitted under the law.

The statute (Public Law 104-191) and Department of Health and Human Services (HHS) regulations are lengthy and complex. In summary: Patients may now find out how their information has been used and what disclosures have been made. They have a right to examine and obtain a copy of their own health records and request corrections in such records. Written authorizations to use or disclose, containing an expiration date, must specifically describe the material to be shared and the purpose in doing so. In most instances providers must maintain an "accounting of disclosures log".

The "minimum necessary rule" generally limits release of information to the minimum reasonably needed for the purpose of the disclosure. Covered entities, however, may use or disclose information without written authorization if such use or disclosure is required by law—for example, in public health and police matters or in the reporting of child abuse and neglect.

HIPAA generally defers to state law concerning the relative rights of parents and minors. Legal guardians will ordinarily exercise the HIPAA rights of their minor children. On the other hand, patients 18 years or older, or with emancipated or "mature minor" status, may exercise their own rights with respect to such matters as the diagnosis and treatment of venereal diseases, drug dependency, and pregnancy.

SEXUAL ABUSE

Reporting statutes exist in every state that require various professionals to report sexual abuse to state agencies, usually a department of social services or its equivalent. Physicians, nurses, and other medical professionals are *mandated* reporters. The standard employed for determining whether the state agency should be notified is reasonable belief or suspicion that a child has suffered sexual abuse. Knowledge of incest or sexual abuse is not required because very rarely is a professional certain that sexual abuse has occurred. Symptoms such as fear of men, nightmares and sleep disturbances, stomachaches, and headaches are symptomatic but not diagnostic of sexual exploitation and may require reporting.

Generally, reports of abuse have no statute of limitations requirement. State child protection agencies, however, are understandably reluctant to accept filings that are difficult to investigate because the alleged events occurred in the past. They may also refuse to accept reports in which the suspected perpetrator is a stranger to the child rather than a care provider (e.g., a parent or family member, babysitter, or school bus driver) with legitimate authority over him/her. Under these circumstances, the professional may defer to the agency's decision, documenting in the patient's chart the agency's refusal to become involved, or file the report regardless, requesting protective services to forward it to law enforcement.

From a legal point of view, if a mandated reporter has concerns about sexual abuse of a patient, it is generally safer to file a report than to withhold filing. Most states, for example, have an immunity provision protecting from suit or liability those professionals who file a report that is later proved erroneous. On the other hand, there are sanctions for mandated reporters who fail to fulfill their statutory responsibility to report.

After child abuse reports are received by state agencies, the agency must investigate the allegedly abusive family to determine whether a child is at risk. Assuming that a report is corroborated, the state agency has an obligation to monitor the child's safety, to provide services that may protect a child from future harm and, in certain circumstances, to refer the case for possible criminal prosecution or to remove the child from biologic parents for placement in foster care. Most states waive any privileges that otherwise may exist between the professional and patient in order to encourage reporting; in other words, the confidentiality that usually exists within a relationship is waived by law in the case of child abuse.

In addition to mandatory reporting statutes, states may have other legislation relevant to the management of sexual abuse. For example, statutes often exist that allow a health care provider serving in a hospital or health center to prevent a child from being removed by his or her caretaker if the child is in imminent and serious danger because of abuse and neglect. Legislation may also exist that allows professionals to petition juvenile or family courts if they feel that parental unfitness is causing harm to a child. Under such circumstances, the courts may remove legal or physical custody from biologic parents, place it with the state, and order that such children be placed in foster care or another more secure environment.

Because sexual abuse is more often criminally prosecuted than physical abuse, physicians and medical personnel may need to testify in prosecutions of alleged abusers. Sometimes they serve as expert witnesses who, though uninvolved in the direct care of the child, have reviewed records and will offer opinions to the court. At other times, though having expertise, they essentially serve as fact witnesses who communicate what they did or observed in their professional role (e.g., the diagnostic tests performed and treatment given). Clearly, these two categories of testimony overlap.

It is imperative for health care providers to keep complete and accurate records of any examinations conducted on children who have been victimized. Before testifying, health care providers should "refresh their recollection" of the case by reviewing their notes and should seek legal consultation and advice, if it is available. The professional should also make certain that no privileges exist that impede communication without the consent of patient or parent.

On the witness stand the physician should not use jargon or overly complex language; if professional terms are necessary, they require clarification. A witness should answer only the specific question asked, should not respond to a question beyond his/her knowledge or expertise, and should refrain from argumentative or clearly partisan communications.

It should be understood that cases of child sexual abuse can be very difficult to prosecute successfully because of the child's age and frequent lack of physical evidence. In criminal matters, the state must prove a defendant guilty beyond a reasonable doubt, and this standard can be difficult to reach in sexual abuse cases.

CONTRACEPTION

The provision of contraception to minors raises two legal issues: consent and the need for parental notification. In regard to consent, in 1977 the US Supreme Court in *Carey v. Population Serv Intl* (3) invalidated a New York statute that prohibited the distribution or sale of contraceptives to minors under the age of 16. The court ruled that the New York law violated the privacy rights of minors, which included the right to make procreative decisions. Such decisions, of course, should be based on informed consent, and a medical practitioner should review state law to ascertain whether additional requirements need to be met before contraceptives are prescribed. With the subdermal implant contraceptives, for example, consent of the parent/guardian of a minor patient is generally recommended, because insertion requires a surgical procedure and, practically, because the device is unlikely to go unnoticed.

Even if unemancipated minors can obtain contraceptives without parental consent, state law may require a provider to notify parents of the provision of contraceptives. In 1980, a US Appeals Court in the case of *Doe v. Irwin* (4) found that parents did not have a right to notification when minors voluntarily sought contraceptive devices from publicly operated family planning centers. This decision finds support in more recent cases that find it is not in the best interest of the minor to breach a confidential relationship between the minor and the family planning service.

Since some contraceptives can have harmful side effects, it is important to assess possible risks, to communicate them to the patient, to properly implement the contraceptive, and to monitor the patient for adverse reactions.

Many states now require insurance companies to provide coverage for prescription contraceptives. Among the arguments for this mandate is gender discrimination—the fact that only women can get pregnant and that only women can use prescription contraception to prevent it. Additionally, states have passed statutes providing for so-called emergency contraception, methods that women may use in the first few days following unprotected intercourse to prevent unwanted pregnancy. Because of budgetary constraints and the unfortunate link by some political groups between emergency contraception and abortion, it is possible that government and the private sector may become increasingly reluctant to support these efforts.

STERILIZATION

The sterilization of minors is almost exclusively a matter of state law. Because sterilization, if successful, ends the minor's reproductive capability, it is strictly regulated or prohibited outright. In some states, a mentally retarded child or adult may be sterilized, but only after a formal judicial determination to ensure protection of the incompetent's best interest. In other states, there is no legal basis for performing sterilization procedures on incompetents. The general rule is that neither courts nor a guardian can authorize voluntary sterilization of minors without specific statutory authority.

A private hospital may prohibit its medical staff from performing voluntary sterilization. Some states, moreover, have so-called conscience clauses that allow individual physicians or nurses to refuse participation in sterilization or abortion procedures if such procedures are performed in the facility in which they work.

ABORTION

In 1973, the US Supreme Court in *Roe v. Wade* (5) held that the "fundamental right" of privacy included the right of abortion. It then developed a trimester system that made the woman's health and viability of the fetus key decision points. In the first trimester of pregnancy, the abortion decision is primarily between a woman and her health care provider. In the second trimester, the state has an increasing interest in the woman's health and can regulate the conditions under which an abortion is performed. In the third trimester, because the fetus is viable and can generally survive separate and apart from its mother, the state develops a "compelling interest" in the life of the fetus and can prohibit abortions except if the mother's life or health is endangered.

In the case of *Webster v. Reproductive Health Services* (6), the Court upheld a Missouri statute requiring doctors to test for fetal viability in any fetus thought to be at least 20 weeks old and forbidding public facilities and employees (doctors, nurses, and other health care providers) from performing abortions other than those to save the life of the mother. Though not specifically overruling the *Roe v. Wade* decision, Chief Justice Rehnquist, writing for a plurality of the Court, attacked its trimester structure as "unsound" and "unworkable": He said there is "no reason why the state's compelling interest in protecting potential human life should not extend throughout pregnancy rather than coming into existence only at the point of viability." While the Roe case functioned to keep states from restricting most abortions, the Webster decision allows states much greater license to regulate and curtail abortions.

Prior to Webster, the Supreme Court had consistently struck down regulations and procedures that limited a woman's access to abortion. Impermissible restrictions included requirements that all second trimester abortions be performed in a hospital, that minors obtain either parental or judicial consent for abortions, and that women wait a minimum of 24 hours after signing a consent form before an abortion can occur. The Seventh Circuit US Court of Appeals, for example, struck down an Illinois statute imposing a 24-hour waiting period on minors seeking abortion (7).

In the 1992 case of *Planned Parenthood of Southeastern Pennsylvania v. Casey* (8), however, the US Supreme Court declared that a 24-hour waiting period between information disclosed for a woman's "informed consent" and the performance of an abortion is constitutional as long as the delay may be voided in a medical emergency and does not create any appreciable health risk to the patient. Generally, statutes requiring parental consent as a precondition to abortion have been struck down. In the case of *Planned Parenthood of Central Missouri v. Danforth* (9), the Supreme Court held unconstitutional a statute requiring parental consent to abortions for unmarried women under age 18. Some states, however, have enacted legislation allowing minors seeking abortions to apply for judicial consent as an alternative to parental consent. In the Massachusetts case of *Bellotti v. Baird* (10), the court ruled that the state must provide a pregnant minor with a timely and confidential court hearing to show she is mature and informed enough to make her own abortion decision in consultation with her health care provider. If the court finds the minor not sufficiently mature to give consent, it must authorize an abortion if this is found to be in her best interest. If state legislation contains these two provisions, then according to the Baird case, requiring parental consent would not constitute the absolute and arbitrary veto that was found unconstitutional in *Danforth.*

In addition to the issue of parental consent for a minor's abortion is the question of parental notification. In *H. L. v. Matheson* (11), the Supreme Court upheld a Utah statute that required physicians to "notify if possible" the parents or guardian of an unmarried minor who sought an abortion. The Court stated that the statute served an important state interest in protecting family integrity, safeguarding adolescents, and providing parents the opportunity to supply essential psychological and medical information to their child's physician. Although most parental notification statutes have been found constitutional, those that require more than simple notification have been struck down. For example, in *Hodgson v. Minnesota* (12), the US Court of Appeals for the Eighth Circuit ruled that a judicial consent alternative must be an option in abortion statutes that require parental notification. The court wished to ensure that the notice requirement was not unduly burdensome to the pregnant minor attempting to obtain an abortion. To ensure that the parental notification requirement is not unduly burdensome, the minor must be given the option of an alternative court procedure in which she can show her maturity or demonstrate that performance of an abortion is in her best interest.

Given the current Congressional balance and the political strength of some antiabortion groups, abortions may be increasingly restricted or curbed. Controversial issues include a ban on abortions in overseas military hospitals, the prohibition of abortion coverage in federal employees' health insurance except in cases of life endangerment, state authorization to eliminate Medicaid funding for abortions for low-income women who are pregnant from rape or incest, the ending of federal funding for human embryo research, and the outlawing of late-term abortions. The ultimate fate of these measures depends on the responses of the US House of Representatives and Senate, the willingness of the President to exercise his veto, and, assuming constitutional challenge, the ultimate holdings of the Supreme Court.

It is possible that this political–legal trend will continue and that the US Supreme Court will ultimately overturn Roe. Abortion and its implementation will become increasingly limited. In early 2003 the Supreme Court in the case of A Woman's Choice—*East Side Women's Clinic v. Newman* (02-935)—upheld mandatory preabortion counseling, rejecting a challenge to an Indiana statute that requires women to receive in-person guidance about risks and alternatives at least 18 hours before an abortion. Appellants' attorneys had argued that state law imposed an undue constitutional burden, especially on poor women who must travel long distances.

The Court also ruled in *Scheidler v. National Organization for Women* (01-1118) and *Operation Rescue v. National Organization for Women* (01-1119) that antiabortion protesters cannot be punished for civil disobedience under a federal antiracketeering law. Chief Justice William H. Rehnquist, writing for the majority, held that political activity did not qualify as extortion, providing a victory to Operation Rescue and nullifying a previous order compelling it to pay damages to abortion clinics and barring it from interfering with their businesses for 10 years.

Congress, moreover, passed the Partial Birth Abortion Ban Act, which prohibits the performance of late-term abortion procedures ("partial birth", "dilation and extraction," and "intact dilation and evacuation") that entail (a) delivery of the torso, (b) piercing the undelivered skull, (c) collapsing the skull via suction curate, and then (d) completing delivery.

In 2000, by a five-to-four margin, the US Supreme Court in *Stenberg v. Carhart* (530 US 914) affirmed an Eighth Circuit decision nullifying a Nebraska "partial birth abortion" statute that proscribed both the D&E and D&X procedures. The Court based its decisions on two Constitutional defects: lack of an exception for the mother's health and restriction of more than the D&X procedure. As of early 2003 at least 30 states have passed limiting legislation on this issue.

SEXUALLY TRANSMITTED DISEASES

States commonly require that health care professionals report cases of venereal disease or diseases dangerous to the public health to a state or local board of health. For example, in Massachusetts, a physician treating a patient with acquired immunodeficiency syndrome (AIDS) must report the fact of AIDS to the local board of health. Gonorrhea and syphilis, on the other hand, are reported directly to the state Department of Public Health. As indicated earlier, a minor who believes that he or she is suffering from a sexually transmitted disease usually can consent to treatment without the authorization of a parent or guardian.

HIV AND AIDS

The statutes on HIV infection and AIDS are of recent origin and, like other laws, vary by state. Four important issues that arise are testing, confidentiality, universal precautions, and documentation. To test for the presence of HIV antibody, voluntary and informed consent of the patient and/or parent/guardian usually is required. As a matter of public policy, many states prohibit mandatory, coerced, or secret testing of individual patients for AIDS.

Many states, moreover, require that HIV testing and test results be maintained in confidence. In these states, the fact and the results of such testing cannot be disclosed without the subject's written informed consent. This confidentiality requirement may conflict with the professional's perceived duty to warn a party who may be exposed to HIV or AIDS. For example, a teenager who has used drugs and tests positive on an HIV test may request that her boyfriend not be informed of the test results. The health care provider may feel strongly that the boyfriend is entitled to the test information so that he also may be tested, receive medical and psychiatric intervention, and take prophylactic action regarding other sexual partners. The health care provider should learn whether a state confidentiality statute exists for HIV infection or AIDS.

The Occupational Safety and Health Administration of the US Department of Labor requires the implementation of universal precautions in health care settings. Use of universal precautions makes mandatory testing less necessary to protect hospital staff. If professionals assume that blood and body fluids of all patients need to be avoided, the rationale for universal mandatory testing becomes less salient.

Though health care providers need to maintain the confidentiality of HIV testing and results, it is necessary to document the fact and the results of testing in hospital and private patient records. Documentation is necessary so that professionals can provide the best and most appropriate care for a patient. The confidentiality concern is not met by failing to record medical information. It is fulfilled by giving access only to those who have a clinical or administrative need to know.

SUMMARY

Minors are generally not capable of consenting to their own health care. In an emergency situation, however, consent of a parent or a guardian is not required. Furthermore, if a minor is mature (close to the age of majority and capable of reasonable decision making), he or she may consent to care without parental involvement if the mature minor doctrine is recognized by the state courts. If the minor is emancipated under state statute (has an adult status or a condition that is health endangering, such as pregnancy, venereal disease, or drug dependency), the teen is empowered to consent to treatment.

Parents generally have access to the medical and other information of their children. However, if a statutory privilege exists such as between social worker and client or psychotherapist and patient or if common law requires that a physician not disclose patient data, the confidential relationship between the professional and minor must be maintained. Confidentiality also must be respected if the minor is defined as mature or emancipated.

All 50 states have child-abuse reporting statutes that require professionals to report cases of incest and sexual abuse to government agencies. State law may also allow or require professionals to obtain restraining orders to protect victims of sexual exploitation who are in imminent and serious danger. Legislation may also exist that allows minors to be placed in the temporary custody of the state for their protection.

The Supreme Court has upheld the right of minors to make procreative decisions and has forbidden states from prohibiting the distribution of contraceptives to them. In terms of notification, a US Court of Appeals has ruled that parents have no constitutional right to be advised when a public facility distributes contraceptives to their children.

In the case of *Peck v. Califano* (13), it was held that sterilization of persons under 21 years of age may not lawfully be funded with federal money. This decision supports social policy restricting a minor's access to sterilization.

The Supreme Court decisions in *Roe v. Wade* (5) and *Doe v. Bolton* (14) essentially permit abortions to occur during the first two trimesters of pregnancy. States may not promulgate regulations or procedures that restrict the constitutionally protected right of privacy unless a compelling state interest overrides that right. Generally, statutes requiring parental consent as a precondition to an abortion have been struck down by courts. Some states, however, have passed laws allowing minors seeking abortions to apply for the consent of a judge as an alternative to parental consent.

Certain sexually transmitted diseases must be reported to local or state public health agencies. HIV testing generally requires the voluntary informed and written consent of the patient and/or parent/guardian. The testing itself and the test results usually are confidential, but a duty to warn may exist if someone is in danger of contagion. Universal precautions as specified by the federal Centers for Disease Control and Prevention should be followed, and HIV or AIDS testing and treatment should be properly documented in a medical record.

REFERENCES

1. Massachusetts General Law, C112, sec 12F.
2. Bourne R. Coerced treatment of adolescents. In: Ventrell MR, ed. *Children's law, policy and practice.* Denver: National Association of Counsel for Children, 1995.
3. *Carey v. Population Serv Intl,* 431 US 678, 97 SCt 2010 (1977).
4. *Doe v. Irwin,* 615 F2d 1162 (6th Cir 1980).
5. *Roe v. Wade,* 410 US 113, 93 SCt 705 (1973).
6. *Webster v. Reproductive Health Services,* 109 SCt 3040 (1989).
7. *Zbarez v. Hartigan,* 763 F2d 1532 (7th Cir 1985).
8. *Planned Parenthood of Southeastern Pennsylvania v. Casey,* 120 LEd 2d 674 (1992).
9. *Planned Parenthood of Central Missouri v. Danforth,* 428 US 52, 96 SCt 2831 (1976).
10. *Bellotti v. Baird,* 443 US 622, 99 SCt 3035 (1979).
11. *H.L. v. Matheson,* 450 US 398, 1101 SCt 1164 (1981).
12. *Hodgson v. Minnesota,* 827 F2d 1191 (8th Cir 1987).
13. *Peck v. Califano,* 454 F Supp 484 (1977).
14. *Doe v. Bolton,* 410 US 179, 93 SO 739 (1973).

FURTHER READING

English A, Kenney KE. State minor consent laws: a summary, 2nd ed. Center for Adolescent Health & the Law, 2003.

Appendix 1

Resources

Clinicians interested in providing educational materials for their patients and parents on a wide variety of topics related to pediatric and adolescent gynecology should consult their public library and peruse the materials available for parents, children, and adolescents to become familiar with the content. The internet has become a major source of information, and identifying accurate information from the plethora of sites can be challenging. Our Center for Young Women's Health (CYWH) resource center and website www.youngwomenshealth.org can be a great starting place for girls, their families, and providers. Funded by the Children's Hospital League, the Cabot Family Charitable Trust, the Office of Women's Health, the Maternal Child Health Bureau, and multiple other benefactors, we are grateful to be able to provide resources. The CYWH is physically located at Children's Hospital Boston (www.childrenshospital.org). Pamphlets for the office can be obtained from local Planned Parenthood clinics, the Sexuality Information and Education Council of the United States (SIECUS), the American Academy of Pediatrics (AAP), and the American College of Obstetricians and Gynecologists (ACOG). Physicians working with developmentally disabled patients will find the SIECUS bibliographies helpful.

SELECTED WEBSITES

P: Professionals; Y: Youth; F: Parents/Families

The Center for Young Women's Health, Children's Hospital, Boston (Y, P, F)—The Center for Young Women's Health offers information resource and clinical care for young women ages 12–22, as well as resources for parents, educators, and health professionals. www.youngwomenshealth.org

The Boston Leadership Education in Adolescent Health (LEAH) training program (P, F, Y)—The LEAH Program hosts a site with links to many of the resources listed below. The LEAH program is funded by the Maternal and Child Health Bureau to provide training in adolescent health to physicians, nurses, nutritionists, social workers, and psychologists, to work collaboratively with the State Adolescent Health

Coordinators to improve adolescent health in the states, and to disseminate research and best practices. www.bostonleah.org

Association of Reproductive Health Professionals (P, Y, F)—The web site of the Association of Reproductive Health Professionals offers reproductive health information for parents, youth, and professionals. www.arhp.org

Contraceptive Technology (P)—The Contraceptive Technology web site offers information and publications for health professionals involved in contraception education. www.managingcontraception.com

Contraceptive Report (P)—The Contraceptive Report is part of the Contraception online web site and provides up-to-date information on contraception and review of the latest developments. www.contraceptiononline.org

Planned Parenthood (P, F)—Planned Parenthood offers reproductive health information and clinical care. www.plannedparenthood.org

National Campaign to Prevent Teen Pregnancy (F, Y, P)—The National Campaign to Prevent Teen Pregnancy offers a wealth of information, educational materials, and other resources for preventing teen pregnancy. www.teenpregnancy.org

Alan Guttmacher Institute (P)—The Alan Guttmacher Institute is a nonprofit organization focused on sexual and reproductive health and the rights of individuals as they pertain to these issues. www.agi-usa.org

National Organization on Adolescent Pregnancy, Parenting, and Prevention (P)—NOAPP provides a wealth of information and resources for individuals and organizations involved in adolescent pregnancy, parenting, and prevention. www.noappp.org

Advocates for Youth (Y, F, P)—Advocates for Youth offers information and resources around issues of adolescent reproductive and sexual health. www.advocatesforyouth.org

Sexuality Information and Education Council of the United States (P, F, Y)—SIECUS offers a wealth of information and educational resources around sex and sexuality. www.siecus.org

CDC's Reproductive Health Information Source (P)—The CDC's Reproductive Health Information Source offers reports, information, and statistics on adolescent pregnancy and births, contraception, and more. www.cdc.gov/nccdphp/drh/up_adol preg.htm

Child Trends (P)—Child Trends collects, conducts, and disseminates a wealth of data related to children's research. www.childtrends.org

Planned Parenthood's Teen Wire (Y)—Teen Wire web site offers teens straightforward information about sexuality and sexual health. www.teenwire.com/home_content.asp

Go Ask Alice! (Y)—Go Ask Alice! is a wide-ranging health question and answer web site maintained by Columbia University's Health Education Program. www.goaskalice.columbia.edu/index.html

The North American Society for Pediatric and Adolescent Gynecology (NASPAG) (P). This site provides information regarding their mission of education of health care providers and patients relating to pediatric and adolescent gynecology. www.naspag.org

The AWARE Foundation (Y, F, P)—The AWARE Foundation offers information and resource in support of empowering adolescents to make responsible decisions with regard to sexual and reproductive health and wellness. www.awarefoundation.org

The Intersex Society of North America (P, F, Y)—This site is a resource for addressing issues for intersexed individuals and providing support and medical information. www.isna.org

The MRKH website (P, F, Y)—This site is an excellent resource for young women with MRKH looking for information and support. www.MRKH.org

The American Society for Reproductive Medicine (P)—This site is an excellent resource regarding up-to-date information regarding reproductive medical issues. www.asrm.org

Resolve (P, F, Y)—Resolve is an organization for patients and health care providers regarding the treatment and options for individuals with infertility. www.resolve.org

The Endometriosis Association (P, F, Y)—The Endometriosis Association is an international organization committed to the diagnosis and treatment of endometriosis. The organization has been in existence for over 20 years and recently has focused on endometriosis in teens. www.endometriosisassn.org

Fertile Hope (P, F, Y)—Fertile Hope is a non-profit organization addressing fertility issues for cancer patients and survivors. www.fertilehope.org

Outlook Life (P, F, Y)—This is a website for childhood cancer survivors and provides information for patients, families, and health care providers. www.outlook-life.org

Turner Syndrome Society of the United States (Y, F, P)—The Turner Syndrome Society of the United States offers information for young women, adult women, families, and professionals. www.turner-syndrome-us.org

ADOL: Adolescence Directory On-Line (P, Y, F)—Adolescence Directory Online is a collection of Internet resources dedicated to issues of adolescent health and wellness. www.education.indiana.edu/cas/adol/adol.html

CYFERnet: Children, Youth, and Families Education and Research Network (P, Y, F)—CYFERnet offers a wealth of information and resources relating to all aspects of child and family health. www.cyfernet.org

OUTProud (Y, P)—OUTProud is the web site of the National Coalition for Gay, Lesbian, Bisexual & Transgender Youth; the site offers information and resources for both youth and educators. www.outproud.org

PFLAG (F)—PFLAG is the web site of Parents, Families, and Friends of Lesbians and Gays. The site offers information, advocacy, support resources, and more. www.pflag.org

Girl Power! (Y, F, P)—Girl Power! is a national health education campaign for young women ages 9 to 13 from the U.S. Department of Health and Human Services. www.girlpower.gov

4 Girls Health (Y, F)—4 Girls Health is a health information web site for young women ages 10 to 16 offered by the Office on Women's Health in the U.S. Department of Health and Human Services. www.4girls.gov

Connect for Kids (P, F)—Connect for Kids is an information resource devoted to helping adults provide kids with the tools and support they need for healthy development physically, mentally, and emotionally. www.connectforkids.org

Learning Disabilities Online (F, P)—Learning Disabilities Online offers a wide range of information resources for families and educators concerned with learning disabilities. www.ldonline.org

National Information Center for Children and Youth with Disabilities (F, Y, P)—NICHCY is an information clearinghouse concerned with disabilities information for children birth through age 22. www.nichcy.org

KidsHealth.org (F, Y)—KidsHealth.org offers a wide variety of health and wellness information for children, youth, and parents. www.kidshealth.org

National Eating Disorder Association (F, Y, P)—NEDA is a comprehensive resource for information about eating disorders. www.nationaleatingdisorders.org

Henry J Kaiser Family Foundation (P, F)—This site provides updates on reproductive health information, recent surveys, and policy in addition to their other missions. www.kff.org

Tufts Nutrition Navigator (F, Y, P)—The Nutrition Navigator rates the best nutrition-related web sites for a variety of specific target audiences. www.navigator.tufts.edu

About Our Kids (F, P)—About Our Kids is a mental health and parenting resource for parents and professionals working with children and youth. www.aboutourkids.org/

AskERIC (F, P)—AskERIC is an internet-based clearinghouse of education information for parents and professionals. www.eduref.org and www.eric.ed.gov

RAND (P)—RAND is a non-profit organization offering research and analysis to help improve policy. Children and adolescents are one of RAND's primary research areas. www.rand.org

National Adolescent Health Information Center (P)—NAHIC offers a wealth of information and research on issues in adolescent health. http://youth.ucsf.edu/nahic

National Network for Health (F, P)—The National Network for Health is dedicated to educating and empowering consumers and families to make healthy lifestyle choices and informed health care decision. www.nnh.org/

SAMHSA's National Mental Health Information Center (P, F, Y)—The National Mental Health Information Center offers a wealth of mental health information for professionals and consumers, and includes a special section for youth. www.mental health.org/

Partnership Against Violence Network (P)—PAVNET is an online library of information about violence and at-risk youth comprised of information and statistics from 7 different federal agencies. www.pavnet.org

Resource Center for Adolescent Pregnancy Prevention (P)—ReCAPP offers information and resources for educators and health professionals to support practical approaches to adolescent pregnancy prevention. www.etr.org/recapp

Sex Education Coalition (P, F, Y)—The Sex Education Coalition offers information and resources promoting informed discussion on the topic of sexuality education and provides professionals involved in sexual and reproductive health education with educational and informational materials. www.sexedcoalition.org

American Academy of Pediatrics (AAP) (P)—This site provides health information for providers to give to patients on a wide variety of topics and links to the Bright Futures materials as noted later. www.aap.org

Bright Futures (P, F)—Bright Futures is dedicated to promoting and improving infant, child, and adolescent health through publications, training tools, and distance education for professionals through the American Academy of Pediatrics website. http://brightfutures.aap.org/web Twenty nine Bright Futures cases with facilitators' guides written by Children's Hospital Boston faculty and fellows for teaching residents and other health care providers are linked through this site to www.pedi cases.org

American Medical Women's Association (P)—This site provides an innovative reproductive health initiative and model curriculum (2nd) edition, which has been used for the education of medical students and other health professionals. www.amwa-doc.org/RHI.htm

American College of Obstetrics and Gynecology (ACOG) (P, F, Y)—This site provides policy statements for professionals and educational materials for teens and families. The site also provides practice guidelines and committee opinions relating to clinical care in obstetrics and gynecology. www.acog.org

American Medical Association (P, F, Y)—This site has an adolescent specific section with educational resources. www.ama-assn.org/ama/pub/category/1979.html

Institute for Youth Development (P, F, Y)—IYD information and advice to professionals, families, and teens interested in promoting adolescent avoidance of key risk behaviors. www.youthdevelopment.org

Center for Substance Abuse Prevention (P, F, Y)—CSAP offers a wealth of information for professionals, parents, families, and teens about alcohol and drugs, including facts and statistics, prevention resources, and more. http://prevention. samhsa.gov

National Institute on Media and the Family (P, F)—The National Institute on Media and the Family is a non-profit, non-partisan organization dedicated to maximizing the benefits and minimizing the harm of mass media through research, education, and advocacy. www.mediafamily.org

ETR Associates (P)—This site provides countless pamphlets for the health education of youth and families. www.etr.org

Channing Bete Company (P)—This site also provide educational materials for the education of youth and families www.channing-bete.com

Autism Resources (F, P)—Autism Resources offers a wealth of resources related to autism and Asperger's syndrome. www.autism-resources.com

SELECTED VIDEOTAPES (P)

Ortho Pharmaceutical Corporation

The pelvic examination: a practical guide
From childhood through adolescence: issues in gynecologic care
The Victim of Rape
Terrorism in the home: responding to the victim of domestic violence
Patients with mental retardation: Issues in gynecologic care
Patients with physical disabilities: Issues in gynecologic care
On the threshold of sadness: Emotional issues surrounding preterm labor
Helping mothers nurse successfully
Breaking the silence: Issues in lesbian healthcare

SELECTED BOOKS

Books for Parents

1. Ames L, Ilg F, Baker S. *Your 10- to 14-year-old.* New York: Dell Publishing, 1988.
2. Faber A, Mazlish E. *How to talk so kids will listen and listen so kids will talk.* New York: Rawson, Wade Publishers, 1980.
3. Ginsburg K, Jablow M. *"But I'm almost 13!": An action plan for raising a responsible adolescent.* New York: McGraw-Hill/ Contemporary Books, 2002.

4. Kaufman M. *Understanding the adolescent years: Mothering teens.* Charlottetown, Canada: Gynergy Books, 1997.
5. Riera M. *Uncommon sense for parents with teenagers.* Berkeley, CA: Celestial Arts, 1995.
6. Wolf A. *"Get out of my life but first could you drive me and Cheryl to the mall?": A parent's guide to the new teenager.* New York: Farrar, Straus, & Giroux, 1991.
7. Apter T. *Altered loves: Mothers and daughters during adolescence.* New York: Ballantine Books, 1990.
8. Marks A, Rothbart B. *Healthy teens, body and soul: A parent's complete guide.* New York: Skylight Press Book/Fireside Book, 2003
9. Lopez, R. *The teen health book: A parents' guide to adolescent health and well being.* New York, W.W. Norton, 2003
10. Gillooly JB. *Before she gets her period: talking with your daughter about menstruation.* Los Angeles: Perspective Publishing, 1998.
11. Greydanus DE, and Bashe, P, (eds.) *Caring for your teenager: the complete and authoritative guide.* New York: Bantam Books, 2003.
12. Richardson J. *Everything you never wanted your kids to know about sex, but were afraid they'd ask: the secrets to surviving your child's sexual development from birth to the teens.* New York: Crown Publishers, 2003.

Reading for adolescents:

1. CityKids. *CityKids speak on relationship.* New York: Random House, Inc, 1994
2. McCoy K, Wibbelsman C. *Life happens: A teenager's guide to friends, failure, sexuality, love, rejection, addiction, peer pressure, families, loss, depression, change, and other challenges of living.* New York: The Berkley Publishing Group, 1996. (out of print)
3. Packer A. *Bringing up parents: The teenager's handbook.* Minneapolis, MN: Free Spirit Publishing Inc 1992.
4. Packer A. *How rude!: The teenagers' guide to good manners, proper behavior, and not grossing people out.* Minneapolis, MN: Free Spirit Publishing Inc, 1997.
5. Scott S. *How to say no and keep your friends: Peer pressure reversal for teens and preteens,* 2nd ed. Amherst, MA: Human Resources Development Press, Inc, 1997.
6. Basso MJ. *The underground guide to teenage sexuality: an essential handbook for today's teens and parents.* Minneapolis: Fairview Press, 2nd edition, 2003. (Also good for parents)
7. Bell R, et al. *Changing bodies, changing lives: a book for teens on sex and relationships.* New York: Times Books, 3rd edition, 1998.
8. Boston Women's Health Book Collective. *Our Bodies, ourselves. For the new century.* New York: Touchstone, 1998.
9. Columbia University's Health Education Program. *The "Go ask Alice" book of answers: a guide to good physical, sexual, and emotional health.* New York: Henry Holt and Company, 1998.
10. McCoy K, Wibblesman C. *The teenage body book.* New York: Perigree, 1999.
11. Stoppard M. *Sex ed: growing up, relationships, and sex.* New York: DK Publishing, 1998.
12. Vitkus J. *Smart sex: honest, expert information to answer all your questions.* New York: Pocket Books, 1998.
13. The Young Women's Editorial Group. *It's about time! A book by and for young women about our relationships, rights, futures, bodies, minds, and souls.* San Francisco: Girlsource Inc., 2000.

Reading for pre-teens to young teens (10–13):

1. Madams L. *What's happening to my body? book for girls: a growing up guide for parents and daughters.* New York: Newmarket Press, 3rd edition, 2000.
2. Gravelle K, Gravelle J. *The period book: Everything you don't want to ask (but need to know).* New York: Walker and Company, 1996.

3. Weston C. *Girltalk: all the stuff your sister never told you. No soapboxes, no sermons, no nonsense.* New York: Harper Collins Publishers, 1997.
4. Thomson R. *Have you started yet? All about getting your period...period.* New York: Price Stern Sloan, 1996.
5. Jukes M. *It's a girl thing: how to stay healthy, safe, and in charge.* New York: Alfred A. Knopf, 1996.
6. McCoy K, Wibbelsman C. *Growing and changing.* New York: Berkley Publishing Group, 2003.

For children under 10:

1. Mayle P. *Where did I come from?: the facts of life without any nonsense and with illustrations.* New Jersey: Carol Publishing Group, 1997.
2. Jukes M. *Growing up: it's a girl thing. Straight talk about first bras, first periods, and your changing body.* New York: Alfred A. Knopf, 1998.
3. Nilsson M, Swanberg LK. *How was I born?* New York: Delacorte Press, 1996.
4. Cole, J. *How you were born.* New York: Mulberry Books, 1994 (revised edition).
5. Johnston A. *Girls speak out: finding your true self.* New York: Scholastic Press, 1997.
6. Schaefer VL. *The care & keeping of you: the body book for girls.* Middleton, WI: Pleasant Company Publications, 1998.

Appendix 2

World Health Organization, Medical Eligibility Criteria for Contraceptive Use, 3rd edition, 2004.

Summary Tables

Adapted from:
http://www.who.int/reproductive-health/publications/RHR_00_2_medical_eligibility_criteria_3rd/index.htm
Summary tables:
http://www.who.int/reproductive-health/publications/MEC_3/mec.pdf

by permission

Summary Tables

Condition	COC P/R	CIC	POP	DMPA NET-EN	LNG/ETG Implants	Cu-IUD	LNG-IUD
PERSONAL CHARACTERISTICS AND REPRODUCTIVE HISTORY							
PREGNANCY	NA	NA	NA	NA	NA		
AGE	Menarche to <40 = 1, ≥40 = 2	Menarche to <40 = 1, ≥40 = 2	Menarche to <18 = 1, 18–45 = 1, >45 = 1	Menarche to <18 = 2, 18–45 = 1, >45 = 2	Menarche to <18 = 1, 18–45 = 1, >45 = 1	<20 = 2, ≥20 = 1	<20 = 2, ≥20 = 1
PARITY							
a) Nulliparous	1	1	1	1	1	2	2
b) Parous	1	1	1	1	1	1	1
BREASTFEEDING							
a) <6 weeks postpartum	4	4	3	3	3		
b) 6 weeks to < 6 months (primarily breastfeeding)	3	3	1	1	1		
c) ≥ 6 months postpartum	2	2	1	1	1		
POSTPARTUM (in non-breastfeeding women)							
a) <21 days	3	3	1	1	1		
b) ≥21 days	1	1	1	1	1		
POSTPARTUM (breastfeeding or non-breastfeeding)							
a) <48 hours						2	3
b) ≥48 hours to <4 weeks						3	3
c) ≥4 weeks						1	1[a]
d) Puerperal sepsis						4	4

[a] if the women is breastfeeding

COC = Combined oral contraceptive
P/R = Patch/Ring
CIC = Combined injectable contraceptive
POP = progestin only pills; DMPA NET-EN = depotmedroxyprogesterone acetate, norethindrone enanthate; Cu-IUD = Copper IUD;
LNG IUD = Levonorgestrol IUD; LNG/ETG Implants = Levonorgestrol, Etonogestrol Implants

Summary Tables

Condition	COC P/R	CIC	POP	DMPA NET-EN	LNG/ETG Implants	CU-IUD	LNG-IUD
POST-ABORTION							
a) First trimester	1	1	1	1	1	1	1
b) Second trimester	1	1	1	1	1	2	2
c) Immediate post-septic abortion	1	1	1	1	1	4	4
PAST ECTOPIC PREGNANCY	1	1	2	1	1	1	1
HISTORY OF PELVIC SURGERY (see also postpartum section) (including caesarean section)	1	1	1	1	1	1	1
SMOKING							
a) Age <35	2	2	1	1	1	1	1
b) Age ≥35							
(i) <15 cigarettes/day	3	2	1	1	1	1	1
(ii) ≥15 cigarettes/day	4	3	1	1	1	1	1
OBESITY ≥30 kg/m^2 body mass index (BMI)	2	2	1	1	1	1	1
ANATOMICAL ABNORMALITIES							
a) That distort the uterine cavity						4	4
b) That do not distort the uterine cavity						2	2
BLOOD PRESSURE MEASUREMENT UNAVAILABLE	NA	NA	NA	NA	NA	NA	NA
CARIOVASCULAR DISEASE							
MULTIPLE RISK FACTORS FOR ARTERIAL CARDIOVASCULAR DISEASE (such as older age, smoking, diabetes and hypertension)	3/4	3/4	2	3	2	1	2

[a] if the women is breastfeeding

COC = Combined oral contraceptive
P/R = Patch/Ring
CIC = Combined injectable contraceptive
POP = progestin only pills; DMPA NET-EN = depotmedroxyprogesterone acetate, norethindrone enanthate; Cu-IUD = Copper IUD;
LNG IUD = Levonorgestrel IUD; LNG/ETG Implants = Levonorgestrel, Etonogestrel Implants

Summary Tables

Condition	COC P/R	CIC	POP	DMPA NET-EN	LNG/ETG Implants	CU-IUD	LNG-IUD
HYPERTENSION							
a) History of hypertension where blood pressure CANNOT be evaluated (including hypertension during pregnancy)	3	3	2	2	2		2
b) Adequately controlled hypertension, where blood pressure CAN be evaluated	3	3	1	2	1	1	1
c) Elevated blood pressure levels (properly taken measurements)							
(i) systolic 140–159 or diastolic 90–99	3	3	1	2	1	1	1
(ii) systolic ≥160 or diastolic ≥100	4	4	2	3	2	1	1
d) Vascular disease	4	4	1	3	2	1	2
HISTORY OF HIGH BLOOD PRESSURE DURING PREGNANCY (where current blood pressure is measurable and normal)	2	2	1	1	1	1	1
DEEP VENOUS THROMBOSIS (DVT)/ PULMONARY EMBOLISM (PE)							
a) History of DVT/PE	4	4	2	2	2	1	2
b) Current DVT/PE	4	4	3	3	3	1	3
c) Family history (first-degree relatives)	2	2	1	1	1	1	1
d) Major surgery							
(i) with prolonged immobilization	4	4	2	2	2	1	2
(ii) without prolonged immobilization	2	2	1	1	1	1	1
e) Minor surgery without immobilization	1	1	1	1	1	1	1

COC = Combined oral contraceptive
P/R = Patch/Ring
CIC = Combined injectable contraceptive
POP = progestin only pills; DMPA NET-EN = depotmedroxyprogesterone acetate, norethindrone enanthate; Cu-IUD = Copper IUD;
LNG IUD = Levonorgestrol IUD; LNG/ETG Implants = Levonorgestrol, Etonogestrol Implants

Summary Tables

Condition	COC P/R	CIC	POP	DMPA NET-EN	LNG/ETG Implants	CU-IUD	LNG-IUD
SUPERFICIAL VENOUS THROMBOSIS							
a) Varicose veins	1	1	1	1	1	1	1
b) Superficial thrombophlebitis	2	2	1	1	1	1	1
CURRENT AND HISTORY OF ISCHAEMIC HEART DISEASE	4	4	I=2, C=3	3	I=2, C=3	1	I=2, C=3
STROKE (history of cerebrovascular accident)	4	4	I=2, C=3	3	2	1	2
KNOWN HYPERLIPIDAEMIAS (screening is NOT necessary for safe use of contraceptive methods)	2/3[b]	2/3[b]	2	2	2	1	2
VALVULAR HEART DISEASE							
a) Uncomplicated	2	2	1	1	1	1	1
b) Complicated (pulmonary hypertension, atrial fibrillation, history of subacute bacterial endocarditis)	4	4	1	1	1	2	2
KNOWN THROMBOGENIC MUTATIONS	4	4	2	2	2	1	2
NEUROLOGIC CONDITIONS							
HEADACHES							
a) Non migrainous (mild or severe)	I=1, C=2	I=1, C=2	I=1, C=1	1	I=1, C=1	1	I=1, C=1
b) Migraine							
(i) without aura							
Age <35	I=2, C=3	I=2, C=3	I=1, C=2	2	2	1	2
Age ≥35	I=3, C=4	I=3, C=4	I=1, C=2	2	2	1	2
(ii) with focal aura (at any age)	4	4	I=2, C=3	I=2, C=3	I=2, C=3	1	I=2, C=3

[b] Depending on severity of condition
I = initiation
C = continuation
P/R = Patch/Ring
CIC = Combined injectable contraceptive
POP = progestin only pills; DMPA NET-EN = depotmedroxyprogesterone acetate, norethindrone enanthate; Cu-IUD = Copper IUD;
LNG IUD = Levonorgestrel IUD; LNG/ETG Implants = Levonorgestrel, Etonogestrel Implants

Summary Tables

Condition	COC P/R	CIC	POP	DMPA NET-EN	LNG/ETG Implants	CU-IUD	LNG-IUD
EPILEPSY	1	1	1	1	1	1	1
DEPRESSION	1	1	1	1	1	1	1
REPRODUCTIVE TRACT INFECTIONS AND DISORDERS							
VAGINAL BLEEDING PATTERNS							
a) Irregular pattern without heavy bleeding	1	1	2	2	2	1	I 1 / C 1
b) Heavy or prolonged bleeding (include regular and irregular patterns)	1	1	2	2	2	2	2
UNEXPLAINED VAGINAL BLEEDING (suspicious for serious condition)							
Before evaluation	2	2	2	3	3	I 4 / C 2	I 4 / C 2
ENDOMETRIOSIS	1	1	1	1	1	2	1
BENIGN OVARIAN TUMOURS (including cysts)	1	1	1	1	1	1	1
SEVERE DYSMENORRHOEA	1	1	1	1	1	2	1
TROPHOBLAST DISEASE							
a) Benign gestational trophoblastic disease	1	1	1	1	1	3	3
b) Malignant gestational trophoblastic disease	1	1	1	1	1	4	4
CERVICAL ECTROPION	1	1	1	1	1	1	1
CERVICAL INTRAEPITHELIAL NEOPLASIA (CIN)	2	2	1	2	2	1	2

I = initiation
C = continuation
P/R = Patch/Ring
CIC = Combined injectable contraceptive
POP = progestin only pills; DMPA NET-EN = depotmedroxyprogesterone acetate, norethindrone enanthate; Cu-IUD = Copper IUD;
LNG IUD = Levonorgestrel IUD; LNG/ETG Implants = Levonorgestrel, Etonogestrel Implants

Summary Tables

Condition	COC P/R	CIC	POP	DMPA NET-EN	LNG/ETG Implants	CU-IUD I	CU-IUD C	LNG-IUD I	LNG-IUD C
CERVICAL CANCER (awaiting treatment)	2	2	1	2	2	4	2	4	2
BREAST DISEASE									
a) Undiagnosed mass	2	2	2	2	2	1		2	
b) Benign breast disease	1	1	1	1	1	1		1	
c) Family history of cancer	1	1	1	1	1	1		1	
d) Cancer									
(i) current	4	4	4	4	4	1		4	
(ii) past and no evidence of current disease for 5 years	3	3	3	3	3	1		3	
ENDOMETRIAL CANCER	1	1	1	1	1	4	2	4	2
OVARIAN CANCER	1	1	1	1	1	3	2	3	2
UTERINE FIBROIDS									
a) Without distortion of the uterine cavity	1	1	1	1	1	1		1	
b) With distortion of the uterine cavity	1	1	1	1	1	4		4	
PELVIC INFLAMMATORY DISEASE (PID)									
a) Past PID assuming no current risk factors of STIs									
(i) with subsequent pregnancy	1	1	1	1	1	1	1	1	1
(ii) without subsequent pregnancy	1	1	1	1	1	2	2	2	2
b) PID-current or within the last 3 months	1	1	1	1	1	4	2	4	2

I = initiation
C = continuation
COC = Combined oral contraceptive
P/R = Patch/Ring
CIC = Combined injectable contraceptive
POP = progestin only pills; DMPA NET-EN = depotmedroxyprogesterone acetate, norethindrone enanthate; Cu-IUD = Copper IUD; LNG IUD = Levonorgestrol IUD; LNG/ETG Implants = Levonorgestrol, Etonogestrol Implants

Summary Tables

Condition	COC P/R	CIC	POP	DMPA NET-EN	LNG/ETG Implants	CU-IUD		LNG-IUD	
						I	C	I	C
STIs[c]									
a) Current purulent cervicitis or chlamydial infection or gonorrhea	1	1	1	1	1	4	2	4	2
b) Other STIs (excluding HIV and hepatitis)	1	1	1	1	1	2	2	2	2
c) Vaginitis (including trichomonas vaginalis and bacterial vaginosis)	1	1	1	1	1	2	2	2	2
d) Increased risk of STIs	1	1	1	1	1	2/3	2	2/3	2
HIV/AIDS[c]									
HIGH RISK OF HIV	1	1	1	1	1	2	2	2	2
HIV-POSITIVE	1	1	1	1	1	2	2	2	2
AIDS	1	1	1	1	1	3	2	3	2
Clinically well on ARV therapy	1	1	1	1	1	2	C	2	C
OTHER INFECTIONS									
SCHISTOSOMIASIS									
a) Uncomplicated	1	1	1	1	1	1		1	
b) Fibrosis of the liver	1	1	1	1	1	1		1	
TUBERCULOSIS									
a) Non-pelvic	1	1	1	1	1	1	C	1	C
b) Known pelvic	1	1	1	1	1	4	3	4	3
MALARIA	1	1	1	1	1	1		1	

[c] Barrier methods, especially condoms, are always recommended for prevention of STI/HIV/PID.

I = initiation

C = continuation

COC = Combined oral contraceptive

P/R = Patch/Ring

CIC = Combined injectable contraceptive

POP = progestin only pills; DMPA NET-EN = depotmedroxyprogesterone acetate, norethindrone enanthate; Cu-IUD = Copper IUD;

LNG IUD = Levonorgestrel IUD; LNG/ETG Implants = Levonorgestrel, Etonogestrel Implants

Summary Tables

Condition	COC P/R	CIC	POP	DMPA NET-EN	LNG/ETG Implants	CU-IUD	LNG-IUD
ENDOCRINE CONDITIONS							
DIABETES							
a) History of gestational disease	1	1	1	1	1	1	1
b) Non-vascular disease							
(i) non-insulin dependent	2	2	2	2	2	1	2
(ii) insulin dependent	2	2	2	2	2	1	2
c) Nephropathy/retinopathy/neuropathy	3/4	3/4	2	3	2	1	2
d) Other vascular disease or disease or diabetes of >20 years' duration	3/4	3/4	2	3	2	1	2
THYROID							
a) Simple goitre	1	1	1	1	1	1	1
b) Hyperthyroid	1	1	1	1	1	1	1
c) Hypothyroid	1	1	1	1	1	1	1
GASTROINTESTINAL CONDITIONS							
GALL BLADDER DISEASE							
a) Symptomatic							
(i) treated by cholecystectomy	2	2	2	2	2	1	2
(ii) medically treated	3	2	2	2	2	1	2
(iii) current	3	2	2	2	2	1	2
b) Asymptomatic	2	2	2	2	2	1	2
HISTORY OF CHOLESTASIS							
a) Pregnancy-related	2	2	1	1	1	1	1
b) Past COC-related	3	2	2	2	2	1	2

COC = Combined oral contraceptive
P/R = Patch/Ring
CIC = Combined injectable contraceptive
POP = progestin only pills; DMPA NET-EN = depotmedroxyprogesterone acetate, norethindrone enanthate; Cu-IUD = Copper IUD;
LNG IUD = Levonorgestrol IUD; LNG/ETG Implants = Levonorgestrol, Etonogestrol Implants

Summary Tables

Condition	COC P/R	CIC	POP	DMPA NET-EN	LNG/ETG Implants	CU-IUD	LNG-IUD
VIRAL HEPATITIS							
a) Active	4	3/4	3	3	3	1	3
b) Carrier	1	1	1	1	1	1	1
CIRRHOSIS							
a) Mild (compensated)	3	2	2	2	2	1	2
b) Severe (decompensated)	4	3	3	3	3	1	3
LIVER TUMOURS							
a) Benign (adenoma)	4	3	3	3	3	1	3
b) Malignant (hepatoma)	4	3/4	3	3	3	1	3
ANAEMIAS							
THALASSAEMIA	1	1	1	1	1	2	1
SICKLE CELL DISEASE	2	2	1	1	1	2	1
IRON DEFICIENCY ANAEMIA	1	1	1	1	1	2	1
DRUG INTERACTIONS							
DRUGS WHICH AFFECT LIVER ENZYMES							
a) Rifampicin	3	2	3	2	3	1	1
b) Certain anticonvulsants (phenytoin, carbamazepine, barbiturates, primidone)	3	2	3	2	3	1	1
ANTIBIOTICS (EXCLUDING RIFAMPICIN)							
a) Griseofulvin	2	1	2	1	2	1	1
b) Other antibiotics	1	1	1	1	1	1	1
ANTIRETROVIRAL THERAPY	2	2	2	2	2	I 2/3 C 2	I 2/3 C 2

I = initiation
C = continuation
COC = Combined oral contraceptive
P/R = Patch/Ring
CIC = Combined injectable contraceptive
POP = progestin only pills; DMPA NET-EN = depotmedroxyprogesterone acetate, norethindrone enanthate; Cu-IUD = Copper IUD;
LNG IUD = Levonorgestrol IUD; LNG/ETG Implants = Levonorgestrol, Etonogestrol Implants

Appendix 3

Instructions for Cyclic and Continuous Birth Control Pills

CHILDREN'S HOSPITAL BOSTON
INSTRUCTIONS FOR PATIENTS TAKING 28 DAY CYCLIC BIRTH
CONTROL PILLS

1. The name of your birth control pill is _____
2. A. Sunday Start:

   If you are taking pills for the first time, take the first pill of your first package on the **Sunday** following the first day of your next period, even if you have stopped bleeding before that day. If your period begins on Sunday, start taking the pill on that same day.

If menstrual flow starts on	Tablet taking begins on
Monday Tuesday Wednesday Thursday Friday Saturday	Following Sunday
Sunday	**that** Sunday

   B. First day start:

   Start your pills on the **first day** of your next period, then take one pill a day at the same time. Because you start the pill on the first day of your period, you will have two periods your first package (1st week and 4th week). After that you will have only one period each package (4th week).

   C. Quick start:

   Your health care provider may instruct you to start the same day you are seen. Then take one pill a day at the same time. You may be irregular the first cycle.
3. Take one pill every day at the same time without fail. When you finish your last pill in the package, start the first pill in a new package the next day. This means that you will be taking the pills even during the days you are having a period. **Never skip a day.**

4. Always take the pill at approximately the same time each day. The best time is 1/2 hour after a good meal or snack or at bedtime. Try to think of something you do everyday so you can take your pill at the same time (such as brushing your teeth). You may have mild nausea the first month. This usually disappears with time. You are less likely to have this problem if you take your pills in the evening with food.

5. **If you forget pills:**

   If you forget 1 pill—take the pill you forgot as soon as you remember, then take your regular pill for that day at your usual time.

   If you forget 2 pills in a row in the first 2 weeks—take 1 pill every 12 hours until you catch up. That means that you take 2 pills on the day you remember and 2 pills the next day. Take 1 pill per day until the pack is finished. Use condoms for at least 7 days.

   If you forget 2 pills in a row in the third week. OR you miss 3 pills or more in a row at any time— **Sunday starter:** Keep taking a pill every day until Sunday. On Sunday throw away the unused portion of the pack and start a new pack. Use condoms for at least 7 days and until your next menstrual period. **Non-Sunday starter:** throw out the rest of the current pack. Start a new pack the same day. Use condoms for at least 7 days and until your next menstrual period.

   If you have had intercourse during the time of missed pills, you should strongly consider taking emergency contraception (EC) pills. Call our clinic for instructions. You will take the EC pills and resume your birth control pills the next day.

6. If you have vomiting or diarrhea or are taking a course of antibiotics, the pill may be less effective. Use a back-up method such as a condom.

7. **Remember the pill does not protect you from AIDS or sexually transmitted diseases, and we advise that you always use condoms.**

8. If you miss a period and have taken every pill on time, begin your next pack as usual, but call or come into the clinic for a pregnancy test. If you miss a period and may have forgotten or been late with one or more pills, call the clinic and talk to the nurse immediately to make arrangements to come in.

9. **Extra bleeding while taking the 21 hormone tablets**

   Breakthrough bleeding is very common in the first 3 months of taking birth control pills; especially if pills are missed or taken late. The bleeding usually occurs during the second week of taking the hormone tablets and may be light (spotting for a few days) or heavy (like a normal menstrual period). The bleeding can usually be ignored and will become less of a problem by the third cycle. If you develop extra bleeding after several months and have not missed pills, you may need to be checked for STDs. Please call your nurse or doctor with any questions.

10. **Danger signals**

    1. Severe abdominal pain

2. Severe chest pain
3. Severe headaches
4. Blurred vision, loss of sight, flashing lights
5. Yellowing of whites of your eyes (jaundice)
6. Severe leg pain or leg swelling in the calf or thigh.
    Please call clinic and ask to speak to a doctor or nurse.

11. Benefits of the Pill—Birth control pills lower your chance of acquiring cancer of the uterus or ovary and make you less likely to have anemia, ovarian cysts, or menstrual cramps. They also improve acne.

12. If you purchase your pills in 3-month supplies, you must keep the pharmacy label from the first package and bring it with you when you go to the pharmacy to get refills. This label has your prescription number on it.

CHILDREN'S HOSPITAL BOSTON INSTRUCTIONS FOR PATIENTS TAKING CONTINUOUS PILLS

* Your pill is _____.

* We want you to take the pill continuously. This means that you will be taking one pill that contains the female hormones, estrogen and progesterone, every day. Taking the pill this way helps keep the lining of the uterus very thin. The goal is for you to have no periods.

  Unlike women who take these birth control pills only for contraception or for some other gynecological problems, you will not take a week of placebo pills (pills without hormones) and will not have a regular monthly menstrual period. You may have some irregular spotting or bleeding as your body gets adjusted to this new medication, especially in the first six months. If you are bleeding heavily (soaking a large pad or super tampon more than every 2 hours) and it does not slow down with 4 hours of bedrest, then call us at the numbers listed below. In addition, please call us if you are experiencing a heavy menstrual flow (a soaked pad or tampon every 2 or 3 hours) for more than 7 days.

* Taking the birth control pill continuously does protect you from pregnancy if you are sexually active. However, you are not fully protected until you have finished your first pack and have not missed any pills in that pack. The pill does not protect you from HIV or other sexually transmitted diseases. Therefore, if you are sexually active, you should <u>always</u> use condoms.

* In addition to treating your gynecological problem, these birth control pills have some other important benefits for your health. Taking the pill can lower your risk of getting cancer of the uterus or ovary. It also reduces your chances of anemia (low blood count), ovarian cysts, and menstrual cramps. For some women, it reduces acne, premenstrual syndrome (PMS) symptoms, and period-associated headaches.

Important Instructions and Warnings

1) Take one pill at the same time every day. When you finish one pack of the hormone pills, begin another pack of pills the following day.

   —**21 Day Pill Pack:** start a new pack the day after you finish all the pills in your current pack.

   —**28 Day Pill Pack:** take the three weeks of hormone pills but not the week of placebo pills (the last seven pills that are a different color). When you finish the hormone pills, throw the pack away and start a new pack the next day.

   If you are going to run out of pills before your next appointment, call us so we can call in one refill.

2) If is common when you first start the pill to have mild nausea. If you do, try taking the pill after some food or in the evening before bed.

3) If you forget to take a pill at the usual time, take it as soon as you remember. If you do not remember until the next day, then take the "forgotten" pill in the morning and the pill for that day 12 hours later. This will get you back on schedule.

   If you are sexually active, your risk of pregnancy increases when you miss a pill. Therefore, if you miss a pill, you MUST use condoms until you start your next pack of pills. If you have intercourse at the time of missed pills, you should strongly consider taking emergency contraception. Call our clinic for instructions.

4) If you have vomiting or diarrhea the pill may be less effective. Use a back-up method such as a condom.

5) **DANGER SIGNALS**
   1. Severe abdominal pain
   2. Severe chest pain
   3. Severe headaches
   4. Blurred vision, loss of sight, flashing lights,
   5. Yellowing of whites of your eyes (jaundice)
   6. Severe leg pain or leg swelling in the calf or thigh

If you are experiencing any of the **DANGER SIGNS** or if you are experiencing **heavy bleeding** that is not getting better, call us immediately. For other problems or any questions, please call us Monday through Friday, 9:00am to 5:00pm.

Appendix 4

Definitions of Anatomical Terms Used in Child Sexual Abuse Evaluations

The forensic medical evaluation of suspected child sexual abuse victims has developed significantly over the past two decades. Pediatricians, gynecologists, family practitioners, nurse practitioners, and physician assistants may be called on to examine children for suspected sexual abuse and describe their findings. The records of such examinations then become medicolegal documents. Precision in documentation is critical for all who must communicate and understand medical findings. In the early 1990s, the American Professional Society on the Abuse of Children (APSAC) developed terminology guidelines to assist professionals involved in the medical diagnosis and treatment of child sexual abuse so that they would have a shared vocabulary. This vocabulary has enabled those in child protection, law enforcement, and the courts to understand previously confusing and at times inconsistent terminology. The terminology presented below are selected, shortened and/or adapted from the APSAC *Glossary of Terms and the Interpretation of Findings for Child Sexual Abuse Evidentiary Examinations* or the *Descriptive Terminology in Child Sexual Abuse Medical Evaluations;* only those most commonly applied to girls are included in this gynecology text. Clinicians doing sexual abuse evaluations are encouraged to obtain the references from APSAC (www.apsac.org). The definitions emanate from medical dictionary definitions including *Stedman's medical dictionary* and *Dorland's illustrated medical dictionary,* anatomy texts, peer-reviewed papers, and clinicians actively involved in the care of sexually abused children. As experience and scientific knowledge expand, further revision of the terminology is expected.

ANATOMICAL STRUCTURES

Anal skin tag A protrusion of anal verge tissue that interrupts the symmetry of the perianal skin folds.

Anal verge The tissue overlying the subcutaneous external anal sphincter at the most distal portion of the anal canal (anoderm) and extending exteriorly to the margin of the anal skin.

Anterior commissure The union of the two labia minora anteriorly (toward the clitoris).

Anus The anal orifice, which is the lower opening of the digestive tract, lying in the fold between the buttocks, through which feces are extruded.

Clitoris A small cylindrical erectile body situated at the anterior (superior) portion of the vulva, covered by a sheath of skin called the clitoral hood.

Fossa navicularis/posterior fossa Concavity on the lower part of the vestibule, situated posteriorly (inferiorly) to the vaginal orifice and extending to the posterior fourchette (posterior commissure).

Genitalia (external) The external sexual organs, which include the contents of the vulva.

Hymen A membrane that partially, or rarely completely, covers the vaginal orifice. This membrane is located at the junction of the vestibular floor and the vaginal canal.

Labia majora ("outer lips") Rounded folds of skin forming the lateral boundaries of the vulva.

Labia minora ("inner lips") Longitudinal thin folds of tissue enclosed within the labia majora. In the pubertal child, these folds extend from the clitoral hood to approximately the midpoint on the lateral wall of the vestibule. In the adult, they enclose the structures of the vestibule.

Median raphe A ridge or furrow that marks the line of union of the two halves of the perineum.

Mons pubis The rounded, fleshy prominence created by the underlying fat pad that lies over the symphysis pubis (pubic bone) in females.

Pectinate/dentate line The saw-toothed line of demarcation between the distal (lower) portion of the anal valves and the pectin, the smooth zone of stratified epithelium that extends to the anal verge. This line is apparent when the external and internal anal sphincters relax and the anus dilates.

Perianal folds Wrinkles or folds of the anal verge skin radiating from the anus, created by contraction of the external anal sphincter.

Perineal body The central tendon of the perineum located between the vulva and the anus in females.

Perineum The external surface or base of the perineal body, lying between the vulva and the anus in females. Underlying the external surface of the perineum is the pelvic floor and its associated structures occupying the pelvic outlet, which is bounded anteriorly by the pubic symphysis, laterally by the ischial tuberosity, and posteriorly by the coccyx.

Posterior commissure The union of the two labia majora posteriorly (toward the anus).

Posterior fourchette The junction of two labia minora posteriorly (inferiorly). This area is referred to as a posterior commissure in the prepubertal child, as the labia minora are not completely developed to connect inferiorly until puberty, when it is referred to as the fourchette.

Urethral orifice External opening of the canal (urethra) from the bladder.

Vagina The uterovaginal canal in females that extends from the uterine cervix to the inner aspect of the hymen.

Vaginal vestibule An anatomic cavity containing the opening of the vagina, the urethra, and the ducts of Bartholin's glands, bordered by the clitoris anteriorly, the labia laterally, and the posterior commissure (fourchette) posteriorly (inferiorly). The vestibule encompasses the fossa navicularis immediately posterior (inferior) to the vaginal introitus.

Vulva The external genitalia or pudendum of females; includes the mons pubis, clitoris, labia majora, labia minora, vaginal vestibule, urethral orifice, vaginal orifice, hymen, and posterior fourchette (or commissure).

HYMENAL MORPHOLOGY

Annular Circumferential; hymenal membrane tissue extends completely around the circumference of the entire vaginal orifice.

Crescentic Hymen with attachments at approximately the 11 and 1 o'clock positions without tissue being present between the two attachments.

Cribriform Hymen with multiple small openings.

Imperforate Hymenal membrane with no opening.

Septate A hymen that is bisected by a band of hymenal tissue creating two or more orifices.

DESCRIPTIVE TERMS RELATING TO THE HYMEN

Estrogenized Effect of the female sex hormone estrogen on the genitalia: the hymen takes on a thickened, redundant, pale appearance. These changes are observed in neonates, with the onset of puberty, and as the result of exogenous estrogen.

Fimbriated/denticular Hymen with multiple projections and indentations along the edge, creating a ruffled appearance.

Membrane thickness The relative amount of tissue between the internal and external surfaces of the hymenal membrane.

Narrow/wide hymenal rim The width of the hymenal membrane as viewed in the coronal plane, i.e., from the edge of the hymen to the muscular portion of the vaginal introitus.

Redundant Abundant hymenal tissue that tends to fold back on itself or protrude.

OTHER STRUCTURES OR FINDINGS

Acute laceration A tear through the full thickness of the skin or other tissue.

Attenuated Used to describe areas where the hymen is narrow. However, the term should be restricted to indicate a documented change in the width of the posterior portion of the hymen following an injury.

Clock position reference A method by which the location of structures or findings may be designated by using the positions of the numerals on the face of a clock. The 12 o'clock position is always superior (up). The 6 o'clock position is always inferior (down). The position of a patient must be indicated when using this designation.

Caruncula myrtiformis (hymenales) Small elevations of rounded mounds of hymen encircling the vaginal orifice, found in sexually active and postpartum females.

Concavity (Depression) A curved or hollowed "U"-shaped depression on the edge of the hymenal membrane.

Diastasis ani A congenital midline smooth depression that may be V or wedge shaped, located either anterior or posterior to the anus; due to a failure of fusion of the underlying corrugator external anal sphincter muscle.

Erythema Redness of tissues.

External hymenal ridge A midline longitudinal ridge of tissue on the external surface of the hymen. May be either anterior or posterior. Usually extends to the edge of the membrane.

Friability of the posterior fourchette/commissure A superficial breakdown of the skin in the posterior fourchette (commissure) when gentle traction is applied, causing slight bleeding.

Hymenal cleft An angular or V-shaped indentation on the edge of the hymenal membrane.

Hymenal cyst A fluid-filled elevation of tissue, confined within the hymenal tissue.

Hymenal mound/bump A solid, localized, rounded and thickened area of tissue on the edge of the hymenal membrane. This structure may be created by the hymenal attachment of a longitudinal intravaginal ridge.

Hymenal tag An elongated projection of tissue rising from any location on the hymenal rim. Commonly found in the midline and may be an extension of a posterior vaginal ridge.

Intravaginal Longitudinal Ridges (ILR) Narrow, mucosa-covered ridges of tissue on the vaginal wall that may be attached to the inner surface of the hymen.

Labial agglutination (labial adhesion) The result of adherence (fusion) of the adjacent edges of the mucosal surfaces of the labia minora. This may occur at any point along the length of the vestibule, although it most commonly occurs posteriorly (inferiorly).

Linea vestibularis (midline sparing) A vertical pale/avascular line across the posterior fourchette and/or fossa, which may be accentuated by putting lateral traction on the labia majora.

Perineal groove Developmental anomaly, also called "failure of midline fusion". This skin and mucosal defect may be located anywhere from the fossa to the anus.

Scar Fibrous tissue that replaces normal tissue after the healing of a wound.

Synechiae Any adhesion that binds two anatomic structures through the formation of a band of fibrous or scar tissue.

Transection of hymen (complete) A tear or laceration through the entire width of the hymenal membrane extending from the hymenal edge to (or through) the attachment to the vaginal wall.

Transection of hymen (partial) A tear or laceration through a portion of the hymenal membrane not extending to its attachment to the vaginal wall. The term "partial tear" is preferred.

Vaginal columns (columnae rugarum vaginae) Raised (sagittally oriented) columns, most prominent on the anterior wall with less prominence on the posterior wall. May also be observed laterally.

Vaginal rugae (rugae vaginales) Folds of epithelium (rugae) running circumferentially from vaginal columns. These rugae account in part for the ability of the vagina to distend.

Vascularity (increased) Dilatation of existing superficial blood vessels.

Vestibular bands
1. **Perihymenal bands (pubovaginal)** Bands lateral to the hymen connecting to the vestibular wall.
2. **Periurethral bands** Small bands lateral to the urethra that connect the periurethral tissues to the anterior lateral wall of the vestibule. These bands are usually symmetrical and frequently create a semilunar-shaped space between the bands on either side of the urethral meatus. Also called urethral supporting ligaments.

DESCRIPTIVE TERMS FOR VARIATIONS IN PERIANAL ANATOMY

Anal dilatation Opening of the external (and possibly internal) anal sphincters with minimal traction on the buttocks.

Anal fissure A superficial break (split) in the perianal skin that radiates out from the anal orifice.

Flattened anal folds A reduction or absence of the perianal folds or wrinkles, noted when the external anal sphincter is partially or completely relaxed.

Venous congestion The collection of venous blood in the venous plexus of the perianal tissues creating a flat, purple discoloration. May be localized or diffuse.

REFERENCES

1. American Professional Society on the Abuse of Children, Interpretation of Physical Findings in Sexual Abuse subcommittee (chaired by John McCann). Glossary of Terms and the Interpretations of Findings for Child Sexual Abuse Evidentiary Examinations. 1998.
2. American Professional Society on the Abuse of Children, Terminology Subcommittee of the APSAC Taskforce on the Medical Evaluation of Suspected Child Abuse (chaired by Joyce Adams). Descriptive Terminology in Child Sexual Abuse Medical Evaluations. 1995.
3. *Stedman's medical dictionary,* 22nd ed. Baltimore, MD: Williams & Wilkins, 1972.
4. *Dorland's ilustrated medical dictionary,* 27th edition. Philadelphia: W.B. Saunders, 1988.
5. Berenson A, Heger A, Andrews S. Appearance of the hymen in newborns. *Pediatrics* 1991;87:458.
6. Berenson AB, Heger AH, Hayes JM, et al. Appearance of the hymen in prepubertal girls. *Pediatrics* 1992;89:387.
7. Emans S, Woods E, Flagg N, et al. Genital findings in sexually abused, symptomatic and asymptomatic girls. *Pediatrics* 1987;79:778.
8. Muram D. Classification of genital findings in prepubertal girls who are victims of sexual abuse. *Adolesc Pediatr Gynecol* 1988;1:151.
9. Adams J, Harper K, Knudson S, et al. Examination findings in legally confirmed child sexual abuse: it's normal to be normal. *Pediatrics* 1994;94:310.
10. Finkel, M. Medical findings in child sexual abuse. In: Reece R, ed. *Child abuse.* Baltimore, MD: Williams & Wilkins, 1994.
11. Kellogg N, Parra J. Linea vestibularis: a previously undescribed normal genital structure in female neonates. *Pediatrics* 1991;87:926.
12. Heger A, Ticson L, Guerra L, et al. Appearance of the genitalia in girls selected for nonabuse: Review of hymenal morphology and nonspecific findings. *J Pediatr Adolesc Gynecol* 2002;15:27.
13. Kerns D, Ritter M, Thomas R. Concave hymenal variations in suspected child sexual abuse victims. *Pediatrics* 1992;90:265.

Appendix 5

Sexual Assault Forensic Medical Report

Adapted from the Forensic Medical Report Suspected Acute Adult/Adolescent
Sexual Assault State of California, Office of Criminal Justice Planning
OCJP 923

PATIENT DEMOGRAPHIC INFORMATION

Name of patient	Age
Patient ID number	Date of birth
Address	Gender
City	Ethnicity
County	Race
State	Date/time of arrival
Telephone number	Date/time of examination
	Date/time of discharge

Presence of interpreter?
  If so, name?
  Language?

LAW ENFORCEMENT INFORMATION

Law enforcement information will be dictated by local protocol and may document:
  Name of officer who took the report and the responding office
  Agency
  ID number
  Telephone number

PATIENT NOTIFICATION

Patients may be notified about duty of medical personnel to report to law enforcement in cases of sexual assault (as dictated by local protocol). Patients should be informed that victims of crime are eligible to submit crime victim compensation claims and that Family Code sections address the ability of minors to consent to medical examination treatment and evidence collection related to sexual assault without parental consent, as dictated by state and local laws.

PATIENT CONSENT

Consent for the following:
    Medical legal examination for evidence of sexual assault
    Collection of evidence including photographs
Consent for release of information to health authorities and qualified persons
Consent for patient advocate to attend
Other consent as dictated by local needs/requirements

DISTRIBUTION FORM OR FORENSIC MEDICOLEGAL REPORT

Multiple legible copies of the medical report should be made available to law enforcement, forensic laboratory, and the medical facility. The medicolegal record should be maintained separately from the patient's other medical records to ensure limited access.

PATIENT HISTORY

Name of person providing history (document relationship to patient)
Document if an interpreter is used, including name and language
Pertinent medical history
    Last normal menstrual period (document any recent anogenital injuries, operations, diagnostic procedures, or medical treatment that may affect physical findings)
Other pertinent medical condition(s)
Preexisting physical injuries
Pertinent history related to the encounter
    History of other intercourse within the past 72 hours (document time course in detail, such as when did ejaculation occur and whether a condom was used)
    Drug and alcohol use before the assault?
    Drug and alcohol use after the assault?

Post-assault hygiene activity: Document whether the patient did any of the following after the encounter:

Urinated	Gargled/brushed teeth
Defecated	Smoked
Vomited	Ate or drank
Douched	Chewed gum
Removed/inserted tampon/diaphragm	Changed clothing
Wiped/cleaned genital area	Took medications
Bathed/showered	

ASSAULT HISTORY

Document patient's description of the encounter in direct quotes if at all possible:
Date of assault(s)
Time of assault(s)
Physical surrounding of assault(s)
Lapse of consciousness
    Anterograde amnesia
Nongenital injury, pain, and/or bleeding
Anogenital injury, pain, and/or bleeding
Verbal coercion (No threats, but fear of injury experienced by patient)
Force or coercion used
    Weapons: threatened or used
    Physical assault
    Grabbing/holding/pinching
    Physical restraints
    Drugs used to facilitate sexual assault; voluntary ingestion; clandestine drugging of patient
    Choking
    Burns
    Threat(s)
    Target of threat
    Ingestion of a substance (including alcohol or suspected drugs)
Injuries inflicted on assailant(s) during assault (Describe.)
Acts described by patient (Note that any penetration, however slight, constitutes the act)
Oral copulation requires only contact
If more than one assailant, identify by number
Document the following acts and whether a penis, finger, or other object was used:
Penetration of labia majora (vulva or deeper structures)
Penetration of anus or deeper structures
Oral copulation of genitals

Oral copulation of anus
Nongenital acts
   Biting of patient or by patient on perpetrator
   Licking
   Kissing
Other acts
Did ejaculation occur? If yes, note location:

Vulva or deeper structures	Bedding
Anus or deeper structures	Mouth
Body surface	Other
Clothing	

Contraceptives or lubricant products used
   Document use of foam, jelly, lubricant, and/or condom, and the brand, if known
Recent consensual intercourse

GENERAL PHYSICAL EXAMINATION AND FINDINGS

Vital signs
Date and time of examination
General physical appearance
General demeanor/behavior/orientation
Description of clothing on arrival
Conduct physical examination and document, draw, number injuries/findings, including size and appearance, on a diagram (Figure 1) and use a legend for abbreviations or numbers (be specific)

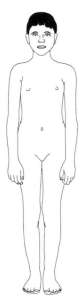 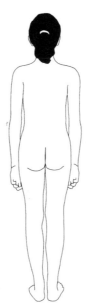 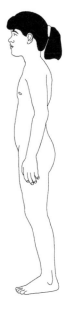

Alternative light source examination (such as Wood's lamp)

Collect dry and moist secretions, stains, and foreign materials from the body, including head, hair, and scalp

Collect fingernail scrapings or cuttings according to local policy

Examine the oral cavity for injury

Collect dried and moist secretions, stains, and foreign materials from the lips, perioral region, and nares

Collect reference samples per local protocol (Module—Adult/Adolescent Patient)

Swab the areas the suspect kissed, licked, or sucked

GENITAL EXAMINATION—FEMALE

Perform an external examination and document findings (Figure 2) of the external genitalia and perineal area specifically for injury, foreign materials, and other findings in the following areas:

Abdomen

Thighs

Perineum

Labia majora

Labia minora

Clitorial hood and surrounding area

Periurethral tissue/urethral meatus

Perihymenal tissue (vestibule)

Hymen

Fossa navicularis

Posterior fourchette

Follow procedure noted in the sexual assault kit or evidence collection kit

Examine the vagina and cervix for injury, foreign materials, and foreign bodies. Use colposcope or other magnification, if available (Module—Use of Colposcope)

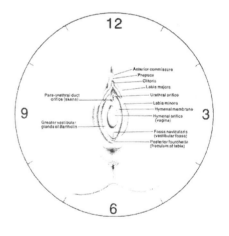

Examine the buttocks, perianal skin, and anal folds for injury, foreign materials, and other findings

Consider anoscopy if rectal injury is suspected

GENITAL EXAMINATION—MALE

Examine the external genitalia and perineal area (Figure 3) for injury, foreign materials, and other findings; include the following body areas:

Abdomen

Buttocks
Thighs
Foreskin
Urethral meatus
Shaft
Scrotum
Perineum
Glans
Testes
Document whether the patient
is circumcised (Figure 3)

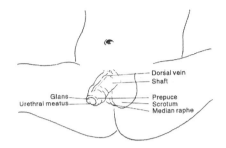

DOCUMENT EVIDENCE SUBMITTED TO THE FORENSIC LABORATORY

Document all materials sent to the forensic laboratory, including the following:
Clothing
Foreign materials on the body
  Blood
  Dried secretions
  Fiber/loose hairs
  Vegetation
  Soil/debris
  Swabs of suspected semen
  Swabs of suspected saliva
  Swabs of areas highlighted by alternative light source (such as Wood's lamp)
Body cavity samples
Oral sample
Vaginal/anal sample
Fingernail scrapings/cuttings
Matted hair cuttings
Pubic hair combing/brushing
Intravaginal foreign body
Intrarectal foreign body
Oral genital samples
Reference samples
  Buccal swabs/blood
  Toxicology samples: blood and/or urine
Photodocumentation (Module-Medicolegal Photography in Sexual Assaults)
Document use of toluidine blue (Module-Use of Toluidine Blue)
Document all examination methods used

PERSONNEL INVOLVED IN SEXUAL ASSAULT EVALUATION

Document all personnel involved in taking the history, performing the physical examination, and handling specimens; include times.

OVERALL CLINICAL ASSESSMENT

Please note that history of sexual assault with no physical findings may still be consistent with the sexual assault. Avoid legal terms such as "rape" or "abuse."

Please accurately document the assessment of the patient, remembering that the lack of obvious injuries does not preclude the possibility that sexual assault took place.

Name of health care provider

Signature of health care provider performing the examination

LAW ENFORCEMENT INFORMATION

Document the name and ID number of the officer to whom the kit is given and the officer's agency and the date the kit is transferred to the officer. Include a comprehensive list of the evidence collected.

At the conclusion of the examination, brief the law enforcement person on findings, interpretation, and assessment. Anything found during the examination, such as foreign fibers like dirt, carpet, and so on, should be discussed.

From: American College of Emergency Physicians. Evaluation and Management of the Sexually Assaulted or Sexually Abused Patient. Dallas, TX: American College of Emergency Physicians; 1999.

Appendix 6

Methods for Estimating Percentage Body Fat from Skinfold Measurements in Girls

TABLE 6-1. *The use of the sum of triceps plus subscapular skinfolds in girls to estimate body fat percentage*

Skinfolds (mm)	% Fat	
5	4	Very Low
10	10	
		Low
15	15	
20	20	Optimal Range
25	24	
30	28	Moderately High
35	30	
40	33	High
45	33.5	
50	38	
		Very High
55	40	
60		

(Adapted from Lohman TG. The use of skinfold to estimate body fatness in children and youth. *JOPERD* 1987:98.)

TABLE 6-2. *Percentage body fat estimated from the sum of biceps, triceps, suprailiac, and subscapular skinfolds in girls of different maturation levels*[a]

Sum of skinfolds	Prepubertal 10.5 yr (SE 1.6)		Pubertal 13.1 yr (SE 1.3)		Postpubertal 16.8 yr (SE 2.1)	
	Mean	*95% CI*	*Mean*	*95% CI*	*Mean*	*95% CI*
15	9.2	8.3–10.1	9.3	8.6–10.0	—	
20	13.0	12.1–13.9	12.3	9.6–13.0	—	—
25	15.9	15.0–16.8	14.6	13.9–15.3	11.1	9.9–12.3
30	18.2	17.3–19.1	16.5	15.8–17.2	14.1	12.9–15.3
35	20.2	19.5–21.1	18.1	17.4–18.8	16.8	15.6–18.0
40	22.0	21.1–22.9	19.5	18.8–20.2	19.0	17.8–20.2
45	23.5	22.6–24.4	20.7	20.0–21.4	21.0	19.8–22.2
50	24.8	23.9–25.7	21.8	21.1–22.5	22.8	21.6–24.0
55	26.1	25.2–27.0	22.8	22.1–23.5	24.4	23.2–25.6
60	27.2	26.3–28.1	23.7	23.0–24.4	25.9	24.7–27.1
65	28.2	27.3–29.1	24.5	23.8–25.2	27.2	26.0–28.4
70	29.2	28.3–30.1	25.3	24.6–26.0	28.5	27.3–29.7
75	30.1	29.2–31.0	26.0	25.3–26.7	29.7	28.5–30.9
80	30.9	30.0–31.8	26.7	26.0–27.4	30.8	29.6–32.0
85	31.7	30.8–32.6	27.3	26.6–28.0	31.8	30.6–33.0
90	32.5	31.6–33.4	27.9	27.2–28.6	32.8	31.6–34.0
95	33.2	32.3–34.1	28.5	27.8–29.2	33.7	32.5–34.9

[a]95% CI, 95% confidence interval; SE, standard error.
(From: Duerenberg P, Pieters JJL, Hautvast JG. The assessment of the body fat percentage by skinfold thickness measurements in childhood and young adolescence. *Br J Nutr* 1990;63: 293; with permission.)

Appendix 7

Percentages and Estimated Mature Heights for Girls, Using Skeletal Age

TABLE 7-1. *Average girls: Percentages and estimated mature heights for girls with skeletal ages within 1 year of their chronological ages:*
Skeletal ages 6–11 years

Skeletal age (yr-mo)

Height (inches)	6-0	6-3	6-6	6-10	7-0	7-3	7-6	7-10	8-0	8-3	8-6	8-10	9-0	9-3	9-6	9-9	10-0	10-3	10-6	10-9	11-0	11-3	11-6	11-9
% of mature height	72	72.9	73.8	75.1	75.7	76.5	77.2	78.2	79	80.1	81	82.1	82.7	83.6	84.4	85.3	86.2	87.4	88.4	89.6	90.6	91	91.4	91.8
37	51.4																							
38	52.8	52.1	51.5																					
39	54.2	53.5	52.8	52.0	51.5	51.0																		
40	55.6	54.9	54.2	53.3	52.8	52.3	51.8	51.2																
41	56.9	56.2	55.6	54.6	54.2	53.6	53.1	52.4	51.9	51.2														
42	58.3	57.6	56.9	55.9	55.5	54.9	54.4	53.7	53.2	52.4	51.9	51.2												
43	59.7	59.0	58.3	57.3	56.8	56.2	55.7	55.0	54.4	53.7	53.1	52.4	52.0	51.4										
44	61.1	60.4	59.6	58.6	58.1	57.5	57.0	56.3	55.7	54.9	54.3	53.6	53.2	52.6	52.1	51.6	51.0							
45	62.5	61.7	61.0	59.9	59.4	58.8	58.3	57.5	57.0	56.2	55.6	54.8	54.4	53.8	53.3	52.8	52.2	51.5						
46	63.9	63.1	62.3	61.3	60.8	60.1	59.6	58.8	58.2	57.4	56.8	56.0	55.6	55.0	54.5	53.9	53.4	52.6	52.0	51.3				
47	65.3	64.5	63.7	62.6	62.1	61.4	60.9	60.1	59.5	58.7	58.0	57.2	56.8	56.2	55.7	55.1	54.5	53.8	53.2	52.5	51.9	51.6	51.4	51.2
48	66.7	65.8	65.0	63.9	63.4	62.7	62.2	61.4	60.8	59.9	59.3	58.5	58.0	57.4	56.9	56.3	55.7	54.9	54.3	53.6	53.0	52.7	52.5	52.3
49	68.1	67.2	66.4	65.2	64.7	64.1	63.5	62.7	62.0	61.2	60.5	59.7	59.3	58.6	58.1	57.4	56.8	56.1	55.4	54.7	54.1	53.8	53.6	53.4
50	69.4	68.6	67.8	66.6	66.1	65.4	64.8	63.9	63.3	62.4	61.7	60.9	60.5	59.8	59.2	58.6	58.0	57.2	56.6	55.8	55.2	54.9	54.7	54.5
51	70.8	70.0	69.1	67.9	67.4	66.7	66.1	65.2	64.6	63.7	63.0	62.1	61.7	61.0	60.4	59.8	59.2	58.4	57.7	56.9	56.3	56.0	55.8	55.6
52	72.2	71.3	70.5	69.2	68.7	68.0	67.4	66.5	65.8	64.9	64.2	63.3	62.9	62.2	61.6	61.0	60.3	59.5	58.8	58.0	57.4	57.1	56.9	56.6
53	73.6	72.7	71.8	70.6	70.0	69.3	68.7	67.8	67.1	66.2	65.4	64.6	64.1	63.4	62.8	62.1	61.5	60.6	60.0	59.2	58.5	58.2	58.0	57.7
54		74.1	73.2	71.9	71.3	70.6	69.9	69.1	68.4	67.4	66.7	65.8	65.3	64.6	64.0	63.3	62.6	61.8	61.1	60.3	59.6	59.3	59.1	58.8
55			74.5	73.2	72.7	71.9	71.2	70.3	69.6	68.7	67.9	67.0	66.5	65.8	65.2	64.5	63.8	62.9	62.2	61.4	60.7	60.4	60.2	59.9
56				74.6	74.0	73.2	72.5	71.6	70.9	69.9	69.1	68.2	67.7	67.0	66.4	65.7	65.0	64.1	63.3	62.5	61.8	61.5	61.3	61.0
57						74.5	73.8	72.9	72.2	71.2	70.4	69.4	68.9	68.2	67.5	66.8	66.1	65.2	64.5	63.6	62.9	62.6	62.4	62.1
58								74.2	73.4	72.4	71.6	70.6	70.1	69.4	68.7	68.0	67.3	66.4	65.6	64.7	64.0	63.7	63.5	63.2
59									74.7	73.7	72.8	71.9	71.3	70.6	69.9	69.2	68.4	67.5	66.7	65.8	65.1	64.8	64.6	64.3
60										74.9	74.1	73.1	72.6	71.8	71.1	70.3	69.6	68.7	67.9	67.0	66.2	65.9	65.6	65.4
61												74.3	73.8	73.0	72.3	71.5	70.8	69.8	69.0	68.1	67.3	67.0	66.7	66.4
62														74.2	73.5	72.7	71.9	70.9	70.1	69.2	68.4	68.1	67.8	67.5
63															74.6	73.9	73.1	72.1	71.3	70.3	69.5	69.2	68.9	68.6
64																	74.2	73.2	72.4	71.4	70.6	70.3	70.0	69.7
65																		74.4	73.5	72.5	71.7	71.4	71.1	70.8
66																			74.7	73.7	72.8	72.5	72.2	71.9
67																				74.8	74.0	73.6	73.3	73.0
68																						74.7	74.4	74.1

(From: Bayley N, Pinneau SR. Tables for predicting adult height from skeletal age: Revised for use with the Greulich-Pyle hand standards. *J Pediatr* 1952;40:423; with permission.)

TABLE 7-2. Average girls: Percentages and estimated mature heights for girls with skeletal ages within 1 year of their chronological ages: Skeletal ages 12–18 years

Skeletal age (yr-mo)	12-0	12-3	12-6	12-9	13-0	13-3	13-6	13-9	14-0	14-3	14-6	14-9	15-0	15-3	15-6	15-9	16-0	16-3	16-6	16-9	17-0	17-6	18-0
% of mature height	92.2	93.2	94.1	95	95.8	96.7	97.4	97.8	98	98.3	98.6	98.8	99	99.1	99.3	99.4	99.6	99.6	99.7	99.8	99.9	99.95	100
Height (inches)																							
47	51.0																						
48	52.1	51.5	51.0																				
49	53.1	52.6	52.1	51.6	51.1																		
50	54.2	53.6	53.1	52.6	52.2	51.7	51.3	51.1	51.0														
51	55.3	54.7	54.2	53.7	53.2	52.7	52.4	52.1	52.0	51.9	51.7	51.6	51.5	51.5	51.4	51.3	51.2	51.2	51.2	51.1	51.1	51.0	51.0
52	56.4	55.8	55.3	54.7	54.3	53.8	53.4	53.2	53.1	52.9	52.7	52.6	52.5	52.5	52.4	52.3	52.2	52.2	52.2	52.1	52.1	52.0	52.0
53	57.5	56.9	56.3	55.8	55.3	54.8	54.4	54.2	54.1	53.9	53.8	53.6	53.5	53.5	53.4	53.3	53.2	53.2	53.2	53.1	53.1	53.0	53.0
54	58.6	57.9	57.4	56.8	56.4	55.8	55.4	55.2	55.1	54.9	54.8	54.7	54.5	54.5	54.4	54.3	54.2	54.2	54.2	54.1	54.1	54.0	54.0
55	59.7	59.0	58.4	57.9	57.4	56.9	56.5	56.2	56.1	56.0	55.8	55.7	55.6	55.5	55.4	55.3	55.2	55.2	55.2	55.1	55.1	55.0	55.0
56	60.7	60.1	59.5	58.9	58.5	57.9	57.5	57.3	57.1	57.0	56.8	56.7	56.6	56.5	56.4	56.3	56.2	56.2	56.2	56.1	56.1	56.0	56.0
57	61.8	61.2	60.6	60.0	59.5	58.9	58.5	58.3	58.2	58.0	57.8	57.7	57.6	57.5	57.4	57.3	57.2	57.2	57.2	57.1	57.1	57.0	57.0
58	62.9	62.2	61.6	61.1	60.5	60.0	59.5	59.3	59.2	59.0	58.8	58.7	58.6	58.5	58.4	58.3	58.2	58.2	58.2	58.1	58.1	58.0	58.0
59	64.0	63.3	62.7	62.1	61.6	61.0	60.6	60.3	60.2	60.0	59.8	59.7	59.6	59.5	59.4	59.4	59.2	59.2	59.2	59.1	59.1	59.0	59.0
60	65.1	64.4	63.8	63.2	62.6	62.0	61.6	61.3	61.2	61.0	60.9	60.7	60.6	60.5	60.4	60.4	60.2	60.2	60.2	60.1	60.1	60.0	60.0
61	66.2	65.5	64.8	64.2	63.7	63.1	62.6	62.4	62.2	62.1	61.9	61.7	61.6	61.6	61.4	61.4	61.2	61.2	61.2	61.1	61.1	61.0	61.0
62	67.2	66.5	65.9	65.3	64.7	64.1	63.7	63.4	63.3	63.1	62.9	62.8	62.6	62.6	62.4	62.4	62.2	62.2	62.2	62.1	62.1	62.0	62.0
63	68.3	67.6	67.0	66.3	65.8	65.1	64.7	64.4	64.3	64.1	63.9	63.8	63.6	63.6	63.4	63.4	63.3	63.3	63.2	63.1	63.1	63.0	63.0
64	69.4	68.7	68.0	67.4	66.8	66.2	65.7	65.4	65.3	65.1	64.9	64.8	64.6	64.6	64.4	64.4	64.3	64.3	64.2	64.1	64.1	64.0	64.0
65	70.5	69.7	69.1	68.4	67.8	67.2	66.7	66.5	66.3	66.1	65.9	65.8	65.7	65.6	65.5	65.4	65.3	65.3	65.2	65.1	65.1	65.0	65.0
66	71.6	70.8	70.1	69.5	68.9	68.3	67.8	67.5	67.3	67.1	66.9	66.8	66.7	66.6	66.5	66.4	66.3	66.3	66.2	66.1	66.1	66.0	66.0
67	72.7	71.9	71.2	70.5	69.9	69.3	68.8	68.5	68.4	68.2	68.0	67.8	67.7	67.6	67.5	67.4	67.3	67.3	67.2	67.1	67.1	67.0	67.0
68	73.8	73.0	72.3	71.6	71.0	70.3	69.8	69.5	69.4	69.2	69.0	68.8	68.7	68.6	68.5	68.4	68.3	68.3	68.2	68.1	68.1	68.0	68.0
69	74.8	74.0	73.3	72.6	72.0	71.4	70.8	70.6	70.4	70.2	70.0	69.8	69.7	69.6	69.5	69.4	69.3	69.3	69.2	69.1	69.1	69.0	69.0
70			74.4	73.7	73.1	72.4	71.9	71.6	71.4	71.2	71.0	70.8	70.7	70.6	70.5	70.4	70.3	70.3	70.2	70.1	70.1	70.0	70.0
71				74.7	74.1	73.4	72.9	72.6	72.4	72.2	72.0	71.9	71.7	71.6	71.5	71.4	71.3	71.3	71.2	71.1	71.1	71.0	71.0
72						74.5	73.9	73.6	73.5	73.2	73.0	72.9	72.7	72.7	72.5	72.4	72.3	72.3	72.2	72.1	72.1	72.0	72.0
73							74.9	74.6	74.5	74.3	74.0	73.9	73.7	73.7	73.5	73.4	73.3	73.3	73.2	73.1	73.1	73.0	73.0
74												74.9	74.7	74.7	74.5	74.4	74.3	74.3	74.2	74.1	74.1	74.0	74.0

(From: Bayley N, Pinneau SR. Tables for predicting adult height from skeletal age: Revised for use with the Greulich-Pyle hand standards. *J Pediatr* 1952;40:423; with permission.)

TABLE 7-3. *Accelerated girls—percentages and estimated mature heights for girls with skeletal ages 1 year or more advanced over their chronological ages: Skeletal ages 7–11 years*

Skeletal age (yr-mo)

Height (inches)	7-0	7-3	7-6	7-10	8-0	8-3	8-6	8-10	9-0	9-3	9-6	9-9	10-0	10-3	10-6	10-9	11-0	11-3	11-6	11-9
% of mature height	71.2	72.2	73.2	74.2	75.0	76.0	77.1	78.4	79.0	80.0	80.9	81.9	82.8	84.1	85.6	87.0	88.3	88.7	89.1	89.7
37	52.0																			
38	53.4	51.2																		
39	54.8	52.6	51.9	51.2																
40	56.2	54.0	53.3	52.6	52.0	51.3														
41	57.6	55.4	54.6	53.9	53.3	52.6	51.9	51.0												
42	59.0	56.8	56.0	55.3	54.7	53.9	53.2	52.3	51.9	51.3										
43	60.4	58.2	57.4	56.6	56.0	55.3	54.5	53.6	53.2	52.5	51.9	51.3								
44	61.8	59.6	58.7	58.0	57.3	56.6	55.8	54.8	54.4	53.8	53.2	52.5	51.9	51.1						
45	63.2	60.9	60.1	59.3	58.7	57.9	57.1	56.1	55.7	55.0	54.4	53.7	53.1	52.3	51.4					
46	64.6	62.3	61.5	60.6	60.0	59.2	58.4	57.4	57.0	56.3	55.6	54.9	54.3	53.5	52.6	51.7	51.0			
47	66.0	63.7	62.8	62.0	61.3	60.5	59.7	58.7	58.2	57.5	56.9	56.2	55.6	54.7	53.7	52.9	52.1	51.9	51.6	51.3
48	67.4	65.1	64.2	63.3	62.7	61.8	61.0	59.9	59.5	58.8	58.1	57.4	56.8	55.9	54.9	54.0	53.2	53.0	52.7	52.4
49	68.8	66.5	65.6	64.7	64.0	63.2	62.3	61.2	60.8	60.0	59.3	58.6	58.0	57.1	56.1	55.2	54.4	54.1	53.9	53.5
50	70.2	67.9	66.9	66.0	65.3	64.5	63.6	62.5	62.0	61.3	60.6	59.8	59.2	58.3	57.2	56.3	55.5	55.2	55.0	54.6
51	71.6	69.3	68.3	67.4	66.7	65.8	64.9	63.8	63.3	62.5	61.8	61.1	60.4	59.5	58.4	57.5	56.6	56.4	56.1	55.7
52	73.0	70.6	69.7	68.7	68.0	67.1	66.1	65.1	64.6	63.8	63.0	62.3	61.6	60.6	59.6	58.6	57.8	57.5	57.2	56.9
53	74.4	72.0	71.0	70.1	69.3	68.4	67.4	66.3	65.8	65.0	64.3	63.5	62.8	61.8	60.7	59.8	58.9	58.6	58.4	58.0
54		73.4	72.4	71.4	70.7	69.7	68.7	67.6	67.1	66.3	65.5	64.7	64.0	63.0	61.9	60.9	60.0	59.8	59.5	59.1
55		74.8	73.8	72.8	72.0	71.1	70.0	68.9	68.4	67.5	66.7	65.9	65.2	64.2	63.1	62.1	61.2	60.9	60.6	60.2
56				74.1	73.3	72.4	71.3	70.2	69.6	68.8	68.0	67.2	66.4	65.4	64.3	63.2	62.3	62.0	61.7	61.3
57					74.7	73.7	72.6	71.4	70.9	70.0	69.2	68.4	67.6	66.6	65.4	64.4	63.4	63.1	62.8	62.4
58							73.9	72.7	72.2	71.3	70.5	69.6	68.8	67.8	66.6	65.5	64.6	64.3	64.0	63.5
59								74.0	73.4	72.5	71.7	70.8	70.0	69.0	67.8	66.7	65.7	65.4	65.1	64.7
60									74.7	73.8	72.9	72.0	71.3	70.2	68.9	67.8	66.8	66.5	66.2	65.8
61											74.2	73.3	72.5	71.3	70.1	69.0	68.0	67.6	67.3	66.9
62												74.5	73.7	72.5	71.3	70.1	69.1	68.8	68.5	68.0
63													74.9	73.7	72.4	71.3	70.2	69.9	69.6	69.1
64														74.9	73.6	72.4	71.3	71.0	70.7	70.2
65															74.8	73.6	72.5	72.2	71.8	71.3
66																74.7	73.6	73.3	72.9	72.5
67																	74.7	74.4	74.1	73.6

(From: Bayley N, Pinneau SR. Tables for predicting adult height form skeletal age: revised for use with the Greulich-Pyle hand standards. *J Pediatr* 1952;40:423; with permission.)

TABLE 7-4. Accelerated girls—percentages and estimated mature heights for girls with skeletal ages 1 year or more advanced over their chronological ages: skeletal ages 12–17 years

	Skeletal age (yr-mo)																					
	12-0	12-3	12-6	12-9	13-0	13-3	13-6	13-9	14-0	14-3	14-6	14-9	15-0	15-3	15-6	15-9	16-0	16-3	16-6	16-9	17-0	17-6
% of mature height	90.1	91.3	92.4	93.5	94.5	95.5	96.3	96.8	97.2	97.7	98.0	98.3	98.6	98.8	99.0	99.2	99.3	99.4	99.5	99.7	99.8	99.95
Height (inches)																						
46	51.1																					
47	52.2	51.5	50.9																			
48	53.3	52.6	51.9	51.3																		
49	54.4	53.7	53.0	52.4	51.9	51.3	50.9															
50	55.5	54.8	54.1	53.5	52.9	52.4	51.9	51.7	51.4	51.2	51.0	50.9										
51	56.6	55.9	55.2	54.5	54.0	53.4	53.0	52.7	52.5	52.2	52.0	51.9	51.7	51.6	51.5	51.4	51.4	51.3	51.3	51.2	51.1	51.0
52	57.7	57.0	56.3	55.6	55.0	54.5	54.0	53.7	53.5	53.2	53.1	52.9	52.7	52.6	52.5	52.4	52.4	52.3	52.3	52.2	52.1	52.0
53	58.8	58.1	57.4	56.7	56.1	55.5	55.0	54.8	54.5	54.2	54.1	53.9	53.8	53.6	53.5	53.4	53.4	53.3	53.3	53.2	53.1	53.0
54	59.9	59.1	58.4	57.8	57.1	56.5	56.1	55.8	55.6	55.3	55.1	54.9	54.8	54.7	54.5	54.4	54.4	54.3	54.3	54.2	54.1	54.0
55	61.0	60.2	59.5	58.8	58.2	57.6	57.1	56.8	56.6	56.3	56.1	56.0	55.8	55.7	55.6	55.4	55.4	55.3	55.3	55.2	55.1	55.0
56	62.2	61.3	60.6	59.9	59.3	58.6	58.2	57.9	57.6	57.3	57.1	57.0	56.8	56.7	56.6	56.5	56.4	56.3	56.3	56.2	56.1	56.0
57	63.3	62.4	61.7	61.0	60.3	59.7	59.2	58.9	58.6	58.3	58.2	58.0	57.8	57.7	57.6	57.5	57.4	57.3	57.3	57.2	57.1	57.0
58	64.4	63.5	62.8	62.0	61.4	60.7	60.2	59.9	59.7	59.4	59.2	59.0	58.8	58.7	58.6	58.5	58.4	58.4	58.3	58.2	58.1	58.0
59	65.5	64.6	63.9	63.1	62.4	61.8	61.3	61.0	60.7	60.4	60.2	60.0	59.8	59.7	59.6	59.5	59.4	59.4	59.3	59.2	59.1	59.0
60	66.6	65.7	64.9	64.2	63.5	62.8	62.3	62.0	61.7	61.4	61.2	61.0	60.9	60.7	60.6	60.5	60.4	60.4	60.3	60.2	60.1	60.0
61	67.7	66.8	66.0	65.2	64.6	63.9	63.3	63.0	62.8	62.4	62.2	62.1	61.9	61.7	61.6	61.5	61.4	61.4	61.3	61.2	61.1	61.0
62	68.8	67.9	67.1	66.3	65.6	64.9	64.4	64.0	63.8	63.5	63.3	63.1	62.9	62.8	62.6	62.5	62.4	62.4	62.3	62.2	62.1	62.0
63	69.9	69.0	68.2	67.4	66.7	66.0	65.4	65.1	64.8	64.5	64.3	64.1	63.9	63.8	63.6	63.5	63.4	63.4	63.3	63.2	63.1	63.0
64	71.0	70.1	69.3	68.4	67.7	67.0	66.5	66.1	65.8	65.5	65.3	65.1	64.9	64.8	64.6	64.5	64.4	64.4	64.3	64.2	64.1	64.0
65	72.1	71.2	70.3	69.5	68.8	68.1	67.5	67.1	66.9	66.5	66.3	66.1	65.9	65.8	65.7	65.5	65.5	65.4	65.3	65.2	65.1	65.0
66	73.3	72.3	71.4	70.6	69.8	69.1	68.5	68.2	67.9	67.6	67.3	67.1	66.9	66.8	66.7	66.5	66.5	66.4	66.3	66.2	66.1	66.0
67	74.4	73.4	72.5	71.7	70.9	70.2	69.6	69.2	68.9	68.6	68.4	68.2	68.0	67.8	67.7	67.5	67.5	67.4	67.3	67.2	67.1	67.0
68		74.5	73.6	72.7	72.0	71.2	70.6	70.2	70.0	69.6	69.4	69.2	69.0	68.8	68.7	68.5	68.5	68.4	68.3	68.2	68.1	68.0
69			74.7	73.8	73.0	72.3	71.7	71.3	71.0	70.6	70.4	70.2	70.0	69.8	69.7	69.6	69.5	69.4	69.3	69.2	69.1	69.0
70				74.9	74.1	73.3	72.7	72.3	72.0	71.6	71.4	71.2	71.0	70.8	70.7	70.6	70.5	70.4	70.3	70.2	70.1	70.0
71						74.3	73.7	73.3	73.0	72.7	72.4	72.2	72.0	71.9	71.7	71.6	71.5	71.4	71.4	71.2	71.1	71.0
72							74.8	74.4	74.1	73.7	73.5	73.2	73.0	72.9	72.7	72.6	72.5	72.4	72.4	72.2	72.1	72.0
73										74.7	74.5	74.3	74.0	73.9	73.7	73.6	73.5	73.4	73.4	73.2	73.1	73.0
74														74.9	74.7	74.6	74.5	74.4	74.4	74.2	74.1	74.0

(From: Bayley N, Pinneau SR. Tables for predicting adult height from skeletal age: revised for use with the Greulich-Pyle hand standards. *J Pediatr* 1952;40:423; with permission.)

TABLE 7-5. Retarded girls: Percentages and estimated mature heights for girls with skeletal ages 1 year or more retarded for their chronological ages: Skeletal ages 6–11 years

Skeletal age (yr-mo)	6-0	6-3	6-6	6-10	7-0	7-3	7-6	7-10	8-0	8-3	8-6	8-10	9-0	9-3	9-6	9-9	10-0	10-3	10-6	10-9	11-0	11-3	11-6	11-9
% of mature height	73.3	74.2	75.1	76.3	77.0	77.9	78.8	79.7	80.4	81.3	82.3	83.6	84.1	85.1	85.8	86.6	87.4	88.4	89.6	90.7	91.8	92.2	92.6	92.9
Height (inches)																								
38	51.8	51.2																						
39	53.2	52.6	51.9	51.1																				
40	54.6	53.9	53.3	52.4	51.9	51.3																		
41	55.9	55.3	54.6	53.7	53.2	52.6	52.0	51.4																
42	57.3	56.6	55.9	55.0	54.5	53.9	53.3	52.7	52.2	51.7	51.0													
43	58.7	58.0	57.3	56.4	55.8	55.2	54.6	54.0	53.5	52.9	52.2	51.4	51.1											
44	60.0	59.3	58.6	57.7	57.1	56.5	55.8	55.2	54.7	54.1	53.5	52.6	52.3	51.7	51.3									
45	61.4	60.6	59.9	59.0	58.4	57.8	57.1	56.5	56.0	55.4	54.7	53.8	53.5	52.9	52.4	52.0	51.5							
46	62.8	62.0	61.3	60.3	59.7	59.1	58.4	57.7	57.2	56.6	55.9	55.0	54.7	54.1	53.6	53.1	52.6	52.0	51.3					
47	64.1	63.3	62.6	61.6	61.0	60.3	59.6	59.0	58.5	57.8	57.1	56.2	55.9	55.2	54.8	54.3	53.8	53.2	52.5	51.8	51.2	51.0		
48	65.5	64.7	63.9	62.9	62.3	61.6	60.9	60.2	59.7	59.0	58.3	57.4	57.1	56.4	55.9	55.4	54.9	54.3	53.6	52.9	52.3	52.1	51.8	51.7
49	66.9	66.0	65.2	64.2	63.6	62.9	62.2	61.5	60.9	60.3	59.5	58.6	58.3	57.6	57.1	56.6	56.1	55.4	54.7	54.0	53.4	53.1	52.9	52.7
50	68.2	67.4	66.6	65.5	64.9	64.2	63.5	62.7	62.2	61.5	60.8	59.8	59.5	58.8	58.3	57.7	57.2	56.6	55.8	55.1	54.5	54.2	54.0	53.8
51	69.6	68.7	67.9	66.8	66.2	65.5	64.7	64.0	63.4	62.7	62.0	61.0	60.6	59.9	59.4	58.9	58.4	57.7	56.9	56.2	55.6	55.3	55.1	54.9
52	70.9	70.1	69.2	68.2	67.5	66.8	66.0	65.2	64.7	64.0	63.2	62.2	61.8	61.1	60.6	60.0	59.5	58.8	58.0	57.3	56.6	56.4	56.2	56.0
53	72.3	71.4	70.6	69.5	68.8	68.0	67.3	66.5	65.9	65.2	64.4	63.4	63.0	62.3	61.8	61.2	60.6	60.0	59.2	58.4	57.7	57.5	57.2	57.1
54	73.7	72.8	71.9	70.8	70.1	69.3	68.5	67.8	67.2	66.4	65.6	64.6	64.2	63.5	62.9	62.4	61.8	61.1	60.3	59.5	58.8	58.6	58.3	58.1
55		74.1	73.2	72.1	71.4	70.6	69.8	69.0	68.4	67.7	66.8	65.8	65.4	64.6	64.1	63.5	62.9	62.2	61.4	60.6	59.9	59.7	59.4	59.2
56			74.6	73.4	72.7	71.9	71.1	70.3	69.7	68.9	68.0	67.0	66.6	65.8	65.3	64.7	64.1	63.3	62.5	61.7	61.0	60.7	60.5	60.3
57				74.7	74.0	73.2	72.3	71.5	70.9	70.1	69.3	68.2	67.8	67.0	66.4	65.8	65.2	64.5	63.6	62.8	62.1	61.8	61.6	61.4
58						74.5	73.6	72.8	72.1	71.3	70.5	69.4	69.0	68.2	67.6	67.0	66.4	65.6	64.7	63.9	63.2	62.9	62.6	62.4
59							74.9	74.0	73.4	72.6	71.7	70.6	70.2	69.3	68.8	68.1	67.5	66.7	65.8	65.0	64.3	64.0	63.7	63.5
60									74.6	73.8	72.9	71.8	71.3	70.5	69.9	69.3	68.7	67.9	67.0	66.2	65.4	65.1	64.8	64.6
61											74.1	73.0	72.5	71.7	71.1	70.4	69.8	69.0	68.1	67.3	66.4	66.2	65.9	65.7
62												74.2	73.7	72.9	72.3	71.6	70.9	70.1	69.2	68.4	67.5	67.2	67.0	66.7
63													74.7	74.0	73.4	72.7	72.1	71.3	70.3	69.5	68.6	68.3	68.0	67.8
64															74.6	73.9	73.2	72.4	71.4	70.6	69.7	69.4	69.1	68.9
65																	74.4	73.5	72.5	71.7	70.8	70.5	70.2	70.0
66																		74.7	73.7	72.8	71.9	71.6	71.3	71.0
67																			74.8	73.9	73.0	72.7	72.4	72.1
68																					74.1	73.8	73.4	73.2
69																						74.8	74.5	74.3

(From: Bayley N, Pinneau SR. Tables for predicting adult height from skeletal age: revised for use with the Greulich-Pyle hand standards. *J Pediatr* 1952;40:423; with permission.)

TABLE 7-6. Retarded girls: Percentages and estimated mature heights for girls with skeletal ages 1 year or more retarded for their chronological ages: Skeletal ages 12–17 years

Skeletal age (yr-mo)	12-0	12-3	12-6	12-9	13-0	13-3	13-6	13-9	14-0	14-3	14-6	41-9	15-0	15-3	15-6	15-9	16-0	16-3	16-6	16-9	17-0
% of mature height	93.2	94.2	94.9	95.7	96.4	97.1	97.7	98.1	98.3	98.6	98.9	99.2	99.4	99.5	99.6	99.7	99.8	99.9	99.9	99.95	100.0
Height (Inches)																					
48	51.5	51.0																			
49	52.6	52.0	51.6	51.2																	
50	53.6	53.1	52.7	52.2	51.9	51.5	51.2	51.0													
51	54.7	54.1	53.7	53.3	52.9	52.5	52.2	52.0	51.9	51.7	51.6	51.4	51.3	51.3	51.2	51.2	51.1	51.1	51.1	51.0	51.0
52	55.8	55.2	54.8	54.3	53.9	53.6	53.2	53.0	52.9	52.7	52.6	52.4	52.3	52.3	52.2	52.2	52.1	52.1	52.1	52.0	52.0
53	56.9	56.3	55.8	55.4	55.0	54.6	54.2	54.0	53.9	53.8	53.6	53.4	53.3	53.3	53.2	53.2	53.1	53.1	53.1	53.0	53.0
54	57.9	57.3	56.9	56.4	56.0	55.6	55.3	55.0	54.9	54.8	54.6	54.4	54.3	54.3	54.2	54.2	54.1	54.1	54.1	54.0	54.0
55	59.0	58.4	58.0	57.5	57.1	56.6	56.3	56.1	56.0	55.8	55.6	55.4	55.3	55.3	55.2	55.2	55.1	55.1	55.1	55.0	55.0
56	60.1	59.4	59.0	58.5	58.1	57.7	57.3	57.1	57.0	56.8	56.6	56.5	56.3	56.3	56.2	56.2	56.1	56.1	56.1	56.0	56.0
57	61.2	60.5	60.1	59.6	59.1	58.7	58.3	58.1	58.0	57.8	57.6	57.5	57.3	57.3	57.2	57.2	57.1	57.1	57.1	57.0	57.0
58	62.2	61.6	61.1	60.6	60.2	59.7	59.4	59.1	59.0	58.8	58.6	58.5	58.3	58.3	58.2	58.2	58.1	58.1	58.1	58.0	58.0
59	63.3	62.6	62.2	61.7	61.2	60.8	60.4	60.1	60.0	59.8	59.7	59.5	59.4	59.3	59.2	59.2	59.1	59.1	59.1	59.0	59.0
60	64.4	63.7	63.2	62.7	62.2	61.8	61.4	61.2	61.0	60.9	60.7	60.5	60.4	60.3	60.2	60.2	60.1	60.1	60.1	60.0	60.0
61	65.5	64.8	64.3	63.7	63.3	62.8	62.4	62.2	62.1	61.9	61.7	61.5	61.4	61.3	61.2	61.2	61.1	61.1	61.1	61.0	61.0
62	66.5	65.8	65.3	64.8	64.3	63.9	63.5	63.2	63.1	62.9	62.7	62.5	62.4	62.3	62.2	62.2	62.1	62.1	62.1	62.0	62.0
63	67.6	66.9	66.4	65.8	65.3	64.9	64.5	64.2	64.1	63.9	63.7	63.5	63.4	63.3	63.3	63.2	63.1	63.1	63.1	63.0	63.0
64	68.7	67.9	67.4	66.9	66.4	65.9	65.5	65.2	65.1	64.9	64.7	64.5	64.4	64.3	64.3	64.2	64.1	64.1	64.1	64.0	64.0
65	69.7	69.0	68.5	67.9	67.4	66.9	66.5	66.3	66.1	65.9	65.7	65.5	65.4	65.3	65.3	65.2	65.1	65.1	65.1	65.0	65.0
66	70.8	70.1	69.5	69.0	68.5	68.0	67.6	67.3	67.1	66.9	66.7	66.5	66.4	66.3	66.3	66.2	66.1	66.1	66.1	66.0	66.0
67	71.9	71.1	70.6	70.0	69.5	69.0	68.6	68.3	68.2	68.0	67.7	67.5	67.4	67.3	67.3	67.2	67.1	67.1	67.1	67.0	67.0
68	73.0	72.2	71.7	71.1	70.5	70.0	69.6	69.3	69.2	69.0	68.8	68.6	68.4	68.3	68.3	68.2	68.1	68.1	68.1	68.0	68.0
69	74.0	73.2	72.7	72.1	71.6	71.1	70.6	70.3	70.2	70.0	69.8	69.6	69.4	69.3	69.3	69.2	69.1	69.1	69.1	69.0	69.0
70		74.3	73.8	73.1	72.6	72.1	71.6	71.4	71.2	71.0	70.8	70.6	70.4	70.4	70.3	70.2	70.1	70.1	70.1	70.0	70.0
71		74.8		74.2	73.7	73.1	72.7	72.4	72.2	72.0	71.8	71.6	71.4	71.4	71.3	71.2	71.1	71.1	71.1	71.0	71.0
72					74.7	74.1	73.7	73.4	73.2	73.0	72.8	72.6	72.4	72.4	72.3	72.2	72.1	72.1	72.1	72.0	72.0
73							74.7	74.4	74.3	74.0	73.8	73.6	73.4	73.4	73.3	73.2	73.1	73.1	73.1	73.0	73.0
74											74.8	74.6	74.4	74.4	74.3	74.2	74.1	74.1	74.1	74.0	74.0

(From: Bayley N, Pinneau SR. Tables for predicting adult height from skeletal age: Revised for use with the Greulich-Pyte hand standards. *J Pediatr* 1952;40:423; with permission.)

Appendix 8

Calcium Information for Teens

See also http://www.youngwomenshealth.org/calciuminfo.html
Adequate calcium intake is needed during adolescence to minimize facture risk and to prevent osteoporosis later in life. The Recommended Adequate Intake for adolescents 9 to 18 years old is 1300 mg per day. Dietary sources of calcium can be found in most food groups, although most of the calcium in the American food supply comes from foods in the milk group.

MILK GROUP

It is difficult to get the required intake of calcium without eating milk group foods. Calcium found in foods from the milk group is generally well absorbed because of the added vitamin D.

Foods in this group provide riboflavin and protein, in addition to calcium and vitamin D.

Milk group	Calcium (mg)
Yogurt, plain, nonfat (1 cup)	488
Yogurt, plain, low-fat (1 cup)	448
Milkshake, chocolate (10 fl oz)	375
Yogurt, fruit-flavored, low-fat (1 cup)	372
Cheese, Swiss (1 1/2 oz)	336
Cheese, mozzarella, part skim (1 1/2 oz)	333
Milk, skim (1 cup)	316
Milk 2% (1 cup)	314
Milk, 1% (1 cup)	313
Cheese, cheddar (1 1/2 oz)	307
Milk, whole (1 cup)	290
Milk, chocolate, 2% (1 cup)	285
Buttermilk, low-fat (1 cup)	284
Milk, chocolate, whole (1 cup)	280
Cheese, American (1 1/2 oz)	239
Ice cream, hardened, 16% fat (1/2 cup)	125
Ice cream, soft serve (1/2 cup)	113
Yogurt, frozen, vanilla (1/2 cup)	103
Pudding (1/2 cup)	99
Ice cream, hardened, 10% fat (1/2 cup)	92
Cheese, cottage 2% low-fat (1/2 cup)	78

MEAT, VEGETABLE, AND GRAIN GROUPS

Foods in the meat group are major sources of protein, niacin, iron, and thiamin, but also provide a small amount of calcium. The vegetable and grain groups supply even less calcium than the meat group. However, vegetables are a major source of vitamin A, vitamin C, and fiber, and grains are a major source of carbohydrate, thiamin, iron, niacin, and fiber. A few foods in each of these groups contain calcium. For example, canned salmon and sardines supply calcium when the bones are eaten. Components found in some of the foods from these groups may inhibit calcium absorption. For example, phytates, found in some grains, nuts, and seeds, and oxalates, found in some vegetables, interfere with the absorption of calcium.

Meat group	Calcium (mg)
Tofu, with calcium sulfate (1/2 cup)	434
Sardines, canned, with bones (3 oz)	325
Salmon, canned, with bones (3 oz)	203
Tofu, without calcium sulfate (1/2 cup)	125
Almonds (1/3 cup)	118
Perch, baked (3 oz.)	116

Vegetable group**	Calcium (mg)
Spinach, fresh, cooked (1/2 cup)	122
Turnip greens, fresh, cooked (1/2 cup)	99
Okra, frozen, cooked (1/2 cup)	88
Beet greens, fresh, cooked (1/2 cup)	82

**The calcium found in vegetables is poorly absorbed

Grain group	Calcium (mg)
Waffle, homemade (7-in waffle)	191
Biscuit, from mix (1 biscuit)	82

COMBINATION FOODS

Combination foods are made with foods from more than one food group. Ingredients from the milk group make these combination foods good sources of calcium. Combination foods are also good sources of many other nutrients.

Combination foods	Calcium (mg)
Cheese pizza (1/4 of 14 inch pie)	332
Macaroni and cheese (1/2 cup)	181
Taco, beef with cheese (1 small)	174
Cream of tomato, made with milk (1 cup)	168
Spaghetti, meatballs, sauce, and cheese (1 cup)	124
Chili con came with beans, canned (1 cup)	82

CALCIUM-FORTIFIED FOODS

Calcium is sometimes added to juice, bread, energy bars, cereal bars, soft drinks, dairy substitutes (like soy milk and cheese), cereal, and other foods. Additional calcium is also added to some milk and yogurt to increase calcium content. The amount of calcium in these foods is listed on the label. Keep in mind that calcium-fortified foods can increase calcium intake, but they may not provide the body with other nutrients supplied by dairy foods. For example, calcium-fortified juices contain as much as milk, but some brands do not have the added vitamin D needed for calcium absorption, and no juice contains the protein found in milk.

CALCIUM AND VITAMIN D SUPPLEMENTS

There are a wide variety of calcium supplements on the market, each containing different calcium compounds and amounts of calcium. The amount of calcium in these supplements is listed on the label, along with the form of calcium. Calcium carbonate and calcium citrate are the most frequently used calcium supplements because they are relatively inexpensive and well absorbed. Calcium supplements are more efficiently absorbed when consumed in divided doses, each containing less than 500 mg of calcium. Vitamin D stimulates absorption of calcium and, therefore, adolescents usually benefit from taking a daily multivitamin to provide adequate vitamin D or a calcium supplement that contains vitamin D.

There are no benefits for taking more than your recommended daily allowance (RDA) for calcium. In addition, high intakes of calcium may interfere with the absorption of other nutrients. Talk to your health care provider or dietitian before taking a calcium supplement.

AT RISK POPULATIONS

Certain adolescent populations are at increased risk for inadequate calcium intake, including vegans/vegetarians and individuals with lactose intolerance. Vegans and some vegetarians avoid foods from the milk group. In addition, consumption of vegetarian/vegan diets may influence the calcium requirement because of the their relatively high contents of oxalates and phytates. Individuals with lactose intolerance absorb calcium normally from milk, but they are at risk for calcium deficiency because of avoidance of dairy products. Both of these populations must rely on non-dairy sources of calcium, calcium-fortified foods, and calcium supplements to meet calcium requirements.

Appendix 9

Nonsteroidal Anti-Inflammatory Agents

APPENDIX 9. *Nonsteroidal anti-inflammatory agents*

Drug	Chemical Classification	Dose Available dosages (mg)	Common dosing intervals
Aspirin (Ecotrin®, Ascriptin®)	Salicylate Group	325 500	BID-QID
Celecoxib (Celebrex®)	Benzenesulfonamide Group	100	QD-BID
Choline magnesium trisalicylate (Trilisate®)	Salicylate Group	500 750 1,000	BID-TID
Diclofenac DR (Voltaren®)	Acetic Acid Group	25 50 75	BID-TID
Diclofenac XR (Voltaren XR®)		100	QD-BID
Etodolac (Lodine®)	Acetic Acid Group	200 300 400	BID-TID
Etodolac XL (Lodine XL®)		400 500 600	QD
Fenoprofen (Nalfon Pulvules®)	Propionic Acid Group	200 300	TID-QID
Flurbiprofen (Ansaid®)	Propionic Acid Group	50 100	BID-QID
Ibuprofen (Motrin®)	Propionic Acid Group	400 600 800	TID-QID
Indomethacin (Indocin®)	Acetic Acid Group	25 50	BID-TID
Indomethacin (Indocin SR®)		75	QD-BID

Drug	Group	Dose (mg)	Frequency
Ketoprofen (Orudis®)	Propionic Acid Group	50	TID-QID
Ketoprofen XR (Oruvail®)		75	
Meclofenamate	Fenamate Group	100	TID
		50–100	Q6H
Meloxicam (Mobic®)	Oxicam Group	7.5	QD
Nabumetone (Relafen®)	Acetic Acid Group	500	QD-BID
		750	
Naproxen (Naprosyn®)	Propionic Acid Group	250	BID
		375	
		500	
(Naprelan®)		375	QD
		500	
Oxaprozin (Daypro®)	Propionic Acid Group	600	QD-BID
Piroxicam (Feldene®)	Oxicam Group	10	QD
		20	
Rofecoxib (Vioxx®)	Furanone Group	12.5	QD
		25	
		50	
Sulindac (Clinoril®)	Acetic Acid Group	150	BID
		200	
Tolmetin (Tolectin®)	Acetic Acid Group	400	TID
		600	
Valdecoxib (Bextra®)	Benzenesulfonamide Group	10	QD
		20	

[Adapted from: Smith RP. Cyclic pelvic pain and dysmenorrhea. *Obstet Gynecol Clin North Am* 1993;20:753 and Ansani NT, Starz, TW. Effective use of nonsteroidal anti-inflammatory drugs. *The Female Patient* 2002;27:25.]

Subject Index

Page numbers in *italic* indicate figures; page numbers followed by t indicate tables